XIE'S CHINESE VETERINARY HERBOLOGY

兽医中草药及方剂学

XIE'S CHINESE VETERINARY HERBOLOGY

兽医中草药及方剂学

EDITED BY
Huisheng Xie, DVM, PhD, MS
Vanessa Preast, DVM, CVA

ILLUSTRATED by Barbara Jean Beckford

WILEY-BLACKWELL
A John Wiley & Sons, Ltd., Publication

Edition first published 2010

Blackwell Publishing was acquired by John Wiley & Sons in February 2007. Blackwell's publishing program has been merged with Wiley's global Scientific, Technical, and Medical business to form Wiley-Blackwell.

Editorial Office
2121 State Avenue, Ames, Iowa 50014-8300, USA

For details of our global editorial offices, for customer services, and for information about how to apply for permission to reuse the copyright material in this book, please see our website at www.wiley.com/wiley-blackwell.

NOTICE
This book is intended to be a reference for veterinarians trained to practice Traditional Chinese Veterinary Medicine (TCVM). This text is **not** a substitute for a sound medical education. Veterinarians are strongly advised to seek a comprehensive TCVM training program before using herbal medicine. Several certification programs in the United States and other countries are available to veterinarians. Nonveterinarians should not practice medicine on animals, unless permitted by law. Individuals who are untrained or inadequately trained in TCVM are unable to accurately assess a patient's health status or make appropriate therapeutic recommendations.

Library of Congress Cataloging-in-Publication Data

Xie's Chinese veterinary herbology / edited by Huisheng Xie, Vanessa Preast ; illustrated by Barbara Beckford.
p. ; cm.
Includes bibliographical references and index.
ISBN 978-0-8138-0369-2 (hardback : alk. paper)
1. Alternative veterinary medicine. 2. Herbs–Therapeutic use. 3. Herbs–Therapeutic use–China. 4. Traditional veterinary medicine–China. 5. Medicine, Chinese. I. Xie, Huisheng. II. Preast, Vanessa. III. Title: Chinese veterinary herbology. [DNLM: 1. Phytotherapy–veterinary. 2. Veterinary Medicine–methods. 3. Drugs, Chinese Herbal. SF 745.5 X6 2010]
SF745.5.X543 2010
636.089'5321–dc22

2009041420

A catalog record for this book is available from the U.S. Library of Congress.

Set in 9.5 on 12pt ITC Stone Serif-Medium by Toppan Best-set Premedia Limited
Printed and bound by CPI Group (UK) Ltd, Croydon, CR0 4YY

C9780813803692_310724

Contents

About the Editors

Huisheng Xie, DVM, PhD, MS

Dr. Xie is an associate professor at the University of Florida (UF), director of the Veterinary Acupuncture Program at the UF Veterinary Medical Center, and president and head instructor of the Chi Institute. He has been teaching and practicing Traditional Chinese Veterinary Medicine (TCVM) since 1983.

Huisheng Xie (pronounced "shay") is a third-generation Traditional Chinese Medicine (TCM) practitioner. He grew up watching his father and grandfather treat people using traditional Chinese herbal medicines. He thought he was going to follow in his father's footsteps, but his plans changed when his beloved dog Shan-Shan (meaning "mountain") died. The heartbroken 8-year-old boy decided that he would pursue veterinary school rather than medical school when he entered college.

Dr. Xie received his Doctor of Veterinary Medicine at the Sichuan College of Animal Science and Veterinary Medicine in Sichuan, China, in 1983. He worked as a faculty member in TCVM at the Beijing Agricultural University College of Veterinary Medicine from 1983 to 1987. After receiving his Master of Veterinary Science in Veterinary Acupuncture in 1988, he served as an associate professor in the college until 1994. During this time, he continued his advanced training in human acupuncture at the Beijing College of Traditional Chinese Medicine and the National Academy of Traditional Chinese Medicine. He completed his advanced training in 1992.

To explore different approaches for studying and advancing TCVM, he moved to the United States in 1994 and began his doctoral training at the University of Florida. He investigated using acupuncture as pain control mechanisms in horses and received his PhD in 1999. Believing that TCVM should be available to more veterinarians, Dr. Xie founded the Chi Institute of Chinese Medicine in 1998. The Chi Institute trains veterinarians in the various branches of TCVM, including acupuncture, herbal medicine, Tui-na, and food therapy.

Dr. Xie's academic accomplishments are extensive. He has received Achievement Awards from several Chinese institutions including the Ministry of Agriculture, the National Science and Technology Committee, and the Beijing Agricultural University. As an invited speaker in the United States, Japan, Thailand, Mexico, Brazil, and Europe, he has lectured about veterinary acupuncture and herbal medicine around the world. He has authored 10 books and 100 scientific papers. His textbooks, including *Xie's Veterinary Acupuncture* and *Traditional Chinese Veterinary Medicine—Fundamental Principles,* have been used for TCVM training programs in China, Japan, Europe, South America, and the United States.

Vanessa Preast, DVM, CVA

Dr. Preast received her DVM from the University of Florida in 2000. As a graduate of the Chi Institute, she became certified in small animal acupuncture. She incorporated acupuncture into her practice of small animal medicine and surgery until returning to school as a full-time doctoral student in Curriculum and Instructional Technology at Iowa State University (ISU). She is interested in using her training in teaching and learning methods to improve college-level education, especially veterinary medicine.

Her professional accomplishments include coauthoring and editing *Xie's Veterinary Acupuncture* and *Traditional Chinese Veterinary Medicine—Fundamental Principles* with Dr. Xie. She also helped design a computer-based interactive tutorial to teach veterinary students how to make blood smears. Her study reporting the tutorial's effectiveness was published in *Veterinary Clinical Pathology.*

She has applied her instructional design skills to a wide range of topics, including teaching classes on Servant Leadership to ISU honors students and developing a hands-on workshop teaching community members how to make effective sandbag levees. Along with three other graduate students, she cofounded an instructional design service center, Learning Design Solutions. This student-led center provides services such as evaluation, assessment, usability, and instructional design and development.

Contributors

Michael Bartholomew, DVM, CVA, CVCH, CVTP, CVFT
South Salem, NY

Barbara Jean Beckford, BS
Alachua, FL 32615

Kelly Chandler, DVM, CVA
Foresthill, CA

Cheryl Chrisman, DVM, MS Eds, DACVIM-neurology, CVA
Gainesville, FL

Xiaolin Deng, MD, OMD
Gainesville, FL

Constance DiNatale, DVM, CVA, CVCH, CVFT
Winter Park, FL

Bruce Ferguson, DVM, MS, CVA, CVCH, CVTP, CVFT
Murdoch, WA, AUSTRALIA

Elizabeth Fernandez, DVM, CVA
Newbury Park, CA

Songhua Hu, DVM, PhD
Hanzhou, Zhejiang, CHINA

Min Su Kim, DVM, PhD
DuckJin-dong, DuckJin-gu, JeonJu Jeonbuk, KOREA

Li Lin, PhD, OMD
Merritt Island, FL

Hanru Liu, DVM, MS
Chongqing, CHINA

Chaoying Luo, DVM
Lanzhou, Gansu, CHINA

Vanessa Preast, DVM, PhD, CVA
Ames, IA

Tiffany Rimar, DVM, CVA, CVCH, CVFT
St. Petersburg Beach, Fl

Dayou Shi, DVM, MS, PhD
Guangzhou, Guangdong Province, CHINA

Justin Shmalberg, DVM, CVA, CVCH, CVFT
Gainesville, FL

Sara Jane Skiwski, DVM, CVA, CVCH
San Jose, CA

Dalu Song, DVM, Professor
Nanjing, Jiangsu CHINA

Lisa Trevisanello, DVM, CVA
Reddick, FL

Xiujun Wang, DVM, MS
Zhengzhou, Henan, CHINA

Huisheng Xie, DVM, PhD
Reddick, FL

Yasu Xie, MD
Gaoxin District, Chongqing, China

Xuguang Yang, OMD, MD
Gainesville, FL

Preface

Traditional Chinese Veterinary Medicine (TCVM) has been practiced routinely in China for more than 2,000 years. This medical system incorporates both acupuncture and Chinese Herbal Medicine (CHM). Although many people associate Chinese therapies with acupuncture only, most patients in China (about 70%) are actually treated with Chinese herbs or a combination of herbs and acupuncture. Only about 30% of all traditional Chinese medicine patients receive acupuncture alone.

As early as 4,000 years ago, the Chinese recorded their knowledge of herbal medicines on bones and tortoise shells. Because archeologists excavated ancient bones from the Shang Dynasty (16th to 11th century BCE) containing inscriptions for "herbal wine," they believe herbal wine was one of the earliest ways to use Chinese herbal medicine. Today's modern preparation methods, which are still guided by the historical wisdom underlying CHM, effectively release the healing powers stored within the herbs. Many clinical studies have indicated that CHM is extremely effective for treating medical disorders in a wide variety of areas including cardiology, dermatology, endocrinology, gastroenterology, reproduction, oncology, behavior, respiratory problems, and sports medicine. For example, new evidence supports using herbal remedies to treat and even prevent gastric ulcers in horses. Herbal medicine has helped increase the quality of life in geriatric patients, especially those diagnosed with terminal cancer, because CHM can help shrink the tumor when chemotherapy is not an option.

As more veterinarians learn about TCVM and use acupuncture, they are seeking Chinese Herbal Medicine texts to increase their TCVM knowledge and to expand their treatment options with herbal medicine. Unfortunately, the literature about veterinary Chinese herbal medicine is primarily written in Chinese. Furthermore, the few English-language CHM books that are available focus on human rather than veterinary patients. Thus, we created this text to provide Western veterinarians with a clear, practical guide to the theory and application of CHM in veterinary hospitals.

This book is intended to serve as a quick reference for practicing veterinarians and as a textbook for continuing education courses in TCVM. To assist the readers, the book is presented in three parts: Part 1, Chinese Veterinary Materia Medica; Part 2, Chinese Veterinary Herbal Formulation; and Part 3, Clinical Application of Chinese Veterinary Herbology.

Chinese Veterinary Materia Medica: Part 1 discusses 381 herbs and divides them into chapters by herbal categories. The actions, properties, and applications of the herbs are compared at the end of each chapter. This section lists the original reference, part used, name (pharmaceutical, common, Wade-Giles, translation), energy/taste, channel-organ, actions, form and preparation, dosage, cautions and contraindications, and side effects for every herb. Additional details and illustrations are provided for the 133 most commonly used herbs. The illustrations help readers visually identify the herbs. These herbs include information about their clinical applications, history, related research, and pharmaceutical ingredients.

Chinese Veterinary Herbal Formulation: Detailed information is provided in Part 2 for 222 herbal formulas including nomenclature, source, ingredients, preparation, actions, indications, dosage and usage, formula analysis, and cautions and contraindications. Additionally, Dr. Xie provides commentary on most of the formulas. Some of the herbal formulas also list recent clinical and pharmacological studies related to those formulas.

Some classical formulas contain ingredients that were used historically but are not available for use in modern times. For example, the ingredients Xi Jiao

(Rhinoceros) and Hu Gu (Tiger bone) come from endangered species, so their use is prohibited. In these cases, the classical formulas are included in the text for educational purposes, but acceptable substitutes for the unavailable ingredients are also listed with the formula.

Clinical Application of Chinese Veterinary Herbology: The three chapters within Part 3 present detailed information on how to apply Chinese herbal medicine in veterinary practice, especially for the most common diseases in dogs, cats, and horses. This section also teaches how to select an herbal formula based on the TCVM Pattern diagnosis.

Acknowledgments

This book was born from a superb team's work. We greatly appreciate the efforts of all who helped make this book possible. First, we recognize the chapter contributors: Drs. Michael Bartholomew, Kelly Chandler, Cheryl Chrisman, Xiaolin Deng, Constance DiNatale, Bruce Ferguson, Elizabeth Fernandez, Songhua Hu, Min Su Kim, Lin Li, Hanru Liu, Chaoying Luo, Tiffany Rimar, Dayou Shi, Justin Shmalberg, Sara-Jane Skiwski, Dalu Song, Lisa Trevisanello, Xiujun Wang, Yasu Xie, and Xuguang Yang. They wrote about their subjects with exceptional skill. We also thank Drs. Cheryl Chrisman, Kelly Chandler, Linda Boggie, Elizabeth Fernandez, Chester Wheeler, Anita Weiss, Maria Gore, and Dazhi Xie for intensively proofreading and editing all the chapters. Thank you to Drs. Wen Liu and Dayou Shi, Allen Dong, and Wei Zhang for translating the historical stories for each herb. We acknowledge Dr. Minsu Kim for adding the pharmaceutical ingredients for each herb. We sincerely appreciate the patience of Wiley-Blackwell as we have slowly brought this text together. Finally, special thanks go to Barbara Beckford and Zhen Zhao for their wonderful illustrations.

XIE'S CHINESE VETERINARY HERBOLOGY

兽医中草药及方剂学

Part 1 Chinese Veterinary Materia Medica
兽医中草药

Table I.1. Five types of energy and their actions.

5 Energies	TCM Actions	Physiological Effects	Examples
Cold	Purge Heat and Fire, cool Blood	Antiinflammatory, antispasmodic, sedative	Coptis *Huang Lian* Scutellaria *Huang Qin*
Cool	Relieve Heat, resolve toxin, nourish *Yin*	Reduces fevers, detoxifies, lowers blood pressure, soothes nerves	Bupleurum *Chai Hu* Morus *Sang Ye* Glehnia *Bei Sha Shen*
Neutral	Mediate Cold, Cool, Hot and Warm herbs	Gentle effects, regulations	Glycyrrhiza *Gan Cao* Jujube *Da Zao*
Warm	Warm the Interior, disperse Cold, tonify *Qi-Yang*	Promotes circulation, alleviates chills	Ledebouriella *Fang Feng* Ginseng *Ren Shen*
Hot	Tonify *Yang Qi*, activate the Channels	Improves organ functions, stimulates and strengthens	Zingiberis *Gan Jiang* Cinnamomum *Rou Gui*

Table I.2. Five tastes and their actions.

5 Tastes	TCM Actions	Physiological Effects	Examples	Others
Sour	Astringent effect	Contract flaccid tissues; stop abnormal secretions or discharges; promote digestion, enzyme secretion, and liver function; alter blood conditions	Schisandra *Wu Wei Zi,* Mume *Wu Mei,* Apricot, grape, mango, peach, pineapple, plum, vinegar, tomato	Green, yellowish-green Liver Wood
Bitter	Eliminate Heat-Damp, purge the intestines	Antiinflammatory; antipyretic; detoxifying; antiviral; antiparasitic; enhances secretion of bile through the liver; promotes the secretion of hydrochloric acid by the stomach; anticholesterolemic action	Coptis *Huang Lian*, Rheum *Da Huang*, Asparagus, celery, coffee, pork and sheep gallbladder	Red Heart Fire
Sweet	Tonify *Qi* or *Yang*, nourish Blood or *Yin*, Soothe the Liver, Regulate *Qi* and Blood	Soothe acute diseases; regulate internal organ functions	Ginseng *Ren Shen,* Glycyrrhiza *Gan Cao,* Apple, banana, corn, egg, carrot, yam, sugar, wine	Yellow, brown Spleen Earth
Pungent	Diaphoresis, activate *Qi* and Blood	Stimulate blood circulation; distribute energy from the interior to the surface	Cinnamomum *Rou Gui,* Saussurea *Mu Xiang,* Cloves, chives, fennel, garlic, ginger, nutmeg, radish, pepper, wine	White, pale Lung Metal
Salty	Soften hardness, purge the intestines	Diuretic; soften hard masses and resolve bumps; relieve constipation through purgation; help maintain fluid balance	Mirabilitum *Mang Xiao* Abalone, barley, clam, crab, duck, ham, kelp, pork kidney, oyster, mussel, human milk	Black, dark Kidney Water

chloride, potassium, and magnesium salts in Sargassum *Hai Zao* make this herb taste salty. Pungent or acrid herbs, such as Cinnamomum *Rou Gui*, usually contain high percentages of terpenoid volatile oil or complex aromatic compounds from which essential oils can be distilled. Glycyrrhiza *Gan Cao* and Ginseng *Ren Shen*, which are rich in saponin glycosides, have a sweet taste.

Tastes can also be described as 1) Light and 2) Bland. Herbs with a light taste, such as Poria *Fu Ling* and Polyporus *Zhu Ling*, will excrete Damp and cause diuresis. Herbs with a bland taste, such as mushrooms, have calming, soothing, and diuretic actions.

Four Directions of Herbal Energy: Ascending, Descending, Floating, and Sinking

Herbs send their energy in a specific direction in the body. Chinese herbal medicines are described by four directions of herbal energy: 1) Ascending (up) or toward the head in animals, 2) Descending (down) or toward the tail in animals, 3) Floating (toward the Exterior of the body) or 4) Sinking (toward the Interior of the body. These energy directions affect the herb's activity and how it can treat disease.

Generally speaking, herbs with a warm/hot temperature and pungent/sweet taste possess ascending/

floating tendencies, and herbs with a cold/cool temperature and sour, bitter, or salty taste possess descending/sinking tendencies. The herbs with ascending and floating tendencies have upward and outward effects and are categorized as *Yang*. These herbs are effective for elevating *Yang Qi*, causing diaphoresis, dispersing Wind or Cold, warming the body's Exterior, and inducing vomiting. On the other hand, herbs with descending and sinking tendencies have downward and inward effects, which relate to *Yin*. These inhibitory herbs will have an astringent effect, stop coughing and asthma, eliminate Heat, excrete Damp, and purge accumulations from the intestines. In some cases, herbs may have both ascending/floating and descending/sinking tendencies. For instance, Ephedra *Ma Huang* is able to disperse Wind-Cold (diaphoresis, ascending) and is able to stop asthma and excrete water (descending).

The herbal energy direction is also related to which parts of the plant, animal or mineral are used for the herbal medicine. The light parts of a plant, such as flowers (Chrysanthemum *Ju Hua)* and leaves (Perilla leaf *Zi Su Ye*), have ascending/floating energy. The herbs with ascending/floating energy can elevate *Yang Qi* to warm the Exterior, and have a diaphoretic effect to disperse Wind or Cold. On the other hand, the heavy parts of a plant, such as the fruit (Immature bitter orange Aurantium *Zhi Shi)* and seed (Perilla seed *Zi Su Zi)*, have descending/sinking energy.

Minerals have descending energy. The Chinese herbal medicines with descending/sinking energy have an astringent effect, which can stop cough/asthma, eliminate Heat, excrete Damp, and purge the intestines.

The processing technique used while manufacturing the herbal medication can alter the herbal energetic properties. Cooking an herb in wine or with ginger will cause its energy to become ascending and floating. On the other hand, herbal energy becomes descending and sinking when herbs are cooked in a salt or vinegar solution.

When treating specific conditions, a practitioner may select medications based on the herbal energy direction. A practitioner may choose an herb that moves energy in the opposite direction of that which the disease moves. In this case, herbs that move the energy down are indicated for diseases that move upward in the body, and herbs with an ascending tendency are used to treat diseases with a downward direction. Alternatively, a practitioner may choose herbs whose energy acts in the same region as the disease condition. In this case, herbs with floating tendencies may treat anterior/upper body or exterior/superficial conditions while descending herbs may assist lower body or interior conditions.

The following conditions illustrate herbal selections based on the disease and herbal energy direction. When Liver *Yang* is rising and the patient has red eyes and dizziness, the disease energy is upward. Thus, herbs such as Ostrea *Mu Li* and Coptis *Huang Lian*, are appropriate selections because they move the energy downward and inward (sinking and descending). For uterine prolapse, which results from pathologic sinking of *Zhong Qi*, herbs to raise the *Zhong Qi* and hold up the inner organs, such as Astragalus *Huang Qi* and Codonopsis *Dang Shen*, are used. Ephedra *Ma Huang* and Cinnamomum *Gui Zhi* have floating tendencies and are used for external Wind Cold problems. On the other hand, the descending tendency of Rhubarb/Rheum *Da Huang* is used for lower body problems such as constipation (Tables I.3, I.4).

Table I.3. Four directions of the herbal energy.

Energy Direction	Category	Actions	Examples
Up or ascending Floating (to the exterior)	*Yang* warm/hot pungent/sweet flower and leaf in wine or ginger	Elevate *Yang Qi*, diaphoresis Disperse Wind or Cold warming the Exterior Cause vomit	Cimicifuga *Sheng Ma* Cinnamomum *Rou Gui* Ginseng *Ren Shen* Perilla *Zi Su Ye* Zingiberis *Sheng Jiang*
Down or descending Sinking (to the interior)	*Yin* cold/cool sour, bitter, salty fruit and seed in salt or vinegar	Astringent effect Stop cough/asthma Eliminate heat Excrete dampness purging the intestines	Schisandra *Wu Wei Zi* Armenica *Xing Ren* Coptis *Huang Lian* Poria *Fu Ling* Rheum *Da Huang*

Table I.4. Clinical application of herbal energy directions.

Disease Direction		Symptoms	Herbal Energy Direction	Herbs
Up or floating	Liver *Yang* Rising; hypertension	Headache, Dizziness, Red eyes	Down or sinking	Ostrea *Mu Li* Coptis *Huang Lian*
Down or sinking	Uterine prolapse	Sinking of Zhong *Qi*	Up or floating	Astragalus *Huang Qi* Cimicifuga *Sheng Ma*

Table I.5. Entering Channel-Organ (*Gui Jing*) of the herbs.

Herb	Pin *Yin*	Entering Channel(s)	Category
Gentiana	*Long Dan Cao*	LIV/GB	Heat-clearing
Atractylodes	*Bai Zhu*	SP/ST	*Qi* tonic
Platycodon	*Jie Geng*	LU	Phlegm-transforming
Bupleurum	*Chai Hu*	LIV/GB/PC	Wind-heat clearing
Anemarrhena	*Zhi Mu*	Upper Burner	Heat-clearing
Phellodendron	*Huang Bai*	Lower Burner	Heat-clearing
Achyranthes	*Niu Xi*	Stifle/rear limbs	*Yang* tonic
Ligusticum	*Gao Ben*	Head	Wind-cold clearing

Entering Channel-Organ

Herbal formulas are capable of targeting specific Channels or body areas. Some herbs have physiological effects primarily on the internal organs associated with a specific Channel. The Channel that an herb specifically affects is that herb's "entering Channel" (Table I.5). Because Gentian *Long Dan Cao* acts only on the Liver and Gallbladder Channels without affecting the other Channels, it is "entering the Liver and Gallbladder Channels."

Some herbs in a formula are able to coordinate the other herbs' activities and direct them to a particular Channel or Burner (*Jiao*) and their associated organs. For example, Bupleurum *Chai Hu* directs all the herbs in the formula to the Liver, Gallbladder, and Pericardium Channels, and Anemarrhena *Zhi Mu* directs the whole formula to the Upper Burner (*Shang Jiao*). Other herbs can direct the formula to a specific anatomical area. For example, Achyranthes *Niu Xi* directs herbal actions to the stifle.

COMBINATION OF CHINESE HERBS

Chinese herbal medicine generally involves combining two or more herbs into a formula that treats a specific disease Pattern. The herbs within a formula may combine to produce four different effects: 1) summative, 2) synergistic, 3) antagonistic, and 4) toxic (side effect). A summative effect occurs when the formula's activity equals the sum of each component herb's activity. A synergistic effect occurs when the activity of the formula exceeds the sum of the component herbs. An antagonistic effect occurs when the activity of the formula is less than the activity of one or more component herbs. A toxic effect occurs when there is an undesirable side effect of the herbal formula. Figure I.1 demonstrates the four possible effects when two herbs with a certain effect on their own are combined into a formula. When formulating a Chinese herbal recipe, an herbalist tries to attain the summative or synergistic effect and avoid any antagonistic or toxic effects.

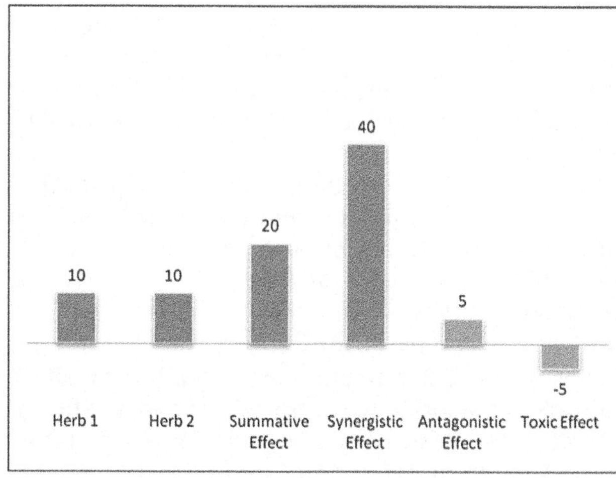

Figure I.1. *Possible outcomes when combining two herbs.*

Seven Types of Combinations

Traditionally, herbs are combined in seven different ways, which are called the Seven Features or the Seven Effects of Herbs. These combinations are as follows: 1) Potentiation, 2) Enhancement, 3) Antagonism, 4) Suppression, 5) Counterdrive, 6) Incompatibility, and 7) Single Action.

Potentiation (*Xiang Xu*)

Xiang Xu literally means mutual necessity. In this case, two or more Chinese herbs that are similar in effect, nature, or taste are combined so that they can enhance each other. When Gypsum fibrosum *Shi Gao* and Anemarrhena rhizome *Zhi Mu* are combined, they have an increased ability to eliminate Heat and Fire. Combining Rheum *Da Huang* and Mirabilitum *Mang Xiao* can enhance the formula's ability to purge accumulation from the intestines.

Enhancement (*Xiang Shi*)

Xiang Shi literally means mutual employment. Herbs are combined in such a way that one herb is the main ingredient while the other herbs act to enhance the primary herbs' effect. A formula with Astragalus root *Huang Qi* as the main ingredient may include Poria *Fu Ling*, which excretes water and Dampness in order to

Table I.6. Nineteen traditional antagonisms.

Chinese Herb	Herbal Antagonist
Ginseng *Ren Shen*	Trogopterus dung *Wu Ling Zhi*
Cinnamomum *Rou Gui*	Halloysite *Chi Shi Zhi*
Aconite *Chuan Wu*	Rhinoceros horn *Xi Jiao*
Aconite *Cao Wu*	Rhinoceros horn *Xi Jiao*
Caryophylli *Ding Xiang*	Sparganium *San Leng*
Croton *Ba Dou*	Pharbitis *Qian Niu Zi*
Sulphur *Liu Huang*	Mirabilitum *Mang Xiao*
Mercury *Shui Yin*	Arsenic *Pi Shuang*
Stellera chamaejasme *Lang Du*	Lithargyrum *Mi Tuo Seng*

enhance the Astragalus root's ability to tonify *Qi* and excrete water. Combining the purging effect of Rheum *Da Huang* with the diuretic effect of Akebia stem *Mu Tong* into a formula containing Scutellaria root Rheum *Huang Qin* will enhance the Scutellaria root's ability to eliminate Heat and Fire.

Antagonism (*Xiang Wu*)

Xiang Wu literally means mutual aversion. This occurs when one herb in a formula decreases or eliminates the curative effects of another. For instance, Scutellaria root *Huang Qin* can decrease the warming effect of fresh ginger Zingiberis *Sheng Jiang*, and Radish seed Raphanus *Lai Fu Zi* can decrease the ability of Ginseng *Ren Shen* to tonify *Qi*. Generally, using herbs that demonstrate antagonism in a formula is contraindicated. Table I.6 lists the 19 traditional antagonisms; however, many of the herbs in this group are no longer used.

Suppression (*Xiang Sha*)

Xiang Sha literally means mutual killing. One Chinese herb can decrease or eliminate the toxicity or side effects of another herb in the formula. For example, Zingiberis *Sheng Jiang* can eliminate or decrease the toxicity and side effects of fresh Pinellia *Ban Xia* and Arisaema tuber *Tian Nan Xing*. Similarly, Ledebouriella root *Fang Feng* suppresses the toxic effect of Arsenic *Pi Shuang*, and Mung bean Phaseolus *Lu Dou* can suppress the toxic effect of Croton seed *Ba Dou*. Suppression is similar to Counterdrive, but Suppression is active and Counterdrive is passive.

Counterdrive (*Xiang Wei*)

Xiang Wei literally refers to mutual fear. One herb counteracts or eliminates the toxic or side effects of another herb. The toxic effects of fresh Pinellia *Ban Xia* and fresh Arisaema tuber *Tian Nan Xing* are counteracted by Zingiberis *Sheng Jiang*. Again, Counterdrive (*Xiang Wei*) is the same as Suppression (*Xiang Sha*), but Counterdrive is passive while Suppression is active.

Incompatibility (*Xiang Fan*)

Xiang Fan literally means mutual opposition. Incompatibility occurs when an herb can cause severe toxicity or side effects when used with another herb. For instance, Licorice root Glycyrrhiza *Gan Cao* causes toxicity when combined with Kansui root Euphorbia *Gan Sui*. When creating herbal formulas, a practitioner should avoid incompatible herbs. The ancient veterinary practitioners identified 18 herbs that could be incompatible with some others (Table I.7); however, recent clinical trials indicate that this list may not be accurate for certain herbs.[1,2] For example, no side effects or discomfort were noted in bovine cases of respiratory diseases[1] and gastrointestinal disorders[2] after orally administering the water extract of Licorice Glycyrrhiza *Gan Cao* combined with Kansui Euphorbia *Gan Sui* or Euphorbia *Da Ji*.

Table I.7. Eighteen incompatibilities (*Shi Ba Fan*).

Herb	Incompatible Herbs
Glycyrrhiza *Gan Cao*	Euphorbia *Gan Sui*
	Euphorbia *Da Ji*
	Genkwa *Yuan Hua*
	Sargassum *Hai Zao*
Aconite *Wu Tou* (including *Chuan Wu* and *Chuan Wu*)	Pinellia *Ban Xia*
	Trichosanthes *Gua Lou*
	Fritillaria *Bei Mu*
	Bletilla *Bai Ji*
	Ampelopsis *Bai Lian*
Veratrum *Li Lu*	Ginseng *Ren Shen*
	Glehnia *Bei Shan Shen*
	Salvia *Dan Shen*
	Asarum *Xi Xin*
	Sophora *Ku Shen*
	Paeonia *Bai Shao Yao*

Single Action (*Dan Xing*)

Dan Xing literally means single action. In this case, a single herb is used to treat a disease. For instance, Licorice root Glycyrrhiza *Gan Cao* alone is used to eliminate a poisonous disease, and Dandelion Taraxacum *Pu Gong Ying* is the only ingredient in a prescription for hot swelling of the skin.

Contraindications During Pregnancy

Some herbs might harm a fetus or result in miscarriage. These toxic or very strong herbs should be avoided during pregnancy (Table I.8).

Interaction and Incompatibility of Western and Chinese Medicine

Chinese herbal medicines can usually be used safely with Western pharmaceuticals. In fact, treatment with Western medications can cause imbalances in the body, so herbal formulas may be used to treat the Patterns resulting from the side effects of the pharmaceutical. However, there are some situations in which Chinese herbal and Western medicines should not be used together (Table I.9).

Table I.8. Herbs contraindicated during pregnancy.

Herb Name	Category	Commonly Used?
Persica *Tao Ren*	Blood Stasis–breaking herbs	+++ yes
Carthamus *Hong Hua*	Blood Stasis–breaking herbs	+++ yes
Akebia *Mu Tong*	Dampness-dispelling herbs	+++ yes
Tetrapanax *Tong Cao*	Dampness-dispelling herbs	+ yes
Dianthus *Qu Mai*	Dampness-dispelling herbs	+ yes
Pinellia *Ban Xia*	Phlegm-transforming herbs	++ yes
Aconite *Fu Zi*	Warming herbs	++ yes
Cinnamomum *Rou Gui*	Warming herbs	+++ yes
Zingiberis *Gan Jiang*	Warming herbs	+++ yes
Mirabilitum *Mang Xiao*	Purgative herbs	+ yes
Pharbitis *Qian Niu Zi*	Purgative herbs	no
Sparganium *San Leng*	Blood Stasis–breaking herbs	no
Arisaema *Tian Nan Xing*	Phlegm-transforming herbs	no
Mylabris *Ban Mao*	Topical application herbs	no
Hirudo *Shui Zhi*	Blood Stasis–breaking herbs	no
Horsefly *Meng Chong*	Blood Stasis–breaking herbs	no
Croton *Ba Dou*	Purgative herbs	no
Euphorbia *Da Ji*	Purgative herbs	no
Genkwa *Yuan Hua*	Purgative herbs	no
Moschus *She Xiang*	Orifice-opening herbs	no

Table I.9. Cautions of combination of herbs and Western pharmaceutical drugs.

Chinese Herb		Incompatible Western Drug	Possible Side Effect
Herbs containing flavonoids	Scutellaria *Huang Qin* Lonicera *Jin Yin Hua* Citrus *Chen Pi* Inula *Xuan Fu Hua*	Aluminum hydroxide Magnesii trisilicas Calcium carbonate	Chemical interactions create metal complexes that reduce the herbal effect.
Charred herbs	Sanguisorba *Di Yu* Acacia *Er Cha* Melaphis *Wu Bei Zi* Polygonum *Hu Zhang* Rheum *Da Huang*	Vitamin B family Vit B12 Vit B6 Vit B complex	The vitamin B effects are reduced.
Special patients	Cardiac medication Diuretics Antidiabetic medication Antihypertensive medications Blood thinners		When Chinese Herbs and Western drugs have similar effects, it is possible to overdose the patient.

Herbs containing flavonoids (Scutellaria *Huang Qin*, Lonicera *Jin Yin Hua*, Citrus *Chen Pi*, and Inula *Xuan Fu Hua*) should not be used with aluminium hydroxide, magnesii trisilicas and calcium carbonate. The metal ions in these Western medications interact with the flavonoids in the herbs to form metal complexes. This changes the herbs' original properties and can significantly reduce their effect.

Charred herbs (Sanguisorba *Di Yu*, Acacia *Er Cha*, Melaphis *Wu Bei Zi*, Polygonum *Hu Zhang*, and Rheum *Da Huang*) should not be used with vitamin B because the herbal charcoal combines with the vitamin B, and this complex is then eliminated from the body. Therefore, efficiency of both the herbs and the vitamin B is decreased.

It is important to carefully monitor patients who are receiving Western cardiac drugs, diuretics, antidiabetic drugs, antihypertensive medications and blood thinners in addition to herbal formulas with similar actions. These patients are more susceptible to overdose.[3,4]

Cautions and Contraindication with Food

Generally, any herbal medicine should be cautioned with raw, spicy, or greasy foods, and with poultry and fish because they could irritate the Stomach, and retain the *Xie Qi* (Evil *Qi*). Selected foods should be avoided in patients with certain Traditional Chinese Medicine disease diagnoses (Tables I.10, I.11).[5]

Federal Drug Administration (FDA) Regulations

In the United States, the federal government regulation of Chinese Herbal Medicines falls under the Dietary Supplement Health and Education Act (DSHEA), which

Table I.10. Food contraindications for special Patterns.

Special Pattern	Contraindicated Foods
Spleen *Qi* Deficiency patients	Raw, cold, fried, or oily foods, hard and solid foods, cheese or other dairy products
Cold Pattern	Cold and raw foods
Yang excess (Heat) Pattern	Pungent, hot, oily or fried foods, wine (alcohol)
Liver *Yang* Rising	Garlic, liquor (Chinese white wine), pepper
Congested chest disorders	Fatty foods, alcohol, coffee
Liver *Yang* rising	Hot pepper, onion, alcohol, coffee
Spleen/stomach deficiency	Deep-fried food or hard, cold frozen food
Skin disorders	Fish, shrimp, crab
Exterior Pattern	Oily or greasy food
Cancer or tumors	Shrimp, crab, poultry

Table I.11. Food contraindications for special herbs.

Special Herb	Contraindicated Foods
Salvia *Dan Shen*, or Poria *Fu Ling*	Vinegar
Rehmannia *Shu* or *Sheng Di Huang* or Polygonum *He Shou Wu*	Onion, garlic, or horseradish
Ginseng *Ren Shen*	Radish, or horseradish
Mentha *Bo He*	Crab
Smilax *Tu Fu Ling*, or Quisqualis *Shi Jun Zi*	Tea
Honey *Feng Mi*	Onion

was initiated by the 103rd Congress in 1994 and signed into law by President Clinton. According to this law, herbs are considered a dietary supplement and are regulated as such by the new law. Unlike pharmaceuticals, dietary supplements are regulated using food standards for adulteration, and the burden of proof rests with the federal government when finding a product or ingredient to be adulterated or having an unreasonable risk of injury.[6,7] The FDA does not approve the safety and effectiveness of dietary supplements before they are available to consumers.[8]

Since this law passed, some herbal ingredients have come under scrutiny of the FDA. On May 16, 2000, the FDA posted a warning to the industry about herbs containing aristolochic acid.[9] Products containing aristolochic acid were associated with life-threatening adverse effects due to its nephrotoxicity. On April 9, 2001, the FDA posted a revised list of botanical ingredients, which are known or suspected to contain aristolochic acid (http://www.cfsan.fda.gov/~dms/ds-bot2.html).

The following are examples of herbs that definitely or possibly contain aristolochic acid:

1. Aristolochia spp. (*Guan Mu Tong* or *Guang Mu Tong*)
2. Aristolochia contorta (*Ma Dou Ling* or *Tian Xian Teng*)
3. Aristolochia debilis (*Ma Dou Ling, Tian Xian Teng,* or *Qing Mu Xiang*)
4. Aristolochia fangchi (*Guang Fang Ji* or *Fang Ji*)

The following are examples of Chinese herbal medications that may be adulterated by aristolochic acid:

1. Akebia spp. (*Mu Tong, Ku Mu Tong, Zi Mutong,* or *Bai Mu Tong*)
2. Asarum heterotropoides (*Bei Xi Xin* or *Xi Xin*)
3. Asarum sieboldii (*Xi Xin* or *Hua Xi Xin*)
4. Clematis chinensis (*Wei Ling Xian*)
5. Sinomenium acutum (*Xun Feng Teng* or *Da Feng Teng*)
6. Stephania tetrandra (*Fen Fang Ji, Fang Ji,* or *Han Fang Ji*)

Another herbal medication that came under federal scrutiny is Ephedra *Ma Huang*, which had often been used in weight loss supplements. Ephedra *Ma Huang* can cause increased heart rate and blood pressure and may cause a stroke or heart attack. At least 155 death reports were associated with Ephedra *Ma Huang*. In 2004, the FDA issued a final rule that prohibited the sale of dietary supplements containing ephedrine alkaloids due to the unreasonable risk of illness those products presented to the consumer.[10]

CHINESE HERBAL FORMULAS

During the early development of herbal medicine, the ancient practitioners used individual Chinese herbs (*Zhong-yao*) to treat diseases. When the herbal healers later found that combining several Chinese herbs was more effective, the concept of Chinese herbal formulas was born. A traditional Chinese veterinary formula contains different quantities of several Chinese medicinal components as guided by TCM principles. Although minerals and animal-origin products may be components in some formulas, the formulas are comprised primarily of plants or herbs; thus, these formulas are labeled as Chinese herbal formulas. A typical Chinese herbal formula contains between 4 and 15 herbs, each of which may have an assigned role within the formula.

There are four roles in an herbal formula: 1) King (Emperor), 2) Ministers, 3) Adjuvant (Assistant), and 4) Messenger (Servant or Transporter) (Table I.12). The King (Emperor) is the main part of a formula. These roles generate the formula's major therapeutic effects in addressing the primary Patterns or causes of disease. Ministers are the Chinese medicine components that assist or enhance the effects of the King. The Adjuvant (Assistant) plays three roles: 1) treating adjunct Patterns

Table I.12. Roles of a Chinese herbal formula.

Member	Roles/Actions	# of Members
King *Jun*	Address the major cause of a disease or major Pattern	1–2
Minister *Cheng*	Assist/enhance the King	1–5
Adjuvant *Zuo*	Address the minor cause of a disease or a secondary Pattern Suppress toxic or drastic activities of King/Minister Balance the energy of the whole formula	1–6
Messenger *Shi*	Transportation Harmonization; a peacemaker and coordinator among herbal components	1–3

Table I.13. The analysis of *Ping Wei San* (neutralizing-stomach powder).

Ingredients	Actions	Dose (Ratio)	Role
Atractylodes *Cang Zhu*	Dry up Damp, strengthen Spleen	8	King
Magnolia *Hou Po*	Clear Damp	5	Minister
Citrus *Chen Pi*	Move *Qi* to clear stagnation	5	Adjuvant
Glycyrrhiza *Gan Cao*	Coordination of other herbs	3	
Zingiberis *Sheng Jiang*	Regulate the Middle, transporter	3	Messenger
Jujube *Da Zao*	Regulate the Middle, transporter	3	

or complications, 2) suppressing the toxic or extreme activities of the King and Minister, and 3) counteracting. Counteracting is adding small quantities of cool or cold herbal components to warming or heating formulas or warm or hot herbs to cool or cold formulas. This helps to balance the formula's overall temperature. The Messenger (Servant or Transporter) is the component of the formula that distributes the formula's effects to the diseased areas or organs and coordinates the effects of the other ingredients in the formula. Table I.13 demonstrates how each of the components of the formula *Ping Wei San* takes on one of these four roles.

FORMS AND ADMINISTRATION OF CHINESE HERBAL PRODUCTS

Processed herbs are available in various forms, including powder, capsule, decoction, patent pill and extract granule, paste, and wine.

Powder, *San*

The herbs are ground into powder, which can be administered orally or applied topically. Simple preparation, easy administration, and rapid absorption make herbal powders one of the most commonly used forms in veterinary clinics.

Oral Administration

Tubing: Mix the powder with hot water and administer with a gastric tube. This approach may be used for large animals.

Top-dressing on food: Use this method for either small or large animals.

Topical Application

Mix the herbal powder with wine, vinegar, or honey and apply to the surface of wounds, boils, swellings, or locally affected areas.

Decoction, *Tang*

The herbs are mixed with an appropriate amount of water, added to a metal or porcelain container, and boiled for about 1–2 hours. Next, the liquid is poured or filtered out so that the herbs are kept inside the container. More water is added to the herbs and they are again boiled for 1–2 hours and drained twice more in the same way. The final result is a mixture of the filtered liquid from all three boilings, and this is stored in a refrigerator 4°C/39.21°F for later use. It can be stored for up to 7 days and still be effective.

A decoction can be administered orally by tubing (horses) or syringing (small animals), or can be applied topically. Because of its fast absorption with superior therapeutic outcomes, this form is commonly used to treat acute or severe diseases. However, as it is very time consuming to prepare and palatability is a big problem, this form is not commonly used in the veterinary practice (Fig. I.2).

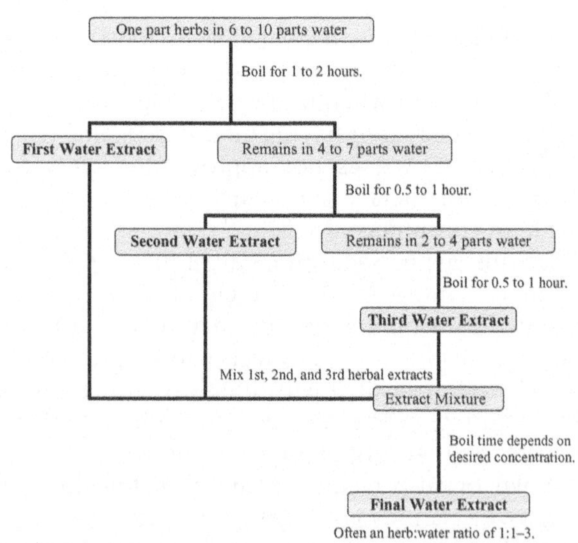

Figure I.2. *Diagram of formulation of an herbal decoction.*

Patent Pills or Extract Granules

Patented pills (teapills) or extract granules are the modern form of the Chinese herbal medicine (Fig. I.3). Teapills are the popular forms used in small animal practice because the teapill is easy to administer orally due to its small size and palatable coating. Extract granules, often concentrated, are easily disguised in food with less. However, potency may be lost during processing of either teapills or extract granules so it requires prolonged administration to achieve good clinical results.

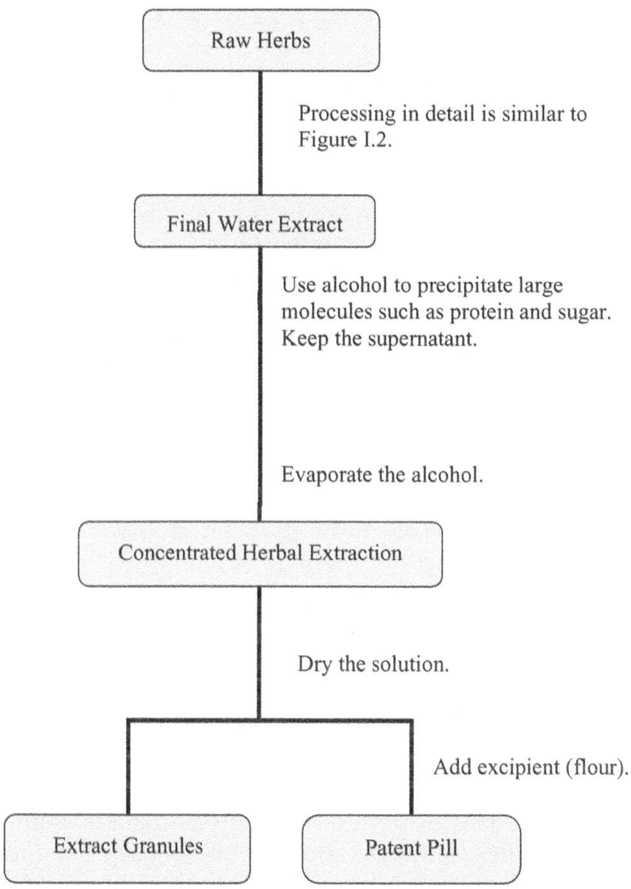

Figure I.3. *Diagram of formulation of an herbal pill or extract granules.*

Capsules, *Jiao Nang*

When powder forms or extract granules are given in small animals, including cats and dogs, palatability is always a major challenge. Thus, powder or extract granules can be encapsulated. Capsules can be administered orally in a similar manner to either powder or extract granules.

Paste, *Gao*

Pastes are used only topically. Beeswax is added to sesame seed, cottonseed or peanut oil. This is heated until it melts, and then finely powdered herbs are added while stirring constantly to form a paste as it cools. This is mostly used to treat skin lesions such as wounds, boils, and swellings.

Herbal Wine/Alcohol Tincture

Herbal wine is commonly used for arthritis, *Bi* syndrome, chronic pain, or as a general tonic. This form can be used topically and rubbed in around the pain area in veterinary practice. When it is given orally, boiling water is used to dispel and dilute the alcohol for 10–15 minutes. The obtained low-alcohol herbal tea can then be added into food or directly administered into the patient's mouth.

Regardless of the herb's form, palatability is always a major consideration in veterinary practice. Pills, powder, and capsules can be administered in a similar manner as typical pharmaceuticals. Honey, molasses, clam juice, tuna juice, or other highly palatable foods may help to conceal the taste and texture of the herbal medicine from the patients.

Decoction used to be the most commonly used form of Chinese herbs in ancient times (Table I.14). Due to the inconvenience in administration, decoction is now used only for acute or severe problems, such as high fever and acute infections in horses. The oral administration of raw herbal powder placed in capsules is widely accepted by patients in small animal practice.

Today's busy lifestyle also favors the "pop-a-pill" approach. The Chinese herbal patent pill is popular.

Table I.14. Comparison between the different forms of Chinese herbs.

Form of Herbs	Absorption	Dosage	Excipient	Effective Ingredient Loss During Processing	Convenience of Administration	Application
Decoction	Fast	High	No	Low	Not good	Horses
Raw powder	Good	Middle	No	No	OK	Horses/Dogs/Cats
Capsule (raw powder)	Good	Middle	No	No	OK	Dogs/Cats
Patent pill	Slow	Middle	High	High	Good	Dogs/Cats
Extract granules	Good	Low	No	High	OK	Dogs/Cats/Horses
Capsule (extract granules)	Good	Low	Small	High	OK	Dogs/Cats

The patent pill, however, contains a high percentage of excipient and risks losing the effectiveness of the ingredients during processing. Extract granules also have a similar high risk of losing the effective agents during their processing.

STORAGE REQUIREMENTS AND CONDITIONS

In general, the powder form of herbal formulas has a minimum 1-year shelf life, if stored in a dry and air-conditioned room. The capsule form has a minimum 2-year shelf life and the teapill form should have a minimum 3-year shelf life.

Dryness

Without water, microorganisms are unable to grow and reproduce. Dryness is the most important requirement for storage of herbs and herbal productions. This is especially true of herbs containing high concentrations of sugar. For example, Rehmannia *Di Huang*, Astragalus *Huang Qi*, Codonopsis *Dang Shen* and Achyranthes *Niu Xi* need very dry conditions. Hydroscopic agents such as silicon gel can help herbs keep dry.

Low Temperature

The storage place for herbs and herbal products should be air-conditioned (20°C/68°F or lower with adequate ventilation).

Avoiding Direct Sunlight

Direct sunlight can cause the herbs to change color and deteriorate.

Sealed Container Herbal containers may be made of glass, wood, or pottery. To prevent deliquescing and oxidizing, herbs should be stored in sealed containers.

DOSAGE OF FORMULAS

The correct dosage is critical for the successful use of Chinese herbal medicines in the treatment of veterinary patients. Giving the appropriate dose of herbal medicines at an appropriate frequency of administration is as important as making an accurate diagnosis and selecting the appropriate herbal formula. Healing will not start unless the patient gets an adequate amount of the herbal medication and at the appropriate time of the day. This may be true for other pharmaceutical medications as well.

Generalizing the amount of any particular ingredient in an herbal formula is very difficult, because the amount needed varies with the part of the plant part, the herbs' actions, the disease's characteristics, the species of the patient, and individual animal differences in response to therapy. Flowers, leaves, and aromatic herbs are used in relatively small amounts. Roots, fruits, heavy substances, minerals, and shells are added in larger amounts.

Excessive Patterns (Heat, *Yang* conditions) need relatively higher dosages; whereas, Deficient Patterns need lower dosages. Sensitive individuals may need lower dosages initially and gradually have the dosage increased to the optimal amount. Also, some species are sensitive to specific herbs. For example, feline patients are very sensitive to Lily *Bai He*; thus, avoid using Lily *Bai He* in cats or use very small doses if necessary.

Small Animal Herbal Dosage Instructions

When beginning a new herbal formula in a small animal patient, it is recommended to begin at one-third the dose and slowly increase it. For the first 2 days, 33% of the recommended herbal dose is administered twice a day. If the patient has no adverse signs (nausea, vomiting, diarrhea, lethargy, anorexia, or drooling) after 2 days, the dose is increased to 66% of the recommended dosage twice daily for 3 days. If the patient still has no adverse signs after 3 days, the standard recommended dose is administered twice daily for 2–4 weeks.

If there is improvement, but some clinical signs are still present after 4 weeks, the standard dose is continued twice daily until the clinical signs resolve (up to 6 months). If there is no improvement in one month or sooner, or if new clinical signs appear, the patient is reevaluated to detect the presence of an underlying previously undiagnosed Pattern or a misdiagnosis of the original Pattern. Then an appropriate different herbal medication is selected and administered at 33% of the dose and increased as described above.

If the patient exhibits adverse effects (nausea, vomiting, diarrhea, lethargy, anorexia, or drooling) in the first 2–5 days of beginning a new herbal formula at 33% or 66% of the recommended dose, the herbal medication is discontinued for 2 days and the patient is evaluated for other problems not related to the herbal medication. If the signs resolve after 48 hours off the herbal medication, a second attempt is made and 33% of the standard dose twice daily is again administered. If the patient appears to have no adverse effects this time, the medication is increased after 2–3 days and continued as described above.

If the adverse signs (nausea, vomiting, diarrhea, lethargy, anorexia, or drooling) improve when the herbal medication is discontinued but reappear when the medication is reintroduced at 33% or 66% of the standard dose, another herbal formula is selected and administered at 33% of the standard dose and slowly increased, as described above.

Table I.15. General standard dosage of herbal formulas for large and small animals.

Herbal Form	Species	Size	Dosage
Capsule	Canine	Small	1 to 2 capsules (0.5 to 1 g), once to twice daily
		Medium	3 to 5 capsules (1.5 to 3 g), once to twice daily
		Large	6 to 10 capsules (3 to 5 g), once to twice daily
	Feline	1 to 3 capsules (0.2 to 0.6 g) once to twice daily	
Raw powder	Equine	Foal	Top-dressing with food 3 to 8 g twice daily
		Pony	Top-dressing with food 10 to 20 g, twice daily; or tubing, 150 to 250 g, once daily
		Horse	Top-dressing with food 15 to 30 g, twice daily; or tubing, 200 to 400 g, once daily
Patent pills	Canine	Small	1 to 3 pills, once to twice daily
		Medium	3 to 5 pills, once to twice daily
		Large	6 to 10 pills, once to twice daily
	Feline	1 to 3 pills, once to twice daily	
Extract granules	Canine	Small	1/4 tsp, twice daily
		Medium	1/2 tsp, twice daily
		Large	1 tsp, twice daily
	Feline	Small	1/8 tsp, twice daily
		Large	1/4 tsp, twice daily
	Equine	Foal	1 to 2 tsp, twice daily
		Pony	2 to 4 tsp, twice daily
		Horse	3 to 5 tsp, twice daily

Equine Herbal Dosage Instructions

For equine patients there is no need to begin at 33% of the dose as in small animals (Table I.15). The total recommended dose is begun twice a day in horses. If the medication is administered as a top-dressing on grain, it is usually continued for at least 4–8 weeks. If the medication is administered by nasogastric tube, it is usually continued for only 5–7 days.

If a patient on herbal medication administered with the top-dressing with food has improved after 2 weeks, but clinical signs are still present, the standard dose is continued twice a day for 4–8 weeks. If the patient completely recovers in 4 weeks, the herbal medicine with the top-dressing with food is often continued at 50% of the recommended dose for another 4 weeks to ensure that healing is complete.

If the horse has not improved within 1 month or has more clinical signs within 2 weeks, the patient should be reevaluated to detect another Pattern or a Pattern misdiagnosis, and an additional or different herbal therapy is prescribed.

REFERENCES

1. Gong QL. Study on eighteen incompatibilities (*Shi Ba Fan*). Journal of Traditional Chinese Veterinary Medicine 1983;1: 14–16.
2. Editorial. Clinical application of eighteen incompatibilities in veterinary medicine. Journal of Traditional Chinese Veterinary Medicine 1974;2:33.
3. Bensky D, Clavey S, Stoger E. Chinese Herbal Medicine Materia Medica (3rd Edition). Seattle, WA: Eastland Press, Inc., 2004.
4. Xu XY. Pharmacology of Chinese Herbal Materia Medica. Beijing: People's Health Press, 2005.
5. Gao XM. Chinese Herbal Materia Medica. Beijing: China Traditional Chinese Medicine Publishing House, 2002: 39–41.
6. http://www.fda.gov/opacom/laws/dshea.html#sec4
7. http://www.health.gov/dietsupp/ch1.htm
8. http://www.cfsan.fda.gov/~dms/ds-oview.html#safe
9. http://www.cfsan.fda.gov/~dms/ds-botl1.html
10. http://www.cfsan.fda.gov/~lrd/fpephed6.html

1 Herbs to Tonify Deficiency 补益药

Huisheng Xie, Min Su Kim, Cheryl Chrisman

INTRODUCTION

Identifying a Deficiency Pattern

Treating a Deficiency with herbs first requires recognizing which Deficiency Pattern is present. Deficiency Patterns are collections of disease signs that occur when there are certain kinds of imbalances in the body. As stated in the ancient text, *Huang Di Nei Jing*, "no disease occurs if *Yin* and *Yang* maintain a relative balance" but "disease occurs when there is loss of the balance between *Yin* and *Yang*." The Eight Principles method further characterizes disease by using pairs of opposite Patterns, which include Exterior or Interior, Heat or Cold, Excess or Deficiency, and *Yang* or *Yin*. Deficiency Patterns are then divided into four categories: *Qi* Deficiency, Blood Deficiency, *Yin* Deficiency and *Yang* Deficiency (Table 1.1).

Deficiency Patterns are often seen in geriatric patients with chronic illnesses. Patients with Deficiency Patterns usually exhibit general weakness, fatigue, lethargy, a weak pulse, and a pale or red tongue. An individual patient's specific combination of clinical signs, tongue appearance, and pulse quality help pinpoint which of the four Deficiency categories are occurring in the patient, indicating which treatments are most appropriate.

Treating a Deficiency Pattern

According to the *Huang Di Nei Jing*, "Deficiency is treated with tonification" to restore the equilibrium of *Yin* and *Yang*. There are four categories of Chinese herbs that tonify Deficiency: *Qi* Tonic, Blood Tonic, *Yin* Tonic and *Yang* Tonic (Table 1.1). Each herb category treats a specific Deficiency Pattern because the properties of the herbs counteract the particular deficiencies within that Pattern.

A *Qi* tonic focuses on the Upper Burner (*Shang Jiao*) and Middle Burner (*Zhong Jiao*) Deficiencies (Lung, Heart, and Spleen), which are often present in a *Qi* Deficiency Pattern. The Spleen generates *Qi* and the Lung distributes the *Qi*, so strengthening these two organs will promote the production and distribution of *Qi*, counteracting the *Qi* Deficiency. The herb Astragalus *Huang Qi* falls in the *Qi* Tonic category because it can tonify Spleen *Qi*, Lung *Qi*, and Heart *Qi*. A Blood tonic focuses on the Lower and the Middle Burners (Kidney and Liver) because the Kidney stores Essence (*Jing*) and the Liver stores Blood. This herbal tonic strengthens the Kidney and enriches the *Jing* stored there, and then the *Jing* transforms into Blood. This strengthening of the Liver further increases its supply and availability of Blood. The herb Rehmannia *Shu Di Huang* is a basic Blood tonic, because it tonifies Kidney *Jing* and Liver Blood, resulting in increased Blood. A *Yang* tonic, such as Morinda *Ba Ji Tian*, uses warm tonification because it needs to replace the missing Heat due to insufficient *Yang*. A *Yin* tonic, such as Lily *Bai He*, uses cool tonification because it replaces the missing coolness due to insufficient *Yin*. In all these cases, the tonic herbs increase the deficient component in order to bring it back into balance with the other components.

Generally speaking, tonifying herbs have several possible actions, including 1) enhancing the physiological activities of internal organs (*Qi* tonic), 2) moistening and nourishing the body (Blood and *Yin* tonic), 3) increasing disease resistance, 4) improving the healing process, 5) enhancing the immune response, and 6) promoting absorption of and better utilization of nutrients. Some of these herbs act similarly to western pharmaceuticals such as epinephrine, corticosteroids, hormones, and digoxin.

Tonic herbal formulas frequently include other herbs in addition to the tonic herbs. First, a pure tonic may generate Stagnation because it increases essential substances (*Qi*, Blood, *Yin*, or *Yang*). For this reason, tonic herbs are often combined with one or more herbs that move *Qi*-Blood to resolve Stagnation. For example, *Si Wu Tang*, a basic Blood tonic herbal formula, consists

Table 1.1. Tonic and indications.

Deficiency Category	Clinical Signs	Tonic Category	Tonic Characteristics
Qi Deficiency	Weakness, fatigue, or shortness of breath Depression, anorexia Chronic diarrhea, urinary leakage Tongue: pale/wet Pulse: weak	*Qi* Tonic	Energy: Warm/neutral Taste: Sweet Activity: Tonify the Upper/Middle Burner
Blood Deficiency	Dry and cracked paws/hooves Flaky skin (large dandruff) Poor stamina Tongue: pale/dry Pulse: thin/weak	Blood Tonic	Energy: Neutral Taste: Sweet Activity: Tonify the Lower/ Middle Burner
Yin Deficiency	Cool-seeking, hot, panting, thirsty Flaky skin (fine dandruff) Hyperactivity Tongue: red/dry Pulse: thin/fast	*Yin* Tonic	Energy: Cool Taste: Sweet/bitter Activity: Moisten Body Fluids/clear Heat
Yang Deficiency	*Qi* Deficiency with Cold signs (warm-seeking, Cold ear/nose/back/extremity) Tongue: pale purple/swollen/wet Pulse: deep/slow/weak	*Yang* Tonic	Energy: Warm/hot Taste: Sweet Activity: Tonify *Yang*/warm the Interior

of Rehmannia *Shu Di Huang*, Angelica *Dang Gui*, Paeonia *Bai Shao Yao*, and Ligusticum *Chuan Xiong*. In this formula, Rehmannia, Angelica, and Paeonia act as Blood tonics while Ligusticum prevents Stagnation by acting as a Blood mover. Second, Deficiency Patterns are often combined with Excess Patterns. Thus, a tonic herbal formula will often contain one or more herbs that address the pathogenic Excess factors (Damp, Heat, Cold, Dryness, Summer Heat and Wind). For example, the basic *Qi* tonic formula *Si Jung Zi Tang* contains the herb Poria *Fu Ling* to drain Excessive Dampness.

HERBS TO TONIFY *QI*

Qi Tonic Herbs treat *Qi* Deficiency Patterns by stimulating and invigorating the *Zang-fu* organs, especially the Spleen and Lung. *Qi* Deficiency Patterns are most commonly found in the Spleen and Lung because these two *Zang* organs are primarily responsible for 1) forming *Qi* (including *Gu Qi* and *Zong Qi*) from the food and air (universe) and 2) transporting and distributing *Qi* within the body. Table 1.2 describes the clinical signs of Spleen and Lung *Qi* Deficiency Patterns.

Most *Qi* tonic herbs have a neutral or warm temperature and a sweet taste, and they affect the Spleen and Lung Channels. Some *Qi* tonic herbs taste bitter and work to clear Heat or dry Dampness. Because *Qi* is partly responsible for generating and moving Blood, *Qi* tonic herbs are also used in treating Blood Deficiency Patterns. However, if a patient has a *Qi* Deficiency Pattern accompanied by Blood, *Yin*, or *Yang* Deficiency, additional herbs are combined with the *Qi* tonic herbs to tonify these other substances.

Table 1.2. *Qi* Deficiency and *Qi* tonic herbs.

Pattern	Clinical Signs	Examples of *Qi* Tonic Herbs
Spleen *Qi* Deficiency	Poor appetite, fatigue or lethargy Diarrhea Muscle atrophy, or body weight loss Abdominal distention or fullness Edema, prolapsed rectum	Atractylodes *Bai Zhu*
Lung *Qi* Deficiency	Cough/asthma, dyspnea, shortness of breath Weak voice Exercise intolerance Recurrent influenzas, spontaneous sweat in horses	Astragalus *Huang Qi*

Use caution when administering *Qi* tonic herbs because they can promote several side effects, including 1) *Qi* Stagnation in the Upper Burner or the Middle Burner, 2) loss of appetite or nausea, and 3) creation or aggravation of Heat. *Qi* tonic herbs are contraindicated in patients with Heat conditions or Excess exogenous conditions. These herbs are also not recommended for patients with signs of Exterior conditions unless they are combined with herbs to release the Exterior.

Ginseng *Ren Shen* 人参

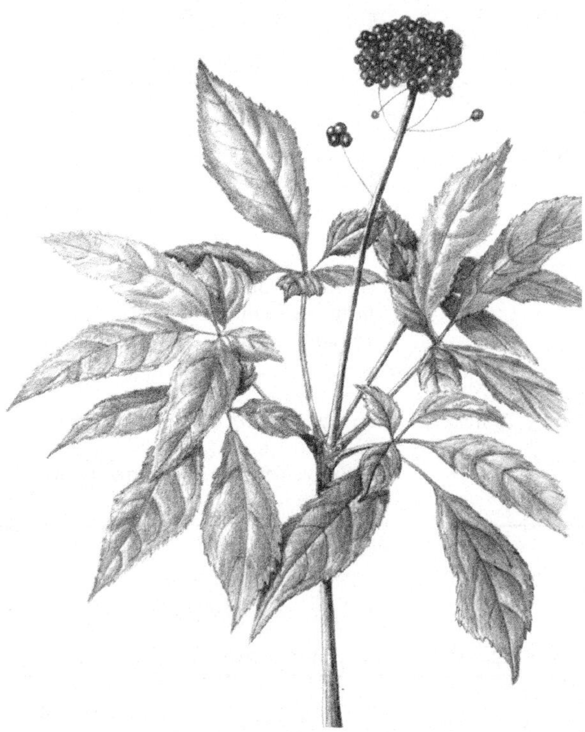

a

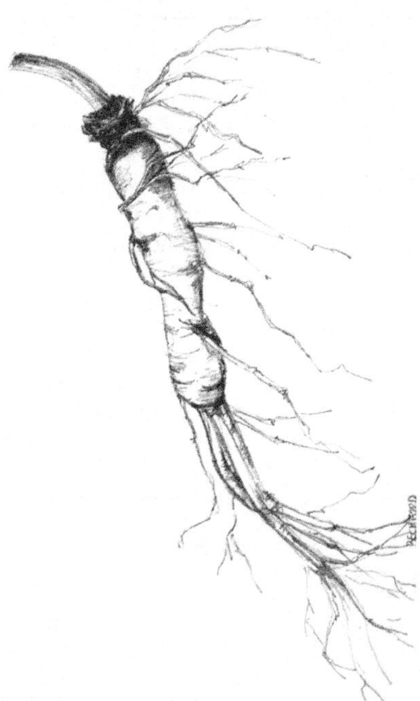

b

Original Reference: *Shen Nong Ben Cao Jing* (*Shen Nong's Materia Medica*, 1st century BCE) 神农本草经

Part Used: Root

Name:
Pharmaceutical: Ginseng, Radix
Botanical: Panax ginseng
Common: Chinese ginseng
Wade-Giles: *Jen-Shen*
Translation: Man Root or Root of Person

Energy/Taste: Warm, sweet, slightly bitter

Channel-Organ: Spleen, Lung, Heart

Actions:
1. Replenish *Qi*, rescue *Yuan Qi* collapse, and strengthen *Yang*
2. Tonify Spleen, Lung, and Heart *Qi*
3. Promote fluid and relieve thirst
4. Calm *Shen*

Form and Preparation: Powder or decoction; when administering this herb alone, it is best to double-boil and save the fluid instead of boiling it off.

Dosage:
Use double the dose for patients in shock.
Horses and Cattle: 15–30 g
Llamas, Alpacas, Goats, Sheep, and Pigs: 5–10 g
Dogs: 1–3 g
Cats and Rabbits: 0.2–1 g

Cautions and Contraindications:
1. Avoid in patients with Heat, False (deficient) Heat, or Damp-Heat.
2. Avoid in patients with *Yang* rising clinical signs, including high blood pressure. Instead, use Codonopsis *Dang Shen* as a substitute.
3. The herb is incompatible with iron, tea, caffeine, and turnips, so avoid diets that contain these substances.
4. Rhaphanus *Lai Fu Zi* or Trogopterus *Wu Ling Zhi* may reduce Ginseng *Ren Shen*'s effect.

Side Effects:
1. Bleeding is a common sign of acute toxicity.
2. Overdose or mistakenly using this herb for patients with *Yin* Deficiency or *Yang* rising can lead to headache or head-shaking, sweating, nosebleeds, insomnia (behavior issues at night), palpitations, and elevated blood pressure.
3. Skin rash
4. Restlessness; barking or behavior changes at night
5. Depression or mania

Clinical Applications:
1. Collapse of *Qi*, Yuan *Qi*, and *Yang* due to severe Deficiency, loss of Blood, severe vomiting, or severe diarrhea

Clinical signs: Sweating, cold limbs, shortness of breath, weak and fading pulse
Use: Use alone or combine with Aconite *Fu Zi*
Classical herbal formula: Shen Fu Tang

2. Weakness of Stomach and Spleen *Qi*
   Clinical signs: Poor appetite, lassitude, abdominal distension, diarrhea
   Combine with: Atractylodes *Bai Zhu*, Poria *Fu Ling*, Glycyrrhiza *Gan Cao*
   Classical herbal formula: Si Jun Zi Tang
3. Deficiency of Lung and Kidney *Qi*
   Clinical signs: Shortness of breath due to asthma, spontaneous sweating, fatigue
   Combine with: Gecko *Ge Jie*
   Classical herbal formula: Ren Shen Ge Jie San
4. Deficiency of Lung and Heart *Qi* and *Yin*
   Clinical signs: Dry throat, fatigue, palpitations
   Combine with: Ophiopogon *Mai Men Dong* and Schisandra *Wu Wei Zi*
   Classical herbal formula: Sheng Mai San
5. Deficiency of Spleen and Heart *Qi*
   Clinical signs: Fatigue, palpitations, anxiety, *Shen* disturbance, edema or diarrhea
   Combine with: Polygala *Yuan Zhi* and Poria *Fu Ling*
   Classical herbal formula: Gui Pi Tang
6. Deficiency of Kidney *Qi* and *Yang*
   Clinical signs: Male impotence or female infertility
   Combine with: Cervus *Lu Rong*

History and Comments:

1. Ginseng *Ren Shen* was discovered thousands of years ago by accident. Two brothers were trapped on the big mountain *Chang Bai Shan* (Long White) in Northeast China because of a sudden snowstorm while they were hunting in the late fall. The snow was so heavy that there was no way for them to go home, and they had to stay on the deep mountain. Many days later, after they had eaten all their food, they dug in the soil to search for new food supplies. Surprisingly, they found a big root, which became their only food for the entire winter. After the snow melted the following spring, the brothers brought this herbal root home where they were welcomed by the villagers who had thought that they were dead. Since then, the people named this special plant with green leaves *Ren Shen*, which translates literally as "man root," because this herb can reinforce *Qi* and empower a person. Therefore, this herb is the root of man and Essence of the body. The best quality *Ren Shen* is called *Ye Shan Shen*. *Ye* means "wild" and *Shan* means "a big mountain," which is where Ginseng naturally grows. *Shen* is *Ren Shen*. Although *Ye Shan Shen* produces the best results, nearly all Ginseng on the market is cultivated because wild Ginseng is now rare due to overharvesting.
2. During the *Qin* Dynasty (221–206 BC), Dr. Fei Bai Xiong attended to a patient named Zhen. Despite his strong body and strong constitution, Zhen loved to take tonic herbs. He had consumed a special meal consisting of duck cooked with about 65 grams of Ginseng *Ren Shen*. Five days later, his vision significantly declined. Ten days later, he lost his vision completely. After many other doctors' treatments failed, *Zhen* turned to Dr. Fei. Dr. Fei told Zhen that overeating Ginseng caused *Qi* Stagnation and *Qi* Stasis, which led to his blindness. Dr. Fei used *Xie-fa* (a reducing method) to treat Zhen. He instructed Zhen to drink pear juice. At first, Zhen had two to three loose bowel movements each day. After 10 days, the patient's vision had increased. One month later, his vision was completely restored. This is the early story of the side effect of *Ren Shen*.
3. Chinese Ginseng is native to China, and the root of this slow-growing plant has been valued in Chinese medicine for more than 2,000 years. According to *Shen Nong's Materia Medica*, Ginseng was known to "fill the five internal organs, calm the spirit of the soul, eliminate the evil influences, keep fitness level, maintain youthful appearance, and improve mental and physical performance."
4. There are two types of Ginseng: Chinese Ginseng *Ren Shen* and American Ginseng *Xi Yang Shen*. They are both popular, but expensive, tonic herbs that taste sweet and bitter. Chinese Ginseng *Ren Shen* is the root of Panax Ginseng *C.A. Mey*, which originated in Northeastern China. Chinese Ginseng is one of the most powerful *Qi* tonic herbs in traditional Chinese medicine. Most Chinese Ginseng is produced in *Ji Lin* Province and thus called *Ji Lin Shen*. Ginseng produced in North Korea is called Korean Ginseng, *Gao Li Shen*. Red Ginseng (*Hong-Shen*) has been steamed in rice wine and molasses to increase the effect of tonify*ing* *Qi* and *Yang* and prolonging the shelf life. Otherwise, it is White Ginseng (*Bai Shen*).
5. American Ginseng *Xi Yang Shen*, which is the root of Panax quinquefolium L., is a powerful *Yin* tonic herb in addition to *Qi* tonic. This herb is primarily produced in North America, especially Wisconsin. Chinese Ginseng *Ren Shen* is warm and used to tonify *Qi* and to rescue *Yuan* (Source) *Qi* from collapse. When entering the Spleen, Lung, and Heart channels, it both tonifies the Spleen and Lung as well as calms *Shen* with cardiotonic effects. Chinese Ginseng is classically used to promote secretion of Body Fluids and relieve thirst. Because of its warm energy and potency, it is often used at a lower dosage or short-term duration. High dosage or chronic usage can lead to nosebleeds, hypertension, and *Yin* Deficiency. It is contraindicated for use in *Yin*-Deficient and hypertensive patients. On the other hand, American Ginseng *Xi Yang Shen* is cool and used to nourish *Yin*, replenish Body Fluids, and Clear Deficient Heat in addition to tonification of *Qi*.

Pharmaceutical Ingredients:[1–4]

1. Volatile oils, triterpene saponins, Aglycone (20S)-protopanaxadiol (Ginsenosides: Ra_0, Ra_1, Ra_2, Ra_3, Rb_1, Rb_2, Rb_3; Notoginsenosides: R_4, Rs_1, Rs_2, Rs_3, Rs_4; Malonylginsedosides: Rb_1, Rb_2, Rc, Rd)
2. Aglycone (20S)-protopanaxytriol (Ginsenosides: Re, Rf, Rg_1; Notoginsenosides
3. Aglycone oleanolic acid (Ginsenoside R_0; Chikusetsusasaponin-V Rb_1, Rb_2, Rc, Rd, Re, Rg_1)
4. Water-soluble polysaccarides (panaxane A to U)
5. Polyynes (falcarinol, falcarintriol)
6. Antioxidants
7. Fatty acids
8. Salicylic acid
9. Vanillin acid
10. Vitamins C, B1, B2, B12, and niotinic acid
11. Small quantity of minerals (Mn, Cu, Co, As, Al, P, K)
12. Flavonoids

Research: Abstracts of over 3,000 scientific studies on Ginseng can be found on PubMed, a scientific article database. The research demonstrates the saponins called *ginsenosides* (panaxosides) to be the primary active ingredients in Panax species. Thus far, 13 saponins have been identified and given names such as Ra_1, Rb_1, and Rg_1. Not surprisingly, this powerful tonic herb has a large variety of positive effects: promoting tissue healing,[5] decreasing the body weight and total serum cholesterol,[6] inhibiting cancer cells,[7] and increasing endurance and performance.[8]

Codonopsis *Dang Shen* 党参

Original Reference: *Ben Cao Chong Xin* (*Thoroughly Revised Materia Medica* by *Wu Yi-Luo*, 1751) 本草从新

Part Used: Root

Name:
Pharmaceutical: Radix Codonopsis Pilosulae
Botanical: Codonopsis pilosula
Common: Pilose
Wade-Giles: *Tang-Shen*
Translation: Relative Root

Energy/Taste: Neutral, sweet

Channel-Organ: Spleen, Lung

Actions:
1. Tonify the Middle Burner, strengthen *Qi*
2. Produce Body Fluids, nourish Blood

Form and Preparation:
Decoction or powder

Dosage:
Horses and Cattle: 20–60 g
Llamas, Alpacas, Goats, Sheep, and Pigs: 5–10 g
Dogs: 2–5 g

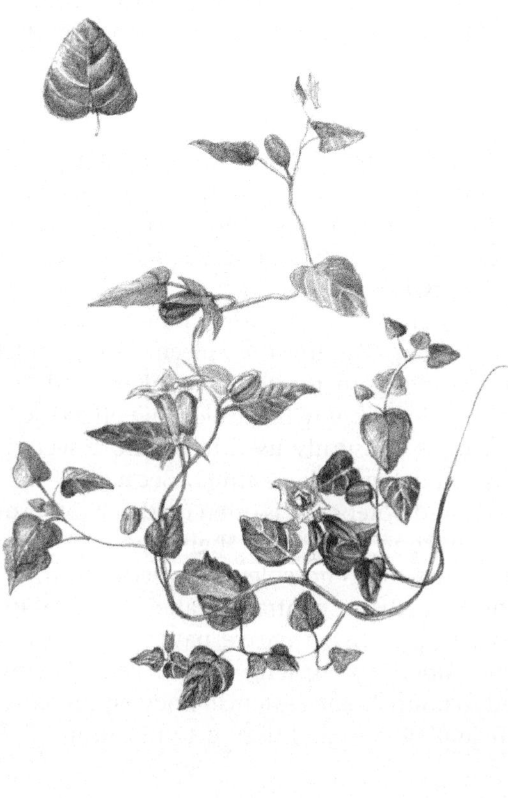

a

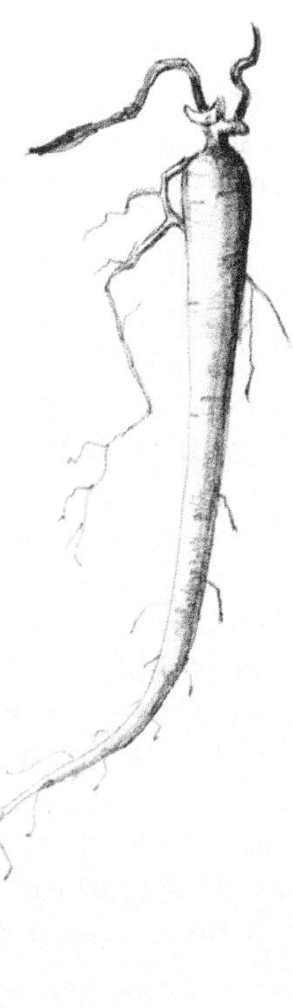

b

Cats: 0.5–1 g
Rabbits: 0.5–1 g
Birds: 0.2–1.5 g

Cautions and Contraindications:

1. None known
2. Due to its neutral energy, Codonopsis *Dang Shen* may be used for *Yin* Deficiency (False Heat).

Side Effects:

1. Side effects are rare.
2. With an overdosage, a patient may experience discomfort in the chest or an irregular pulse.

Clinical Applications:

1. Deficient *Qi* of Stomach and Spleen
   Clinical signs: Poor appetite, diarrhea, tired limbs, fatigue, vomiting, organ prolapse
   Combine with: Atractylodes *Bai Zhu* and Poria *Fu Ling*
   Classical herbal formula: Shen Ling Bai Zhu San
2. Deficient Lung *Qi*
   Clinical signs: Short breath, lassitude, cough, loss of voice, weak pulse
   Combine with: Astragalus *Huang Qi*
   Classical herbal formula: Bu Fei San
3. *Qi* and *Yin* Deficiency
   Clinical signs: Dizziness or disorientation, weakness, lassitude, increased thirst, cool seeking
   Combine with: Astragalus *Huang Qi* and Schisandra *Wu Wei Zi*

History and Comments:

1. *Dang Shen* was so named because it was first discovered at *Shang Dang* in *Shanxi* Province and its root looked like *Ren Shen*. The *Shang Dang* area was originally famous for its *Ren Shen* production, but by the Ming Dynasty (1368–1644 CE) *Ren Shen* was rare due to excessive harvesting. When the price of *Shang Dang Ren Shen* skyrocketed, unethical businessmen began to pass *Dang Shen* off as *Ren Shen*. Over decades, doctors realized *Dang Shen* was wonderful for tonifying *Qi*, even though it did not have *Ren Shen*'s warming and nourishing effects. Today, *Dang Shen* is used much more than *Ren Shen* in Chinese medicine. Who would have expected a fake to become the primary Chinese herb! Codonopsis *Dang Shen* is a neutral *Qi* tonic and is good as a general *Qi* Tonic.
2. Codonopsis *Dang Shen* may be used as a general substitute for Ginseng in most tonic formulas. Generally, Codonopsis *Dang Shen* acts similarly to Ginseng *Ren Shen*, but not as strongly. When substituting Codonopsis *Dang Shen* for Ginseng *Ren Shen*, use Codonopsis *Dang Shen* at 3–4 times the Ginseng *Ren Shen* standard dose. In serious cases of collapsed *Qi* with devastated *Yang*, Ginseng is preferred over Codonopsis *Dang Shen*.

Pharmaceutical Ingredients:[1–4]

1. Saponins
2. α-spinasterol, amino acid, Stimastereol
3. Alkalois (codonopsine, codonopsinine)
4. Glycosides (inulin, fructose, syringin, gludopyranoside, fructofuranoside, tangshenoside I, II, III, IV)
5. Flavonoids (luteolin-7-glucoside, apigenin, apigenin-7-glucoside, luteolin, aynaroside, luteotin-7-rotinoside, luteoin-7-galactoside)
6. Triterpenoids (oleanolic acid, echino cystic acid, albigenic acid, taraxeryl acetate, taraxerol, friedelin)
7. Essential oils (palmitic acid, hexanoic acid, octanoic acid, dodecanoic acid, tetradecoic acid, octadecadiecoic acid)

Astragalus *Huang Qi* 黄芪

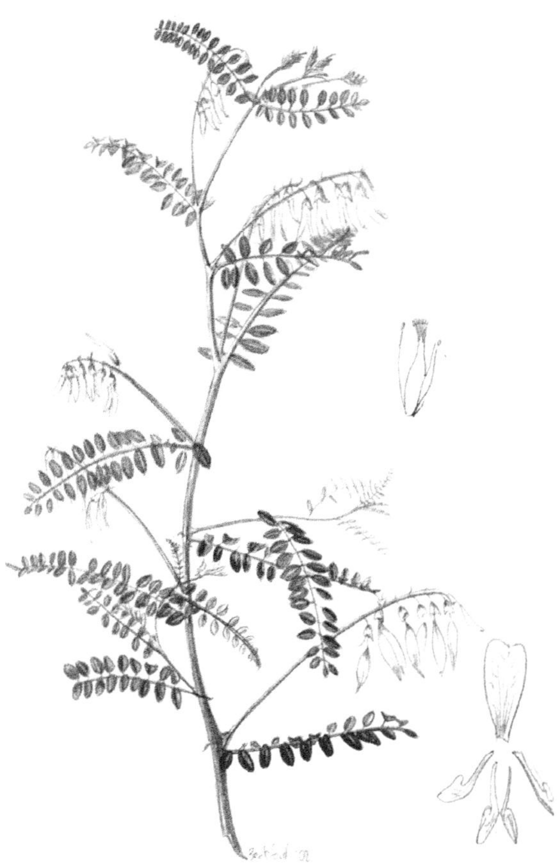

a

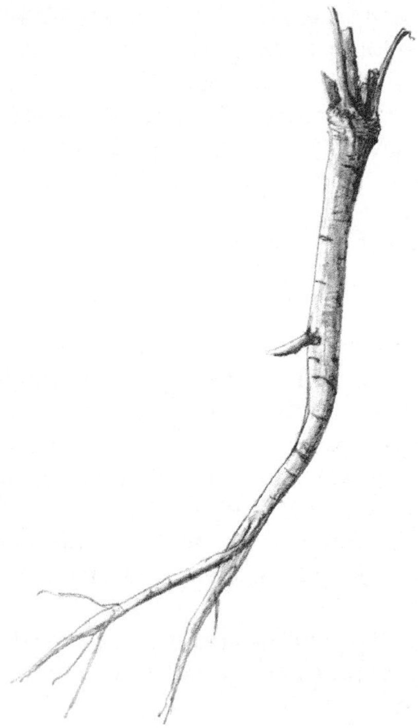

b

Original Reference: *Shen Nong Ben Cao Jing* (*Shen Nong*'s *Materia Medica*, 1st century BCE) 神农本草经

Part Used: Root

Name:
Pharmaceutical: Radix Astragali Membranaceus
Botanical: Astragalus membranaceus; A. mongolicus; A. mongholicus
Common: Astragalus root
Wade-Giles: *Huang-Ch'i*
Translation: Yellow Herb

Energy/Taste: Warm, sweet

Channel-Organ: Spleen, Lung

Actions:
1. Replenish *Qi* and raise *Yang* to strengthen Spleen
2. Tonify *Wei Qi*, stabilize the Exterior, and stop sweating
3. Clear toxins and pus, promote healing
4. Circulate water to reduce edema

Form and Preparation: Powder or decoction; stirring with honey enhances its actions to tonify Spleen *Qi*.

Dosage:
Horses and Cattle: 20–60 g
Camels: 30–80 g
Llamas, Alpacas, Goats, Sheep, and Pigs: 5–15 g
Dogs: 3–10 g
Cats: 1–2 g
Rabbits: 0.5–1.5 g
Birds: 0.3–2 g

Cautions and Contraindications:
1. *Yin* Deficiency with Excess Heat
2. Food retention
3. Exterior Excess Patterns

Side Effects:
1. May cause skin rashes
2. May extend the gestational period
3. May increase body weight of the fetus

Clinical Applications:
1. Deficiency of Lung and Spleen *Qi*
   Clinical signs: Poor appetite, diarrhea, short breath, fatigue, weakness and lassitude
   Combine with: Codonopsis *Dang Shen* (or Ginseng *Ren Shen*) and Atractylodes *Bai Zhu*
   Classical herbal formula: Si Jun Zi Tang
2. *Qi* sinking due to Deficiency of Spleen *Qi*
   Clinical signs: Prolapse of the uterus, anus, and Stomach; excessive uterine bleeding
   Combined with: Codonopsis *Dang Shen*, Atractylodes *Bai Zhu*, Bupleurum *Chai Hu*, Cimicifuga *Sheng Ma*
   Classical herbal formula: Bu Zhong Yi Qi Tang
3. Deficiency of *Wei Qi*
   Combined with: Ledebouriella *Fang Feng*
   Classical herbal formula: Yu Ping Feng San
4. Edema due to Spleen dysfunction
   Clinical signs: Swelling of face or extremities due to superficial floating edema
   Combine with: Cinnamomum *Gui Zhi*, Stephania *Han Fang Ji*, Poria *Fu Ling*, Atractylodes *Cang Zhu*
5. Slowing-healing ulcerated wounds with pus
   Clinical signs: Suppurative, difficult to drain but once perforated will produce only a thin clear discharge
   Combine with: Manitis *Chuan Shan Jia*, Angelica *Dang Gui*
   Classical herbal formula: Yang He Tang

History and Comments:
1. During the *Qing* Dynasty (1644–1911), Dr. Xu treated a patient in critical condition. The patient had edema from head to foot, shortness of breath, and loss of voice, and was unable to urinate or have a bowel movement. Dr. Xu made Astragalus *Huang Qi* wine, which is 120 grams of Astragalus soaked in 1 cup of sweet rice wine. After drinking the herbal wine, the patient was able to breathe normally and

he began urinating profusely, which significantly decreased the edema. Two months later, all clinical signs had resolved except edema in the patient's foot. The patient lost patience and saw a different doctor. The new doctor criticized Dr. Xu's therapy and gave the patient a stronger Damp-remover. The new herbal medicine almost killed the patient, so he returned to Dr. Xu's clinic. Dr. Xu prescribed 2 kg of *Huang Qi* and the foot edema completely resolved.
2. According to *Tang Shu* (The Book of the *Tang* Dynasty, 618–907 CE), Astragalus *Huang Qi* was used to treat the Emperor's mother. One day, Mother Liu suffered from a stroke and was unable to speak. The emperor hired a dozen doctors, but none could cure her. Finally the emperor called Dr. Xu Yin Zong, who was believed to possess immortal medical abilities. Mother Liu's pulse was too deep to be felt. Dr. Xu diagnosed the Emperor's Mother with a *Yang* Deficiency because the *Qi* and Blood could not flow well. She was unable to drink, so large quantities of an Astragalus *Huang Qi* and Ledebouriella *Fang Feng* herbal decoction were steamed underneath her bed until the herbal steam filled the whole room like a sauna. Mother Liu absorbed the herbs through her nose, mouth, and skin and made a complete recovery after the herbal sauna. Dr. Zhenheng Zhu, one of the greatest Traditional Chinese Medicine (TCM) masters of the *Jin-Yuan* Dynasty, later commented on this case that "Man's mouth is connected to the ground and man's nose is connected to the sky. The sky is light and clear, so the nose only receives shapeless things; the ground is deep and heavy, so the mouth only receives matters with shapes and forms. If the patient's mouth channel is blocked, herbal soup which has a shape cannot pass through, but steam can enter the mouth and the nose and dissolve the illness. The Emperor's mother could not have been saved if it weren't for Dr. Xu's great wisdom."
3. *Huang Qi* has broad-ranged immunotonic and adaptagenic effects. It has been useful in cancer. For chronic nephrosis with proteinuria, a combination of *Huang Qi* and *Dang Shen* can decrease proteinuria.

Pharmaceutical Ingredients:[1–4]
1. Isoastragaloside I–II, Cycloastragenol, Cyclosiversigenin, Fomononectic, kumatakenin
2. Astramembrannin II, Acetylastragaloside I, Soyasaponin I, tragacantha
3. Palmitic acid, linoleic acid, linolenic acid
4. Polysaccharide: astraglalan I–III
5. Protein (6.16–9.9%)
6. Selenium, Fe, Ca, O, Mg

Atractylodes *Bai Zhu* 白术

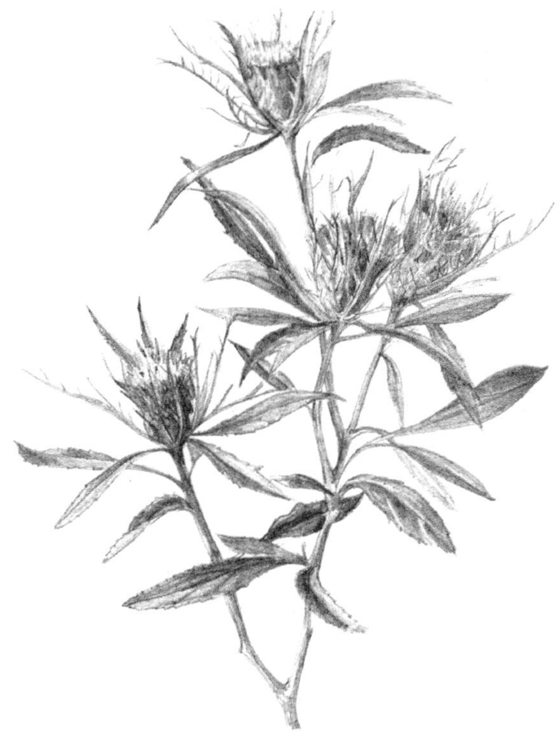

Original Reference: *Shen Nong Ben Cao Jing* (*Shen Nong*'s *Materia Medica*, 1st century BCE) 神农本草经

Part Used: Root

Name:
Pharmaceutical: Radix Atractylodes Macrocephalae
Botanical: Atractylodes macrocephalae
Common: White atractylodes
Wade-Giles: *Pai-Chu*
Translation: White Atractylodes

Energy/Taste: Warm, bitter, sweet, pungent

Channel-Organ: Spleen, Stomach

Actions:
1. Replenish Spleen *Qi*
2. Resolve Spleen Damp and circulate water
3. Calm the fetus
4. Stabilize the Exterior and stop sweating

Form and Preparation: Decoction or powder; stir-frying enhances its action to tonify Spleen *Qi* and stop diarrhea.

Dosage:
Horses and Cattle: 20–60g
Camels: 30–90g
Llamas, Alpacas, Goats, Sheep, and Pigs: 10–15g
Dogs: 3–10g
Cats: 1–2g
Rabbits: 0.5–1.5g
Birds: 0.3–2g

Cautions and Contraindications: Caution in *Yin* Deficiency with Internal Dryness due to Heat

Side Effects: None known

Clinical Applications:

1. Spleen *Qi* Deficiency
   Clinical signs: Poor appetite, diarrhea, epigastric distension, fatigue, vomiting, abdominal distension, fullness
   Combine with: Codonopsis *Dang Shen* (or Ginseng *Ren Shen*), Poria *Fu Ling*, and Glycyrrhiza *Gan Cao*
   Classical herbal formula: *Si Jun Zi Tang*
2. Water retention due to Spleen Deficiency
   Clinical signs: Edema, ascites, decreased urine
   Combine with: Areca *Da Fu Pi* and Poria *Fu Ling*
3. Prevention of abortion or restless fetus due to Spleen *Qi* Deficiency
   Combine with: Condonopsis *Dang Shen* and Scutellaria *Huang Qin*
   Classical herbal formula: Bai Zhu San

History and Comments:

1. *Ge Hong* wrote about Atractylodes *Bai Zhu* in *Bao Po Zi*. During the last years of the *Han* Dynasty (206 BCE–220 CE), a young woman fled into the secluded mountains to escape her abusive husband. Wandering for many days and nights, she could not find any food. Dying from hunger and exhaustion, a mysterious old man appeared before her. He gave her a piece of *Bai Zhu* and taught her how to find it in the wild. Her body was filled and regained its strength after she had eaten the *Bai Zhu* for a few days. For 20 years, she continued to live in the mountains and eat the *Bai Zhu*. One day, she was picking berries by a lake when she saw a beautiful girl with flawless skin and radiant eyes. To her surprise, she realized this girl was her own reflection in the water. The woman went back to her home town, which caused quite a fright in her family. Her husband thought she was a ghost coming back for revenge, for how could she grow younger after 20 years?
2. During the *Qing* Dynasty (China's last Dynasty, 1644–1912 CE) there was a governor of *Hebei* Province who suffered from Heart *Qi* Deficiency when he was young. Whenever he worked, doing even small errands, he would quickly collapse with fatigue and begin shivering. His doctor prescribed *Da Zao Ren* and *Yuan Zhi*, which caused some improvement but did not prevent the shivering from recurring. His condition would be good at one moment and poor in the next. One day, the young man happened to see a Taoist performing a Chinese game called *Fu Ji* (扶乩) at his friend's home. The Taoist, while lightly holding a willow stylus that stood on a sand tray, murmured some mantras. After a while, the stylus started moving automatically, as if some divine force was answering the prayer. The Taoist asked several questions that had been perplexing his friend. In response, the stylus slowly drew symbols and Chinese characters on the sand. The Taoist interpreted the wise and insightful answers to each question. Amazed, the man begged the Taoist to consult the Spirit about his long-lingering illness. The Taoist read from the sand tray, "The symptoms occur in your Heart, but the source of the illness is rooted in your Spleen. The Spleen is so deficient that it stole its Mother's *Qi* (the Heart). Take *Bai Zhu* frequently (to tonify Spleen *Qi*) and you will be fine." He followed the instruction diligently and soon recovered completely.
3. The raw herb is best for resolving Damp. The fried herb is best for tonifying Spleen *Qi*. The carbonized herb is best for stopping diarrhea.
4. Atractylodes *Cang Zhu* is used mostly for diaphoresis and drying Dampness. Atractylodes *Bai Zhu* is used when Spleen *Qi* is weak but Dampness is not predominant.
5. There is a saying that "*Ren Shen* is in the North while *Bai Zhu* is in the South." This refers to the highest quality Ginseng *Ren Shen* coming from Northern China while Southern China produces better Atractylodes *Bai Zhu*.
6. *Bai Zhu* can mildly decrease blood sugar levels. It also increases the white blood cell count in cancer patients with leukopenia due to chemotherapy or radiotherapy.

Pharmaceutical Ingredients:[1–4]

1. Atractylon, Hydroxyactyldide,8-β-ethoxyatractylenolide, Atractylol, β-eudesmol, hinesol
2. Palmitic acid, anhydroatractyloide, Junipercamphor, Atractylolide, fructose, Synanthrin, Sesquiterpenelon
3. Aspartic acid, serine, glutamic acid, glycine, alanice, valine, isoleucine, leucine
4. Tyrosine, phenylalanine, lysine, histidine, arginine, proline

Dioscorea *Shan Yao* 山药

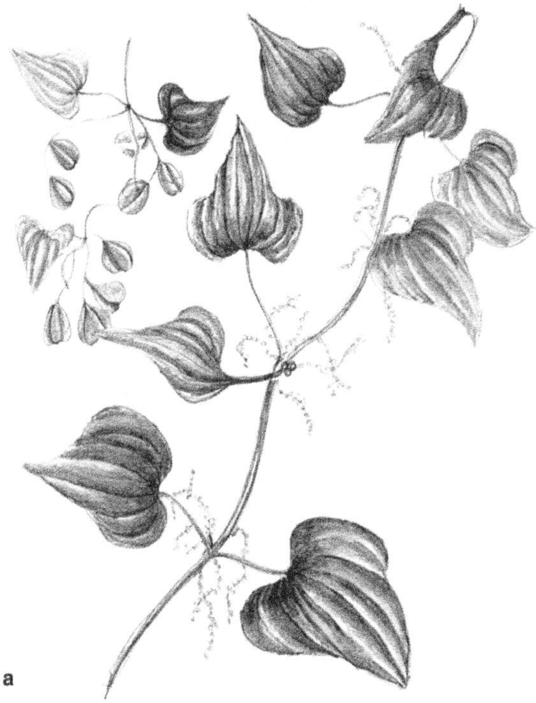

a

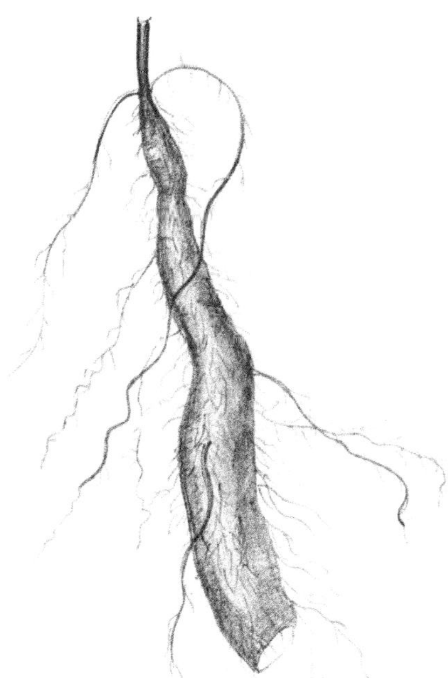

b

Original Reference: *Shen Nong Ben Cao Jing* (*Shen Nong*'s *Materia Medica*, 1st century BCE) 神农本草经

Part Used: Root

Name:
Pharmaceutical: Rhizome Dioscoreae
Botanical: Dioscorea opposita
Common: Batatatis, Chinese yam
Wade-Giles: *Shan-Yao*
Translation: Mountain Medicine
Alternate: *Shao Yu* (Mountain Encountering)

Energy/Taste: Neutral, sweet

Channel-Organ: Spleen, Lung, Kidney

Actions:
1. Tonify the Spleen *Qi*
2. Tonify the Kidney *Qi* and *Jing*
3. Tonify the Lung *Yin*

Form and Preparation: Decoction or powder; stir-frying with wheat bran enhances its action to tonify Spleen to stop diarrhea; raw will Tonify *Yin*.

Dosage:
Horses and Cattle: 30–90 g
Llamas, Alpacas, Goats, Sheep, and Pigs: 10–30 g
Dogs: 5–15 g
Cats: 1–3 g
Rabbits: 1–1.5 g
Birds: 1–5 g

Cautions and Contraindications: Caution for Excessive Dampness and Stagnation

Side Effects: None known

Clinical Applications:
1. Spleen *Qi* Deficiency
   Clinical signs: Poor appetite, diarrhea, fatigue
   Combine with: Ginseng *Ren Shen* or Codonopsis *Dang Shen*, Atractylodes *Bai Zhu*, Poria *Fu Ling*
   Classical herbal formula: Shen Ling Bai Zhu San
2. Chronic cough due to deficient Lung *Yin* and Kidney *Qi*
   Combine with: Ophiopogon *Mai Men Dong*, Glehnia *Bei Sha Shen*, Schisandra *Wu Wei Zi*
3. Diabetes (Wasting and Polydipsea)
   Clinical signs: Extreme thirst, hunger, urination, fatigue
   Combine with: Astragalus *Huang Qi*, Trichosanthes *Tian Hua Fen*, Rehmannia *Sheng Di Huang*, Pueraria *Ge Gen*
   Herbal formula: Xiao Ke Fang

4. Urinary leakage due to Kidney Deficiency
   Combine with: Alpinia *Yi Zhi Ren* and Mantidis *Sang Piao Xiao*

History and Comments:

1. The City of *Jiao Zuo* in the *Henan* Province was the home of the Kingdom of Ye in the early Ming Dynasty (1368–1644 CE). The Kingdom Ye was often bullied by its neighbors. In one winter battle, Ye's army was heavily outnumbered by the enemy and was chased deep into the mountains. The weather was bitterly cold, snow swirled through the air, and the provisions had run out. Despair began growing in the troops. Out of desperation, a soldier dug up some roots from a snow-covered field and gulped them down. To his surprise, the roots were sweet, juicy, and quite delicious. This news was greeted with cheers as it spread quickly through the army. The soldiers consumed the roots for several days, and they found their strength and vigor had returned. Many wounded soldiers had healed. Even the horses that had eaten the vines of the plant became much sturdier than before. The army rushed down from the mountain like lions, broke though the enemy's encirclement, and recovered their lost lands. At the celebration dinner, the soldiers named the plant *Shan* (山, "mountain") *Yu* (遇, "encounter"). Somehow this later changed into *Shao Yao* because *Yao* means medicine and sounds more proper. Today, *Jiao Zuo* still produces the best quality *Shan Yao* in the world. This area was also famous for its Rehmannia *Sheng Di Huang*, Achyranthes *Huai Niu Xi* (Cyathula *Chuan Niu Xi*) and Chrysanthemum *Ju Hua* production.
2. This herb is neutral, neither hot nor cold. It can treat both Kidney *Yin* and *Yang* Deficiency. It can be used long-term, often in foods as well as teas, powders, and pills. It is often used in Spleen tonics with Atractylodes *Bai Zhu* and Ginseng *Ren Shen* and in Kidney tonics with Poria *Fu Ling*.
3. *Shan Yao* has been very effective for neonatal diarrhea and has successfully treated ulcers in the gums and mouth. *Shan Yao* also improves the digestive system, promotes urination, lowers blood sugar, lowers blood pressure, and has antiaging effects.

Pharmaceutical Ingredients:[1–4]

1. Saponin, choline, allantoin, batasine
2. Manna, Choline, Abscisin, Phytic acid, 16% Starch, Dopamine
3. Amylase, glycoprotein
4. Vitamin C, polyphenoloxidase
5. Arginine, glutamic acid, aspartic acid
6. Fe, Cu, Zn, Co, Cy

Glycyrrhiza *Gan Cao* 甘草

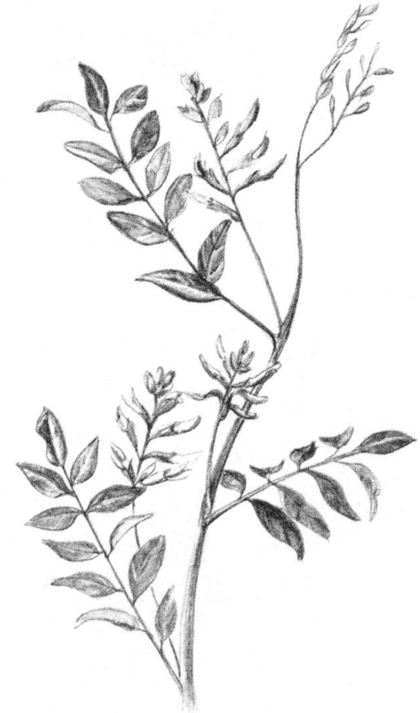

a

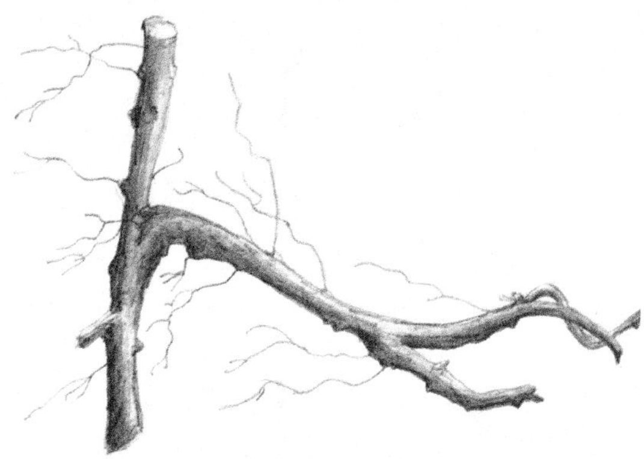

b

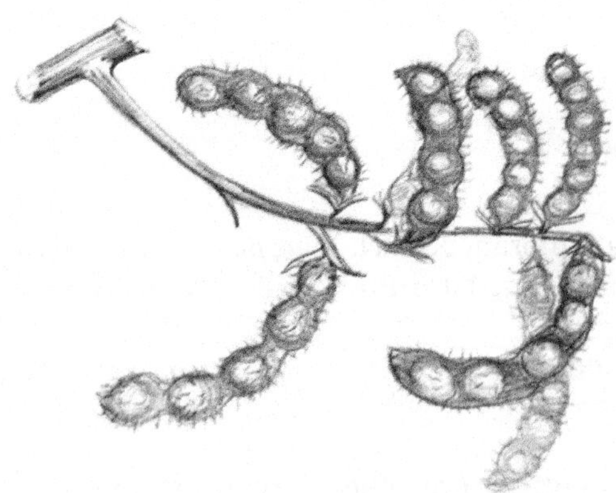

c

Original Reference: *Shen Nong Ben Cao Jing* (*Shen Nong's Materia Medica*, 1st century BCE) 神农本草经

Part Used: Root

Name:
Pharmaceutical: Radix Glycyrrhiza
Botanical: Glycyrrhiza uralensis; G. inflata; G. glabra Licorice)
Common: Licorice Root
Wade-Giles: *Kan-Tsao*
Translation: Sweet Herb
Alternate: *Guo* Lao

Energy/Taste: Neutral, sweet

Channel-Organ: Heart, Lung, Spleen, Stomach, and all other organs (12 Channels)

Actions:
1. Tonify the Spleen and *Qi*
2. Moisten the Lung and stop coughing
3. Moderate spasms and relieve pain
4. Regulate and harmonize herbs
5. Clear Heat and relieve toxicities

Form and Preparation: Decoction or powder; stir-fry with honey to tonify Spleen *Qi* and moisten Lung; raw is slightly cold to clear Heat and remove toxins.

Dosage:
Horses and Cattle: 15–60 g
Camels: 45–100 g
Llamas, Alpacas, Goats, Sheep, and Pigs: 3–10 g
Dogs: 1–5 g
Cats: 0.5–2 g
Rabbits: 0.5–1.5 g
Birds: 0.3–3 g

Cautions and Contraindications:
1. Excessive Damp; nausea, abdominal distension
2. Do not use in diuretic formulas for the Lower Burner.
3. Incompatible with Genkwa *Yuan Hua*, Sargassum *Hai Zao*, Euphorbia *Da Ji*, and Euphorbia *Gan Sui*

Side Effects:
1. Long-term use or overdose causes edema because it contains potassium and leads to a potassium/sodium imbalance. It also causes hypertension, weakness of the limbs, spasm or numbness, headache or head-shaking, and dizziness or disorientation.
2. Long-term use or overdose may cause hypertension and congestive heart failure in geriatric patients, especially those that have heart disease or renal disease.
3. Chronic usage causes milk production in non-pregnant animals.

Clinical Applications
1. Spleen and Stomach *Qi* Deficiency
   Clinical signs: Poor appetite, diarrhea, fatigue
   Combine with: Codonopsis *Dang Shen* (or Ginseng *Ren Shen*), Atractylodes *Bai Zhu*, Poria *Fu Ling*
   Classical herbal formula: Si Jun Zi Tang
2. Heart *Qi* Deficiency
   Clinical signs: Palpitations, irregular pulse, pale tongue
   Combine with: Ginseng *Ren Shen*
   Classical herbal formula: Zhi Gan Cao Tang
3. Cough and asthma due to either Heat or Cold in the Lungs
   Combine with: Armeniaca *Xing Ren* and Ephedra *Ma Huang*
   Classical herbal formula: Ma Xing Shi Gan Tang
4. Used raw for carbuncles, furuncles, and sore throat due to toxic Heat
   Combine with: Platycodon *Jie Geng*, Scrophularia *Xuan Shen*, Arctium *Niu Bang Zi*, Lonicera *Jin Yin Hua* and Forsythia *Lian Qiao*.
5. Abdominal pain due to Stomach spasms or muscle spasms of the limbs
   Combine with: Paeonia *Bai Shao Yao*
   Classical Herbal formula: Shao Yao Gan Cao Tang
6. Moderating and harmonizing the actions of other herbs
   For example: Glycyrrhiza *Gan Cao* can reduce the warm and harsh effects of Aconite *Fu Zi* and the cold and purgative effect of Rheum *Da Huang*. Because of its strong sweet taste, *Gan Cao* makes any herbal formula more palatable.
7. An antidote for general food or drug poisons
   Combine with: Phaseolus *Lu Dou*

History and Comments:
1. In the *Ming* Dynasty (1368–1644 CE), Emperor Chengzu greatly trusted Sheng Yin, his personal physician. When Sheng Yin cured the Emperor's severe rheumatism, the emperor appointed him as the head of the imperial physicians for more than 30 years. When walking into the imperial palace pharmacy early one morning, Sheng Yin suddenly developed a headache and dizziness. He then collapsed and lost consciousness. Because the doctors at the Emperor's Hospital did not know what had happened to him, they did not know what to administer to him. The Emperor made a public request for immediate assistance with Dr. Sheng Yin's treatment. A folk doctor showed up at the palace and offered to treat Dr. Sheng by administering an herbal decoction. After a while, Dr. Sheng woke up. The surprised Emperor asked the folk doctor about his

treatment. The folk doctor answered, "Dr. Sheng had not eaten breakfast before entering the herbal pharmacy. He collapsed because his Stomach *Qi* was too weak to resist the various herbal and poison *Qi*. Only *Gan Cao* can relieve various kinds of evil *Qi* and harmonize the herbal medicines. I used a high concentration of *Gan Cao* to treat Dr. Sheng. That was not a secret prescription." Dr. Sheng confirmed what the folk doctor said, including not having eaten yet that morning. To show his appreciation for what this folk doctor had accomplished, the Emperor gave the folk doctor a full bag of money.

2. *Gan Cao* has both mineralocorticoid and glucocorticoid effects and increases both the duration and strength of the effects of cortisone. *Gan Cao* also decreases secretion of gastric acid and has anti-ulcer effects.

Pharmaceutical Ingredients:[1–4]

1. Triterpenoids (6–14% glycyrrhizin of the herb, glycyrrhizic acid, glycyrrhetinic acid, glyyrrhetic acid)
2. Flavonoids (liguiritin, isoliquiritin, liquiritigenin, uralenol-3-methylether, uralene)
3. Deoxyglycyrrhetic acid I,II, liquiritic acid, glycyrrhetol, glabrolide
4. Herniarin, umbelliferone, ferulic acid
5. Biotic, mannitol

Jujube *Da Zao* 大枣

Original Reference: *Shen Nong Ben Cao Jing* (*Shen Nong's Materia Medica*, 1st century BCE) 神农本草经

Part Used: Fruit

Name:
Pharmaceutical: Fructus Ziziphi Jujubae (Fructus Ziziphus Sativae)
Botanical: Ziziphus jujube; Z. sativa
Common: Date
Wade-Giles: *Ta-Ts'ao*
Translation: Big Date

Energy/Taste: Neutral, sweet

Channel-Organ: Spleen, Stomach

Actions:

1. Tonify Spleen *Qi*
2. Moderate the actions of other herbs
3. Nourish Blood, calm the mind, clear Heat, and relieve toxicities

Form and Preparation: Decoction or powder; slice before water decoction.

Dosage:
Horses and Cattle: 30–60 g
Llamas, Alpacas, Goats, Sheep, and Pigs: 10–15 g
Dogs: 1–5 g
Cats: 0.5–2 g
Rabbits: 0.5–1.5 g
Birds: 0.5–3 g

Cautions and Contraindications: Use caution in Excessive Damp conditions, which present with nausea, abdominal distension, food retention, cough due to Phlegm-Heat, intestinal parasites, and Damp Phlegm

Side Effects: None known

Clinical Applications:

1. Spleen *Qi* Deficiency
   Clinical signs: Lassitude, poor appetite, diarrhea
   Combine with: Ginseng *Ren Shen* or Codonopsis *Dang Shen*, Atractylodes *Bai Zhu*
2. Moderates the actions of other herbs
   Combine with: Diuretic purgatives (Euphorbia *Da Ji*, Euphorbia *Gan Sui*) to moderate harshness and prevent injury to the Spleen and Stomach
   Classical herbal formula: Shi Zao Tang
3. *Shen* Disturbance due to Heart Blood/*Yin* Deficiency
   Combine with: Asinum Gelatinum *E Jiao*

Comments: Two types of Jujubes are available: *Hong Zao* (red date) and *Hei Zao* (black date). The black date has a stronger action.

Ganoderma *Ling Zhi* 灵芝

Original Reference: *Shen Nong Ben Cao Jing*, the oldest and most famous medical herbal text ranked Ganoderma *Ling Zhi* as the number one herb, ahead of Ginseng *Ren Shen*.

Part Used: Spore

Name:
Pharmaceutical: Ganoderma
Botanical: Ganoderma lucidum
Common: Ganoderma, or reishi mushroom
Wade-Giles: *Ling-Chih*
Translation: Spiritual Mushroom

Energy/Taste: Neutral, sweet

Channel-Organ: Heart, Lung, Liver, Kidney

Actions:
1. Nourish Heart to calm *Shen*
2. Tonify *Qi* and Blood
3. Stop cough and asthma

Form and Preparation: Syrup, tincture, tablet, or powder

Dosage:
Horses and Cattle: 15–30 g
Llamas, Alpacas, Goats, Sheep, and Pigs: 5–10 g
Dogs: 1–3 g
Cats and Rabbits: 0.2–1 g

Cautions and Contraindications: None known

Side Effects:
1. No side effects have been found with oral administration.
2. The injectable form of *Ling Zhi* may cause an acute allergic reaction (hives, shortness of breath, vomiting) 20–30 minutes after injection.

Clinical Applications:
1. Restlessness due to Heart *Qi*/Blood Deficiency
2. Chronic cough and asthma
3. Fatigue, congestive heart failure, immunodeficiency, irregular pulse
4. Prevention of heart or brain diseases

Comments:
1. There are wild, cultivated, or synthetic forms of *Ling Zhi*, which is an herbal mushroom known to have great health benefits.
2. Polysaccharides of *Ling Zhi* have antitumor, immune modulating, blood pressure lowering and antiaging effects. Ganoderic acids help alleviate common allergies by inhibiting histamine release and improving oxygen utilization and Liver functions.

Pseudostellaria *Tai Zi Shen* 太子参

Original Reference: *Zhong Guo Yao Yong Zhi Wu Zi* (*China Medical Botanical Encyclopedia*, by *Pei Jian* in 1939) 中国药用植物志

Part Used: Root

Name:
Pharmaceutical: Radix Pseudostellariae Heterophyllae
Botanical: Pseudostellaria heterophylla
Common: Prince's Ginseng
Wade-Giles: *Tieh-Tzu-Shen*
Translation: Prince Root

Energy/Taste: Neutral, sweet, slightly bitter

Channel-Organ: Spleen, Heart, Lung

Actions:
1. Tonify *Qi* and replenish Body Fluids
2. Strengthen the Spleen

Form and Preparation: Decoction or powder

Dosage:
Horses and Cattle: 30–60 g
Llamas, Alpacas, Goats, Sheep, and Pigs: 10–30 g
Dogs: 2–5 g
Cats and Rabbits: 0.5–1 g

Cautions and Contraindications: None known

Side Effects: None known

Clinical Applications:
Deficiency of *Qi* and *Yin* of Heart and Lungs
Clinical signs: Fatigue, difficulty breathing, thirst
Combine with: Ophiopogon *Mai Men Dong* and Schisandra *Wu Wei Zi*

Comments:
1. Like Codonopsis *Dang Shen*, *Tai Zi Shen* is a neutral *Qi* tonic, but it is less tonic and more fluid generating.
2. Similar to American Ginseng *Xi Yang Shen*, *Tai Zi Shen* has *Qi* and *Yin* tonic effects, but *Tai Zi Shen* is milder and more often used for young patients.
3. *Tai Zi Shen* is often used for Deficiency cough, especially with Dryness (and *Yin* Deficiency). It can stimulate the production and activities of lymphocytes.

Gynostemma *Jiao Gu Lan* 绞股蓝

Original Reference: *Jiu Huang Ben Cao* (*Materia Medica for Relief of Famine*) by *Zhu Su* in 1404 救荒本草

Part Used: Root, stem, or whole herb

Name:
Pharmaceutical: Herba Gynostemma
Botanical: Gynostemma pentaphllam Makino
Common: Gynostemma
Wade-Giles: *Chiao-Gu-lan*
Translation: Binding Band Blue

Energy/Taste: Cold, sweet, bitter

Channel-Organ: Spleen, Lung

Actions:
1. Tonify *Qi* and strengthen the Spleen
2. Transform Phlegm and stop cough
3. Clear Heat, detoxify

Form and Preparation: Decoction or powder

Dosage:
Horses and Cattle: 20–60 g
Camels: 30–80 g
Llamas, Alpacas, Goats, Sheep, and Pigs: 5–15 g
Dogs: 3–10 g
Cats: 0.5–2 g
Rabbits: 0.5–1.5 g
Birds: 0.2–2 g

Cautions and Contraindications: None known

Side Effects: None known

Clinical Applications:
1. Spleen *Qi* Deficiency
   Clinical signs: Fatigue, anorexia, diarrhea
   Combined with: Atractylodes *Bai Zhu*, Poria *Fu Ling*
2. Stomach *Yin* Deficiency and Spleen *Qi* Deficiency
   Clinical signs: Increased thirst, red tongue, Stomach ulcers, fatigue, diarrhea
   Combined with: Pseudostellaria *Tai Zi Shen*, Dioscorea *Shan Yao*
3. Cough or asthma due to Lung *Qi* Deficiency and Lung *Yin* Deficiency
   Clinical signs: Dry cough, red tongue, general weakness, shortness of breath
   Combined with: Fritillaria *Chuan Bei Mu* and Lily *Bai He*

Comments:
1. *Jiao Gu Lan* increases performance, longevity, and immune response, and has anticancer effects.
2. *Jiao Gu Lan* is useful for the treatment of hyperlipoproteinemia in renal disease patients and thrombocytopenia.

Rhodiola *Hong Jing Tian* 红景天

Original Reference: *Si Bu Yi Dian* (*The Four Medical Tantras*) by Elder *Yuthog Yonten Gonpo* in 708–833 四部医典

Part Used: Root, stem

Name:
Pharmaceutical: Radix et Rhizoma Rhodiola
Botanical: Rhodiola rosea Limn
Common: Rhodiola
Wade-Giles: *Hong-Ching-Tien*
Translation: Red Sight Sky

Energy/Taste: Cold, sweet

Channel-Organ: Spleen, Lung

Actions:
1. Tonify *Qi* and strengthen the Spleen
2. Clear the Lung and transform Phlegm
3. Activate Blood and resolve Stagnation

Form and Preparation: Decoction or syrup

Dosage:
Horses and Cattle: 30–60 g
Llamas, Alpacas, Goats, Sheep, and Pigs: 10–30 g
Dogs: 2–5 g
Cats and Rabbits: 0.5–1 g

Cautions and Contraindications: None known

Side Effects: None known

Clinical Applications:
1. Spleen *Qi* Deficiency
   Clinical signs: Fatigue, weakness of limbs
   Combined with: Other *Qi* tonics but often used alone
2. Excessive genital/uterine discharge due to Spleen Deficiency
   Combined with: Atractylodes *Bai Zhu* and Dioscorea *Shan Yao*
3. Dry cough due to Lung *Yin* Deficiency with Heat
   Combined with: Adenophora *Nan Sha Shen* and Lily *Bai He* or used alone

Comments:
1. *Hong Jing Tian* has antihypoxia, antifatigue, and anticold effects.
2. *Hong Jing Tian* is useful for the treatment of hyperlipoproteinemia in patients with renal disease and also high altitude sickness.
3. *Hong Jing Tian* can be used for the treatment of Blood Stagnation due to traumatic injuries.

Maltose *Yi Tang* 饴糖

Original Reference: *Ming Yi Bie Lu* (*Miscellaneous Records of Famous Physicians*) by *Tao Hong-Jing*, North and South Kingdoms (5th century) 名医别录

Part Used: Whole part of maltose

Name:
Pharmaceutical: Maltosum
Botanical: Oryza sativa; Triticum aestivum; Granorum saccharon
Common: Maltose, barley malt sugar
Wade-Giles: *I-T'ang*
Translation: Happy Sugar

Energy/Taste: Slightly warm, sweet

Channel-Organ: Spleen, Stomach, Lung

Actions:
1. Tonify *Qi* of the Middle Burner
2. Relax spasms to relieve pain
3. Moisten the Lung and alleviate cough

Form and Preparation: Decoction or powder form

Dosage:
Horses and Cattle: 20–60 g
Camels: 30–80g
Llamas, Alpacas, Goats, Sheep, and Pigs: 5–15 g
Dogs: 3–10 g
Cats: 0.5–2 g
Rabbits: 0.5–1.5 g
Birds: 0.2–2 g

Cautions and Contraindications: Excessive Damp in the Middle Burner (abdominal fullness, vomiting, and diarrhea)

Side Effects: None known

Clinical Applications:
1. Deficiency Cold and colic in the Middle Burner
   Clinical signs: Abdominal pain that responds well to pressure and is alleviated after eating
   Combine with: Cinnamomum *Gui Zhi*, Paeonia *Bai Shao*, Glycyrrhiza *Gan Cao*
   Classical herbal formula: *Xiao Jiao Zhong Tang*
2. Wind-Cold Exterior Pattern
   Clinical signs: Nasal congestion and discharge, colds
   Combine with: Zingiberis *Sheng Jiang Pi*

Honey *Feng Mi* 蜂蜜

Original Reference: *Shen Nong Ben Cao Jing* (*Shen Nong's Materia Medica*, 1st century BCE) 神农本草经

Part Used: Bee honey

Name:
Pharmaceutical: Apis cerana
Common: Honey
Zoological: Apis mellifera
Wade-Giles: *Feng-Mi*
Translation: Bee honey

Energy/Taste: Neutral, sweet

Channel-Organ: Lung, Large Intestine, Spleen

Actions:
1. Tonify *Qi* of the Middle Burner, relieve pain
2. Moisten the Lung to stop cough
3. Detoxify

Form and Preparation: Raw or infusion

Dosage:
Horses and Cattle: 30–90 g
Camels: 50–100 g
Llamas, Alpacas, Goats, Sheep, and Pigs: 15–45 g
Dogs: 4–10 g
Cats: 1–4 g
Rabbits: 0.5–1.5 g
Birds: 0.5–3 g

Cautions and Contraindications: Excessive Damp in the Middle Burner (abdominal fullness, vomiting, and diarrhea)

Side Effects: None known

Clinical Applications:
1. Spleen *Qi* Deficiency with colic
   Clinical signs: Abdominal pain that responds to pressure and is alleviated after eating
   Combine with: Paeonia *Bai Shao* and Glycyrrhiza *Gan Cao*, or use alone
2. Chronic cough due to Lung *Qi* and/or Lung *Yin* Deficiency
   Combine with: Fritillaria *Chuan Bei Mu* and Morus *Sang Ye*
3. Constipation
   Combine with: Angelica *Dang Gui* and Cannabis *Huo Ma Ren* or use alone
4. Antidote to poisoning with Aconite *Chuan Wu* or Aconite *Cao Wu*

Comments:
1. Oral administration of honey is a good adjunct therapy for asthma, constipation, and ulcerated gingivitis and stomatitis.
2. Topical application of honey promotes healing of wounds due to ulceration, burns, and trauma.
3. Honey increases gastrointestinal motility, inhibits bacteria, promotes healing of wounds, and protects the Liver.

HERBS TO TONIFY BLOOD

Herbs that tonify Blood are used for Blood Deficiency Patterns. The general clinical signs of Deficient Blood include anemia, dry skin or dandruff, pale gums and lips, diminished vision, lethargy, lack of stamina, poor hoof or toenail growth, palpitations, pale and dry tongue, and thin pulse. Blood Deficiency Patterns are

Table 1.3. Blood Deficiency and Blood tonic herbs.

Pattern	Clinical Signs	Examples of Blood Tonics
Basic Blood Deficiency	Anemia Dry skin or dandruff Pale gums and lips Dizziness or vertigo (disorientation) Diminished vision Lack of stamina or lethargy Palpitation Tongue: pale/dry Pulse: thin	Angelica *Dang Gui*
Liver Blood Deficiency	Poor growth of toenails/hooves or tendons/ligaments Dry or cracked paws/hooves Poor vision and spots before eyes (fly-biting seizure activities) Irregular estrus or short estrous cycle Internal Wind (seizure activities)	Paeonia *Bai Shao Yao*
Heart Blood Deficiency	Palpitations Insomnia (behavior issue at night) Poor memory, forgetfulness, or disorientation Fatigue Anxiety and nervousness	Longan *Long Yan Rou*

not always associated with anemia, but they may arise from a variety of problems, including emotional stress, Kidney Deficiency (renal failure), Spleen *Qi* Deficiency, hemorrhage (trauma, parturition), heart failure, and chronic hepatitis. The Liver and Heart are most affected by Blood Deficiency (Table 1.3). Liver Blood Deficiency may cause poor growth of toenails/hooves or tendons/ligaments, dry paws/hooves, poor vision and seeing spots (fly-biting seizure activity), or Internal Wind (seizure activity). Animals with Heart Blood Deficiency often present with palpitations, insomnia (behavior issues at night), fatigue, anxiety, and nervousness.

A few Blood tonic herbs can directly stimulate red Blood cell production; however, most work by strengthening the body and improving nutrition, indirectly increasing the number of circulating Blood cells.[9]

The close relationship between *Qi* and Blood is represented by these sayings: "*Qi* is the General of Blood" and "Blood is the mother of *Qi*." In health, *Qi* generates Blood and causes it to circulate while Blood is the vehicle transporting *Qi* to the whole body. In disease, deficient *Qi* fails to move and generate Blood, leading to Blood Deficiency and Blood Stagnation. For this reason, a Blood Deficiency Pattern may be treated with Blood tonic formulas, which include *Qi* tonic herbs. Blood tonic formulas may also contain *Yin* tonic herbs, because nourishing *Yin* and Body Fluid can also reinforce Blood.

Herbs to tonify Blood are rich and excessively sweet. Long-term use or overdosage can easily cause Stagnation and Spleen *Qi* Deficiency. These herbs may have side effects such as indigestion, poor appetite, diarrhea, and epigastric distension. Thus, herbs to move *Qi*-Blood and strengthen the Spleen are often added to counteract these effects.

Angelica *Dang Gui* 当归

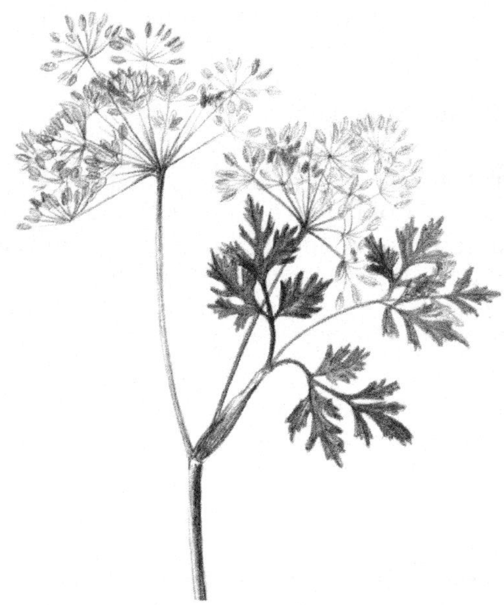

a

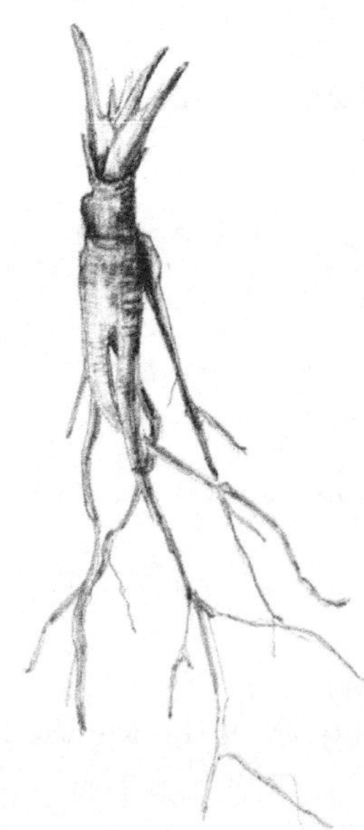

b

Original Reference: *Shen Nong Ben Cao Jing* (*Shen Nong's Materia Medica*, 1st century BCE) 神农本草经

Part Used: Root

Name:
Pharmaceutical: Angelicae Sinensis, Radix
Botanical: Angelica sinensis
Common: Angelica
Wade-Giles: *Tang-Kuei*
Translation: Should Return

Energy/Taste: Warm, sweet, pungent

Channel-Organ: Liver, Heart, Spleen

Actions:
1. Nourish and replenish Blood
2. Invigorate Blood, stop pain
3. Moisten intestines
4. Regulate female reproductive organs

Form and Preparation: Decoction, powder form, Food Therapy

Dosage:
Horses and Cattle: 15–60 g
Camels: 35–75 g
Llamas, Alpacas, Goats, Sheep, and Pigs: 5–15 g
Dogs: 1–5 g
Cats: 0.5–1 g
Rabbits: 0.5–1.5 g
Birds: 0.3–2 g

Cautions and Contraindications:
1. Spleen *Qi* Deficiency with diarrhea
2. Excess Damp leads to nausea and diarrhea
3. Prohibited during heavy bleeding

Side Effects: None known

Clinical Applications:
1. General Blood Deficiency
   Clinical signs: Pale complexion, dizziness or disorientation, palpitations, poor vision, dry skin, insomnia (behavior issues at night)
   Combine with: Paeonia *Bai Shao*, Rehmannia *Shu Di Huang*, and Astragalus *Huang Qi*
   Classical herbal formula: Si Wu Tang
2. Blood Stagnation due to traumatic injury
   Combine with: Carthamus *Hong Hua*, Persica *Tao Ren*, Olibanum *Ru Xiang*, and Myrrh *Mo Yao*
   Classical herbal formula: Tao Hong Si Wu Tang
3. Constipation due to Dryness in the intestines
   Combine with: Cistanche *Rou Cong Rong*, Cannabis *Huo Ma Ren*, and Polygonum He *Shou Wu*
   Classical herbal formula: Dang Gui Cong Rong Tang
4. Pain due to Wind-Damp obstruction in the channels (chronic arthritis)
   Combine with: Cinnamomum *Gui Zhi*, Paeonia *Bai Shao*, and Millettia *Ji Xue Teng*
   Classical herbal formula: Du Huo Ji Sheng Tang

History and Comments:
1. Angelica *Dang Gui* is a key herb for maintaining women's health and well-being, due to its ability to nourish Blood and resolve Stagnation. The name *Dang Gui* came from a romantic story: Once upon a time, a young boy named Ji fell in love with a beautiful girl, *Qin*. They married and lived happily together where the *Wei* River originated from the Mountain *Min* in the *Si-chuan* Province. In time, *Qin* gave birth to their child, but *Qin* suffered serious postpartum hemorrhaging. They visited many doctors, but none could help them. One day, *Ji* ran into an old Taoist from the Mountain *E-mei* (one of the four mountain ranges in China that Buddhists consider sacred) in *Si-chuan* Province. The old Taoist told *Ji* that he cultivated hundreds of herbs in his garden at *E-mei*. These herbs could cure hundreds of diseases, including Qin's hemorrhaging. Ji said farewell to his wife and joined the old Taoist on the thousand-mile hike to the garden. After a seemingly endless journey, they arrived at *E-mei*. Ji was immediately enchanted by the view. Mountain peaks rose from the enveloping sea of clouds and the exotic flowers and grasses adorning the valley filled the air with a pleasant aroma. The old Taoist showed Ji a plant with purple stems and white flowers. He said to Ji, "This is the herb you need, but you must follow my instructions carefully. Any tiny mistake will ruin the whole plant. You must gather the seeds after the flowers wither and plant them at the beginning of autumn. Then, dig out the seedlings at the end of autumn, preserve them through the winter and transplant them in the spring. Water, weed and fertilize with extreme caution." For 3 years, Ji followed the instructions devotedly, nursing the plants day and night until they were mature. One day the old Taoist came to Ji telling him, "Your wife needs you. You should go home now!" Thus, the herb's name comes from the word *Dang* (当: meaning

"should") and *Gui* (归: meaning "return"). When *Ji* arrived home, he saw his wife was dying. *Ji* immediately prepared *Dang Gui* soup and fed it to his wife. Upon drinking, her eyes brightened and she soon recovered. The couple cultivated many acres of *Dang Gui* and generously shared the herb. Ever since, *Dang Gui* has grown along the Wei River, and its sweet fragrance can be smelled many miles away every summer.

2. Different portions of the herb have differing therapeutic properties. The root tails (Angelica *Dang Gui Wei*) are better for moving Blood, but they are prohibited during pregnancy. The root head (Angelica *Dang Gui Tou*) is used for nourishing Blood. The whole root (Angelica *Quan Dang Gui*) is most commonly used for both invigorating and nourishing Blood.
3. Soaking the herb in wine enhances the herb's invigorating function. Frying the herb in vinegar enhances its ability to move Blood. Toasting the herb into ash increases its ability to warm the channels and stop bleeding.
4. Angelica *Dang Gui* is best combined with Astragalus *Huang Qi* to build Blood.
5. *Dang Gui* causes an increase in uterine contractions. This may be the mechanism underlying its effectiveness in treating uterine retention. The herb does not appear to have any estrogenic effect.

Pharmaceutical Ingredients:[1–4]

1. Essential oils (ligustilide, n-butylidenephthalide, n-butylphthalide, n-valero-phenone-O-carboxylic acid, β-pinene, α-pinene, camphene, p-cymene, β-phillandrene, mycene, β—ocimene-X, allo-ocimene, 6-n-butyl-cycloheptadiene-1, 4, acetophenone, β-bisabolene, isoacroraene, acoradiene, chamigrene, α-cedrene, n-butyl-tetrahydrophthalide, n-butyl-phthalide, n-butylidene-phthalide, 4-dihydrophthalic anhydride, dodecanol, bergapten)
2. Ferulic acid, scopletin, butanedioic acid, uracil, adenine
3. Vitamins A, B12, E
4. Palmitic acid, stearic acid, myristic acid, oleic acid, linoleic acid

Rehmannia *Shu Di Huang* 熟地黄

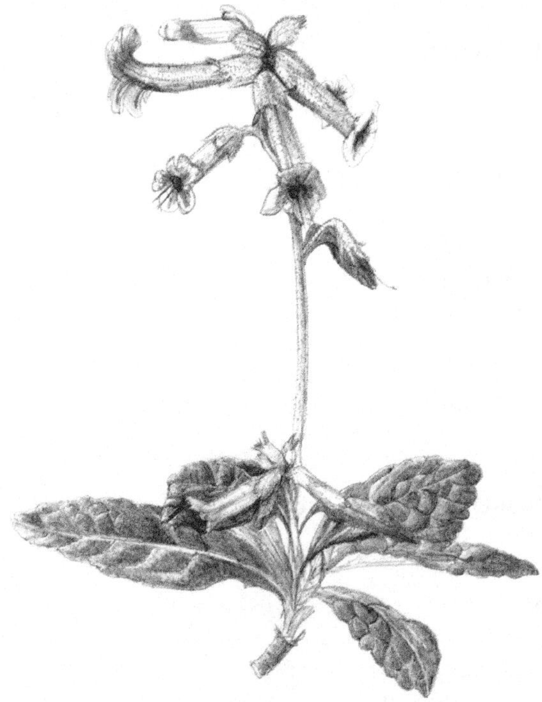

a

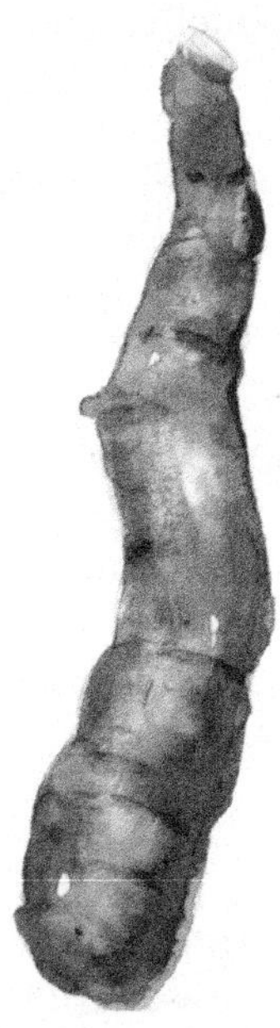

b

Original Reference: *Ben Cao Shi Yi* (*Supplement to Materia Medica*) by *Chen Cang-Qi* in 8th century 本草拾遺

Part Used: Root; steam the herb in wine until both the inside and outside turn black and moist.

Name:
Pharmaceutical: Rehmanniae Glutinosae Conquitae, Radix
Botanical: Rehmannia glutinosa Libosch
Common: Prepared Rehmannia
Wade-Giles: *Shu-Ti-Hwang*
Translation: Cooked Earth Yellow

Energy/Taste: Warm, sweet

Channel-Organ: Liver, Kidney

Actions:
1. Nourish Blood
2. Nourish *Yin*
3. Tonify Essence and marrow

Form and Preparation: Decoction or powder form

Dosage:
Horses and Cattle: 45–60 g
Llamas, Alpacas, Goats, Sheep, and Pigs: 5–15 g
Dogs: 2–10 g
Cats: 1–3 g

Cautions and Contraindications:
1. Profuse Phlegm or Damp due to Spleen *Qi* Deficiency
2. Traditionally avoided with garlic, onions, or turnips

Side Effects: Overuse can lead to loss of appetite, abdominal distention, and diarrhea.

Clinical Applications:
1. Deficiency of Blood
   Clinical signs: Pale gums/lips, dry skin/paws/hooves, vertigo or dizziness (disorientation), palpitation, insomnia (behavior issues at night)
   Combine with: Angelica *Dang Gui* and Paeonia *Bai Shao*, Ligusticum *Chuan Xiong*
   Classical herbal formula: Si Wu Tang
2. Deficiency of Kidney and Liver *Yin*
   Clinical signs: Cool-seeking, panting, poor vision, ear-ringing (head-shaking), dizziness or disorientation, diabetes, back pain, impotence, or afternoon fever
   Combine with: Cornus *Shan Zhu Yu* and Dioscorea *Shan Yao*
   Classical herbal formula: Liu Wei Di Huang Wan
3. Deficiency of *Jing* and Blood
   Clinical signs: Back pain, weakness of the hindquarters, dizziness or disorientation, ear-ringing (head-shaking), diminished hearing function, premature graying of the hair, infertility.
   Combine with: Epimedium *Yin Yang Huo*
   Herbal formula: Yin Yang Huo San

History and Comments:
1. Rehmannia *Di Huang* was called *Di Shui* (Essence of the Earth) in *Ben Cao Gang Mu* (*Materia Medica Compendium*) by Dr. Li Shi Zhen in 1590. During the *Ming* Dynasty, the famous doctor Zhang Jing-yue was particularly fond of using *Di Huang* to treat illnesses. His 1624 text *Jing-Yue Quan Shu* (*Collected Treatises of* Zhang Jing-Yue) included many references to *Di Huang*. "Disturbed *Shen* caused by *Yin* Deficiency cannot be consolidated without *Di Huang*. Raised Fire caused by *Yin* Deficiency cannot be restrained without *Di Huang*. Restlessness caused by *Yin* Deficiency cannot be eased without *Di Huang*. Irritability caused by *Yin* Deficiency cannot be calmed without *Di Huang*. Water metabolism disorders caused by *Yin* Deficiency cannot be controlled without *Di Huang*. Dispersed *Yuan* (Source) *Qi* caused by *Yin* Deficiency cannot be restored without *Di Huang*. Deprived *Jing* and Blood caused by *Yin* Deficiency cannot be nourished without *Di Huang*." It is not surprising that he earned his reputation as "*Master Di Huang*" in his later years!
2. The prepared herb is commonly referred to as Rehmannia *Shu Di Huang* to distinguish it from unprepared Rehmannia *Sheng Di Huang*. *Shu Di Huang* is warm and good for Blood tonification, while *Sheng Di Huang* is cool and good for Blood Heat, but both nourish *Yin*.
3. *Shu Di Huang*, or Prepared Rehmannia, is soaked, steamed, and dried in wine numerous times until it is soft and pliable.
4. Rehmannia *Di Huang* is a very heavy, greasy herb that causes Stagnation. Amomum *Sha Ren*, Alisma *Ze Xie*, or Leonurus *Yi Mu Cao* can neutralize this effect.
5. *Shu Di Huang* can lower blood sugar levels significantly, protect neurons, and improve memory and brain function.

Pharmaceutical Ingredients:[1–4]
1. Catalpol, 6-o-acetylcatalpol, aucubin, melittoside, rehmanniosides A, B, C, D
2. Rehmaglutins A, B, C, D
3. Glutinoside, rehmannans A, B, C
4. Stachyose, D-mannitol
5. Leonuride, monomelittoside, dyhydrocatalpol

Paeonia *Bai Shao Yao* 白芍药

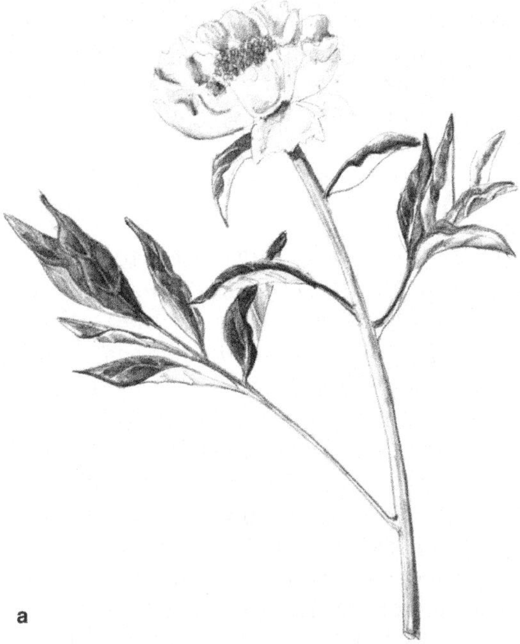

a

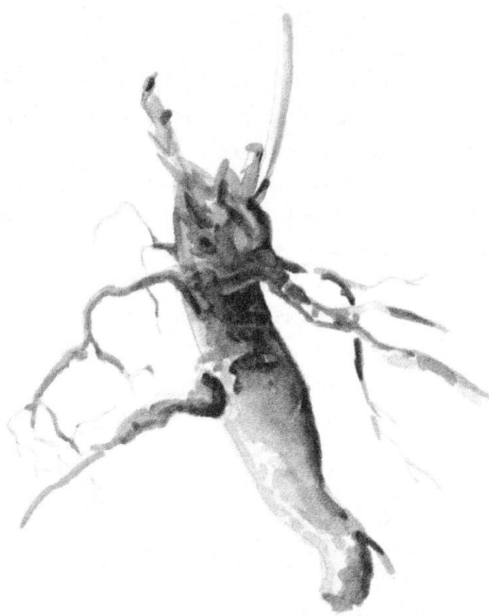

b

Original Reference: *Shen Nong Ben Cao Jing* (*Shen Nong's Materia Medica*, 1st century BCE) 神农本草经

Part Used: Root

Name:
Pharmaceutical: Paeoniae Lactiflorae, Radix
Botanical: Paeonia lactiflora
Common: White peony
Wade-Giles: *Pai-Shao*
Translation: White Peony

Energy/Taste: Slightly cold, bitter, sour

Channel-Organ: Liver, Spleen

Actions:
1. Tonify Blood, consolidate *Yin*
2. Smoothen Liver *Qi* and stop pain
3. Cool Blood and suppress the Liver *Yang*

Form and Preparation: Decoction or powder

Dosage:
Horses and Cattle: 15–60 g
Camels: 30–100 g
Llamas, Alpacas, Goats, Sheep, and Pigs: 6–15 g
Dogs: 1–3 g
Cats: 0.5–1 g
Rabbits: 0.5–1.5 g
Birds: 0.2–2g

Cautions and Contraindications:
1. Caution in cases of diarrhea due to Spleen or Kidney *Yang* Deficiency
2. Incompatible with Veratrum *Li Lu*
3. Antagonizes Dendrobium *Shi Hu* and Mirabilitum *Mang Xiao* and counteracts Amyda *Bie Jia* and Cirsium *Da Ji*

Side Effects: None known

Clinical Applications:
1. Blood Deficiency Patterns
   Clinical signs: Dry skin, dry pale tongue, anemia
   Combine with: Angelica *Dang Gui*, Rehmannia *Shu Di Huang*, Ligusticum *Chuan Xiong*
   Classical herbal formula: Si Wu Tang
2. Liver *Qi* Stagnation and Liver *Qi* Stagnation with Heat
   Clinical signs: Purple tongue, wiry pulse, depression, breast distension, hypochondriac pain, spasms or pain in extremities
   Combine with: Bupleurum *Chai Hu* and Cyperus *Xiang Fu*
   Classical herbal formula: Chai Hu Shu Gan San

3. Liver *Yang* Rising
   Clinical signs: Headache or head-shaking, ear-ringing or fly-biting seizure, irritability, aggression, quick anger, dizziness or disorientation
   Combine with: Cyathula *Niu Xi*, Uncaria *Gou Teng*, Chrysanthemum *Ju Hua*, and Rehmannia *Shu Di Huang*
   Classical herbal formula: Tian Ma Gou Teng Yin
4. Muscle pain and spasms, epigastric and abdominal pain
   Combine with: Glycyrrhiza *Gan Cao*
   Classical herbal formula: Shao Yao Gan Cao Tang
5. Deficiency of *Yin* and Blood leading to floating *Yang* and *Shen* disturbance
   Combine with: Draconis *Long* Gu and Ostrea *Mu Li*
   Classical herbal formula: An Shen Fang

History and Comments:

1. Paeonia *Bai Shao Yao* is often called *Bai Shao*. Paeonia *Bai Shao* comes from the inner part of the root. Paeonia *Chi Shao* comes from the outer part of the root and is used for Blood invigoration.
2. Paeonia *Bai Shao* is one of only two cool Blood tonics. It is an important herb for regulating the Liver.
3. Hua Tuo, a famous physician during the Eastern *Han* Dynasty and Three Kingdoms (25 CE–280 CE), was so widely respected that his name and image adorn numerous medical products in China. A group of frequently used acupuncture points (*Hua Tuo Jia Ji*) also includes his name. The *Qi Gong* exercise he invented (the Frolics of the Five Animals) involves imitating the movements of tigers, deer, bears, apes, and birds. *Hua Tuo* is considered to be China's first surgeon. Unfortunately, he had no significant successors until the modern era, when surgery was reintroduced by Western doctors. *Hua Tuo* was also known to plant thousands of herbs in his garden to study their medicinal properties. When he received a pot of pretty white flowers (called *Bai Shao Hua*) from a friend, he planted it under his window. The next spring, when the flowers blossomed, *Hua Tuo* tasted the flowers and leaves. He found nothing indicating any medical usefulness, so he ignored the plant. One autumn night, while *Hua Tuo* was writing a book, he heard someone crying outside his window. He looked out and saw a beautiful girl dressed in green and white standing in his yard and weeping. He hurried outside, but he couldn't find the girl anywhere. All he saw was *Bai Shao Hua* growing where he had seen the girl standing. When he returned to his desk, he heard the cry again, and again he stepped out to find the girl had disappeared. After this occurred several times, he was completely confused. So he woke up his wife, who said to him, "By your hand, almost all the plants around our house have become useful medicines and have saved numerous lives. Only the plant with white flowers has remained idle and lonely. Maybe you have wrongfully judged it." Hua Tuo said, "I have tested it many times and found no use for its flowers, leaves, and stems." "Then what about its root?" asked his wife. The exhausted Hua Tuo did not respond and fell right to sleep. The next morning, Hua Tuo's wife accidentally cut her hand while cooking. Blood gushed out like a small fountain. Hua Tuo immediately used his best medicine with little success. His wife suggested, "why not try the root of *Bai Shao Hua*?" The suggestion was taken seriously this time. Hua Tuo smashed the root of *Bai Shao Hua* and applied it to the wound. The bleeding stopped and the pain diminished rapidly. After a few days, the wound healed with no scar. *Hua Tuo* renamed the plant *Bai Shao Yao* because *Yao* literally means "medicine." *Bai Shao Yao* remained the name from then on.
4. *Shao Yao* has a strong analgesic and antispasm effect. The classical Herbal Formula *Shao Yao Gan Cao Tang* was effective for the treatment of facial spasms. It is also a basic formula for muscle spasms and muscle pain with the following modification:
   a. For the forelimbs: add Cinnamomum Gui *Zhi* and Morus *Sang Zhi*
   b. For the hind limbs: add Dipsacus *Xu Duan* and Cyathula *Niu Xi*
   c. For the neck: add Pueraria *Ge Gen* and Ligusticum *Chuan Xiong*
   d. For the chest: add Bupleurum *Chai Hu* and Platycodon *Jie Geng*
   e. For the abdominal area: add Citrus *Fo Shou* and Atractylodes *Bai Zhu*

Pharmaceutical Ingredients:[1–4]

1. Paeoniflorin, albiflorin, oxypaeoniflorin, benzoylpaeoniflorin, paeonin, hydroxypaeoniflorin, triterpenoids

Polygonum *He Shou Wu* 何首乌

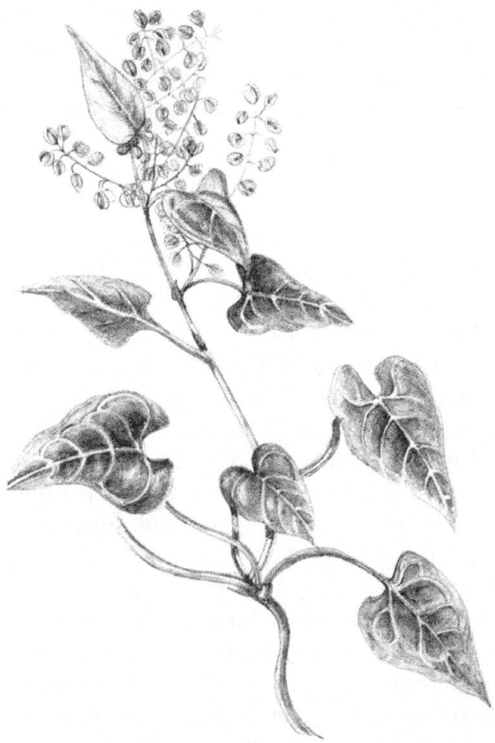

a

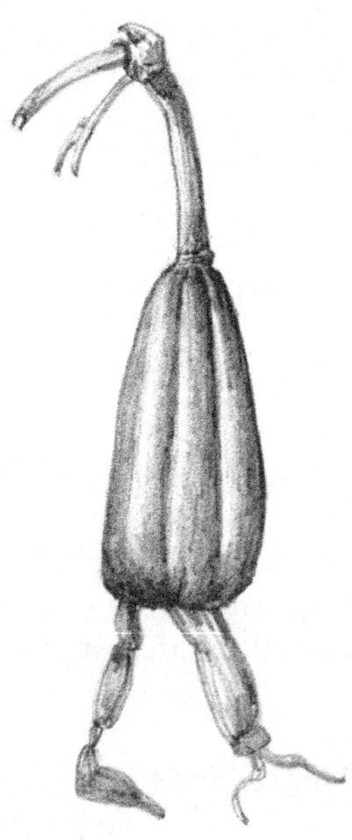

b

Original Reference: *Ri Hua-Zi Ben Cao* (*Materia Medica* of *Ri Hua-Zi*) by *Ri Hua-Zi* in 713 日华子本草

Part Used: Root

Name:
Pharmaceutical: Polygoni Multiflori, Radix
Botanical: Polygonum multiflorum
Common: Fleece flower root
Wade-Giles: *Ho-Shou-Wu*
Translation: Mr. Head Black

Energy/Taste: Slightly warm, bitter, sweet, astringent

Channel-Organ: Liver, Kidney

Actions:
1. Tonify the Liver Blood and replenish the Kidney *Jing* (prepared)
2. Dispel toxins, moisten intestines to benefit bowel movements (raw)

Form and Preparation: Steam with black soy bean juice until it turns black.

Dosage:
Horses and Cattle: 30–90 g
Camels: 30–100 g
Llamas, Alpacas, Goats, Sheep, and Pigs: 10–15 g
Dogs: 1–6 g
Cats: 0.5–2 g
Rabbits: 0.5–1.5 g
Birds: 0.3–3 g

Cautions and Contraindications:
1. Excessive Phlegm or Damp or Spleen *Qi* Deficiency with diarrhea
2. Do not cook in iron or steel pots.
3. According to some traditional sources, this herb should not be taken with onions, chives, or garlic.

Side Effects: It may cause diarrhea, colic, nausea, and vomiting.

Clinical Applications:
1. Deficiency of Blood Patterns
   Clinical signs: Dandruff, dry or cracked hooves or feet, pale gums and lips, dizziness or disorientation, poor vision, spots before eyes (fly-biting seizure activities) or ear-ringing (head-shaking), insomnia (behavior issues at night), premature gray hair, weakness in the lower back and stifles, numbness and soreness in the extremities
   Combine with: Rehmannia *Shu Di Huang*, Ligustrum *Nü Zhen Zi*, Lycium *Gou Qi Zi*, Cuscuta *Tu Si Zi*, Loranthus *Sang Ji Shen*, and Cyathula *Niu Xi*
2. Deficiency of *Jing*
   Clinical signs: Early graying of hair, weak lower back and stifles, weak limbs, reduced sexual function, premature aging, infertility
   Combine with: Rehmannia *Shu Di Huang*, Ligustrum *Nü Zhen Zi*, Lycium *Gou Qi Zi*, Cuscuta *Tu Si Zi*, Psoralea *Bu Gu Zhi*, and Angelica *Dang Gui*
   Classical herbal formula: Yin Yang Huo San

3. Constipation due to Dryness in the intestines and Deficiency of Blood
   Clinical signs: Constipation in older patients
   Combine with: Angelica *Dang Gui* and Cannabis *Huo Ma Ren*
4. Toxic carbuncles
   Clinical signs: Carbuncles, sores, scrofula, goiter, neck lumps
   Combine with: Prunella *Xia Ku Cao*, Scrophularia *Xuan Shen*, Forsythia *Lian Qiao*, and Fritillaria *Chuan Bei Mu*

History and Comments:

1. Polygonum *He Shou Wu* was discovered during the *Tang* Dynasty (618–907 CE) in Shun-yi County, Beijing, by a drunkard named He Tian-Er. Tian-Er had various health problems and a weak constitution. This 58-year-old man still did not have a child. Frustrated with himself one night, he drank too much and fell face down on his way home through the mountains. As if in a dream, he saw two vines, 3 feet apart, reaching out and caressing each other. Their branches intertwined together for a while, then loosened, and then intertwined again. Tian-Er couldn't believe his eyes and dug out the vines. He was even more astonished to see the roots: One looked exactly like an adult male and the other like an adult female. Tian-Er showed the roots to everyone passing by but no one knew what they were. Finally, an old wise man who came from the heart of the mountain told him, "These incredible vines may be gifts from God. Why don't you use them since you are unable to have children?" So Tian went back home, ground the roots into power, and took 5 grams (1 *Qian*) with wine every day. After 7 days, his sexual desire improved. He doubled the dosage and felt increasingly vigorous. After several years, all his old illnesses were gone and his white hair had turned black. Within 10 years, he fathered a number of sons and changed his name to *Neng-si* (which means "capable of reproduction"). One of his sons, Yan-xiu, continued to take this herbal medication. Yan-xiu also had a son he named Shou-wu. Father and son lived to be 160 years old and the grandson lived to be 130. The herb was named *Shou Wu* after the grandson to honor the family for their discovery of this magical plant.
2. Polygonum *He Shou Wu* is often called *Shou Wu*. *Shou Wu* is honored for its benefit for longevity and sexual vitality. It is a good tonic for Liver and Kidney *Yin* as well as Liver Blood. Polygonum *He Shou Wu* is also a good tonic for geriatric animals.
3. Combine Polygonum *He Shou Wu* with Longan *Long Yan Rou* and Lycium *Gou Qi Zi* and soak them in *Beijing* White Wine *Bai Jiu* for 49 days. Use this to prevent graying hair and premature aging.
4. Polygonum *He Shou Wu* reduces the Blood cholesterol level in rabbits with experimentally induced hypercholesterolemia. It also reduces the absorption of cholesterol from the intestinal tract of rabbits.
5. As a daily food additive of 0.4–2.0%, *He Shou Wu* powder increases longevity in birds.

Pharmaceutical Ingredients:[1–4]

1. Chrysophanol, emodin, senniside, physcion, questin, citrosein questinol, 2-acetylemodin, chein, chrysophanol anthrone, rhapontin, tricin, calcium
2. Fe, Zn, Cu
3. Polygonimitin B, C

Asinum Gelatinum *E Jiao* 阿胶

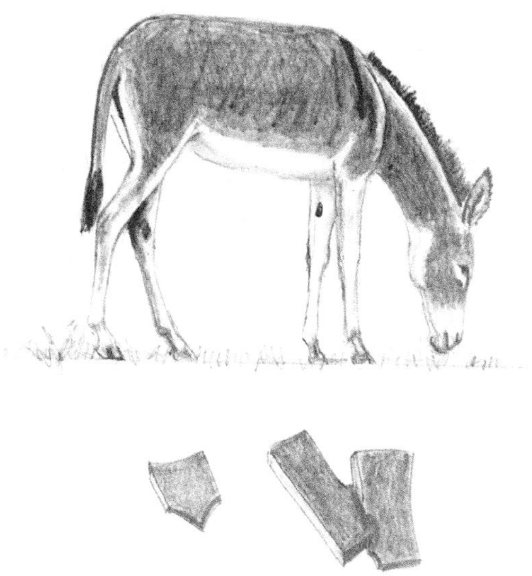

Original Reference: *Shen Nong Ben Cao Jing* (*Shen Nong's Materia Medica*, 1st century BCE) 神农本草经

Part Used: Glue or gelatin made from inner tallow of donkey skin

Name:
Pharmaceutical: Asini, Gelatinum Corii (previously: Gelatinum Asini; Colla corii asini)
Zoological: Equus asinus
Common: Donkey-hide gelatin
Wade-Giles: *A-Chiao*
Translation: Ass-hide glue

Energy/Taste: Neutral, sweet

Channel-Organ: Lung, Liver, Kidney

Actions:
1. Tonify Blood
2. Stop bleeding
3. Nourish *Yin* and moisten the Lung

Form and Preparation: Dissolve first and then add into decoction, melt by boiling water, or dissolve in yellow rice wine.

Dosage:
Horses and Cattle: 15–60 g
Camels: 30–100 g
Llamas, Alpacas, Goats, Sheep, and Pigs: 10–15 g
Dogs: 2–8 g
Cats: 1–2 g
Rabbits: 0.5–1.5 g
Birds: 0.3–3 g

Cautions and Contraindications:
1. Exterior Pattern with Interior Stagnation
2. Counteracts Rheum *Da Huang*, according to traditional sources

Side Effects: Overuse may cause poor appetite, diarrhea, and indigestion.

Clinical Applications:
1. Blood Deficiency
   Clinical signs: Anemia, dizziness or disorientation, poor vision, palpitations
   Combine with: Ginseng *Ren Shen* or Codonopsis *Dang Shen*, Angelica *Dang Gui*, Rehmannia *Shu Di Huang* and Astragalus *Huang Qi*
2. Various types of bleeding
   Clinical signs: Epistaxis, Lung bleeding, uterine bleeding, bleeding during pregnancy, vomiting Blood, bloody stool
   Combine with: Agrimony *Xian He Cao* and Imperata *Bai Mao Gen* for epistaxis
   Combine with: Bletilla *Bai Ji* for the Lung bleeding
   Combine with: Artemisia *Ai Ye*, Rehmannia *Sheng Di Huang*, Angelica *Dang Gui* for uterine bleeding
   Combine with: Sophora *Huai Hua* and Sanguisorba *Di Yu* for intestinal bleeding
   Combine with: Artemisia *Ai Ye* for fetus restlessness and uterine bleeding during pregnancy
3. *Yin* consumed by fever
   Clinical signs: Irritability, insomnia (behavior issues at night), spasms in the limbs
   Combine with: Coptis *Huang Lian*, Paeonia *Bai Shao*, egg yolk
   Classical herbal formula: Huang Lian E Jiao Tang
4. Chronic cough due to Deficiency of *Yin*
   Clinical signs: Dry cough, dry mouth, Bloody or sticky Phlegm
   Combine with: Ophiopogon *Mai Men Dong*, Morus *Sang Ye*, Armeniaca *Xing Ren*
   Classical herbal formula: Qing Zao Jiu Fei Tang
5. *Yin* Deficiency with muscle spasms and contractures
   Combine with: Testudines *Gui Ban*, Ostrea *Mu Li*
   Classical Formula: Da Ding Feng Zhu

History and Comments:
1. Asinum Gelatinum *E Jiao* comes in prepared blocks. It can be taken alone, cooked with other herbs, or dissolved in boiling water before adding to other herbs.
2. Asinum Gelatinum *E Jiao* is greasy and can cause Stagnation.
3. Over two thousand years ago, an unusual epidemic swept the *Shan-dong* province. The disease symptoms started with a pale face and loss of body weight and then progressed to mobility loss. Those affected also developed dyspnea and coughing, which was rapidly followed by vomiting Blood until death. Hundreds of prosperous towns and villages quickly turned into deserted and forlorn areas. After her parents died due to this disease, a smart and brave girl named E-Jiao vowed to find a cure to help her fellow villagers. She journeyed alone to the *Tai* Mountain, one of the four sacred mountain ranges in China. In the mountains, she met an old man with white hair and ruddy cheeks. He told her, "The disease is curable, but the medicine is difficult to obtain. It is extracted from the skin of the vicious black donkey." E-Jiao was so happy to hear about a cure that she knelt down to the old man saying, "I am willing to stop the disease even if I must risk my life. Master, please accept me as your student!" With a smile, the old man nodded his approval. In 49 days, E-Jiao learned 49 sword movements. She waved farewell to the master and journeyed toward the isolated mountain where the black donkey was hiding. When E-Jiao encountered the black donkey, they fought a long hard battle. The sky darkened and obscured everything on the ground, but E-Jiao was victorious at last. E-Jiao stewed the donkey skin for 49 days, using up 64 buckets of spring water and 81 bundles of mulberry firewood, until the precious, sparkling donkey-skin gelatin was revealed. When she returned home, E-Jiao dispensed the gelatin to every patient she encountered. The gelatin cured them all and the *Shan-dong* area gradually recovered its prosperity. Donkey-skin gelatin was later named *E Jiao* to show the people's deep gratitude toward this courageous, lovely girl.
4. *E Jiao* increases the concentration of RBCs and hemoglobin. It also increases the absorption and retention of calcium in the Blood.

Pharmaceutical Ingredients:[1–4]
1. Collagen
2. Amino acid (lysine, arginine, histadine, glycine, cysteine)
3. Na, K, Ca, Mg, Al, Zn

Longan *Long Yan Rou* 龙眼肉

Original Reference: *Shen Nong Ben Cao Jing* (*Shen Nong's Materia Medica*, 1st century BCE) 神农本草经

Part Used: Fleshy part of the fruit

Name:
Pharmaceutical: Euphoriae Longanae, Arillus
Botanical: Euphoria Longan
Common: Longan
Wade-Giles: *Lung-Yen-Jou*
Translation: Dragon Eyes Meat
Alternate: *Gui Yuan* (*Rou*)

Energy/Taste: Warm, sweet

Channel-Organ: Heart, Spleen

Actions:
1. Tonify Heart Blood and calm *Shen*
2. Tonify Spleen *Qi* and strengthen postpartum weakness

Form and Preparation: Slice before adding to decoction, soak in wine, and use as Food Therapy.

Dosage:
Horses and Cattle: 25–60 g
Llamas, Alpacas, Goats, Sheep, and Pigs: 10–15 g
Dogs: 2–8 g
Cats: 0.5–2 g
Rabbits: 0.5–1.5 g
Birds: 0.3–3 g

Cautions and Contraindications:
1. Phlegm-Damp in the Stomach
2. Phlegm-Heat in the Stomach

Side Effects:
1. Overeating can cause nausea or nosebleeds.
2. Excessive consumption will damage the Spleen.

Clinical Applications:
1. Heart Blood Deficiency and Spleen *Qi* Deficiency
   Clinical signs: Insomnia (behavior issues at night), poor memory, palpitations, nervousness, dizziness or disorientation, anemia
   Combine with: Ginseng *Ren Shen* or Codonopsis *Dang Shen*, Astragalus *Huang Qi*, Angelica *Dang Gui*, Ziziphus *Suan Zao Ren* or Acorus *Shi Chang Pu*
   Classical herbal formula: Gui Pi Tang
2. General weakness for geriatric patients
   Combine with: Other tonics or use alone soaked in wine or as Food Therapy

Morus *Sang Shen* 桑椹

Original Reference: *Tang Ben Cao* (*Tang Materia Medica*) by Su *Jing* et al. in *Tang* Dynasty (618–907 CE) 唐本草

Part Used: Mature fruit, whole fruit clusters

Name:
Pharmaceutical: Mori Albae, Fructus
Botanical: Morus Alba
Common: Mulberry fruit
Wade-Giles: *Sang-Chen*
Translation: Morus Fruit

Energy/Taste: Sweet, cold

Channel-Organ: Heart, Liver, Kidney

Actions:
1. Nourish *Yin* and Blood
2. Generate Body Fluids to reduce thirst
3. Moisten intestines to move feces

Form and Preparation: Powder or decoction; single or combined with other tonics or as Food Therapy

Dosage:
Horses and Cattle: 30–90 g
Llamas, Alpacas, Goats, Sheep, and Pigs: 10–30 g
Dogs: 2–8 g
Cats: 0.5–2 g
Rabbits: 0.5–1.5 g
Birds: 0.3–3 g

Cautions and Contraindications: Caution with diarrhea due to Spleen Deficiency or Cold

Side Effects: Overuse may cause diarrhea.

Clinical Applications:
1. Deficiency of *Yin*, Blood, and *Jing*
   Clinical signs: Dizziness or disorientation, poor vision, headache (head-shaking), ear-ringing (fly-biting seizure), insomnia (behavior issues at night), premature graying of hair

Combine with: Polygonum *He Shou Wu*, Ligustrum *Nü Zhen Zi*, and Eclipta *Han Lian Cao*
Classical herbal formula: Shou Wu Yan Shou Dan

2. Deficient Body Fluid or Diabetes causing thirst and dry mouth
   Clinical signs: Thirst, fatigue, increased urination
   Combine with: Trichosanthes *Tian Hua Fen*, Ophiopogon *Mai Men Dong*, Ligustrum *Nü Zhen Zi*
3. Constipation from dry intestines due to *Yin* and Blood Deficiency
   Combine with: Polygonum *He Shou Wu*, Cannabis *Huo Ma Ren*, and Sesame *Hei Zhi Ma*

HERBS TO NOURISH *YIN*

The herbs to nourish *Yin* are used primarily to tonify the *Yin* of the Lung, Stomach, Liver, or Kidney. Most are sweet and cold. Therefore, the herbs in this section are also called Sweet-Cold *Yin* Tonics. In addition to tonification of *Yin*, they can promote Body Fluid production to alleviate thirst, moisten the Interior (Large Intestines) to resolve Dryness, nourish Blood, calm *Shen*, stop bleeding, and clear Heat. Because *Yin* tonic herbs are sweet, cold, enriching, and stagnant, they are inappropriate for patients with Spleen *Qi* Deficiency, internal Dampness or Phlegm, and abdominal distention or diarrhea, unless these properties are counteracted by other herbals in the formula. Contraindications of *Yin* Tonic herbs include 1) Deficient Spleen *Qi*, 2) Internal Phlegm or Damp, 3) Abdominal distension, and 4) Diarrhea.

These cold *Yin* tonic herbs may be used to treat Internal-Heat Patterns caused by Deficient *Yin* such as *Yin* Deficiency with Heat (False Heat, or Deficient Heat) Patterns. *Yin* Deficiency generally occurs after chronic febrile disorders, during other chronic diseases, or as a side effect of other therapies (including corticosteroid and interferon therapy, radiotherapy, or chemotherapy). *Yin* Deficiency can affect the Lung, Stomach, Liver, Kidney, and Heart. Common *Yin* Deficiency signs are cool-seeking, panting, red/dry tongue, thin pulse, hot ears and body, and low-grade fever. Table 1.4 lists each organ's *Yin* Deficiency clinical signs.

Practitioners have observed organ-specific effects with *Yin* tonics. Some *Yin* tonic herbs can have a dual-organ effect. Herbs that tonify Lung *Yin* may also tonify

Table 1.4. Comparison of common *Yin* Deficiency Patterns and *Yin* tonic herbs.

Pattern	Clinical Signs	Examples of *Yin* Tonic
Lung *Yin* Deficiency	Dry cough Loss of voice Thirst, dry mouth Scanty Phlegm, thick and sticky sputum in some cases Dry skin Sore throat If progressed, bloody cough, low-grade fever	Glehnia *Bei Sha Shen*
Heart *Yin* Deficiency	Insomnia (behavioral changes at night) Muscle spasms or crying during sleep Restlessness or anxiety Palpitations Poor memory, forgetfulness, or disorientation	Lily *Bai He*
Stomach *Yin* Deficiency	Poor appetite or hungry all the time Thirst Nonproductive vomit Constipation Dry mouth and throat Peeling coating of the tongue	Dendrobium *Shi Hu*
Liver *Yin* Deficiency	Poor vision, or night blindness Dry and dull eyes Dry nails or skin Headache or tinnitus (head-shaking or fly-biting seizure) Vertigo or disorientation Insomnia or behavior issue at night	Lycium *Gou Qi Zi*
Kidney *Yin* Deficiency	Dizziness or disorientation Tinnitus (head-shaking or fly-biting seizure) Weak back and knees Hot feet Low-grade fevers Diminished sexual function or infertility Chronic degenerative joint disease (DJD), degenerative disc disease, or bony changes Involved in many chronic diseases	Testudinis *Gui Ban*

the Stomach, and herbs that nourish Kidney *Yin* may also nourish Liver *Yin*. Because *Yin* is derived from *Yang*, using a small amount of *Yang* tonic herbs in combination with the *Yin* tonic may produce superior results when tonifying Kidney *Yin*.

Glehnia *Bei Sha Shen* 北沙参

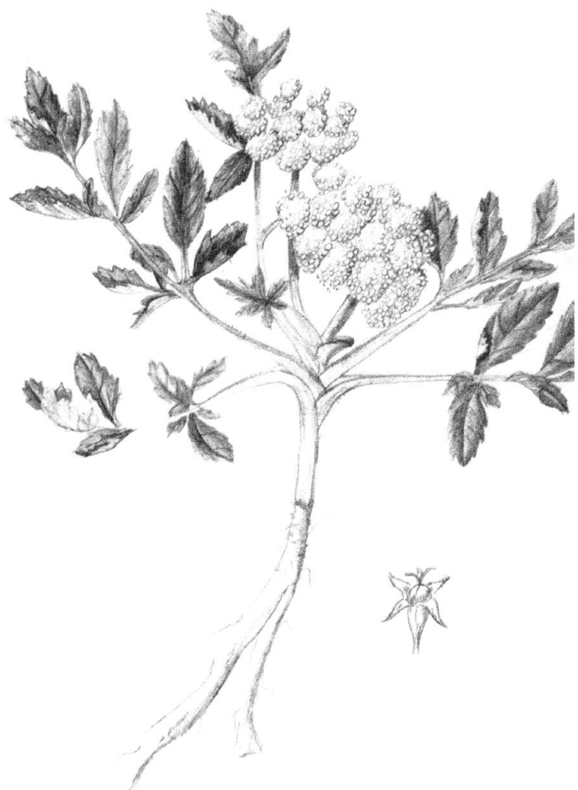

Original Reference: *Ben Cao Hui Yan* (*Treasure of Words on the Materia Medica*) by *Ni Zhu-Mo* in *Ming* Dynasty 本草汇言

Part Used: Root

Name:
Pharmaceutical: Glehniae, Radix
Botanical: Glehnia littoralis
Common: Glehnia root
Wade-Giles: *Pei-Sha-Shen*
Translation: Northern Sand Root

Energy/Taste: Slightly cold, sweet

Channel-Organ: Lung, Stomach

Actions:
1. Moisten the Lung, nourish *Yin*
2. Reinforce the Stomach, generate Body Fluids

Form and Preparation: Decoction or powder

Dosage:
Horses and Cattle: 30–60 g
Camels: 35–75 g
Llamas, Alpacas, Goats, Sheep, and Pigs: 10–15 g
Dogs: 1–5 g
Cats: 0.5–1 g
Rabbits: 0.5–1.5 g
Birds: 0.3–2 g

Cautions and Contraindications:
1. Damp Phlegm due to Lung *Qi* Deficiency and Cold
2. Incompatible with Veratrum *Li Lu*
3. According to traditional sources, this herb antagonizes Stephania *Han Fang Ji*.

Side Effects: Contact dermatitis (skin rash, itching, ocular discharge, fever) has resulted after exposure to *Bei Shan Shen* powder in a few cases.

Clinical Applications:
1. Dry cough due to Heat in the Lung with *Yin* Deficiency
   Clinical signs: Dry and chronic cough that is worse at night, Bloody cough, dry and red tongue, thirst, decreased appetite or constipation in the aftermath of febrile disease
   Combine with: Ophiopogon *Mai Men Dong*, Rehmannia *Sheng Di Huang*, and Polygonatum *Yu Zhu* and Dendrobium *Shi Hu*
   Classical herbal formula: Bai He Gu Jin Tang
2. Stomach *Yin* Deficiency
   Clinical signs: Dry tongue, thirst, constipation, peeled coating of the tongue, constant hunger or poor appetite
   Combine with: Dioscorea *Shan Yao*, Polygonatum *Huang Jing* and Pseudostellaria *Tai Zi Shen*

History and Comments:
1. Glehnia (*Bei Sha Shen*) and Adenophora (Adenophora tetraphylla, *Nan Sha Shen*t) are both called *Sha Shen* and may be used interchangeably. Both can be used for Lung and/or Stomach *Yin* Deficiency. The two types of *Sha Shen* were not clearly differentiated until the 17th century by Zhang Lu. *Bei Sha Shen* (Northern sand root) has a stronger *Yin* tonic effect. *Nan Sha Shen* (Southern sand root) is better at transforming Phlegm and stopping cough.
2. If just *Sha Shen* is given, it is referred to as Glehnia (*Bei Sha Shen*).
3. *Sha Shen*, Ginseng *Ren Shen*, Scrophularia *Xuan Shen*, Salvia *Dan Shen*, and Sophora *Ku Shen* are the Five *Shen*s. According to Tao Hong-Jing (456–536 CE, a

famous Taoist and pharmacologist in the Northern and Southern Dynasties), these herbs had different shapes but similar effects; therefore, all were named *Shens*. However, the medical saint Li Shi-zhen (1368–1644 CE), who lived during the *Ming* Dynasty, had very different opinions on this issue. He commented, "*Ren Shen* is sweet, bitter and warm. It is also heavy and dense. It can replenish Spleen and Stomach and tonify *Yuan* (Source) *Qi*, therefore is best for treating Internal *Qi* Deficiency. By contrast, *Sha Shen* is sweet, bland and cold. It is light in weight. *Sha Shen* can tonify Lung and thereby benefit the Kidney. The former reinforces *Yang* and cultivates *Yin*; the latter reinforces *Yin* to restrain *Yang*. The difference is too great to be ignored."

Pharmaceutical Ingredients:[1–4]
Phellopterin, bergapten, psoralen, xanthotoxin, marmesin, bergaptin, imperatorin, isoimperatorin, cnidilin

Adenophora *Nan Sha Shen* 南沙参

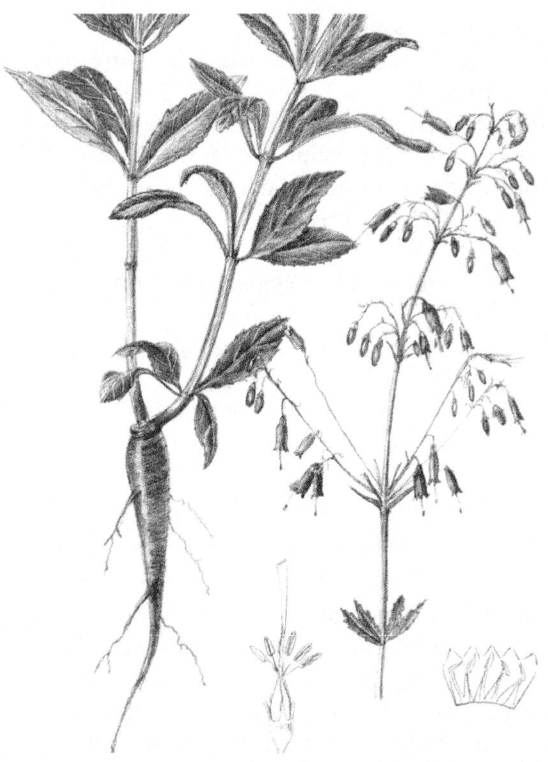

Original Reference: *Shen Nong Ben Cao Jing* (*Shen Nong's Materia Medica*, 1st century BCE) 神农本草经

Part Used: Root

Name:
Pharmaceutical: Adenophorae, Radix
Botanical: Adenophora tetraphylla (Thunb.)
Common: Adenophora root
Wade-Giles: *Nan-Sha-Shen*
Translation: South Sand Root

Energy/Taste: Slightly cold, sweet

Channel-Organ: Lung, Stomach

Actions:
1. Moisten the Lung, nourish *Yin*
2. Clear the Stomach, generate Body Fluids
3. Tonify *Qi* and transform Phlegm

Form and Preparation: Decoction or powder

Dosage:
Horses and Cattle: 30–60 g
Camels: 35–75 g
Llamas, Alpacas, Goats, Sheep, and Pigs: 10–15 g
Dogs: 1–5 g
Cats: 0.5–1 g
Rabbits: 0.5–1.5 g
Birds: 0.3–2 g

Cautions and Contraindications: Incompatible with Veratrum *Li Lu*

Side Effects: None known

Clinical Applications:
1. Dry cough with sticky Phlegm due to Lung *Yin* and *Qi* Deficiency
   Clinical signs: Dry cough, hoarse voice, sticky Phlegm, dry throat, shortness of breath, dyspnea, fatigue
   Combine with: Ophiopogon *Mai Men Dong* and Fritillaria *Chuan Bei Mu*
2. Stomach *Yin* Deficiency with *Qi* Deficiency
   Clinical signs: Dry tongue, poor appetite or hunger, general weakness after chronic febrile diseases
   Combine with: Ophiopogon *Mai Men Dong*, Rehmannia *Sheng Di Huang*, and Polygonatum *Yu Zhu* and Dendrobium *Shi Hu*

History and Comments:
1. Glehnia (*Bei Sha Shen*) and Adenophora (Adenophora tetraphylla, *Nan Sha Shen*) are both called *Sha Shen* and may be used interchangeably. Both can be used for Lung and/or Stomach *Yin* Deficiency. *Nan Sha Shen* has a weaker *Yin* tonifying effect than Glehnia *Bei Sha Shen, but Nan Sha Shen* also tonifies *Qi* and transforms Phlegm. Glehnia *Bei Sha Shen* is more suitable for *Yin* Deficiency with Heat, whereas Adenophora *Nan Sha Shen* seems preferable when there is sticky Phlegm with both *Yin* and *Qi* Deficiency.

2. *Bei Sha Shen* is brittle. *Nan Sha Shen* is pliable and has properties similar to Quinquefolium *Xi Yang Shen*.
3. *Nan Sha Shen* combined with Ophiopogon *Mai Men Dong* and Lonicera *Jin Yin Hua* is very effective for the treatment of esophagitis.

Pharmaceutical Ingredients:[1–4]
1. Taraxerone, β-sitosterol, β-sitostereol-o-β-d-gluco-pyranoside
2. Syringinoside, linoleic acid, ikshusterol, sessile folic 3-o-isovalerate, camphene, eucalyptol, camphor, azulene, bornyl acetate, daucosterol

Lycium *Gou Qi Zi* 枸杞子

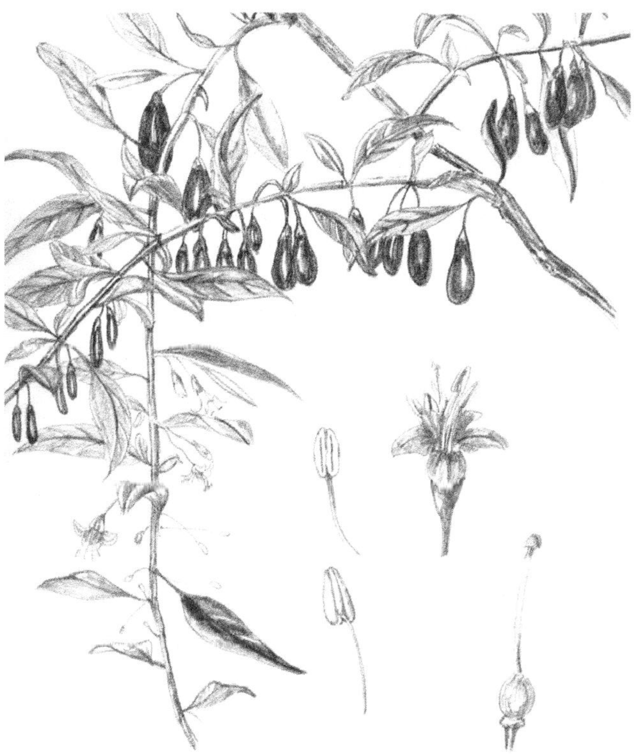

Original Reference: *Shen Nong Ben Cao Jing* (*Shen Nong's Materia Medica*, 1st century BCE) 神农本草经

Part Used: Fruit

Name:
Pharmaceutical: Lycii, Fructus
Botanical: Lycium barbarum; L. chinense
Common: Wolfberry
Wade-Giles: *Kou-Chi-Tzu*
Translation: Wolfberry fruit

Energy/Taste: Neutral, sweet

Channel-Organ: Liver, Kidney, Lung

Actions:
1. Tonify Kidney *Yin* and *Jing*
2. Nourish Liver *Yin* and Blood, brighten the eyes
3. Moisten the Lung

Form and Preparation: Single use, combined with others, or use as Food Therapy treats

Dosage:
Horses and Cattle: 30–60 g
Camels: 35–75 g
Llamas, Alpacas, Goats, Sheep, and Pigs: 10–15 g
Dogs: 2–8 g
Cats: 1–2 g
Rabbits: 0.5–1.5 g
Birds: 0.2–3 g

Cautions and Contraindications:
1. Spleen *Qi* or *Yang* Deficiency with Damp and diarrhea
2. Excess Heat Patterns

Side Effects: It may cause diarrhea.

Clinical Applications:
1. Eye problems due to Deficiency of *Yin*, *Jing*, and Blood
   Clinical signs: Dizziness or disorientation, poor eye vision, dry eyes, uveitis, cataracts, glaucoma
   Combine with: Chrysanthemum *Ju Hua* and Rehmannia *Shu Di Huang*
   Classical herbal formula: Qi Ju Di Huang Wan
2. Endocrine disorder due to Liver and Kidney *Yin* Deficiency
   Clinical signs and Disorders: Diabetes, Cushing's disease, hot feet
   Combine with: Rehmannia *Shu Di Huang*, Polygonum *He Shou Wu*, and Eucommia *Du Zhong*, Asparagus *Tian Men Dong* and Cuscuta *Tu Si Zi*
   Herbal formula: Xiao Ke Fang
3. Premature aging due to Kidney *Jing* Deficiency
   Clinical signs: Infertility, early onset of intervertebral disc disease and degenerative joint disease, sore back, weakness in the hind limbs, dizziness or disorientation, urinary incontinence, premature graying of hair

Combine with: Polygonum *He Shou Wu*, Epimedium *Yin Yang Huo*, and Cuscuta *Tu Si Zi*
Herbal formula: *Yin Yang Huo San*

4. Consumptive cough due to the Lung *Yin* Deficiency
Clinical signs: Dry cough, barking cough, sticky Phlegm
Combine with: Ophiopogon *Mai Men Dong*, Anemarrhena *Zhi Mu*, Fritillaria *Chuan Bei Mu*
5. Liver *Qi* Stagnation with Liver *Yang* Rising due to *Yin* Deficiency
Clinical signs: Flank pain, acid regurgitation, dry mouth and bitterness in mouth, hypertension
Combine with: Angelica *Dang Gui*, Glehnia *Bei Sha Shen*, Melia *Chuan Lian Zi*

History and Comments:

1. During the Northern *Song* Dynasty (618–907 CE), an emissary from the court went to the West River, *Ning-xia*, on a governmental business trip. On his way he met a pretty girl about 17 years old. The girl held a long cane in her hands and was chasing a gray-haired old man. The emissary stopped the girl and asked her, "How can you insult an old man like this?" "This is my great-grandson," answered the girl angrily. "He disregarded the family rules, and I must give him a lesson." The emissary asked, "What rule has he violated?" The lady replied, "We have a traditional family medicine, but he refused to take it. As you can see, he became so senile and doddering at such a young age." "May I ask how old you are?" the emissary questioned in awe. "I am already 372." "What's the secret of your longevity?" the emissary asked, eager to know the answer. "No big secret—just taking a single herb frequently. It has different names in each season. In spring, we call it *Tian Jin*. In summer, it is called *Gou Qi*. In fall, the folks call it *Di Gu*; In winter its name is *Xian Ren Zang*. You can obtain and take it in all four seasons and experience longevity with nature." The emissary jotted it down and this secret has been handed down to present times.
2. Lycium *Gou Qi Zi* is honored as a tonic for longevity. It is a good tonic for Liver and Kidney *Yin* and *Jing* as well as Liver Blood. It is combined with Polygonum *He Shou Wu* and Longan *Long Yan Rou* and soaked in wine for 2 weeks to use as a tonic.
3. Lycium *Di Gu Pi* is the root bark of this plant. *Di Gu Pi* is sweet and cold. Because it cools Blood and clears Heat, it is a good treatment for *Yin* Deficiency Bi syndrome.
4. *Gou Qi Zi* has a protective effect on the hepatic cells, reduces Blood cholesterol, and lowers blood pressure. It also induces a therapeutic effect for the treatment of hyperlipidemia and chronic hepatitis, obesity, and male infertility.

Pharmaceutical Ingredients:[1–4]

1. Betaine, solavetivone, zeaxanthin, physalien, β-sitosterol, linoleic acid
2. Na, Ca, K, Mg, Cu, Zn, Fe
Vitamins B1, B2, C, carotene

Lily *Bai He* 百合

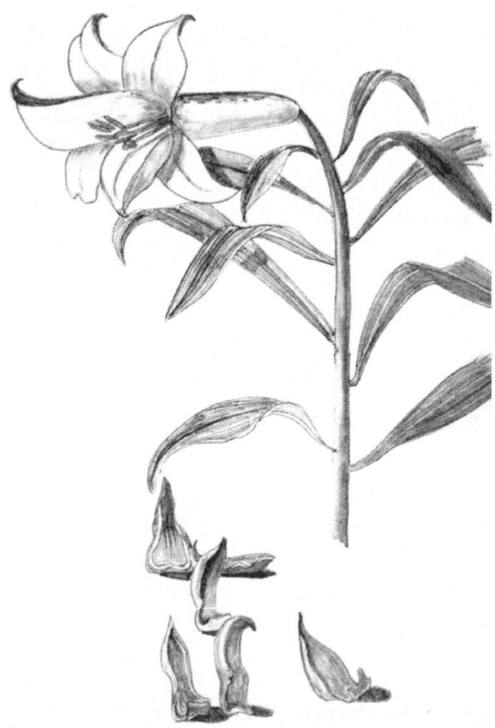

a

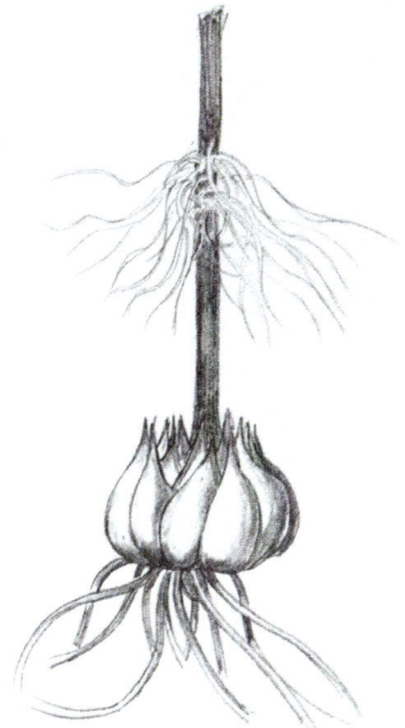

b

Original Reference: *Shen Nong Ben Cao Jing* (*Shen Nong's Materia Medica*, 1st century BCE) 神农本草经

Part Used: Pulpy bulb

Name:
Pharmaceutical: Lilii, Bulbus
Botanical: Lilium lancifolium; L. brownii; L. pumilum; L. longiflorum
Common: Lily bulb
Wade-Giles: *Pai-Ho*
Translation: Hundred Closing

Energy/Taste: Slightly cold, sweet

Channel-Organ: Lung, Heart

Actions:
1. Moisten the Lung to stop cough
2. Clear Heart Heat and calm *Shen*

Form and Preparation: Powder or decoction; stirring with honey enhances its effect to moisten the Lung.

Dosage:
Horses and Cattle: 30–60g
Camels: 35–75g
Llamas, Alpacas, Goats, Sheep, and Pigs: 5–10g
Dogs: 2–5g
Rabbits: 0.5–1.5g
Birds: 0.2–2g

Cautions and Contraindications:
1. Cough due to Wind-Cold invasion because it is cold
2. Diarrhea due to Spleen *Qi*/*Yang* Deficiency

Side Effects: It may cause diarrhea.

Clinical Applications:
1. Lung *Yin* Deficiency with Heat
   Clinical signs: Very chronic cough, dry cough, Bloody or sticky, stubborn Phlegm
   Combine with: Scrophularia *Xuan Shen*, Fritillaria *Chuan Bei Mu*, Rehmannia *Sheng Di Huang*, Tussilago *Kuan Dong Hua*
   Classical herbal formula: Bai He Gu Jin Tang
2. Residual Heat following fever
   Clinical signs: Irritability, palpitations, insomnia (behavior issues at night), restlessness
   Combine with: Rehmannia *Sheng Di huang* and Anemarrhena *Zhi Mu*

History and Comments:
1. *Bai* (百), means a hundred, *He* (合) means harmony. The name *Bai He* means everything has peace and harmony. *Bai He* has had an important role in several societies. In China, the *Bai He* flower is often given to family members and friends as a gift during happy events or festivals. In ancient France, *Bai He* represented the majesty of the royal house. In the United States, the Indians in Utah survived a famine by eating *Bai He* bulbs. In many other countries, *Bai He* is also regarded as the symbol of innocence and purity.
2. *Bai He* consists of the scales from the bulb. It has an antiallergenic effect and alleviates histamine-induced asthma. It can be applied externally to treat swellings and ulcers.

Pharmaceutical Ingredients:[1–4]
1. Colchicine, starch, protein, lipids, polysaccharides
2. Regaloside A, D, 3, 6-O-diferuloysucrose, 1-O-feruloyglycerol, 1-O-p-coumaroylglycerol, 26-O-β-d-glucopyranosylnuatigenin-3-O-α-l-rhamnopyranosyl-β-d-glucopyranoside, brownnioside, deacylbrownoside, β1-solamargine
3. Sugars, organ acids
4. Ca, Mg, Fe, Al, K, Zn

Ophiopogon *Mai Men Dong* 麦门冬

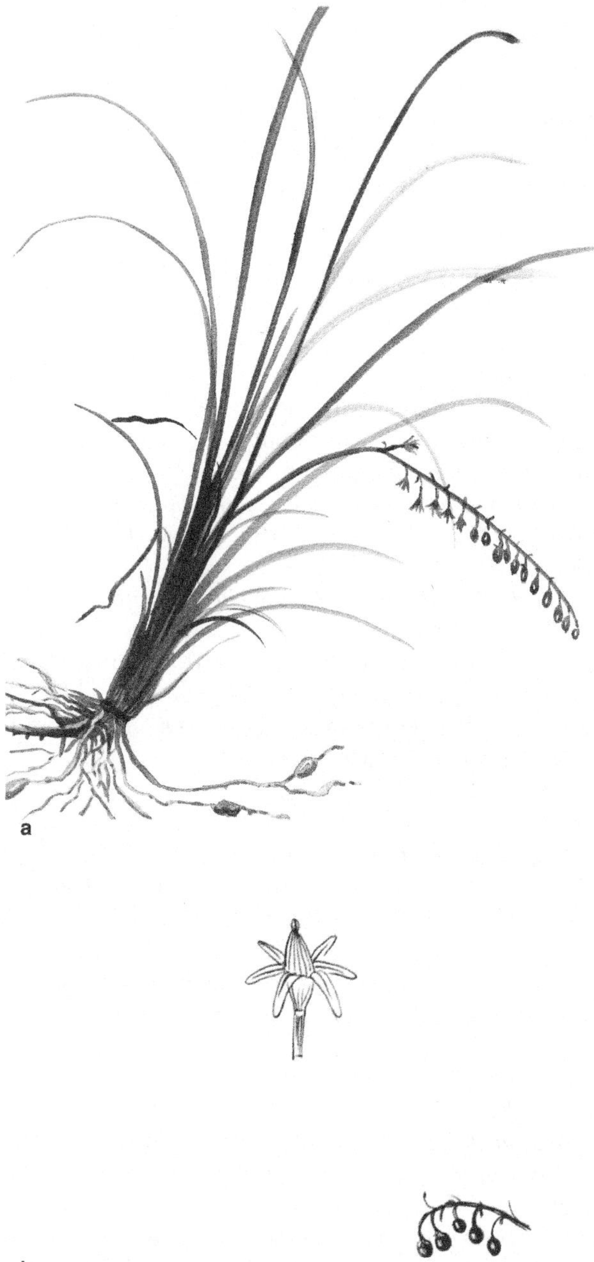

Original Reference: *Shen Nong Ben Cao Jing* (*Shen Nong's Materia Medica*, 1st century BCE) 神农本草经

Part Used: Root (tuber); sliced tuber with core removed

Name:
Pharmaceutical: Ophiopogonis Japonici, Tuber
Botanical: Ophiopogon japonicus
Common: Ophiopogon tuber
Wade-Giles: *Mai-Men-T'ung*
Translation: Wheat Door of Winter

Energy/Taste: Slightly cold, sweet, slightly bitter

Channel-Organ: Lung, Heart, Stomach

Actions:
1. Moisten Lung, nourish *Yin*
2. Nourish Stomach *Yin* and generate Body Fluids
3. Eliminate Heart Heat and irritability
4. Moisten intestines and promote bowel movements

Form and Preparation: It is sold as whole tubers or cut with the center removed to reduce bitterness. It is considered more potent when sliced because the core is inactive as a *Yin* tonic. The core is actually slightly agitating.

Dosage:
Horses and Cattle: 20–60 g
Camels: 35–75 g
Llamas, Alpacas, Goats, Sheep, and Pigs: 10–20 g
Dogs: 2–8 g
Cats: 0.5–1 g
Rabbits: 0.5–1.5 g
Birds: 0.2–2 g

Cautions and Contraindications:
1. Cough due to Wind-Cold invasion
2. Excessive Phlegm or Damp
3. Diarrhea
4. According to some traditional sources, this herb antagonizes Tussilago *Kuan Dong Hua* and counteracts Sophora *Ku Shen* and Tremella *Bai Mu Er.*

Side Effects: It may cause diarrhea.

Clinical Applications:
1. Dryness and Heat in the Lung due to Lung *Yin* Deficiency
   Clinical signs: Dry cough with scanty or sticky sputum, or Blood
   Combine with: Adenophora *Nan Sha Shen*, Asparagus *Tian Men Dong*, Fritillaria *Chuan Bei Mu*, Rehmannia *Sheng Di Huang*, and Glehnia *Sha Shen*, Loranthus *Sang Ji Sheng*, Armeniaca *Xing Ren*, Asinum Gelatinum *E Jiao*
   Classical herbal formula: Qing Zao Jiu Fei Tang
2. Stomach *Yin* Deficiency
   Clinical signs: Vomiting, colic, gastric ulcers, constant hunger or no appetite, dry tongue, thirst, sore throat
   Combine with: Polygonatum *Yu Zhu*, Glehnia *Sha Shen*, Rehmannia *Sheng Di Huang*
   Classical herbal formula: Yu Nü Jian (Jade Lady)
3. Pathological Heat in *Ying* level or in the later stage of a febrile disease with *Yin* Deficiency

Clinical signs: Systemic fever, irritability, insomnia (behavior issues at night), with dry mouth and increased thirst
Combine with: Rehmannia *Sheng Di Huang* and Coptis *Huang Lian*, Bambusa *Zhu Ye*
Classical herbal formula: Qing Ying Tang
4. Heart *Yin* Deficiency
Clinical signs: Irritability, restlessness, behavioral changes (especially at night), arrhythmia
Combine with: Rehmannia *Sheng Di Huang* and Ziziphus *Suan Zao Ren*, Scrophularia *Xuan Shen*
Classical herbal formula: An Shen Fang
5. Constipation due to Dryness and Heat in the intestines or with fever
Combine with: Scrophularia *Xuan Shen* and Rehmannia *Sheng Di Huang*
Classical herbal formula: Zeng Ye Tang

History and Comments:

1. The first story about *Mai Men Dong* includes Qin Shi Huang, the first emperor who united China during *Qin* Dynasty (221 to 209 BCE). One day, a small bird carrying a plant in its beak flew into the palace and dropped the herb right onto Emperor Qin's desk. The elegant herb had beautiful lavender flowers and long, narrow green leaves. The emperor asked Gui Gu Zi about the herb. Gui Gu Zi, a famous military tactician and sly diplomat, answered carefully: "This is the herb of immortality from the *Ying* Island of the East Sea. When a person dies, cover him with this herb on the third day, and he will come back to life immediately. One herb can revive one person." Because the Emperor Qin believed Gui Gu Zi, he sent his emissary Xu Fu along with three thousand virgin boys and three thousand virgin girls to the East Sea to search for the herb of immortality. They finally found and brought this plant back to the emperor.
2. Although *Mai Men Dong* cannot bring a dead emperor to life, it is able to moisten the Metal (Lung) and purify the Water (Kidney). When *Mai Men Dong* is combined with *Ren Shen* and *Wu Wei Zi*, it forms the classical herbal formula *Sheng Mai Yin*, which translates literally as "reviving the pulse."
3. Good quality Ophiopogon *Mai Men Dong* is thick, large, soft, aromatic, chewy, sweet, and light yellowish white in color. The herb may be stir-fried in wine to reduce its coolness.
4. *Mai Men Dong* is the best herb for thirst, whether used alone or combined with *Lu Gen*. It is often combined with other herbs for the following treatments:
    a. Treat deficient Lung *Yin*: Combine with Asparagus *Tian Men Dong* or Lily *Bai He*
    b. Benefit Liver *Yin*: Combine with Glehnia *Bei Sha Shen*
    c. Treat uprising *Qi* (headache or head-shaking, neurosis, coughing): Combine with Pinellia *Ban Xia*

Pharmaceutical Ingredients:[1–4]

1. Steroid saponin (Ophiopogonin A, B, C, D, ruscogenin, β-sitosterol, stigmasterol, β-sitosterol-β-glucoside
2. Ophioside, kaempferol-3-galactoglucoside
3. Isoflavonoids (6-aldehydo-isoophiopogonanone A and B, methylophiopogonanone A and B, 6-aldehydopogonone A
4. Amino acid, vitamin A

Asparagus *Tian Men Dong* 天门冬

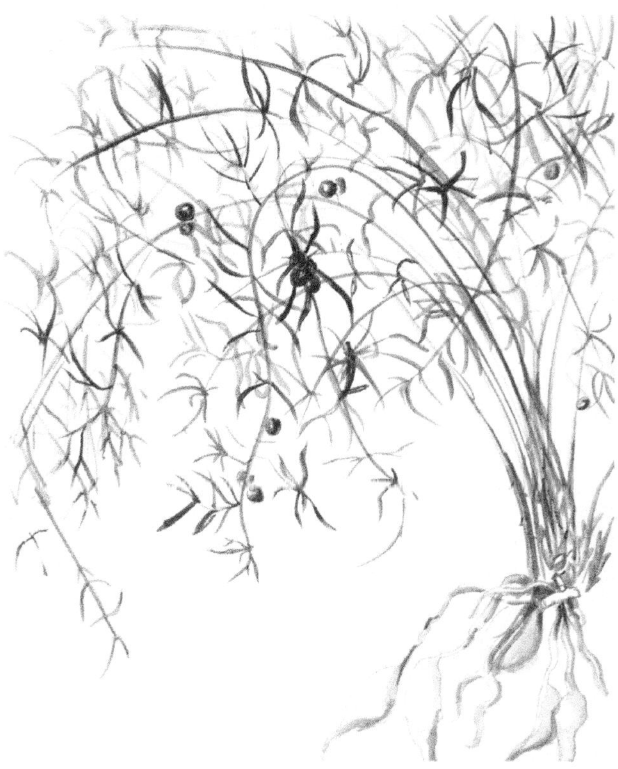

Original Reference: *Shen Nong Ben Cao Jing* (*Shen Nong's Materia Medica*, 1st century BCE) 神农本草经

Part Used: Root

Name:
Pharmaceutical: Asparagi Cochinchenensis, Tuber
Botanical: Asparagus cochinchinensis
Common: Asparagus root
Wade-Giles: *T'ien-Men-Tung*
Translation: Heaven's Door to Winter

Energy/Taste: Very cold, sweet, bitter

Channel-Organ: Lung, Kidney

Actions:
1. Nourish *Yin* and clear Heat
2. Moisten the Lung and nourish the Kidney

Form and Preparation: Powder or decoction

Dosage:
Horses and Cattle: 30–60 g
Camels: 45–90 g
Llamas, Alpacas, Goats, Sheep, and Pigs: 5–20 g
Dogs: 1–3 g
Cats: 0.5–1 g
Rabbits: 0.5–1.5 g
Birds: 0.2–2 g

Cautions and Contraindications:
1. Spleen *Qi* Deficiency or Interior Dampness or Phlegm (poor appetite and/or diarrhea)
2. Cough due to Wind-Cold invasion

Side Effects: It may cause diarrhea.

Clinical Applications:
1. Lung *Yin* and Kidney *Yin* Deficiency
   Clinical signs: Dry cough with scanty or sticky sputum or Blood, chronic cough in a geriatric patient
   Combine with: Ophiopogon *Mai Men Dong*
2. Thirst and dry mouth due to consumption of *Yin* by fever or diabetes
   Combine with: Rehmannia *Sheng Di Huang* and Codonopsis *Dang Shen*, or Pseudostellaria *Tai Zi Shen*, Ginseng *Ren Shen*
3. Constipation due to Dryness in intestines
   Combine with: Angelica *Dang Gui*, Cistanche *Rou Cong Rong*, Rehmannia *Sheng Di Huang*, Cannabis *Huo Ma Ren*
4. Stomatitis due to Deficient Stomach *Yin* with Fire
   Combine with: Coptis *Huang Lian* or Scutellaria *Huang Qin*

History and Comments:
1. Because Taoists considered *Tian Men Dong* to have similar functions as *Mai Men Dong*, they gave it a similar name. This herb is described in the highly influential text *Bao Pu Zi* (*The Master Embracing Simplicity*) written by Ge Hong, an early 4th century Taoist master. Ge Hong researched the art of transcendence and immortality, including topics such as alchemy, health preservation, meditation, breathing techniques, exorcism, sexual practices, and talismanic charms. He advised Taoists to start taking *Tian Men Dong* beginning with their very first stage toward transcendence. *Tian Men Dong* could be steamed or boiled and then consumed twice daily to completely replace rice, wheat, beans, corn, and millet in the diet. It could also be pounded into a powder and drunk in wine. Alternatively, one could squeeze out the juice and condense it into an ointment. Taking *Tian Men Dong* for 100 days continuously can significantly improve one's stamina and vitality, which is much faster than using other herbs such as Atractylodes *Bai Zhu* and Polygonatum *Huang Jing*. Taking the herb for 200 days in a row can strengthen bones and muscles, and preserve one's youth.
2. Another story about *Tian Men Dong* was recorded in *Lie Xian Zhuan* (*Biographies of the Ranked Immortals*) written by Liu Xiang in the West *Han* Dynasty (206 BCE–25 CE). According to this text, when the Immortal named Chi-song-zi used *Tian Men Dong* persistently, his teeth and hair regenerated at 150 years of age and he lived over 300 years.
3. *Er Dong* (Two Winters) is the combination of Asparagus *Tian Men Dong* (Heaven's Door to Winter) and Ophiopogon *Mai Men Dong* (Wheat Door of Winter). Both these herbs have similar actions of nourishing Lung and Stomach *Yin*, moistening the Lung to stop cough, and clearing Heat. A practitioner may combine these herbs or may substitute each for the other. However, these herbs do have some differences. *Tian Men Dong* is much colder, clears Heat more strongly, nourishes Kidney *Yin*, and treats False Heat. *Mai Men Dong*, on other hand, nourishes Heart *Yin*, calms *Shen*, and treats *Shen* Disturbance due to Heart *Yin* Deficiency.
4. Good quality *Tian Men Dong* is thick, dense, translucent, and yellow-white. It is often combined with honey to moisten the Lung and relieve cough. It is also used with other *Yin* tonics to treat False Heat in the Upper Burner (*Shang Jiao*).
5. *Tian Men Dong* has an antimutation and anticancer effect. It can also be effective for the treatment of uterine bleeding.

Pharmaceutical Ingredients:[1–4]
1. Asparagine, β-sitosterol, 5-methoxy-methylfurfural
2. Steroidal saponin, smilagenin, xylose, glucose, neoketose

Quinquefolium *Xi Yang Shen* 西洋参

Original Reference: *Ben Cao Cong Xin* (*Thoroughly Revised Materia Medica*) by *Wu Yi-Luo* in 1751 本草从新

Part Used: Root

Name:
Pharmaceutical: Panacis Quinquefolii, Radix
Botanical: Panax quinqueflium
Common: American Ginseng
Wade-Giles: *Hsi-Yang-Shen*
Translation: Western (Foreign) Ginseng

Energy/Taste: Cool, bitter, slightly sweet

Channel-Organ: Heart, Lung, Kidney

Actions:
1. Tonify *Qi*
2. Nourish *Yin*
3. Clear Heat and generate Body Fluids

Form and Preparation: Powder or decoction; single use or combined with other herbs, but cooked separately

Dosage:
Horses and Cattle: 20–60 g
Llamas, Alpacas, Goats, Sheep, and Pigs: 5–20 g
Dogs: 0.5–3 g
Cats: 0.5–1 g
Rabbits: 0.5–1.5 g
Birds: 0.2–2 g

Cautions and Contraindications:
1. Incompatible with Veratri *Li Lu*
2. During exogenous invasions (Wind-Cold or Wind-Heat)
3. Do not cook in iron pots.

Side Effects: Oral medication may cause skin allergic reaction.

Clinical Applications:
1. Deficiency of both *Qi* and *Yin* due to fever or other chronic illness
   Clinical signs: Thirst, fatigue, irritability and restlessness, shortness of breath, weak pulse
   Combine with: Rehmannia *Sheng Di Huang*, Ophiopogon *Mai Men Dong*, Dendrobium *Shi Hu*
2. Cough or asthma due to both Lung *Yin* and *Qi* Deficiency
   Clinical signs: Difficult breathing, dry cough
   Combine with: Ophiopogon *Mai Men Dong*, Asinum Gelatinum *E Jiao*, Anemarrhena *Zhi Mu* and Fritillaria *Chuan Bei Mu*
3. Heart *Qi* and *Yin* Deficiency
   Clinical signs: Palpitations, restlessness, insomnia (behavior issues at night), anxiety, chest pain
   Combine with: Ophiopogon *Mai Men Dong* and Glycyrrhiza *Gan Cao*
4. Diabetes due to *Qi* and *Yin* Deficiency
   Clinical signs: Polyuria, urination immediately after drinking water, glucosuria, fatigue, weak back and rear limbs, cool-seeking behavior
   Combine with: Atractylodes *Bai Zhu*, Astragalus *Huang Qi*, and Glehnia *Bei Sha Shen*
5. Spleen *Qi* and *Yin* Deficiency
   Clinical signs: Poor appetite, fatigue, diarrhea, thirst, excessive worry
   Combine with: Pseudostellaria *Tai Zi Shen*, Dioscorea *Shan Yao* and Massa Fermentata *Shen Qu*
6. Blood in stool due to intestinal Heat
   Combine with: Longan *Long Yan Rou*

History and Comments:
1. American Ginseng Quinquefolium *Xi Yang Shen* has been used in TCM since 1716. About 90% of American Ginseng *Xi Yang Shen* comes from Wisconsin. Cultivated roots are harvested when the plants are from 3 to 6 years old. Wild roots can be found in Wisconsin, New York, and North Carolina. Wild Ginseng is best used as a general tonic and is more tonifying than cultivated Ginseng. Cultivated Ginseng is good for treating Heat conditions.
2. Both American Ginseng *Xi Yang Shen* (Quinquefolium) and Chinese Ginseng *Ren Shen* tonify *Qi* and are used for *Qi* Deficiency. *Ren Shen*, a warm herb, is a strong *Qi* tonic frequently used to treat severe *Qi* Deficiency and to resuscitate patients with *Yang* collapse. Quinquefolium *Xi Yang Shen*, a cool herb, is a first choice *Qi* and *Yin* tonic for long-term use due to its adaptogenic properties. American Ginseng *Xi Yang Shen* is typically preferred in patients who develop aggravated Heat and *Qi* congestion when using Chinese Ginseng *Ren Shen*.
3. Quinquefolium *Xi Yang Shen* is as expensive as Chinese Ginseng *Ren Shen*. Practitioners may substitute Pseudostellaria *Tai Zi Shen* for *Xi Yang Shen* and use Codonopsis *Dang Shen* to replace *Ren Shen*.
4. The roots of *Ren Shen* and *Xi Yang Shen* look similar, but there are some distinguishing characteristics. A 6–7-year-old Chinese Ginseng root is about 60 cm long with fewer branches (accessory roots) than the shorter (about 30 cm) American Ginseng root. Chinese Ginseng leaves are round-oval, and American Ginseng leaves appear more long-oval. Chinese Ginseng seeds are larger (1,000 seeds weigh 32–35 grams) than American Ginseng seeds (1,000 seeds weigh 23–25 grams).

Pharmaceutical Ingredients:[1–4]
1. Quinquenoside R_1, ginsenoside Rb_1, Rb_2, Rb_3, Rc, Rd, Re, Rf_2, Rg, R_0
2. Pseudo-ginsenoside F_{11}, quinquefolans A, B, C
3. Essential oils, rutin

Dendrobium *Shi Hu* 石斛

Original Reference: *Shen Nong Ben Cao Jing* (*Shen Nong's Materia Medica*, 1st century BCE) 神农本草经

Part Used: Stem

Name:
Pharmaceutical: Dendrobii, Herba
Botanical: Dendrobium loddidesii; D. chrysanthym; D. fimbriatum; D. nobile; D. candium; D. officinale

Common: Dendrobium
Wade-Giles: *Shih-Hu*
Translation: Stone Bushel

Energy/Taste: Cool, sweet, bitter

Channel-Organ: Lung, Stomach, Kidney

Actions:
1. Tonify *Yin* and clear Heat
2. Promote production of Body Fluids
3. Nourish Stomach *Yin* Deficiency
4. Brighten the vision and strengthen the lower back

Form and Preparation: Powder or decoction; cook first for 10 minutes before adding other herbs.

Dosage:
Horses and Cattle: 15–60g
Camels: 30–100g
Llamas, Alpacas, Goats, Sheep, and Pigs: 5–20g
Dogs: 2–5g
Cats: 0.5–3g
Rabbits: 0.5–1.5g
Birds: 0.2–2g

Cautions and Contraindications:
1. In early stage of fever because it preserves/retains external Pathogenic *Qi*
2. Abdominal distention and thick greasy tongue coating, because it assists Dampness
3. According to some traditional sources, this herb antagonizes Croton *Ba Dou* and counteracts Omphalia *Lei Wan*.

Side Effects: It may cause diarrhea.

Polygonatum *Yu Zhu* 玉竹

Original Reference: *Shen Nong Ben Cao Jing* (*Shen Nong's Materia Medica*, 1st century BCE) 神农本草经

Part Used: Rhizome; this rhizome has a yellow color, whereas Polygonatum *Huang Jing* is black and has an appearance very similar to cooked Rehmannia *Shu Di Huang*.

Name:
Pharmaceutical: Polygonati Odorati, Rhizoma
Botanical: Polygonatum officinalis; P. odoratum
Common: Solomon's seal
Wade-Giles: *Yu-Chu*
Translation: Jade Bamboo

Energy/Taste: Slightly cool, sweet

Channel-Organ: Lung, Stomach

Actions:
1. Nourish *Yin* and moisten the Lung
2. Generate Body Fluids and assist the Stomach
3. Extinguish Wind and soften and moisten the sinews

Form and Preparation: Powder or decoction

Dosage:
Horses and Cattle: 15–60g
Camels: 30–100g
Llamas, Alpacas, Goats, Sheep, and Pigs: 5–20g
Dogs: 2–5g
Cats: 0.5–3g
Rabbits: 0.5–1.5g
Birds: 0.2–2g

Cautions and Contraindications:
1. Spleen *Qi* Deficiency
2. Phlegm-Damp in the Stomach or Lung
3. Stomach *Qi* Stagnation

Side Effects: It may cause diarrhea.

Polygonatum *Huang Jing* 黄精

Original Reference: *Ming Yi Bie Lu* (*Miscellaneous Records of Famous Physicians*) by *Tao Hong-Jing* during North and South Kingdoms (5th century) 名医别录

Part Used: Rhizome

Name:
Pharmaceutical: Rhizoma Polygonati
Botanical: Polygonatum sibiricum; P. kingnianum; P. cyrtonema
Common: Polygonatum
Wade-Giles: *Huang-Ching*
Translation: Yellow Essence

Energy/Taste: Neutral, sweet

Channel-Organ: Lung, Spleen, Kidney

Actions:
1. Nourish Lung *Yin*
2. Tonify the Spleen *Qi*
3. Tonify the Kidneys and augment the Essence

Form and Preparation: Powder or decoction

Dosage:
Horses and Cattle: 15–60g
Camels: 30–100g

Llamas, Alpacas, Goats, Sheep, and Pigs: 5–20 g
Dogs: 2–5 g
Cats: 0.5–3 g
Rabbits: 0.5–1.5 g
Birds: 0.3–3 g

Cautions and Contraindications:
1. Spleen *Qi* Deficiency with Damp and poor digestion or diarrhea due to Cold in the Spleen and Stomach
2. Cough with profuse sputum

Side Effects: It may cause diarrhea.

Clinical Applications:
1. Deficiency of *Qi* and *Yin* following febrile diseases
   Clinical signs: Exhaustion, poor appetite, dry cough, dry throat and mouth with thirst
   Combine with: Ginseng *Ren Shen* or Codonopsis *Dang Shen*, Ophiopogon *Mai Men Dong*, Adenophora Nan *Sha Shen*, Pseudostellaria *Tai Zi Shen*, and Fritillaria *Chuan Bei Mu*
2. General debility due to Deficiency of *Qi* and Blood
   Clinical signs: Decreased appetite, weakness and soreness of the back and stifles, jaundice, muscular atrophy, fatigue
   Combine with: Lycium *Gou Qi Zi*, Angelica *Dang Gui*, and Ligustrum *Nu Zhen Zi* for Heat in feet and low back pain.
3. Diabetes
   Combine with: Astragalus *Huang Qi* and Dioscorea *Shan Yao*, Ophiopogon *Mai Men Dong*, Trichosanthes *Tian Hua Fen*, and Rehmannia *Sheng Di Huang*
4. Deficiency of Liver and Kidney *Yin*
   Combine with: Dipsacus *Xu Duan*
5. Spleen and Stomach *Yin* Deficiency
   Combine with: Glehnia *Sha Shen*, Ophiopogon *Mai Men Dong*, Oryza *Gu Ya*

Comments: Most often used for treatment of general debility and recovery from chronic disease (i.e., bronchitis, diabetes, renal failure).

Ligustrum *Nü Zhen Zi* 女贞子

Original Reference: *Shen Nong Ben Cao Jing* (*Shen Nong's Materia Medica*, 1st century BCE) 神农本草经

Part Used: Seed

Name:
Pharmaceutical: LiGustri Lucidi, Fructus
Botanical: Ligustrum lucidum
Common: Ligustrum
Wade-Giles: *Nü-Chen-Tzu*
Translation: Female Virtue Seed

Energy/Taste: Cool, sweet

Channel-Organ: Liver, Kidney

Actions:
1. Tonify Liver and Kidney *Yin*
2. Clear Liver Heat to brighten eyes
3. Darken the hair
4. Strengthen the stifles
5. Preserve *Jing*

Form and Preparation: Decoction or powder

Dosage:
Horses and Cattle: 15–60 g
Camels: 30–100 g
Llamas, Alpacas, Goats, Sheep, and Pigs: 5–20 g
Dogs: 2–5 g
Cats: 0.5–3 g
Rabbits: 0.5–1.5 g
Birds: 0.3–3 g

Cautions and Contraindications:
1. Diarrhea due to Spleen *Qi* Deficiency
2. *Yang* Deficiency

Side Effects: It may cause diarrhea.

Clinical Applications:
1. Deficient Liver and Kidney *Yin*
   Clinical signs: Dry eyes, poor vision, ear-ringing (head-shaking), sore back and legs, nocturnal emissions, graying of hair
   Combine with: Morus *Sang Shen*, Lycium *Gou Qi Zi*, Eclipta *Han Lian Cao*, Rehmannia *Shu Di Huang*
2. Deficiency of *Yin* with Heat, including Blood Heat
   Clinical signs: Dry mouth, hot palms and soles, dry eyes, rashes, bleeding
   Combine with: Lycium *Di Gu Pi*, Moutan *Mu Dan Pi*, Rehmannia *Sheng Di Huang*
3. Kidney *Yin* Deficiency
   Clinical signs: Dizziness or disorientation, weakness, soreness of the lower back and stifles
   Combine with: Psoralea *Bu Gu Zhi* or Cuscuta *Tu Si Zi*

Comments:
1. Ligustrum *Nü Zhen Zi* is often combined with Eclipta *Han Lian Cao*, Morus *Sang Shen,* or Lycium *Gou Qi Zi* to benefit Liver *Yin*. It is also combined with Psoralea *Bu Gu Zhi* or Cuscuta *Tu Si Zi* to tonify Kidney *Qi*.
2. It is used to enhance immune function, when combined with Astragalus *Huang Qi* during chemotherapy, and also as a longevity herb in folk medicine.
3. It is useful to treat cataracts and retinitis.

Testudinis *Gui Ban* 龟板

Original Reference: *Shen Nong Ben Cao Jing* (*Shen Nong*'s *Materia Medica*, 1st century BCE) 神农本草经

Part Used: Plastron (tortoise underbelly)

Name:
Pharmaceutical: Plastrum Testudines
Zoological: Chinemys reevesii (freshwater tortoise)
Common: Fresh-water turtle shell
Wade-Giles: *Kuei-Pan*
Translation: Tortoise Hard Plank

Energy/Taste: Cool, sweet, salty

Channel-Organ: Liver, Kidney

Actions:
1. Nourish *Yin* to anchor *Yang*
2. Tonify Kidney to strengthen bones
3. Stop bleeding due to *Yin* Deficiency with Heat
4. Nourish Blood and tonify Heart

Form and Preparation: Powder or decoction; cook 10–20 minutes before adding other herbs to decoction.

Dosage:
Horses and Cattle: 15–60 g
Camels: 30–100 g
Llamas, Alpacas, Goats, Sheep, and Pigs: 5–20 g
Dogs: 2–5 g
Cats: 0.5–3 g
Rabbits: 0.5–1.5 g
Birds: 0.2–2 g

Cautions and Contraindications:
1. Caution during pregnancy
2. Do not use during Wind invasions.
3. Phlegm conditions
4. Cold Damp in Stomach or diarrhea due to *Yang* Deficiency
5. According to some traditional sources, this substance antagonizes Glehnia *Sha Shen* and Ginseng *Ren Shen*.

Side Effects: None known

Comments:
1. *Gui Ban* is available cooked into glue as *Gui Ban Jiao*. It has a stronger effect for tonifying *Yin* and Blood.
2. *Gui Ban* is an important tonic because it aids the upward flow of *Qi* from the Lower Burner (*Xia Jiao*) while tonifying *Yin* and settling the unruly *Yang*. It is often combined with Cervus *Lu Rong* (deer antler) as a Kidney *Qi* tonic.

Amyda *Bie Jia* 鳖甲

Original Reference: *Shen Nong Ben Cao Jing* (*Shen Nong*'s *Materia Medica*, 1st century BCE) 神农本草经

Part Used: Bony shell

Name:
Pharmaceutical: Amyda sinensis, Carapax (*Trionyx sinensis*)
Zoological: Carapax Amydae; C. Trionycis
Common: Turtle shell
Wade-Giles: *Pieh-chia*
Translation: Chinese Soft-shelled Turtle Shell

Energy/Taste: Cold, salty

Channel-Organ: Liver, Kidney

Actions:
1. Nourish *Yin*, anchor *Yang*
2. Soften hardness, remove nodules

Form and Preparation: Powder or decoction; cook 30 minutes before adding other ingredients.

Dosage:
Horses and Cattle: 15–60 g
Camels: 30–100 g
Llamas, Alpacas, Goats, Sheep, and Pigs: 5–20 g
Dogs: 2–5 g
Cats: 0.5–3 g
Rabbits: 0.5–1.5 g
Birds: 0.2–2 g

Cautions and Contraindications:
1. Caution during pregnancy
2. Deficiency and Cold in the Spleen leading to diarrhea
3. When an Exterior disorder has not been fully restored
4. According to some traditional sources, this substance antagonizes Alum *Ming Fan*.

Side Effects: None known

Comments:
1. Good quality *Bie Jia* is large, clean, and without meat. It is very useful for diabetes.
2. Raw *Bie Jia* enriches *Yin* and anchors *Yang*; fried *Bie Jia* in vinegar softens and reduces hard swellings or nodules.

Eclipta *Han Lian Cao* 旱莲草

Original Reference: *Xin Xiu Ben Cao* (*Newly Revised Materia Medica*) by *Su Jing* et al. during *Tang* Dynasty (618–907 CE) 新修本草

Part Used: Aboveground parts of the plant

Name:
Pharmaceutical: Ecliptae Prostratae, Herba
Botanical: Eclipta prostrata
Common: Eclipta
Wade-Giles: *Han-Lien-Ts'ao*
Translation: Lotus Grass

Energy/Taste: Cold, sweet, sour

Channel-Organ: Liver, Kidney

Actions:
1. Nourish Kidney *Yin*
2. Cool Blood, stop bleeding

Form and Preparation: Decoction or powder

Dosage:
Horses and Cattle: 15–60 g
Camels: 30–100 g
Llamas, Alpacas, Goats, Sheep, and Pigs: 5–20 g
Dogs: 2–5 g
Cats: 0.5–3 g
Rabbits: 0.5–1.5 g
Birds: 0.2–2 g

Cautions and Contraindications:
1. It can damage Spleen and Stomach *Qi*.
2. It is contraindicated in diarrhea due to Cold and *Qi* Deficiency in Spleen or Kidney.

Side Effects: It may cause diarrhea.

Comments: It is useful for autoimmune diseases.

Tremella *Bai Mu Er* 白木耳

Original Reference: *Tang Ben Cao (Tang Materia Medica)* by *Su Jing* et al in *Tang* Dynasty (618–907 CE)

Part Used: Fruiting body

Name:
Pharmaceutical: Tremellae Fuciformis, Fructificatio
Botanical: Tremella Fuciformus
Common: White wood ear fungus
Wade-Giles: *Pai–Mu-Erh*
Translation: White Wood Ear

Energy/Taste: Neutral, sweet, bland

Channel-Organ: Lung, Stomach

Actions:
1. Nourish Stomach *Yin* and generate fluids
2. Moisten the Lung

Form and Preparation: Decoction or powder; often used as a Food Therapy

Dosage:
Horses and Cattle: 15–60 g
Camels: 30–100 g
Llamas, Alpacas, Goats, Sheep, and Pigs: 5–20 g
Dogs: 2–5 g
Cats: 0.5–3 g
Rabbits: 0.5–1.5 g
Birds: 0.2–2 g

Cautions and Contraindications: None known

Side Effects: None known

Clinical Applications:
1. Lung *Yin* Deficiency with Heat
   Clinical signs: Coughing Blood, Lung abscesses
   Combine with: Lily *Bai He*, Glehnia *Sha Shen*, crystal sugar *Bing Tang*
2. Debility after a long illness
   Combine with: Jujube *Da Zao*
3. Palpitations and shortness of breath
   Combine with: Pseudostellaria *Tai Zi Shen*, crystal sugar *Bing Tang*

Comments: *Bai Mu Er* is a mild *Yin* tonic for Lung *Yin* and Stomach *Yin* Deficiencies. It is often used as Food Therapy and may take time to achieve a therapeutic effect.

Sesame *Hei Zhi Ma* 黑芝麻

Original Reference: *Shen Nong Ben Cao Jing* (*Shen Nong's Materia Medica*, 1st century BCE)

Part Used: Seed

Name:
Pharmaceutical: Sesami Indici, Semen
Botanical: Sesamum indicum (Black Sesame)
Common: Black sesame seed
Wade-Giles: *Hei-Chih-Ma*
Translation: Black Sesame

Energy/Taste: Neutral, sweet

Channel-Organ: Liver, Kidney, Lung, Large Intestine

Actions:
1. Nourish *Yin, Jing,* and Blood
2. Moisten the intestine and promote bowel movements

Form and Preparation: Decoction or powder; often used as a Food Therapy

Dosage:
Horses and Cattle: 15–60 g
Camels: 30–100 g
Llamas, Alpacas, Goats, Sheep, and Pigs: 5–20 g
Dogs: 2–5 g
Cats: 0.5–3 g
Rabbits: 0.5–1.5 g
Birds: 0.2–2 g

Cautions and Contraindications: Diarrhea due to Spleen *Qi* Deficiency

Side Effects: None known

Clinical Applications:
1. Deficient *Yin, Jing,* and Blood
   Clinical signs: Dry and dandruff skin, gray hair, premature aging, seizure, behavioral changes, poor vision
   Combine with: Morus *Sang Ye*, Angelica *Dang Gui*, and Cistanche *Rou Cong Rong*
2. Constipation due to deficient *Yin*
   Combine with: Biota *Bai Zi Ren* or Cannabis *Huo Ma Ren*
   Combine with: Angelica *Dang Gui*, Cistanche *Rou Cong Rong*, Biota *Bai Zi Ren*

Comments: Sesame *Hei Zhi Ma* can be combined with chicken egg as Food Therapy for chronic constipation due to deficient *Yin*.

HERBS TO TONIFY *YANG*

The herbs to tonify *Yang* are also known as herbs that warm or assist the *Yang*. They are used for *Yang* Deficiency Patterns, which include Heart *Yang* Deficiency, Spleen *Yang* Deficiency, and Kidney *Yang* Deficiency. Because the Kidney controls the *Ming-Men* (the gate of life), which is the basis of the whole body's *Yang* (or global *Yang*), various *Yang* Deficiency Patterns originate from or at least are associated with the Kidney. Therefore, tonifying *Yang* generally means tonifying Kidney *Yang*.

The main clinical signs of Kidney *Yang* Deficiency include 1) cold back or extremities, aversion to cold, withdrawal into oneself, or warm-seeking behavior; 2) sore or weak lower back, stifles, bones, or muscles; 3) exhaustion, impotence, or infertility; 4) polyuria or urinary incontinence; 5) asthma, dyspnea, or wheezing; 6) pale tongue with a white coating; and 7) deep, weak pulse. Kidney *Yang* is the source of the global *Yang*. Kidney *Yang* Deficiency may lead to Heart or Spleen *Yang* Deficiency. On the other hand, chronic Deficient Heart or Spleen *Yang* gradually consumes Kidney *Yang*, which leads to Kidney *Yang* Deficiency. *Yang* Deficiency Pattern differentiation and examples of *Yang* tonic herbs are listed in Table 1.5.

Generally, the herbs to tonify the *Yang* are warm and dry in nature. They regulate adrenal cortex functions and energy metabolism, promote growth and sexual function, and strengthen the immune system. *Yang* tonic herbs can include animal, plant, and mineral sources:

1. Animal products generally have a strong effect but are expensive. Examples include Gecko, Deer horn, Cordyceps fungi, and Pipefish. Some animals such as seahorses are endangered and prohibited for use.

Table 1.5. Comparison of common *Yang* Deficiency Patterns and *Yang* tonic herbs.

Pattern	Clinical Signs	Examples of *Yang* Tonic Herbs
Kidney *Yang* Deficiency	Cold back or extremities, aversion to Cold, withdrawal into oneself, or warm-seeking behavior Sore or weak lower back knees, or bones and muscles; Exhaustion, impotence, or infertility Polyuria or incontinence of urine Asthma, dyspnea, or wheezing Tongue: pale or purple with white coating Pulse: slow/deep/weak	Morinda *Ba Ji Tian*
Heart *Yang* Deficiency	Shortness of breath, worse if exercise Palpitation Restlessness, or anxiety Coolness of ears, nose, trunk/limbs Ascites Tongue: pale or purple Pulse: feeble, irregularly or regularly intermittent	Eleutherococcus *Wu Jia Shen*
Spleen *Yang* Deficiency	Anorexia Daybreak diarrhea Chronic loose stools, colic Tongue: wet, swollen with teeth marks	Psoralea *Bu Gu Zhi*

2. Examples of plant sources include Psoralea *Bu Gu Zhi*, Morinda *Ba Ji Tian*, and Eucommia *Du Zhong*.
3. Mineral sources include Actinolite *Yang Qi Shi*.

The warm, dry nature of herbs to tonify *Yang* can damage Body Fluids and consume *Yin*. Overuse of *Yang* tonics may generate internal Heat, which leads to *Yin* Deficiency. Therefore, these herbs are contraindicated in patients with Heat conditions and *Yin* Deficiency unless other herbs are included in a formula to counteract these effects.

Epimedium *Yin Yang Huo* 淫羊藿

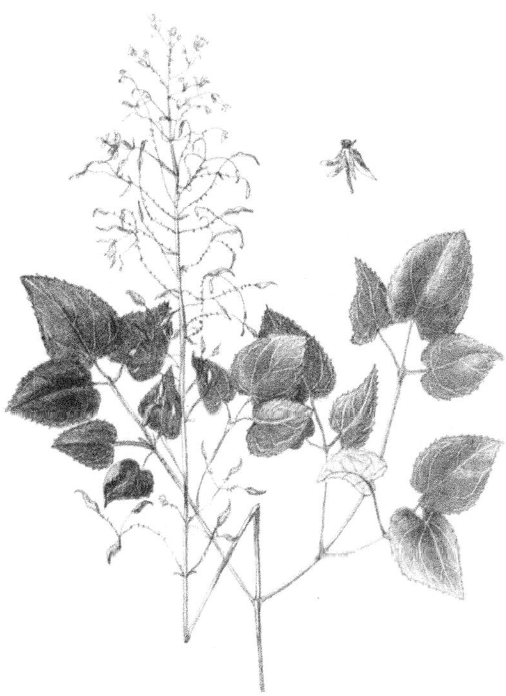

a

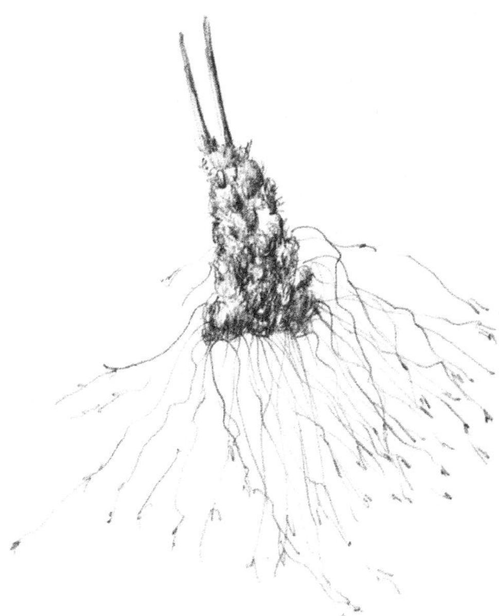

b

Original Reference: *Shen Nong Ben Cao Jing* (*Shen Nong's Materia Medica*, 1st century BCE) 神农本草经

Part Used: Above-ground part, or leaf and stem

Name:
Pharmaceutical: Epimedii, Herba
Botanical: Epimedium brevecornum; E. grandiflorum; E. sagitatum
Common: Epimedium
Wade-Giles: *Yin-Yang-huo*
Translation: Horny Goat Plant
Alternate: *Xian Ling Pi*

Energy/Taste: Warm, pungent, sweet

Channel-Organ: Liver, Kidney

Actions:
1. Tonify Kidney *Yang*, strengthen *Yang-Qi*
2. Expel Wind-and eliminate Dampness

Form and Preparation: Powder or decoction

Dosage:
Horses and Cattle: 15–30 g
Llamas, Alpacas, Goats, Sheep, and Pigs: 5–10 g
Camels: 30–50 g
Dogs: 1–3 g
Cats: 0.3–1 g
Rabbits: 0.5–1.5 g
Birds: 0.1–1.5 g

Cautions and Contraindications:
1. Caution during pregnancy
2. Deficient *Yin* with Heat
3. This herb should not be taken as a decoction over prolonged periods.

Side Effects:
1. In very large doses it can cause respiratory arrest.
2. Long-term use may lead to Heat and Dryness.

Clinical Applications:
1. Kidney *Yang* Deficiency
   Clinical signs: Infertility, frequent urination (dribbling)
   Combine with: Schisandra *Wu Wei Zi*, Lycium *Gou Qi Zi*, and Astragalus *Huang Qi* or use as a single herb
   Herbal formula: Yin Yang Huo San
2. Wind-Damp-Cold *Bi* syndromes
   Clinical signs: Pain; numbness in the back, stifles, and limbs; arthritis
   Combine with: Clematis *Wei Ling Xian*, Loranthus *Sang Ji Sheng*, Eucommia *Du Zhong*, Cinnamomum *Gui Zhi*

3. Accumulation of Lung Phlegm with difficulty breathing
   Combine with: Platycodon *Jie Geng*
4. Ascites due to Heart *Yang* and Kidney *Yang* Deficiency
   Clinical signs: Shortness of breath, cold limbs
   Combine with: Curculigo *Xian Mao*, Ginseng *Ren Shen*, Aconite *Fu Zi* and Angelica *Dang Gui*

History and Comments:

1. During the *Tang* Dynasty (618–907 CE), a goat farmer owned 1 buck and 15 does that had not produced offspring for many years. Annoyed by this situation, the farmer asked a wise man for advice. The wise man suggested that the farmer feed an herb called *Xian Ling Pi* to his goats. The farmer fed the herb to the goats and was pleased when the animals began to breed. However, his enthusiasm waned a little when the animals' libido responded too positively. The male goat became so lustful that he mated with the female goats relentlessly day and night hundreds of times. Thus, he had to discontinue the herbal medication to balance the buck's libido. Upon hearing the news, other farmers also began feeding *Xian Ling Pi*, in smaller amounts, to encourage their goats to mate. The farmers changed the herb's name to *Yin Yang Huo* because its leaves looked like *Huo* (ageratum) and it could stimulate *Yin* (libido) in the *Yang* (goat).
2. Epimedium *Yin Yang Huo* is also called *Xian Ling Pi*. When combined with Curculigo *Xian Mao*, *it* is called *Er Xian Tang* and may be a component of a larger prescription.
3. When prepared, the leaf edges of *Yin Yang Huo* should be trimmed because they are considered slightly toxic. Good quality Epimedium *Yin Yang Huo* is intact, yellow green, and has many leaves.
4. *Yin Yang Huo* increases semen production. It increases sexual activity, increases sperm production, stimulates the sensory nerves, and increases sexual desire.
5. *Yin Yang Huo* increases the immune response. It is externally used for eye infections. It is also very useful for sports injuries with spasms or fractures.

Pharmaceutical Ingredients:[1–4]

1. Flavonoids (icariine, des-o-methyicariine, β-anhydroicaritine, des-o-methy-β-anhydroicaritine, icarisid I, Isoquercetin, icariin, icariin-3-o-d-rhamnoside)
2. Epimedin A, B, C, querceti, epimedokoreanoside, campesterol
3. β-sitosterol, ikarisoside A
4. Hyperin, sagittatoside A, B, C

Cistanche *Rou Cong Rong* 肉苁蓉

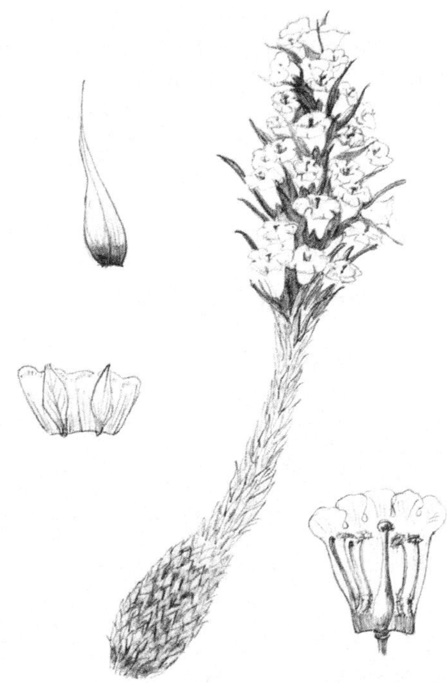

Original Reference: *Shen Nong Ben Cao Jing* (*Shen Nong's Materia Medica*, 1st century BCE) 神农本草经

Part Used: Stem

Name:
Pharmaceutical: Cistanches Deserticolae, Rhizoma
Botanical: Cistanche deserticola; C. salsa
Common: Broomrape
Wade-Giles: *Jou-Tsung-Jung*
Translation: Natural Compliant Flesh
Alternate: *Dian Da Yun*

Energy/Taste: Warm, sweet, salty

Channel-Organ: Kidney, Large Intestine

Actions:

1. Tonify Kidney *Jing*, strengthen *Yang*
2. Moisten Large Intestine to promote bowel movements
3. Warm uterus, strengthen reproductive functions

Form and Preparation: Powder or decoction

Dosage:

It can tonify *Yang* without drying the body, and its actions are moderate and smooth. Therefore, the dosage should be large.

Horses and Cattle: 30–60 g
Llamas, Alpacas, Goats, Sheep, and Pigs: 5–30 g
Camels: 30–90 g
Dogs: 2–5 g
Cats: 1–3 g
Rabbits: 0.5–1.5 g
Birds: 0.3–2 g

Cautions and Contraindications:

1. Deficiency of *Yin* with Heat
2. Diarrhea
3. Constipation due to Excess Heat

Side Effects: It may cause diarrhea.

Clinical Applications:

1. Constipation due to Dryness in intestines and *Yin* Deficiency, especially in geriatric animals
   Combine with: Cannabis *Huo Ma Ren*, and Angelica *Dang Gui*
   Herbal formula: Dang Gui Cong Yong San
2. Kidney *Yang* Deficiency
   Clinical signs: Female or male infertility, lack of sexual desire, impotence, premature ejaculation, frequent urination or urinary dribbling, pale and swollen tongue, deep and weak pulse
   Combine with: Rehmannia *Shu Di Huang*, Cornus *Shan Zhu Yu*, Cuscuta *Tu Si Zi*, and Schisandra *Wu Wei Zi*
3. Cold (Painful) Bi syndrome in the lower back or hind limbs, with hindquarter weakness
   Combine with: Morinda *Ba Ji Tian* and Eucommia *Du Zhong*
4. Prevention for threatened abortion due to deficient Kidney *Qi*
   Combine with: Eucommia *Du Zhong*

History and Comments:

1. In 1190 CE, 13 tribes headed by Zha Mu He were attacking Mongolia. During the fighting, the great King Genghis Khan and his 30,000-man army were trapped on a sandy hill covered with *Suo Suo*, a common desert shrub. Meanwhile, Zha Mu He tortured captives by tossing them into 70 large caldrons filled with boiling water. God, infuriated by Zha Mu He's cruelty, sent his horse to help Genghis Khan. The divine horse leapt down from the heaven and appeared above the sandhill. Looking skyward, the horse gave a long neigh and caused his blood to sprinkle the roots of the *Suo Suo* shrubs. Suddenly, some purple plants sprouted from the spot and within minutes, these plants grew into armlike fleshy stems about 1 foot tall. King Genghis Khan and his soldiers knelt down to thank God and then ate the plant. They immediately felt a burst of power flow through their bodies. The King and his army rushed down the sandhill and effortlessly destroyed the enemy. Subsequently, King Genghis Khan and his mounted Mongol army swept out from the steppes of Asia to conquer two-thirds of the known world. Today, *Rou Cong Rong* is classified as a Class-Two Rare and Endangered Plant in China; however, lucky travelers can still spot it occasionally in the desert of Northwest China.
2. *Rou* literally means "meat" or "flesh" because of its nature to provide rich nourishment. *Cong Rong* means "staying relaxed and comfortable." *Rou Cong Rong* is a warm tonic herb that can replenish Blood and Kidney *Qi* without harsh actions, demonstrating the *Cong Rong* part of its name. Because Cistanche *Rou Cong Rong* is a very mild tonic for both *Yang* and *Yin*, *it* is commonly used in geriatric patients.
3. *Rou Cong Rong* is an effective immune stimulant when combined with Epimedium *Yin Yang Huo*.

Pharmaceutical Ingredients:[1–4]

1. β-sitosterol, succinic acid, caffeic acid, amino acids
2. Potassium, sodium, calcium, zinc, magnesium, and iron

Morinda *Ba Ji Tian* 巴戟天

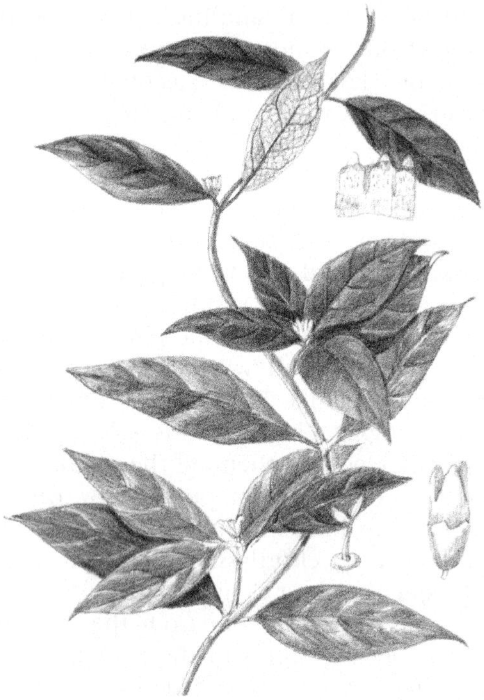

a

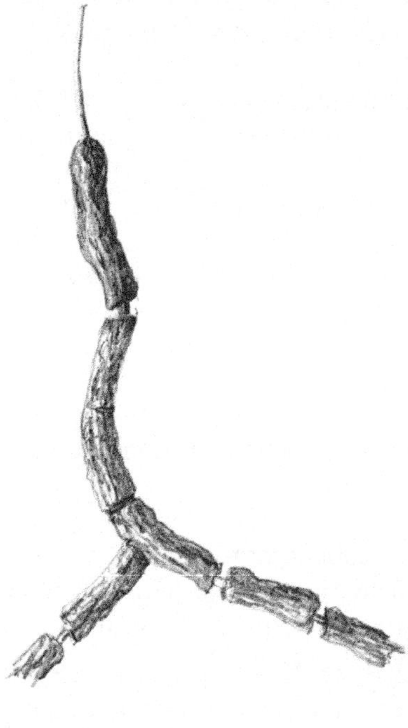

b

Original Reference: *Shen Nong Ben Cao Jing* (*Shen Nong's Materia Medica*, 1st century BCE) 神农本草经

Part Used: Root

Name:
Pharmaceutical: Morindae Officinalis, Radix
Botanical: Morinda officinalis
Common: Morinda root
Wade-Giles: *Pa-Chi-T'ien*
Translation: Clinging Halberd of Heaven

Energy/Taste: Slightly warm, pungent, sweet

Channel-Organ: Kidney, Liver

Actions:
1. Tonify the Kidney and strengthen *Yang*
2. Dispel Wind and transform Damp
3. Strengthen the sinews and bones
4. Increase mental powers
5. Quiet and soothe the Five Organs

Form and Preparation: Powder or decoction

Dosage:
Horses and Cattle: 15–30g
Llamas, Alpacas, Goats, Sheep, and Pigs: 5–10g
Camels: 30–60g
Dogs: 1–5g
Cats: 0.5–2g
Rabbits: 0.5–1.5g
Birds: 0.1–1.5g

Cautions and Contraindications:
1. Deficient *Yin* with Heat or Damp-Heat
2. According to some traditional sources, this herb antagonizes Salvia *Dan Shen*.
3. It is considered slightly toxic and is often combined with Glycyrrhiza *Gan Cao* to help neutralize its toxicity.

Side Effects: It may cause Internal Fire or Heat.

Clinical Applications:
1. Soreness and weakness of the back and hind limbs due to a Deficiency of Kidney *Yang*
   Combine with: Dipsacus *Xu Duan* and Eucommia *Du Zhong*
   Classical herbal formula: Ba Ji San
2. Wind-Cold-Damp pain in lumbar region, hip, stifle, and hock, with difficulty walking
   Combine with: Cibotium *Gou Ji*, Loranthus *Sang Ji Sheng* and Cyathula *Niu Xi*; or Eucommia *Du Zhong*, Dipsacus *Xu Duan* and Cyathula *Niu Xi*.
3. Deficiency of Kidney *Yang*
   Clinical signs: Infertility, impotence, premature ejaculation, infertility, ear-ringing (head-shaking)
   Combine with: Ginseng *Ren Shen*, Cistanche *Rou Cong Rong*, and Cuscuta *Tu Si Zi* or Epimedium *Yin Yang Huo*, Dioscorea *Shan Yao*

4. Urinary incontinence or increased frequency
   Combine with: Psoralea *Bu Gu Zhi* and Rubus *Fu Pen Zi*, Alpinia *Yi Zhi Ren*
5. To strengthen bone degeneration and help in repair of bone fractures
   Combine with: Dipsacus *Xu Duan*

History and Comments:

1. *Ba Ji Tian* was accidentally used and helped Zhuge Liang's army. Zhuge Liang (181–234 CE) was the most famous statesman and strategic general in Chinese history. He was the Chief Chancellor of the *Shu* Kingdom (known as *Si-chuan* today) during the Three Kingdoms period (220–280 CE). Zhuge Liang marched south to conquer the barbaric tribes and devised a clever plan to capture the tribal King. He commanded General Zhang Yi to lead one thousand soldiers to hide in a valley. The troops were to move in behind the barbarian tribes entering the valley and prevent their escape, trapping them. Zhuge Liang sent Zhang Yi to his task with a final warning that "Anyone who fails to execute the plan will be beheaded." When the troops failed their task, Zhang Yi was afraid that he and his subordinates would all be killed. Attempting to avert mortal punishment, he wrote a report explaining the reason for the failure. He explained that a 3-day storm cut off provisions from the troops waiting in ambush in the valley. The cold and hungry soldiers ate the roots of the nearby grasses. One herb (*Ba Ji Tian*) with a white and purple root, tender texture, fleshy appearance, and a sweet, slightly spicy taste was particu larly popular among the men. It deterred hunger and kept them warm, so everyone enjoyed eating it. However, after eating the herb for several days, all the soldiers suffered from an embarrassing ailment. Every man had a long-lasting erection he could hardly bear, and he could not stop groaning. The groaning sound from the one thousand soldiers reverberated in the valley like a roaring wind, which scared away the enemy. Thus, the army won the battle but did not capture all the barbaric tribe members. When Zhuge Liang heard the story, he summarized the battle by writing: "*Ba Ji* pointed to the sky, gave man's power, and made the enemy run away. We all would enjoy having this problem." *Ba Ji* literally refers to a halberd, which is an ancient spearlike weapon. When the two characters are reversed to form "*Ji Ba*," it becomes a Chinese slang term referring to a man's penis. "*Tian*" literally means sky. Therefore the herb's name "*Ba Ji Tian*" became a testament to the Chief Counselor's sense of humor. Since that time, "*Ba Ji Tian*" has often been used in formulas that tonify the Kidney *Yang*.
2. Good quality *Ba Ji Tian* is thick, large, interconnected, and purple. *Ba Ji Tian* is taken as a tonic to strengthen the mind and vertebral column. It also is good for both female and male fertility.
3. It lowers blood pressure.
4. Combined with Cornus *Shan Zhu Yu*, it can be effective for renal diseases.

Pharmaceutical Ingredients:[1–4]

1. Rudiadin, rudiadin-1-methylether, physcion, monotropein, asperulosidetetraacetate, palmitic acid, nonadecane
2. Morindin, monotropein, asperuloside tertraacetate, β-sitosterol, vitamin C
3. Monosaccharide, polysaccharide
4. Cardiac glycoside, flavone, amino acid, anthraquinone
5. K, Ca, Mg

Psoralea *Bu Gu Zhi* 补骨脂

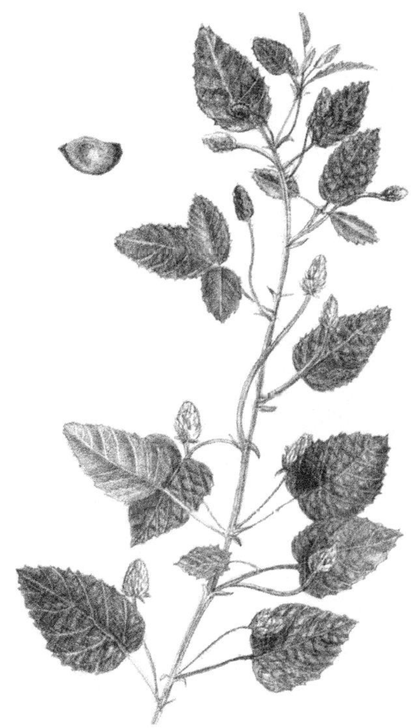

Original Reference: *Kai Bao Ben Cao* (*Materia Medica of the Kai Bao Era*) by *Ma Zhi* in 973 开宝本草

Part Used: Fruit-seed

Name:
Pharmaceutical: Psoraleae Corylifoliae, Fructus
Botanical: Psoralea corylifolia

Common: Psoralea seed
Wade-Giles: *Pu-Ku-Chih*
Translation: Tonify Bone Resin

Energy/Taste: Very warm, pungent, bitter

Channel-Organ: Kidney, Spleen

Actions:
1. Tonify the Kidney and strengthen *Yang*
2. Hold Essence and prevent incontinence
3. Warm Spleen and stop diarrhea

Form and Preparation: Powder or decoction

Dosage:
Horses and Cattle: 15–45 g
Llamas, Alpacas, Goats, Sheep, and Pigs: 5–10 g
Camels: 30–60 g
Dogs: 1–5 g
Cats: 0.5–2 g
Rabbits: 0.5–1.5 g
Birds: 0.3–2 g

Cautions and Contraindications:
1. Deficiency of *Yin* with Heat
2. Constipation

Side Effects:
1. It may cause constipation.
2. In very large doses, it may cause Kidney toxicity.

Clinical Applications
1. Diarrhea due to Deficiency of Kidney and Spleen *Yang*
   Clinical signs: Chronic diarrhea, or diarrhea before dawn (daybreak diarrhea)
   Combine with: Evodia *Wu Zhu Yu*, Myristica *Rou Dou Kou*, and Schisandra *Wu Wei Zi*
   Classical herbal formula: Si Shen Wan
2. Weakness of limbs and bones, difficulty moving, getting up, or laying down
   Combine with: Cuscuta *Tu Si Zi*, Cistanche *Rou Cong Rong*, Eucommia *Du Zhong*
   Classical herbal formula: Ba Ji San
3. Urinary or fecal incontinence (or dribbling) due to Kidney and Spleen *Yang* Deficiency
   Combine with: Cuscuta *Tu Si Zi* and Alpinia *Yi Zhi Ren*
4. Failure of the Kidneys to grasp Lung *Qi*
   Clinical signs: Shortness of breath, wheezing, heaves, asthma
   Combine with: Ginkgo *Bai Guo* and Juglans *Hu Tao Ren*

History and Comments:
1. During the *Tang* Dynasty (618–907 CE), a 75-year-old senior court officer named Zheng was sent to the *Hai-nan* Province as a new governor. *Hai-nan*'s chilly and damp environment made the governor very sick. The local TCM doctors diagnosed *Zheng* with a severe *Yang Qi* Deficiency. Based on this diagnosis, he took many tonic *Yang* herbal medicines, but he did not improve. Seven years later (812 CE), a barefoot monk recommended a new herbal medicine. The governor doubted the remedy and did not take it. Recognizing Mr. Zheng's suspicions, the monk made three more visits to persuade *Zheng* to try the medication. The governor finally relented and started taking the new herbal medication. One week later, Mr. Zheng's energy level improved. After another month of medication, all of his clinical signs disappeared. He recovered completely, returning to the same health status he enjoyed when he had first arrived in *Hai-nan*. In 815 CE, Mr. Zheng left *Hai-nan* for Beijing. He continued using this herbal recipe (*Gu Tao San)*, and he shared his experiences with others. *Gu Tao San* can be made by grinding 10 ounces each of Psoralea *Bu Gu Zhi* and Walnut *He Tao Ren* into a fine powder and mixing it with honey. Mix 1 teaspoon of this recipe with 1 teaspoon of warm wine or water, and administer orally once daily in the morning. Feed rice after the medication to harmonize the Stomach. *Gu Tao San* can extend the life span, tonify *Qi*, benefit the Liver and Heart, and strengthen tendons and bones.
2. Psoralea *Bu Gu Zhi* is a common *Yang* tonic for geriatric patients. It is often stir-fried in salt to increase its tonification effect on the Kidney.
3. Psoralea *Bu Gu Zhi* contracts the uterus, shortens bleeding time and prevents excessive loss of Blood, and it is often used for uterine bleeding.

Pharmaceutical Ingredients:[1–4]
1. Angelicin, psoralen, isopsoralen, psoralidin, isopsoralidin
2. Corylifolinin, corylidin, isobavahin, bavachinin, bavachalcone, bavachromenn, isoneobavachalion
3. Dihydrofuranochalcone, bakuchalcone, chalcone
4. Coumestrol, daidzin, 8-methoxyporalen, bakuchiol, psoraldehyde, limonene, terpineol

Eucommia *Du Zhong* 杜仲

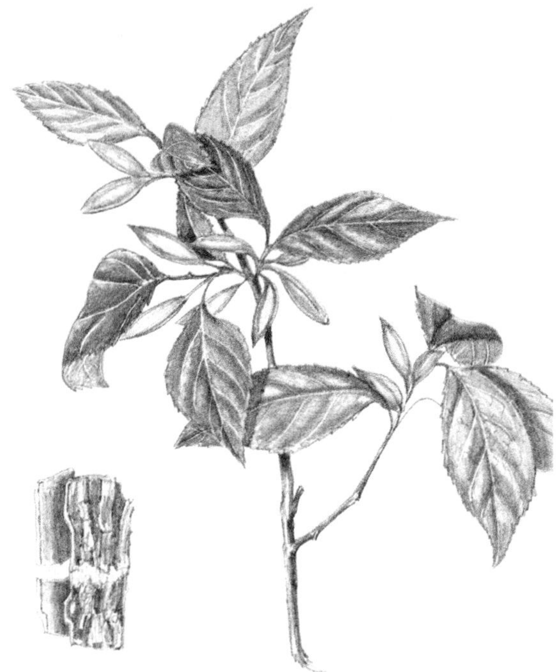

a

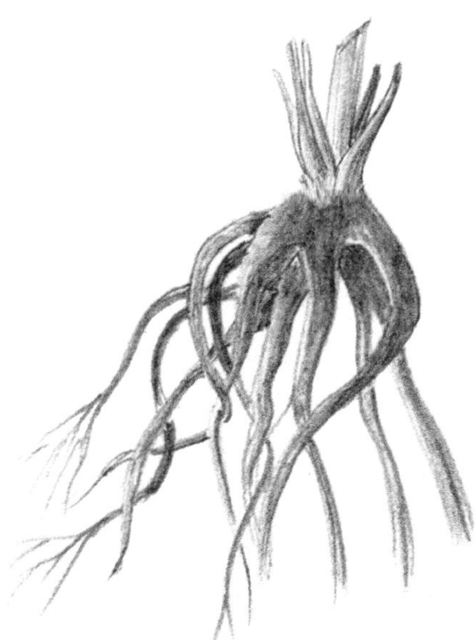

b

Original Reference: *Shen Nong Ben Cao Jing* (*Shen Nong*'s *Materia Medica*, 1st century BCE) 神农本草经

Part Used: Bark

Name:
Pharmaceutical: Eucommiae Ulmoidis, Cortex
Botanical: Eucommia ulmoides
Common: Eucommia bark
Wade-Giles: *Tu-Chung*
Translation: Eucommia bark

Energy/Taste: Warm, sweet, pungent

Channel-Organ: Liver, Kidney

Actions:
1. Tonify the Liver and Kidney
2. Strengthen the tendons, sinews, and bones
3. Calm the fetus to prevent abortion

Form and Preparation: Powder or decoction; stir-fried is better than raw Eucommia.

Dosage:
Horses and Cattle: 15–60 g
Llamas, Alpacas, Goats, Sheep, and Pigs: 5–10 g
Dogs: 2–5 g
Cats: 1–2 g
Rabbits: 0.5–1.5 g
Birds: 0.3–2 g

Cautions and Contraindications:
1. Deficiency of *Yin* with Heat
2. Antagonizes Scrophularia *Xuan Shen*

Side Effects: It may injure *Yin*.

Clinical Applications:
1. Weakness and pain in the back and hind limbs due to the Liver-Kidney Deficiency
   Clinical signs: Sore or painful lower back and stifles, fatigue, urinary incontinence
   Combine with: Psoralea *Bu Gu Zhi*, Cyathula *Niu Xi*, and Juglans *Hu Tao Ren* or Morinda *Ba Ji Tian* and Cistanche *Rou Cong Rong*. To reinforce effect on tendons, combine with Polygonum *He Shou Wu*.
   Classical herbal formula: Ba Ji San
2. Threatened abortion or restless fetus, due to weak Kidney *Qi*
   Clinical signs: Lower abdominal pain, uterine bleeding
   Combine with: Dipsacus *Xu Duan*, Loranthus *Sang Ji Sheng* and Dioscorea *Shan Yao* or Cuscuta *Tu Si Zi*, Loranthus *Sang Ji Sheng*
3. Hypertension due to Liver *Yin* Deficiency with rising *Yang*
   Combine with: Cyathula *Niu Xi*, Prunella *Xia Ku Cao*, Loranthus *Sang Ji Sheng*, and Paeonia *Bai Shao*

History and Comments:
1. Long ago in the mountainous region of West *Sichuan*, the barren soil frequently failed to produce sufficient

food for the farmers to make a living with their harvest. A farmer named Du Zhong suffered from chronic lower back pain, but he took a job chopping wood in order to supplement his income. After 2 hours, he was sore and soaked with sweat. Taking a break, he took off his clothes and leaned his back against a tree. To his surprise, his lower back pain was significantly relieved after leaning on the tree. Every day after work he repeated the same routine. Eventually, his lower back pain completely disappeared. Remembering that his 80-year-old mother also had chronic back soreness, but was too weak to walk to the tree, he removed bark from the tree and took it home. He wrapped this bark around his mother's lumbar area. Sure enough, his mother's sore back also improved. The herb was named after the man who discovered it.
2. During the *Ming* Dynasty (1368–1644 CE), a young boy complained of leg and hip pain soon after getting married. His legs felt too weak to walk. A local doctor diagnosed Dampness in his hip and leg and gave the boy herbs to take. After experiencing no improvement with this doctor, the boy saw Dr. Suan, who diagnosed the boy with Kidney *Qi* Deficiency, resulting in leg and hip pain. Only one herb was needed to cure the patient. Dr. Suan prescribed an herbal decoction containing 30 grams of Eucommia *Du Zhong* sliced 1 inch long and cooked in a mixture of half wine and half water. After taking this herbal soup for 3 days, this boy was able to walk. After another 3 days of treatment, all his clinical signs were gone and the boy was completely cured. Dr. Suan explained that due to his new marriage and young age, the young boy's excessive sexual activity damaged his Kidney *Qi*, which led to pain and weakness of his limbs. *Du Zhong* is the best choice for this condition.
3. Eucommia *Du Zhong* is a primary *Yang* tonic for treating the back, hindquarters, and rear limbs. The four big indications for using Du Zhong are Lower Burner Deficiency, Lower Burner Dampness. stifle pain, and back weakness and pain.
4. When good quality *Du Zhong* (bark) is cracked, it will reveal a dense mass of strong, thin, white fibers. The leaves of this plant have the same white stretchy fibers and the same active ingredients, but in a smaller quantity than the bark.
5. Eucommia *Du Zhong* is safe during pregnancy for weakness and back pain.
6. Eucommia *Du Zhong* can lower blood pressure significantly. Its leaves are especially good for high blood pressure.

Pharmaceutical Ingredients:[1–4]

1. Syrigaresinol, pinoresinol, eucommin A, Gutta-percha, eucommiol
2. Iridoidal glycosides (aucubin, ulmoside, genipin, geniposide)
3. Triterpenoides (betulin, ursoic acid, β-sitosterol)
4. Alkaloids, proteins, amino acid, organic acid, vitamins, microelements

Dipsacus *Xu Duan* 续断

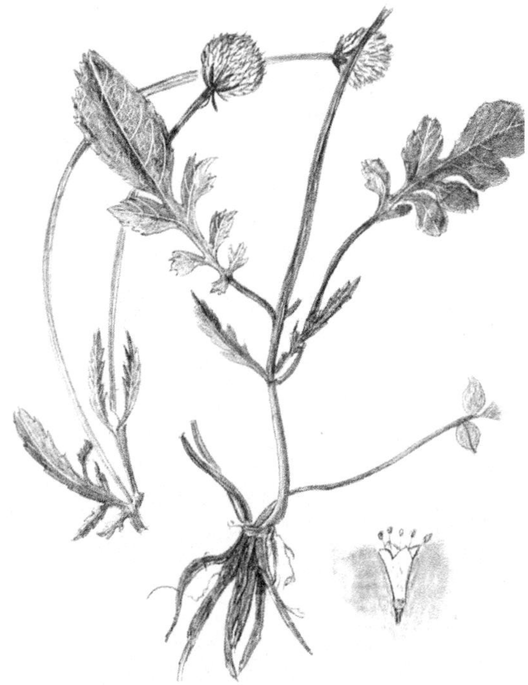

Original Reference: *Shen Nong Ben Cao Jing* (*Shen Nong's Materia Medica*, 1st century BCE) 神农本草经

Part Used: Root

Name:
Pharmaceutical: Radix Dipsaci Asperi
Botanical: Dipsacus asper
Common: Dipsacus root
Wade-Giles: *Hsu-Tuan*
Translation: Restore the Broken
Alternate: *Chuan Duan*

Energy/Taste: Slightly warm, bitter, sweet, pungent

Channel-Organ: Liver, Kidney

Actions:
1. Tonify the Liver and Kidney to strengthen the sinews/tendons and bones
2. Promote Blood circulation
3. Stop uterine bleeding and calm the fetus

Form and Preparation: Decoction, powder, or topical application as tincture or paste

Dosage:
Horses and Cattle: 25–60g
Llamas, Alpacas, Goats, Sheep, and Pigs: 5–15g
Camels: 30–60g
Dogs: 1–5g
Cats: 0.5–2g
Rabbits: 0.5–1.5g
Birds: 0.3–2g

Cautions and Contraindications:
1. *Yin* Deficiency with Heat
2. According to some traditional sources, it antagonizes *Lei Wan.*
3. Caution during pregnancy and cases of diarrhea, because it stimulates bowel movements

Side Effects: None known

Clinical Applications:
1. Pain in the back and weakness of the hindquarters due to Liver and Kidney *Yang Qi* Deficiency
   Combine with: Eucommia *Du Zhong*, Loranthus *Sang Ji Sheng*, Cyathula *Niu Xi*, and Dioscorea *Bei Xie*
2. Derangement of *Chong* and *Ren* channels due to Deficiency of Liver and Kidney
   Clinical signs: Uterine bleeding, excessive genital discharge during the estrous cycle, restless fetus and abortion threat
   Combine with: Eucommia *Du Zhong*, Loranthus *Sang Ji Sheng*, Cuscuta *Tu Si Zi*, Asinum Gelatinum *E Jiao*, Artemisia *Ai Ye*, Astragalus *Huang Qi* and Angelica *Dang Gui*, and Sanguisorba *Di Yu*
3. Joint pain or stiffness, deformed bones, bone fractures, and injuries to bone and tendons
   Combine with: Morinda *Ba Ji Tian* or Eucommia *Du Zhong*, Polygonum *He Shou Wu*, Drynaria *Gu Sui Bu*, and Eupolyphaga *Tu Bie Chong*

History and Comments:
1. *Xu Duan* is the root of Dipsacus. It is also called *Shu Zhe* (restoring what is broken) and *Jie Gu* (setting broken bones). As its name suggests, the herb's main functions are stimulating Blood circulation, strengthening bones and tendons, and tonifying *Qi*. These indications are familiar to most TCM practitioners, but few know that *Xu Duan* can also be used to treat diarrhea and control bleeding during pregnancy. Li Shi-zhen recorded a story about *Xu Duan* in the *Materia Medica Compendium* (*Ben Cao Gang Mu*). During the *Song* Dynasty in China (about one thousand years ago), the governor of the *Jian* County, Zhang Su-Qian, suffered from chronic bloody diarrhea for a very long time. He visited many local doctors and tried numerous formulas, but he did not improve. One of the best TCM doctors was traveling around the country and handling difficult cases, as was common for the best doctors in ancient China to do. He visited the governor's region and the governor became his patient. This unnamed doctor prescribed the following recipe: 2 grams of *Xu Duan* powder and 5 grams of *Peng Wei San*, decocted, and taken twice a day. Governor Zhang's diarrhea stopped after taking this herbal soup for 1 day. The governor was so happy that he gave the doctor 10 pounds of gold to express his thanks. Five years later, a diarrhea epidemic outbreak occurred in *Hui Ji* County. Thousands of people were affected and hundreds lost their lives. Upon hearing this news, Governor Zhang sent his son out on the fastest horse they could find to deliver the formula to the *Hui Ji* officials. Once again, the herbal soup worked amazingly well. Most people were cured after about 2 weeks of treatment. For children especially, the diarrhea usually ceased after drinking the herbal soup once or twice. The people in *Hui Ji* were very grateful to Governor Zhang and they recorded his good deeds in the county's epic book. From these records, Dr. Li Shi-zhen rediscovered the function of *Xu Duan*, 500 years later.
2. Good quality Dipsacus *Xu Duan* is thick, pliant, yellowish red on the outside, and gray-green on the inside.
3. Toasting *Xu Duan* in vinegar enhances its actions of moving Blood. Stir-frying the herb in salt increases its actions of tonifying the Kidney. Stir-frying it with wine aids tonification of the Liver and Kidney. The fried herb is used for uterine bleeding.
4. *Xu Duan* promotes healing and repairs of tendons and bones and is often used for pain due to trauma or degenerative joint disease, because it tonifies the Kidney and Liver without causing Stagnation.

Pharmaceutical Ingredients:[1–4]
1. β-sitosterol, hederagenin, ursol aldehyde, ursolic acid
2. Sucrose, daucosterol, triterpenoidal saponin
3. Ca, Mg, Fe, Mn, Zn, Cu

Cuscuta *Tu Si Zi* 菟丝子

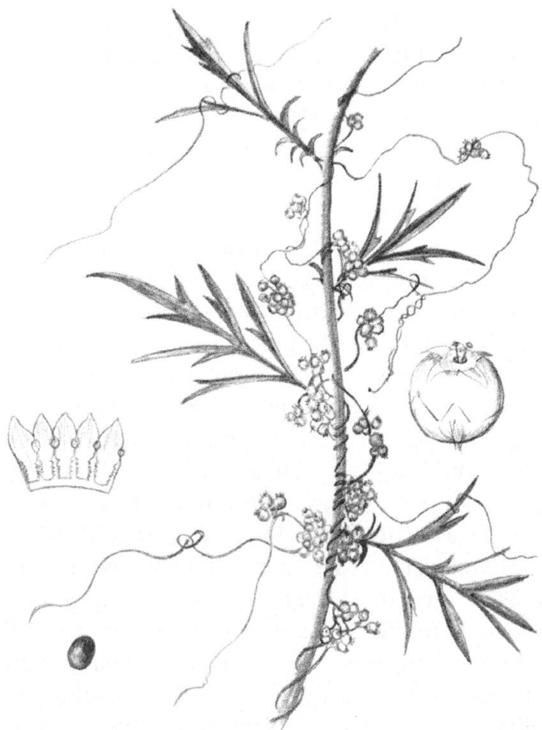

Original Reference: *Shen Nong Ben Cao Jing* (*Shen Nong's Materia Medica*, 1st century BCE) 神农本草经

Part Used: Seed

Name:
Pharmaceutical: Cuscutae Chinensis, Semen
Botanical: Cuscuta chinensis
Common: Dodder Seed
Wade-Giles: *T'u-Su-Tzu*
Translation: Rabbit Silky Seed

Energy/Taste: Neutral pungent, sweet

Channel-Organ: Liver, Kidney

Actions:
1. Tonify both Kidney *Yang* and *Yin*
2. Anchor the Essence, calm the fetus
3. Nourish the Liver and brighten the eyes
4. Benefit the Spleen and Kidney and stop diarrhea

Form and Preparation: Powder or decoction

Dosage:
Horses and Cattle: 15–45 g
Llamas, Alpacas, Goats, Sheep, and Pigs: 5–15 g
Dogs: 1–5 g
Cats: 0.5–2 g
Rabbits: 0.5–1.5 g
Birds: 0.1–1.5 g

Cautions and Contraindications: It can tonify both *Yang* and *Yin*, but is slightly more of a *Yang* tonic than a *Yin* tonic. Therefore, it is not recommended to use this herb in *Yin* Deficiency, dry stool, or concentrated urine Patterns.

Side Effects: None known

Clinical Applications:
1. Deficiency of Kidney *Yang*, *Yin*, and *Jing*
   Clinical signs: Sore back, weakness of the hind limbs, urinary incontinence, infertility, impotence, premature ejaculation
   Combine with: Eucommia *Du Zhong*, Dioscorea *Shan Yao*, Psoralea *Bu Gu Zhi*, Cibotium *Gou Ji*, and Cervus *Lu Rong*
   Herbal formula: Yin Yang Huo San.
2. Deficient Kidney and Liver causing vision disorders
   Clinical signs: Weak vision, red eyes, an early stage of glaucoma or cataracts
   Combine with: Lycium *Gou Qi Zi*, Plantago *Che Qian Zi*, and Ligustrum *Nü Zhen Zi*
3. Chronic diarrhea due to Deficiency of Spleen *Yang*
   Combine with: Codonopsis *Dang Shen*, Atractylodes *Bai Zhu* and Dioscorea *Shan Yao*

History and Comments:
1. According to legend, *Tu Si Zi* was accidentally discovered by a man who was hired to care for some rabbits. A greedy farmer raised many kinds of rabbits ranging from white to black and long-haired to short-haired. He hired a man to care of the rabbits. The hired man's contract stated that the farmer would deduct a quarter of his wages if one rabbit died. One day the hired man found a rabbit with a broken back, and fearing lost wages, he hid the injured rabbit in a soy bean field. However, the farmer realized a rabbit was missing. He told the hired man to find the rabbit or face lost wages. The rabbit caretaker brought back the injured rabbit from the soy bean field. Surprisingly, he found the rabbit was almost healed. One day, while investigating this miracle, the caretaker followed the injured rabbit to the soy bean field. The rabbit began eating the seeds of a yellow, silky plant. A couple of days later, the rabbit had completely healed. The rabbit man realized that he had just discovered a miracle drug to treat lumbar injuries. He took some seeds to his father who had been bedridden for 3 years following a lumbar injury. His father started walking

again just 10 days after eating the seeds. The rabbit caretaker later specialized in treating lumbar injuries. He called the miracle drug *Tu* (Rabbit) *Si* (Silky) *Zi* (Seed).
2. *Tu Si Zi* was recorded as a tonic herbal medicine in *Sheng Nong Ben Cao Jing*: "It can tonify Deficiency, move *Qi*, balance health, brighten eyes."
3. It has therapeutic effects on cataracts in rats.

Pharmaceutical Ingredients:[1–4]
1. Sterols (Cholesterol, campesterol, β-sitosterol, stigmasterol, βamyrin)
2. Glycosides, saccharides, alkaloids, anthraquinone, coumarin
3. Flavonoids (quercetin, astragaline, hyperin)
4. Ca, Mg, Fe, Mn, Zn, Cu

Cervus *Lu Rong* 鹿茸

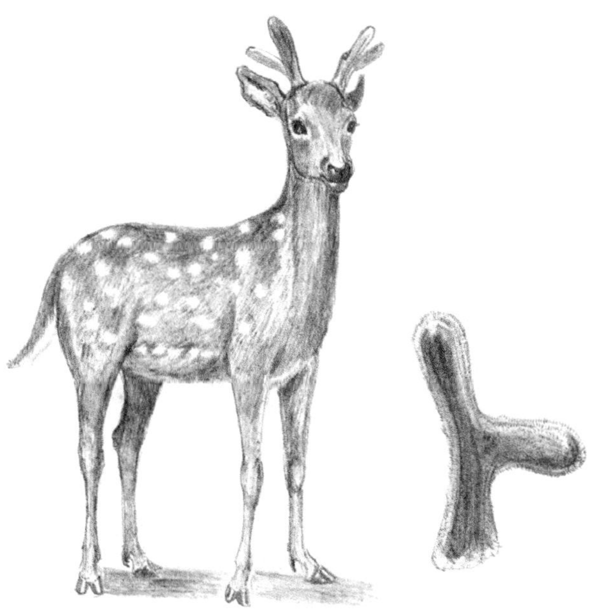

Original Reference: *Shen Nong Ben Cao Jing* (*Shen Nong*'s *Materia Medica*, 1st century BCE) 神农本草经

Part Used: Hairy young horn of male deer over 3 years old (that starts to have new velvet)

Name:
Pharmaceutical: Cornu Parvi, Cervi (previously: Cornu Cervi Pantotrichum)
Zoological: Cervus nippon; C. elaphus
Common: Deer antler
Wade-Giles: *Lu-Jung*
Translation: Hairy deer horn

Energy/Taste: Warm, sweet, salty

Channel-Organ: Liver, Kidney

Actions:
1. Tonify the Kidney *Yang*
2. Nourish Essence and Blood
3. Strengthen tendons and bones

Form and Preparation: Often use fine powder; start with a low dose and slowly increase to avoid Liver *Yang* Rising.

Dosage:
Horses and Cattle: 5–15 g
Dogs: 0.5–1 g
Cats: 0.1–0.5 g
Birds: 0.1–1 g

Cautions and Contraindications:
1. Deficient *Yin* with hyperactive *Yang*
2. Excess Heat, Blood Heat, Stomach fire, Lung Phlegm-Heat, and Fever

Side Effects:
1. Overdose leads to *Yin* Deficiency (red eyes, panting, cool-seeking, dizziness, disorientation).
2. It assists and raises *Yang*, or Heat in the Blood; thus, it may cause bleeding.

Clinical Applications:
1. Kidney *Yang* Deficiency
   Clinical signs: Weak body, cold extremities, warm-seeking behavior, infertility, impotence, frequent urination, sore back and limbs, loss of hearing
   Combine with: Ginseng *Ren Shen*, Rehmannia *Shu Di Huang*, and Cuscuta *Tu Si Zi*
   Classical herbal formula: *Shen Rong Gu Ben Wan*
2. Deficiency of *Jing* and Blood
   Clinical signs: Sore and weak bones and tendons, impotence, poor growth or development of young
   Combine with: Dioscorea *Shan Yao*, Cornus *Shan Zhu Yu*, and Rehmannia *Shu Di Huang*

History and Comments:
1. There are four products from deer horn: *Lu Rong, Lu Jiao, Lu Jiao Jiao, Lu Jiao Shuang*:
   - *Lu Rong* is a young deer antler.
   - *Lu Jiao* is a mature deer antler. It tonifies the Kidney and assists *Yang*, but is weaker than Lu Rong.
   - *Lu Jiao Jiao* is the glue or gelatin made from cooking the deer horn for a long time. This herb can stop bleeding and tonify the Liver and the Kidney. Its *Yang* tonic action is weaker than *Lu Jiao*.

- *Lu Jiao Shuang* is the residual frosting after making *Lu Jiao Jiao*. It is similar in function to *Lu Jiao Jiao* and is cheaper, but it is less effective.

2. Cervus *Lu Rong* is harvested from captive deer in the spring when Blood is rushing through the antlers and they are covered in felt. The deer are not killed. The horn is boiled and dried twice, and the hairs are burned off. It is then soaked in white wine and sliced into very thin pieces.
3. Cervus *Lu Rong* is highly valued for its ability to promote *Yang*, Blood, and *Jing*. It is very expensive. It is often administered alone, double-boiled as a tonic. The powder remaining after cutting Cervus *Lu Rong* into thin slices is available in capsule form.
4. Cervus *Lu Rong* is the tender, unossified horn of the male spotted deer or red deer. Kou Zong-shi (a master of herbal medicine in the *Song* Dynasty (960–1279 CE) once commented, "Among all the things that contain Blood, flesh grows the fastest, tendons come second, and bones grow the slowest; that's why it takes a human being 20 years to have his bones fully formed. But, the deer's horn is an exception. The horns can grow to over 20 lbs within 2 months, which is 2 oz a day. No other bones can grow as fast. Grass and trees cannot even grow that fast. The deer's horn is able to tonify Blood in the bones, strengthen *Yang*, and nourish marrow. All the *Yang* Channels converge at the head and then flow up to the angle. How can any other Blood compare to that in the horns?"
5. The medical value of *Lu Rong*, according to folklore, was found by three brothers. The eldest of the three was mean, the second eldest was sly, and the youngest was kind and brave. One day they went hunting. The youngest walked in front. The second was in the middle, and the eldest followed. Suddenly, a strange sound came out from the forest. The eldest and the second eldest brothers fled as fast as they could to hide behind a tree. The youngest brother went forward and saw a red deer in the high grass. He took out his bow and caught the deer. The second eldest brother suggested, "Our eldest brother is the head of our family and should get the head of the deer; our little brother came last to our family and should get the tail; I am in the middle so I should get the body." After the middle and eldest argued, they finally divided the deer's body and left only the head to their youngest brother. According to the village rules, the quarry is shared with the neighbors. The youngest brother made soup with the deer head and horns. He had not removed the horns as was typically done because the head was too small. He offered soup to all his neighbors. After drinking the soup, everyone felt invigorated and energized. With many repeated testings, they confirmed that the tender horns of the deer did have tonifying medical effects. Since these horns are usually covered with a coat of *Rong* (dense, fluffy hairs), they were called *Lu* (deer) Rong by the villagers.

Pharmaceutical Ingredients:[1–4]

1. Proline, lysine, serine, uracil, hypoxanthine, urea, uridine, niacin
2. Gelatin 25%, calcium phosphate 50–60%, calcium carbonate, amino acid
3. Lysophosphatidylcholine (myristic acid, palmitic acid, pentadecanoic acid, palmitoleic acid, stearic acid, oleic acid, linoleic acid, daturic acid
4. Amines (spermine, spermidine, putrescine)
5. Chondroitin sulfate A
6. Gangliosides
7. Androgen, estradiol

Cervus *Lu Jiao Jiao* 鹿角胶

Original Reference: *Shen Nong Ben Cao Jing* (*Shen Nong*'s *Materia Medica*, 1st century, BCE) 神农本草经

Part Used: Deer horn glue, made from cooking for a long time

Name:
Pharmaceutical: Cervi, Gelatinum Cornu
Common: Deer antler glue
Wade-Giles: *Lu-chiao-chiao*
Translation: Deer Antler Glue

Energy/Taste: Warm, salty, sweet

Channel-Organ: Kidney, Liver

Actions:

1. Tonify Liver and Kidney
2. Replenish Blood and *Jing*
3. Stop bleeding

Form and Preparation: Use in melted form; it is usually melted in yellow wine.

Dosage:
Horses and Cattle: 15–30 g
Llamas, Alpacas, Goats, Sheep, and Pigs: 5–10 g
Camels: 30–60 g
Dogs: 1–5 g
Cats: 0.5–2 g
Rabbits: 0.5–1.5 g
Birds: 0.1–1.5 g

Cautions and Contraindications: *Yin* Deficiency with Heat

Side Effects: Overdose leads to *Yin* Deficiency (red eyes, panting, cool-seeking, dizziness, disorientation).

Gecko *Ge Jie* 蛤蚧

Original Reference: *Lei Gong Pao Zhi Lun* (*Lei's Method of Preparing Drugs*) by Lei Xiao, 5th century 雷公炮炙论

Part Used: Dried body

Name:
Pharmaceutical: Gecko
Botanical: Gecko gecko L. (Toad headed lizard)
Common: Gecko lizard
Wade-Giles: *Ko-Chieh*
Translation: Male Female

Energy/Taste: Neutral, salty,

Channel-Organ: Lung, Kidney

Actions:
1. Tonify Lung *Qi* and Kidney *Yang*
2. Stop asthma and cough
3. Nourish Essence and Blood

Form and Preparation: Use powder often.

Dosage: Horse and Cattle: 1–2 pairs

Cautions and Contraindications:
1. Cough or asthma due to Internal Heat or invasion of Wind-Cold or Wind-Heat
2. Do not use in large doses over a long period.

Side Effects: None known

Clinical Applications:
1. Cough and asthma due to Lung *Qi* and Kidney *Yang* Deficiency
   Combine with: Ginseng *Ren Shen* or Codonopsis *Dang Shen*, Armeniaca *Xing Ren*, and Fritillaria *Chuan Bei Mu*
   Classical herbal formula: Ren Shen Ge Jie San
2. Infertility or urinary dribbling due to Deficiency of Kidney *Yang* and *Qi*
   Combine with: Ginseng *Ren Shen* or Codonopsis *Dang Shen*, Cervus *Lu Rong*, Epimedium *Yin Yang Huo* and Lycium *Gou Qi Zi*; or take alone

History and Comments:
1. *Ge-Jie* is like singing, in which the male's voice forms the *"Ge"* note and the female's voice creates the *"Jie"* note. Therefore, the male gecko is called *"Ge"* (brother) and usually has coarse scales, a big mouth, a small body, and a big tail. The female gecko is called *"Jie"* (sister) and often has fine scales, a pointed mouth, a big body, and a small tail. Male and female geckos mate for life and are called *"Ge Jie"*, which sounds like the English word gecko. Ancient Chinese people thought that Gecko *Ge Jies* possessed some mythical power and called them "the heavenly toads."
2. The adult Gecko *Ge Jie* can grow up to 4 to 5 inches long, half of which is the tail. They have a unique defense mechanism whereby they can drop off their tail, if they feel threatened or are grabbed by the tail. Traditional Chinese medicine considers the tail the most important part of a Gecko *Ge Jie*. Without an intact tail, a Gecko *Ge Jie* does not have much medical effect. Gecko *Ge Jies* are also loyal lovers. The *Ge* and the *Jie* may chirp at each other for days before they mate. Totally absorbed in their love, they will not notice anything else, even if someone approaches and catches them during mating. Their embracing bodies are very difficult to separate after death. It is said that some curious people had caught a pair of *Ge Jies* and made two candles using their ground powder: one candle with the male and the other with the female. The flames of the two candles would not remain separate but instead converged into one!
3. The internal organs and eyes are removed from the gecko lizard and are spread wide on bamboo pieces to dry. The head and feet are removed prior to preparation. The gecko can be cooked with rice or mixed in decoction, but is commonly used in powder form.
4. Gecko *Ge Jie* is slightly toxic. It should not be used in large quantities over extended periods of time.
5. Gecko *Ge Jie* is clinically proven to aid male and female infertility.

Pharmaceutical Ingredients:[1–4]
1. Cholesterol, cholesterol ester, triglyceride, glycolipid, lecithin, steroids
2. Lectins (phosphatidylethanolamine, phosphatidyl acid, lysophosphatidyl cholin)
3. Alcholes (glysin, proline, glutamate, alanine, arginine, aspartic acid, lysine)
4. Carnoside, carnitine, Guanine, albumen
5. Fatty acid, Ca, Mg, Fe, Zn, P, Na

Drynaria *Gu Sui Bu* 骨碎补

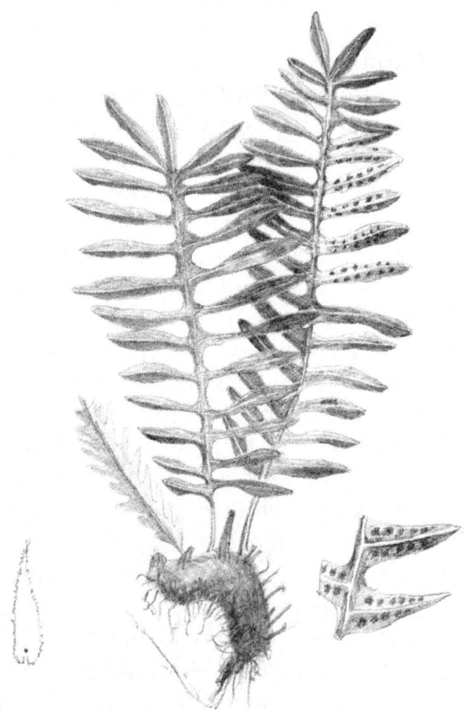

Original Reference: *Kai Bao Ben Cao* (*Materia Medica of the Kai Bao Era*) by *Ma Zhi* in 973 开宝本草

Part Used: Rhizome

Name:
Pharmaceutical: Drynariae, Rhizoma
Botanical: Drynaria fortunei; D. baronii
Common: Drynaria rhizome
Wade-Giles: *Ku-Sui-Pu*
Translation: Bone Broken Mender
Alternate: *Mao Jiang*

Energy/Taste: Warm, bitter

Channel-Organ: Liver, Kidney

Actions:
1. Tonify the Kidney and nourish the Liver
2. Invigorate the Blood to promote healing of wounds and mending of the sinews and bones

Form and Preparation: Orally or topically

Dosage:
Horses and Cattle: 15–45 g
Llamas, Alpacas, Goats, Sheep, and Pigs: 5–10 g
Camels: 30–60 g
Dogs: 1–5 g
Cats: 0.5–2 g
Rabbits: 0.5–1.5 g
Birds: 0.3–3 g

Cautions and Contraindications:
1. Deficient *Yin* with Heat
2. Do not use without clinical signs of Blood Stagnation.

Side Effects: It may injure *Yin*.

Clinical Applications:
1. Kidney *Yang* Deficiency
   Clinical signs: Back pain and weak limbs, arthritic joints, hip dysplasia, deafness, loose tooth or toothache, chronic diarrhea
   Combine with: Psoralea *Bu Gu Zhi*, Cyathula *Niu Xi*, Juglans *Hu Tao Ren*, Rehmannia *Shu Di Huang*, Dioscorea *Shan Yao* and Cornus *Shan Zhu Yu*
2. Swelling, pain or fractures due to external trauma or tendon-bone injury
   Combine with: Dipsacus *Xu Duan*, Olibanum *Ru Xuang*, Myrrh *Mo Yao*, and Testudines *Gui Ban*
   Classical herbal formula: Jie Gu San

History and Comments:
1. As the name indicates, *Gu* (bone) *Sui* (broken) *Bu* (mend) is mainly used for mending fractures and broken bones. During the *Tang* Dynasty (618–907 CE), Emperor Li and his Queen were out hunting. Suddenly, a leopard ran out from the forest. The startled Queen fell from her horse. Her ankle was fractured and bleeding. A local folk doctor picked an herb from the ground and applied it topically around the Queen's wound. This herb stopped the bleeding and immediately relieved the pain. A month later, the Queen's fracture had also healed from applying the herb topically. Emperor Li was so happy and named this herb *Gu Shui Bu*.
2. Li Shi-Zhen records a case about *Bu Gui Bu* in the *Materia Medica Compendium* (*Ben Cao Gang Mu*). During the *Wei* Dynasty (220–265 CE), a governor's young son was dying from persistent diarrhea. He had not responded to any of the many Spleen tonic treatments they tried thus far. So they tried a new treatment strategy in which *Gu Sui Bu* powder was put into a pig kidney, which was then stewed over a low fire. After the child ate the kidney with the herb, his diarrhea immediately stopped. *Li Shi-zhen* analyzed this case and stated that, "The Kidney was in charge of both fecal and urinary excretion. Persistent diarrhea must be caused by Kidney Deficiency, so it couldn't be cured by targeting the Spleen and Stomach alone."

3. Drynaria *Gu Sui Bu* is known for treating tendon and bone injuries. It can be used topically for corns and warts as well as bleeding wounds. It also stimulates the growth of hair and can be topically applied for the treatment of alopecia as a tincture.

Pharmaceutical Ingredients:[1–4]
1. Naringin, naringenin
2. Sugar

Alpinia *Yi Zhi Ren* 益智仁

Original Reference: *Ben Cao Shi Yi* (*Supplement to Materia Medica*) by *Chen Cang-Qi*, 8th century 本草拾遗

Part Used: Mature seed

Name:
Pharmaceutical: Alpiniae Oxyphyllae, Fructus
Botanical: Alpinia oxyphylla (Black Cardamon)
Common: Black cardamon
Wade-Giles: *I-Chih-Jen*
Translation: Benefit Intelligence Nut

Energy/Taste: Warm, pungent

Channel-Organ: Spleen, Kidney

Actions:
1. Warm the Spleen to stop diarrhea and excessive salivation
2. Warm the Kidney to stop urinary incontinence

Form and Preparation: Powder or decoction

Dosage:
Horses and Cattle: 15–45 g
Llamas, Alpacas, Goats, Sheep, and Pigs: 5–10 g
Dogs: 1–5 g
Cats: 0.5–2 g
Rabbits: 0.5–1.5 g
Birds: 0.3–3 g

Cautions and Contraindications:
1. Deficient *Yin* with Heat
2. Uterine bleeding due to Heat

Side Effects: It may damage *Yin* and assist *Yang* Fire.

Astragalus *Sha Yuan Zi* 沙苑子

Original Reference: *Ben Cao Yan Yi* (*Extension of the Materia Medica*) by *Kou Zong*-Shi, 1116 本草衍义

Part Used: Seed

Name:
Pharmaceutical: Astragali Complanati, Semen
Botantical: Astragalus companatus (Flattened Milkvetch)
Common: Flattened milkvetch seed
Wade-Giles: *Sha-Yuan-Tzu*
Translation: Sandy Garden Seed
Alternate: *Sha Yuan Ji Li*

Energy/Taste: Warm, sweet

Channel-Organ: Liver, Kidney

Actions:
1. Tonify the Kidney and astringe the Essence
2. Nourish the Liver and brighten the eyes

Form and Preparation: Powder or decoction

Dosage:
Horses and Cattle: 15–45 g
Llamas, Alpacas, Goats, Sheep, and Pigs: 5–10 g
Dogs: 1–5 g
Cats: 0.5–2 g
Rabbits: 0.5–1.5 g
Birds: 0.1–1.5 g

Cautions and Contraindications:
1. Dysuria
2. Deficiency of *Yin* with Heat

Side Effects: It may damage *Yin* and assist *Yang*-Fire.

Cordyceps *Dong Chong Xia Cao* 冬虫夏草

Original Reference: *Ben Cao Cong Xin* (*Thoroughly Revised Materia Medica*) by *Wu Yi-Luo*, 1751 本草从新

Part Used: Fungus and the caterpillar larva carcass on which it grows

Name:
Pharmaceutical: Cordyceps sinensis
Botanical: Sclerotium Cordycipitas Sinensis
Common: Chinese caterpillar fungus
Zoological: Hepialus varians
Wade-Giles: *Tung-Ch'ung-Hsia-Ts'ao*
Translation: Winter Bug Summer Herb

Energy/Taste: Warm, sweet

Channel-Organ: Kidney, Lung

Actions:
1. Tonify the Kidney and Lung
2. Stop bleeding and remove Phlegm

Form and Preparation: Single or combined; it is also a good tonic Food Therapy; cook in a stew with fish, chicken, duck, or pork for a good tonic.

Dosage:
Horses and Cattle: 5–20 g
Dogs: 0.5–3 g
Cats: 0.2–0.5 g
Rabbits: 0.1–0.5 g
Birds: 0.1–0.5 g

Cautions and Contraindications: It should be used with caution during exogenous invasions.

Side Effects: Because it strengthens both the *Yin* and *Yang* and is a very safe substance, it can be taken over a long period of time. No side effects have been noted.

History and Comments:
1. A fungus (Cordyceps sinensis Sacc.) parasitizes the caterpillar larvae (Hepialus armoricanus or Holotrichia koraiensis). The larva with the cordyceps fungus becomes a carcass in the winter and hibernates in the ground. The fruiting body of the fungus emerges from the head of the larva in the summertime and resembles a grass sprout; thus, it is called "winter-bug, summer-grass," or *Dong Chong Xie Cao.*
2. It is often harvested in the early summer when the fungus has merged but before the larval body has disintegrated. It is found on high mountain peaks over 3,800 meters above sea level. It is one of the very few Chinese medicines that consists of two symbiotic living substances (fungus and larva). It is known in English as the Chinese Caterpillar Mushroom. Originating in loose, leafy fertile soils in the cool forested hills and mountains of Sichuan and southern Tibet, it is now also found in other provinces, such as *Yunnan* and *Shaanxi*. In autumn, this mushroom grows underground from the anterior end of previously infected host larvae and eventually surfaces during the course of the following summer, when it can be harvested as a remedy. Cultivated mycelia (cordyceps biomass) are also available today and have been shown to be equally as effective therapeutically as the natural mushroom.
3. Good quality is indicated by the fungus being intact with a short, sticklike appearance and a bright yellow, fat, full, and round insect part with a yellowish white cross-section.
4. It is commonly used for back pain, hindquarter weakness, and infertility due to Kidney *Yang* Deficiency and also asthma and cough due to Lung *Qi* and Kidney *Yang* Deficiency. It also enhances immune functions.

Cynomorium *Suo Yang* 锁阳

Original Reference: *Ben Cao Cong Xin* (*Thoroughly Revised Materia Medica*) by *Wu Yi-Luo*, 1751 本草从新

Part Used: Fleshy stem

Name:
Pharmaceutical: Cynomorii Songarici, Herba
Botanical: Cynomorium Songaricum
Common: Cynomorium stem
Wade-Giles: *Suo-Yang*
Translation: Lock *Yang*

Energy/Taste: Warm, sweet

Channel-Organ: Liver, Kidney, Large Intestine

Actions:
1. Tonify Kidney *Yang*
2. Moisten Intestines

Form and Preparation: Powder or decoction

Dosage:
Horses and Cattle: 20–45 g
Llamas, Alpacas, Goats, Sheep, and Pigs: 5–15 g
Camels: 30–60 g
Dogs: 2–6 g
Cats: 0.5–2 g
Rabbits: 0.5–1.5 g
Birds: 0.3–3 g

Cautions and Contraindications:
1. Deficient Kidney *Yin* with Heat
2. Diarrhea from Spleen *Qi* Deficiency or constipation from Excess Heat

Side Effects: It may increase internal Fire, cause diarrhea, and damage *Yin.*

Curculigo *Xian Mao* 仙茅

Original Reference: *Kai Bao Ben Cao* (*Materia Medica of the Kai Bao Era*) by *Ma Zhi* in 973 CE
开宝本草

Part Used: Rhizome

Name:
Pharmaceutical: Curculiginis Orchioidis, Rhizoma
Botanical: Curculigo orchioides
Common: Golden eye-grass rhizome
Wade-Giles: *Hs'ian Mao*
Translation: Immortal Grass

Energy/Taste: Hot, pungent, toxic

Channel-Organ: Kidney, Liver

Actions:
1. Warm Kidney and strengthen *Yang*
2. Dispel Cold and Damp

Form and Preparation: Powder or decoction

Dosage: Because of toxicity, long-term use is not recommended.
Horses and Cattle: 15–30 g
Llamas, Alpacas, Goats, Sheep, and Pigs: 5–10 g
Dogs: 0.5–2 g
Cats: 0.2–0.5 g
Rabbits: 0.1–0.5 g
Birds: 0.1–1.0 g

Cautions and Contraindications:
1. Deficient *Yin* with Heat
2. It should not be used during pregnancy.

Side Effects: Toxic reactions such as swelling of the tongue can occur and can be alleviated by taking a decoction of Rheum *Da Huang*, Coptis *Huang Lian*, and Scutellaria *Huang Qin*.

Walnut *He Tao Ren* 核桃仁

Original Reference: *Kai Bao Ben Cao* (Materia Medica *of the Kai Bao Era*) by *Ma Zhi*, 973 CE 开宝本草

Part Used: Nut

Name:
Pharmaceutical: Juglandis Regiae Semen
Botanical: Juglans regia L.
Common: Walnut nut
Wade-Giles: *He-Tao-Ren*
Translation: Core peach pit
Alternate: *Hu Tao Ren*

Energy/Taste: Warm, sweet

Channel-Organ: Kidney, Lung, Large Intestine

Actions:
1. Tonify Kidney and warm Lung
2. Moisten intestines to benefit bowel movements

Form and Preparation: Single or combined; good tonic Food Therapy; stir-fry and use for urinary tract stones or crystals.

Dosage:
Horses and Cattle: 15–45 g
Llamas, Alpacas, Goats, Sheep, and Pigs: 5–10 g
Camels: 30–90 g
Dogs: 1–5 g
Cats: 0.5–2 g
Rabbits: 0.5–1.5 g
Birds: 0.1–1.5 g

Cautions and Contraindications: Use with caution during diarrhea

Side Effects: None known

Trigonella *Hu Lu Ba* 胡芦巴

Original Reference: *Jia You Ben Cao* (*Materia Medica of the Jia You Era*) by *Zhang Yu-xi* and *Su Song*, 1061 嘉佑本草

Part Used: Seed

Name:
Pharmaceutical: Trigonellae Foeni-graeci Semen
Botanical: Trigonella Foenum-graecum L.
Common: Fenugreek seed
Wade-Giles: *Fu-Lu-Pa*

Energy/Taste: Warm, bitter

Channel-Organ: Kidney

Actions:
1. Tonify Kidney and warm *Yang*
2. Dispel Cold and stop pain

Form and Preparation: Decoction or powder

Dosage:
Horses and Cattle: 15–45 g
Llamas, Alpacas, Goats, Sheep, and Pigs: 5–10 g
Camels: 30–60 g
Dogs: 1–5 g
Cats: 0.5–2 g
Rabbits: 0.5–1.5 g
Birds: 0.1–1.5 g

Cautions and Contraindications: Caution during Damp-Heat or False Heat

Side Effects: None known

Actinolite *Yang Qi Shi* 阳起石

Original Reference: *Shen Nong Ben Cao Jing* (*Shen Nong's Materia Medica*, 1st century BCE) 神农本草经

Part Used: Mineral

Name:
Pharmaceutical: Actinolitum
Common: Actinolite
Wade-Giles: *Yang-Chee-She*
Translation: *Yang*-raising Stone

Energy/Taste: Warm, salty

Channel-Organ: Kidney

Actions:
1. Warm Kidney and strengthen *Yang*
2. Dispel Cold and stop pain

Form and Preparation: Decoction or powder

Dosage:
Horses and Cattle: 15–45 g
Llamas, Alpacas, Goats, Sheep, and Pigs: 5–10 g
Dogs: 1–5 g
Cats: 0.5–2 g

Table 1.6. Herbs to tonify Deficiency: A quick overview and comparison.

Qi Tonics	Special Actions	Common Characteristics
Ren Shen	The number 1 power of *Qi* Tonic Rescue Yuan *Qi* for resuscitation	Taste: Sweet Channel-organ: Spleen, Lung
Dang Shen	Neutral *Qi* tonic, safer to use Often substitute for *Ren Shen*	Action: Tonify *Qi*; Indication: *Qi* Deficiency
Huang Qi	Raise *Yang* for prolapse of Spleen *Qi* Strengthen Wei *Qi* to promote wound healing	Energy: Neutral *Dang Shen*
Bai Zhu	The number 1 herb of tonifying Spleen *Qi* Dry up Dampness	*Gan Cao* *Shau Yao*
Shan Yao	Neutral *Qi* Tonic, can be a long-term usage Tonify Kidney Jing and Lung *Yin*	*Da Zao* *Ling Zhi*
Gan Cao	Harmonize other herbs General antidote to food or drug poisons	*Tai Zi Shen* *Feng Mi*
Da Zao	Nourish Heart Blood, calm Shen Protect Stomach *Qi* from other harsh herbs	Energy: Warm *Ren Shen*
Ling Zhi	Nourish Heart Blood to calm Shen Stop cough and asthma	*Huang Qi* *Bai Zhu*
Tai Zi Shen	Promote production of Body Fluids Nourish *Yin*	*Yi Tang* Energy: Cold
Jiao Gu Lan	Transform Phlegm to stop cough Clear Heat, detoxify	*Jiao Gu Lan* *Hong Jing Tian*
Hong Jing Tian	Nourish Lung *Yin* Activate Blood to relieve pain	
Yi Tang	Relax the GI spasm to relieve colic Moisten Lung to stop cough	
Feng Mi	Moisten Lung to stop cough Moisten large intestine to benefit bowel movements	

Blood Tonics	Special Actions	Common Characteristics
Angelica *Dang Gui*	Activate Blood to relieve pain Moisten large intestine to benefit bowel movements	Taste: Sweet and rich, may cause *Qi* Stagnation, generate Damp
Rehmannia *Shu Di Huang*	Tonify Kidney *Jing* Tonify Global *Yin*	Energy: Warm except for the following E Jiao: neutral
Paeonia *Bai Shao Yao*	Soothe Liver to relieve spasm Nourish *Yin* to tranquilize Liver *Yang*	*Bai Shao Yao*: Slightly Cold *Sang Shen*: Cold
Polygonum *He Shou Wu*	Tonify Kidney Jing Moisten large intestine to benefit bowel movements	Action: Tonify Blood Indications: Blood Deficiency anemia,
Asinum Gelatinum *E Jiao*	Stop Bleeding, calm fetus Moisten Lung to stop cough	dizziness, ear-ringing, dry/cracked paws/ hooves, poor memory, pale tongue, thin
Longan *Long Yan Rou*	Nourish Heart and calm Shen Tonify Spleen *Qi*	pulse Combine with *Qi* or *Yin* Tonic, or *Qi* mover
Morus *Sang Shen*	Nourish *Yin* to resolve thirst Moisten large intestine to benefit bowel movements.	Caution: Spleen *Qi* Deficiency

Table 1.6. *(Continued)*

Yin Tonics	Special Actions	Common Characteristics
Lung and Stomach *Yin* Tonics		
Bei Sha Shen	Is a strong Lung *Yin* tonic	Taste: Sweet
Nan Sha Shen	Tonify Spleen *Qi* and transform Phlegm	Energy: Cool or Cold
Bai He	Nourish Heart *Yin* to calm Shen	Action: Tonify *Yin*, Generate Body Fluids, Clear Heat
Mai Men Dong	Nourish Heart *Yin* and calm Shen	
Tian Men Dong	Tonify Kidney *Yin*	Indication: *Yin* Deficiency, Internal Dryness, False Heat
Xi Yang Shen	Tonify *Qi* of Lung, Heart, and Spleen	
Shi Hu	Is a strong Stomach *Yin* tonic	Cautions: Spleen *Qi* Deficiency, internal Dampness, loose stool
Yu Zhu	Nourish Heart *Yin*	
Huang Jing	Tonify Kidney Jing, tonify Spleen *Qi*	
Bai Mu Er	Mild *Yin* tonic, often used for food therapy	
Kidney *Yin* and Liver Tonics		
Gou Qi Zi	Tonify Kidney Jing, brighten eyes	
Nü Zhen Zi	Tonify Kidney Jing, brighten eyes	
Gui Ban	Strengthen bones, nourish Heart Blood	
Bie Jia	Clear False Heat, soften the lumps	
Han Lian Cao	Cool Blood and stop bleeding	
Hei Zhi Ma	Moisten large intestine to benefit bowel movements	

Yang Tonics	Special Actions	Common Characteristics
Tonify Kidney *Yang Qi* and promote sexual functions		
Yin Yang Huo	Dispel Wind-Damp, strengthen tendons and bones	Taste: Sweet
Rou Cong Rong	Tonify *Yin*, Moisten intestines	Energy: Warm and dry
Tu Si Zi	Nourish *Jing* and Liver, brighten the eyes	Action: Tonify *Yang*, Warm Kidney
Lu Rong	Nourish *Jing* and Blood, strong *Yang* tonic	Indication: *Yang* Deficiency
Lu Jiao Jiao	Nourish Kidney *Jing* and Liver Blood	Contraindication: *Yin* Deficiency, Excess Heat
Suo Yang	Moisten intestines, benefit bowel movements	
Yang Qi Shi	Warm uterus and hindquarter	Cautions: May damage *Yin*
Tonify Liver and Kidney, strengthen tendons and bones		Generally regulates functions of adrenal cortex, regulates energy metabolism, promotes sexual functions, promotes growth and strengthens resistance
Du Zhong	Strengthen back, calm fetus	
Xu Duan	Strengthen joints, repair broken bones and tendons	Kidney dominates the *Yang* of the whole body; the therapy of tonifying *Yang* always begins with tonifying the Kidney.
Gu Sui Bu	Move Blood, repair broken bones and tendons	
Tonify Lung and Kidney, stop asthma and cough		
Ge Jie	Tonify Lung *Qi* and Kidney *Jing*	
He Tao Ren	Moisten intestines and benefit bowel movements	
Dong Chong Xia Cao	Strengthen back and hind limbs, stop bleeding	
Tonify Kidney, dispel Cold, relieve Bi syndrome		
Ba Ji Tian	Strengthen back	
Xian Mao	Tonify *Jing*, nourish Liver	
Hu Lu Ba	Dispel internal Cold and stop colic	
Tonify Kidney *Qi* to stop urinary incontinence and anchor *Jing*		
Bu Gu Zhi	Tonify Spleen *Yang* to stop diarrhea	
Yi Zhi Ren	Warm Spleen *Yang* to relieve excessive salivation	
Sha Yuan Zi	Nourish Liver and brighten the eyes	

Rabbits: 0.5–1 g
Birds: 0.1–1.5 g

Cautions and Contraindications:

1. Caution in False Heat
2. Long-term usage is not recommended.

Side Effects: None known

History and Comments: It is good for infertility due to Kidney *Yang Qi* Deficiency or Cold Bi syndrome.

SUMMARY OF HERBS THAT TONIFY DEFICIENCY

Table 1.6 summarizes and compares the herbs that tonify Deficiency.

REFERENCES

1. Chen JK, Chen TT. Chinese Medical Herbology and Pharmacology. City of Industry, CA: Art of Medicine Press, 2004.
2. Brinker, FJ. The Toxicology of Botanical Medicines. Sandy, OR: Eclectic Medical Publications, 2000.
3. Duke, JA. Handbook of Medicinal Herbs. New York: Chemical and Rubber Company Press, 2001.
4. Huang, KC. The Pharmacology of Chinese Herbs, 2nd Edition. New York: Chemical and Rubber Company Press, 1999.
5. Kanzaki T, Morisaki N, Shiina R, Saito Y. Role of transforming growth factor-beta pathway in the mechanism of wound healing by saponin from Ginseng Radix rubra. British Journal of Pharmacology 1998;125(2):255–262.
6. Kim JH, Kang SA, Han SM, Shim I. Comparison of the anti-obesity effects of the protopanaxadiol- and protopanaxatriol-type saponins of red ginseng. Phytotherapeutical Research 2009;23(1):78–85.
7. Li QF, Shi SL, Liu QR, Tang J, Song J, Liang Y. Anticancer effects of ginsenoside Rg1, cinnamic acid, and tanshinone IIA in osteosarcoma MG-63 cells: nuclear matrix down regulation and cytoplasmic trafficking of nucleophosmin. International Journal of Biochemical Cell Biology 2008;40(9): 1918–1929.
8. Liang MT, Podolka TD, Chuang WJ. Panax notoginseng supplementation enhances physical performance during endurance exercise. Journal of Strength Conditioning Research. 2005;19(1):108–114.
9. Wang XJ, Liu H, Guo SN. Clinical Applications and Research of Si Wu Tang: A Review. American. Journal of Traditional Chinese Veterinary Medicine 2006;1(1):22–29.

2 Herbs to Release the Exterior 解表药

Xuguang Yang, Li Lin, Huisheng Xie

The Chinese herbs in this chapter treat Exterior Patterns by clearing external pathogenic factors from the surface or upper parts of body. Targeting these locations is important with Exterior Patterns because the surface and upper body—which includes the skin, muscles, head, eyes, ears, nose, mouth, and throat—are attacked first when the external pathogenic factors invade the body. Attacks by external pathogenic factors can result in either Wind-Cold or Wind-Heat Patterns, which are described in Table 2.1.

Most herbs that release the Exterior taste pungent or spicy and are light in quality. The pungent or spicy taste helps to dispel the surface and the light quality has lifting and floating effects. The *Huang Di Nei Jing* describes when to use these spicy herbs by stating, "when the pathogen is lodged in the skin, induce sweat to expel it." These herbs are also mainly attributed to Channels going to the surface and upper body, especially the Lung, Bladder, and Liver Channels. The clinical signs benefited by such herbs can include fever, chills, pain or body aches, absent or slight sweating, superficial pulse, edema, cough, wheezing, skin rashes, hives, measles, rubella, rubeolla, arthritis, *Bi* syndrome, early boils, and disorders of the eyes, ears, nose, mouth, and throat.

Various factors influence herb selection, including the herb's temperature, the diagnosis (Pattern of disease), the herb's actions and the environmental conditions. The herb's temperature should counteract the disease present in the patient. Use Pungent-Warm herbs for Wind-Cold conditions, and use Pungent-Cool herbs for Wind-Heat. If other diseases are simultaneously present in the patient, one may combine these herbs with herbs that target the other disease conditions. Sometimes the disease conditions relate to the environmental conditions and seasonal changes. In this case, one may select herbs that relate to the time of year. The predominant conditions for winter, spring, summer, and fall are, respectively, Wind-Cold, Wind-Heat, Damp Heat, and Dryness. Thus, it is beneficial to use herbs that treat Wind-Cold in the winter, clear Wind-Heat in the spring, drain Damp-Heat in the summer, and moisten Dryness in the fall. When Exterior pathogenic factors invade patients with weak body constitutions, the specific herbal treatment depends on the particular Deficiency Pattern present: *Qi* Deficiency, Blood Deficiency, *Yin* Deficiency, or *Yang* Deficiency. The general treatment plan is to treat both the Exterior and the Deficiency by combining herbs that will eliminate the external pathogenic factors and strengthen the constitution through tonifying the *Qi*, Blood, *Yin*, or *Yang*. Early-stage febrile diseases that are at the Wei (defense) level require a combination of herbs that clear heat and eliminate toxins.

Herbs that release the Exterior will cause sweating. If these herbs are used inappropriately, the profuse sweating could consume Body Fluids and *Yin* or could damage *Yang* and *Qi*. Use these herbs cautiously in patients with the following conditions: 1) spontaneous sweating due to an Exterior Pattern with Deficiency, 2) night sweating due to *Yin* Deficiency, 3) late-stage febrile disease with *Yin* or Body Fluid Deficiency, 4) Exterior Pattern with *Yang* or *Qi* Deficiency, 5) Exterior Pattern with bleeding or Blood Deficiency, 6) *Lin Zheng* (dysuria syndrome), and 7) prolonged sore and abscess. Also, dosing these herbs may depend upon the environmental conditions present. During summer or on hot days, sweating occurs easily, so the dosage of herbs that release the Exterior should be lowered. On the other hand, the body surface is less prone to sweating in winter or on a cold day, so the dosage should be slightly increased. This principle also extends to cold and warm climates. Patients living in frigid areas require larger doses, but patients living in temperate zones need lower doses.

The chemical composition of herbs to release the Exterior can make herbal formula preparation challenging. Most of these pungent or spicy herbs contain

Table 2.1. Exterior Patterns and their herbal characteristics.

Exterior Patterns	Clinical Signs	Herbal Categories	Herbal Characteristics
Wind-Cold	Chills/aversion to cold Fever/no fever Headache, pain or aching of body, stiff neck Nasal congestion, clear discharge Absence of sweating Tongue: pale/pale, red/thin, and white coating Pulse: superficial/tight	Pungent-Warm Herbs to Clear the Surface	Energy: Warm Taste: Pungent Action: Clear Wind-Cold in the surface
Wind-Heat	Fever Slight aversion to wind/cold, or slight chills, headache Sweating Thirst or sore throat Tongue: red in tip/sides body/thin and yellow coating Pulse: superficial/rapid	Pungent-Cool Herbs to Clear the Surface	Energy: Cool Taste: Pungent Activity: Clear Wind-Heat in surface

volatile oils that could be lost with incorrect preparation. When decocting a formula containing these herbs, cook the formula for a short time (about 10 to 15 minutes) and add the herbs to release the Exterior at the end of the process. Extended decoction can reduce the herbs' therapeutic effects.

These herbs are divided into the Pungent-Warm or Pungent-Cool categories depending on their taste, energy, actions, and indications. The following sections describe each category in detail.

PUNGENT-WARM HERBS TO RELEASE THE EXTERIOR

Pungent-Warm herbs are primarily used to treat Exterior Patterns with Wind-Cold (Table 2.2). Most of the herbs in this category have a pungent taste, are warm in temperature, and have an affinity for the Lung and Bladder Channels. These properties allow Pungent-Warm herbs to release the Exterior and to disperse Wind-Cold in the surface, muscle, skin, and upper body, including the head, eyes, ears, nose, mouth, and throat.

To understand how these herbs work, consider the relationship between the Channels, body areas and pathogenic factors. Both the Lung and Bladder Channels are connected to superficial areas of the body, and the Lung is specifically related to the skin, nose and throat. Wind and Cold are pathogenic factors that affect the body in particular ways. Wind attacks the upper body and the superficial areas of the body while Cold causes congestion of muscle, skin, eyes, ears, nose, and throat. These body areas happen to be the same as those related to the Lung and Bladder. Thus, Wind and Cold commonly cause imbalance within those two meridians. The Pungent-Warm herbs are particularly beneficial for treating Exterior Patterns with Wind-Cold, because the pungent taste disperses Wind, the warm energy clears the Cold, and the affinity for the Lung and Bladder Channels directs the herbal effects toward body areas most affected by Wind and Cold pathogens.

Table 2.2. Exterior Pattern: Wind-Cold and Pungent-Warm herbs.

Pattern	Clinical Differentiations	Examples of Pungent-Warm Herbs
Wind-Cold	Chills or aversion to cold Fever, no sweating or slight sheen to skin Headache (head-shaking), body pain or aches Nasal congestion with discharge No significant thirst or sore throat Tongue: thin and white tongue coating Pulse: superficial and tight	Ephedra *Ma Huang* Cinnamomum *Gui Zhi* Ledebouriella *Fang Feng*

Some Pungent-Warm herbs have additional therapeutic actions including relief from pain, coughing, asthma, edema, itching, and rashes. Thus, these herbs are used to treat *Bi* syndrome, arthritis, cough, wheezing, edema, skin disorders, carbuncles, and boils in addition to treating an Exterior Pattern with Wind-Cold. However, Pungent-Warm herbs are contraindicated in patients with the following conditions: 1) profuse sweating due to *Qi* or *Yang* Deficiency; 2) night sweating due to *Yin* Deficiency; 3) *Yin* Deficiency with Heat, Blood Heat, or excessive Fire; 4) dehydration; 5) blood loss due to injury, parturition, or surgery; 6) weak constitutions; 7) high blood pressure, convulsions, seizures, or heart failure; 8) Liver *Yang* rising or Liver Wind; and 9) bleeding, epistaxis, or hematemesis.

Cinnamomum *Gui Zhi* 桂枝

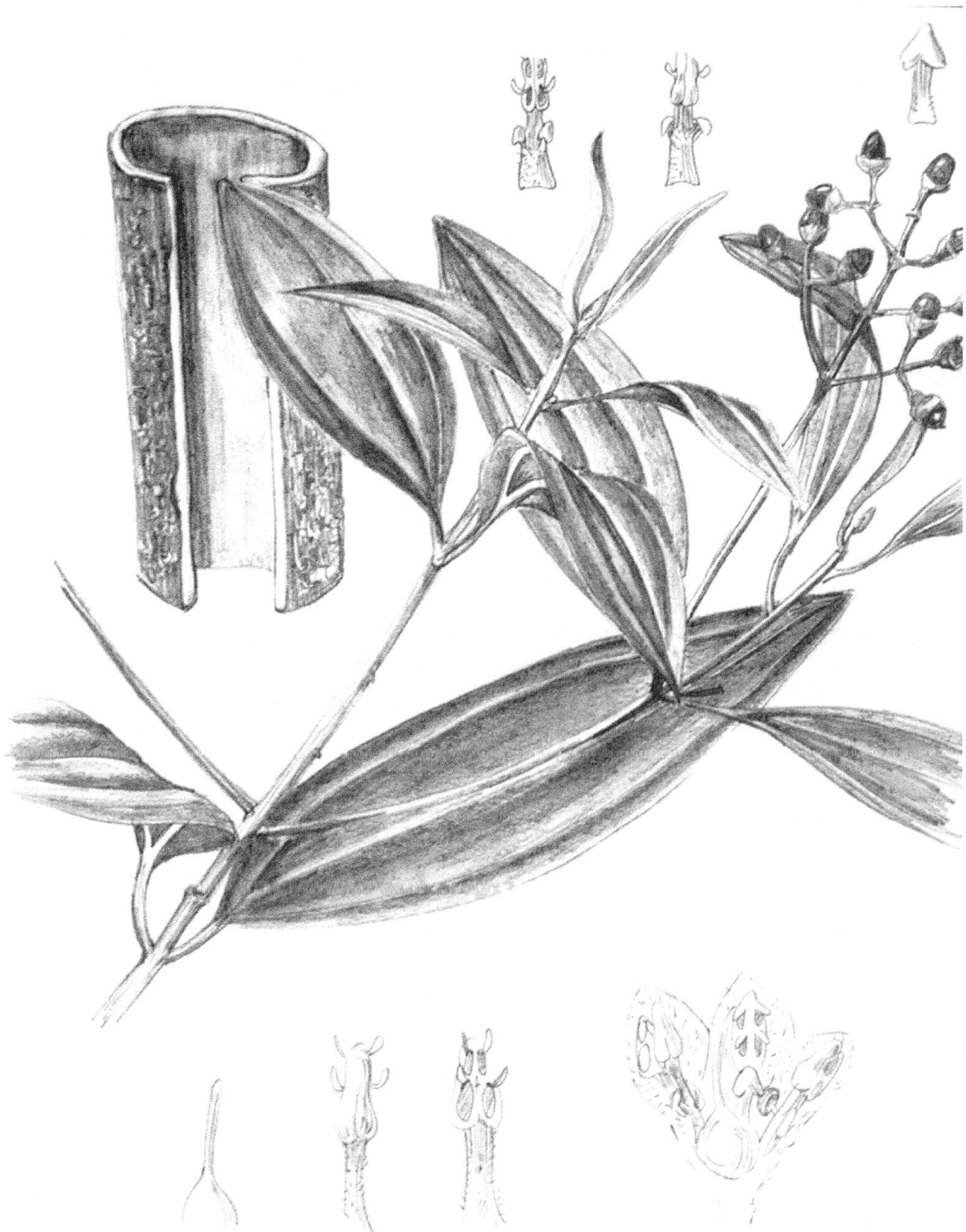

Original Reference: *Shen Nong Ben Cao Jing* (*Shen Nong's Materia Medica*, 1st century BCE) 神农本草经

Part Used: Twig

Name:
Pharmaceutical: Cinnamomi Cassiae, Ramulus
Botanical: Cinnamomum cassia Presl
Common: Cinnamon twig
Wade-Giles: *Kuei-Chih*
Translation: Cinnamon Twig

Energy/Taste: Warm, pungent, sweet

Channel-Organ: Heart, Lung, Bladder

Actions:
1. Promote sweating and clear the surface
2. Promote Blood circulation
3. Warm the Channels and dispel Cold
4. Relieve surface pain, especially in the upper body
5. Regulate the *Ying* and *Wei*

Form and Preparation: Powder, decoction, or pill

Dosage:
Horses and Cattle: 15–45 g
Camels: 30–60 g
Llamas, Alpacas, Goats, and Pigs: 3–10 g
Dogs: 3–5 g
Cats and Rabbits: 0.5–1 g
Birds: 0.2–1.5 g

Cautions and Contraindications:
1. Caution during pregnancy
2. Contraindicated for *Yin* Deficiency with Heat, Blood Heat, or Excessive Fire

Side Effects: Overdose or long-term use may cause dryness of the throat and mouth.

Clinical Applications:
1. Wind-Cold invasion
   Clinical signs: Chills, fever, general pain, nasal obstruction, absence of sweating, superficial tight pulse
   Combine with: Ephedra *Ma Huang*
   Classical herbal formula: *Ma Huang Tang*
2. Wind-Cold invasion with Deficiency
   Clinical signs: Sweating, slight fever, superficial weak pulse
   Combine with: Paeonia *Bai Shao*, Codonopsis *Dang Shen*, Zingiberis *Sheng Jiang*
   Classical herbal formula: *Gui Zhi Tang*
3. Wind-Cold-Damp invasion
   Clinical signs: Joint pain, body aches
   Combine with: Aconite *Fu Zi*
4. *Yang* Deficiency of Heart and Spleen
   Clinical signs: Palpitations, edema, shortness of breath, cold feeling in the back, hypochondriac distention, cough, dyspnea, vertigo
   Combine with: Poria *Fu Ling*, Atractylodes *Bai Zhu*, Aconite *Fu Zi*, Ostrea *Mu Li*
5. Poor circulation in the extremities
   Combine with: Paeonia *Chi Shao Yao*
   Skin numbness: add Scolopendra *Wu Gong*
   Classical herbal formula: *Dang Gui Si Ni San*
6. Deficiency of *Ying* and *Wei*
   Clinical signs: Arthralgia, numbness
   Combine with: Astragalus *Huang Qi*, Paeonia *Bai Shao*
7. False Cold Pattern due to *Yang* Deficiency in Middle Burner
   Clinical signs: Vague pain in the abdomen region, which can be ameliorated by warmth and pressing
   Combine with: Paeonia *Bai Shao*, Astragalus *Huang Qi*
   Classical herbal formula: *Huang Qi Jian Zhong Tang*
8. Stagnation of *Qi* in Lower Burner
   Clinical signs: Difficult urination, edema
   Combine with: Poria *Fu Ling*, Polyporous *Zhu Ling*
   Classical herbal formula: *Wu Ling San*

History and Comments:
1. *Shen Nong Ben Cao Jing* classifies *Gui Zhi* as a superb grade. *Gui* Zhi has been an important herb in Chinese medicine since ancient times, as demonstrated by its frequent appearance in Chinese classic formulas. In the textbook *Shang Han Lun*, 38 of the 112 formulas described include *Gui Zhi*.
2. *Yi Yu Lu* described how a man with a painful, red, swollen eye was successfully treated. The man's Traditional Chinese Medical diagnosis was Liver *Yang* rising with Spleen *Qi* Deficiency. This caused a treatment dilemma for the doctors because cold herbs would further weaken Spleen *Qi* and warm herbs would push Liver *Yang* to an even higher level. The doctors used an herbal formula with extra *Gui Zhi* to ease the Liver while simultaneously tonifying the Spleen. The patient recovered quickly with this herbal recipe.
3. Good quality Cinnamomum *Gui Zhi* is fragrant and has a brownish red color.
4. *Gui Zhi* and cinnamaldehyde have antipyretic effects. The ethanol extract of Cinnamomum *Gui Zhi* has an inhibitory effect on influenza viruses, dermatophytes, and certain bacteria, including *Staphylococcus aureus*, *Staphylococcus epedermidis*, *Salmonella typhi*, *Bacillus dysenteriae*, *Salmonella enteritidis*, and *Vibrio cholera*. Cinnamyl acetate and cinnamaldehyde have an inhibitory effect on *Mycobecterium Tuberculosis*. The essential oil of *Gui Zhi* can stop coughing and clear Phlegm.
5. *Gui Zhi* has a cardiotonic effect and promotes urination.

Pharmaceutical Ingredients:[1–4]
1. Essential oils: cinnamic aldehyde, cinnamic acid, cinnamyl acetate, benzyl benzoate, phenylpropyl acetate, calamenene, terpinon-4-ol
2. Tannin, mucus, resin
3. Trans-cinnamic acid, coumarin, protocatechuic acid

Ephedra *Ma Huang* 麻黄

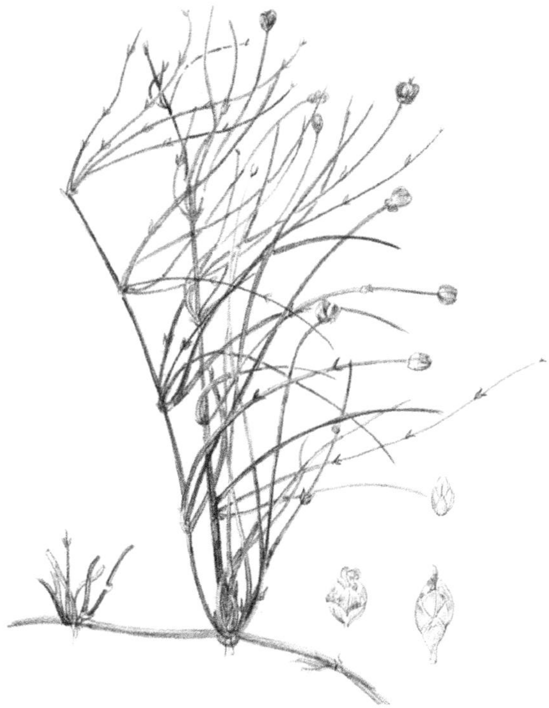

Original Reference: *Shen Nong Ben Cao Jing* (*Shen Nong's Materia Medica*, 1st century BCE) 神农本草经

Part Used: Leaf and stem

Name:
Pharmaceutical: Ephedrae, Herba
Botanical: Ephedra sinica; E. intermedia; E. equisetina
Common: *Ma Huang*
Wade-Giles: *Ma-Huang*
Translation: Hemp Yellow

Energy/Taste: Warm, pungent, bitter

Channel-Organ: Lung, Bladder

Actions:
1. Promote sweating and clear the surface
2. Stop asthma and relieve cough
3. Benefit urination and reduce edema

Form and Preparation: Powder, decoction, or pill

Dosage:
Horses and Cattle: 15–30g
Goats and Pigs: 3–5g
Dogs: 1–3g

Cautions and Contraindications:
1. Contraindicated in patients with weak constitutions or with Deficiency of *Yin*, *Yang*, *Qi*, and Blood
2. Contraindicated in patients with night sweating and spontaneous sweating
3. Contraindicated in patients with *Yang* Rising or False Fire or Excessive Fire, bleeding, epistaxis, or hematemesis
4. Contraindicated in patients with high blood pressure, convulsions, epilepsy, seizure, and heart failure
5. Caution in patients with wheezing, cough, and edema due to Deficiency
6. Use caution during pregnancy.

Side Effects:
1. Poor appetite, nausea, vomiting, fatigue
2. Red face, insomnia, restlessness, dizziness, tremors, rising blood pressure
3. Sweating or excessive sweating, palpitations
4. Excessively rapid or irregular heartbeat and rapid or irregular pulse
5. Severe effects may be epilepsy or convulsions.

Clinical Applications:
1. Wind-Cold invasion
   Clinical signs: Chills, fever, general pain, nasal obstruction, absence of sweating, superficial tight pulse
   Combine with: Cinnamomum *Gui Zhi*
   Classical herbal formula: *Ma Huang Tang*
2. Wind-Cold in the Channels, or Cold and edema associated with *Yang* Deficiency
   Clinical signs: Cold, painful joints, *Bi* Syndrome
   Combine with: Aconite *Fu Zi*
   Classical herbal formula: *Ma Huang Fu Zi Xi Xin Tang*
3. *Yin* furuncles caused by Damp/Cold obstructing the Channels
   Combine with: Rehmannia *Shu Di Huang*
   Classical herbal formula: *Yang He Tang*
4. Cough and asthma with profuse thin clear sputum due to obstruction of the Lung by Cold Phlegm
   Combine with: Asarum *Xi Xin*, Zingiberis *Gan Jiang*, Pinellia *Ban Xia*
   Classical herbal formula: *Xiao Qing Long Tang*
5. Cough with dyspnea and fever due to retention of pathogenic Heat in the Lungs
   Combine with: Gypsum *Shi Gao*, Armeniaca *Xing Ren*, Glycerrhiza *Gan Cao*
   Classical herbal formula: *Ma Xing Shi Gan Tang*

History and Comments:
1. During the *Liang* Dynasty, doctor Tao Hong-Jing called *Ma Huang* the best medicine for treating colds.

2. A Chinese Doctor named Fan Wenfu (1870–1936) was famous for prescribing high-dosage herbal treatments. One day, a boy was rushed in for emergency treatment. Several other doctors' initial attempts at treatment had been unsuccessful. When Wenfu took the case, he heard that the boy's father disapproved of high dosage treatments and that he always reduced a high-dose prescription in half without the doctor's knowledge. Wenfu told the father to boil 24 g *Ma Huang* and have the boy drink it until he sweated. The boy completely recovered with just one dose of *Ma Huang* herb soup. When father and son returned the next day for a checkup, Wenfu asked the father, "How much did you reduce the *Ma Huang* dose?" Surprised, the boy's father answered, "Half, but how did you know about it?" Wenfu replied, "I knew you would reduce it, that's why I doubled the dose."
3. Use raw Ephedra *Ma Huang* for Exterior disorders, but fry Ephedra *Ma Huang* to reduce its dispersing effect. Honey-frying the herb increases the moistening effects in the Lungs and is better for asthma and cough.
4. *Ma Huang* contains ephedrine alkaloids, which can raise the heart rate and blood pressure and can cause stroke, heart attack, or death. As a result, the United States Food and Drug Administration (FDA) banned dietary supplements containing ephedrine alkaloids in April 2004.
5. The root, Ephedra *Ma Huang Gen*, can counteract the negative effects of *Ma Huang* (leaf and stem).
6. If Heat is generated from the use of Ephedra *Ma Huang*, Gypsum *Shi Gao* and Scutellaria *Huang Qin* may be added for their cooling effect.
7. The essential oil of Ephedra *Ma Huang* has a diaphoretic effect, thereby acting as an antipyretic. Ephedrine can increase the secretion of sweat glands in high temperature environments. Both ephedrine and pseudoephedrine have a relaxing effect on bronchial smooth muscle. Pseudoephedrine has remarkable diuretic effects. Pseudoephedrine can stimulate the heart, constrict the blood vessels, and raise blood pressure.
8. Pseudoephedrine also has an excitatory effect on the central nervous system (CNS). It causes excitement, insomnia, and restlessness.

Pharmaceutical Ingredients:[1–4]

1. Ephedrine alkaloids: (l-ephedrine, d-pseudoephedrine, l-norephedrine, d-norpseudoephedrine, l-methylephedrine, l-N-methylephedrine, d-methylpseudoephedrine, d-N-methylpseudoephedrine, ephedrine
2. Phedroxane, 2,3,4-trimethyl-5-phenyloxazolidine benzylmethylamine, 2,3,5,6-tetramethylpyrazine
3. Essential oils (l-α-terpineol), tannin

Ledebouriella *Fang Feng* 防风

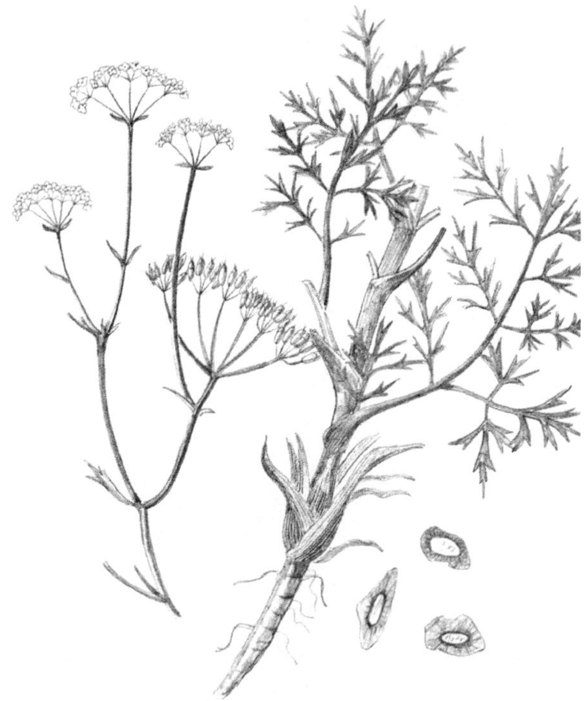

Original Reference: *Shen Nong Ben Cao Jing* (*Shen Nong's Materia Medica*, 1st century BCE) 神农本草经

Part Used: Root

Name:
Pharmaceutical: Ledebouriellae Divaricatae, Radix
Botanical: Siler divaricatum; Ledebouriella divaricata
Common: Siler
Wade-Giles: *Fang-Feng*
Translation: Guard (against) Wind

Energy/Taste: Warm, pungent, sweet

Channel-Organ: Bladder, Liver, Spleen

Actions:
1. Promote sweating and clear the surface
2. Expel Wind and stop pain
3. Alleviate spasms

Form and Preparation: Powder, decoction, or pill

Dosage:
Horses and Cattle: 15–60 g
Camels: 45–100 g
Llamas, Alpacas, Goats, and Pigs: 5–15 g
Dogs: 3–8 g

Cats and Rabbits: 0.5–2 g
Birds: 0.3–3 g

Cautions and Contraindications:
1. Caution in patients with spasms due to Blood Deficiency
2. Caution in patients with *Yin* Deficiency with Heat or dizziness due to Liver *Yang* rising or Liver Wind
3. Ledebouriella *Fang Feng* may antagonize Zingiberis *Gan Jiang* and counteract Dioscorea *Bei Xie*.

Side Effects: None known

Clinical Applications:
1. Wind-Cold invasion
   Clinical signs: Chills, fever, general body aches, superficial tight pulse
   Combine with: Schizonepeta *Jing Jie* and Notopterygium *Qiang Huo*
   Classical herbal formula: *Jing Fang Bei Du San*
2. Wind-Heat invasion
   Clinical signs: Fever, sore throat, red eyes, joint pain
   Combine with: Schizonepeta *Jing Jie*, Scutellaria *Huang Qin*, Mentha *Bo He*, and Forsythia *Lian Qiao*
   Classical herbal formula: *Fang Feng Tong Shen San*
3. Wind-Cold-Damp *Bi* syndrome
   Clinical signs: Joint pain, spasm of limbs, sudden contracture
   Combine with: Notopterygium *Qiang Huo*, Angelica *Dang Gui*, and Clematis *Wei Ling Xian*
4. Hives and pruritis
   Clinical signs: Red raised welts or allergic skin rash
   Combine with: Sophora *Ku Shen* and Cicada *Chan Tui*
   Classical herbal formula: *Xiao Feng San*
5. Diarrhea due to Spleen Damp
   Combine with: Atractylodes *Cang Zhu*, Citrus *Chen Pi*
   Classical herbal formula: *Tong Xie Yao Fang*
6. Wind Damp in patients suffering from Blood Deficiency
   Combine with: Gentiana *Qin Jiao*

History and Comments:
1. *Shen Nong Ben Cao Jing* (*Shen Nong's Materia Medica*) classifies *Fang Feng* as a superior medicinal.
2. *Fang* means defense and *Feng* means wind. The name *Fang Feng* originates from a folk story. Once upon a time, Mang Shan, the most beautiful mountain in central China, concealed many hidden treasures. One day, a greedy monster, who dwelled in the South China Sea, heard about the treasures in the mountain. He desired to own the entire mountain. In an attempt to transport the mountain, he called forth his most powerful witchcraft. Suddenly dark clouds moved across the sky, blocking out the sun. Strong winds filled the air with sand, stones shot through the sky like arrows, but the mountain did not move a bit. Puzzled, the monster drew close to the mountain to see what had thwarted his magic. He was stunned to find that it had been a green grass that stopped his power. This grass, called *Fang Feng* (Defend Wind) by local inhabitants, has been used to treat diseases of Wind invasion ever since.
3. Good quality Ledebouriella *Fang Feng* is coarse and strong with a tight, thin cortex. The cross section should have brown rings with a light yellow center.
4. Ledebouriella *Fang Feng* has antipyretic, antiinflammatory, antiallergic, analgesic, and tranquilizing effects. The fresh juice of *Fang Feng* has an antibiotic effect against *Pseudomonas aeruginosa* and *Staphylococcus aureus*. The water decoction has inhibitory effects against *Bacillus dysenteriae* and *Streptoccus hemolyticus* to different degrees.

Pharmaceutical Ingredients:[1–4]
1. Polysaccharides: saposhnikovan A, B, C
2. Essential oils: α-pinene, β-pinene, limonene, palmitic acid, bisabolene
3. Coumarins: imperatorin, phellopterin, ledeboriello, hamaudol, 3-o-angeloyl-hamaudol, ledebouriellol, cimifugin, prim-o-glycosylcimifugin, anomalin, xanthotoxin, scopoletin, falcarindiol

Schizonepeta *Jing Jie* 荆芥

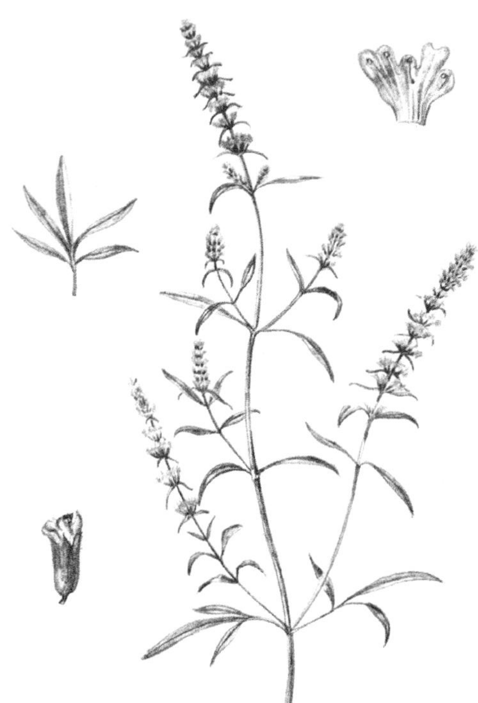

Original Reference: *Shen Nong Ben Cao Jing* (*Shen Nong's Materia Medica*, 1st century BCE) 神农本草经

Part Used: Stem, leaf, and flower

Name:
Pharmaceutical: Schizonepetae Tenuifoliae, Herba seu Flos
Botanical: Schizonepeta tenuifolia
Common: Schizonepeta
Wade-Giles: *Ching-Chieh*

Energy/Taste: Warm, pungent, aromatic

Channel-Organ: Lung, Liver

Actions:
1. Clear Wind from the surface and promote sweating
2. Stop bleeding
3. Clear skin eruptions

Form and Preparation: Powder, decoction, or pill

Dosage:
Horses and Cattle: 15–60 g
Llamas, Alpacas, Goats, and Pigs: 3–10 g
Dogs: 3–5 g
Cats and Rabbits: 0.5–1 g
Birds: 0.2–1.5 g

Cautions and Contraindications: Caution in Internal Liver Wind, or sweating with *Yin* Deficiency

Side Effects: None known

Clinical Applications:
1. Wind-Cold invasion
   Clinical signs: Chills, fever, general body aches, superficial tight pulse
   Combine with: Ledebouriella *Fang Feng* and Notopterygium *Qiang Huo*, and Mentha *Bo He*
   Classical herbal formula: *Jing Fang Bei Du San*
2. Wind-Heat invasion
   Clinical signs: Fever, swollen sore throat, red eyes, joint pain
   Combine with: Lonicera *Jin Yin Hua*, Forsythia *Lian Qiao*, Mentha *Bo He*, and Platycodon *Jie Geng*, and Morus *Sang Ye*
   Classical herbal formula: *Yin Qiao San*
3. Wind-Heat eye inflammations
   Combine with: Chrysanthemum *Ju Hua*, Scutellaria *Huang Qin*
4. Skin eruptions with itching
   Clinical signs: Accompanying fever
   Combine with: Mentha *Bo He*, Forsythia *Lian Qiao*, Ledebouriella *Fang Feng*
   Or, combine with: Mentha *Bo He*, Cicada *Chan Tui*, Arctium *Niu Bang Zi*
5. Carbuncles and boils
   Combine with: Mentha *Bo He*, Arctium *Niu Bang Zi*, and Cicada *Chan Tui*
   Or, combine with: Equisetum *Mu Zei*
   Contraindication: Carbuncles that have opened
6. Bleeding disorders; preparation is charred or carbonized
   Clinical signs: Epistaxis, bloody stool, uterine bleeding

History and Comments:
1. *Jing Jie* has been used in many classic formulas, among which *Hua Tuo Yu Feng San* is the most famous. According to the text *Ben Shi Fang* by Xu Shu Wei (*Song* Dynasty, 1080), a woman fell into a coma after giving birth. Eventually she slightly improved, but she remained in a semicomatose state. After taking the herbal recipe *Hua Tuo Yu Feng San*, she fell asleep right away and scratched her head while sleeping, and then she gradually recovered.
2. Li Shizhen (1518–1593 CE, *Ming* Dynasty) wrote about *Jing Jie* in his text *Ben Cao Gong Mu* (*Compendium of Materia Medica*). "*Jing Jie* goes through the Liver Channel. It can dispel Wind, dissolve trauma, break Stasis, and resolve toxin because the Liver belongs to Wood, which governs Blood. That is why *Jing Jie* is the most important ingredient for any disease with Wind invasion, Blood Stasis and trauma."
3. Historically *Jing Jie* is contraindicated with fish and crab. *Jing Jie* with fish may cause vomiting. *Jing Jie* with crab may result in seizures.
4. Good quality Schizonepeta *Jing Jie* is light purple and has a thin stem with dense spikes.
5. *Jing Jie Sui*, the flower of Schizonepeta, can strongly dispel Wind invasion of the head.
6. Fried Schizonepeta *Jing Jie* is a special herb to stop bleeding. It is used to treat uterine bleeding and dizziness following delivery. Raw Schizonepeta *Jing Jie* strongly dispels the Exterior.
7. The water decoction of *Jing Jie* can promote the blood circulation at the skin level and increase the secretion of sweat glands. It has antibiotic effects against *Salmonella typhi*, *Bacillus dysenteriae*, *Pseudomonas aeruginosa*, and *Mycobacterium tuberculosis*.

Pharmaceutical Ingredients:[1–4]
1. Essential oils (pulegone, menthone, d-menthone, isomenthone, isopulegone, limonene, d-limonene)

2. Monosaccaride (schizonepetoside A, B, C, D, E, schizonol, schizonodiol)
3. Flavonoids (hesperidine, luteolin, leteolin 7β-d-glucopyranosiduronic acid, luteolin 7-o-β-d-glucopyranoside, diosmetin)

Perilla *Zi Su Ye* 紫苏叶

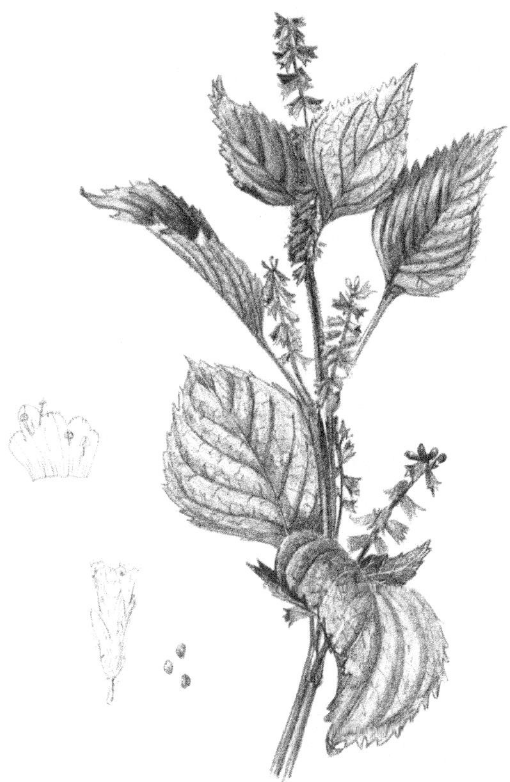

Original Reference: *Ming Yi Bie Lu* (*Miscellaneous Records of Famous Physicians*) by *Tao Hong-Jing*, North and South Kingdoms (5th century) 名医别录

Part Used: Leaf

Name:
Pharmaceutical: Perillae Frutescentis, Folium
Botanical: Perilla fructescens
Common: Perilla leaf
Wade-Giles: *Tzu-Su-Yeh*
Translation: Purple Perilla Leaf

Energy/Taste: Warm, pungent, aromatic

Channel-Organ: Lung, Spleen

Actions:
1. Clear the surface and dispel Cold
2. Invigorate *Qi* and harmonize Stomach
3. Counter fish and crab poisoning
4. Calm the fetus

Form and Preparation: Powder, decoction, or pill

Dosage:
Horses and Cattle: 15–60 g
Camels: 25–80 g
Llamas, Alpacas, Goats, and Pigs: 3–15 g
Dogs: 3–8 g
Cats and Rabbits: 0.5–2 g
Birds: 0.3–3 g

Cautions and Contraindications: Caution in Damp-Heat conditions or Exterior Deficiency with pronounced sweating

Side Effects: None known

Notopterygium *Qiang Huo* 羌活

Original Reference: *Shen Nong Ben Cao Jing* (*Shen Nong's Materia Medica*, 1st century BCE) 神农本草经

Part Used: Root and stem

Name:
Pharmaceutical: Notopterygii, Rhizoma et Radix
Botanical: Notopterygium incisium; N. forbesii
Common: *Notopterygium*
Wade-Giles: *Ch'iang-Huo*

Energy/Taste: Warm, pungent, bitter, aromatic

Channel-Organ: Bladder, Kidney

Actions:
1. Clear the surface and dispel Cold
2. Dispel Wind-Damp
3. Stop pain
4. Guide *Qi* to *Tai Yang* and *Du* Channels

Form and Preparation: Powder, decoction, or pill

Dosage:
Horses and Cattle: 15–45 g
Llamas, Alpacas, Goats, and Pigs: 3–10 g
Dogs: 2–4 g
Cats and Rabbits: 0.5–1 g
Birds: 0.2–1.5 g

Cautions and Contraindications: Caution in *Yin* or Blood Deficiency

Side Effects: Nausea and vomiting

Zingiberis *Sheng Jiang* 生姜

Original Reference: *Ming Yi Bie Lu* (*Miscellaneous Records of Famous Physicians*) by *Tao Hong-Jing*, North and South Kingdoms (5th century) 名医别录

Part Used: Root and stem

Name:
Pharmaceutical: Rhizoma Zingiberis
Botanical: Zingiber officinale
Common: Fresh ginger
Wade-Giles: *Sheng-Chiang*
Translation: Fresh Ginger

Energy/Taste: Warm, pungent

Channel-Organ: Lung, Spleen, Stomach, Kidney, Heart

Actions:
1. Promote sweating and clear the surface
2. Warm the Spleen and Stomach, relieve vomiting
3. Warm the Lung and alleviate cough
4. Regulate *Ying* and *Wei Qi*
5. Neutralize toxic herbs including Pinellia *Ban Xia* and Arisaema *Tian Nan Xing*

Form and Preparation: Powder, decoction, or pill

Dosage:
Horses and Cattle: 15–60 g
Camels: 30–90 g
Llamas, Alpacas, Goats, and Pigs: 5–15 g
Dogs: 1–5 g
Cats and Rabbits: 0.5–1 g
Birds: 0.2–1.5 g

Cautions and Contraindications: Caution in *Yin* Deficiency with Heat

Side Effects: None known

Angelica *Bai Zhi* 白芷

Original Reference: *Shen Nong Ben Cao Jing* (*Shen Nong's Materia Medica*, 1st century BCE) 神农本草经

Part Used: Root

Name:
Pharmaceutical: Angelicae Dahuricae, Radix
Botanical: Angelica dahurica
Common: Angelica root
Wade-Giles: *Pai-Chih*
Translation: White Angelica

Energy/Taste: Warm, pungent

Channel-Organ: Lung, Stomach

Actions:
1. Clear the surface and dispel Wind
2. Reduce swelling and discharge pus
3. Open nasal passages and stop pain

Form and Preparation: Powder, decoction, or pill

Dosage:
Horses and Cattle: 15–30 g
Camels: 25–45 g
Llamas, Alpacas, Goats, and Pigs: 3–10 g
Dogs: 1–5 g
Cats and Rabbits: 0.5–1 g
Birds: 0.2–1.5 g

Cautions and Contraindications:
1. Caution in *Yin* Deficiency with Heat
2. May antagonize Inula *Xuan Fu Hua*

Side Effects:
1. Nausea, vomiting, poor appetite
2. Dizziness
3. Numbness of limbs and convulsions

Magnolia *Xin Yi Hua* 辛夷花

Original Reference: *Shen Nong Ben Cao Jing* (*Shen Nong's Materia Medica*, 1st century BCE) 神农本草经

Part Used: Flower (bud)

Name:
Pharmaceutical: Magnoliae, Flos
Botanical: Magnolia biondii; M. denudata; M. liliflora
Common: Magnolia flower
Wade-Giles: *Hsing-I-Hua*
Translation: Pungent Smooth Flower

Energy/Taste: Warm, pungent

Channel-Organ: Lung, Stomach

Actions:
1. Dispel Wind and Cold
2. Open the nasal orifice

Form and Preparation: Powder, decoction, or pill

Dosage:
Horses and Cattle: 15–60 g
Llamas, Alpacas, Goats, and Pigs: 5–15 g
Dogs: 1–5 g
Cats and Rabbits: 0.5–1 g
Birds: 0.2–1.5 g

Cautions and Contraindications: Caution in *Qi* Deficiency or Excessive Fire in the Upper Burner

Side Effects: An overdose leads to red eyes and dizziness.

Xanthium *Cang Er Zi* 苍耳子

Original Reference: *Shen Nong Ben Cao Jing* (*Shen Nong's Materia Medica*, 1st century BCE) 神农本草经

Part Used: Ripe fruit involving the entire bud

Name:
Pharmaceutical: Fructus Xanthii Sibirici
Botanical: Xanthium Sibiricum Patr. ex widd
Common: Xanrhium, Cocklebur fruit
Wade Giles: *Tsang-Erh-Tzu*
Translation: Old Ear Seed

Energy/Taste: Warm, pungent, bitter

Channel-Organ: Lung

Actions:
1. Dispel Wind-Cold and promote sweat
2. Open the nasal orifice
3. Eliminate Wind-Damp

Form and Preparation: Powder, decoction, or pill

Dosage:
Horses and Cattle: 15–45 g
Llamas, Alpacas, Goats, and Pigs: 3–10 g
Dogs: 1–3 g
Cats and Rabbits: 0.5–1 g
Birds: 0.1–1 g

Cautions and Contraindications:
1. Caution during pregnancy
2. Contraindicated in renal or liver failure

Side Effects:
1. Poor appetite, nausea, vomiting, abdominal pain, diarrhea, or constipation
2. Fatigue, dizziness, excessive sweating, red face, restlessness, unconsciousness, convulsions
3. Chest tightness, jaundice
4. Heart palpitations, excessively rapid or irregular heartbeat, and rapid or irregular pulse
5. May damage Liver and Kidney

Asarum *Xi Xin* 细辛

Original Reference: *Shen Nong Ben Cao Jing* (*Shen Nong's Materia Medica*, 1st century BCE) 神农本草经

Part Used: Entire plant

Name:
Pharmaceutical: Asari, Herba cum Radice
Botanical: Asarum heterotropoides; A. sieboldii (Wild Ginger)
Common: Wild ginger
Wade-Giles: *Hsi-Hsin*
Translation: Delicate and Pungent

Energy/Taste: Warm, pungent, toxic

Channel-Organ: Heart, Lung, Kidney

Actions:
1. Clear the surface and dispel Cold
2. Dispel Wind and stop pain
3. Warm the Lung and resolve Phlegm

Form and Preparation: Powder, decoction, or pill

Dosage:
Horses and Cattle: 10–15 g
Camels: 15–30 g
Llamas, Alpacas, Goats, and Pigs: 1–5 g
Dogs: 0.2–1 g

Cautions and Contraindications:
1. Caution during pregnancy or in Deficiency conditions
2. It may cause Kidney toxicity; contraindicated in any renal diseases
3. May antagonize Cornus *Shan Zhu Yu*, Astragalus *Huang Qi*, and counteracts Talcum *Hua Shi*

Side Effects:
1. Dizziness, red face, hot flush, excessive sweating, insomnia, restlessness, dizziness, and heart palpitations
2. Chest tightness, nausea, and vomiting
3. Severe overdose may produce an excessively rapid or irregular heartbeat and a rapid or irregular pulse.

Ligusticum *Gao Ben* 藁本

Original Reference: *Shen Nong Ben Cao Jing* (*Shen Nong's Materia Medica*, 1st century BCE) 神农本草经

Part Used: Stem and root

Name:
Pharmaceutical: Rhizome Ligustici
Botanical: Liusticum sinense Oliv.
Common: Ligusticum
Wade Giles: *Kao-Pen*

Energy/Taste: Warm, pungent

Channel-Organ: Bladder

Actions:
1. Release the surface and dispel Wind-Cold
2. Remove Damp and release pain

Form and Preparation: Powder, decoction, or pill

Dosage:
Horses and Cattle: 15–30 g
Llamas, Alpacas, Goats, and Pigs: 3–10 g
Dogs: 1–3 g
Cats and Rabbits: 0.5–1 g
Birds: 0.2–1.5 g

Cautions and Contraindications: Caution in Blood Deficiency or Heat

Side Effects: None known

Centipeda *E Bu Shi Cao* 鹅不食草

Original Reference: *Shi Xing Ben Cao* (*Materia Medica of Food Therapy*) by *Meng Shen* in the 7th century 食性本草

Part Used: Entire plant

Name:
Pharmaceutical: Herba Centipedae
Botanical: Centipeda herb, small centipede herb
Common: Centipedae
Wade-Giles: *E-Bu-Shih-Ts'ao*
Translation: Goose Not Eating Herb

Energy/Taste: Warm, pungent

Channel-Organ: Lung, Liver

Actions:
1. Dispel Wind-Cold, open the nasal orifices
2. Relieve cough and remove toxins

Form and Preparation: Powder, decoction, or pill

Dosage:
Horses and Cattle: 15–30 g
Llamas, Alpacas, Goats, and Pigs: 3–10 g
Dogs: 0.5–5 g
Cats and Rabbits: 0.2–1 g
Birds: 0.2–1 g

Cautions and Contraindications: Caution in weak digestive systems, gastritis, or duodenal ulcers

Side Effects: It may cause diarrhea.

PUNGENT-COOL HERBS TO RELEASE THE EXTERIOR

Pungent-Cool herbs are primarily used to treat Exterior Patterns with Wind-Heat (Table 2.3). Most of the herbs in this category have a pungent taste, are cool in temperature, and have an affinity for the Lung and Liver Channels. These properties allow Pungent-Cool herbs to release the Exterior and to dispel Wind-Heat in the surface, skin, muscle, and upper body including the head, eyes, ears, nose, mouth, and throat.

As with the Pungent-Warm herbs, consider the relationship between the Channels, body areas, and pathogenic factors to understand how the Pungent-Cool herbs function. The Lung Channel is connected to the skin, nose, and throat; and the Liver Channel is connected to the eyes, ears, sides, and top of the body. The pathogenic factors Wind toxin and Heat toxin target particular body areas. Wind attacks the upper body and superficial areas of the body, and Heat attacks the muscle, skin, eyes, ears, nose, mouth, and throat. These body areas happen to be the same as

Table 2.3. Exterior Pattern: Wind-Heat and Pungent-Cool herbs.

Pattern	Clinical Differentiations	Examples of Pungent-Cool Herbs
Wind-Heat	Fever, slight aversion to cold Headache (head-shaking) Significant thirst Dry throat or sore throat Dry cough Red eye Tongue: red tip or side with thin, yellow coating Pulse: superficial and rapid	Bupleurum *Chai Hu* Mentha *Bo He* Chrysanthemum *Ju Hua*

those related to the Lung and Liver; thus, the pathogenic factors commonly cause clinical signs relating to those two Channels. For these reasons, the Pungent-Cool herbs are particularly beneficial for treating Exterior Patterns with Wind-Heat and early-stage febrile diseases at the *Wei* (defense) level. The pungent taste helps disperse Wind, the cool energy clears Heat or eliminates toxins, and the affinity for the Lung and Liver Channels directs the herbal effects toward the body areas most affected by the Wind and Heat pathogens.

Some Pungent-Cool herbs have additional therapeutic actions, which include clearing the head, brightening the eyes, soothing the throat, stopping cough, promoting the eruption of urticaria or skin lumps, and stopping itching. Thus, these herbs are commonly used to treat eye redness and pain, sore throat, swollen tonsils, cough, urticaria or skin lumps, and pruritis or redness due to an Exterior Pattern with Wind-Heat. However, Pungent-Cool herbs are contraindicated in patients with the following conditions: 1) Deficiency conditions including *Yang* Deficiency, *Qi* Deficiency, Blood Deficiency, or *Yin* Deficiency; 2) *Yin* Deficiency with Heat and Exterior Deficiency; 3) Spleen *Qi* Deficiency, Stomach Cold, poor appetite, or diarrhea; 4) Cold in the Interior; and 5) Internal Wind.

Mentha *Bo He* 薄荷

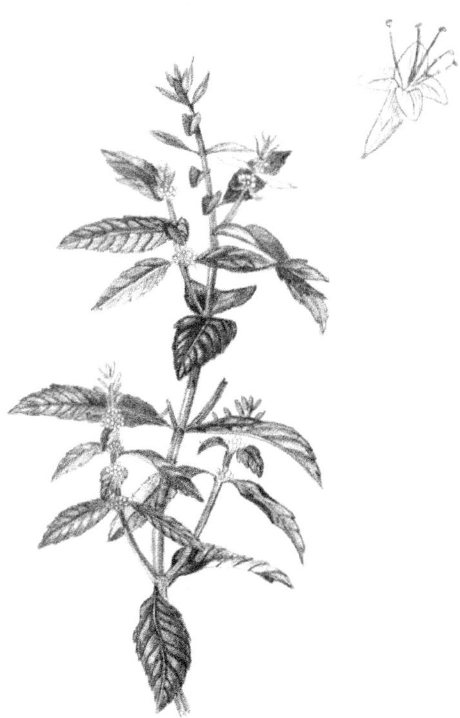

Original Reference: *Tang Ben Cao* (*Tang Materia Medica*) by *Su Jing* et al., in *Tang* Dynasty 唐本草

Part Used: Leaf and stem

Name:
Pharmaceutical: Menthae Haplocalycis, Herba
Botanical: Mentha haplocalyx (Peppermint)
Common: Mint
Wade-Giles: *Po-He*
Translation: Field Mint

Energy/Taste: Cool, pungent

Channel-Organ: Lung, Liver

Actions:
1. Disperse Wind-Heat and clear the eyes
2. Smooth Liver *Qi* and clear Liver Heat
3. Promote eruption of rashes
4. Clear the head and benefit the throat

Form and Preparation: Powder, decoction, or pill; must not be overcooked. Add the herb to the decoction 5 minutes before finishing.

Dosage:
Horses and Cattle: 15–45 g
Llamas, Alpacas, Goats, and Pigs: 5–10 g
Dogs: 2–5 g
Cats and Rabbits: 0.5–1 g
Birds: 0.2–1.5 g

Cautions and Contraindications: Caution in *Yin* Deficiency with Heat or spontaneous sweating due to *Qi* Deficiency

Side Effects: None known

Clinical Applications:
1. Wind-Heat invasion
   Clinical signs: Fever, sore throat, dry cough, red eyes; also swelling in the eyes due to excessive Liver fire

Combine with: Platycodon *Jie Geng*, Arctium *Niu Bang Zi*, and Chrysanthemum *Ju Hua* or combine with Forsythia *Lian Qiao*, Schizonepeta *Jing Jie*, and Lonicera *Jin Yin Hua*
Classical herbal formula: *Yin Qiao San*
Caution: Deficiency Exterior conditions

2. Stagnation of Liver *Qi* with Heat
   Clinical signs: Fullness in costal region, chest distention, irritability, red eyes, purple tongue, wiry pulse
   Combine with: Bupleurum *Chai Hu* and Paeonia *Bai Shao*
   Classical herbal formula: *Xiao Yao San;* for red eyes, combine with Prunella X*ia Ku Cao* or Scrophularia *Xuan Shen*
3. Skin rash and itching due to Blood Heat
   Combine with: Schizonepeta *Jing Jie*
4. Painful swollen throat
   Combine with: Schizonepeta *Jing Jie*, Bombyx *Jiang Can*
5. Neonatal convulsions and/or pruritic rash
   Combine with: Patrinia *Bai Jiang Cao*, Cicada *Chan Tui*, Buthus *Quan Xie*
6. Externally contracted Wind Heat
   Clinical signs: Sores, dry mouth, cough with yellow sputum, pruritic rash
   Combine with: Arctium *Niu Bang Zi*
7. Summer Heat
   Clinical signs: Fever, dizziness, increased thirst, scant dark urine
   Combine with: Talcum *Hua Shi*, Glycerrhiza *Gan Cao*
   Classical herbal formula: *Ji Su San*

Comments:

1. Good quality Mentha *Bo He* is dry, green, fragrant, and has no roots.
2. The essential oil of Mentha *Bo He* can excite the central nervous system, dilate the skin capillaries, and increase secretion of sweat glands. Therefore, it has diaphoretic and antipyretic effects. The essential oil of Mentha *Bo He* can also inhibit the constriction of the smooth muscle of the gastrointestinal tract. The decoction of Mentha *Bo He* has antibacterial and antiviral effects. The external application of the essential oil can protect the skin from burn. It also has antiinflammatory, antipruritic, and locally analgesic effects.

Pharmaceutical Ingredients:[1–4]

1. Essential oils (menthol, methacamphor, menthone, isomenthol, isomenthone, menthenone, neomenthol, camphene, α-pinene, myrcene, limonene, p-cymene, 3-octanol, menthyl acetate, pulegone, piperitone)
2. Monogalactosyl diglycerides, rosmarinic acid, azulen, 1-carboxy-2-(3, 4-dihydroxyphenyl) ethyl-1, 2-dihydroxy-naphthalene-2, 3-dicarboxylic acid
3. Lipoflavones, coumarins

Chrysanthemum *Ju Hua* 菊花

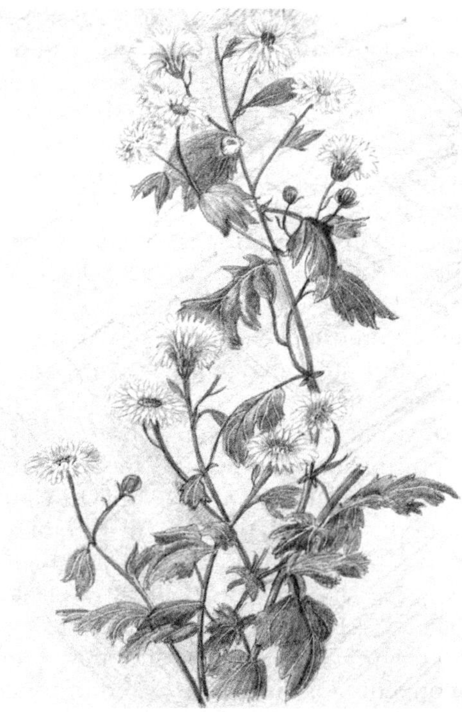

Original Reference: *Shen Nong Ben Cao Jing* (*Shen Nong's Materia Medica*, 1st century BCE) 神农本草经

Part Used: Flower

Name:
Pharmaceutical: Chrysanthemi Morifolii, Flos
Botanical: Chrysanthemum morifolium
Common: Chrysanthemum flower
Wade-Giles: *Chu-Hua*
Translation: Chrysanthemum flower

Energy/Taste: Cool, sweet, bitter

Channel-Organ: Lung, Liver

Actions:

1. Disperse Wind-Heat
2. Clear Liver Heat and brighten the eyes
3. Remove toxins

Form and Preparation: Powder, decoction, or pill

Dosage:
Horses and Cattle: 15–60 g
Camels: 30–60 g
Llamas, Alpacas, Goats, and Pigs: 5–15 g

Dogs: 2–8 g
Cats and Rabbits: 0.5–2 g
Birds: 0.3–3 g

Cautions and Contraindications: Caution in *Yang* Deficiency

Side Effects: None known

Clinical Applications:

1. Wind-Heat invasion
   Clinical signs: Fever, sore throat, dry cough, red eyes
   Combine with: Morus *Sang Ye*, Platycodon *Jie Geng*, and Mentha *Bo He*; for dry cough or throat, combine with Imperata *Bai Mao Gen*
   Classical herbal formula: *Sang Ju Yin*
2. Liver Fire affecting the eyes
   Clinical signs: Red, swollen, painful eyes, excessive tearing
   Combine with: Morus *Sang Ye*, Prunella *Xia Ku Cao*, and Cicada *Chan Tui*
3. Liver and Kidney *Yin* Deficiency
   Clinical signs: Poor night vision or red eyes, dizziness
   Combine with: Lycium *Gou Qi Zi*, Ligustrum *Nü Zhen Zi*, and Rehmannia *Shu Di Huang*
   Classical herbal formula: *Qi Ju Di Huang Wan*
4. Hyperactive Liver *Yang*, hypertension
   Clinical signs: Dizziness, vertigo, or seizures
   Combine with: Halitois *Shi Jue Ming*, Uncaria *Gou Teng*, Gastrodia *Tian Ma*, Paeonia *Bai Shao*, and Cassia *Jue Ming Zi*; or combine with Antelopis *Ling Yang Jiao*, Uncaria *Gou Teng*
   Classical herbal formula: *Ling Jiao Gou Teng Tang*
5. To clear skin rashes due to Blood Heat
   Combine with: Schizonepeta *Jing Jie*
6. Poor circulation in extremities
   Combine with: Paeonia *Chi Shao Yao*; for skin numbness combine with Scolopendra *Wu Gong*
7. Toxic swelling and colorless, painless, flat, slow-healing suppurative inflammations of the soft tissue
   Combine with: Lonicera *Jin Yin Hua*

History and Comments:

1. *Ju Hua* is a popular perennial flower that grows wild and is a cultivated ornamental plant in China. When dried, the pale yellow flowers are used medicinally and have a bittersweet taste. *Shen Nong Ben Cao Jing* (*Shen Nong's Materia Medica*), the first text to classify Chinese medicinals, characterizes *Ju hua* as a superior herb. *Shen Nong Ben Cao Jing* classifies all medicinals in one of three grades: 1) superior medicinal, 2) medium medicinal, and 3) inferior medicinal. Superior medicinals correspond to heaven, maintain life, and are nontoxic. Medium medicinals correspond to humankind, benefit human nature, and have some medicinal functions. Inferior medicinals correspond to the earth, cure disease, and have some toxicity.
2. There are three types of *Ju Hua* on the market. The one with a large, white flower and sweet taste is called *Bai Ju Hua* or *Tian Ju Hua*. The small yellow flower is called *Huang Ju Hua*, and the smallest flower with a bitter taste is called *Ye Ju Hua*. White Chrysanthemum *Bai Ju Hua* is most suitable for soothing the liver and benefiting the eyes, and thus it is preferred for eye problems. Yellow Chrysanthemum flower *Huang Ju Hua* is most suitable for clearing Heat and is used for Wind-Heat dispersion. Wild Chrysanthemum *Ye Ju Hua* may be used for toxic carbuncles, furuncles, sore throat, and external applications. Wild Chrysanthemum *Ye Ju Hua* is usually combined with Taraxacum *Pu Gong Ying* and Lonicera *Jin Yin Hua*. Wild Chrysanthemum *Ye Ju Huang* is extremely bitter and hard on Stomach *Qi*.
3. *Fang Su Tong Yi*, a *Han* Dynasty folk storybook, tells about a village named Gangu in *Ne Xiang* county of *He Nan* province. A stream flowed from the surrounding *Ju Hua* mountains and through *Ju Hua* bushes before it reached the village. This stream was the water source for the villagers and they could taste *Ju Hua* in the water whenever the *Ju Hua* flowers fell into the stream. Coincidentally, everyone from the 30 families in the village lived to 130 years of age. During the *Han* period, the Great Emperor Wu often held a *Ju Hua* wine tasting during the *Chong Yang* festival because *Ju Hua* was believed to extend peoples lives.
4. Many Chinese folk stories report people turning into immortals after consuming *Ju Hua*. During the East *Han* Dynasty, a Taoist priest named Fei told his follower, Heng Jing, that a disaster would occur in the village named *Runan* on September 9th. Fei advised climbing the mountain and drinking *Ju Hua* wine to prevent the disaster. Heng Jing and his family followed his mentor's advice, and when they returned from the mountain they found everyone remaining in the village had died. Since this day, September the 9th has been celebrated as the *Chong Yang* Festival during which people will climb a mountain and drink *Ju Hua* wine.
5. Chrysanthemum *Ju Hua* is a popular summer tea in southern China. It is used alone in folk medicine for skin rashes.
6. Good quality *Ju Hua* has a good shape, is bright in color, and is fragrant.
7. The water extract and decoction of Chrysanthemum *Ju Hua* has inhibitory effects against *Staphylococcus aureus* and dermatophytes. It also shows inhibitory effects against influenza virus PR3 and leptospirosis. The extract of Chrysanthemum *Ju Hua* can dilate the coronary arteries, increase the blood flow of the coronary arteries, and increase the oxygen consumption of the cardiac muscle. It has antihypertensive and anticoagulative effects.

Pharmaceutical Ingredients:[1–4]

1. Essential oils (camphor, borneol, chrysanthenone, bornyl acetate)
2. Flavonoids (chrysanthemin, acacetin, luteolin, apigenin)
3. Sesquiterpenoids (chrysanthemin A, B, chrysandiol, chlorochrymorin)
4. Chlorogenic acid, quinic acid-4-o-caffeic acid, vitamin E, Mg

Bupleurum *Chai Hu* 柴胡

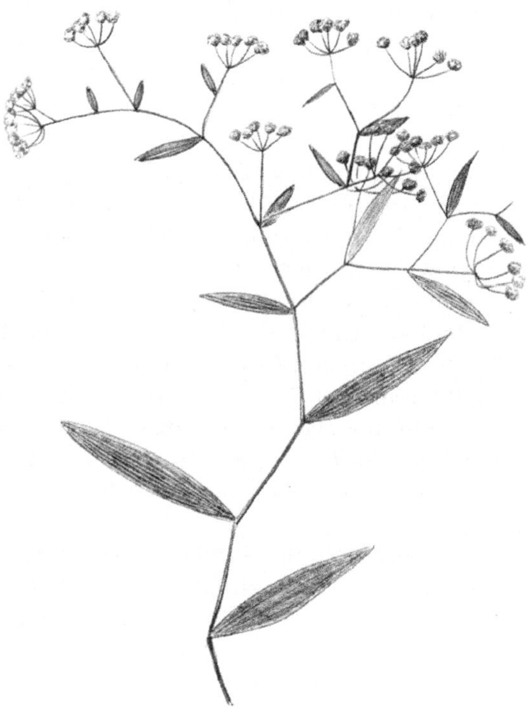

a

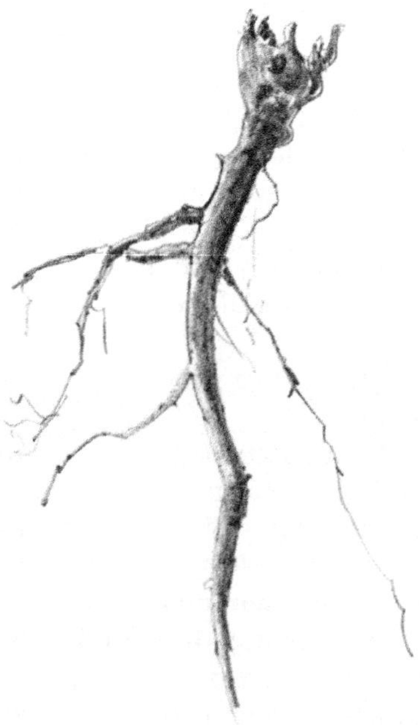

b

Original Reference: *Shen Nong Ben Cao Jing* (*Shen Nong's Materia Medica*, 1st century BCE) 神农本草经

Part Used: Root

Name:
Pharmaceutical: Bupleuri, Radix
Botanical: Bupleurum chinense; B. scrozonerifolim
Common name: Bupleurum
Wade-Giles: *Ch'ai-Hu*

Energy/Taste: Slightly cold, bitter, pungent

Channel-Organ: Liver, Gallbladder

Actions:

1. Dispel Wind-Heat
2. Smooth Liver *Qi*
3. Raise *Yang*
4. Resolve *Shao Yang* disorder and reduce fever

Form and Preparation: Powder, decoction, or pill

Dosage:
Horses and Cattle: 15–45 g
Llamas, Alpacas, Goats, and Pigs: 5–10 g
Dogs: 2–5 g
Cats and Rabbits: 0.5–1 g
Birds: 0.3–3 g

Cautions and Contraindications: Caution in *Yin* Deficiency

Side Effects:

1. Nausea
   Combine with: Zingiberis *Sheng Jiang* to reduce nausea
2. Long-term usage can cause liver enlargement.
3. Can cause dizziness

Clinical Applications:

1. Fever due to Wind invasion
   Combine with: Glycerrhiza *Gan Cao*
   Classical herbal formula: *Chai Hu San*
2. *Shao Yang* Pattern of Cold invasion
   Clinical signs: Alternative chills and fever, costal pain, nausea
   Combine with: Scutellaria *Huang Qin*, Pinellia *Ban Xia*, and Codonopsis *Dang Shen*
   Classical herbal formula: *Xiao Chai Hu Tang*
3. Stagnation of Liver *Qi*
   Clinical signs: Distension in costal region, breast distension, irritability, digestive disturbances, red or painful eyes

Combine with: Cyperus *Xiang Fu*, Aurantium *Zhi Ke*, Citrus *Qing Pi*, Paeonia *Bai Shao*, and Ligusticum *Chuan Xiong*

Classical herbal formula: *Si Ni San*

Contraindications: Liver Fire causing dizziness, ear-ringing

To harmonize the Blood: add Ligusticum *Chuan Xiong* and Angelica *Dang Gui*

To fortify Qi, add: Codonopsis *Dang Shen* and Atractylodes *Bai Zhu*

With Blood Deficiency or Blood Stagnation: combine with Angelica *Dang Gui* and Paeonia *Bai Shao*

Classical herbal formula: *Xiao Yao San*

With heat: combine with Scutellaria *Huang Qin* and Mentha *Bo He*

4. Sinking of Spleen *Qi* and *Yang*

   Clinical signs: Chronic diarrhea; prolapses of uterus, intestine, or rectum; hemorrhoids

   Combine with: Cimicifuga *Sheng Ma*, and Codonopsis *Dang Shen* or Ginseng *Ren Shen*, Astragalus *Huang Qi*, and Atractylodes *Bai Zhu*

   Classical herbal formula: *Bu Zhong Yi Qi Tang*

5. Hepatitis

   Combine with: Gentiana *Long Dan Cao*, Gardenia *Zhi Zi* and Glycerrhiza *Gan Cao*

History and Comments:

1. *Shen Nong Ben Cao Jing* characterizes *Chai Hu* as a Superior medicinal. Zhang Zhong Jing, the sage of Chinese medicine, used *Chai Hu* extensively in his formulas for treating Cold diseases. Consequently, *Chai Hu* is considered one of the most important medicines for treating Cold diseases.
2. *Chai Hu* usually grows in mountainous regions. Young *Chai Hu* plants can be eaten as a vegetable. The older, woody plants are also used as firewood. *Chai Hu* roots are used as medicine. *Ying Zhou* (currently known as *Tie Ling* in China's *Liao Ning* Province) grows the best *Chai Hu* in the nation. *Ying Zhou Chai Hu* roots can grow up to 2 feet long, appear like a large mouse tail, and have a pleasant taste.
3. During the *Song* Dynasty, the historian Pong Yuan Yin recorded a story about a Governor in his book *Tang Shu* (*Historical Book of Tang Dynasty*). For more than a year, Governor Zhang suffered from malaria with alternating chills and fever, which made him sweat constantly. Zhang became very weak and skinny. One doctor treated him for *Qi* Deficiency with Cervus *Lu Rong* and Aconite *Fu Zi*. These hot herbs added Heat to the fever and Zhang's constant sweating worsened. Pong called a royal doctor named Sun Ling for assistance. Sun Ling prescribed *Xiao Chai Hu Tang*, which contains *Chai Hu* as the King ingredient. One dose reduced the fever syndrome 90%. Three doses later, Zhang recovered completely. Then Sun Ling explained that "The symptom of Malaria is the Heat. The first doctor treated him with potent herbs like *Lu Rong* and *Fu Zi* whose hot properties supplement Essence and increase Blood circulation, increasing sweating. Excessive sweating can deplete *Qi* leading to *Qi* Deficiency. That is why the Governor became so weak. Heat in the Exterior and Interior (*Zhang Fu* organs) should be treated differently. In this case, the Governor's Heat is in the Exterior, *Chai Hu* is the essential ingredient. Three doses of *Chai Hu* were necessary because the *Chai Hu* was produced in southern China. If the Governor had used *Ying Zhou* (northern China) *Chai Hu*, only one dose would have cured him."
4. Bupleurum *Chai Hu* can release pent-up anger and Heat. To moderate this effect, Paeonia *Bai Shao* is commonly included in the formula. A large dose of raw Bupleurum *Chai Hu* is used to dispel the Exterior and relieve fever. A moderate dosage of the herb stir-fried with vinegar is used to soothe the Liver. A small dose of raw herb is used to lift *Yang Qi*.
5. Bupleurum *Chai Hu* has antiinflammatory, antipyretic, tranquilizing, and analgesic effects. Saikosaponin from *Chai Hu* lowers serum cholesterol levels. Therefore, *Chai Hu* can protect the Liver from damage. The water decoction of Bupleurum *Chai Hu* has an antibiotic effect against *Mycobacterium Tuberculosis*. It also has an antiviral effect against influenza viruses.

Pharmaceutical Ingredients:[1–4]

1. Saponin (saikosaponin A, B, C, D, E, saikogenin F, G, E, saikoside)
2. Sterols (α-spinasterol, stigmasterol)
3. Essential oils (r-heptalactone, r-decalactone, bupleurmol, eugenol, hexoic acid, r-lactone undecylate, p-methoxy phenyl diketone)
4. Oleic acid, linolenic acid, palmitic acid, stearic acid. Polysaccharide, carbohydrates, alkaloids, glucose, amino acids, coumarin, flavone

Pueraria *Ge Gen* 葛根

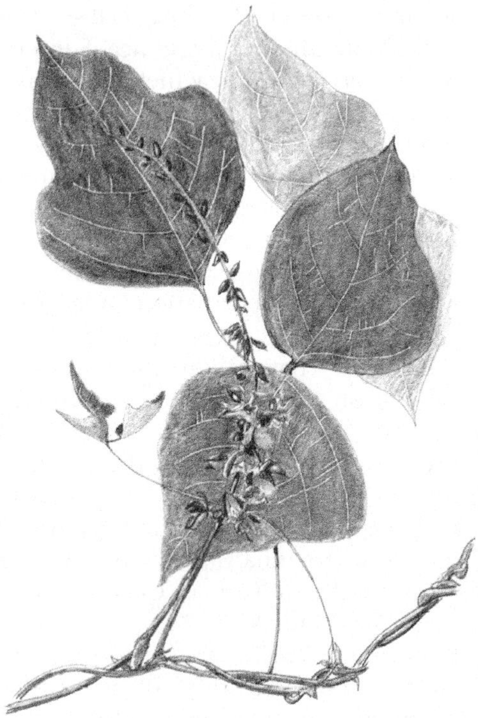

a

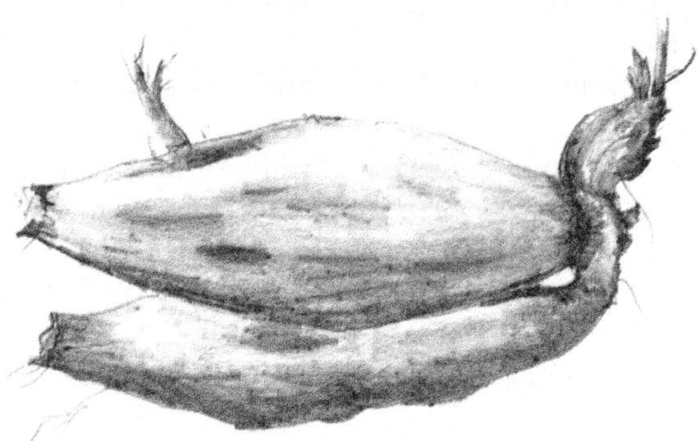

b

Original Reference: *Shen Nong Ben Cao Jing* (*Shen Nong*'s *Materia Medica*, 1st century BCE) 神农本草经

Part Used: Root

Name:
Pharmaceutical: Puerariae, Radix
Botanical: Pueraria lobata; P. thomsanii (Kudzu root)
Common: Kudzu root
Wade-Giles: *Ko-Ken*
Translation: Kudzu root; pueraria

Energy/Taste: Cool, pungent, sweet

Channel-Organ: Spleen, Stomach, Bladder

Actions:
1. Clear the surface and release muscles
2. Promote Body Fluids and relieve thirst
3. Raise *Yang* to relieve diarrhea
4. Clear Heat and treat hypertension

Form and Preparation: Powder, decoction, or pill

Dosage:
Horses and Cattle: 20–60 g
Llamas, Alpacas, Goats, and Pigs: 3–15 g
Dogs: 2–5 g
Cats and Rabbits: 0.5–1 g
Birds: 0.3–3 g

Cautions and Contraindications: None known

Side Effects: None known

Clinical Applications:
1. Wind-Cold invasion, following perspiration
   Clinical signs: Stiffness and pain in neck and upper back, chills, fever
   Combine with: Ephedra *Ma Huang*, Cinnamomum *Gui Zhi*, and Paeonia *Bai Shao*
   Classical herbal formula: *Ge Gen Tang*
   For neck pain: combine with Notopterygium *Qiang Huo*
2. Wind-Heat invasion affecting Liver
   Clinical signs: Fever, nausea, painful eyes, dry throat
   Combine with: Bupleurum *Chai Hu*, Scutellaria *Huang Qin*, and Talcum *Hua Shi*
   Classical herbal formula: *Chai Ge Jie Ji Tang*
3. Thirst due to diabetes or fever
   Combine with: Ophiopogon *Mai Men Dong*, Trichosanthes *Tian Hua Fen*, and Rehmannia *Shu Di Huang*
   Classical herbal formula: *Yu Quan Wan*
4. Damp-Heat dysentery
   Combine with: Coptis *Huang Lian* and Scutellaria *Huang Qin*
   Classical herbal formula: *Ge Gen Qin Lian Tang*

5. Diarrhea due to Spleen Deficiency or diarrhea due to Heat where Body Fluids are injured
   Combine with: Codonopsis *Dang Shen*, Atractylodes *Bai Zhu*, Dioscorea *Shan Yao*, Saussurea *Mu Xiang*, and Poria *Fu Ling*
   Classical herbal formula: *Qi Wei Bai Zhu San*
   Preparation: Roasted; use smaller dosage, 4–6 g
6. Normalize Stomach *Qi*
   Clinical signs: Nausea, vomiting, diarrhea
   Combine with: Pinellia *Ban Xia* and Zingiberis *Sheng Jiang*

History and Comments:
1. Long ago in China, a man fell in love with a native girl and wanted to marry her. Parents on both sides disapproved of the marriage. The lovers ran away together to live in the wild mountains. One day the man fell ill. His whole body was covered with a rash, his face was dark red, and he was unconscious. His beloved girlfriend felt powerless as she watched her lover dying, and she began to cry. A monk passing by heard her sobbing and investigated the situation. The monk handed the woman a stick, which was white on the inside and purple on the outside. The monk said, "This is *Ge Gen*. Make juice out of it, feed it to your man, and he shall live." The woman followed these instructions and the man recovered quickly after drinking the *Ge Gen* juice. The couple continued using *Ge Gen* as a supplement and they lived a long and happy life together.
2. Good quality Pueraria *Ge Gen* is big, solid, white, and powdery. It should not be very fibrous.
3. The water decoction and alcohol extract of Pueraria *Ge Gen* can reverse acute myocardial ischemia. The flavonoids from *Ge Gen* can dilate the coronary artery and brain blood vessels and increase the blood flow and oxygen supply.

Pharmaceutical Ingredients:[1–4]
1. Flavonoids (daidzin, daidzein, puerarin, daidzin-4′, 7-diglycoside, pueranin-7-xyloside, 4′, 6″-o-diacethy puerarin, formononetin, genistein, 4′-methoxypuerarin)
2. Tritertenoidal sapogenol (sophoradiol, soyasapogenol A, B)
3. Allantoin, β-sitosterol, starch

Arctium *Niu Bang Zi* 牛蒡子

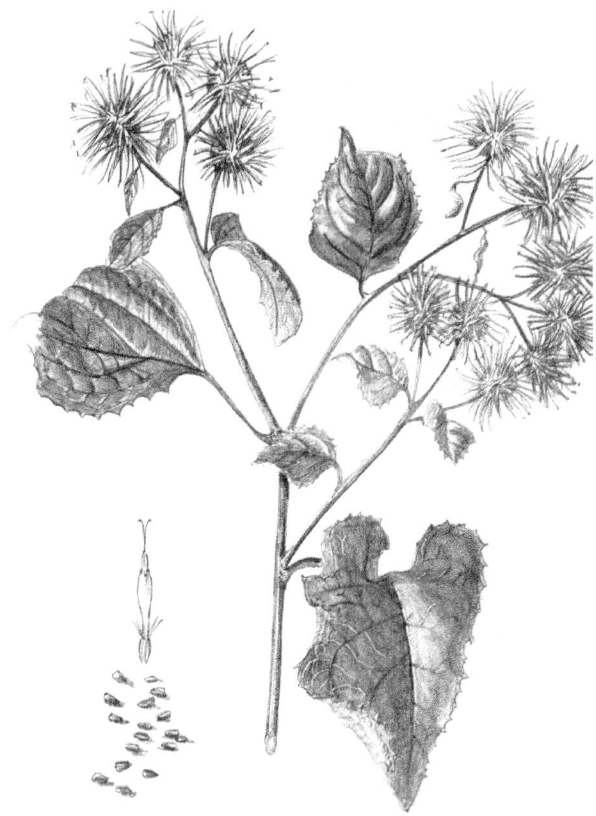

Original Reference: *Ming Yi Bie Lu* (*Miscellaneous Records of Famous Physicians*) by *Tao Hong-Jing*, North and South Kingdoms (5th century) 名医别录

Part Used: Seed

Name:
Pharmaceutical: Arctii Lappae, Fructus
Botanical: Arctium lappa (Burdock)
Common: Burdock seed
Wade-Giles: *Niu-Pang-Tzu*

Energy/Taste: Cold, pungent, bitter

Channel-Organ: Lung, Stomach

Actions:
1. Disperse Wind-Heat and benefit the throat
2. Relieve toxin and reduce swelling
3. Moisten Intestines

Form and Preparation: Powder, decoction, or pill

Dosage:
Horses and Cattle: 15–30 g
Llamas, Alpacas, Goats, and Pigs: 3–15 g

Dogs: 2–5 g
Cats and Rabbits: 0.5–2 g
Birds: 0.2–1.5 g

Cautions and Contraindications: Caution in Spleen Deficiency with diarrhea, or *Qi* and Blood Deficiency. Not appropriate with open sores and oozing.

Side Effects: It may cause diarrhea.

Clinical Applications:

1. Sore throat due to Wind-Heat invasion
   Clinical signs: Sore throat accompanied by fever, dry cough, constipation
   Combine with: Platycodon *Jie Geng*, Mentha *Bo He*, and Schizonepeta *Jing Jie*
   Classical herbal formula: *Niu Bang Tang*
   Also useful for: Swollen tonsils
   Combine with: Scutellaria *Huang Qin* and Forsythia *Lian Qiao*
2. Toxic Heat causing carbuncles or mumps
   Combine with: Chrysanthemum *Ye Ju Hua*, Angelica *Bai Zhi*, Lonicera *Jin Yin Hua*, Viola *Zi Hua Di Ding*, and Isatis *Ban Lan Gen*
3. Topically for carbuncles, hives, and toxic ulcerations
4. Pain and swelling associated with carbuncles or boils that have not yet erupted or ulcerated
   Combine with: Angelica *Bai Zhi*, Platycodon *Jie Geng*, Lonicera *Jin Yin Hua*
5. Pain and swelling of the throat, ulcerations, and abscesses of the tongue and mouth
   Combine with: Forsythia *Lian Qiao*

Comments:

1. Depending on its preparation, the herb can have different actions. When Arctium *Niu Bang Zi* is fried, it is called *Chao Niu Bang Zi*. Arctium *Niu Bang Zi* is stronger than *Chao Niu Bang Zi* for dispelling Wind Heat, reducing toxins, and purging stools. It is used for sore throat, carbuncles, mumps, and constipation. The frying decreases the Cold energy of *Chao Niu Bang Zi* (Arctium) and makes this herb stronger for removing Phlegm and better for the throat. This herb is suitable for treating cough and sore throat with stagnation of Heat Phlegm.
2. Arctium *Niu Bang Gen* is the root of the same plant as Arctium *Niu Bang Zi* (seed). The root is used for carbuncles, mumps, and toxic ulcerations.
3. The water extract of *Niu Bang Zi* has an antibacterial effect against *Diplococcus pneumonia*. It also has an antihyperglycemic effect.

Pharmaceutical Ingredients:[1–4]

1. Arctinin, arctigenin, isoarctigenin, matairesinol, vitamin A, B_1, gobostenin, arctiin, lappaol A~H
2. Essential oils

Cicada *Chan Tui* 蝉蜕

Original Reference: *Ming Yi Bie Lu* (*Miscellaneous Records of Famous Physicians*) by *Tao Hong-Jing*, North and South Kingdoms (5th century) 名医别录

Part Used: Exudated shell/skin

Name:
Pharmaceutical: Cicadae, Periostracum
Botanical: Crytotympana pustulata Fabricius
Common: Cicada molting
Wade-Giles: *Ch'an-T'ui*
Translation: Cicada molting

Energy/Taste: Cold, Sweet, salty

Channel-Organ: Lung, Liver

Actions:

1. Disperse Wind-Heat, stop itching
2. Clear the eyes and remove superficial visual obstruction
3. Stop spasms and extinguish Wind

Form and Preparation: Powder, decoction, or pill

Dosage:
Horses and Cattle: 15–30 g
Llamas, Alpacas, Goats, and Pigs: 2–10 g
Dogs: 1–2 g
Cats and Rabbits: 0.2–1 g
Birds: 0.1–1.5 g

Cautions and Contraindications: None known

Side Effects: None known

Morus *Sang Ye* 桑叶

Original Reference: *Shen Nong Ben Cao Jing* (*Shen Nong's Materia Medica*, 1st century BCE) 神农本草经

Part Used: Leaf

Name:
Pharmaceutical: Mori Albae, Folium
Botanical: Morus alba (Mulberry)
Common: Mulberry leaf
Wade-Giles: *Sang-Yeh*
Translation: Mulberry Leaf

Energy/Taste: Cold, bitter, sweet

Channel-Organ: Lung, Liver

Actions:

1. Dispel Wind-Heat
2. Clear Liver Heat and benefit the eyes

3. Clear Heat from Lung to stop cough
4. Cool Blood and stop bleeding

Form and Preparation: Decoction using low-grade heat; cooked separately in a formula; powder form

Dosage:
Horses and Cattle: 15–30g
Llamas, Alpacas, Goats, and Pigs: 3–10g
Dogs: 2–8g
Cats and Rabbits: 0.5–2g
Birds: 0.3–2.5g

Cautions and Contraindications: None known

Side Effects: None known

Cimicifuga *Sheng Ma* 升麻

Original Reference: *Shen Nong Ben Cao Jing* (*Shen Nong's Materia Medica*, 1st century BCE) 神农本草经

Part Used: Root

Name:
Pharmaceutical: Cimicifugae, Rhizoma et Radix
Botanical: Cimicifuga Foetida; C. dahurica; C. heracleifolia
Common: Black cohosh
Wade-Giles: *Sheng-Ma*
Translation: Ascending Hemp

Energy/Taste: Cool, pungent, sweet, bitter

Channel-Organ: Spleen, Lung, Liver, Stomach

Actions:
1. Release the Exterior
2. Clear Heat and remove toxins
3. Raise *Yang*

Form and Preparation: Powder, decoction, or pill

Dosage:
Horses and Cattle: 15–30g
Camels: 30–60g
Llamas, Alpacas, Goats, and Pigs: 3–10g
Dogs: 1–2g
Cats and Rabbits: 0.5–1g
Birds: 0.3–3g

Cautions and Contraindications: Caution in *Yin* Deficiency with Heat

Side Effects: It is toxic. Overdosage leads to dizziness, nausea, vomiting.

Soja *Dan Dou Chi* 淡豆鼓

Original Reference: *Ming Yi Bie Lu* (*Miscellaneous Records of Famous Physicians*) by *Tao Hong-Jing*, North and South Kingdoms (5th century) 名医别录

Part Used: Seed, prepared

Name:
Pharmaceutical: Sojae Praeparatum, Semen
Botanical: Glysine Max. (Soybean)
Common: Fermented soybean
Wade-Giles: *Tan-Tou-Shih*
Translation: Prepared Soybean

Energy/Taste: Cool, pungent, bitter, sweet

Channel-Organ: Lung, Stomach

Actions:
1. Clear Wind from the surface
2. Relieve restlessness
3. Purge fire

Form and Preparation: Powder, decoction, or pill

Dosage:
Horses and Cattle: 15–30g
Llamas, Alpacas, Goats, and Pigs: 3–10g
Dogs: 1–5g
Cats and Rabbits: 0.5–1g
Birds: 0.2–1.5g

Cautions and Contraindications: None known

Side Effects: None known

SUMMARY OF HERBS THAT RELEASE THE EXTERIOR

Tables 2.4 and 2.5 summarize and compare the herbs that release the Exterior.

Table 2.4. Pungent-Warm herbs to release the Exterior: A quick overview and comparison.

Herbs	Special Actions	Common Characteristics
Dispel Wind-Cold and induce Sweat		Taste: Pungent or spicy
Gui Zhi	Warm the Channels and Move Blood	Energy: Warm
	Relieve surface pain, especially in upper body	Action: 1) Induce sweat to dispel
Ma Huang	#1 potent herb to induce sweat	Wind-Cold; 2) Release the Exterior
	Stop asthma and relieve cough	Indication: Wind-Cold or Exterior
	Benefit urination and reduce edema	Cold
Sheng Jiang	Harmonize Stomach to stop vomiting	Clinical Signs:
Xi Xin	Stop pain and warm Lung to transform Phlegm, **toxic**	Fever without sweating
Release the Exterior and dispel Wind		Aching body
Fang Feng	Dispel Wind and stop pain	Chills and aversion to cold
Jing Jie	Stop bleeding, clear skin eruptions	Coldness in ears and nose
Zi Su Ye	Harmonize Stomach, calm the fetus	Thirst: Decreased
	Counter fish and crab poisoning	Tongue: Wet with thin white
Open to the Nose and nasal passages		coating
and dispel Wind-Cold		Pulse: Superficial/tight
Bai Zhi	Reduce swelling and discharge pus, **mild toxic**	
Xin Yi Hua	#1 herb for the nose, open the Lung	
Cang Er Zi	Eliminate Wind-Damp to stop pain, **toxic**	
E Bu Shi Cao	Relieve cough and reduce toxin	
Expel Wind-Damp		
Qiang Huo	Stop pain, guide *Qi* to *Tai Yang* and *Du* channels	
Gao Ben	Release the surface and stop pain	

Table 2.5. Pungent-Cool herbs to release the Exterior: A quick overview and comparison.

Herbs	Special Actions	Common Characteristics
Dispel Wind-Heat		Taste: Pungent or spicy
Bo He	Potent to induce sweating	Energy: Cool
	Smooth Liver *Qi* and clear Liver heat	Action: 1) Dispel Wind-Heat; 2) Release
	Clear the head and benefit the throat	the Exterior Heat
Ge Gen	Promote body fluids and relieve thirst	Indication: Wind-Cold, or Exterior Cold
	Raise *Yang* to relieve diarrhea	Clinical Signs:
Niu Bang Zi	Benefit the throat, moisten Intestine	Fever and sweating
	Relieve toxin and reduce swelling	Sore throat
Chan Tui	Remove superficial visual obstruction	Red eyes
	Stop spasms, extinguish Wind, stop itching	Warm in ears and nose
Dan Dou Chi	Relieve restlessness, purge fire	Thirst: Increased
Clear Liver Heat and brighten the eyes		Tongue: Red and dry
Ju Hua	Disperse Wind-Heat, remove toxins	Pulse: Superficial and fast
Sang Ye	Clear Heat from Lung to stop cough	
	Cool Blood and stop bleeding	
Release the Exterior and Raise *Yang*		
Chai Hu	Smooth Liver *Qi*	
	Resolve *Shao Yang* disorder and reduce fever	
Sheng Ma	Bring measles rash to the surface, clear Heat	

REFERENCES

1. Chen JK, Chen TT. Chinese Medical Herbology and Pharmacology. City of Industry, CA: Art of Medicine Press, 2004.
2. Brinker FJ. The Toxicology of Botanical Medicines. Sandy, OR: Eclectic Medical Publications, 2000.
3. Duke JA. Handbook of Medicinal Herbs. New York: Chemical and Rubber Company Press, 2001.
4. Huang KC. The Pharmacology of Chinese Herbs, 2nd Edition. New York: Chemical and Rubber Company Press, 1999.

3 Herbs to Transform Phlegm and Relieve Cough and Asthma 化痰止咳平喘药

Huisheng Xie, Yasu Xie, Xiaolin Deng

This chapter describes three categories of herbs: 1) herbs to transform Cold-Phlegm, 2) herbs to transform Heat-Phlegm, and 3) herbs to relieve cough and asthma. Even though they are in different categories, all of these herbs are related to Phlegm. So, what is Phlegm?

Phlegm is called *Tan*, which is a turbid, thick, and Damp material. It is the pathological product of *Zang-Fu* organ dysfunction. Phlegm often results when the Body Fluids fail to circulate adequately and properly, and congeal due to Heat, Cold, Damp, or Spleen *Qi* Deficiency. Diseases due to Phlegm include a variety of syndromes depending upon the body region affected. Phlegm may appear in the Lung, Stomach, Heart, or the Meridians and Channels (Table 3.1). Retention of Phlegm in the Lung, for instance, may lead to cough and asthma. Obstructed Phlegm in the Meridians may give rise to subcutaneous nodules or suppurative inflammation of deep tissues. Phlegm afflicting the Heart may cause *Shen* disturbance, Internal Wind (Seizure or convulsions), loss of consciousness or coma.

Phlegm accumulation may be caused by exogenous Heat or Cold; thus, there are two forms of Phlegm: Heat Phlegm and Cold Phlegm. Cold Phlegm is also called Damp Phlegm because it is often associated with Damp. Herbs to treat Phlegm are divided into three categories based on which form of Phlegm or symptoms they treat: 1) herbs to transform Cold-Phlegm, 2) herbs to transform Heat-Phlegm (Table 3.2), and 3) herbs to relieve cough and asthma, which focus on treating Phlegm-related symptoms, such as the five Patterns in Table 3.3. As necessary, combine these three categories of herbs with the following: 1) Wind-dispersing herbs, 2) *Qi* tonics, 3) herbs to dispel endogenous Wind or to calm *Shen*, 4) herbs to soften hardness, and 5) herbs to dispel Cold and remove stagnation, especially for *Yin* carbuncles.

Pharmacological studies indicate that these herbs may have the following effects: 1) eliminating sputum by increasing respiratory tract secretions and demonstrating strong expectorant effects, 2) antitussive effects and antiasthmatic effects, 3) bronchodilatory effects, and 4) antiemetic effects (for gastrointestinal conditions).[1–4]

HERBS TO TRANSFORM COLD-PHLEGM

Pinellia *Ban Xia* 半夏

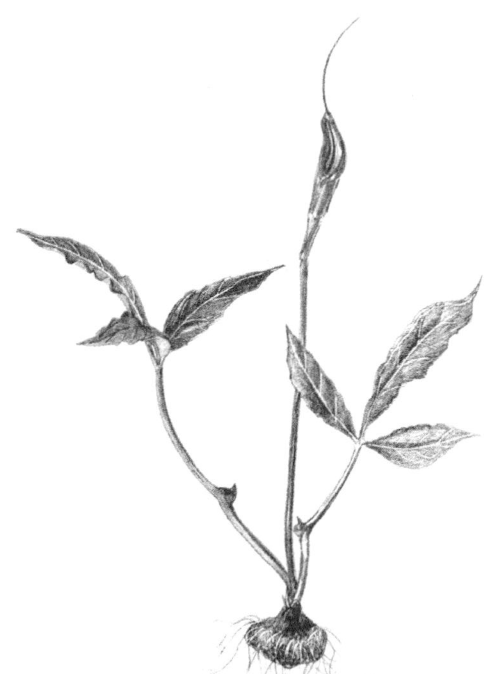

Table 3.1. Location of Phlegm and clinical signs.

Location of Phlegm	Clinical Signs	Treatment Principles and Examples of Herbal Formulas
Phlegm in the Lung	Profuse sputum, or thick sticky sputum, usually clear and white Often accompanied by cough, difficult breathing, heaviness in chest, wheezing, pain in the ribs Nasal congestion or discharge, or sneezing Tongue: thin or thick white, or greasy coating Pulse: slippery, often excess in Lung position	Open Lung, transform Phlegm, stop cough, eliminate Phlegm *Er Chen Tang*
Phlegm retention in the Stomach	Nausea or vomiting Loss of appetite Loose stools or abdominal fullness Tongue: white or greasy coating Pulse: slippery, often excess in Stomach-Spleen positions	Harmonize Stomach, transform Phlegm *Liu Jun Zi Tang*
Phlegm misting the Heart	Dizziness, coma, depression Shen disturbance or behavioral problems Epilepsy, seizure, convulsions Tongue: white or greasy coating Pulse: slippery, often excess in Heart positions	Quell Wind, calm *Shen*, expel Phlegm, disperse Wind *Di Dan Tang*
Phlegm in the Meridians and Channels	Thyroid mass, lipoma Skin growth or masses Chronic pain due to poor circulation Tongue: pale purple with white or greasy coating Pulse: slippery or wiry	Soften the hard, reduce Phlegm, clear the Channels *Hai Zao Yu Hu Tang*
Phlegm in any internal locations	Nodules, lumps, masses, or tumor *Yin* Carbuncles, which are characterized by slow-healing carbuncles and sores Tongue: white or greasy coating Pulse: deep, slippery, or weak	Soften the hard, transform Phlegm, break masses *Nei Xiao Luo Li San*

Table 3.2. Types of Phlegm and Phlegm-transforming herbs.

Type of Phlegm	Clinical Signs	Examples of Herbs
Cold (Damp) Phlegm	Clear nasal discharge Wet cough or productive cough Nodules, nonhealed wound Tongue: pale and wet Pulse: slippery	Pinellia *Ban Xia*
Heat Phlegm	Dry cough or nonproductive cough Fever, seizure Masses Tongue: red and dry Pulse: fast	Fritillaria *Chuan Bei Mu*

Original Reference: *Shen Nong Ben Cao Jing* (*Shen Nong*'s *Materia Medica*, 1st century BCE) 神农本草经

Part Used: Whole underground rhizome and tubers

Name:
Pharmaceutical: Pinelliae Ternatae, Rhizoma
Botanical: Pinellia ternata
Common: Pinellia
Wade-Giles: *Pan-Hsia*
Translation: Half Summer

Energy/Taste: Warm, pungent, toxic (peel removed, processed to reduce toxicity)

Channel-Organ: Spleen, Stomach, Lung

Actions:
1. Dry Dampness and transform Phlegm
2. Descend rebellious *Qi* and stop vomiting or nausea
3. Eliminate nodule and dissipate mass
4. Topical application: dispel swelling and relieve pain

Table 3.3. Patterns of cough and clinical signs.

Patterns	Symptoms	Herbal Formulas	Food
Wind-Cold	Clear sputum Headache or head-shaking Nasal discharge or congestion Aversion to Cold or fever Tongue: pale or purple with thin white coating Pulse: superficial and tight	*Zhi Suo San*	Ginger + radish
Wind-Heat	Fever Dry mouth Sore throat or painful coughing Cough with sputum that is thick and difficult to expectorate Tongue: red Pulse: superficial and fast	*Yin Qiao San*	Pear
Dry-fire	Dry cough Scanty sputum Lip and throat dryness Tongue: dry and red Pulse: fast	*Qing Zao Jiu Fei Tang*	Pawpaw
Phlegm Damp	Wet cough or copious sputum Painful response on palpation in the chest area Fatigue, exercise intolerance Tongue: wet or pale Pulse: slippery	*Er Chen Tang*	Coix
Lung *Yin* Deficiency	Cough that comes and goes Dry cough Rapid respiration Slight fever, even with bleed Tongue: red and dry Pulse: thin and fast	*Bai He Gu Jin Tang*	Honey

Form and Preparation: Powder or decoction; it can be very toxic when fresh. Always prepare or process before use. Its toxicity can be reduced when combined with Zingiberis *Sheng Jiang*.

Dosage:
Horses and Cattle: 15–45 g
Camels: 30–60 g
Llamas, Alpacas, Goats, Sheep, and Pigs: 3–10 g
Dogs: 2–5 g
Cats and Rabbits: 0.5–1 g
Birds: 0.1–1 g

Cautions and Contraindications:
1. Caution in Dry cough due to *Yin* Deficiency, hemorrhages, or Phlegm-Heat
2. Caution during pregnancy
3. Do not combine with Aconite *Chuan Wu* or *Cao Wu*.

Side Effects: May cause loss of voice, vomiting, watery diarrhea, and dyspnea

Clinical Applications
1. Lung Phlegm-Damp due to Deficiency of Spleen *Qi*
   Clinical signs: Cough with thick or watery white Phlegm, nasal discharge, or congestion
   Combine with: Poria *Fu Ling*, Citrus *Chen Pi*, and Zingiberis *Sheng Jiang*
   Classical herbal formula: *Er Chen Wan*
2. Nausea and vomiting due to rebellious Stomach *Qi*
   Combine with: Pogostemon *Huo Xiang*, Poria *Fu Ling*, Citrus *Chen Pi*, and Zingiberis *Sheng Jiang*
   Classical herbal formula: *Liu Jun Zi Tang*
3. Nodules, masses, goiter, scrofula
   Combine with: Sargassum *Hai Zao*, Laminaria *Kun Bu*, and Fritillaria *Chuan Bei Mu*
   Classical herbal formula: *Hai Zao Yu Hu Tang*

History and Comments:
1. *Shen Nong Ben Cao Jing* lists *Ban Xia* as an inferior medicinal because raw *Ban Xia* is toxic. In *Ben Cao Gong Mu*, *Ban Xia* is also described as a toxic herb. *Ban Xia* receives its name from the harvest season. The plant is produced in the South and Southwest regions of China, begins growing in March, but is harvested in mid-May, which is halfway through Summer. Thus, the name is *Ban* (half) *Xia* (summer).
2. Once upon a time during the *Song* Dynasty, a judge named *Yang* Lizhi came back from a trip to southern China. Soon after his return, he developed a swollen throat. The excruciating pain made eating

and sleeping impossible. He saw many doctors, but his symptoms only worsened. One day, *Yang*'s son heard that the famous royal doctor was in town, so he asked the royal doctor for help. The doctor examined *Yang* and stated his diagnosis, "Your father has a mysterious disease. If he wants to live, your father must eat one pound of *Sheng Jiang* (Fresh Ginger) soon. Considering his extreme sore throat, *Yang* was skeptical about the prescription, but he followed the doctor's instructions. Oddly enough, he did not feel the Ginger's pungency while eating, and quickly consumed half a pound of Ginger. *Yang* immediately felt relief from the pain and swelling. After a short while, he felt the pungency of the Ginger, so he began to eat and drink his usual foods. The next day, *Yang* visited the royal doctor to thank him for saving his life. *Yang* asked the doctor about the miracle cure, and the doctor told him, "While traveling in the south, you must have eaten many partridges which like to eat *Ban Xia*. The toxin of *Ban Xia* infused the partridge flesh, and these toxins transferred to your body when you ate the bird. Over time, the accumulated toxin caused the throat swelling. *Shen Nong Ben Cao Jing* states that Fresh Ginger can detoxify the *Ban Xia*'s toxin. That's why I prescribed *Sheng Jiang*."

3. Pinellia *Ban Xia* is commonly combined with Zingiberis *Sheng Jiang* and Poria *Fu Ling*. For Lung Phlegm-Damp, the herb is commonly combined with Fritillaria *Chuan Bei Mu*.
4. Pinellia *Ban Xia is* available in the U.S. and Western countries in a form called *Fa Ban Xia*, which has been prepared with vinegar, Glycerrhiza *Gan Cao*, Alum *Bai Fan*, and Zingiberis *Sheng Jiang* to reduce toxicity.
5. Pinellia *Ban Xia* powder is mixed with egg whites for external application on carbuncles, deep-rooted carbuncles, lumbodorsal cellulitis, and breast furuncles.

Pharmaceutical Ingredients:[1–4]

1. Homogentisic acid, homogenitisic acid gluciside, 3,4-dihydroxybenzaldehyde, 3,4-dihydroxybenzaldehyde diglucoside
2. Choline
3. l-ephedrine, β-sitosterol
4. Aspartic acid, aminobutyric acid, linoleic acid, starch

Platycodon *Jie Geng* 桔梗

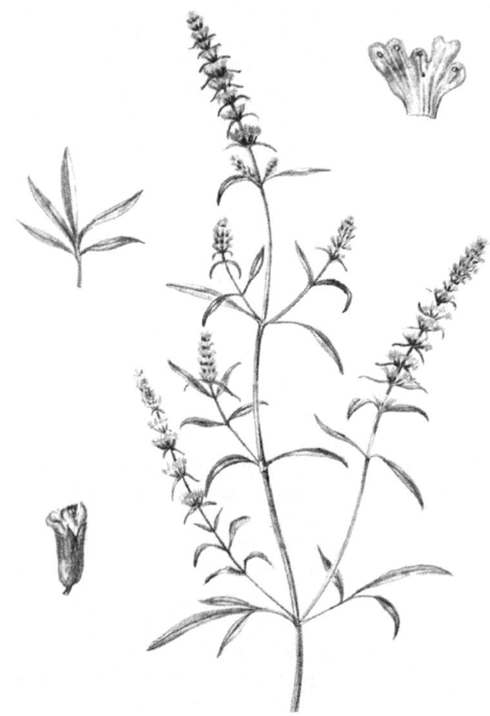

Original Reference: *Shen Nong Ben Cao Jing* (*Shen Nong*'s *Materia Medica*, 1st century BCE) 神农本草经

Part Used: Root

Name:
Pharmaceutical: Platycodi Grandiflori, Radix
Botanical: Platycodon grandiflorum
Common: Platycodon
Wade-Giles: *Chieh-Keng*
Translation: Root of the Balloon Flower

Energy/Taste: Neutral, bitter, pungent

Channel-Organ: Lung

Actions:

1. Open (disperse) the Lung *Qi*
2. Transform Phlegm and expel pus
3. Direct other herbs to upper regions of the body

Form and Preparation: Powder or decoction

Dosage:
Horses and Cattle: 15–45 g
Llamas, Alpacas, Goats, Sheep, and Pigs: 3–10 g
Dogs: 2–5 g
Cats and Rabbits: 0.5–1 g
Birds: 0.2–1.5 g

Cautions and Contraindications:
1. Contraindicated for Hemoptysis
2. Counteracts Gentiana *Long Dan Cao* and Longan *Long Yan Rou*

Side Effects: Overdose may cause mild nausea and vomiting.

Clinical Application
1. Failure of Lung *Qi* to disperse during Exogenous Invasion of Wind-Heat
   Clinical signs: Cough with profuse sputum, fullness in chest, difficulty breathing, sore throat, coarse voice
   Combine with: Lonicera *Jin Yin Hua* and Forsythia *Lian Qiao*
   Classical herbal formula: *Yin Qiao San*
2. Deficiency of Lung *Qi*
   Clinical signs: Weak voice, labored breathing
   Combine with: Codonopsis *Dang Shen* and Astragalus *Huang Qi*
   Classical herbal formula: *Bu Fei San*
3. Lung abscess due to accumulated toxic Heat
   Clinical signs: Cough with Blood, pus, yellow foul sputum, sore throat, suppurative pneumonia, mucus in the Lung
   Combine with: Houttuynia *Yu Xing Cao*, Phragmites *Lu Gen*, Benincasa *Dong Gua Ren*, and Trichosanthes *Gua Lou Ren*, and Coix *Yi Yi Ren*
   Classical herbal formula: *Wei Jing Tang*
4. Transporter to bring formula to the Lung and Upper Burner (*Shang Jiao*) including the chest, neck, and head regions

History and Comments
1. Platycodon *Jie Geng* is also used in treating difficult urination or defecation.
2. When prepared with honey, this herb is good for nourishing the Lung.

Pharmaceutical Ingredients:[1–4]
1. Saponin (Platycodoside, Platycodigenin, polygalaccic acid, platycodin D), α-sinosterol, α-spinasteryl glycosides, platycodonin
2. Terpenes (platycogenic acid A,B,C)
3. Glucose, alkaloids
4. Amino acid

Sinapis *Bai Jie Zi* 白芥子

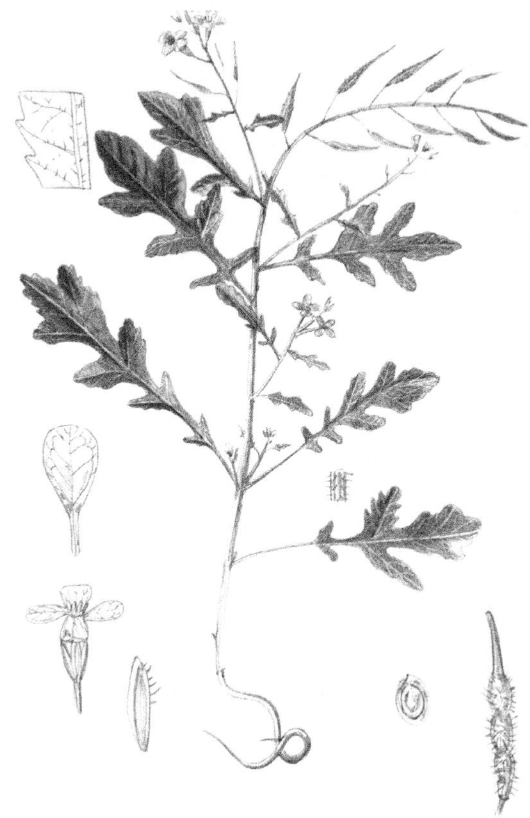

Original Reference: *Tang Ben Cao* (Tang *Materia Medica*) by *Su Jing* et al., *Tang* Dynasty (618–907 CE) 唐本草

Part Used: Seed

Name:
Pharmaceutical: Sinapis Albae, Semen
Botanical: Brassica alba; B. juncea (Mustard Seed)
Common: Brassica, White Mustard Seed
Wade-Giles: *Pai-Chieh-Tzu*
Translation: White Mustard Seed

Energy/Taste: Warm, pungent

Channel-Organ: Lung

Actions:
1. Warm the Lung and transform Phlegm
2. Move *Qi* and dissipate nodule
3. Unblock the Channel and relieve pain

Form and Preparation: Decoction, or may be taken powdered and mixed with vinegar to be taken alone

Dosage:
Horses and Cattle: 15–45 g
Llamas, Alpacas, Goats, Sheep, and Pigs: 2–9 g

Cautions and Contraindications:
1. Caution for patients with allergic skin problems
2. Caution with Deficiency of *Yin* with *Fire*
3. Caution with cough or dyspnea due to Lung *Yin* Deficiency

Side Effects:
1. Topical application may cause skin allergy and blister.
2. Oral medication may cause vomiting, abdominal pain, and diarrhea.

Clinical Application
1. Cold Phlegm obstruction in the Lung and chest
   Clinical signs: Chronic cough with profuse, dilute, frothy mucus, and chest distention and pain
   Combine with: Perilla *Su Zi* and Rhaphanus *Lai Fu Zi*
   Classical herbal formula: *San Zi Yang Qin Tang*
2. Phlegm-Damp obstructs the Channels
   Clinical signs: Pain of joints and limbs and body aches
   Combine with: Saussurea *Mu Xiang*, Cinnamomum *Rou Gui*, and Myrrh *Mo Yao*
3. *Yin* Ju (*Yin* type of carbuncles)
   Clinical signs: Chronic and Cold oozing sores without redness
   Combine with: Cervus *Lu Jiao Jiao*, Cinnamomum *Rou Gui*, and Rehmannia *Shu Di Huang*
   Classical herbal formula: *Yang He Tang*

History and Comments
1. Sinapis *Bai Jie Zi*, Perilla *Su Zi*, and Raphanus *Lai Fu Zi* are all capable of transforming Phlegm, regulating the *Qi*, and pacifying wheezing. However, Sinapsis *Bai Jie Zi* warms the Lung *Qi*, Raphanus *Lai Fu Zi* disperses the Lung *Qi*, and Perilla *Su Zi* directs the Lung *Qi* downward.
2. Topical application of *Bai Jie Zi* at acupoint CV-3 can treat retention of urine.
3. Topical application of *Bai Jie Zi* at BL-13, CV-17, and Ding-Chuan can treat chronic dyspnea or cough.

Pharmaceutical Ingredients:[1–4]
1. Sinalbin, sinapine, myrosin, lipids, protein
2. p-hydroxybenzylisothiocynate, sinapine bisulfate, sinapic acid, choline

Arisaema *Tian Nan Xing* 天南星

Original Reference: *Shen Nong Ben Cao Jing* (*Shen Nong's Materia Medica*, 1st century BCE) 神农本草经

Part Used: Rhizome

Name:
Pharmaceutical: Arisaematis, Rhizoma
Botanical: Arisaema consanguineum; A. heterophyllum; A. Amurense
Common: Arisaema
Wade-Giles: *T'ien-Nan-Hsing*
Translation: Heaven's Southern Star

Energy/Taste: Warm, bitter, pungent, toxic

Channel-Organ: Lung, Liver, Spleen

Actions:
1. Dry up Damp and transform Phlegm
2. Dispel Wind-Phlegm and stop spasm
3. Reduce swelling and alleviate pain in trauma

Form and Preparation: Powder or decoction

Dosage:
Horses and Cattle: 15–25 g
Llamas, Alpacas, Goats, Sheep, and Pigs: 3–10 g
Dogs: 1–2 g
Cats and Rabbits: 0.1–0.5 g
Birds: 0.1–1 g

Cautions and Contraindications:
1. It is toxic, but Zingiberis *Sheng Jiang* can counteract its toxicity.
2. Cautioned in Deficiency of *Yin*
3. Contraindicated during pregnancy and dry cough due to Lung *Yin* Deficiency
4. It counteracts Aconite *Fu Zi*.

Side Effects:
1. Oral medication may cause swelling, pain and numbness of the tongue and throat, and dyspnea.
2. Topical application may cause skin allergy.

Arisaema *Dan Nan Xing* 胆南星

When Arisaema *Tian Nan Xing* is soaked with bile, it becomes *Dan Nan Xing*. Bile enhances the herb's ability to transform Phlegm and clear Heat. Thus, Arisaema *Dan Nan Xing* is often used for treating Heat Phlegm, and *Tian Nan Xing* is used for Damp Phlegm.

Inula *Xuan Fu Hua* 旋覆花

Original Reference: *Shen Nong Ben Cao Jing* (*Shen Nong's Materia Medica*, 1st century BCE) 神农本草经

Part Used: Flower

Name:
Pharmaceutical: Inulae, Flos
Botanical: Inula japonica; I. Britannica
Common: Inula

Wade-Giles: *Hsuan-Fu-Hua*
Translation: Rotated, upturned Flower

Energy/Taste: Warm, bitter, pungent, salty

Channel-Organ: Lung, Liver, Stomach, Spleen, Large Intestine

Actions:
1. Transform Phlegm and promote water metabolism
2. Conduct rebellious *Qi* downward and stop vomiting

Form and Preparation: Powder or decoction

Dosage:
Horses and Cattle: 15–45 g
Llamas, Alpacas, Goats, Sheep, and Pigs: 5–15 g
Dogs: 2–6 g
Cats and Rabbits: 0.5–1 g
Birds: 0.2–1 g

Cautions and Contraindications: Caution in weak patients

Side Effects: May cause allergy in sensitive patients

Cynanchum *Bai Qian* 白前

Original Reference: *Ming Yi Bie Lu* (*Miscellaneous Records of Famous Physicians*) by *Tao Hong-Jing*, North and South Kingdoms (5th century) 名医别录

Part Used: Rhizome

Name:
Pharmaceutical: Cynanchi Baiqian, Radix et Rhizoma
Botanical: Cynanchum stauntonii; Century glaucescens
Common: Cynanchum
Wade-Giles: *Pai-Ch'ien*
Translation: White Before

Energy/Taste: Warm or neutral, pungent, sweet

Channel-Organ: Lung

Actions:
1. Transform Phlegm and stop cough
2. Conduct rebellious *Qi* downward

Form and Preparation: Powder or decoction

Dosage:
Horses and Cattle: 15–45 g
Llamas, Alpacas, Goats, Sheep, and Pigs: 5–15 g
Dogs: 2–6 g
Cats and Rabbits: 0.5–1 g
Birds: 0.2–1 g

Cautions and Contraindications: Contraindicated for cough from Lung *Qi* Deficiency or Kidneys not grasping the *Qi*

Side Effects: None known

Gleditsia *Zao Jiao* 皂角

Original Reference: *Shen Nong Ben Cao Jing* (*Shen Nong's Materia Medica*, 1st century BCE) 神农本草经

Part Used: Fruit

Name:
Pharmaceutical: Gleditsia Fructus
Botanical: Gleditsia sinensis Lam
Common: Gleditea
Wade-Giles: *Tsao-Chiao*
Translation: Soap Angle

Energy/Taste: Warm, pungent, salt, slightly toxic

Channel-Organ: Lung and Large Intestine

Actions:
1. Transform stubborn Phlegm and open the orifices
2. Eliminate Wind and kill parasites

Form and Preparation: Powder or decoction

Dosage:
Horses and Cattle: 20–40 g
Llamas, Alpacas, Goats, Sheep, and Pigs: 3–10 g
Dogs: 1–5 g
Cats and Rabbits: 0.2–0.5 g
Birds: 0.1–1 g

Cautions and Contraindications:
1. Contraindicated during pregnancy or hemorrhage
2. Caution with weakness

Side Effects: Overdose may cause vomiting or diarrhea, or it might damage the central nerve system and cause dyspnea, shock, and death.

Typhonium *Bai Fu Zi* 白附子

Original Reference: *Ming Yi Bie Lu* (*Miscellaneous Records of Famous Physicians*) by *Tao Hong-Jing*, North and South Kingdoms (5th century) 名医别录

Part Used: Rhizome

Name:
Pharmaceutical: Typhonii Gigantei, Rhizoma
Botanical: Typhonium giganteum
Common: Typhonium
Wade-Giles: *Pai-Fu-Tzu*
Translation: White Aconite or White Appendage
Alternative: *Yu Bai Fu*

Energy/Taste: Warm, pungent, sweet, bitter, toxic

Channel-Organ: Stomach, Liver, Spleen

Actions:
1. Dry up Damp and transform Phlegm
2. Dispel Wind and stop spasm
3. Dispel toxic nodules
4. Expel Wind-Cold-Damp and alleviate pain

Form and Preparation: Powder or decoction; the raw herb is toxic. Typhonium *Bai Fu Zi* is prepared when picked by steaming in sulfur, which detoxifies it.

Dosage: Horses and Cattle: 15–30 g

Cautions and Contraindications:
1. Contraindications during pregnancy
2. Caution in Liver *Yang* Rising with Deficiency of *Yin* causing dizziness, or patients with allergies to sulfur (many asthmatics)

Side Effects:
1. It is very drying and may damage *Yin*.
2. Overdose may damage nerve system and cause paresis and paralysis of tongue and limbs, nausea, vomiting, excessive salivation, and death.

HERBS TO TRANSFORM HEAT-PHLEGM

Fritillaria *Chuan Bei Mu* 川贝母 and *Zhe Bei Mu* 浙贝母

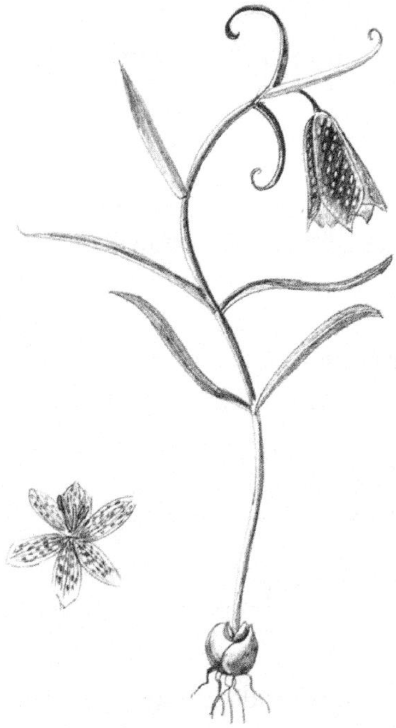

a

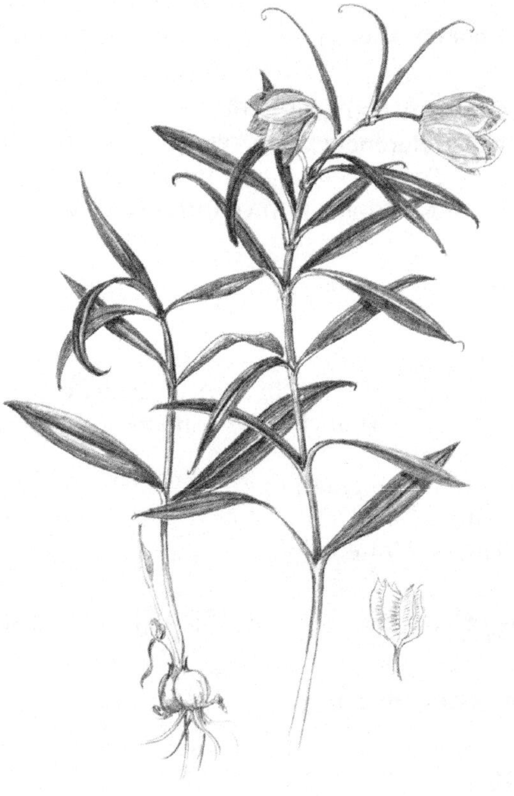

b

Original Reference: *Shen Nong Ben Cao Jing* (*Shen Nong's Materia Medica*, 1st century BCE) 神农本草经

Part Used: Underground bulb

Name:
Pharmaceutical: Fritillaria Bulbus
Botanical: Fritillaria cirrhosa; F. unibracteata; F. przewalskii; F. delavayi
Common: Fritillaria
Wade-Giles: *Ch'uan-Pei-Mu* or *Cheh-Pei-Mu*
Translation: Sichuan Shell Mother or Zhejiang Shell Mother

Energy/Taste: *Chuan Bei Mu*—Cool, bitter, sweet; *Zhe Bei Mu*—Cold, bitter

Channel-Organ: Lung, Heart

Actions:
Chuan Bei Mu (Figure a):
1. Moisten the Lung to treat chronic cough, scanty sputum, and dry throat
2. Transform Phlegm, stop cough
3. Clear Heat and dissipate nodule

Zhe Bei Mu (Figure b):
1. Transform Heat-Phlegm for treatment of Phlegm-*Fire*–induced cough
2. Transform Phlegm, stop cough
3. Clear Heat and dissipate nodule

Form and Preparation: Powder prior to decoction; buy it prepared and then crush and add directly to boiled tea.

Dosage:
Horses and Cattle: 15–30 g
Llamas, Alpacas, Goats, Sheep, and Pigs: 3–10 g
Dogs: 1–2 g
Cats and Rabbits: 0.1–0.5 g
Birds: 0.1–1 g

Cautions and Contraindications:
1. Do not combine with Aconite *Wu Tou* (including *Chuan Wu* and *Cao Wu*).
2. Contraindicated for Cold and Damp Phlegm in Spleen and Stomach
3. Some traditional sources say this herb counteracts Gentiana *Qin Jiao*.

Side Effects: None known

Clinical Application
1. Chronic cough due to Lung *Yin* Deficiency
   Clinical signs: Dry cough with dry throat, red and dry tongue
   Combine with: Lily *Bai He*, Ophiopogon *Mai Men Dong*, Glehnia *Bei Sha Shen*
   Classical herbal formula: *Bai He Gu Jin Tang*
2. Phlegm-Heat cough with thick yellow sputum
   Combine with: Anemarrhena *Zhi Mu*, Scutellaria *Huang Qin*, Trichosanthes *Gua Lou*
3. Mastitis
   Combine with: Taraxacum *Pu Gong Ying* and Forsythia *Lian Qiao*
4. Masses and tumors
   Combine with: Ostrea *Mu Li* and Sparganium *San Leng*
   Classical herbal formula: *Nei Xiao Luo Li San*
5. Sore throat with swollen lymph glands
   Combine with: Forsythia *Lian Qiao*, Scrophularia *Xuan Shen*, and Ostrea *Mu Li*

History and Comments
1. This herb is commonly referred to as Tendrilled Fritillaria.
2. Fritillaria *Chuan Bei Mu* is sweeter, more moistening, and more tonifying than Fritillaria *Zhe Bei Mu*. It is preferred for dry cough with sticky Phlegm and for chronic cough. However, Fritillaria *Chuan Bei Mu* is also four times the price of Fritillaria *Zhe Bei Mu*.

Pharmaceutical Ingredients:[1–4]
Chuan Bei Mu
1. Alkaloids (fritimine, Chinpeimine, fritiminine, beilupeimine, sonpeimine, sipeimine, minpeimine, minpeiminine, verticine, verticinine, fritillarine)
2. Saponin

Zhe Bei Mu
1. Alkaloids (peimine, peiminie, peimidine, peomiphine, peimisine, peimitidine)
2. Peminoside, propeimine
3. Starch

Trichosanthes *Gua Lou* 瓜蒌

Original Reference: *Shen Nong Ben Cao Jing* (*Shen Nong's Materia Medica*, 1st century BCE) 神农本草经

Part Used: Fruit

Name:
Pharmaceutical: Trichosanthes, Fructus
Botanical: Trichosanthes kirilowii; T. uniflora
Common: Trichosanthes Fruit (Snakegourd)
Wade-Giles: *Kua-Lou*
Translation: Trichosanthes Fruit

Energy/Taste: Cool or cold, sweet, bitter

Channel-Organ: Lung, Stomach, Large Intestine

Actions:
1. Clear Heat and transform Phlegm
2. Moisten intestines to move stool
3. Regulate *Qi* in the chest
4. Release nodules

Form and Preparation: Powder or decoction

Dosage:
Horses and Cattle: 30–60 g
Camels: 30–60 g
Llamas, Alpacas, Goats, Sheep, and Pigs: 10–20 g
Dogs: 3–8 g
Cats and Rabbits: 1–2 g
Birds: 0.2–1.5 g

Cautions and Contraindications:
1. Contraindications with Aconite *Wu Tou* (including *Chuan Wu* and *Cao Wu*)
2. Cautions for diarrhea, or Cold Damp Phlegm conditions with deficient Spleen

Side Effects: None known

Trichosanthes *Gua Lou Ren* 瓜蒌仁 and Trichosanthes *Gua Lou Pi* 瓜蒌皮

Both Trichosanthes *Gua Lou Ren* and Trichosanthes *Gua Lou Pi* are from the same plant of Trichosanthes *Gua Lou*. *Gua Lou* is the whole fruit of the plant. *Gua Lou Ren* is the seed, and *Gua Lou Pi* is the peel. Either *Gua Lou Ren* or *Gua Lou Pi* can substitute for Trichosanthes *Gua Lou* because they have the same properties and actions.

Trichosanthes *Tian Hua Fen* 天花粉

Original Reference: *Shen Nong Ben Cao Jing* (*Shen Nong's Materia Medica*, 1st century BCE) 神农本草经

Part Used: Root

Name:
Pharmaceutical: Trichosanthis Kirilowii, Radix
Botanical: Trichosanthes kirilowii; T. uniflora (Snakegourd)
Common: Trichosanthes root
Wade-Giles: *T'ien-Hua-Feng*
Translation: Heaven Flower Powder

Energy/Taste: Cool, sweet, bitter, sour

Channel-Organ: Lung, Stomach

Actions:
1. Clear Heat and promote Body Fluids
2. Reduce swelling and dispel pus

Form and Preparation: Powder, decoction, or pill

Dosage:
Horses and Cattle: 15–45 g
Llamas, Alpacas, Goats, Sheep, and Pigs: 5–15 g
Dogs: 2–5 g
Cats and Rabbits: 0.5–2 g
Birds: 0.2–2 g

Cautions and Contraindications:
1. Cautioned during pregnancy
2. Diarrhea due to Cold from Deficiency of Spleen and Stomach

Side Effects: None known

Bambusa *Zhu Ru* 竹茹

Original Reference: *Ming Yi Bie Lu* (*Miscellaneous Records of Famous Physicians*) by *Tao Hong-Jing*, North and South Kingdoms (5th century) 名医别录

Part Used: Shavings of stalk, after green skin is removed

Name:
Pharmaceutical: Bambusae, Caulis in Taeniam
Botanical: Bambusa breviflora; Phyllostachys nigra; Sinocalamus beecheyanus
Common: Bamboo shavings
Wade-Giles: *Chu-Ju*
Translation: Bamboo Shavings

Energy/Taste: Cool, sweet

Channel-Organ: Stomach, Gallbladder, Lung

Actions:
1. Transform Phlegm and clear Heat
2. Relieve irritability and stop vomiting
3. Cool the Blood and stop bleeding
4. Stop nosebleed and vomiting of Blood

Form and Preparation: Powder or decoction

Dosage:
Horses and Cattle: 15–45 g
Llamas, Alpacas, Goats, Sheep, and Pigs: 3–10 g
Dogs: 2–5 g
Cats and Rabbits: 0.5–1 g
Birds: 0.2–1 g

Cautions and Contraindications:
1. Contraindications in cases with nausea and vomiting due to Stomach Cold or Cold Food Stagnation
2. Cautions with diarrhea caused by Spleen Deficiency or cough caused by Cold

Side Effects: None known

Bambusa *Zhu Li* 竹沥 and *Tian Zhu Huang* 天竺黄

In addition to Bambusa *Zhu Ru*, other Bamboo products used include *Zhu Li* and *Tian Zhu Huang*. They all have similar properties and actions:

1. Bambusa *Zhu Li* (Bamboo Sap) is obtained by Heating fresh bamboo stems and collecting the fluid that extrudes from both ends of the bamboo stems. Its main actions are a) transform Heat-Phlegm and stop cough, and b) stop Epilepsy
2. Bambusa *Tian Zhu Huang* (Bamboo Resin). It is the solidified internal secretions of bamboo. It is formed in the joints of the bamboo that have been aged or damaged. Its actions include a) clear Heat from the Heart, b) stop convulsions, especially infant seizures; and c) transform profuse Phlegm following stroke.

Peucedanum *Qian Hu* 前胡

Original Reference: *Lei Gong Pao Zhi Lun* (*Lei's Method of Preparing Drugs*) by *Lei Xiao*, 5th century 雷公炮炙论

Part Used: Radix

Name:
Pharmaceutical: Peucedani, Radix
Botanical: Peucedanum praeruptorum; P. decursivum
Common: Peucedanum
Wade-Giles: *Ch'ien-Hu*
Translation: Before Barbarians

Energy/Taste: Cool, bitter, pungent

Channel-Organ: Lung, Spleen

Actions:
1. Open and disperse the Lung
2. Transform Phlegm to stop cough
3. Settle up-rebellious *Qi* to stop vomiting

Form and Preparation: Powder, decoction, or pill

Dosage:
Horses and Cattle: 15–45 g
Llamas, Alpacas, Goats, Sheep, and Pigs: 5–10 g
Dogs: 2–5 g
Cats and Rabbits: 0.5–1 g
Birds: 0.3–3 g

Cautions and Contraindications: Counteracts Veratrum *Li Lu*

Side Effects: None known

Lepidium *Ting Li Zi* 葶苈子

Original Reference: *Shen Nong Ben Cao Jing* (*Shen Nong's Materia Medica*, 1st century BCE) 神农本草经

Part Used: Seed

Name:
Pharmaceutical: Descurainiae seu Lepidii, Semen
Botanical: Lepidium apetalum; L. virginicum; Descurainia sophia
Common: Lepidium seed
Wade-Giles: *Ting-Li-Tzu*

Energy/Taste: Cold, bitter, pungent

Channel-Organ: Lung, Bladder

Actions:
1. Transform Phlegm to soothe asthma
2. Promote urination to reduce edema
3. Cardiotonic

Form and Preparation: Powder, decoction, or pill

Dosage:
Horses and Cattle: 15–30 g
Llamas, Alpacas, Goats, Sheep, and Pigs: 6–12 g
Dogs: 2–5 g
Cats and Rabbits: 0.5–2 g
Birds: 0.2–2 g

Cautions and Contraindications: Cautioned for Deficiency conditions: Lung *Qi* Deficiency and edema from Spleen *Qi* Deficiency

Side Effects: May cause skin allergy, nausea, restlessness, dypsnea, hypotension

Sargassum *Hai Zao* 海藻

Original Reference: *Shen Nong Ben Cao Jing* (*Shen Nong's Materia Medica*, 1st century BCE) 神农本草经

Part Used: Whole plant

Name:
Pharmaceutical: Sargassii, Herba
Botanical: Sargassum pallidium; S. fusiforme (Hijiki)
Common: Sargassum
Wade-Giles: *Hai-Tsao*
Translation: Sea Algae

Energy/Taste: Cold, salty, slightly bitter

Channel-Organ: Liver, Spleen, Kidney, Lung

Actions:
1. Transform Phlegm and soften hardness
2. Promote water metabolism

Form and Preparation: Powder, decoction, or pill

Dosage:
Horses and Cattle: 15–45 g
Llamas, Alpacas, Goats, Sheep, and Pigs: 3–10 g
Dogs: 2–5 g
Cats and Rabbits: 0.5–1 g
Birds: 0.2–1 g

Cautions and Contraindications:
1. Contraindications with Glycerrhiza *Gan Cao*, according to traditional sources
2. Cautions with Spleen Cold-Damp

Side Effects: None known

Laminaria *Kun Bu* 昆布

Original Reference: *Ming Yi Bie Lu* (*Miscellaneous Records of Famous Physicians*) by *Tao Hong-Jing* and North and South Kingdoms (5th century) 名医别录

Part Used: Whole plant

Name:
Pharmaceutical: Thallus Laminariae
Botanical: Laminaria japonica; Ecklonia kurome (Kelp)
Common: Kelp
Wade-Giles: *K'un-P'u*
Translation: Kun Cloth

Energy/Taste: Cold, salty

Channel-Organ: Kidney, Liver, Stomach

Actions:
1. Transform Phlegm and soften hardness
2. Promote water metabolism

Form and Preparation: Powder, decoction, or pill

Dosage:
Horses and Cattle: 15–45 g
Llamas, Alpacas, Goats, Sheep, and Pigs: 3–10 g
Dogs: 2–5 g
Cats and Rabbits: 0.5–1 g
Birds: 0.2–1 g

Cautions and Contraindications:
Cautioned with Spleen Cold-Damp

Side Effects: None known

Other Comments: Laminaria *Kun Bu* is one of the best agents for treatment of lymphatic swellings. It is usually combined with Sargassum *Hai Zao* for this purpose.

Sterculia *Pang Da Hai* 胖大海

Original Reference: *Ben Caos Gang Mu Shi Yi* (*Supplement to Materia Medica Compendium*) by *Zhao Xue-Min*, 1765

Part Used: Seed

Name:
Pharmaceutical: Semen Sterculiae Scaphigerae
Botanical: Sterculia scaphigera
Common: Sterculia
Wade-Giles: *P'ang-Ta-Hai*
Translation: Fat, Big Sea

Energy/Taste: Cold, sweet

Channel-Organ: Lung, Large Intestine

Actions:
1. Clear Lung Heat and benefit throat
2. Disperse the Lung to release rashes
3. Moisten intestines to move feces

Form and Preparation: Powder, decoction, or Food Therapy. As the Food Therapy, take a single cracked seed and add 1 cup boiling water. In a good seed, the gelatinous seed cover will expand to fill half the cup. Drink the tea as an excellent remedy for laryngitis or tired vocal chords.

Dosage:
Horses and Cattle: 15–45 g
Llamas, Alpacas, Goats, Sheep, and Pigs: 3–10 g
Dogs: 2–5 g
Cats and Rabbits: 0.5–1 g
Birds: 0.2–1 g

Cautions and Contraindications: None

Side Effects: None known

Cyclina *Hai Ge Ke* 海蛤壳

Original Reference: *Shen Nong Ben Cao Jing* (*Shen Nong's Materia Medica*, 1st century BCE) 神农本草经

Part Used: Shell

Name:
Pharmaceutical: Cyclinae Sinensis, Concha
Botanical: Cyclina sinensis; Century meretrix
Common: Clam shell
Wade-Giles: *Hai-Ke-K'e*
Translation: Sea Clam Shell

Energy/Taste: Cold, salty

Channel-Organ: Lung, Stomach, Kidney

Actions:
1. Clear Lung Heat and transform Phlegm
2. Redirect Lung *Qi* downward to stop asthma
3. Soften hardness to release nodules
4. In calcined form, for epigastric pain and acid regurgitation

Form and Preparation: Powder; or crush and boil 15–20 minutes prior to other herbs

Dosage:
Horses and Cattle: 15–45 g
Llamas, Alpacas, Goats, Sheep, and Pigs: 3–10 g
Dogs: 2–6 g
Cats and Rabbits: 0.5–1 g
Birds: 0.2–2 g

Cautions and Contraindications: Contraindicated for *Qi* Deficiency and Cold

Side Effects: None known

HERBS TO RELIEVE COUGH AND ASTHMA

Armeniaca *Xing Ren* 杏仁

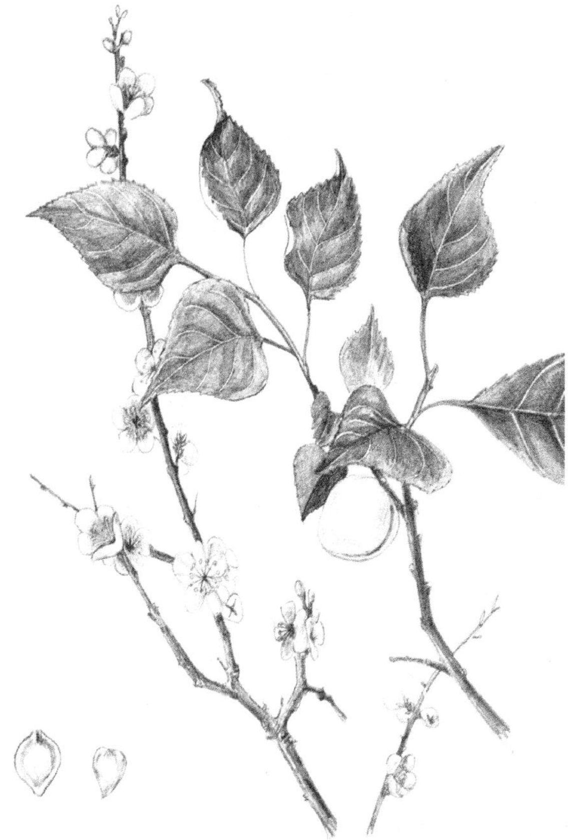

Original Reference: *Shen Nong Ben Cao Jing* (*Shen Nong's Materia Medica*, 1st century BCE) 神农本草经

Part Used: Seed

Name:
Pharmaceutical: Pruni Armeniacae, Semen
Botanical: Prunus armeniaca; P. mandshurica; P. sibirica (Apricot seed)
Common: Apricot seed
Wade-Giles: *Hsing-Jen*
Translation: Apricot Seed

Energy/Taste: Slightly toxic, slightly warm, bitter, sweet

Channel-Organ: Lung, Large Intestine

Actions:
1. Stop cough and relieve asthma
2. Moisten the Intestine to move feces

Form and Preparation: Powder, decoction, or pill

Dosage:
Horses and Cattle: 25–45 g
Camels: 30–60 g
Llamas, Alpacas, Goats, Sheep, and Pigs: 3–15 g
Dogs: 2–8 g
Cats and Rabbits: 0.5–1 g
Birds: 0.2–1 g

Cautions and Contraindications:
1. Prohibited in infants and pediatric patients
2. Caution in coughs due to Deficiency of *Yin*, and diarrhea
3. May antagonize Astragalus *Huang Qi*, Scutellaria *Huang Qin*, and Pueraria *Ge Gen*

Side Effects: It is slightly toxic. Do not use *Ku Xing Ren* in excessive dosages, because it can injure bones and tendons, Liver, and Kidney, as well as inhibit Heart and Lung function. *Tian Xing Ren* is safe.

Clinical Application
1. Cough or asthma
   Combine with: Perilla *Zi Su Ye*
   Classical herbal formula: Ren Shen Ge Jie San
2. Constipation due to dryness in the intestines
   Combine with: Cannabis *Huo Ma Ren* and Angelica *Dang Gui*

History and Comments
1. During the three-kingdom days (AD 221–263), Dong Fong lived on a mountain called *Lu Shan*. This doctor had an illustrious reputation and used his superior medical skills to treat patients at no charge. Rather than accepting payment, Dong Fong let his appreciative patients plant a *Xing* (apricot) tree around his house instead. After several years, there were more than ten thousand apricot trees around the doctor's house, and the area was known as *Dong Xian Xing Ling* (Dr. Dong's Apricot Forest). When the apricots matured, Dr. Dong traded these fruits for rice to help poor people and also kept the seeds of apricots to treat cough or asthma patients without any payment. Since this time, doctors who perform meritoriously are awarded the special name "Apricot Forest" in appreciation for their excellent work.

   One day a tiger came to Dr. Dong's house to ask for help. Dr. Dong carefully examined the tiger. He found a fish bone stuck in the tiger's throat and he risked his life to remove the fish bone. In return for Dr. Dong's help, the tiger became Dr. Dong's "Housekeeper" and "Apricot Forest Keeper" for the rest of his life. Today one can usually find a scroll hanging in the herbal pharmacy lobby that reads: "tiger protects apricot forest."
2. Bitter Armeniaca (*Ku Xing Ren* or *Bei Xing Ren*) is used most often, especially for Heat conditions. This herb comes from the wild plant. When *Xing Ren* is unspecified in a prescription, *Ku Xing Ren* is given, rather than *Tian Xing Ren*.
3. Sweet Armeniaca (*Tian Xing Ren* or *Nan Xing Ren*) can substitute for Bitter Armeniaca. Sweet Armeniaca comes from the cultivated apricot tree and is not considered toxic. These seeds are often used in cooking. This herb is better suited for dry coughing due to *Yin* Deficiency without Heat.

Pharmaceutical Ingredients:[1–4]
1. Fatty acid
2. Amygdalin, amygdalase, emuisin, prunase, hydroxynitrile lyase, amygdalase, punnase
3. Cholesterol, estrone, α-estradiol
4. Hydrocyanic acid, benzaldehyde

Research and Clinical Study
1. Armeniaca *Xing Ren* relaxes chest muscles and muscles in the bronchioles, during spasmodic coughing or labored breathing.
2. Recent Chinese research shows *Xing Ren* to be useful in the treatment of various carcinomas.

Perilla *Su Zi* 苏子

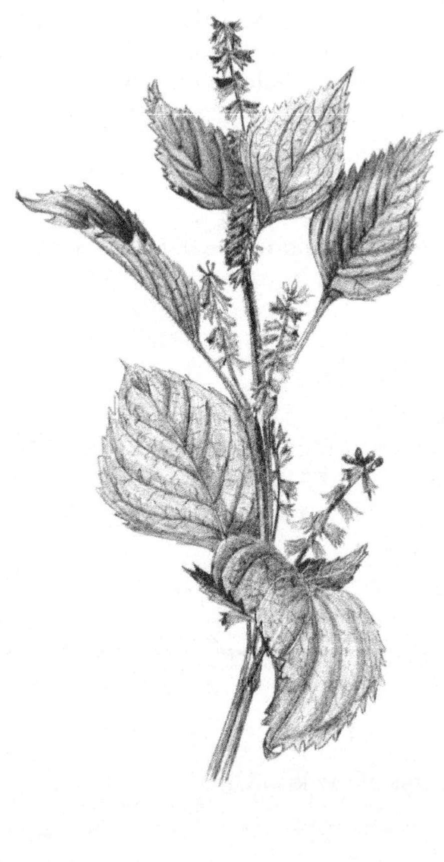

Original Reference: *Ming Yi Bie Lu* (*Miscellaneous Records of Famous Physicians*) by *Tao Hong-Jing*, North and South Kingdoms (5th century) 名医别录

Part Used: Seed

Name:
Pharmaceutical: Perillae Fructescentis, Fructus
Botanical: Perilla fructescens
Common: Perilla leaf
Wade-Giles: *T'se-Su-Ts'e*
Translation: Purple seed

Energy/Taste: Warm, pungent

Channel-Organ: Lung, Large Intestine

Actions:
1. Stop cough and asthma
2. Moisten the Intestines to move feces
3. Redirect the Lung *Qi* downward

Form and Preparation: Powder, decoction, or pill; the essential oil is important for the herb's action, so Perilla seed should not be overcooked.

Dosage:
Horses and Cattle: 15–60 g
Camels: 20–80 g
Llamas, Alpacas, Goats, Sheep, and Pigs: 3–10 g
Dogs: 2–8 g
Cats and Rabbits: 0.5–1 g
Birds: 0.2–1.5 g

Cautions and Contraindications: Cautioned in asthma and cough due to Deficiency of *Qi*

Side Effects: May cause diarrhea

Clinical Application
1. Asthma or cough
   Combine with: Rhaphanus *Lai Fu Zi* and Sinapis *Bai Jie Zi*
   Classical herbal formula: *Su Zi Jiang Qi Tang*
2. Constipation due to dryness in intestine
   Combine with: Cannabis *Huo Ma Ren*, Trichosanthes *Gua Lou Ren*, and Armeniaca *Xing Ren*

History and Comments Perilla *Zi Su Zi* is often called *Su Zi*. Its leaf is called *Zi Su Ye* or *Su Ye*. *Su Zi* is good at stopping cough and asthma; *Su Ye* is often used for colds due to Wind Cold, or nausea and vomiting.

Pharmaceutical Ingredients:[1–4]
1. Fatty acid, linoleic acid, betulinic acid
2. Flavonoids (morusin, mulberrin, mulberrochromene, cyclomulberrin, cyclomuberrochromene, mulberrofuran A, kuwanon A,B, kuwanon D, kuwanon E, kuwanon F, kuwanon H, saggenon A, sanggenon B, morusin A,B,C,D)
3. α-amyrin, β-amyrin, β-sitosterol, stigmasterol, undecaprenol, dodecaprenol
4. Tannins, vitamin B

Morus *Sang Bai Pi* 桑白皮

Original Reference: *Shen Nong Ben Cao Jing* (*Shen Nong's Materia Medica*, 1st century BCE) 神农本草经

Part Used: Cortex of the root (Root bark)

Name:
Pharmaceutical: Mori Albae Radicis, Cortex
Botanical: Morus alba
Common: Mulberry root bark
Wade-Giles: *Sang-Pai-P'i*
Translation: White Mulberry Bark

Energy/Taste: Cold, sweet

Channel-Organ: Lung, Spleen

Actions:
1. Clear Lung Heat
2. Soothe asthma and stop cough
3. Promote urination to reduce edema

Form and Preparation: Powder, decoction, or pill

Dosage:
Horses and Cattle: 15–45 g
Llamas, Alpacas, Goats, Sheep, and Pigs: 3–10 g
Dogs: 2–5 g
Cats and Rabbits: 0.5–1 g
Birds: 0.2–1.5 g

Cautions and Contraindications: It is cautioned for asthma and cough due to Cold or Wind-Cold in Lung

Side Effects: May cause excessive urination.

Stemona *Bai Bu* 百布

Original Reference: *Ming Yi Bie Lu* (*Miscellaneous Records of Famous Physicians*) by *Tao Hong-Jing*, North and South Kingdoms (5th century) 名医别录

Part Used: Root

Name:
Pharmaceutical: Stemonae, Radix
Botanical: Stemona sessilifolia; S. japonica; S. tuberosa
Common: Stemona root
Wade-Giles: *Pai-Pu*
Translation: Hundred Units

Energy/Taste: Slightly warm, sweet, bitter

Channel-Organ: Lung

Actions:
1. Moisten Lung and stop cough
2. Eliminate lice and worms

Form and Preparation: Powder, decoction, or pill

Dosage:
Horses and Cattle: 15–30 g
Llamas, Alpacas, Goats, Sheep, and Pigs: 5–12 g
Dogs: 2–5 g
Cats and Rabbits: 0.5–2 g

Cautions and Contraindications: Caution for Spleen Deficiency

Side Effects: May cause diarrhea

Tussilago *Kuan Dong Hua* 款冬花

Original Reference: *Shen Nong Ben Cao Jing* (*Shen Nong's Materia Medica*, 1st century BCE) 神农本草经

Part Used: Flower

Name:
Pharmaceutical: Tussilaginis Farfarae, Flos
Botanical: Tussilago Farfara (Coltsfoot)
Common: Farfara, coltsfoot
Wade-Giles: *K'uan-Tung-Hua*
Translation: Welcome-Winter Flower

Energy/Taste: Warm, pungent, sweet

Channel-Organ: Lung

Actions:
1. Transform Phlegm to stop cough
2. Moisten the Lung
3. Descend Lung *Qi*

Form and Preparation: Powder, decoction, or pill

Dosage:
Horses and Cattle: 15–45 g
Camels: 30–60 g
Llamas, Alpacas, Goats, Sheep, and Pigs: 3–10 g
Dogs: 2–5 g
Cats and Rabbits: 0.5–1 g
Birds: 0.2–1.5 g

Cautions and Contraindications: Caution for Lung Heat due to Deficiency of *Yin*

Side Effects: None known

Aster *Zi Wan* 紫菀

Original Reference: *Shen Nong Ben Cao Jing* (*Shen Nong's Materia Medica*, 1st century BCE) 神农本草经

Part Used: Root and rhizome

Name:
Pharmaceutical: Asteris Tatarici, Radix et Rhizoma
Botanical: Aster
Common: Aster
Wade-Giles: *T'se-Wan*
Translation: Purple root

Energy/Taste: Slightly Warm, bitter, sweet, pungent

Channel-Organ: Lung

Actions:
1. Transform Phlegm to stop cough
2. Warms the Lung

Form and Preparation: Powder, decoction, or pill

Dosage:
Large dosage or long-term use is *not* recommended.
Horses and Cattle: 15–45 g
Camels: 24–60 g
Llamas, Alpacas, Goats, Sheep, and Pigs: 3–6 g
Dogs: 2–5 g
Cats and Rabbits: 0.5–1 g
Birds: 0.2–1 g

Cautions and Contraindications:
1. Caution in Heat Pattern or *Yin* Deficiency with Heat signs
2. May counteract Artemisia *Yin Chen Hao*

Side Effects: None known

Eriobotrya *Pi Pa Ye* 枇杷叶

Original Reference: *Ming Yi Bie Lu* (*Miscellaneous Records of Famous Physicians*) by *Tao Hong-Jing*, North and South Kingdoms (5th century) 名医别录

Part Used: Leaf

Name:
Pharmaceutical: Eriobotryae Japonicae, Folium
Botanical: Eriobotrya japonica
Common: Loquat leaf
Wade-Giles: *P'i-P'a-Yeh*
Translation: Loquat leaf

Energy/Taste: Slightly cool, bitter

Channel-Organ: Lung, Stomach

Actions:
1. Transform Phlegm to stop cough
2. Clear Lung Heat
3. Harmonize the Stomach to stop nausea
4. Clears Stomach Heat

Form and Preparation: Powder, decoction, or pill; toast in honey prior to decoction to increase moistening effect and to remove hairs on leaf, which can irritate the throat.

Dosage:
Horses and Cattle: 30–60 g
Llamas, Alpacas, Goats, Sheep, and Pigs: 5–20 g
Dogs: 1–5 g
Cats and Rabbits: 0.5–1 g
Birds. 0.2–2 g

Cautions and Contraindications: Caution for vomiting due to Stomach Cold

Side Effects: If it is processed incorrectly (the fine hairs not removed), this may result in itchy throat and dry cough and, if severe, may cause edematous swelling of the throat.

Aristolochia *Ma Dou Ling* 马兜铃

Original Reference: Yao Xing Lun (*Discussion of Medicinal Properties*) by *Chen Zhou*, 19th century, 药性论

Part Used: Fruit

Name:
Pharmaceutical: Aristolochiae, Fructus
Botanical: Aristolochia contorta; A. debilis
Common: Birthwort fruit
Wade-Giles: *Ma-Tou-Ling*
Translation: Horse's Hat Bell

Energy/Taste: Cool, bitter, pungent, toxic

Channel-Organ: Lung, Large Intestine

Actions:
1. Clear the Lung and transform Phlegm
2. Stop cough and soothe asthma

Form and Preparation: Powder, decoction, or pill

Dosage:
Horses and Cattle: 15–30 g
Goats and pigs: 3–10 g

Cautions and Contraindications:
1. Caution for cough due to Cold or Deficiency
2. Caution for Diarrhea
3. Caution in pregnancy

Side Effects: Overdosage causes nausea and vomiting, dyspnea, and nephritis. Its aristolochic acid can lead to nephropathy.

SUMMARY

Table 3.4 summarizes and compares the herbs that transform Phlegm and relieve cough and asthma.

REFERENCES

1. Chen JK, Chen TT. Chinese Medical Herbology and Pharmacology. City of Industry, CA: Art of Medicine Press, 2004.
2. Brinker FJ. The Toxicology of Botanical Medicines. Sandy, OR: Eclectic Medical Publications, 2000.
3. Duke JA. Handbook of Medicinal Herbs. New York: Chemical and Rubber Company Press, 2001.
4. Huang KC. The Pharmacology of Chinese Herbs, 2nd Edition. New York: Chemical and Rubber Company Press, 1999.

Table 3.4. Herbs to transform Phlegm and to relieve cough and asthma: A quick overview and comparison.

Herbs	Special Actions	Common Characteristics
Herbs to Transform Phlegm-Damp		Taste: Pungent, bitter Energy: Warm and dry Action: Warm Lung and dispel Cold Dry Damp and transform Phlegm Indication: Cold/Damp Phlegm Clinical Signs: Productive cough, nodules, wet and pale tongue
Ban Xia	#1 to transform Damp-Phlegm, dissipate nodules Strengthen Stomach and Spleen, stop vomiting	
Jie Geng	Open (disperse) the Lung *Qi* Direct other herbs to upper regions of the body	
Bai Jie Zi	Move *Qi* and dissipate nodule Unblock the Channels and relieve pain	
Tian Nan Xing	**Toxic**, dispel Wind-Phlegm and stop spasm Reduce swelling and alleviate pain in trauma	
Dan Nan Xing	**Toxic**, clear Heat and transform Phlegm	
Xuan Fu Hua	Conduct rebellious *Qi* downward, stop vomiting	
Bai Qian	Conduct rebellious *Qi* downward to stop cough	
Zao Jiao	Open the orifices, eliminate Wind	
Bai Fu Zi	**Toxic**, dispel Wind and stop spasm	
Herbs to Transform Phlegm-Heat		Taste: Moisture and salty Energy: Cool or Cold Action: Clear Heat and transform Phlegm Indication: Heat Phlegm Clinical Signs: Dry cough, seizure, masses
Chuan Bei Mu	Moisten the Lung to treat chronic dry cough	
Zhe Bei Mu	#1 to transform Heat-Phlegm, dissipate nodule	
Gua Lou	Moisten intestines to move stool	
Zhu Ru	Relieve irritability and stop vomiting	
Zhu Li	Stop epilepsy and clear Summer Heat	
Tian Zhu Huang	Clear Heat from the Heart, and stop convulsions, especially infant seizures	
Qian Hu	Open and disperse the Lung, stop vomiting	
Tian Hua Fen	Promote body fluid, reduce swelling	
Ting Li Zi	Promote urination to reduce edema	
Hai Zao	Soften hardness, promote water metabolism	
Kun Bu	Soften hardness, promote water metabolism	
Pang Da Hai	Benefit throat, moisten intestines to move feces	
Hai Ge Ke	Stop asthma, soften hardness to release nodules In calcined form, stop acid regurgitation	
Herbs to Relieve Cough and Asthma		Taste: Pungent, bitter, or sweet Energy: Warm or Cold Action: Relieve cough and stop cough Indication: Symptoms of cough or asthma
Xing Ren	Moisten the Intestine to move feces	
Su Zi	Redirect *Qi* downward, moisten the intestines	
Sang Bai Pi	Clear Lung Heat, reduce edema	
Bai Bu	Eliminate lice and worms	
Kuan Dong Hua	Moisten the Lung, descend Lung *Qi*	
Zi Wan	Warm the Lung and transform Phlegm	
Pi Pa Ye	Clear Lung or Stomach Heat, stop nausea	
Ma Dou Ling	Clear the Lung and transform Phlegm	

4 Herbs to Clear Heat 清热药

Huisheng Xie, Dayou Shi, Min Su Kim

This chapter focuses on the Traditional Chinese Veterinary Medicine (TCVM) therapy principle "cool what is hot" to clear Internal Heat by using cold or cool energy herbs. As expected, herbs to clear Heat are primarily used to treat Heat Pattern or other diseases associated with Heat. In TCVM, Heat has two major meanings. First, Heat may refer to fever, which is elevated body temperature. Second, Heat may be related to Heat Pattern (Table 4.1) in which the patient's temperature is approximately normal, but the patient may have "Heat-related" signs such as dry mouth, dry throat, warm ears, red eyes, constipation, concentrated urine, skin redness, a red tongue with a yellow coating, and rapid pulse.

Heat Patterns are then further divided into Exterior Heat and Interior Heat based on the affected body areas (Table 4.1). Exterior Heat Pattern causes symptoms such as nasal congestion and discharge, sore throat, fever with aversion to cold, and superficial (floating) pulse. Herbs to release Exterior Heat, including Mentha *Bo He* and Chrysanthemum *Ju Hua*, are discussed in Chapter 2. Interior Heat Pattern symptoms include fever without aversion to cold, thirst, irritability, bitter taste in the mouth, rapid respiration, concentrated urination, constipation, bloated abdomen, yellow coating on tongue, strong pulse, coma, insanity, or manic attacks. Interior Heat Pattern can be further divided into Excess and Deficiency Patterns. Excess Heat includes *Qi* level, Blood level, Summer Heat, Damp-Heat and Heat Toxin (Table 4.2).

HERBS TO CLEAR HEAT AND DRAIN FIRE

Herbs to clear Heat and Drain Fire are very cold. They are often used to treat *Qi* level Heat and the *Yang-ming* stage fever whose clinical signs include high fever, sweating, irritability, thirst, and forceful pulse. These herbs are also used to treat Internal organ Heat, including Liver Heat, Stomach Heat, Lung Heat, Heart Heat, and Wind Heat in the eyes. Due to their cold nature, herbs to clear Heat and drain Fire are contraindicated for Cold or *Yang* Deficiency and Spleen *Qi* Deficiency.

Gypsum *Shi Gao* 石膏

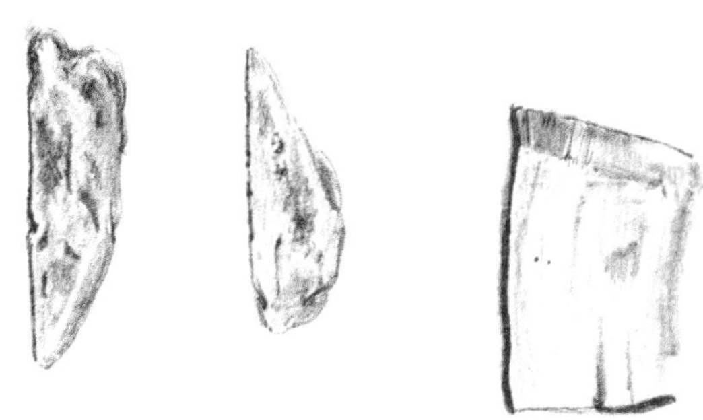

Original Reference: *Shen Nong Ben Cao Jing* (*Shen Nong's Materia Medica*, 1st century BCE) 神农本草经

Part Used: Mineral (main ingredient: $CaSO_3$)

Name:
Pharmaceutical: Gypsum Fibrosum(Calcium Sulphate)
Common: Calcium Sulphate
Wade-Giles: *Shih-Kao*
Translation: Rocky Cream or Stone Paste

Table 4.1. Differentiation of Exterior Heat and Interior Heat.

General Signs of Heat Pattern	Heat in Exterior (Due to Exogenous Wind-Heat)	Heat in the Interior
Red eyes	Acute onset	Fever without chills
Cool-seeking	Fever with chills	Dry mouth and thirst
Warm ears	Nasal discharge or congestion	Irritability
Dry throat or dry stools	Headache and body aching	Scanty and dark urine
Dark scanty urine	Moderate sweating	Constipation or diarrhea
Rapid pulse	Superficial rapid pulse	Red tongue
		Rapid deep pulse

Table 4.2. Summary of Interior Heat Patterns.

Nature	8 Principles	Subgroup	Manifestation	Examples of Herbs
Interior Heat	Excessive	*Qi* Level	Fever, dry mouth	Gypsum *Shi Gao*
		Blood Level	Mental disorder, bleeding	Scrophularia *Xuan Shen*
		Summer Heat	Fever, profuse sweat or nonsweat	Mosla *Xiang Ru*
		Damp-heat	Fever, heavy body, loose stool or diarrhea	Coptis *Huang Lian*
		Heat Toxin	Infectious or virus condition	Lonicera *Jin Yin Hua*
	Deficiency	False Heat	Dry mouth/throat, lower-grade fever	Artemisia *Qing Hao*

Energy/Taste: Very cold, pungent, sweet

Channel-Organ: Lung, Stomach, and Triple Burners (*San Jiao*)

Actions:
1. Clear Heat, drain Fire
2. Clear Heat from the Lung
3. Clear Heat from the Stomach and alleviate thirst

Form and Preparation: Crush into powder; cook 15–20 minutes prior to other herbs. Gypsum *Shi Gao* is sold "raw" or "cooked." The raw form (*Sheng Shi Gao*) is used orally and has actions as described above. Cooked Gypsum (*Shu Shi Gao*) is applied externally to treat inflammation.

Dosage:
Horses and Cattle: 30–120g
Camels: 90–180g
Llamas, Alpacas, Goats, Sheep, and Pigs: 10–30g
Dogs: 2–5g
Cats and Rabbits: 1–2g
Birds: 0.3–3g

Cautions and Contraindications: Caution for Deficiency of Stomach and Spleen or Internal Heat due to *Yin* Deficiency

Side Effects: Overdosage may cause diarrhea.

Clinical Applications:
1. Excess Heat in *Qi* level due to exogenous invasion
   Clinical signs: High fever, intensive thirst, irritability, profuse sweating, red tongue, full pulse
   Combine with: Anemarrhena *Zhi Mu*
   Classical herbal formula: *Bai Hu Tang*
2. Asthma and cough due to Lung Heat
   Combine with: Ephedra *Ma Huang* and Armeniaca *Xing Ren*
   Classical herbal formula: *Ma Xing Shi Gan Tang*
3. Flaring of Stomach Fire
   Clinical signs: Toothache, swollen and painful gums, headache
   Combine with: Rehmannia *Sheng Di Huang*, and Anemarrhena *Zhi Mu*
   Classical herbal formula: *Yu Nü Jian*
4. Infected boils and carbuncles that have opened, nonulcerated sores, burns, or Heat eczema

Combine with (Internally): Isatis *Da Qing Ye* and Phellodendron *Huang Bai; or can be applied externally* (cooked Gypsum *Shi Gao*)

History and Comments:

1. Long ago in ancient China, the mountain named *Tian Ling Shan* was covered with many trees and surrounded by thick mist. An industrious and kind-hearted child lived at the base of *Tian Ling Shan*. He would chop wood in the mountain forests. When he was 14 years old, his parents died. The boy did not have money to buy a coffin, so he had to bury his parents in a nearby mountain cave. For 3 years he mourned for his parents. One day, during his visit to his parents' grave, the young man suffered from a toothache and swollen gums. He saw white light deeper in the cave. The young man followed the light and found a long white mass, which he tasted. The mass was tasty, so he cut it into many small pieces and ate it happily. Surprisingly, the pain in his teeth and gums subsided. The young man called this mass *Shi Gao* (rocky cream) and used it for the treatment of stomatitis and gingivitis.
2. When published in 1918, Zhang Xi Chun's herbal book *Yi Xue Zhong Zhong Can Xi Lu* (*Records of Heartfelt Experiences in Medicine with Reference to the West*) documented using *Shi Gao* in combination with aspirin. Since its introduction to the market in 1899 under the trademark Aspirin®, acetylsalicylic acid has attained a leading position worldwide as an over-the-counter (OTC) medication for pain, inflammation, and fever.
3. *Shi Gao* is the coldest substance in the materia medica. Gypsum is found in drywall and in the sand at White Sands National Monument. Gypsum *Shi Gao* counters the diaphoretic effects of Ephedra *Ma Huang* and helps activate its diuretic effects.
4. If taken for an extended period, Gypsum *Shi Gao* may excessively cool the Stomach and Spleen. Thus, warming digestive aids should be included in the formula if the herbal treatment has prolonged use.
5. Gypsum *Shi Gao* is sold as whole mineral or powder, but only the powder can be extracted in teas.
6. Dehydrated Gypsum (*Duan Shi Gao*) is generally used for abscesses, burns, and eczema.

Pharmaceutical Ingredients:[1–4]

1. $CaSO_4 + 2H_2O$, CaO, SO_3, H_2O
2. Al, Ti, Cu, Fe, Mn, Zn, Cu, Si, Ag, Pb
3. Zn, Co, Cr, Ni

Anemarrhena *Zhi Mu* 知母

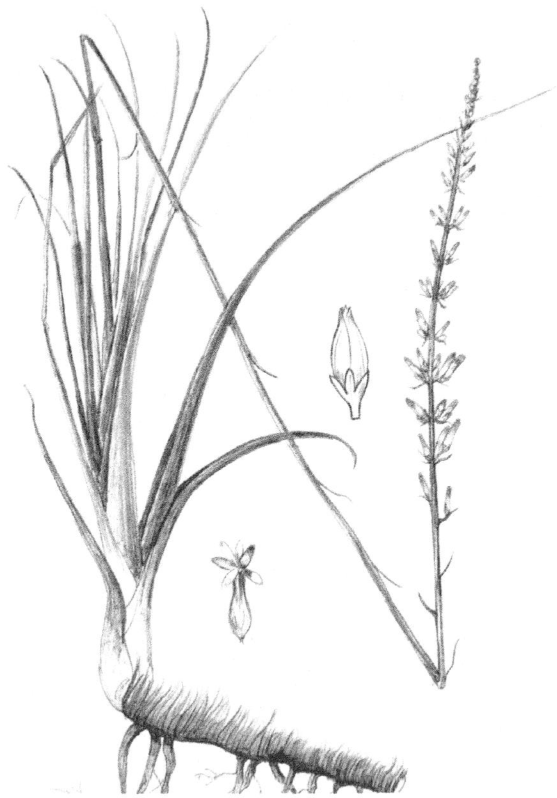

Original Reference: *Shen Nong Ben Cao Jing* (*Shen Nong's Materia Medica*, 1st century BCE) 神农本草经

Part Used: Rhizome

Name:
Pharmaceutical: Anemarrhenae Asphodeloidis, Rhizoma
Botanical: Anemarrhena asphodeloides
Common: Anemarrhena
Wade-Giles: *Chih-Mu*
Translation: Understanding the Mother

Energy/Taste: Cold, bitter, sweet

Channel-Organ: Lung, Stomach, Kidney

Actions:

1. Clear Heat and drain Fire
2. Nourish *Yin* and moisten dryness

Form and Preparation: Powder or decoction

Dosage:
Horses and Cattle: 20–60 g
Camels: 45–100 g

Llamas, Alpacas, Goats, Sheep, and Pigs: 5–15 g
Dogs: 2–8 g
Cats and Rabbits: 0.5–2 g
Birds: 0.2–2 g

Cautions and Contraindications: Contraindications for Spleen Deficiency with diarrhea

Side Effects: High doses may cause loose stool.

Clinical Applications:

1. Excessive Heat in the *Qi* level
   Clinical signs: High fever, irritability, thirst, profuse sweating, red tongue, full pulse
   Combine with: Gypsum *Shi Gao*
   Classical herbal formula: *Bai Hu Tang*
2. Excessive Heat in Stomach, or Stomach *Yin* Deficiency
   Clinical signs: Stomach ulcer, toothache, swollen and painful gums
   Combine with: Ophiopogon *Mai Men Dong*, Coptis *Huang Lian*
   Classical herbal formula: *Yu Nü Jian*
3. Lung and Kidney *Yin* Deficiency with Heat
   Clinical signs: Afternoon fever, night sweats, menopausal hot flashing, Heat in palms and soles
   Combine with: Phellodendron *Huang Bai*, or Testudinis *Gui Ban*
   Classical herbal formula: *Zhi Bai Di Huang Wan*

History and Comments:

1. Once upon a time, there was an old lady who had made her living by collecting medicinal herbs. She had been doing this work since she was a young woman and was now an expert. Because she had no children or apprentices, she was worried that her skill of identifying herbal medicines would be lost when she died. She decided to select a young man and adopt him as her son so he could inherit her skills. With this plan in mind, the old lady went to a village and explained her intent to the villagers. The news spread quickly.

   A rich man found her, took her to his house, and treated her very well. He wanted to get her secrets about identifying valuable herbs, but after a few days, the old lady had still told him nothing. When he realized the old lady wouldn't teach him the skill for a few more years, the impatient rich man became very angry and told the old lady to go away. The old woman again wandered the streets until a merchant found her and told her that he wanted to be her son. Actually, the merchant just wanted to make money by acquiring her skills. He took the old lady to his home and treated her well, but after a month, the lady had still not mentioned a word about the herbal identification skills. The merchant drove her out. Once again on the streets, the old lady kept begging and talking about her plan. Many people regarded her as a crazy woman.

   One cold winter day, she fainted in front of a woodsman's house. The woodsman took her inside and asked his wife to make a meal for the old lady. After finishing the meal, the old lady wanted to leave, but the couple convinced her to stay with them. The old lady thought for a while and agreed. The time flew, and spring soon arrived. The old lady told the woodsman she wanted to leave since she couldn't do anything for them and felt she was a burden. The woodsman was worried about the old woman's safety, so he begged her to stay. He said he would like to regard her as his mother. Hearing the words, the old lady wept.

   Suddenly one summer day, the old lady asked the woodsman to take her to the mountain. Though he didn't know why, he did whatever she asked. When they came to a grassy area, the old lady sat on a stone and pointed to a bunch of leaves with some purple stripes on its flowers. She asked the woodsman to dig out its root, and he obeyed. When he asked what it was, his adopted mother told him that it is an herb that can cure Lung Heat cough and false fever. Then she asked, "My son, do you know why I didn't teach you the skill to identify the herbs until today?" The woodsman answered, "You wanted to find someone kind and honest." The old lady nodded and said, "You are the only one who understands me. This herb has not been given a name yet, so let's call it *Zhi* (*understand*) *Mu* (*mom*)." From then on, they lived a happy life together. The skill of identifying *Zhi Mu* was passed on to the woodsman and was not lost.
2. Anemarrhena *Zhi Mu* can be fried in saltwater to strengthen its ability to nourish the Kidney and to direct the actions of a whole herbal formula downward.
3. Anemarrhena *Zhi Mu* has proven helpful in reducing blood sugar for diabetics.

Pharmaceutical Ingredients:[1–4]

1. Timosaponins A-I, A-II, A-III, A-IV, B-I, B-II (sarsapogenin, markogenin, neogitogenin)
2. Smilagenin, smilagenin 3-β-d-mannopyranoside
3. Mangiferin (chimonin)
4. Flavonoids (isomangiferin)
5. Anemarn A,B,C,D
6. Alkaloids (choline, nicotinamide), tannic acid, nicotinic acid
7. Fe, Zn, Mu, Cu, Cr, Ni

Gardenia *Zhi Zi* 栀子

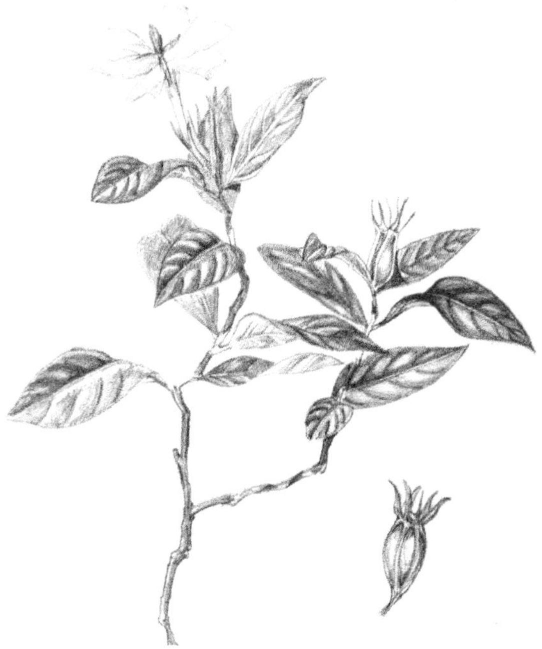

Original Reference: *Shen Nong Ben Cao Jing* (*Shen Nong's Materia Medica*, 1st century BCE) 神农本草经

Part Used: Fruit

Name:
Pharmaceutical: Gardeniae Jasminoidis, Fructus
Botanical: Gardenia jasminoides
Common: Capejasmine
Wade-Giles: *Chih-Tzu*
Translation: Twig Fruit

Energy/Taste: Cold, bitter

Channel-Organ: Liver, Lung, Stomach, Heart, Triple Burner (Triple Heat), Gallbladder

Actions:
1. Drain Fire, eliminate irritability
2. Clear Damp-Heat from the Upper, Middle, and Lower Burners
3. Cool Blood and stop bleeding
4. Move Blood Stasis due to trauma

Form and Preparation: Powder, decoction, or pill; to stop bleeding, charred preparation is required.

Dosage:
Horses and Cattle: 15–60g
Camels: 45–90g
Llamas, Alpacas, Goats, Sheep, and Pigs: 5–10g
Dogs: 2–6g
Cats and Rabbits: 0.5–2g
Birds: 0.2–2g

Cautions and Contraindications: Contraindications for Deficient Spleen with diarrhea or loss of appetite due to Cold from *Yang* Deficiency

Side Effects: None known

Clinical Applications:
1. Excess Heat in whole body
   Clinical signs: High fever, irritability, red tongue, full pulse
   Combine with: Coptis *Huang Lian*, Forsythia *Lian Qiao*, and Scutellaria *Huang Qin*
   Classical herbal formula: *Huang Lian Jie Du Tang*
2. Liver-Gallbladder Damp-Heat causing jaundice with fever
   Combine with: Artemisia *Yin Chen Hao*, Rheum *Da Huang*, and Phellodendron *Huang Bai*
   Classical herbal formula: Yin Chen Hao Tang
3. Liver Heat
   Clinical signs: Red eye, interdigital dermatitis
   Combine with: Paeonia *Bai Shao Yao*
   Classical herbal formula: *Long Dan Xie Gan Tang*
4. Extravasated Blood due to Blood Heat
   Clinical signs: Vomiting of Blood, epistaxis, hematuria
   Combine with: Imperata *Bai Mao Gen*, Rehmannia *Sheng Di Huang*, and Scutellaria *Huang Qin*
5. Bladder Damp-Heat
   Clinical signs: Frequent, painful urination
   Combine with: Dianthus *Qu Mai* and Talcum *Hua Shi*
   Classical herbal formula: *Ba Zheng San*
6. Boils, carbuncles, toxic skin ailments
   Combine with: Coptis *Huang Lian*, Polygonatum *Huang Jing*, Lonicera *Jin Yin Hua*
   Also can apply externally: combine powder with water, or the water decoction
7. Traumatic injury with Heat
   Apply externally: combine powder with egg whites

History and Comments:
1. *Zhi Zi* is the ripe fruit of Gardenia jasminoides Ellis. The fruit acquired its name due to its resemblance to the Chinese character of Zhi, an archaic appliance used to fill wine.
2. *Zhi Zi* is mainly produced in the provinces of *Jiangxi*, *Zhejiang*, and *Hunan*. It is dried in the sunlight after harvesting. This herb may be used without additional preparation or it may be stir-baked until it is brown or turns into charcoal. The stir-baked *Zhi Zi* is often used to treat Blood Heat. The carbonized *Zhi*

Zi is good at stopping bleeding (including hemorrhoids).

3. Gardenia *Zhi Zi* is suitable for treating most Damp Heat conditions and is especially useful for Heat in the pelvic area (including hemorrhoids).

Pharmaceutical Ingredients:[1–4]

1. Iridoidal glycoside (gardenoside, geniposide, jeminoidin, genipin-1-β-D-gentiobioside, shanzhiside, genipin, geniposide acid, gardoside)
2. Chlorogenic acid, gardenin, crocin, crocetin, β-sitosterol, ursolic acid

Research and Clinical Study: Topical application of *Zhi Zi* (fine powder mixed with egg whites) was used for the treatment of 300 cases of non-open traumatic injuries in the soft tissues. After 1 topical treatment, 298 cases were clinically cured.[5]

Prunella *Xia Ku Cao* 夏枯草

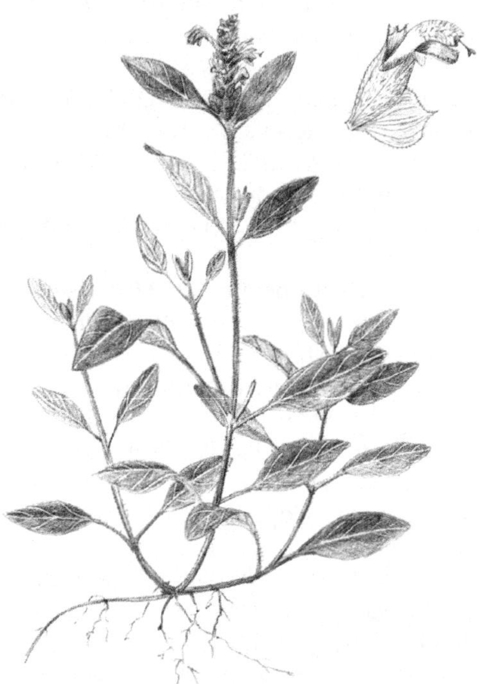

Original Reference: *Shen Nong Ben Cao Jing* (*Shen Nong*'s *Materia Medica*, 1st century BCE) 神农本草经

Part Used: Whole plant above the ground (spike)

Name:
Pharmaceutical: Prunellae Vulgaris, Spica
Botanical: Prunella vulgaris
Common: Prunella
Wade-Giles: *Hsia-K'u-Tsao*
Translation: Summer Dried-up Herb

Energy/Taste: Cold, bitter, pungent

Channel-Organ: Liver, Gallbladder

Actions:

1. Clear Liver Fire and brighten eyes
2. Dissipate nodule and promote urination

Form and Preparation: Powder, decoction, or pill

Dosage:
Horses and Cattle: 15–60 g
Llamas, Alpacas, Goats, Sheep, and Pigs: 5–10 g
Dogs: 2–5 g
Cats and Rabbits: 0.5–2 g
Birds: 0.2–2 g

Cautions and Contraindications: Caution for Deficiency of Spleen and Stomach

Side Effects: Overdose may raise the value of ALT and AST and can be toxic to the Liver.

Clinical Applications:

1. Flaring Liver Fire
   Clinical signs: Red, painful, swollen eyes, headaches, dizziness, hypertension
   Combine with: Haliotis *Shi Jue Ming*, Cyperus *Xiang Fu*, and Chrysanthemum *Ju Hua*
2. Lumps due to accumulation of Phlegm-Fire
   Clinical signs: Masses, nodules, scrophula, swollen lymph glands, mastitis, goiter
   Combine with: Ostrea *Mu Li*, Bupleurum *Chai Hu*, Scrophularia *Xuan Shen*, and Laminaria *Kun Bu*
3. Eye pain *with excessive tearing*
   Combine with: Cyperus *Xiang Fu*
   With pain that increases during night due to Liver Deficiency: combine with Angelica *Dang Gui*, Paeonia *Bai Shao*

History and Comments:

1. Long ago, a literature scholar and writer's mother had tuberculosis, which caused her neck to become swollen and ooze a watery discharge. A doctor told the scholar about an herb on the mountain that could cure his mother. The scholar asked the doctor to make the medicine for his mother. The doctor went to the mountain where he cut the violet spikes from the plants he found. He decocted the spikes and administered the herbal soup to the scholar's mother. After several doses, her illness was cured. She was overjoyed and invited the doctor to stay with them; the doctor accepted. During the day, the doctor would collect medicines and treat

patients, and at night he would stay in the writer's house. After a year the doctor decided to return to his home, but he wanted to demonstrate his appreciation for the scholar's hospitality by sharing his herbal knowledge. The herbalist took the scholar to the mountain where he pointed at some plants with long round leaves and violet flowers. The doctor said, "Study this plant carefully and remember it. This is the medicine that cures tuberculosis. But, remember that this herb disappears after summer." The scholar memorized the plant's appearance.

At the end of summer that year, the county magistrate's mother got tuberculosis. Knowing that he could identify the herb that cured his mother, the scholar told the magistrate he could cure his mother's disease with some herbs. Accepting the scholar's offer, the county magistrate sent some men to accompany the scholar to the mountain. Upon arrival, the scholar searched diligently, but he could not find the herbs. The scholar returned to the County Government Office with the magistrate's men. When the county magistrate heard the report from his men, he called the scholar a liar and punished him severely by beating him on the back 50 times with a board.

The doctor returned the next year. The scholar grabbed the doctor roughly and shouted, "You trapped me!" The puzzled doctor asked what had happened to the scholar. The literature expert explained everything. The doctor realized what had happened and took the scholar back to the mountain. The writer was surprised to find the herbs all over the mountain. The doctor said, "I told you that these herbs will die at the end of the summer. If you wanted them, you had to pick them before the summer ends." Hearing this, the writer suddenly got an idea. His own forgetfulness resulted in a severe beating. To help others remember the lesson, the skillful writer named the herb *Xia* (summer) *Ku* (withered) *Cao* (herb).

2. Protect the aromatic principles contained in Prunella *Xia Ku Cao* by using a short cooking time.
3. Well-preserved Prunella *Xia Ku Cao* has a vibrant purple flower.

Pharmaceutical Ingredients:

1. Triterpenoidal saponin, aglycone (oleanolic acid, ursolic acid)
2. Carotene, camphor, fenchone, hyperin, delphinidin, cyaniding, rosmarinic acid, deucosterol, β-amyrin, rutin, hyperside, caffeic acid, alkaloids
3. Methyl ursolate, methyl oleanolate, methyl 2α, 3α-dihydroxyursen-12-en-28-oate, methyl-2α-hydroxyursoate, methyl 2α, 3α, 28-trihydroxyuena-12-en-28-oate, methyl betulinate
4. 1,8-ieole, β-pinene, myrcene, linalool, α-phellandrene

Phragmites *Lu Gen* 芦根

Original Reference: *Shen Nong Ben Cao Jing* (*Shen Nong*'s *Materia Medica*, 1st century BCE) 神农本草经

Part Used: Rhizome

Name:
Pharmaceutical: Phragmititis Communis, Rhizoma
Botanical: Phragmites communis
Common: Reed grass
Wade-Giles: *Lu-Ken*
Translation: Reed Rhizome

Energy/Taste: Cold, sweet

Channel-Organ: Lung, Stomach

Actions:

1. Clear Heat to relieve irritability
2. Generate Body Fluids to relieve thirst and promote urination
3. Clear Heat from the Lung and Stomach and stop vomiting

Form and Preparation: Powder, decoction, or pill

Dosage:
Horses and Cattle: 30–60 g
Camels: 60–100 g
Llamas, Alpacas, Goats, Sheep, and Pigs: 5–20 g
Dogs: 2–6 g
Cats and Rabbits: 0.5–3 g
Birds: 0.2–2 g

Cautions and Contraindications: Contraindications for Cold and deficient Stomach or Spleen

Side Effects: None known

Lophatherum *Dan Zhu Ye* 淡竹叶

Original Reference: *Shen Nong Ben Cao Jing* (*Shen Nong*'s *Materia Medica*, 1st century BCE) 神农本草经

Part Used: stem and leaf

Name:
Pharmaceutical: Lophatheri Gracilis, Herba
Botanical: Lophatherum gracile
Common name: Lophatheum leaves
Wade-Giles: *Tan-Chu-Yeh*
Translation: Bland Bamboo Leaf

Energy/Taste: Cold, pungent, sweet

Channel-Organ: Heart, Stomach, Small Intestine

Actions:
1. Clear Damp-Heat and benefit urination
2. Clear Heart Heat and lessen irritability

Form and Preparation: Powder, decoction, or pill

Dosage:
Horses and Cattle: 15–45 g
Llamas, Alpacas, Goats, Sheep, and Pigs: 3–15 g
Dogs: 2–5 g
Cats and Rabbits: 0.5–1 g
Birds: 0.2–2 g

Cautions and Contraindications: Do not use in patients with *Yang* Deficiency.

Side Effects: None known

HERBS TO CLEAR HEAT AND COOL BLOOD

Because herbs to clear Heat and cool Blood are often used to treat Blood Heat, they are also called Herbs to Clear Blood Heat. Pathogenic Heat may affect the body at four levels (stages): *Wei*, *Qi*, *Ying*, and *Xue* (Blood). When pathogenic Heat initially invades the body, it lodges in the surface and is considered Heat in the *Wei* Level (Exterior Heat, or Wind Heat). The Heat then migrates into the deep level, *Qi* Stage, which is related to Lung Heat and *Yang*-ming Heat (including Stomach and Large Intestine Heat). The deepest level for Heat to penetrate is the *Xue* (Blood) stage, where it is often called Blood Heat.

The primary clinical signs of Blood Heat include 1) bleeding [nose, gums, Stomach, intestines, or under the skin]; 2) purple, deep red, or dark tongue; 3) skin rashes; 4) vomiting or coughing up Blood; 5) bloody feces or urine; and 5) rapid and thin pulse. Additional signs may include nighttime or low-grade fevers and dry throat. The herbs to clear Blood Heat are cold and may be sweet, salty, and bitter. Some can nourish *Yin* and invigorate the Blood. These herbs cool the Blood and reduce fever. They can also lower the capillary permeability and promote coagulation. These herbs are often combined with other Heat dispersing herbs, astringent herbs, herbs to stop bleeding, or *Yin* tonifying herbs.

Rehmannia *Sheng Di Huang* 生地黄

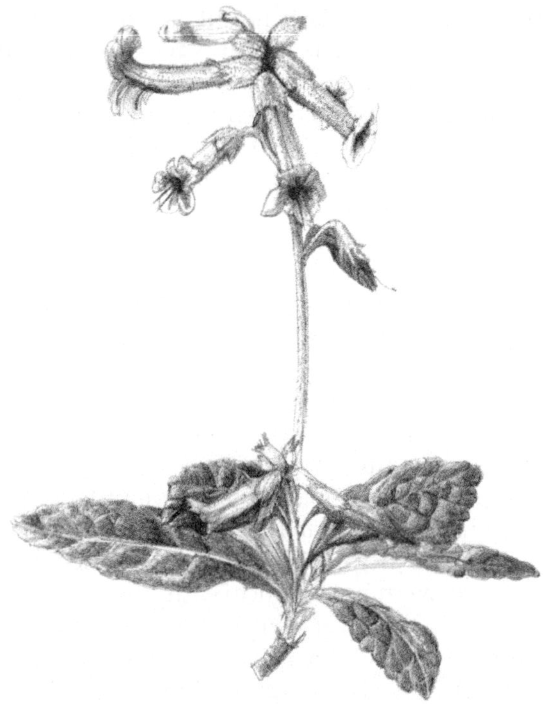

a

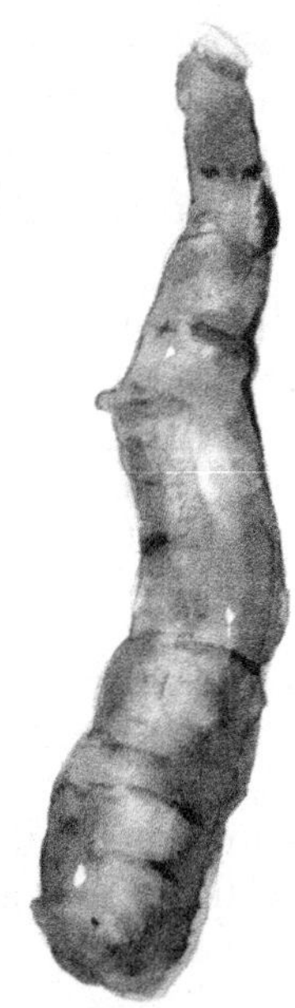

b

Original Reference: *Shen Nong Ben Cao Jing* (*Shen Nong's Materia Medica*, 1st century BCE) 神农本草经

Part Used: Root

Name:
Pharmaceutical: Rehmanniae glutinosae, radix
Botanical: Rehmannia glutinosa
Common: Raw rehmannia

Wade-Giles: *Sheng-Ti-Hwang*
Translation: Raw Earth Yellow

Energy/Taste: Cold, bitter, sweet

Channel-Organ: Heart, Liver, Kidney

Actions:
1. Clear Heat and cool Blood
2. Nourish *Yin* and generate Body Fluids
3. Nourish Kidney *Jing* and tonify Blood

Form and Preparation: Powder, decoction, or pill

Dosage:
Horses and Cattle: 30–60 g
Llamas, Alpacas, Goats, Sheep, and Pigs: 5–15 g
Dogs: 2–6 g
Cats and Rabbits: 0.5–2 g
Birds: 0.2–2 g

Cautions and Contraindications: Cautions for Spleen Deficiency or excessive Dampness or Phlegm

Side Effects: May cause loose stool

Clinical Applications:
1. *Ying* and Xue (Blood) levels invaded by exogenous Heat
   Clinical signs: Red eyes, dry mouth, fever, deep red tongue
   Combine with: Scrophularia *Xuan shen*, Ophiopogon *Mai Men Dong*, and Bubali *Shui Niu Jiao* water buffalo)
   Classical herbal formula: *Qing Ying Tang*
2. Prolonged fever consuming *Yin* and Body Fluids (bone-steaming fever)
   Clinical signs: Panting at night, cool-seeking, fevers, dry throat with thirst, constipation
   Combine with: Anemarrhena *Zhi mu*, Artemisia *Qing Hao*, and Amyda *Bie jia*
   Classical herbal formula: *Xiao Ke Fang*
3. Hemorrhages due to Blood Heat
   Clinical signs: Vomiting of Blood, epistaxis, Blood in urine or stool, uterine bleeding
   Combine with: Cephalanoplos *Xiao Ji*, Biota *Ce Bai Ye* and *Nelumbo He Ye:* or Asinum Gelatinum *E Jiao*
   Classical herbal formula: *Xiao Ji Yin Zi*
4. Deficiency of *Jing*, *Yin*, and Blood
   Clinical signs: Weak lower back and knees, spermatorrhea, deafness or ear-ringing, blurred vision, restless sleep
   Combine with: Cornus *Shan Zhu Yu*
5. False Heat due to *Yin* Deficiency of *Yin* with Heat
   Combine with: Ophiopogon *Mai Men Dong*, Anemarrhena *Zhi Mu*, Phellodendron *Huang Bai*

History and Comments
1. Both Rehmannia *Sheng Di Huang* (*Sheng Di*) and *Shu Di Huang* (*Shu Di*) are from the root of the same plant. *Sheng Di* is raw Rehmannia and *Shu Di* is cooked Rehmannia with wine. It is possible to visually distinguish between raw and cooked Rehmannia by the color. *Shu Di* is blacker, and *Sheng Di* is brown. *Shu Di* also has a greasier, sweet quality. Energetically, *Sheng Di* differs from *Shu Di* in that it is cold. *Sheng Di* is cold and good at clearing Heat conditions and *Shu Di* is warm and good at nourishing Blood. However, these herbs may be substituted for each other when there are shortages.
2. Combine Rehmannia *Sheng Di* with Amomum *Sha Ren* to offset excess sweetness, which can cause nausea and diarrhea.

Pharmaceutical Ingredients:[1–4]
1. Iridoidal glycosides (Catalpol, 6-o-acetylcatapol, aucubin, melittoside, dihydrocatapol, rehmanniosides A,B,C,D)
2. Glutinoside, rehmannans A,B,C
3. Daucosterol, stachyose, amino acid, minenal, β-sitosterol, D-mannitol

Scrophularia *Xuan Shen* (*Yuan Shen*) 玄参

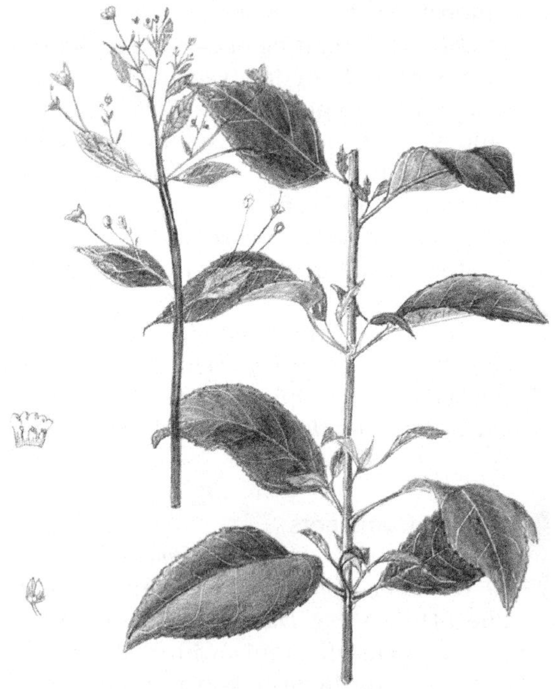

a

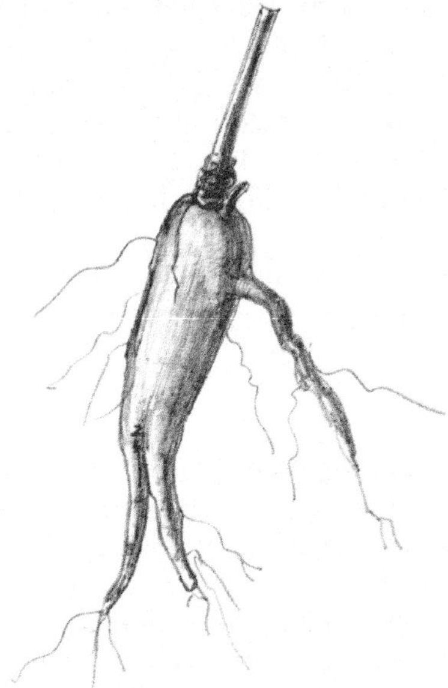

b

Original Reference: *Shen Nong Ben Cao Jing* (*Shen Nong's Materia Medica*, 1st century BCE) 神农本草经

Part Used: Root

Name:
Pharmaceutical: Scrophulariae ningpoensis, radix
Botanical: Scrophularia ningpoenis (figwort)
Common: Scrophularia
Wade-Giles: *Hsuan-Shen*
Translation: dark root
Alternate: *Yuan Shen*

Energy/Taste: Cold, bitter, sweet, salty

Channel-Organ: Lung, Stomach, Kidney

Actions:
1. Clear Heat and cool Blood
2. Nourish *Yin* and release Toxins
3. Soften hardness and dissipate nodules

Form and Preparation: Powder, decoction, or pill

Dosage:
Horses and Cattle: 15–45 g
Camels: 30–60 g
Llamas, Alpacas, Goats, Sheep, and Pigs: 5–15 g
Dogs: 2–5 g
Cats and Rabbits: 0.5–2 g
Birds: 0.2–2 g

Cautions and Contraindications:
1. Cautions For Spleen Deficiency with Damp and diarrhea
2. May antagonize Astragalus *Huang Qi*, Zingiberis *Gan Jiang*, Jujube *Da Zao*, Cornus *Shan Zhu Yu*
3. Is incompatible with Veratrum *Li Lu*

Side Effects: May cause loose stool

Clinical Applications:
1. Heat in *Ying* or Blood levels
   Clinical signs: Fever, thirst, restlessness, severe throat pain and swelling, dry mouth, irritability, or unconsciousness, deep red tongue
   Combine with: Rehmannia *Sheng Di Huang* and Ophiopogon *Mai Men Dong*
   Classical herbal formula: *Qing Ying Tang*
2. *Yin* Deficiency with Heat, or following fever
   Clinical signs: Sore throat, dry throat, dry cough, thirst, Shen disturbance, separation anxiety
   Combine with: Rehmannia *Sheng Di* and Ophiopogon *Mai Men Dong*
   Classical herbal formula: *Er Yin Jian*
3. Sore throat due to Heat
   Combine with: Arctium *Niu Bang Zi*, Platycodon *Jie Geng*, and Mentha *Bo He*
4. Blood Heat causing skin diseases
   Clinical signs: Boils, carbuncles, eruptive red rashes and lesions
   Combine with: Lonicera *Jin Yin Hua*, Moutan *Mu Dan Pi*, and Glycerrhiza *Gan Cao*

5. Mass due to Phlegm
   Signs: Lumps, nodules, scrophula or mass, goiter, swollen lymph glands
   Combine with: Fritillaria *Zhe Bei Mu*, Ostrea *Mu Li*, and Prunella *Xia Ku Cao*
   Classical herbal formula: *Nei Xiao Luo Li San*

History and Comments

1. Scrophularia *Xuan Shen* is the black root, hence called *Hei Xuan Shen*. It is produced chiefly in *Zhejiang* and *Sichuan* provinces and harvested in winter when the aboveground part has withered. The roots are dried in the sunlight until the inside becomes black, and then they are sliced. The herb's main effects are to clear Heat, nourish *Yin*, purge Fire, and remove toxins.
2. Scrophularia *Xuan Shen* can be greasy. Combine it with Amomum *Sha Ren* or Citrus *Chen Pi* to offset cloying.
3. Scrophularia *Xuan Shen* is excellent for tonsillitis and strep throat.
4. Scrophularia *Xuan Shen* can be stir-fried with salt to increase its ability to nourish *Yin*.

Pharmaceutical Ingredients:[1–4]

1. Scrophularin, iridioid, iridoisa, harpagoside
2. 8-(o-methyl-p-coumaroyl)-harpagide
3. Steroids, l-asparagine, oleic acid, linoleic acid, stearic acid

Moutan *Mu Dan Pi* 牡丹皮

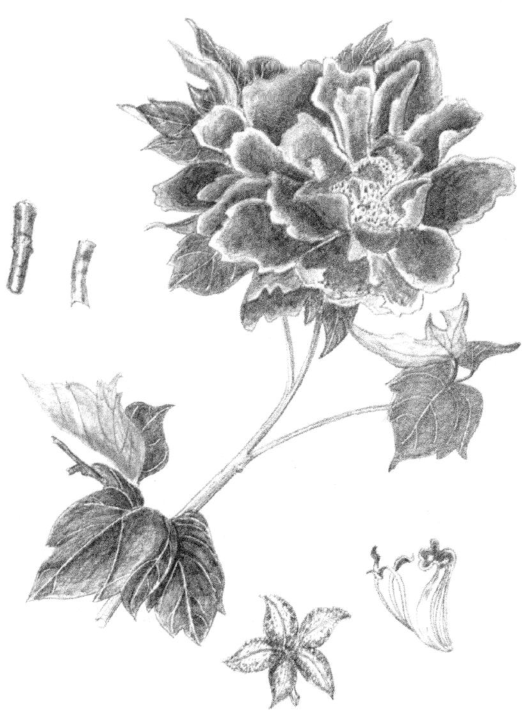

Original Reference: *Shen Nong Ben Cao Jing* (*Shen Nong's Materia Medica*, 1st century BCE) 神农本草经

Part Used: Root bark

Name:
Pharmaceutical: Moutan radicis, cortex
Botanical: Paeonia suffructicosa
Common: Moutan root bark
Wade-Giles: *Mu-Tan-P'i*
Translation: Male Red Bark

Energy/Taste: Slight Cold, bitter, pungent

Channel-Organ: Heart, Liver, Kidney

Actions:

1. Clear Heat and cool Blood
2. Invigorate Blood and resolve Blood Stagnation
3. Clear ascending Liver Fire

Form and Preparation: Powder, decoction, or pill; to stop bleeding, charred herb

Dosage:
Horses and Cattle: 20–45 g
Llamas, Alpacas, Goats, Sheep, and Pigs: 6–12 g
Dogs: 2–6 g
Cats and Rabbits: 0.5–1 g
Birds: 0.2–2 g

Cautions and Contraindications: Cautions during pregnancy or weakness and cold in Spleen; diarrhea

Side Effects: None known

Clinical Applications:

1. Blood level invaded by exogenous Heat
   Clinical signs: Fever, hemorrhage and rash, measles, Blood in urine, vomiting Blood, coughing Blood, deep red tongue
   Combine with: Rehmannia *Sheng Di Huang*, Paeonia *Chi Shao* and Scrophularia *Xuan Shen*
   Classical herbal formula: *Qing Ying Tang*
2. Prolonged fever consuming *Yin* and Body Fluids (bone-steaming fever)
   Clinical signs: Night fevers, fever without sweat, dry throat with thirst, sore throat
   Combine with: Anemarrhena *Zhi Mu*, Artemisia *Qing Hao*, Rehmannia *Sheng Di Huang*, and Testudinus *Gui Ban*

3. Blood Stagnation and pain
   Clinical signs: Internal or External abscess, abdominal masses, lumps or bruises due to traumatic injury
   Combine with: Persica *Tao Ren*, Cinnamomum *Gui Zhi:* Paeonia *Chi Shao* and Poria *Fu Ling*
4. Liver Stagnation with Heat
   Combine with: Paeonia *Bai Shao:* Angelica *Dang Gui and* Chrysanthemum *Ju Hua*
5. Kidney *Yin* Deficiency with Heat
   Combine with: Cornus *Shan Zhu Yu*
   Classical herbal formula: *Liu Wei Di Huang Wan*

History and Comments

1. Over a thousand years ago, a woman named Liu Chun was a well-known weaver of silk fabric. She could create flowers and birds that looked almost real. A rich landlord, who was preparing for his daughter's marriage, requested that Liu Chun weave 24 natural silk quilt blocks inlayed with Moutan flowers. Liu Chun had never seen this flower and did not know how to weave its image into the fabric. Half a month elapsed and Liu Chun still had not woven any flowers. She was so worried that she stopped eating and gradually became emaciated. Working late one night, she became faint and fell down on the loom. At midnight, a red creature shaped like a boy flew to her and poured a bottle of medicinal liquor into Liu Chun's mouth. Liu Chun woke up immediately. The boy told her that he was the moutan fairy. He then gestured outside the window where there were many moutan flowers in full bloom in the court. Staring at the flowers, Liu Chun began to weave. Shortly, Liu Chun wove the moutan flower Pattern into the 24 quilt blocks. As soon as she completed her weaving, all the flowers withered and disappeared; only the moutan root bark remained. This bark was later discovered to be a medicine to cool Blood and clear Heat. Since the red boy led to this discovery, the people called this medicine *Mu* (male) *Dan* (red) *Pi* (bark).
2. Use raw *Mu Dan Pi* for Blood Heat. Stir-bake it for Blood Stagnation. Use the carbonized herb to stop bleeding.
3. Moutan *Mu Dan Pi* is a principle herb in treating gynecological problems associated with Blood Stasis.
4. Moutan *Mu Dan Pi* has antibacterial and antiallergic effect, and also is useful for high blood pressure.

Pharmaceutical Ingredients:[1–4]

1. Paeonol, paeonoside, paeonolide, paeoniflorin, benzoylpaeoniflorin, oxypaeoniflorin, benzoyl-oxypaeoniflorin, apiopaeonoside, benzoylpaeoniflorin
2. Gallic acid, glucopyronose gallates

Lithospermum *Zi Cao* 紫草

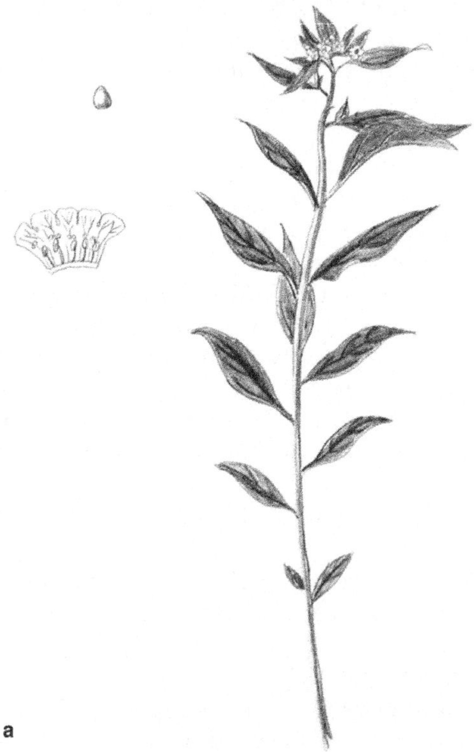

a

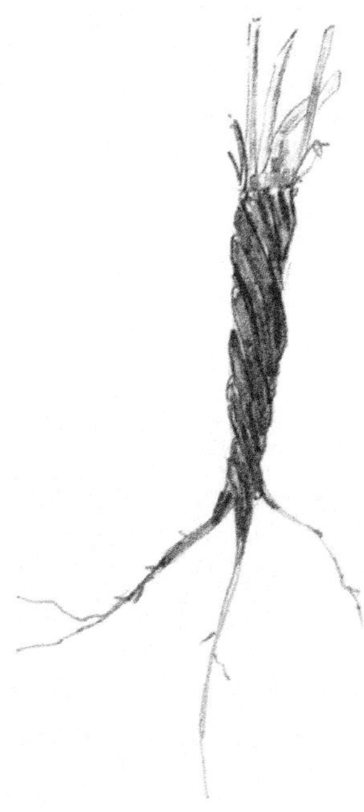

b

Original Reference: *Shen Nong Ben Cao Jing* (*Shen Nong's Materia Medica*, 1st century BCE) 神农本草经

Part Used: Root

Name:
Pharmaceutical: Radix arnebiae seu lithospermi, radix

Botanical: Lithospermum erythrorhizon; arnebia euchroma; macrotomia Euchroma
Common: Lithospermum root
Wade-Giles: *Tzi-Cao*
Translation: Purple Herb

Energy/Taste: Cold, sweet

Channel-Organ: Heart, Liver

Actions:
1. Cool Blood and eliminate toxin
2. Invigorate Blood to relieve rashes and measles
3. Moisten intestines to promote bowel movement

Form and Preparation: Powder, decoction, or pill for oral use; or cream or with oil extract for topical application.

Dosage:
Horses and Cattle: 15–45 g
Camels: 20–60 g
Llamas, Alpacas, Goats, Sheep, and Pigs: 3–10 g
Dogs: 1–5 g
Cats and Rabbits: 0.5–1 g
Birds: 0.2–1.5 g

Cautions and Contraindications:
1. Cautions for cold or deficient Spleen leading to diarrhea
2. Contraindicated for mares trying to get pregnant

Side Effects: It can cause mild diarrhea.

Clinical Applications:
1. Eruption, measles, or chicken pox due to Heat in the Blood Level
   Combine with: Forsythia *Lian Qiao*
   To prevent measles: combine with Glycyrrhiza *Gan Cao*
2. Boils, carbuncles, and skin Heat rashes due to Blood Heat
   Combine with: Isatis *Da Qing Ye*
3. Externally for sore, burns, skin lesions, or vaginal itching
   Combine with: Phellodendron *Huang Bai*
4. Constipation due to Heat in the Blood Level

History and Comments
1. Red lithospermum is used as the base for burn ointments.
2. Long, long ago, two lovers lived in a small town. Sadly, the boy suddenly fell ill and lay unconscious in his bed. The girl, searching for help, kneeled down before a Buddha statue every day. She prayed so often that Buddha would cure the boy that her knees grew calluses. The Buddha was moved to pity for the girl and asked her if she would willingly give her life to cure the boy. The girl agreed without hesitation. Buddha gave the girl an herb and said, "Each day you must water this herb with your own Blood. When the herb blooms with a purple flower, dig up the root and decoct it into a soup for your lover to drink. He will be cured." Happy to have a remedy for her boyfriend, she cut her wrist every day and irrigated the herb with her Blood. She cared for the plant lovingly and hoped it would bloom quickly. One summer day, the girl gasped when she saw purple flowers on the herb. Excitedly, she dug out the herb's root and decocted it into a soup. She carefully fed the soup to her boyfriend, and he gradually awakened. The girl, however, died with a happy smile. Since this time, the people have called the herb *Zi* (purple) *Cao* (herb).

Pharmaceutical Ingredients:[1–4]
1. Lithospermidin A, B
2. Deoxyshikonin, dimethylacrylalkannin, acetylshikonin, dl-acetylalkannin, β-acetoxyisovaleryalkannin, dl-shikonin,β-hydroxyisovalerylalkannin,1-methoxyacetylshikonin

Research and Clinical Study: Lithospermum *Zi Cao* has been clinically used in treating Stomach, thyroid, and Blood and skin cancer, and has been shown to act as a contraceptive, inhibiting female fertility.[4,5,6]

Rhinoceros *Xi Jiao* 犀角

Rhinoceros horn Xi Jiao had been used for centuries to counter life-threatening fever and seizures. However, Rhinoceros horn is currently prohibited because the species is endangered. Bubali *Shui Niu Jiao* is now substituted for Rhinoceros horn in classical herbal formulas. The following information is just for educational purposes.

Original Reference: *Ming Yi Bie Lu* (*Miscellaneous Records of Famous Physicians*) by *Tao Hong-Jing*, North and South Kingdoms (5th century CE) 名医别录

Part Used: Horn

Name:
Pharmaceutical: Rhinoceri (asiatici), cornu
Zoological: Rhinoceros unicornis; r. sondaicus; r. sumatrenis
Common: Rhinoceros horn
Wade-Giles: *Hsi-Chiao*
Translation: Rhinoceros horn

Energy/Taste: Cold, bitter, sour, salty

Channel-Organ: Heart, Liver, Stomach

Actions:
1. Clear fever and stop convulsion
2. Cool Blood and release Toxin

Form and Preparation: Powder, decoction, or pill

Dosage: Horses and Cattle: 15–50g

Cautions and Contraindications:
1. This substance is prohibited as the rhinoceros is an endangered species.
2. Historically, it is contraindicated during pregnancy.

Side Effects: None known

Bubali *Shui Niu Jiao* 水牛角

Original Reference: *Ming Yi Bie Lu* (*Miscellaneous Records of Famous Physicians*) by *Tao Hong-Jing*, North and South Kingdoms (5th century CE) 名医别录

Part Used: Horn

Name:
Pharmaceutical: Bubali, cornu
Zoological: Bubalis bubalis L.
Common: Water Buffalo Horn
Wade-Giles: *Shui-Niu-Chiao*
Translation: Water Buffalo Horn

Energy/Taste: Cold, salty

Channel-Organ: Heart, Liver

Actions:
1. Clear Heat and cool Blood
2. Release Toxins

Form and Preparation: Powder, decoction, or pill

Dosage:
Horses and Cattle: 90–150g
Llamas, Alpacas, Goats, Sheep, and Pigs: 15–50g
Dogs: 3–10g
Cats and Rabbits: 0.5–3g
Birds: 0.2–2g

Cautions and Contraindications: None

Side Effects: None known

Paeonia *Chi Shao Yao* 赤芍药

Original Reference: *Kai Bao Ben Cao* (*Materia Medica of the Kai Bao Era*) by *Ma Zhi* in 973 开宝本草

Part Used: Root

Name:
Pharmaceutical: Paeoniae Rubra, Radix
Botanical: Paeonia lactifloria; P. veitchii; P. obovata
Common: Red Peony
Wade-Giles: *Ch'ih-Shao-Yao*
Translation: Red Peony

Energy/Taste: Cold, bitter

Channel-Organ: Liver, Spleen

Actions:
1. Clear Heat and cool Blood
2. Invigorate Blood and reduce swelling

Form and Preparation: Powder, decoction, or pill

Dosage:
Horses and Cattle: 30–60g
Camels: 60–100g
Llamas, Alpacas, Goats, Sheep, and Pigs: 5–20g
Dogs: 2–6g
Cats and Rabbits: 0.5–3g
Birds: 0.2–2g

Cautions and Contraindications: Cautions in Blood Cold Pattern or during pregnancy

Side Effects: None known

HERBS TO CLEAR HEAT AND DRY DAMPNESS

The herbs to clear Heat and dry Dampness are used to treat Damp-Heat Patterns. Damp-Heat Pattern is a combination of pathogenic A Damp and Heat. Damp-Heat is often associated with Lung/skin, Spleen/Stomach, Liver/Gallbladder, and Bladder (Table 4.3).

All the herbs to clear Heat and dry Damp are cold and bitter. They are often combined with herbs for Internal Heat to "Drain Fire" or toxic Heat. Due to their cold nature, these herbs should not be used in cases of Spleen or Stomach Deficiency. Their general indications include fever, scanty urine, turbid urine, jaundice, bloody diarrhea or dysentery, yellow or foul genital discharge, eczema or moisture dermatitis, furuncles, and sticky tongue coating.

Table 4.3. Brief review of Damp-Heat Patterns.

Zang-Fu Organs		Patterns	Main Signs	Examples of Herbs
Metal/Lung system	Lung	Heat-Phlegm	Cough, pneumonia	Scutellaria *Huang Qin*
	Skin	Damp-Heat	Moisture dermatitis	Sophora *Ku Shen*
Spleen/Gastrointestinal tract		Damp-Heat	Bloody, mucous diarrhea, IBD	Coptis *Huang Lian*
Liver/Gallbladder		Damp-Heat	GB stone, jaundice, hepatitis, otitis	Gentiana *Long Dan Cao*
Bladder		Damp-Heat	Cystitis, UTI	Akebia *Mu Tong*

Scutellaria *Huang Qin* 黄芩

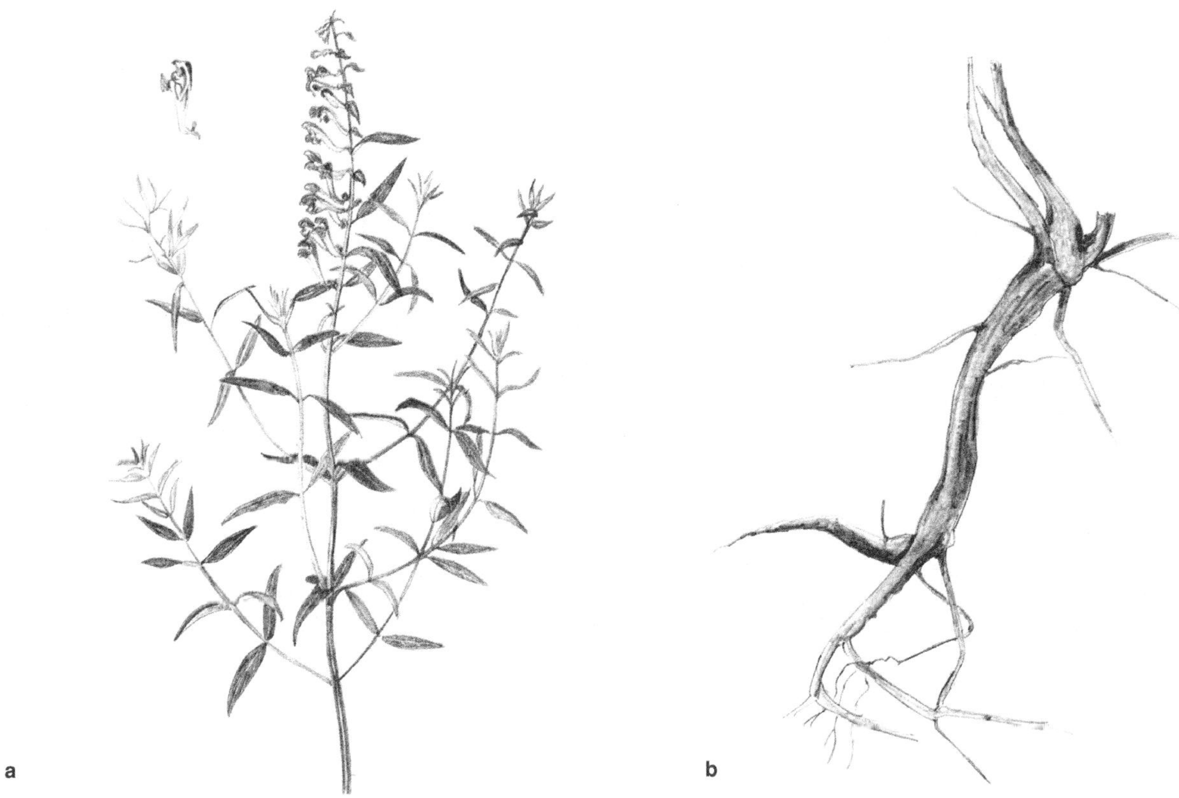

Original Reference: *Shen Nong Ben Cao Jing* (*Shen Nong's Materia Medica*, 1st century BCE) 神农本草经

Part Used: Root

Name:
Pharmaceutical: Radix, Scutellariae Baicalensis
Botanical: Scutellaria Baicalensis (Skullcap)
Common: Scute, Skullcap
Wade-Giles: *Huang-Ch'in*
Translation: Yellow Root

Energy/Taste: Cold, bitter

Channel-Organ: Lung, Gallbladder, Stomach, Large Intestine

Actions:
1. Clear Heat and dry Dampness
2. Drain Fire and release Toxins
3. Stop bleeding
4. Calm the fetus
5. Sedate ascendant Liver *Yang*

Form and Preparation: Powder, decoction, or pill

Dosage:
Horses and Cattle: 20–60 g
Camels: 30–100 g
Llamas, Alpacas, Goats, Sheep, and Pigs: 5–15 g
Dogs: 2–5 g

Cats and Rabbits: 0.5–2 g
Birds: 0.2–2.5 g

Cautions and Contraindications:
1. Cautions for Deficiency and Cold of Stomach and Spleen
2. May counteract Moutan *Mu Dan Pi* and Veratrum *Li Lu*

Side Effects: None known

Clinical Applications:
1. Damp-Heat or Heat-Toxin in the Upper Burner
   Clinical signs: Fever, thirst, irritability, hot sore and swelling in the head or neck, greasy coating
   Combine with: Lonicera *Jin Yin Hua*, Forsythia *Lian Qiao* and Coptis *Huang Lian*
   Classical herbal formula: *Pu Ji Xiao Du Yin*
2. Cough due to Heat or Heat-Phlegm in the Lung
   Clinical signs: Stifling chest, cough with thick, yellow sputum
   Combine with: Morus *Sang Bai Pi* and Anemarrhena *Zhi Mu*
3. Damp-Heat jaundice and hepatitis
   Combine with: Gardenia *Zhi Zi*, Artemisia *Yin Chen Hao*, Bambusa *Zhu Ye*
   Classical herbal formula: *Long Dan Xie Gan Tang*
4. Hemorrhage due to Heat in the Blood
   Clinical signs: Vomiting with Blood, epistaxis, hematuria, uterine bleeding
   Combine with: Rehmannia *Sheng Di*, Imperata *Bai Mao Gen*, and Biota *Ce Bai Ye*
5. Threatened miscarriage, restless fetus
   Combine with: Angelica *Dang Gui* and Atractylodes *Bai Zhu*
   Classical herbal formula: *Bai Zhu San*

History and Comments
1. *Huang Qin* is the root of Scutillaria. It is grown mainly in the provinces of *Hebei*, *Shanxi*, and *Inner Mongolia*. The herb is collected in spring or autumn, dried in sunlight, and sliced. It may be used with no further preparation after stir-baking with wine or after stir-baking into charcoal. Its primary effects are clearing away Heat and Dampness, purging Fire, detoxifying, stopping bleeding, and preventing miscarriage.
2. The raw herb is used to calm the fetus. Use the fried herb to stop bleeding. Fry the herb with wine to treat Heat in Upper Burner.
3. *Huang Qin* is currently used with Houttuynia *Yu Xing Cao* to inhibit pneumonia.

Pharmaceutical Ingredients:[1–4]
1. Flavonoids (baicalein, baicalin, chrysin, oroxylin-A, oroxylin-A-glucuronide, skullcapflavone, oroxylin-β-7-o-glucuronide, wogonin, wogonoside, skullcapflavone, dihydrobaicalin)
2. Tenaxin, koganebanacin, 7-melhoxy-baicalein, 2,5,8-trihydroxy-7-dimefhoxyflarone
3. Stigmasterol, amino acid

Coptis *Huang Lian* 黄连

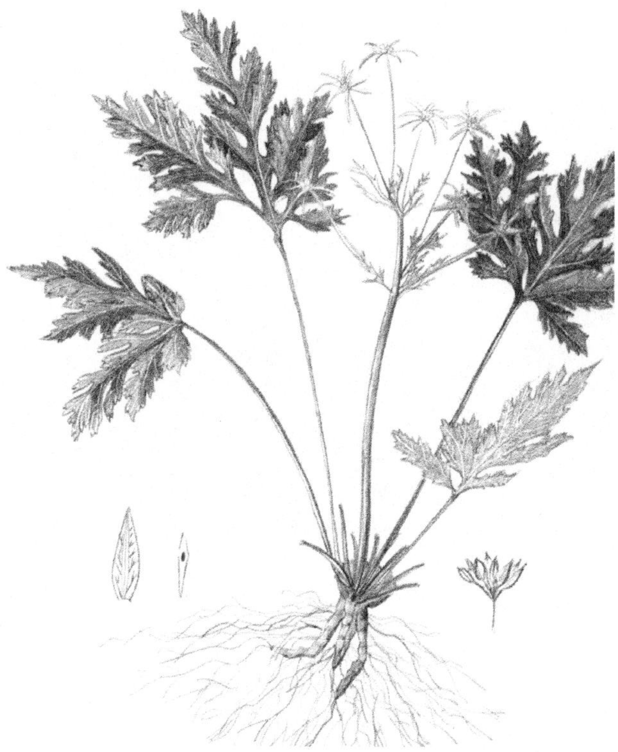

Original Reference: *Shen Nong Ben Cao Jing* (*Shen Nong*'s *Materia Medica*, 1st century BCE) 神农本草经

Part Used: Rhizome and root

Name:
Pharmaceutical: Coptidis, Rhizoma
Botanical: Coptis Chinensis; C. Deltoidea; D. Teetoides (Golden Thread)
Common: Coptis Root
Wade-Giles: *Huang-Lien*
Translation: Yellow Links

Energy/Taste: Cold, bitter

Channel-Organ: Heart, Stomach, Liver, Large Intestine

Actions:
1. Clear Heat and dry Dampness
2. Clear Heart Fire, release Toxins
3. Drain Fire in the Stomach

Form and Preparation: Powder, decoction, or pill

Dosage: Do not overdose or use long-term.
Horses and Cattle: 15–30 g
Camels: 25–45 g
Llamas, Alpacas, Goats, Sheep, and Pigs: 5–10 g
Dogs: 2–8 g
Cats and Rabbits: 0.5–1 g
Birds: 0.1–1 g

Cautions and Contraindications:
1. Contraindications for Deficient Spleen with Diarrhea; Blood Deficiency, including postpartum; or Deficiency of *Jing*
2. May antagonize Chrysanthemum *Ju Hua*, Scrophularia *Xuan Shen*, Dictamnus *Bai Xian Pi*, Bombyx *Jiang Can*, Tussilago *Kuan Dong Hua*, and Achyranthes *Niu Xi*
3. May not be taken with pork

Side Effects: Large doses or long-term use can injure Stomach and Spleen.

Clinical Applications:
1. Damp-Heat in the whole body
   Clinical signs: Fever, open sore in the skin, red tongue, yellow coating
   Combine with: Scutellaria *Huang Qin* and Gardenia *Zhi Zi*
   Classical herbal formula: *Huang Lian Jie Du Tang*
2. Damp-Heat accumulated in the intestines
   Clinical signs: Bloody mucous diarrhea, dysentery, Tenesmus
   Combine with: Saussurea *Mu Xiang*
   Classical herbal formula: *Da Xiang Lian Wan*
3. Shen disturbance due to Heart Fire
   Clinical signs: Anxiety, restlessness, hyperactivity, red tongue
   Combine with: Scutellaria *Huang Qin*, Curcuma *Yu Jin* and Gardenia *Zhi Zi*
   Classical herbal formula: Zhen Xin San
4. Extravasated Blood due to Blood Heat
   Clinical signs: Vomiting of Blood, epistaxis, hematuria, bloody stool
   Combine with: Imperata *Bai Mao Gen*, Rehmannia *Sheng Di*, And Scutellaria *Huang Qin*
5. Lick granuloma, boils, toxic skin ailments
   Take alone and apply topically around and on the open wound with powder
6. Stomach Fire
   Clinical signs: Hunger, burning sensation in Stomach, gastric ulcer, stomatitis, gingivitis, toothache, mouth and tongue ulcers
   Combine with: Cimicifuga *Sheng Ma*, and Rehmannia *Sheng Di Huang*
   Classical herbal formula: *Qing Wei San*

History and Comments:
1. A doctor named Tao lived in a mountain home where he tended a garden with various plants useful for treating his patients. His healing skills were in high demand, even among patients far from his home. When he traveled, he hired Huang Lian to take care of his plants. Doctor Tao's lovely and clever daughter, Meiwa, also liked the plants. The first thing she did every morning was look at the plants. On one cool January morning, when Meiwa checked the plants in the garden, she found no plants with blossoms. As she returned home along a mountain road, she saw some plants with florescent green flowers. She liked them so much she dug them up and planted them in the garden. Under Huang's care, the flowers grew well.

   While her father was treating patients far away, Meiwa developed a strange disease with head-to-foot Dryness-Heat, vomiting, and diarrhea. Meiwa's mother asked another doctor for help. This doctor's treatment did not work; in fact, she worsened after taking three doses. Her worried mother cried every day and couldn't sleep. Seeing the pain of the mother and child, Huang was anxious to help the little girl. He suddenly remembered how he had been feeling sick last month, but when he chewed a leaf of the plant with the green flower he quickly felt better. He had become totally well after chewing another two leaves. He wondered if it could work on Meiwa's illness. He decided to try, so he decocted the stem and leaves of the green flower plant. Then he secretly fed the liquid medicine to Meiwa. After taking three doses, Meiwa got well. Just at that moment, doctor Tao came back. When he learned what had happened while he was gone, he was very thankful for Huang's help. The doctor said, "Meiwa's illness was due to Damp-Heat in her intestines and Stomach. It seems this special plant is effective in reducing the Damp-Heat. To express my appreciation to you for saving my daughter, I will call this herb *Huang Lian*."
2. Good quality Coptis *Huang Lian* is thick, strong, and solid with many interconnections.
3. Coptis *Huang Lian* is known to have strong antibacterial effects. It has been shown effective for streptococcal infections and can be used topically for infected sores and for purulent otitis media.
4. The extreme bitter taste of *Huang Lian* encourages use in pills or capsules as adjunctive to decoction or

powder form. Typically, 1.5g is given in powder form.

Pharmaceutical Ingredients:[1–4]

1. Alkaloids (berberine, coptisine, worenine, palmatine, jatrorrhizine, epiberberinem columbamine, magnoflorine)
2. Ferulic acid, chlorogenic acid

Phellodendron *Huang Bai* 黄柏

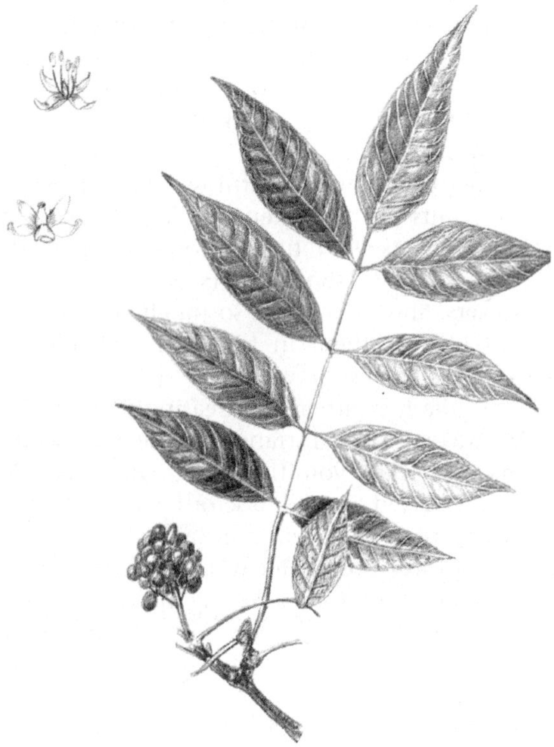

Original Reference: *Shen Nong Ben Cao Jing* (*Shen Nong's Materia Medica*, 1st century BCE) 神农本草经

Part Used: Bark

Name:
Pharmaceutical: Phellodendri, Cortex
Botanical: Phellodendron Chinense; P. Amurense
Common: Phellodendron
Wade-Giles: *Huang-Pai*
Translation: Yellow Fir

Energy/Taste: Cold, bitter

Channel-Organ: Kidney, Bladder, Large Intestine

Actions:

1. Clear Heat and dry up Dampness, particularly in Lower Burner
2. Drain Fire, release Toxins
3. Drain false Fire/Heat from Kidney

Form and Preparation: Powder, decoction, or pill

Dosage:
Horses and Cattle: 10–45g
Camels: 20–50g
Llamas, Alpacas, Goats, Sheep, and Pigs: 5–10g
Dogs: 3–6g
Cats and Rabbits: 0.5–2g
Birds: 0.2–2g

Cautions and Contraindications: Contraindications for Spleen Deficiency with diarrhea

Side Effects: *Huang Bai* may weaken Stomach.

Clinical Applications:

1. Damp-Heat accumulated in intestines
   Clinical signs: Explosive diarrhea or dysentery
   Combine with: Coptis *Huang Lian*, Scutellaria *Huang Qin*, and Pulsatilla *Bai Tou Weng*
2. Damp-Heat jaundice and hepatitis
   Combine with: Gardenia *Zhi Zi* and Artemisia *Yin Chen Hao*
3. Damp-Heat in the uterus and vaginal tract
   Clinical signs: Pyometra, Endometritis, turbid urination, yellow and thick genital discharge
   Combine with: Plantago *Che Qian Zi*, and Leonurus *Yi Mu Cao*
4. Deficiency of Kidney *Yin* with Heat
   Clinical signs: Hot ears/feet, tidal fevers, cool-seeking, night sweats, steaming bone disorder
   Combine with: Rehmannia *Shu Di Huang*, Anemarrhena *Zhi Mu*
   Classical herbal formula: *Zhi Bai Di Huang Wan*
5. External use for open wound, boils, carbuncles, eczema, toxic inflammations
   Combine with: Coptis *Huang Lian* and Rheum *Da Huang*.
   Classical herbal formula: *Ru Yi Jin Huang San*

History and Comments:

1. *Huang Bai* is the bark of Phellodendron, produced chiefly in the provinces of *Liaoning* and *Jilin*. Its main effects include clearing away Heat, removing Dampness, purging Fire, detoxifying, and clearing False (Deficiency) Heat.
2. Phellodendron *Huang Bai* is similar to Coptis *Huang Lian* but is a little weaker.
3. *Huang Bai* can be used for Upper Burner Heat if it is stirred in wine.
4. *Huang Bai* is useful topically or internally for herpes lesions.

Pharmaceutical Ingredients:[1–4]

1. Alkaloids (berberine, palmatine, jatrorrhizine, phellodendrine, α-phellodendrine, β-phellodendrine menisperine, candicine, magnoflorine, limonene, obacunone)
2. Chlorogenic acid, lignan

Gentiana *Long Dan Cao* 龙胆草

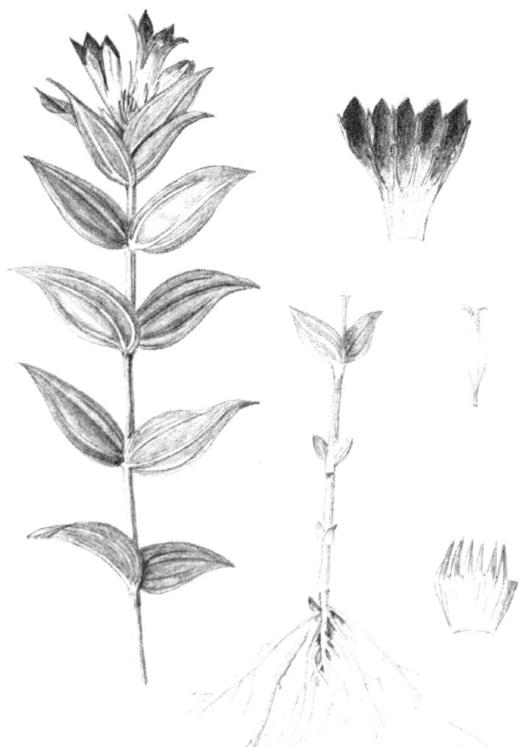

Original Reference: *Shen Nong Ben Cao Jing* (*Shen Nong*'s *Materia Medica*, 1st century BCE) 神农本草经

Part Used: Rhizome and root

Name:
Pharmaceutical: Gentianae Longdancao, Radix
Botanical: Gentiana Manshurica; G. Scabra; G. Trifolia; G. Regescens
Common: Gentian
Wade-Giles: *Lung-Tan-Tsao*
Translation: Dragon Gallbladder Plant

Energy/Taste: Cold, bitter

Channel-Organ: Liver, Gallbladder, Stomach

Actions:

1. Clear Heat and dry Dampness
2. Drain Fire from Liver and Gallbladder

Form and Preparation: Powder, decoction, or pill

Dosage:
Horses and Cattle: 15–45 g
Camels: 30–60 g
Llamas, Alpacas, Goats, Sheep, and Pigs: 5–15 g
Dogs: 2–5 g
Cats and Rabbits: 0.5–2 g
Birds: 0.3–5 g

Cautions and Contraindications:

1. Contraindications for Deficiency of Spleen and Stomach
2. Contraindicated with Rehmannia *Sheng Di Huang*

Side Effects: Overdosage leads to vomiting.

Clinical Applications:

1. Jaundice and hepatitis due to Damp-Heat
   Combine with: Artemisia *Yin Chen Hao* and Gardenia *Zhi Zi*
   Classical herbal formula: *Long Dan Xie Gan Tang*
2. Damp-Heat in lower abdomen
   Clinical signs: Thick and foul vaginal discharge, urinary infections, swollen painful testicles, eczema in genital region
   Combine with: Phellodendron *Huang Bai*, Sophora *Ku Shen* and Plantago *Che Qian Zi*
3. Upward attack of Liver or Gallbladder Fire
   Clinical signs: Headache, sore throat, red eye, eye pressure, tinnitus, costal pain
   Combine with: Scutellaria *Huang Qin*, Gardenia *Zhi Zi*, Bupleurum *Chai Hu*, and Akebia *Mu Tong*
4. High fever leading to convulsion or spasm
   Combine with: Uncaria *Gou Teng* and Bovis *Niu Huang*
5. Toxic and red skin eruptions
   Apply externally
6. Eye inflammations
   Combine with: Coptis *Huang Lian*, Apply externally

History and Comments:

1. *Long Dan Cao* is the root and rhizome of Gentiana. It is grown in every part of Northern and Southern China. The herb is collected in autumn, dried in sunlight, cut into pieces, and used unprepared. Its main effects are clearing away Heat, removing Dampness, and purging Fire in the Liver and Gallbladder.
2. *Long Dan Cao* is a very bitter herb and is the top herb for Liver and Gallbladder Fire and Damp-Heat affecting all Three Burners. It is commonly combined with Scutellaria *Huang Qin*, Bupleurum *Chai Hu*, and Gardenia *Zhi Zi*.

3. To make the effect potent on Liver or Gallbladder Fire, *Long Dan Cao* is stir-fried with pig bile, Suis *Zhu Dan Zhi*.

Pharmaceutical Ingredients:[1–4]
1. Gentiopicrin, gentiopicroside, gentianine, gentianose
2. Sweroside, swetiamarin, amarogentin, amaroswerin, sucrose

Sophora *Ku Shen* 苦参

Original Reference: *Shen Nong Ben Cao Jing* (*Shen Nong's Materia Medica*, 1st century BCE) 神农本草经

Part Used: Root

Name:
Pharmaceutical: Sophorae Flavescentis, Radix
Botanical: Sophora Flavescens
Common: Sophora Root
Wade-Giles: *K'u-Shen*
Translation: Bitter Root

Energy/Taste: Cold, bitter

Channel-Organ: Liver, Kidney, Large Intestine, Small Intestine

Actions:
1. Clear Heat and dry up Dampness
2. Promote urination
3. Disperse Wind to stop itching
4. Kill worms and parasites

Form and Preparation: Powder, decoction, or pill

Dosage:
Horses and Cattle: 15–60g
Llamas, Alpacas, Goats, Sheep, and Pigs: 5–15g
Dogs: 2–8g
Cats and Rabbits: 0.5–1g
Birds: 0.2–1.5g

Cautions and Contraindications:
1. Contraindications for Cold and Deficient Stomach Or Spleen
2. May be incompatible with Veratrum *Li Lu*, antagonizes Cuscuta *Tu Si Zi* and Fritillaria *Chuan Bei Mu*

Side Effects: None known

Dictamnus *Bai Xian Pi* 白鲜皮

Original Reference: *Shen Nong Ben Cao Jing* (*Shen Nong's Materia Medica*, 1st century BCE) 神农本草经

Part Used: Root bark

Name:
Pharmaceutical: Dictamni Dasicarpi Radicis, Cortex
Botanical: Dictamnus Dasycarpus
Common: Dictamnus
Wade-Giles: *Pai-Hsien-P'i*
Translation: White Flesh Bark

Energy/Taste: Cold, bitter

Channel-Organ: Spleen, Stomach

Actions:
1. Clear Heat and release Toxin
2. Remove Damp and stop itching

Form and Preparation: Powder, decoction, or pill

Dosage:
Horses and Cattle: 15–30g
Llamas, Alpacas, Goats, Sheep, and Pigs: 3–10g
Dogs: 2–3g
Cats and Rabbits: 0.5–1g
Birds: 0.2–1.5g

Cautions and Contraindications:
1. Counteract against Platycodon *Jie Geng*, Poria *Fu Ling* and Dioscorea *Bei Xie*
2. Cautions for cold abdomen due to Deficiency of *Qi*

Side Effects: None known

Senecio *Qian Li Guang* 千里光

Original Reference: Ben Cao Gang Mu (*Materia Medica Compendium*) by *Li Shi-Zhen* in 1590 本草纲目

Part Used: Whole plant

Name:
Pharmaceutical: Senecio Herba
Botanical: Senecio scandens Bush, Ham
Common: Senecio
Wade-Giles: *Ch'ien-Li- Kuang*
Translation: Thousand Mile Light

Energy/Taste: Cold, bitter

Channel-Organ: Lung, Liver, Large Intestine

Actions:
1. Clear Damp-Heat, clear Heat Toxin
2. Clear Liver and benefit the eyes

Form and Preparation: Powder, decoction, or pill

Dosage:
Horses and Cattle: 60–120 g
Llamas, Alpacas, Goats, Sheep, and Pigs: 5–30 g
Dogs: 2–7 g
Cats and Rabbits: 0.5–2 g
Birds: 0.2–2 g

Cautions and Contraindications: Contraindications for Spleen Deficiency

Side Effects: May cause nausea, anorexia, diarrhea, or skin allergy

Fraxinus *Qin Pi* 秦皮

Original Reference: *Shen Nong Ben Cao Jing* (*Shen Nong's Materia Medica*, 1st century BCE) 神农本草经

Part Used: Cortex

Name:
Pharmaceutical: Fraxini, Cortex
Botanical: Fraxinus Rhynchophylla Hance, F. Bungeana D.C., or F. Roxb.
Common: Fraxinus
Wade-Giles: *Ch'in-P'i*

Energy/Taste: Cold, bitter

Channel-Organ: Gallbladder, Liver, Large Intestine

Actions:
1. Drain Damp-Heat and stop diarrhea
2. Drain Liver Fire to benefit the eyes
3. Disperse Wind-Dampness

Form and Preparation: Powder, decoction, or pill

Dosage:
Horses and Cattle: 15–60 g
Llamas, Alpacas, Goats, Sheep, and Pigs: 5–10 g
Dogs: 2–6 g
Cats and Rabbits: 0.5–1 g
Birds: 0.2–1.5 g

Cautions and Contraindications:
1. Contraindications for Spleen Deficiency Cold
2. May Antagonize Evodia *Wu Zhu Yu*

Side Effects: None known

HERBS TO CLEAR HEAT AND RELEASE TOXINS

The herbs to clear Heat and release Toxins are used to treat toxic Heat (Heat Toxin) and thus are also called "herbs to clear toxic Heat." Diseases caused by Heat Toxin are often epidemic and infectious in nature. The four main characteristic conditions of Heat Toxin are redness, swelling, Heat, and pain. Heat Toxin Pattern may occur via inflammatory or infectious diseases including influenza, upper airway diseases, inflammatory bowel disease, herpes, and parvovirus. Additional clinical signs include sore throat, boils, carbuncles, abscesses, swollen glands, lumps, or even cancerous masses, which are associated with toxic Heat.

The herbs to clear toxic Heat are cold or cool and are primarily used to treat Excessive Heat Toxin. These herbs can be also used to treat snake bites, cancer, and dysentery. Herbs to clear Heat and release Toxins have varying degrees of antiinflammatory, antiinfectious, antiviral, and antibacterial effectiveness. Some herbs are clinically effective in treating infection, but have not demonstrated antimicrobial function in vitro. Because these herbs tend to be cold or cool, they are contraindicated for Cold conditions. Long-term use can damage *Qi* and *Yang*.

Lonicera *Jin Yin Hua* 金银花

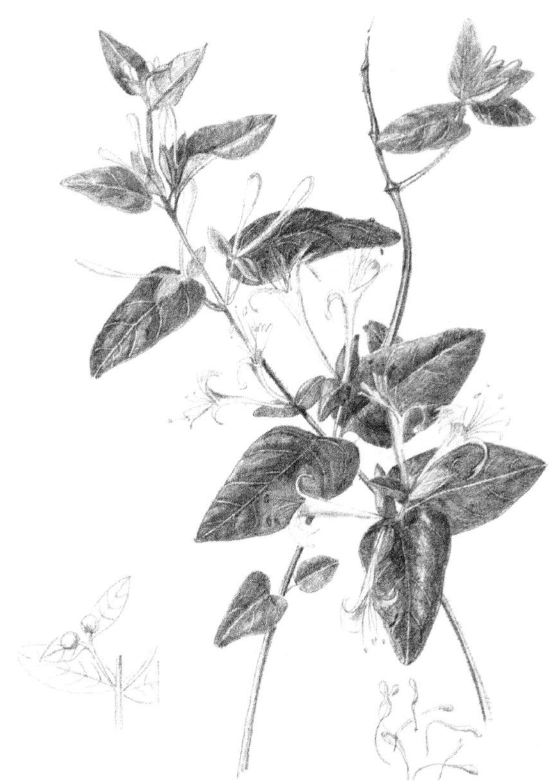

Original Reference: *Tang Ben Cao* (*Tang Materia Medica*) by *Su Jing* et al., *Tang* Dynasty (618–907 CE) 唐本草

Part Used: Flower Bud

Name:
Pharmaceutical: Lonicerae Japonicae, Flos
Botanical: Lonicera Japonica; L. Hypoglauca; L. Confusa; L. Dasystyla
Common: Honeysuckle Flower
Wade-Giles: *Chin-Yin-Hua*
Translation: Gold Silver Flower

Energy/Taste: Cold, sweet

Channel-Organ: Lung, Large Intestine, Stomach

Actions:
1. Clear Heat and release Toxin
2. Expel externally contracted Wind Heat

Form and Preparation: Powder or pill; decoction: steep 10 minutes prior to cooking.

Dosage:
Horses and Cattle: 15–60 g
Llamas, Alpacas, Goats, Sheep, and Pigs: 5–10 g
Dogs: 2–5 g
Cats and Rabbits: 0.5–1 g
Birds: 0.2–2 g

Cautions and Contraindications: Contraindications for Cold type of Diarrhea or *Yin* type of Carbuncles

Side Effects: Topical application may cause skin allergy.

Clinical Applications:
1. Exogenous pathogenic Heat in the *Wei* Level
   Clinical signs: Fever, thirst, sore throat, swollen tonsils and glands
   Combine with: Forsythia *Lian Qiao*, Mentha *Bo He*, and Arctium *Niu Bang Zi*
   Classical herbal formula: *Yin Qiao San*
2. Exogenous pathogenic Heat in the *Ying* and *Blood* Levels
   Clinical signs: Rash, restlessness, anxiety, deep red tongue
   Combine with: Moutan *Mu Dan Pi* And Rehmannia *Sheng Di Huang*
   Classical herbal formula: *Qing Ying Tang*
3. Boils, carbuncles, furuncles
   Combine with: Taraxacum *Pu Gong Ying* and Forsythia *Lian Qiao*
   Can be applied topically
4. Toxic Heat diarrhea and dysentery
   Combine with: Coptis *Huang Lian* and Pulsatilla *Bai Tou Weng* and Paeonia *Chi Shao*
5. Toxic Heat in the Lungs
   Clinical signs: Cough with bloody pus
   Combine with: Houttuynia *Yu Xing Cao* and Phragmites *Lu Gen*

History and Comments:
1. Long, long ago, a kindhearted peasant couple had twin daughters. The older daughter was named Jin Hua (Gold Flower) and the younger was named *Yin* Hua (Silver Flower). The sisters were very similar to each other, including their characters and interests. At 18 years of age, the twins were pursued by many young men, but they did not marry because they were afraid of being apart from each other. The young women swore to live together forever; they would even be buried in the same tomb after dying.

   An unexpected disaster soon hit the family. One day, Jin Hua unexpectedly developed pyrexia, and the disease fiercely spread all over her body. Her parents were very afraid and borrowed money to see a doctor. The doctor said Jin Hua had an infectious pyretic toxicity disease that no medicine could cure. When *Yin* Hua heard this, she cried in extreme pain. Gold Flower asked Silver Flower to stay away from her to avoid infection, but Silver Flower would not leave because she had vowed always to remain with her sister. Within a few days Silver Flower was also ill and had to lie in bed. The sisters told their parents their fate was God's will and they would turn to an herbal medicine that could heal patients with pyretic toxicity diseases. The sisters died and their parents buried them in a tomb as they requested. Unexpectedly, a small plant with many green leaves burst from the sisters' tomb the following summer. Over the next 3 years, the small plant gradually grew and bloomed with yellow (golden) and white (silver) flowers. When herbalists used those flowers to treat patients with pyretic toxicity disease, they found the herbal medicine really had a marvelous effect. The people called the flower *Jin* (Gold) *Yin* (Silver) *Hua* (Flower) in memory of the twin sisters.
2. Lonicera *Jin Yin Hua* is combined with Forsythia *Lian Qiao* to reinforce its effect. The stem, *Ren Dong Teng*, is also used similarly to Jin *Yin* Hua.
3. *Jin Yin Hua* is made into a sweet tonic tea and taken in summertime for protection from the effects of Heat.
4. A clinical trial indicated that a combination of Lonicera *Jin Yin Hua* and Coptis *Huang Lian* had a strong effect for numerous viral and bacterial infections.

Pharmaceutical Ingredients:[1–4]
1. Chlorogenoids (chlorogenic acid, isochlorogenic acid)
2. Flavonoids (luteolin, luteolin-7-glycosides, lonicein, loniceraflavone, loganin, tannin)
3. Aromadendrene, linalool, geraniol, octanal, α-pinene, β-pinene, myrcene, 1,8-cineole, β-terpinene, hexenol, α-terpineol, neral, linalyl acetate, geranial, citronellol, terpinyl acetate, β-eudesmol, geranyl acetate, eugenol, α-copene, patchoulene, α-caryophyllene, β-caryophyllene, iso-bornyl aceate, farnesol, nerolidol
4. Ionositol, saponins

Forsythia *Lian Qiao* 连翘

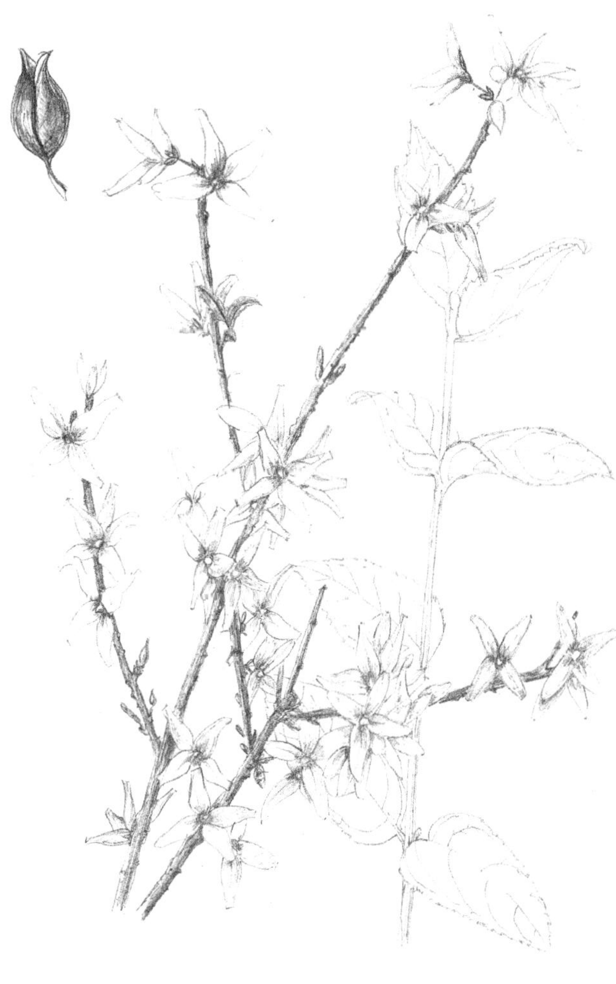

Original Reference: *Shen Nong Ben Cao Jing* (*Shen Nong's Materia Medica*, 1st century BCE) 神农本草经

Part Used: Seed Shells (or capsules)

Name:
Pharmaceutical: Forsythiae Suspensae, F.
Botanical: Forsythia Suspena
Common name: Forsythia fruit
Wade-Giles: *Lien-Ch'iao*
Translation: Connected Capsules

Energy/Taste: Cool, bitter, slightly pungent

Channel-Organ: Lung, Heart, Gallbladder

Actions:
1. Clear Heat and release Toxins
2. Eliminate swelling and dissipate nodule or mass
3. Discharge Pus

Form and Preparation: Powder, decoction, or pill; the seeds are removed during the drying process

Dosage:
Horses and Cattle: 20–30g
Llamas, Alpacas, Goats, Sheep, and Pigs: 5–15g
Dogs: 2–6g
Cats and Rabbits: 0.5–2g
Birds: 0.2–2g

Cautions and Contraindications: Cautions for diarrhea due to Spleen Deficiency

Side Effects: None known

Clinical Applications:
1. Exogenous pathogenic Heat entering the *Wei* Level
   Clinical signs: Early stage of febrile disease, fever, sore throat, headache
   Combine with: Lonicera *Jin Yin Hua*, Arctium *Niu Bang Zi*, and Mentha *Bo He*
   Classical herbal formula: *Yin Qiao San*
2. Exogenous pathogenic Heat entering the Pericardium
   Clinical signs: High fever, delirium, coma
   Combine with: Nelumbo *Lian Zi* and Antelopis *Ling Yang Jiao*
   Classical herbal formula: Qing Ying Tang
3. Exogenous Pathogenic Heat causing skin rash or allergenic rash
   Combine with: Paeonia *Chi Shao*, Glycerrhiza *Gan Cao*
4. Boils, carbuncles, furuncles due to Toxic Heat
   Combine with: Lonicera *Jin Yin Hua* and Sophora *Huai Hua*
5. Scrofula and neck lumps
   Combine with: Prunella *Xia Ku Cao*, Scrophularia *Xuan Shen*, Fritillaria *Chuan Bei Mu*

History and Comments
1. *Lian Qiao* is the fruit of Forsythia, which is produced mostly in the provinces of Shanxi and Gansu. Green Forsythia is the unripe fruit and yellow Forsythia is the fully ripe fruit. The green one is a better medicinal and is used without additional preparation.
2. The herb's main effects include clearing Heat, detoxifying, subduing swelling, and dissolving lumps. It

is often combined with Lonicera *Jin Yin Hua* or Isatis *Ban Lan Gen* to reinforce its effect.

Pharmaceutical Ingredients:[1–4]

1. Lignoids (phillyrin, forsythin), phillygenin, (+)-pinoresinol, (+)-pinoresinol-β-d-glycoside)
2. Oleanolic acid, betulic acid, ursolic acid, rutin, forsythoside A, C, D
3. Essential oils (α-pinene, β-pinene, terpinen-4-ol, β-cymene, terpinen-4-ol)

Isatis *Ban Lan Gen* 板蓝根

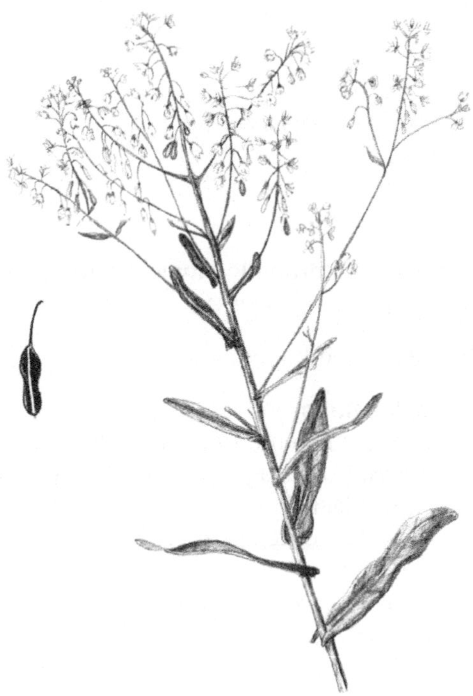

a

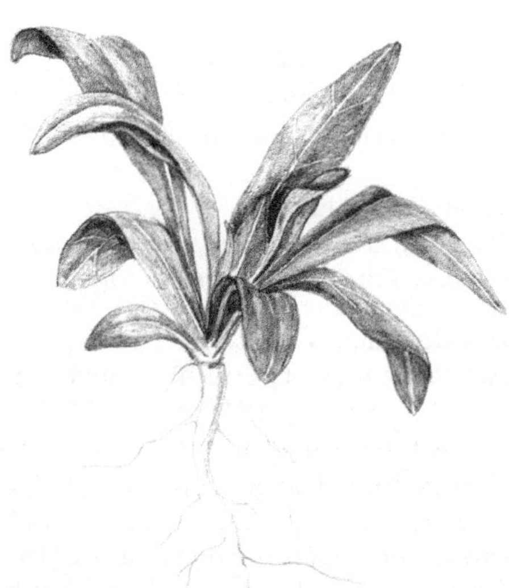

b

Original Reference: *Tang Ben Cao* (*Tang Materia Medica*) by *Su Jing* et al., *Tang* Dynasty (618–907 CE) 唐本草

Part Used: Root

Name:
Pharmaceutical: Isatidis Seu Baphicacanthi, Radix
Botanical: Isatis Tinctoria
Common: Isatis Root
Wade-Giles: *Pan-Leng-Ken*
Translation: Board Orchid Root

Energy/Taste: Cold, bitter

Channel-Organ: Lung, Heart, Stomach

Actions:

1. Clear Heat and release Toxins
2. Clear Heat from the Blood Level
3. Benefit the throat

Form and Preparation: Powder, decoction, or pill

Dosage:
Horses and Cattle: 30–100 g
Camels: 45–120 g
Llamas, Alpacas, Goats, Sheep, and Pigs: 10–30 g
Dogs: 2–5 g
Cats and Rabbits: 0.5–2 g
Birds: 0.3–2 g

Cautions and Contraindications: Contraindications for Deficiency and Cold in Spleen

Side Effects: Overdose may cause diarrhea.

Clinical Applications:

1. Sore throat, swollen glands, carbuncles and boils, rashes
   Combine with: Scrophularia *Xuan Shen*, Lonicera *Jin Yin Hua*, Isatis *Da Qing Ye*, Anemarrhena *Zhi Mu*, Forsythia *Lian Qiao*
2. High fever with rash
   Combine with: Gypsum *Shi Gao* and Moutan *Mu Dan Pi*
3. Hepatitis and Damp-Heat jaundice
   Combine with: Curcuma *Jiang Huang*, Gentiana *Qin Jiao*, Salvia *Dan Shen*, or Artemisia *Yin Chen Hao*
4. Mumps with pain and swelling in throat
   Combine with: Arctium *Niu Bang Zi* And Patrinia *Bai Jiang Cao*

History and Comments:

1. *Ban Lan Gen* is the root of Isatis. It acts primarily to clear Heat, detoxify, remove Heat from the Blood, and relieve throat soreness. *Ban Lan Gen* is excreted within 4 hours of absorption; dosing should be repeated every 4 hours.
2. *Ban Lan Gen* is often combined with *Da Qing Ye* (the leaf of Isatis) to reinforce its effect. Together they have been proven clinically effective against viruses, including encephalitis, pneumonia, hepatitis, shingles, measles, myocarditis, mumps, influenza, and herpes. They also have strong antibacterial effects.

Pharmaceutical Ingredients:[1–4]

1. Indigotin, indigo, indican, isatan B, uridine, hypoxanthine, uracil, salicylic acid, qingdainone, daucosterol, adenosine, kinetin, indirubin
2. β-sitosterol, isatan B

Isatis *Da Qing Ye* 大青叶

Original Reference: *Ming Yi Bie Lu* (*Miscellaneous Records of Famous Physicians*) by *Tao Hong-Jing*, North and South Kingdoms (5th century CE) 名医别录

Part Used: Leaf

Name:
Pharmaceutical: Isatidis Seu Baphicacanthi, Folium
Botanical: Isatis Tinctoria
Common: Isatis leaf
Wade-Giles: *Ta-Ching-Yeh*
Translation: Big Green Leaf

Energy/Taste: Cold, bitter

Channel-Organ: Liver, Stomach, Lung

Actions:

1. Clear Heat and release Toxins
2. Cool Blood and reduce blotches

Form and Preparation: Powder, decoction, or pill

Dosage:
Horses and Cattle: 30–50g
Llamas, Alpacas, Goats, Sheep, and Pigs: 5–10g
Dogs: 2–3g
Cats and Rabbits: 0.5–1g
Birds: 0.2–1.5g

Cautions and Contraindications: Cautions in Cold conditions or Spleen *Qi* Deficiency

Side Effects: Long-term use of overdose may be toxic to the Liver.

Pulsatilla *Bai Tou Weng* 白头翁

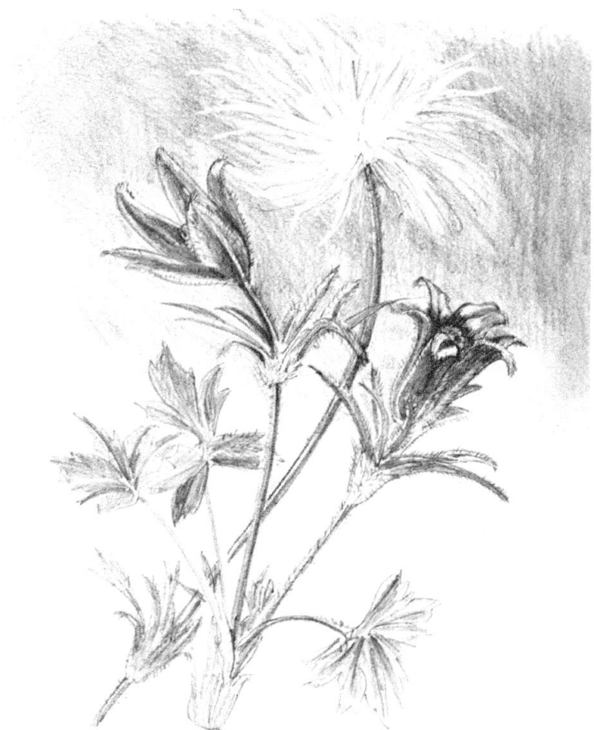

a

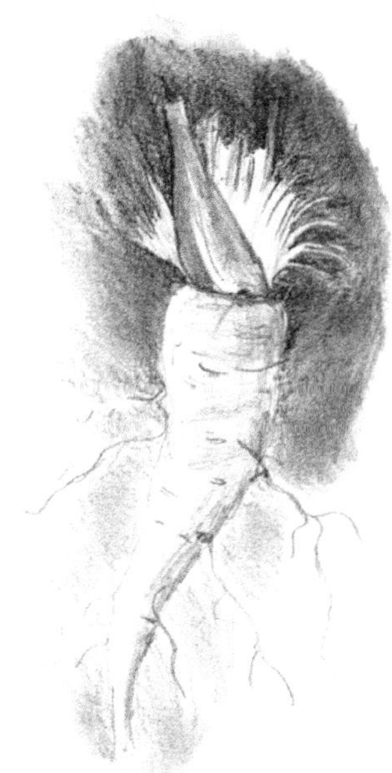

b

Original Reference: *Shen Nong Ben Cao Jing* (*Shen Nong's Materia Medica*, 1st century BCE) 神农本草经

Part Used: Root

Name:
Pharmaceutical: Pulsatillae Chinensis, Radix
Botanical: Pulsatilla Chinensis

Common: *Pulsatilla root*
Wade-Giles: *Pai-T'u-Weng*
Translation: White-Headed Old Man

Energy/Taste: Cold, bitter

Channel-Organ: Stomach, Liver, Large Intestine

Actions:
1. Clear Heat, release Toxins
2. Cool Blood to stop dysentery

Form and Preparation: Powder, decoction, or pill

Dosage:
Horses and Cattle: 15–60 g
Camels: 30–100 g
Llamas, Alpacas, Goats, Sheep, and Pigs: 5–15 g
Dogs: 2–5 g
Cats and Rabbits: 0.5–1 g
Birds: 0.2–3 g

Cautions and Contraindications: Contraindications for diarrhea due to Deficient Cold (or *Yang* Deficiency)

Side Effects: Topical application may cause skin reaction, ocular discharge, sneezing and cough. Overdose of oral medication may cause excessive salivation, vomiting, diarrhea, abdominal pain, hematuria, heart failure, and even death.

Clinical Applications:
1. Dysentery due to Heat in the Stomach or intestines
   Clinical signs: Fever, abdominal pain, Blood and pus in stool, tenesmus
   Combine with: Phellodendron *Huang Bai*, Coptis *Huang Lian*, Fraxinus *Qin Pi*
   Classical herbal formula: *Bai Tou Weng Tang*
2. Warm-Febrile malarial disorders
   Combine with: Bupleurum *Chai Hu*, Areca *Bing Lang*, Scutellaria *Huang Qin*

History and Comments:
1. During the *Qin* Dynasty (221–206 BC), a poor farmer named Wang Gao had abdominal pain and diarrhea after eating a bowl of spoiled rice. Because there was no doctor in his village, he had to bear the pain as he started walking the 3,500-meter road to the nearest doctor. He did not make it far from his village before he fell unconscious due to the pain. At that moment, an old, white-haired gentleman holding a crutch passed by. He helped Wang Gao stand up and asked, "Young man, why are you lying here?" Wang Gao explained his sickness and murmured sadly, "I might pass away soon. Would you be kind enough to take my message to my family?" The old gentleman comforted Wang Gao and then used his crutch to point at a white, hairy fruiting plant growing along the roadside. The old man said, "The root of this plant can save your life," and then he walked away. Wang Gao, though dubious, ripped up the plant and began to chew it. After about half an hour, Wang Gao noticed a decrease in both the pain and diarrhea. He took some plants home with him and continued to use them as medicine. Wang Gao recovered fully after several days' treatment. When people in Wang Gao's village suffered from diarrhea the next year, Wang returned to the place where he met the old gentleman and picked bundles of plants to bring back to the village. The villagers improved after using the medicine. When they asked Wang about the medicine, Wang told his story about meeting the old gentleman on the road. Since that time, the people called the plant *Bai* (white-haired) *Tou* (head) *Weng* (old man) in memory of the old gentleman.
2. *Bai Tou Weng* is effective against both amoebic and bacterial dysentery, and also useful for swelling and hemorrhage due to the rectal growth.

Pharmaceutical Ingredients:[1–4] Anemonin, ranunculin, protoanemonin

Oldenlandia *Bai Hua She She Cao* 白花蛇蛇草

Original Reference: *Guang Xi Zhong Yao Zhi* (*Materia Medica of Guang Xi*) by Guangxi Department of Public Health in 1959

Part Used: Whole Plant

Name:
Pharmaceutical: Oldenlandiae Diffusae, Herba
Botanical: Heydyotis Diffusa; Oldenlandia Diffusa
Common: Hedyotis
Wade-Giles: *Pai-Hua-She-She-Ts'ao*
Translation: White-Patterned Snake's Tongue Herb

Energy/Taste: Cold, slight bitter, sweet

Channel-Organ: Liver, Stomach, Large Intestines

Actions:
1. Clear Heat and release Toxins
2. Resolve Damp
3. Eliminate pus and reduce abscess

Form and Preparation: Powder, decoction, or pill

Dosage:
Horses and Cattle: 50–150 g

Llamas, Alpacas, Goats, Sheep, and Pigs: 20–50 g
Dogs: 5–30 g
Cats and Rabbits: 0.5–3 g
Birds: 0.3–5 g

Cautions and Contraindications: Use with caution in pregnancy

Side Effects: Long-term use may lead to dryness in the mouth.

Clinical Applications:
1. Intestinal abscesses
   Combine with: Patrinia *Bai Jiang Cao*, Sargentodoxa *Hong Teng*
2. Skin infection, boils, and other toxic swellings
   Combine with: Lonicera *Jin Yin Hua*, Forsythia *Lian Qiao*
3. Snakebite (specifically Trimerzourus Steinegeri)
   Combine with: Viola *Zi Hua Di Ding*
4. Hot painful urinary dysfunction
   Combine with: Lobelia *Ban Bian Lian* and Pyrrosia *Shi Wei*
5. Damp-Heat jaundice
   Combine with: Gardenia *Zhi Zi*, Phellodendron *Huang Bai*, Artemisia *Yin Chen Hao*

History and Comments It is often used for treatment of various types of cancer including Stomach cancer, esophageal cancer, and colon cancer.

Pharmaceutical Ingredients:[1–4]
1. Flavonoids
2. Hentriacontane, stigmasterol, ursolic acid, oleanolic acid
3. β-sitosterol, β-sitosterol-D-glucoside

Lobelia *Ban Bian Lian* 半边莲

Original Reference: *Ben Cao Gang Mu* (*Materia Medica Compendium*) by *Li Shi-Zhen* in 1590 本草纲目

Part Used: Whole plant

Name:
Pharmaceutical: Lobeliae chinensis, Herba
Botanical: Lobelia chinensis Lour.
Wade-Giles: *Pan-Pien-Lien*
Common: Chinese lobelia
Translation: Half-Edged Lotus

Energy/Taste: Neutral, pungent

Channel-Organ: Heart, Small Intestine, Lung

Actions:
1. Clear Heat and release Toxins
2. Promote urination and reduce edema

Form and Preparation: Powder, decoction, or pill

Dosage:
Horses and Cattle: 50–150 g
Llamas, Alpacas, Goats, Sheep, and Pigs: 20–50 g
Dogs: 5–30 g
Cats and Rabbits: 0.5–3 g
Birds: 0.3–5 g

Cautions and Contraindications: Caution in edema due to *Qi* or *Yang* Deficiency

Side Effects: Excessive overdose may cause nausea, sweating, excessive salivation, diarrhea, tremor, and hypotension.

Taraxacum *Pu Gong Ying* 蒲公英

Original Reference: *Tang Ben Cao* (*Tang Materia Medica*) by Su Jing et al., *Tang* Dynasty (618–907 CE) 唐本草

Part Used: Whole plant, or aboveground parts of the plant

Name:
Pharmaceutical: Taraxaci Mongolica, Herba Cum Radice
Botanical: Taraxacum Mongolicum; T. Sinicum; T. Officinal
Common Dandelion
Wade-Giles: *P'u-Kung-Ying*
Translation: Cattail Common Flower

Energy/Taste: Cold, bitter, sweet

Channel-Organ: Liver, Stomach

Actions:
1. Clear Heat and release Toxin
2. Resolve Damp and resolve lymphatic swelling
3. Promote lactation

Form and Preparation: Powder, decoction, or pill

Dosage:
Horses and Cattle: 30–90 g
Camels: 45–120 g
Llamas, Alpacas, Goats, Sheep, and Pigs: 10–30 g
Dogs: 2–6 g
Cats and Rabbits: 0.5–3 g
Birds: 0.3–5 g

Cautions and Contraindications: Cautions for Spleen *Qi* Deficiency

Side Effects: Overusage leads to nausea, vomiting, abdominal discomfort, diarrhea, or skin allergy.

Houttuynia *Yu Xing Cao* 鱼腥草

Original Reference: *Ming Yi Bie Lu* (*Miscellaneous Records of Famous Physicians*) by *Tao Hong-Jing*, North and South Kingdoms (5th century CE) 名医别录

Part Used: Aboveground parts of the plant

Name:
Pharmaceutical: Houttuyniae Cordatae, Herba Cum Radice
Botanical: Houttuynia Cordata
Common: Houttuynia
Wade-Giles: *Yu-Hsing-Ts'ao*
Translation: Fishy Smelling Herb

Energy/Taste: Cool, pungent

Channel-Organ: Lung, Liver

Actions:
1. Clear Heat and release Toxin
2. Expel pus
3. Drain Damp Heat and promote urination

Form and Preparation: Powder, decoction, or pill

Dosage:
Horses and Cattle: 30–100 g
Llamas, Alpacas, Goats, Sheep, and Pigs: 5–20 g
Dogs: 2–6 g
Cats and Rabbits: 0.5–1 g
Birds: 0.2–1.5 g

Cautions and Contraindications: Caution for Cold due to *Yang* Deficiency

Side Effects: Skin allergy

Viola *Zi Hua Di Ding* 紫花地丁

Original Reference: *Ben Cao Gang Mu* (*Materia Medica Compendium*) by *Li Shi-Zhen* in 1590 本草纲目

Part Used: Entire plant

Name:
Pharmaceutical: Violae Yedoensis, Herba Cum Radice
Botanical: Viola Yedoensis; V. Japonica
Common: Violet
Wade-Giles: *Tzu-Hua-Ti-Ting*
Translation: Purple Flower Ground Spike

Energy/Taste: Cold, pungent, bitter

Channel-Organ: Heart, Liver

Actions:
1. Clear Toxic Heat, relieve fever
2. Clear hot sores
3. Nourish Blood, regenerate tissues

Form and Preparation: Powder, decoction, or pill

Dosage:
Horses and Cattle: 50–80 g
Camels: 60–120 g
Llamas, Alpacas, Goats, Sheep, and Pigs: 5–30 g
Dogs: 2–6 g
Cats and Rabbits: 0.5–2 g
Birds: 0.2–2 g

Cautions and Contraindications: Caution for Deficient Cold

Side Effects: It may cause diarrhea.

Patrinia *Bai Jiang Cao* 败酱草

Original Reference: *Shen Nong Ben Cao Jing* (*Shen Nong's Materia Medica*, 1st century BCE) 神农本草经

Part Used: Entire plant

Name:
Pharmaceutical: Patriniae, Herba Cum Radice
Botanical: Patrinia Vissosa; P. Scabiosaefolia; Thlaspi Arvense
Common: Patrinia
Wade-Giles: *Pai-Chiang-Cao*
Translation: Spoiled Sauce

Energy/Taste: Cool, pungent, bitter

Channel-Organ: Liver, Stomach, Large Intestine

Actions:
1. Clear Toxic Heat
2. Eliminate pus
3. Invigorate Blood and stop pain

Form and Preparation: Powder, decoction, or pill

Dosage:
Horses and Cattle: 30–60 g
Llamas, Alpacas, Goats, Sheep, and Pigs: 5–20 g
Dogs: 2–5 g
Cats and Rabbits: 0.5–1 g
Birds: 0.2–1.5 g

Cautions and Contraindications: Caution for Deficient Spleen *Qi* or diarrhea

Side Effects: Overdosing leads to thirst, nausea, and dizziness.

Belamcanda *She Gan* 射干

Original Reference: *Shen Nong Ben Cao Jing* (*Shen Nong's Materia Medica*, 1st century BCE) 神农本草经

Part Used: Rhizome

Name:
Pharmaceutical: Belamcandae Chinensis, Rhizoma
Botanical: Belamcanda Chinensis
Common: Belamcanda Rhizome
Wade-Giles: *She-Kan*
Translation: Shooting Stem

Energy/Taste: Cold, bitter

Channel-Organ: Lung, Liver

Actions
1. Clear Heat and release Toxins
2. Transform Phlegm and clear the Lung
3. Benefit throat

Form and Preparation: Powder, decoction, or pill

Dosage:
Horses and Cattle: 15–45 g
Llamas, Alpacas, Goats, Sheep, and Pigs: 5–10 g
Dogs: 1–3 g
Cats and Rabbits: 0.5–1 g
Birds: 0.1–1 g

Cautions and Contraindications: Caution during pregnancy.

Side Effects: It may cause diarrhea.

Lasiosphaera *Ma Bo* 马勃

Original Reference: *Ming Yi Bie Lu* (*Miscellaneous Records of Famous Physicians*) by *Tao Hong-Jing*, North and South Kingdoms (5th century CE) 名医别录

Part Used: Fructifications

Name:
Pharmaceutical: Lasiosphaerae Seu Calvatiae, Frutificatio
Botanical: Lasiophaera Fenslii Reich; L. Nipponica; Calvatia Gigantec; or C. Lilacina
Common: Puffball
Wade-Giles: *Ma-Po*
Translation: Horse Eruption

Energy/Taste: Neutral, pungent

Channel-Organ: Lung

Actions:
1. Clear the Lung, relieve Fire Toxicity
2. Stop bleeding

Form and Preparation: Powder, decoction, or pill

Dosage:
Horses and Cattle: 10–24 g
Llamas, Alpacas, Goats, Sheep, and Pigs: 2–6 g
Dogs: 1–2 g
Cats and Rabbits: 0.2–0.5 g
Birds: 0.2–1 g

Cautions and Contraindications: Caution for Wind Cold and loss of voice

Side Effects: Fever, dizziness, lethargy, vomiting, abdominal pain, frequent urination, and skin allergy

Portulaca *Ma Chi Xian* 马齿苋

Original Reference: *Ben Cao Gang Mu* (*Materia Medica Compendium*) by *Li Shi-Zhen* in 1590 本草纲目

Part Used: Entire plant

Name:
Pharmaceutical: Portulacae Oleraceae, Herba
Botanical: Portulaca Oleracea
Common: Portulaca
Wade-Giles: *Ma-Ch'i-Hsien*
Translation: Horse's Tooth Herb

Energy/Taste: Cold, sour

Channel-Organ: Large Intestine, Liver, Spleen

Actions:
1. Clear Heat and Release Toxin
2. Cool Blood during dysentery
3. Clear Damp Heat and treat sores

Form and Preparation: Powder, decoction, or pill

Dosage:
Horses and Cattle: 100–500 g
Llamas, Alpacas, Goats, Sheep, and Pigs: 50–250 g
Dogs: 2–10 g
Cats and Rabbits: 0.5–3 g
Birds: 0.3–5 g

Cautions and Contraindications: Caution for Cold and Deficiency in the Spleen

Side Effects: None known

Rhaponticum *Lou Lu* 漏芦

Original Reference: *Shen Nong Ben Cao Jing* (*Shen Nong's Materia Medica*, 1st century BCE) 神农本草经

Part Used: Root

Name:
Pharmaceutical: Rhapontici Seu Echinops, Radix
Botanical: Rhaponticum Uniflorum; Echinops Latifolius; E. Ritro
Common: Rhaponticum root
Wade-Giles: *Lou-Lo*
Translation: Leaking Reed

Energy/Taste: Cold, bitter

Channel-Organ: Stomach, Large Intestine

Actions:
1. Clear Heat and release Toxin
2. Reduce swelling
3. Promote lactation

Form and Preparation: Powder, decoction, or pill

Dosage:
Horses and Cattle: 15–30 g
Llamas, Alpacas, Goats, Sheep, and Pigs: 2–9 g
Dogs: 1–3 g
Cats and Rabbits: 0.2–0.5 g
Birds: 0.1–1 g

Cautions and Contraindications:
1. Cautions for Deficiency of *Qi*
2. Prohibited during pregnancy

Side Effects: Overdosage may cause lethargy, lockjaw, and spasm of the limbs.

Andrographis *Chuan Xin Lian* 穿心莲

Original Reference: *Lingnan Cai Yao Lu* (*Records of Picking Herbs in Lingnan*) by *Xiao Bu-dan* in 1936

Part Used: Aboveground parts of the herb

Name:
Pharmaceutical: Andrographitis Paniculatae, Herba
Botanical: Andrographis Paniculata
Common: Andrographis
Wade-Giles: *Ch'uan-Hsin-Lien*
Translation: Threaded Heart Lotus

Energy/Taste: Cold, bitter

Channel-Organ: Lung, Stomach, Large Intestine, Small Intestine

Actions:
1. Clear Heat and release Toxin
2. Dry up Damp

Form and Preparation: Extremely bitter; take in powder form for large animals, in capsules for small animals

Dosage:
Horses and Cattle: 60–120 g
Llamas, Alpacas, Goats, Sheep, and Pigs: 20–60 g
Dogs: 2–10 g
Cats and Rabbits: 0.5–3 g
Birds: 0.3–3 g

Cautions and Contraindications: Contraindicated for Spleen *Qi* Deficiency

Side Effects: Overuse may cause gastrointestinal discomfort and anorexia.

Smilax *Tu Fu Ling* 土茯苓

Original Reference: *Ben Cao Gang Mu* (*Materia Medica Compendium*) by *Li Shi-Zhen* in 1590 本草纲目

Part Used: Rhizome

Name:
Pharmaceutical: Smilacis Glabrae, Rhizoma
Botantical: Smilax Glabra
Common: Smilax
Wade-Giles: *T'u-Fu-Ling*
Translation: Earth Poria

Energy/Taste: Neutral, sweet, bland

Channel-Organ: Liver, Stomach

Actions:
1. Clear Heat and release Toxin
2. Dispel Damp

Form and Preparation: Powder, decoction, or pill

Dosage:
Horses and Cattle: 30–90 g
Llamas, Alpacas, Goats, Sheep, and Pigs: 10–30 g
Dogs: 2–6 g
Cats and Rabbits: 0.5–1 g
Birds: 0.2–2 g

Cautions and Contraindications: Caution in *Yin* Deficiency of Liver or Kidney

Side Effects: None known

Brucea *Ya Dan Zi* 鸭胆子

Original Reference: Ben Cao Gang Mu Shi Yi (*Omissions for the Materia Medica Compendium*) by *Zhao Xue-min* et al. in 1765 本草纲目拾遗

Part Used: Fruit

Name:
Pharmaceutical: Brucea Javanicae, Fructus
Botanical: Brucea Javanica
Common: Java Brucea Fruit
Wade-Giles: *Ya-Tan-Tzu*
Translation: Crow Gallbladder Seed

Energy/Taste: Cold, bitter, toxic

Channel-Organ: Large Intestine, Liver

Actions:
1. Clear toxic Heat to resolve dysenteric disorders
2. Treat intermittent chills and fever (malarial disorders)

Form and Preparation: Powder, decoction, or pill

Dosage:
Horses and Cattle: 5–15 g
Llamas, Alpacas, Goats, Sheep, and Pigs: 1–4.5 g

Cautions and Contraindications:
1. Cautions for Spleen Deficiency
2. Caution in Pregnancy and with pediatric patients
3. Do not take long-term or in large doses.
4. Contraindications for Liver or Kidney Disease

Side Effects:
1. May cause nausea or vomiting, gastrointestinal bleeding
2. Can injure stomach, intestines, liver, and kidneys

Fel Ursi *Xiong Dan* 熊胆

Historically, *Xiong Dan* was used for over thousand years. However, because the bear is a protected and endangered species, this substance is currently prohibited. The following information is merely for educational purposes.

Original Reference: *Tang Ben Cao* (*Tang Materia Medica*) by Su Jing et al., *Tang* Dynasty (618–907 CE) 唐本草

Part Used: Bear Gallbladder

Name:
Pharmaceutical: Ursi, Vesica Fellea
Zoological: Selenarctos thibetanus or Ursus arctos L.
Common: Bear gallbladder
Wade-Giles: *Hsiung-Tan*
Translation: Bear Gallbladder

Energy/Taste: Cold, bitter

Channel-Organ: Gallbladder, Heart, Liver

Actions:
1. Clear Heat and alleviate spasms
2. Relieve Fire toxicity on skin, stop pain
3. Benefit the eyes in Excessive Liver Fire Pattern
4. Reduce swelling and pain

Form and Preparation: Mixed with other herbs to make pill for oral use, or raw for topical use

Dosage:
Horses and Cattle: 6–9 g
Llamas, Alpacas, Goats, Sheep, and Pigs: 3–6 g

Cautions and Contraindications:
1. Because the bear is a protected and endangered species, this substance is prohibited. It can be substituted with Bovis *Niu Huang* or pig gallbladder Suis *Zhu Dan Zhi.*
2. This substance should not be used with either Rehmannia *Sheng Di Huang* or Stephania *Han Fang Ji.*

Side Effects: It may cause skin allergy. Long-time use can be toxic to liver and kidneys.

HERBS TO CLEAR HEAT DUE TO *YIN* DEFICIENCY

Herbs to clear Heat due to *Yin* Deficiency are used to treat false Heat (deficient Heat) that is caused by *Yin* Deficiency. The primary clinical signs of False Heat due to *Yin* Deficiency include fever (low-grade or tidal), dry mouth and throat, night sweating, irritability, red tongue, and a thin-rapid pulse. These herbs are recommended for use in combination with herbs that tonify *Yin* or clear Heat.

Artemisia *Qing Hao* 青蒿

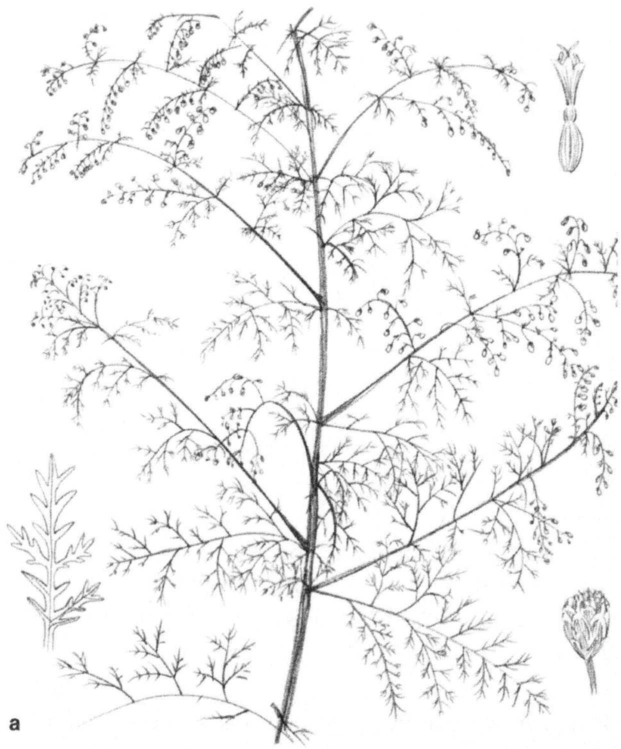

a

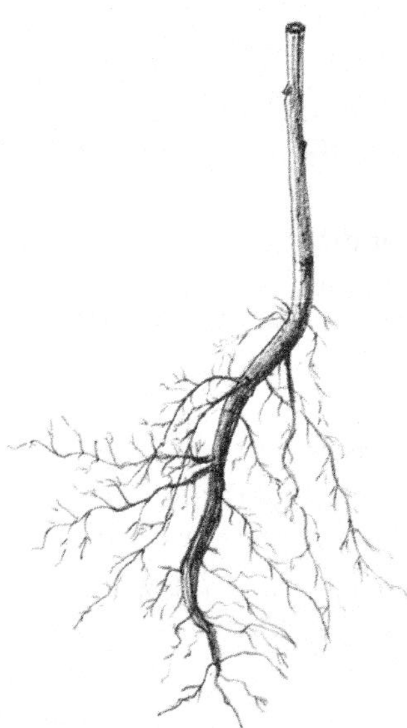

b

Original Reference: *Shen Nong Ben Cao Jing* (*Shen Nong's Materia Medica*, 1st century BCE) 神农本草经

Part Used: Whole herb or aboveground parts

Name:
Pharmaceutical: Artemisiae Annuae, Herba
Botanical: Artemisia Annua; A. Apiacea
Common: Artemisia
Wade-Giles: *Ching-Hao*
Translation: Blue-green artemisia

Energy/Taste: Cold, bitter, pungent

Channel-Organ: Kidney, Liver, Gallbladder

Actions:
1. Clear Heat from *Yin* Deficiency
2. Check malarial disorders and relieve Heat
3. Clear Summer-Heat
4. Cool Blood and stop bleeding

Form and Preparation: Powder, decoction, or pill; for malaria, the best result is from an extract or alcohol extract preparation.

Dosage:
Horses and Cattle: 20–45 g
Llamas, Alpacas, Goats, Sheep, and Pigs: 6–12 g
Dogs: 2–5 g
Cats and Rabbits: 0.5–1 g
Birds: 0.1–1 g

Cautions and Contraindications:
1. Caution for Postpartum mare with Blood Deficiency.
2. Caution for Cold due to Spleen *Yang* Deficiency of Spleen.
3. It should not be used with Rehmannia *Sheng Di Huang* or Angelica *Dang Gui*.

Side Effects: It may cause nausea, vomiting, abdominal pain, and diarrhea.

Clinical Applications:
1. Summer Heat fever
   Clinical signs: Fever without sweating, dizziness
   Combine with: Dolichoris *Bai Bian Dou*, Talcum *Hua Shi*
2. Heat due to *Yin* Deficiency or Blood Deficiency
   Clinical signs: Evening fever, lower-grade fever without sweating
   Combine with: Lycium *Di Gu Pi*, Cynanchum *Bai Wei*
3. Malarial disorders
   Clinical signs: Nausea, intense fevers, or alternative fever and chill of malaria diseases
   Combine with: Scutellaria *Huang Qin*, and Pinellia *Ban Xia*

History and Comments
1. The legends about Artemisia *Qing Hao* can be traced back to a renowned physician during the Eastern *Han* Dynasty and Three Kingdoms era of China (25 CE–280 CE). Earlier in his career, Hua Tuo had repeatedly failed to cure tuberculosis in his patients. When Hua Tuo heard that one tuberculosis patient had

suddenly recovered, he inquired into the case. This patient had used *Qing Hao*, so Hua Tuo collected this herb and used it for other tuberculosis patients. To Hua Tuo's disappointment and puzzlement, the herb had no effect. Upon further investigation, Hua Tuo discovered that the successfully cured patient had taken *Qing Hao* in March. Hua Tuo realized that only the rapidly growing *Qing Hao* harvested in March would be useful because of the rising *Yang Qi*. The next spring, Hua Tuo collected much *Qing Hao* in March and used the herb to treat his tuberculosis patients. All the patients improved. However, after March the *Qing Hao* again lost its effectiveness. The next year, Hua Tuo conducted experiments to determine the effectiveness of each part of *Qing Hao* including the stem, root, and leaf. His clinical trials showed that only the fresh (blue-green) stem and leaf were useful. Hua Tuo named the herb *Qing* (blue-green) *Hao* (artemisia). The legend of Hua Tuo's experience became known as "Hua Tuo's three trials of *Qing Hao*."
2. *Qing Hao* has shown a direct killing effect against the malaria parasite in vitro.
3. The leaves are the most potent part of the herb.

Pharmaceutical Ingredients:[1–4]
1. Terpenoids (artemisinin A, B, C, hydroartemisinin, annulide, arteannuin)
2. Flavonoids (quercetin, chrysosplenol, artemetin, casticin, scopoletic, coumarin
3. Essential oils (artemisia ketone, isoartemisia ketone, camphene, l camphor, β-caryopyllene, β-pinene)

Lycium Di Gu Pi 地骨皮

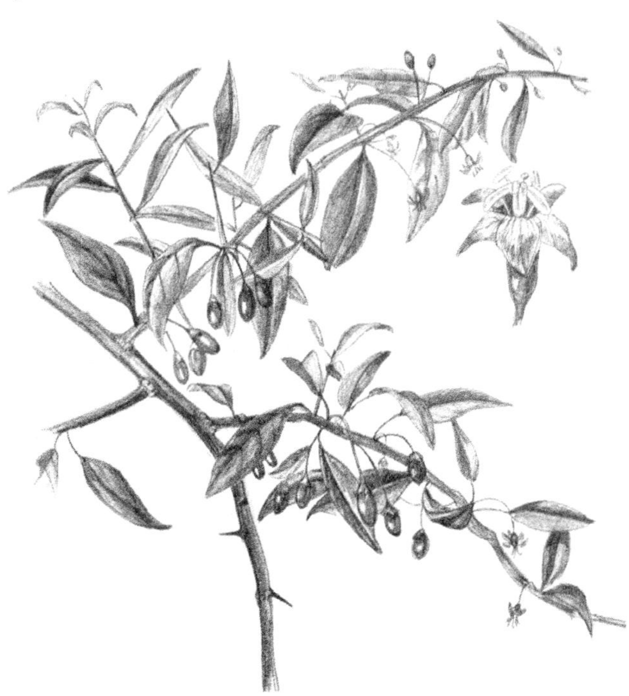

Original Reference: *Shen Nong Ben Cao Jing* (*Shen Nong's Materia Medica*, 1st century BCE) 神农本草经

Part Used: Root Bark

Name:
Pharmaceutical: Lycii Radicis, Cortex
Botanical: Lycium Chinense; L. Barbarum
Common: Wolfberry Root Bark
Wade-Giles: *Ti-Ku-P'i*
Translation: Earth Bone Bark

Energy/Taste: Cold, sweet, bland

Channel-Organ: Lung, Kidney, Liver

Actions:
1. Cool Blood and reduce Deficiency-Heat
2. Clear Lung Heat and stop cough
3. Drain Floating Fire in the Kidney Channel

Form and Preparation: Powder, decoction, or pill; do not cook in iron pots.

Dosage:
Horses and Cattle: 15–60 g
Llamas, Alpacas, Goats, Sheep, and Pigs: 5–15 g
Dogs: 2–5 g
Cats and Rabbits: 0.5–1 g
Birds: 0.2–1.5 g

Cautions and Contraindications:
1. Caution during common colds
2. Caution for diarrhea due to Spleen *Qi* Deficiency

Side Effects: None known

Clinical Applications:
1. Heat in the Blood Level with *Yin* Deficiency (bone-steaming disease)
   Clinical signs: Bi syndrome, night sweating, tidal fever, dry throat, bruising, nosebleeds, fever with rash
   Combine with: Anemarrhena *Zhi Mu*, Testudinis *Gui Ban*, and Stellaria *Yin Chai Hu*
2. Lung Fire with *Yin* Deficiency
   Clinical signs: Dry cough, cough with Blood, difficult breathing, tuberculosis
   Combine with: Ophiopogon *Mai Men Dong*, Gypsum *Shi Gao*, and Morus *Sang Bai Pi*
3. Skin itching due to Heat
   Combine with: Cnidium *She Chuang Zi*, Schisandra *Wu Wei Zi*, and Mentha *Bo He*
   Apply externally

History and Comments

1. *Di Gu Pi* is the root bark of the same plant as Lycium *Gou Qi Zi*, which was originally called *Gou Qi Gen Pi*. *Gou Qi Zi* is the fruit of this plant.
2. During the *Qing* Dynasty (1644–1840 CE), the Empress Dowager Ci Xi (the emperor's mother) felt chest distress and was unable to see clearly. The palace doctors could do nothing. When general Qian told the doctors how his own mother was cured of a similar disease by a local doctor using an herbal root bark, the palace doctors recommended the same prescription for Empress Dowager. Empress Dowager sent General Qian to his hometown to retrieve a big bag of the Wolfberry root bark (*Gou Qi Gen Pi*). The general decocted the medicine himself and sent it to the Empress Dowager. Over several days the Empress Dowager gradually recovered. She asked general Qian for the name of the medicine he had used. General Qian knew that the words *Gou Ji* would make the emperor's mother uncomfortable because *Gou Ji* sounds like "dog's penis," so he chose another lucky name *Di* (Earth) *Gu* (bone) *Pi* (bark) to share with her. Empress Dowager was delighted and said, "That's wonderful. I can live as long as God after eating the *Di Gu Pi*." *Gou Qi Gen Pi* was renamed as *Di Gu Pi* ever since.
3. Lycium *Di Gu Pi* is often used for False (deficient) Fire due to Lung or Kidney *Yin* Deficiency and often combined with Moutan *Mu Dan Pi* or Stellaria *Yin Chai Hu* to reinforce its effect. It is also used in treating malaria.

Pharmaceutical Ingredients:[1–4]

1. Cinnamic acid, phenols, betaine
2. β-sitosterol, linoleic acid, linolenic acid
3. Lyciumins A, B, kukoamine A, lyciumamide

Stellaria *Yin Chai Hu* 银柴胡

Original Reference: *Ben Cao Gang Mu Shi Yi* (*Omissions for the Materia Medica Compendium*) by *Zhao Xue-min* et al. in 1765. 本草纲目拾遗

Part Used: Root

Name:
Pharmaceutical: Stellariae Dichotomae, Radix
Botanical: Stellaria Dichotoma; S. Gypsophiloides
Common: Stellaria Root
Wade-Giles: *Yin-Ch'ai-Hu*
Translation: Silver Bupleurum

Energy/Taste: Cool, sweet

Channel-Organ: Liver, Kidney, Stomach

Actions:

1. Reduce Heat due to *Yin* Deficiency
2. Stop bleeding

Form and Preparation: Powder, decoction, or pill

Dosage:
Horses and Cattle: 15–30 g
Llamas, Alpacas, Goats, Sheep, and Pigs: 2–9 g
Dogs: 1–4 g
Cats and Rabbits: 0.5–1 g
Birds: 0.1–1 g

Cautions and Contraindications:

1. Caution for exogenous fever due to Wind-Cold Invasion.
2. Caution for Deficient Blood without Heat signs.

Side Effects: None known

Cynanchum *Bai Wei* 白薇

Original Reference: *Shen Nong Ben Cao Jing* (*Shen Nong's Materia Medica*, 1st century BCE) 神农本草经

Part Used: Rhizome and root

Name:
Pharmaceutical: Cynanchi Baiwei, Radix
Botanical: Cynanchum Atratum; C. Versicolor
Common: Sallowwort Root
Wade-Giles: *Pai-Wei*

Energy/Taste: Cold, bitter, salty

Channel-Organ: Liver, Stomach, Kidney

Actions:

1. Clear Blood Heat
2. Relieve urinary burning
3. Release Toxins

Form and Preparation: Powder, decoction, or pill

Dosage:
Horses and Cattle: 15–30 g
Llamas, Alpacas, Goats, Sheep, and Pigs: 3–10 g
Dogs: 1–4 g
Cats and Rabbits: 0.5–1 g
Birds: 0.1–1 g

Cautions and Contraindications: Caution for Deficiency of Spleen and Stomach.

Side Effects: Overdosage may cause palpitation, vomiting, dizziness, abdominal pain, and excessive salivation.

Picrorrhiza *Hu Huang Lian* 胡黄连

Original Reference: *Tang Ben Cao* (*Tang Materia Medica*) by Su Jing et al., *Tang* Dynasty (618–907 CE) 唐本草

Part Used: Rhizome/Root

Name:
Pharmaceutical: Picrorhizae, Rhizoma
Botanical: Picrorhiza Scrophulariaeflora Pennell or P. Kurroa Royle Ex Beri
Common: Picrorhiza Rhizome
Wade-Giles: *Hu-Huang-Lien*
Translation: Barbarian Yellow Link

Energy/Taste: Cold, bitter

Channel-Organ: Liver, Stomach, Large Intestine

Actions:
1. Drain Damp-Heat
2. Clear Heat From Deficiency

Form and Preparation: Powder, decoction, or pill

Dosage:
Horses and Cattle: 15–30 g
Llamas, Alpacas, Goats, Sheep, and Pigs: 2–9 g
Dogs: 1–4 g
Cats and Rabbits: 0.5–1 g
Birds: 0.1–1 g

Cautions and Contraindications: Caution with Spleen or Stomach Deficiency.

Side Effects: None known

HERBS TO CLEAR SUMMER HEAT

The herbs in this section are often cold or cool, and bitter. They can clear and resolve Summer Heat and are used for the treatment of Summer Heat Pattern, which is characterized by high fever, heatstroke, profuse sweating or nonsweating, red tongue, and fast pulse.

Mosla *Xiang Ru* 香薷

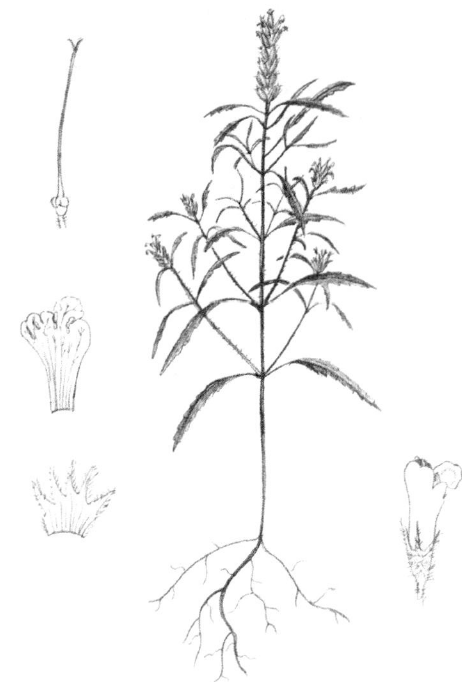

Original Reference: *Ming Yi Bie Lu* (*Miscellaneous Records of Famous Physicians*) by Tao Hong-Jing, North and South Kingdoms (5th century CE) 名医别录

Part Used: Whole plant above the ground

Name:
Pharmaceutical: Moslae Herba or Elsholtzia Herba
Botanical: Mosla chinensis Maxim or Elsholtzia ciliata
Common: Mosla or elsholtzia
Wade-Giles: *Hsiang-Ju*
Translation: Fragrant Mosla

Energy/Taste: Slightly warm, pungent

Channel-Organ: Lung, Stomach

Actions:
1. Clear Summer Heat
2. Induce sweating and release the Exterior
3. Promote urination and reduce edema

Form and Preparation: Powder, decoction, or pill

Dosage:
Horses and Cattle: 15–45 g
Llamas, Alpacas, Goats, Sheep, and Pigs: 3–10 g
Dogs: 2–4 g
Cats and Rabbits: 0.5–1 g
Birds: 0.2–2 g

Cautions and Contraindications: Cautions in weak patients

Side Effects: None known

Clinical Applications:

1. Summer Heat with Damp, or Wind-Cold during the summer
   Clinical signs: Chills and fever, nonsweating, body aches, vomiting, or diarrhea
   Combine with: Dolichos *Bai Bian Dou*, and Magnolia *Hou Po*
   Classical herbal formula: *Xiang Ru San*
2. Edema or urinary difficulty
   Combine with: Atractylodes *Bai Zhu*, and Poria *Fu Ling*

History and Comments *Xiang Ru* is the dried whole plant. It induces sweating to expel Wind-Heat in the Exterior, dispels Summer-Heat, and removes Dampness.

Pharmaceutical Ingredients:[1–4]

1. Essential oils (carvacrol, m-cymene, r-terpinene, humulene, o-cymene, p-cymene, α-phellandrene, α-terpineol, β-ionone, eugenol, cedrol)
2. Apigenin, 2-methylbaicalein, ursolic acid, syringic acid, caffeic acid

Dolichoris *Bai Bian Dou* 白扁豆

Original Reference: *Ming Yi Bie Lu* (*Miscellaneous Records of Famous Physicians*) by *Tao Hong-Jing*, North and South Kingdoms (5th century CE) 名医别录

Part Used: Seed

Name:
Pharmaceutical: Dolichoris Lablab, Semen
Botanical: Dolichos lablab L.
Common: Hyacinth bean, lablab
Wade-Giles: *Pai-Pien-Tou*
Translation: Flat bean

Energy/Taste: Neutral, sweet

Channel-Organ: Spleen, Stomach

Actions:

1. Clear Summer Heat
2. Strengthen the Spleen

Form and Preparation: Powder, decoction, or pill

Dosage:
Horses and Cattle: 15–45 g
Llamas, Alpacas, Goats, Sheep, and Pigs: 5–15 g
Dogs: 2–6 g
Cats and Rabbits: 0.5–1 g
Birds: 0.2–1.5 g

Cautions and Contraindications: Caution for intermittent fevers and chills.

Side Effects: None known

Nelumbo *He Ye* 荷叶

Original Reference: *Shen Nong Ben Cao Jing* (*Shen Nong's Materia Medica*, 1st century BCE) 神农本草经

Part Used: Leaf

Name:
Pharmaceutical: Nelumbinis Nuciferae, Folium
Botanical: Nelumbo nucifera
Common: Lotus leaf
Wade-Giles: *He-Yeh*
Translation: Lotus leaf

Energy/Taste: Neutral, bitter, slightly sweet

Channel-Organ: Heart, Liver, Spleen

Actions:

1. Clear Summer Heat
2. Raise and strengthen the *Yang* of Spleen
3. Stop bleeding

Form and Preparation: Powder, decoction, or pill

Dosage:
Horses and Cattle: 30–90 g
Llamas, Alpacas, Goats, Sheep, and Pigs: 5–30 g
Dogs: 3–9 g
Cats and Rabbits: 0.5–3 g
Birds: 0.2–2 g

Cautions and Contraindications:

1. Caution for bleeding due to Cold or Deficiency.
2. It may counteract Poria *Fu Ling*.

Side Effects: None known

Phaseolus *Lu Dou* 绿豆

Original Reference: *Ri Hua-Zi Ben Cao* (*Materia Medica of Ri Hua-Zi*) by *Ri Hua-Zi* in 713 日华子本草

Part Used: Seed

Name:
Pharmaceutical: Phaseoli Radiati, Semen
Botanical: Phaseolus radiatus or Phaseolus mungo
Common: Mung bean
Wade-Giles: *Lu-Tou*
Translation: Green Bean

Energy/Taste: Cool, sweet

Channel-Organ: Heart, Stomach

Actions:
1. Clear Summer Heat
2. Antidote to Aconite *Fu Zi* and fava beans

Form and Preparation: Powder, decoction, or Food Therapy

Dosage:
Horses and Cattle: 100–500 g
Llamas, Alpacas, Goats, Sheep, and Pigs: 20–100 g
Dogs: 2–6 g
Cats and Rabbits: 0.5–3 g
Birds: 0.2–2 g

Cautions and Contraindications: Caution for diarrhea due to Spleen *Qi* Deficiency.

Side Effects: None known

Citrullus *Xi Gua* 西瓜

Original Reference: Ri Yong Ben Cao (*Household Materia Medica*) by Wu Rui in 1350 日用本草

Part Used: Fruit

Name:
Pharmaceutical: Citrulli Vulgaris, Fructus
Botanical: Citrullus vulgaris Schrad.
Common: Watermelon
Wade-Giles: *Hsi-Kua*
Translation: West Melon

Energy/Taste: Cold, sweet

Channel-Organ: Bladder, Heart, Stomach

Actions:
1. Clear Summer Heat and generate Body Fluids
2. Promote urination and expel jaundice

Form and Preparation: Decoction or Food Therapy

Dosage:
Horses and Cattle: 100–1000 g
Llamas, Alpacas, Goats, Sheep, and Pigs: 50–250 g
Birds: 0.3–5 g

Cautions and Contraindications: Contraindicated for excessive Damp-Cold or Cold from Deficiency of the Middle Burner.

Side Effects: None known

SUMMARY

Tables 4.4–4.9 summarize and compare the herbs that clear Heat.

Table 4.4. Herbs that clear Heat and drain Fire: A quick overview and comparison.

Herbs	Special Actions	Common Characteristics
Shi Gao	Clear Heat from the Lung	Energy: Cold
	Clear Heat from the Stomach to alleviate thirst	Taste: Bitter or sweet
Zhi Mu	Nourish *Yin* and moisten dryness	Action: Strongly Clear Heat and drain Fire
Zhi Zi	Clear Heat from the Upper, Middle, Lower Jiaos	Indication: Heat in *Qi* Stage, Interior Excess Heat
	Cool Blood and stop bleeding	Signs: High fever, thirst, profuse sweat, red tongue with yellow
Xia Ku Cao	Clear Liver Fire, brighten eyes	coating, fast and strong pulse
	Dissipate nodule and promote urination	
Lu Gen	Generate body fluids, promote urination	
	Clear Heat from Lung and Stomach, stop vomiting	
Dan Zhu Ye	Clear Damp-Heat and benefit urination	
	Clear Heart Heat and Lessen irritability	

Table 4.5. Herbs that clear Heat and cool Blood: A quick overview and comparison.

Herbs	Special Actions	Common Characteristics
Sheng Di Huang	Nourish *Yin* and generate body fluid	Energy: Cold
	Nourish Kidney Jing and tonify Blood	Taste: Sweet, salty, or bitter
Xuan Shen	Nourish *Yin* and release Toxins	Action: Clear Heat and cool Blood
	Soften hardness and dissipate nodules	Indication: Heat in *Yin* or Blood stage, or Blood Heat
Mu Dan Pi	Invigorate Blood, resolve Blood Stagnation	Signs: Bleeding in nose, gums, stomach and intestines, or under the
	Clear ascending Liver Fire	skin. Skin rashes, blood in stool or urine, deep red tongue or dark
Zi Cao	Invigorate Blood to relieve rash and measles	purple tongue, rapid and thin pulse
	Moisten intestines to move stool	
Xi Jiao	Clear fever, stop convulsion, release Toxin	
	Prohibited for use now	
Shui Niu Jiao	Clear Heat, cool Blood, release Toxins	
	Substitute *Xi Jiao*	
Chi Shao Yao	Invigorate Blood and reduce swelling	

Table 4.6. Herbs that Clear Heat and dry Dampness: A quick overview and comparison.

Herbs	Special Actions	Common Characteristics
Huang Qin	Drain Fire, release Toxins, stop bleeding Calm fetus, sedate Ascendant Liver *Yang*	Energy: Cold Taste: Bitter Action: Clear Heat and dry up Dampness Indication: Damp-Heat Signs: Fever, scanty urine, turbid urine, jaundice, bloody diarrhea or dysentery, yellow or foul genital discharge, eczema or moisture dermatitis, furuncles
Huang Lian	Clear Heart Fire, release toxins Drain Fire in the Stomach and GI tract	
Huang Bai	Clear Damp-Heat in Lower Burner Drain false Fire/Heat from Kidney	
Long Dan Cao	Drains Fire from Liver and Gallbladder	
Ku Shen	Promote urination, kill worms and parasites Disperse Wind to stop itching	
Bai Xian Pi	Release Toxin and fungus, stop itching	
Qian Li Guang	Clear Liver Heat and benefit the eyes	
Qin Pi	Drain Liver Fire to benefit the eyes Disperse Wind-Dampness	

Table 4.7. Herbs that Clear Heat and release Toxins: A quick overview and comparison.

Herbs	Special Actions	Common Characteristics
Jin Yin Hua	Expel Wind Heat, release the Exterior	Energy: Cold Taste: Bitter Action: Clear toxic Heat Indication: Toxic Heat or Heat Toxin Signs: Redness, swelling, hotness, pain, sore throat, boils, carbuncles, abscesses, swollen glands. May occur in inflammatory or infectious diseases including influenza, upper airway diseases, IBD, herpes, parvovirus
Lian Qiao	Eliminate swelling, dissipate nodule or mass	
Ban Lan Gen	Benefit the throat, cool Blood	
Da Qing Ye	Cool Blood and reduce Blotches	
Bai Tou Weng	Cool Blood to stop dysentery	
Bai Hua She She Cao	Resolve Damp Eliminate pus and reduce abscess	
Ban Bian Lian	Promote urination and reduce edema	
Pu Gong Ying	Resolve Damp, resolve lymphatic swelling Promote lactation	
Yu Xing Cao	Expel pus, drain Damp, promote urination	
Zi Hua Di Ding	Relieve fever, clear hot sores Nourish Blood, regenerate tissues	
Bai Jiang Cao	Eliminate pus, invigorate Blood, stop pain	
She Gan	Transform Phlegm Clear the Lung, benefit the throat	
Ma Bo	Clear the Lung, stop Bleeding	
Ma Chi Xian	Cool Blood during dysentery Clear Damp Heat and treat sores	
Lou Lu	Reduce swelling, promote lactation	
Chuan Xin Lian	Dry up Damp	
Tu Fu Ling	Dispel Damp	
Ya Dan Zi	Treat intermittent chills and fever	
Xiong Dan	Alleviate spasms, benefit the eyes Reduce swelling and pain **Prohibited for use now**	

Table 4.8. Herbs that clear Heat due to *Yin* Deficiency: A quick overview and comparison.

Herbs	Special Actions	Common Characteristics
Qing Hao	Check malarial disorders and relieve heat Clear Summer-heat Cool Blood and stop Bleeding	Energy: Cold or cool Taste: Sweet or bitter Action: Clear false Heat due to *Yin* Deficiency Indication: Fever, low-grade fever or tidal fever, dry mouth and throat, night sweating, irritability, red tongue and thin, rapid pulse
Di Gu Pi	Cool Blood, clear Lung Heat to stop cough Drain Floating Fire in the Kidney Channel	
Yin Chai Hu	Stop Bleeding	
Bai Wei	Clear Blood Heat, relieve urinary burning Release Toxins	
Hu Huang Lian	Drain Damp-Heat Benefit the eyes	

Table 4.9. Herbs that clear Summer Heat: A quick overview and comparison.

Herbs	Special Actions	Common Characteristics
Xiang Ru	Induce sweating and release the Exterior Promote urination and reduce edema	Energy: Cold or cool Taste: Bitter
Bai Bian Dou	Strengthen the Spleen	Action: Clear Summer Heat
He Ye	Raise and strengthen the *Yang* of Spleen Stop bleeding	Indication: Summer Heat Signs: High fever, heatstroke, profuse sweat or nonsweat, red tongue, fast pulse
Lu Dou	Antidote to Aconite *Fu Zi* and general food poisons	
Xi Gua	Generate body fluids Promote urination and expel jaundice	

REFERENCES

1. Chen JK, Chen TT. Chinese Medical Herbology and Pharmacology. City of Industry, CA: Art of Medicine Press, 2004.
2. Brinker FJ. The Toxicology of Botanical Medicines. Sandy, OR: Eclectic Medical Publications, 2000.
3. Duke JA. Handbook of Medicinal Herbs. New York: Chemical and Rubber Company Press, 2001.
4. Huang KC. The Pharmacology of Chinese Herbs, 2nd Edition. New York: Chemical and Rubber Company Press, 1999.
5. Gao XM. Chinese Materia Medica. Beijing: China Publishing House of Traditional Chinese Medicine, 2002:102.
6. Bensky D, Clavey S, Stoger E. Chinese Herbal Medicine Materia Medica (3rd Edition). Seattle, WA: Eastland Press, Inc., 2004.

5 Purgative Herbs 泻下药

Huisheng Xie, Min Su Kim, Elizabeth Fernandez

Purgative herbs are generally used to purge wastes or toxins from the body. Actions of purgative herbs include lubricating the Large Intestine to promote bowel movements, stimulating the Large Intestine to cause diarrhea, draining the Large Intestine of harmful substances or fluids, and draining pathological Heat or Cold from the body. Purgative herbs are divided into three categories: 1) herbs to drain the feces downward (purgatives), 2) herbs to lubricate the intestines (laxatives), and 3) herbs to purge water downward (harsh cathartics).

Considerations When Using Purgative Herbs:

1. When Interior Pattern occurs along with Exterior Pattern in a patient, two methods may be used for treatment. One method is to combine purgative herbs with herbs to release Exterior Patterns. The alternative method is to first use the herbs to treat the Exterior Pattern and then use the herbs to treat the Interior Pattern.
2. If a patient's body resistance (antipathological factor) is weak, combine the purgative herbs with tonic herbs.
3. Purgative herbs should be used cautiously in patients who are weak due to chronic diseases during pregnancy, or postpartum.
4. Many purgative herbs are powerful agents for inducing diarrhea. These herbs should not be used when normal bowel movements have been restored.

HERBS TO DRAIN THE FECES DOWNWARD

Herbs in this category are bitter and cold. They facilitate the expulsion of stool by stimulating or lubricating the intestines. These herbs can remove wastes such as toxins, stasis, parasites, or retained water. Some can clear Heat. Herbs to drain feces downward are used to treat constipation or intestinal obstruction and excessive Heat accumulation. Excessive Heat accumulation signs include high fever, headache, red eyes, sore throat, toothache, or gastric bleeding with/without constipation. In addition to herbal therapy, treatment for constipation also utilizes dietary modifications. For patients with functional constipation, high-fiber diets containing naturally fibrous foods such as fruits, cereals, and vegetables are recommended. The poorly absorbed polysaccharides and cellulose derivatives in these foods absorb H_2O and increase fecal bulk, which promotes bowel movements.

Rheum *Da Huang* 大黄

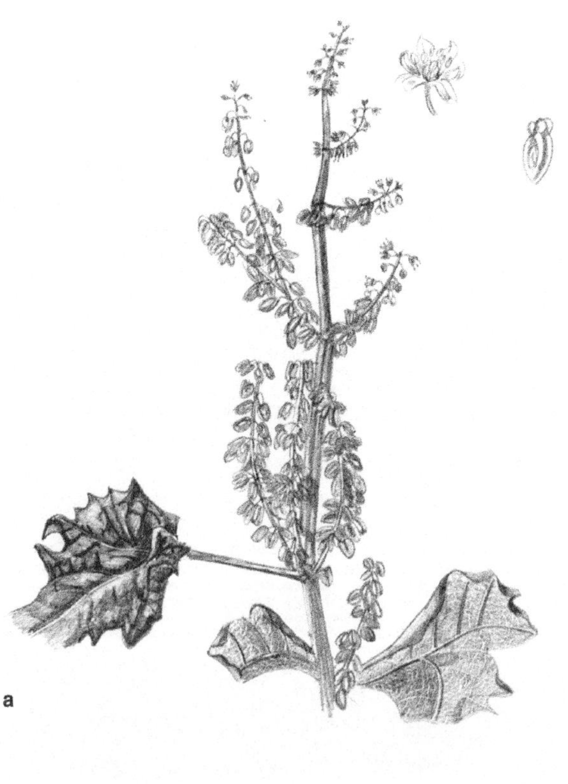

a

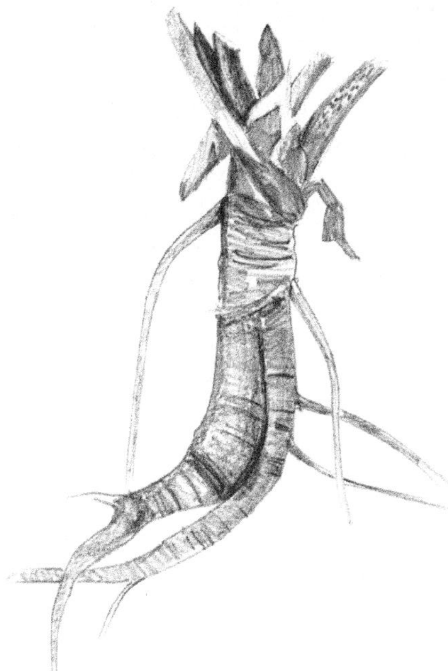

b

Original Reference: *Shen Nong Ben Cao Jing* (*Shen Nong's Materia Medica*, 1st century BCE) 神农本草经

Part Used: Rhizome and root

Name:
Pharmaceutical: Rhei, Radix et Rhizoma
Botanical: Rheum palmatum L.; Rheum officinale baill; Rheum tanguticum maxim, ex Regel.
Common: Rhubarb root
Wade-Giles: *Ta-Huang*
Translation: Big Yellow

Energy/Taste: Cold, bitter

Channel-Organ: Spleen, Stomach, Large Intestine, Liver, Heart

Actions:
1. Remove accumulations and guide out Stagnation
2. Drain Fire and cool Blood
3. Invigorate Blood and eliminate Blood Stagnation
4. Regulate Gallbladder and reduce Jaundices

Form and Preparation: Powder, decoction, or pill; use raw and cook for a short period of time (10 minutes) to move feces strongly; fry with wine to invigorate Blood; longer cooking decreases purgative effects; charred Rhubarb stops bleeding.

Dosage:
Horses and Cattle: 20–90 g
Camel: 35–65 g
Llamas, Alpacas, Goats, Sheep, and Pigs: 5–12 g
Dogs: 2–5 g
Cats and Rabbits: 1–3 g
Birds: 0.3–5 g

Cautions and Contraindications:
1. Contraindication in Deficient *Qi* or Blood, and Cold-Deficient Spleen and Stomach
2. Cautions during pregnancy, nursing, postpartum

Side Effects: Overdose may cause diarrhea and abdominal pain.

Clinical Applications:
1. Constipation
   Combine with: Mirabilitum *Mang Xiao*
   Classical herbal formula: *Da Cheng Qi Tang*
2. Constipation with Heat accumulation and damage to *Yin*
   Combine with: Rehmannia *Sheng Di Huang*, Ophiopogon, *Mai Men Dong*, and Scrophularia *Xuan Shen*
   Classical herbal formula: *Zeng Ye Cheng Qi Tang*
3. Extravasation due to Heat in the Blood: Vomiting with Blood, bleeding from the nose
   Clinical signs: Red, painful swollen eyes, sore throat, painful and swollen gums, vomiting with Blood and epistaxis
   Combine with: Coptis *Huang Lian* and Scutellaria *Huang Qin*
4. Abdominal pain due to Blood Stagnation
   Clinical signs: Amenorrhea, lochia retention, abdom inal pain, abdominal masses, traumatic injury
   Combine with: Ligusticum *Chuan Xiong*, Persica *Tao Ren*, Carthamus *Hong Hua*, Moutan *Mu Dan Pi*, and Angelica *Dang Gui*
5. Jaundice due to Damp Heat
   Combine with: Gardenia *Zhi Zi* and Artemisia *Yin Chen Hao*.
   Classical herbal formula: *Yin Chen Hao Tang*.
6. Burns or skin sores—use as a topical plaster
   Combine with: Gypsum *Shi Gao*

History and Comments:
1. A Poet, Yuan Mei (*Qin* Dynasty, 1716–1798) suffered from a diarrhea disorder. One doctor used Ginseng *Ren Shen* and Astragalua *Huang Qi* to tonify him, but his symptoms became worse. Another doctor diagnosed the poet with dysentery diarrhea due to Damp-Heat and prescribed "Prepared Rhubarb *Da Huang*" for the illness. After 3 doses, the poet's illness was gone. He wrote a poem praising this herb. In the poem, the herb is the "General" and he is the "Peasant":
   Herbs could heal like magic power,
   "General" can save the life of a peasant;

Doctor can make patients' lifespan longer without bias,
Terminal stage could make the "Gallbladder *Qi*" stronger.

2. The famous Dr. Yao Zheng Yuan practiced medicine during the Northern and Southern Dynasties (420–581). When Emperor Lian Wu Di ate Rhubarb *Da Huang* for his fever, Dr. Yao disagreed with this treatment. The doctor said, "You are an elderly patient. Rhubarb *Da Huang* is a strong herb which should be used cautiously." Dr. Yao meant that Rhubarb *Da Huang* could drain away the old Emperor's Yuan *Qi* (Source *Qi*). However, Emperor Lian did not heed Dr. Yao's advice and continued to eat the Rhubarb *Da Huang*. As a result, the Emperor's condition became worse and he died. When the successor to the throne, Emperor Lian Yuan Di, suffered from acute Stomach pain, his doctors gave him an herbal formula intended to harmonize the Stomach. However, Dr. Yao insisted on using Rhubarb *Da Huang* because this new Emperor's pulse was strong and suggested excess. Rhubarb *Da Huang* could relieve the Food Stagnation in his Stomach. This time the Emperor followed Dr. Yao's advice and ate the suggested herbal medication. Afterward, the Emperor's Food Stagnation resolved and his illness disappeared. The new Emperor made Dr. Yao a millionaire.
3. During a party in officer Xu's house, friends discussed Rhubarb *Da Huang*. One friend said he had heard Rhubarb *Da Huang* was so strong that one must use it very carefully. He said, "My friend's friend died from Rhubarb *Da Huang*." Officer Xu responded, "I do not think so. I always eat *Da Huang* and have never had any illness. If you do not believe me, I can show you." The officer immediately asked his housekeeper to buy several ounces of *Da Huang*. Although his friends tried hard to dissuade Officer Xu, he did not listen. Officer Xu ate about 20 g of *Da Huang* at once. At one point, a friend tried to forcibly remove the *Da Huang* from Officer Xu's mouth. The two fought, but eventually officer Xu snatched back the *Da Huang* and put it into his mouth. Officer Xu shouted foul language at the friend who took the Rhubarb. The friend's feelings were hurt and the party ended on an unhappy note. Later that evening after all the guests left, officer Xu developed nonstop diarrhea. When his friends came to check on him the next morning, the housekeeper told them that he had died in the middle of night. Officer Xu played games with an herbal medicine and paid the price with his own life at the age of 44.
4. *Da Huang* was originally called *Huang Gen*, and the name change comes with a story. An ancestor of Dr. Huang had discovered and named five herbs: *Huang Lian* (Coptis), *Huang Qi* (Astragalus), *Huang Jing* (Polygonatum), *Huang Qin* (Scutellaria), and *Huang Gen* (Rheum). He used these herbs extensively in his practice to cure many diseases. When Dr. Huang inherited his ancestor's herbal practice, he continued to use the same five herbs, so everybody called him Mr. Wu Huang (Five Huang Herbs). In March, Dr. Huang made his yearly trip to the mountain to collect medicines. Between March and the end of autumn, he lived in the home of a local farmer named Ma Jun. Over the years, Dr. Huang and Ma Jun became close friends. One year, Dr. Huang traveled to the mountain and discovered that Ma Jun's house was gone. The villagers told Dr. Huang that a big fire in Winter had destroyed the house and had killed Ma Jun's wife. Ma Jun now lived alone in a cave up the hill. Upset by the news, Dr. Huang went to the cave. When Ma Jun saw Dr. Huang, he was moved to tears. Dr. Huang invited Ma Jun to go with him and learn how to collect herbal medicines. Ma Jun was delighted and agreed. From then on, they went everywhere to dig medicine. Within half a year, Ma Jun had learned how to collect the five Huangs. However, Dr. Huang never taught him how to diagnose and treat disease. One day, Ma Jun asked, "Why don't you teach me to treat diseases?" Dr. Huang smiled and said, "Your temperament is not suitable for becoming a Doctor." Dissatisfied with that answer, Ma Jun secretly watched Dr. Huang treat his patients. Over time, Ma Jun felt that he now knew how to cure people. One day, Dr. Huang was away and a pregnant woman came for help. Ma Jun decided to treat her. The woman was weak and thin. Ma Jun asked, "What is your main complaint?" The lady said, "I have had bloody diarrhea for a couple of days." Ma Jun gave her *Huang Gen* accidentally, but he should have given her *Huang Lian*. The woman's condition worsened after taking two doses. She had a miscarriage within two days and then died next day. The woman's family knew Ma Jun had prescribed the wrong herbal medication, so they sent him to court. The court officer looked at the evidence and concluded that Ma Jun was guilty of malpractice. Dr. Huang arrived at the court and told the officer that it was he who should be considered guilty. The officer asked why. Dr. Huang replied, "Ma Jun learned medicine from me. I didn't teach him properly, so I deserve the punishment." Meanwhile, Ma Jun insisted it was his fault. Seeing the two men each offering to take the punishment to save the other, the office was deeply moved by their friendship. The officer took mercy on Ma Jun and let him go, but he sentenced him to pay a fine to the dead woman's family. Feeling ashamed, Ma Jun told Dr. Huang, "I should have listened to you. I won't be

so arrogant anymore." Dr. Huang said, "Doctors must not be too hasty in learning to heal diseases. Even a small mistake can lead to death." From then on, Ma Jun became more stable. Dr. Huang noticed the change in his friend and decided to teach him how to use herbs to treat disease. As a reminder to those who came after him, Dr. Huang changed the name of *Huang Gen* to *Da* (big) *Huang* to be easily recognized.

5. *Da Huang* has strong antimicrobial and antitumor effects. It is also used to decrease Blood cholesterol.

Pharmaceutical Ingredients:[1–4]

1. Anthraquinone, anthracene glycosides, dianthranone glycosides
2. Senoside A, B, C, D, E, F, emodin, aloe-emodin, chrysophanol, rhein, physcion, rhein-8-mono-β-D-glucoside, physcion monoglucoside, aloe-emodin-8-monoglucoside, emodin monoglucoside, chrysophanol monoglycoside
3. Tannin (galloyl glycosides, gallic acid, d-catechinic acid, estrogen)

Mirabilitum *Mang Xiao* 芒硝

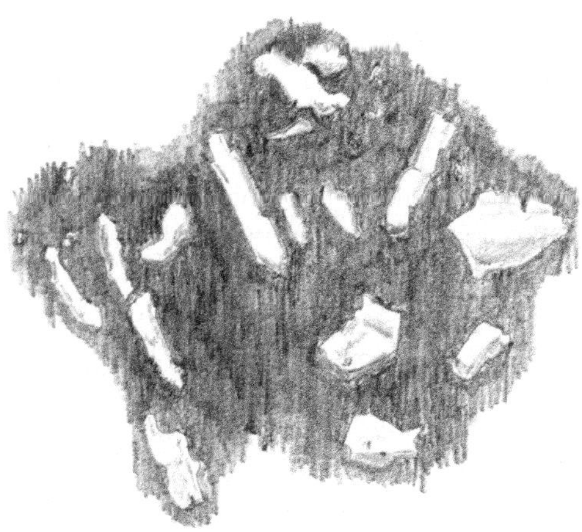

Original Reference: *Ming Yi Bie Lu* (*Miscellaneous Records of Famous Physicians*) by *Tao Hong-Jing*, North and South Kingdoms (5th century) 名医别录

Part Used: Mineral (Sodium sulfate)

Name:
Pharmaceutical: Mirabilitum
Mineral: Mirabilite (Sodium sulfate)
Common: Galuber's salt
Wade-Giles: *Mang-Hsiao*
Translation: Sharp mineral

Energy/Taste: Cold, salty, bitter

Channel-Organ: Stomach, Large Intestine

Actions:

1. Purge feces downward
2. Soften hardness
3. Clear Heat

Form and Preparation: Powder, decoction or pill for oral use; fine powder for topical use

Dosage:
Horses and Cattle: 100–500 g
Llamas, Alpacas, Goats, Sheep, and Pigs: 20–100 g
Dogs: 3–15 g
Cats and Rabbits: 1–3 g
Birds: 0.5–4 g

Cautions and Contraindications:

1. Contraindication in pregnancy and postpartum
2. Cautions in Spleen-Stomach Deficiency Patterns and geriatrics in general

Side Effects: Overdose may cause diarrhea.

Clinical Applications:

1. Constipation with Dryness due to Excess-Heat accumulated in the Intestines
   Combine with: Rheum *Da Huang*
   Classical herbal formula: *Da Cheng Qi Tang*
2. Sore throat, ulcerated mouth, red eyes or boils
   Combine with: Borneol *Bing Pian*, or use alone for external use
3. It can be used to stop lactation.

History and Comments:

1. Mirabilite is not absorbed by the intestines. Its presence in the lumen increases the water in the intestine due to osmotic pressure and it stimulates peristalsis. Thus, it softens up hardened stool. But, addition of Rheum *Da Huang* enhances the purgative effect.
2. It can be used topically for mastitis and pulls out the Heat.

Pharmaceutical Ingredients:[1–4] Hydrated sodium sulfate ($Na_2SO_4 + 10H_2O$), sodium chloride, magnesium chloride, magnesium sulfate, calcium sulfate, NaCl

Senna *Fan Xie Ye* 番泻叶

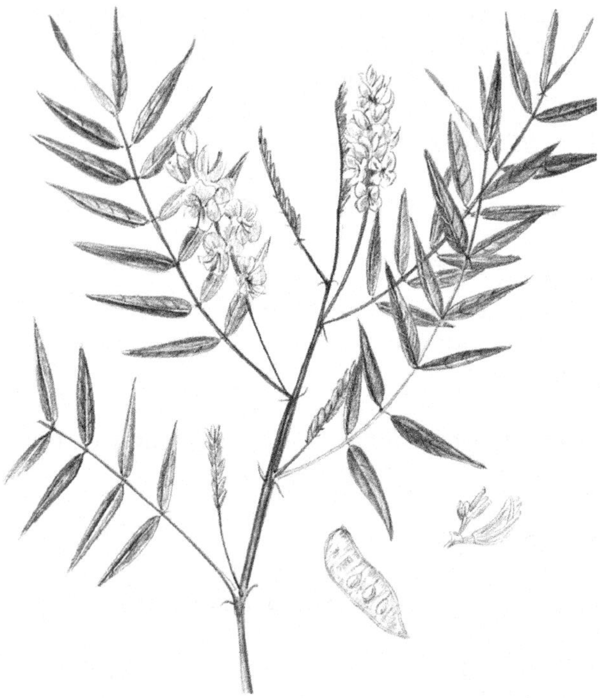

Original Reference: *Zhong Guo Yao Xue Da Ci Dian* (*Great Compendium of Chinese Materia Medica*) 中国药学大辞典

Part Used: Leaf

Name:
Pharmaceutical: Sennae, Folium
Botanical: Cassia angustifolia vahl
Common: Senna leaf
Wade-Giles: *Fan-Hsieh-Yeh*
Translation: Foreign Purgative Leaf

Energy/Taste: Cold, sweet, bitter

Channel-Organ: Large Intestine

Actions: Drain feces downward to guide out Large Intestine Stagnation

Form and Preparation: Powder, decoction, or pill

Dosage:
Horses and Cattle: 30–60 g
Llamas, Alpacas, Goats, Sheep, and Pigs: 5–10 g
Dogs: 1–5 g
Cats and Rabbits: 0.5–1 g
Birds: 0.2–2 g

Cautions and Contraindications: Cautions for lactation and pregnancy

Side Effects: Overdose may result in abdominal pain, nausea, and vomiting.

Clinical Applications:
1. Constipation, especially in weak or elderly patients.
   Use alone or
   Combine with: Magnolia *Hou Po* and Aurantium *Zhi Shi*
2. Constipation due to Heat accumulation in the intestines
   Combine with: Pogostemon *Huo Xiang* and Saussurea *Mu Xiang*

History and Comments:
1. In parts of China, this herb is used as tea to prevent Summer Heat conditions.
2. It is not toxic, but it is only 1/3 as strong as Rhubarb. Thus, this herb is good for elderly and weak patients.

Pharmaceutical Ingredients:[1–4]
1. Sennoside A, B, C, D
2. Rhein, aloe-emodin, chrysophanol

Research and Clinical study:
1. The chemical constituent toxicity and medication safety of *Fan Xie Ye* (Senna) was studied. It was shown in an in vitro study that the high content of a hydroxyanthraquinone derivative may cause gene mutation. However, it was unable to cause gene mutation when *Fan Xie Ye* (Senna) and its active component (e.g., anthraglucosennin) was applied in animals for a long time. *Fan Xie Ye* (Senna) at a normal therapeutical dosage is safe, effective, and has a less adverse reaction; but large doses and extended durational abuse can cause hypokalemia and intestinal mucosal injuries. A short-time application can increase its safety and effectiveness.[5]
2. Feng and Gao have found that there were several mistakes in the application of *Fan Xie Ye* (Senna).[6] **Mistake One**: *Fan Xie Ye* was taken as a tea for a long time. If it is used for a long period in this manner, it may cause abdominal pain and diarrhea. It was also reported that a patient may become dependent upon it if it is taken for extended periods of time and may also make constipation more severe after it is discontinued. So, *Fan Xie Ye* (Senna) must be used under the supervision of a physician and must not be taken as a tea for a long time, especially not as a weight-reducing tea. **Mistake Two**: *Fan Xie Ye* was taken with green tea. Because tannalbain in tea has the function of acting as an astringent on

intestinal mucosa, green tea may work against the purgative effects of *Fan Xie Ye* (Senna). Combining *Fan Xie Ye* (Senna) with tea can affect the overall curative rate of *Fan Xie Ye* (Senna). The correct method is to take 0.5–2 g *Fan Xie Ye* (Senna) and dip it in 100 ml of boiling water for 10 minutes and then drink the senna water extract and abandon the senna leaves. **Mistake Three**: Ignorant of the potential toxicity and side effects. *Fan Xie Ye* (Senna) provides a stronger stimulatory effect to the intestines, and it can cause abdominal pain and diarrhea if abused. *Fan Xie Ye* (Senna) must be applied carefully in young animals and patients exhibiting weakness and malnutrition. The dosage should be decreased or should be no more than 1 g for the weak and malnourished adult patient, and it should be decreased even more for children. It should not be applied during the menstrual period or gestational period of women because it can make the organs in the pelvic cavity hyperemic. This can lead to menstruation disorders, miscarriages, or even premature birth.

Aloe *Lu Hui* 芦荟

Original Reference: Yao Xing Lun *(Discussion of Medicinal Properties)* by *Chen Zhou* in 19th century CE 药性论

Part Used: Juice from the leaves

Name:
Pharmaceutical: Aloes, herba
Botanical name: Aloe vera L.
Common: Aloe
Wade-Giles: *Lu-Huei*

Energy/Taste: Cold, bitter

Channel-Organ: Liver, Large Intestine, Heart, Spleen

Actions:
1. Clear Heat, move stool, guide out accumulations
2. Kill worms and strengthen Stomach, improve digestion
3. Clear Heat from the Liver channel

Form and Preparation: Powder, decoction, or pill

Dosage:
Horses and Cattle: 15–30 g
Llamas, Alpacas, Goats, Sheep, and Pigs: 2–9 g
Dogs: 1–5 g
Cats and Rabbits: 0.5–1 g

Cautions and Contraindications: Caution for pregnancy, weak Spleen, or rectal bleeding

Side Effects: None known

HERBS TO LUBRICATE THE INTESTINES

Most of the lubricating herbs are seeds because the seeds contain oils that lubricate the intestines and move the stool. All the herbs in this category are mild in nature. Lubricating herbs are used for the following conditions: 1) constipation due to Deficient Body Fluids in the elderly, 2) constipation due to weakness from chronic diseases, and 3) constipation due to Dryness following febrile disease or parturition. These herbs are often combined with herbs to nourish Blood or promote circulation of *Qi*.

Cannabis *Huo Ma Ren* 火麻仁

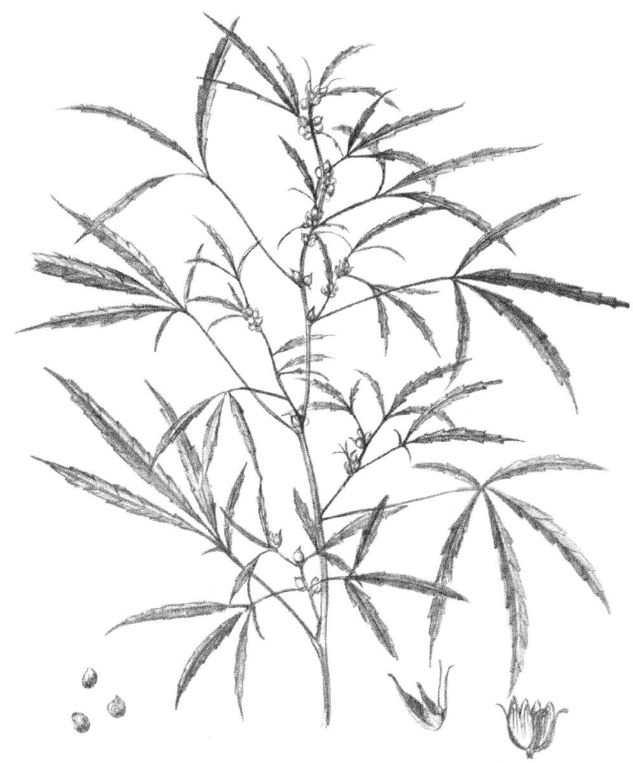

Original Reference: *Shen Nong Ben Cao Jing* (*Shen Nong's Materia Medica*, 1st century BCE) 神农本草经

Part Used: Seed

Name:
Pharmaceutical: Cannabis Sativae, Semen
Botanical: Cannabis sativa L.
Common: Linum, hemp seed
Wade-Giles: *Huo-Ma-Jen*
Translation: Fire Hemp Seeds

Energy/Taste: Neutral, sweet

Channel-Organ: Spleen, Large Intestine

Actions:
1. Lubricate the intestines and move the stool
2. Moisten Dryness and nourish *Yin*
3. Clear Heat and promote healing of sores

Form and Preparation: Powder, decoction, or pill

Dosage:
Horses and Cattle: 120–180 g
Camel: 150–200 g
Llamas, Alpacas, Goats, Sheep, and Pigs: 8–30 g
Dogs: 2–6 g
Cats and Rabbits: 1–2 g
Birds: 0.3–4 g

Cautions and Contraindications: Contraindicated for diarrhea or Spleen *Qi* Deficiency

Side Effects: Overdose or long-term use may result in nausea, vomiting, diarrhea, restlessness, or vaginal discharge or spermatorrhea.

Clinical Applications:
1. Constipation due to intestinal Dryness, *Yin* Deficiency, or Blood Deficiency in elderly or postpartum
   Combine with: Angelica *Dang Gui*, Rehmannia *Sheng Di Huang*, and Armeniaca *Xing Ren*
   Classical herbal formula: *Run Chang Wan*
2. Constipation with hemorrhoid or with Large Intestine Dryness and Heat
   Combine with: Rheum *Da Huang* and Magnolia *Hou Po*
   Classical herbal formula: *Ma Zi Ren Wan*
3. Ulcerations of oral cavity due to Stomach Heat
   Clinical signs: Redness, pain
   Combine with: Lonicera *Jin Yin Hua* and Glycerrhiza *Gan Cao*

History and Comments: Cannabis *Huo Ma Ren* seeds have been processed and can no longer germinate; thus, it is not possible to grow marijuana from this herb. The Cannabis seeds do not contain Tetrahydrocannabinol (THC), the psychoactive component present in the leaves and flowering tops. Therefore, this herb cannot be considered a controlled substance.

Pharmaceutical Ingredients:[1–4]
1. Trigonelline, (d)-isoleucine betaine, cannabinol
2. Oleic acid, linoleic acid, linolenic acid
3. Vitamins E1, B1, B2, lecithin, muscarine
4. Choline, sterol, glucuronic acid, edestinase, phytin
5. - Amides (N-trans-caffeoyltyramine, N-trans-feruloyltyramine, N-p-coumaroyltyramine, grossamide)

Prunus *Yu Li Ren* 郁李仁

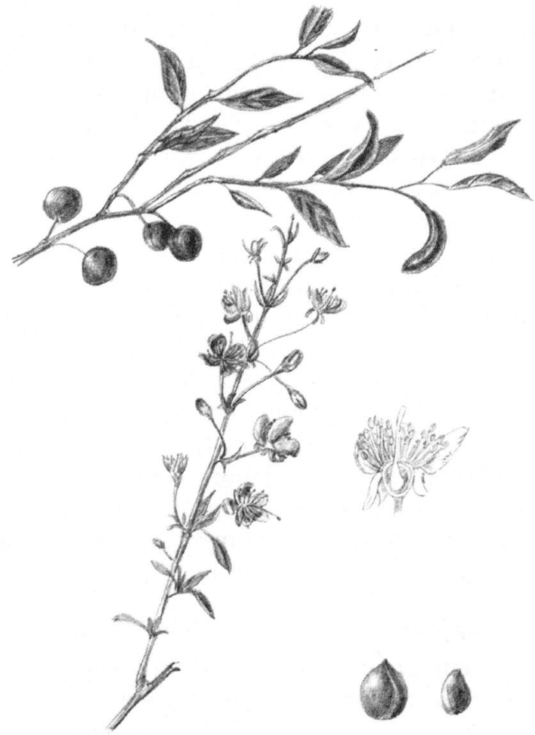

Original Reference: *Shen Nong Ben Cao Jing* (*Shen Nong*'s *Materia Medica*, 1st century BCE) 神农本草经

Part Used: Seed

Name:
Pharmaceutical: Pruni, Semen
Botanical: Prunus japonica Thunb
Common: Bush-cherry pit
Wade-Giles: *Yu-Li-Jen*
Translation: Constrained Plum Pit

Energy/Taste: Neutral, pungent, bitter

Channel-Organ: Small Intestine, Large Intestine

Actions:
1. Lubricate intestine and move stool
2. Promote urination and reduce edema

Form and Preparation: Powder, decoction, or pill

Dosage:
Horses and Cattle: 20–60 g
Llamas, Alpacas, Goats, Sheep, and Pigs: 5–10 g
Dogs: 3–6 g
Cats and Rabbits: 0.5–1 g
Birds: 0.2–2 g

Cautions and Contraindications: Contraindicated for pregnancy or patient with depleted fluids.

Side Effects: None known

Clinical Applications:

1. Constipation due to intestinal Dryness
   Combine with: Persica *Tao Ren*, Biota *Bai Zi Ren*, and Armeniaca *Xing Ren*
   Classical herbal formula: *Wu Ren Wan*
2. Abdominal distention, edema, swollen feet, and urinary retention
   Combine with: Coix *Yi Yi Ren*, Poria *Fu Ling*, Talcum *Hua Shi*
3. Chronic constipation caused by Dryness or *Qi* Deficiency
   Combine with: Cannabis *Huo Ma Ren* and Armeniaca *Xing Ren*

History and Comments:

1. *Yu Li Ren* is the seed of Prunus, which are grown primarily in *Hebei: Liaoning*, and *Inner Mongolia*. The seed is collected in autumn and prepared by crushing the hard stone shell and drying the seed in sunlight. The seed should be broken before using.
2. This herb acts primarily to relieve constipation by moistening the bowels and to eliminate edema by inducing diuresis.

Pharmaceutical Ingredients:[1–4] Amygadin, saponin, lipids, organic acid

Pinus *Song Zi Ren* 松子仁

Original Reference: *Kai Bao Ben Cao* (*Materia Medica of the Kai Bao Era*) by Ma Zhi in 973 CE 开宝本草

Part Used: Seed

Name:
Pharmaceutical: Pinus, Semen
Botanical: Pinus koraiensis Sieb. et Zucc
Common: Red Pine Seed
Wade-Giles: *Sung-Tzu-Jen*
Translation: Pine Seed

Energy/Taste: Warm, sweet

Channel-Organ: Lung, Liver, Large Intestine

Actions:

1. Lubricate intestines to move stool
2. Moisten the Lung to stop cough

Form and Preparation: Powder, decoction, or pill

Dosage:
Horses and Cattle: 20–60 g
Llamas, Alpacas, Goats, Sheep, and Pigs: 5–10 g
Dogs: 3–6 g
Cats and Rabbits: 0.5–1 g
Birds: 0.2–2 g

Cautions and Contraindications: Caution for diarrhea due to Spleen Deficiency or Damp-Phlegm.

Side Effects: Overdose may cause diarrhea.

HERBS TO PURGE WATER DOWNWARD

Herbs to purge water downward are used for four main conditions: 1) constipation due to fluid Stagnation, 2) fluid Stagnation in the thoracic or abdominal cavities (e.g., pleural effusion, ascites, and severe edema), 3) Phlegm fluid in Lung causing asthma, and 4) benign and malignant tumors. These herbs are extremely toxic; their harshness can damage *Yin* and *Qi*. To avoid the severe, harmful effects of overuse, these herbs are only used for a short time; sometimes they are discontinued after one or two doses. These herbs are prohibited during pregnancy.

Pharbitis *Qian Niu Zi* 牵牛子

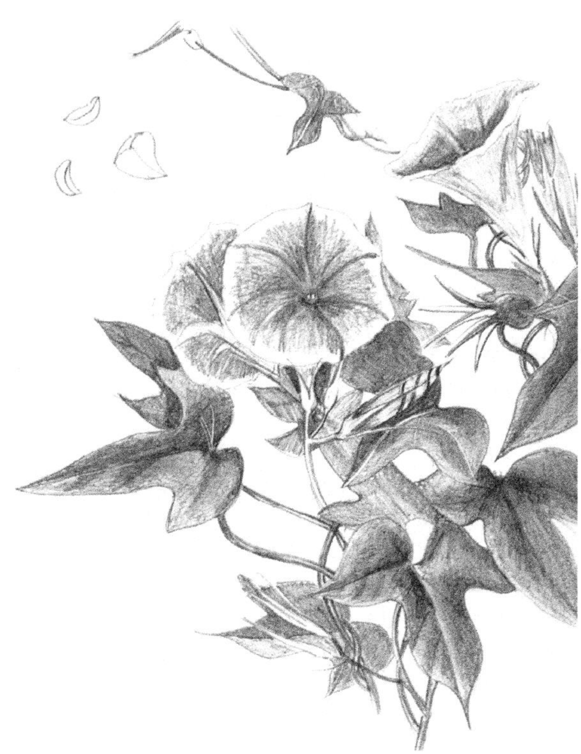

Original Reference: *Ming Yi Bie Lu (Miscellaneous Records of Famous Physicians)* by *Tao Hong-Jing,* North and South Kingdoms (5th century) 名医别录

Part Used: Seed

Name:
Pharmaceutical: Pharbitidis, Semen
Botanical: Pharbitidis purpurea
Common: Morning Glory seeds
Wade-Giles: *Ch'ien-Niu-Tzu*
Translation: Lead Cow Seed

Energy/Taste: Cold, bitter, toxic

Channel-Organ: Lung, Kidney, Large Intestine

Actions:
1. Purge water and Dampness downward
2. Purge accumulation from the GI system
3. Kill worms

Form and Preparation: Powder, decoction, or pill

Dosage:
Horses and Cattle: 15–35 g
Camel: 25–65 g
Llamas, Alpacas, Goats, Sheep, and Pigs: 3–10 g
Dogs: 1–3 g
Cats and Rabbits: 0.2–0.5 g
Birds: 0.2–1 g

Cautions and Contraindications:
1. Contraindication during pregnancy or Deficiency of Spleen *Qi*
2. Do not combine with Croton *Ba Dou.*

Side Effects:
1. It is toxic to the gastrointestinal tract, kidneys, and central nerve system.
2. May cause nausea, vomiting, colic, diarrhea, hemorrhage in urine, coma

Clinical Applications:
1. Edema, ascites, constipation, abdominal swelling
   Combine with: Euphorbia *Gan Sui* or Euphorbia *Da Ji;*
   With Deficiency of Qi: combine with Aquilaria *Chen Xiang* and Cinnamomum *Rou Gui*
2. Cough and asthma due to productive Phlegm or congested fluids
   Combine with: Lepidium *Ting Li Zi* and Armeniaca *Xing Ren*
3. Roundworms and Tapeworms
   Use alone in powder form or combine with Areca *Bing Lang*

History and Comments:
1. A long, long time ago, a penniless father sold his child to a landlord to herd cattle. That autumn the child became ill. The boy was emaciated, had waxy yellow skin, had difficulty urinating, and had an engorged abdomen like a drum. Because the illness prevented him from working, the landlord kicked him off his property. The boy wandered into the open country and then fainted. When the boy regained consciousness, he felt so hungry that he ate the seeds of a plant he found nearby. After a while, he developed watery diarrhea, but his engorged abdomen began to shrink. As he continued to eat the seeds over the next few days, his abdomen gradually flattened and his strength returned. The boy returned to the landlord, who gave him back his job. While herding the cattle, the boy led them to the place where his life was saved by the herb so that he could worship and give thanks for his recovery. Since this time, the herb has been known as *Qian* (lead) *Niu* (cow) *Zi* (boy), which means the boy who leads cows.
2. The herb acts to purge stool and Heat toxin similarly to Rheum *Da Huang*. Dry-frying the herb can attenuate its effects.

Pharmaceutical Ingredients:[1–4]
1. Pharbitin, pharbitic acid C, D
2. Lysegol, chanoclavine, penniclavine, isopenniclavine, elymoclavine
3. Steroids, gibberellin, gibberellin glycosides

Croton *Ba Dou* 巴豆

Original Reference: *Shen Nong Ben Cao Jing* (*Shen Nong's Materia Medica*, 1st century BCE) 神农本草经

Part Used: Seed

Name:
Pharmaceutical: Croton Tiglii, Semen
Botanical: Croton tiglium L.
Common: Croton seed
Wade-Giles: *Pa Tou*
Translation: Clinging Bean

Energy/Taste: Hot, pungent, very toxic

Channel-Organ: Stomach, Large Intestine

Actions:
1. Drain Cold downward
2. Drain water and reduce edema
3. Transform Phlegm and benefit the throat
4. Promote healing of abscesses and ulcers

Form and Preparation: Powder, decoction, or pill

Dosage: Extremely toxic; dose is very sensitive.
Horses and Cattle: 3–6 g
Pig: 0.6–1.8 g
Dogs: 0.1–0.5 g

Cautions and Contraindications:
1. Prohibited during pregnancy and for weak and debilitated patients
2. Not to be taken with hot food or drink; may severely aggravate its laxative effect
3. Do not combine with Pharbites *Qian Niu Zi*.
4. If herb causes unremitting diarrhea, one should take cold rice or a tea made from Coptis *Huang Lian* or Phellodendron *Huang Bai*.

Side Effects:
1. The action of Croton *Ba Dou* is very drastic and can last up to 15 hours. It is extremely toxic and may cause nausea, vomiting, colic, bleeding diarrhea with mucous, sore throat, dizziness, dehydration, dyspnea, and even death.
2. It should be cautioned in skin application because it can irritate the skin and cause blisters.

Phytolacca *Shang Lu* 商陆

Original Reference: *Shen Nong Ben Cao Jing* (*Shen Nong's Materia Medica*, 1st century BCE) 神农本草经

Part Used: Root

Name:
Pharmaceutical: Phytolaccae, Radix
Botanical: Phytolacca acinosa Roxb.; P. esculenta Van Hout.
Common: Poke Root
Wade-Giles: *Shang-Lu*
Translation: Commerce Continent

Energy/Taste: Cold, bitter, toxic

Channel-Organ: Spleen, Lung, Bladder

Actions:
1. Expel water through urination and bowels
2. Reduce sores and carbuncles

Form and Preparation: When treating skin lesions, it is ground up and applied as a paste with Vaseline, honey, or egg white. When used internally it is generally mixed with vinegar.

Dosage:
Horses and Cattle: 15–30 g
Llamas, Alpacas, Goats, Sheep, and Pigs: 2–5 g

Cautions and Contraindications: Contraindicated for pregnancy and all Deficient conditions

Side Effects:
1. A very harsh and toxic herb, the use of which is limited to cases of severe Excess
2. May cause nausea, vomiting, diarrhea, restlessness, muscle spasm, hypotension, coma, and death

Euphorbia *Gan Sui* 甘遂

Original Reference: *Shen Nong Ben Cao Jing* (*Shen Nong's Materia Medica*, 1st century BCE) 神农本草经

Part Used: Tuber

Name:
Pharmaceutical: Euphorbiae Kansui, Radix
Botanical: Euphorbiae kansui Liou
Common: Kansui root
Wade-Giles: *Kan-Sui*
Translation: Sweet Process

Energy/Taste: Cold, bitter, sweet, toxic

Channel-Organ: Lung, Kidney, Large Intestine, Spleen

Actions:
1. Purge water and reduce edema
2. Disperse nodules and reduce swelling

Form and Preparation: Better in pills or powder; use only in severe Patterns of excess in robust patients.

Dosage:
Horses and Cattle: 15–25 g
Llamas, Alpacas, Goats, Sheep, and Pigs: 0.2–1.5 g
Dogs: 0.1–0.5 g

Cautions and Contraindications:
Contraindicated during pregnancy
Cannot be used in combination with Glycerrhiza *Gan Cao* and will antagonize Polygala *Yuan Zhi*

Side Effects: May cause nausea, vomiting, dizziness, palpitation, hypotension, dehydration, dyspnea, lower body temperature, and death

Genkwa *Yuan Hua* 芫花

Original Reference: *Shen Nong Ben Cao Jing* (*Shen Nong's Materia Medica*, 1st century BCE) 神农本草经

Part Used: Flower bud

Name:
Pharmaceutical: Daphnes Genkwa, Flos
Botanical: Daphne Genkwa

Table 5.1. Purgative herbs: A quick overview and comparison.

Herbs	Special Actions	Common Characteristics
Herbs to drain feces downward (purgatives)		Energy: Cold
Da Huang	Remove accumulation, cool Blood Move Blood, eliminate Blood Stagnation Regulate Gallbladder and reduce Jaundices	Taste: Bitter Action: Reduce Fire, promote bowel movements
Mang Xiao	Purge feces downward. Soften hardness, clear Heat	Indication: Constipation, accumulation of Excessive Heat
Fan Xie Ye	Drain feces downward to guide out Large Intestine Stagnation	
Lu Hui	Remove accumulations Kill worms, strengthen Stomach, improve digestion Clear Heat from the Liver channel	
Herbs to lubricate intestines (laxatives)		Part used: Seed
Huo Ma Ren	Moisten dryness and nourish *Yin* Clear Heat and promote healing of sores	Action: Lubricate the intestines and move the stool
Yu Li Ren	Promote urination and reduce edema	Indication: Constipation due to Deficiency of *Yin*, Blood, or Body Fluid
Song Zi Ren	Moisten the Lung to stop cough	
Herbs to purge water downward (harsh cathartics)		Indication: 1) severe constipation,
Qian Niu Zi	Purge accumulation form the GI system Kill worms	2) ascites and Severe edema,
Ba Dou	Drain cold downward Transform Phlegm and benefit the throat	3) cancer mass Toxicity: **Extremely toxic Prohibited during pregnancy**
Shang Lu	Expel water through urination and bowels Reduce sores and carbuncles	
Gan Sui	Disperse nodules and reduce swelling	
Yuan Hua	Resolve Phlegm to stop cough Kill worms and parasites	

Common: Genkwa flower
Wade-Giles: *Yuan-Hua*
Translation: Genkwa flower

Energy/Taste: Warm, pungent, bitter, toxic

Channel-Organ: Lung, Kidney, Large Intestine

Actions:

1. Transform water to reduce edema
2. Resolve Phlegm to stop cough
3. Kill worms and parasites

Form and Preparation: Powder, decoction, or pill

Dosage:

Horses and Cattle: 15–25 g
Llamas, Alpacas, Goats, Sheep, and Pigs: 2–6 g
Dogs: 1–3 g

Cautions and Contraindications:

1. Contraindicated with pregnancy or weak patients
2. Counteracts Glycyrrhiza *Gan Cao*

Side Effects: Watery diarrhea and abdominal pain

SUMMARY

Table 5.1 summarizes and compares the Purgative Herbs.

REFERENCES

1. Duke JA. Handbook of Medicinal Herbs. New York: Chemical and Rubber Company Press, 2001.
2. Huang KC. The Pharmacology of Chinese Herbs, 2nd Edition. New York: Chemical and Rubber Company Press, 1999.
3. Gao XM. Chinese Materia Medica. Beijing: China Publishing House of Traditional Chinese Medicine, 2002:102.
4. Bensky D, Clavey S, Stoger E. Chinese Herbal Medicine Materia Medica (3rd Edition). Seattle, WA: Eastland Press, Inc., 2004.
5. Liu SL, Zhou YC, Li JX. Studies on Chemical Constituent Toxicity and Medication Safety of *Fan Xie Ye* (Senna). Li Shizhen Medicine and Materia Medica Research 2002: 13, No. 11: 693–694. (In Chinese)
6. Feng XQ, Gao GH. Several Mistakes in Application of *Fan Xie Ye* (Senna). Health for the Liberation Army 2005: No. 6: 28. (In Chinese).

6 Herbs to Warm the Interior

Huisheng Xie, Cheryl Chrisman, Min Su Kim

Herbs to warm the Interior are used to treat Interior Cold. *Yang* Deficiency or exogenous invasion of Cold pathogenic factors into the Interior can generate Interior Cold. General signs of Interior Cold include cold extremities, warm-seeking behavior, lack of thirst or attraction to warm water, diarrhea, clear and prolonged urination, pale tongue with a white, thin coating, and deep, slow pulse. Two common Interior Cold Patterns include Spleen Cold and *Yang* Deficiency (Table 6.1).

The pungent or acrid herbs to warm the Interior are warmer and stronger than the sweet *Yang* tonic herbs. Interior warming herbs are associated with the Spleen, Kidney, Heart, Liver, and Lung Channels. These herbs act to warm the Interior, expel Cold, warm the channels to stop pain, build up Fire, and assist *Yang Qi*. Thus, Herbs to warm the Interior treat Cold in the Middle Burner (Spleen and Stomach), pain due to Interior Cold, Spleen *Yang* Deficiency, and Kidney *Yang* Deficiency. Practitioners may combine these herbs with others depending on the patient's condition. Combine Herbs to warm the Interior with 1) herbs to relieve the Exterior for Exterior Patterns, 2) *Qi*-invigorating herbs for *Qi* Stagnation due to Cold, 3) herbs to resolve Spleen Damp for Spleen Damp due to Cold accumulation, 4) Spleen or Kidney tonics for Spleen or Kidney Deficiency, and 5) herbs to tonify source *Qi* for *Yang* collapse. These herbs are contraindicated for Heat Patterns and *Yin* Deficiency with Heat due to their hot and pungent nature. Because they are acrid, dry, and warming, these herbs can easily injure Body Fluids. Use these herbs very cautiously during pregnancy.

Biomedical research indicates that the herbs in this category are cardiotonics that reflexively stimulate the vasoactive centers of the central nervous system, thereby stimulating Blood flow. Some of these herbs are also beneficial for digestive disorders because they increase the intestinal tract's absorptive capability and they alleviate vomiting and diarrhea.

Aconite *Fu Zi* 附子

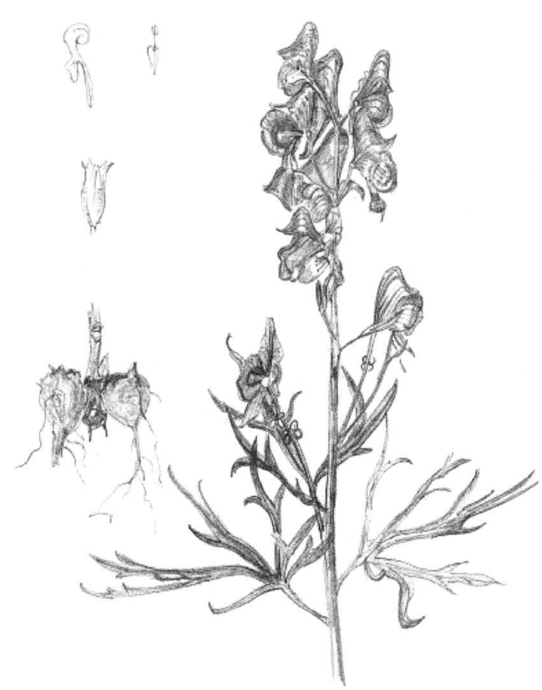

Table 6.1. Differentiation of Spleen Excess Cold and False Cold due to *Yang* Deficiency.

Patterns	Pathology	Clinical Signs
Spleen Cold (Interior Excess Cold)	Cold foods and drinks directly invade the Stomach and Spleen, or exposure to coldness and dampness from environment gradually leads to generation of Cold in the Stomach or Spleen.	Nausea and vomiting Belching Diarrhea Colic or abdominal pain An increase in gut sound
Yang Deficiency (Interior Deficiency Cold)	Long-term invasion of Cold damages *Yang*, or Ming-men Fire weakness because of aging leads to devastated *Yang* or collapsed *Qi*.	Ice cold back or extremities Watery stools or urinary leakage Fading minute pulse Pale, purple, and swollen tongue

Original Reference: *Shen Nong Ben Cao Jing* (*Shen Nong's Materia Medica*, 1st century BCE) 神农本草经

Part Used: Accessory root or branch root

Name:
Pharmaceutical: Aconiti Carmichaeli Praeparata, Radix Lateralis
Botanical: Aconitum carmichaeli
Common: Prepared aconite (detoxified)
Wade-Giles: *Fu-Tzu*
Translation: Branch root

Energy/Taste: Hot, pungent, sweet, toxic

Channel-Organ: Heart, Spleen, Kidney

Actions:
1. Warm and strengthen Kidney *Yang* and Heart *Yang*
2. Expel Cold, and warm Channels to stop pain
3. Resuscitate Collapsed *Yang Qi*
4. Dispel water and Damp

Form and Preparation: Powder or decoction

Dosage:
Horses and Cattle: 15–30g
Llamas, Alpacas, Goats, and Pigs: 3–10g
Dogs: 1–3g
Cats and Rabbits: 0.5–1g
Birds: 0.1–1g

Cautions and Contraindications:
1. Contraindicated during pregnancy
2. Prohibited for young neonatal patients (too *Yang*)
3. Contraindicated for *Yang* Excess or *Yin* Deficiency
4. May antagonize Fritillaria *Bei Mu*, Trichosanthes *Gua Lou*, Trichosanthes *Tian Hua Fen*, Pinellia *Ban Xia*, Bletilla *Bai Ji*, Cynanchum *Bai Wei*, Scolopendra *Wu Gong* and counteract Rhinoceros *Xi Jiao*

Side Effects:
1. It is toxic.
2. Overdosing will cause numb lips, tongue, or extremities, nausea, or coma.
3. Phaseolus *Lu Dou* is used to reduce the toxicity of Aconite *Fu Zi*.

Signs of Toxicity:
1. Lip and tongue numbness, nausea, hands and feet numbness
2. Inability to move
3. Palpitations, pale complexion, cold limbs, congested chest
4. Irritability, decreased sensation
5. Eventually, heart rate and blood pressure decrease, and respiration becomes feeble or patient may die.

Treatment of Aconite Poison:
1. Atropine has been very effective in treating an overdose of this herb.
2. Glycyrrhiza *Gan Cao* and Zingiberis *Gan Jiang* can diminish its toxicity.

Clinical Applications:
1. Collapse of *Yang*
   Clinical signs: Cold extremities, spontaneous difficult breathing, cold sweat, diarrhea with undigested food, minute pulse
   Combine with: Ginseng *Ren Shen*, Glycerrhiza *Gan Cao*, and Zingiberis *Gan Jiang*
   Classical herbal formula: *Si Ni Tang*

2. Kidney *Yang* Deficiency or weakened Kidney *Ming-men* Fire
   Clinical signs: Chills, cold limbs, weak lumbar region, impotence, frequent urination
   Combine with: Cinnamomum *Rou Gui*, Cornus *Shan Zhu Yu*, Rehmannia *Shu Di Huang*
   Classical herbal formula: *Shen Qi Wan*
3. Cold in the Middle Burner due to Spleen *Yang* Deficiency
   Clinical signs: Colic (worse with cold but better with warm), diarrhea
   Combine with: Ginseng *Ren Shen*, Paeonia *Bai Shao*, and Zingiberis *Gan Jiang*, plus Atractylodes *Bai Zhu*
   Classical herbal formula: *Fu Zi Li Zhong Wan*
4. Heart and Kidney Deficiency
   Clinical signs: Palpitations, shortness of breath, ascites, edema
   Combine with: Ginseng *Ren Shen* and Cinnamomum *Gui Zhi*
   Classical herbal formula: Zhen Wu Tang
5. Cold-Damp in the channels
   Clinical signs: Joint pain and chills
   Combine with: Atractylodes *Bai Zhu* and Cinnamomum *Gui Zhi*, Glycyrrhiza *Gan Cao*
   Classical herbal formula: *Gan Cao Fu Zi Tang*

History and Comments:

1. During the *Han* Dynasty (71 BCE), General He Guan and his wife He Xian gave money to their daughter's servant, Chun Yu Hen, so that he would help their daughter, He Chen Jun, to improve her status from concubine to Queen. This meant that the current Queen had to be removed. While Queen Hsu was in labor, Chun Yu Hen gave the Queen *Fu Zi*, an aconite pill, while telling her it would ease her labor pains. However, the pill had its true intended effect shortly. Queen *Hsu* exhibited sweating and irritability right before she died. This is the earliest reported case of a *Fu Zi* (aconite) "accident."
2. Aconite *Fu Zi* is spicy and hot with a potent effect. It can tonify the Heart *Yang* in the Upper Burner, Spleen *Yang* in the Middle Burner, and Kidney *Yang* in the Lower Burner. It is a key herb for treating *Yang* Deficiency or *Yang Qi* collapse.
3. *Fu Zi* is also an excellent herb for severe pain due to Wind-Cold-Damp.
4. *Fu Zi* is poisonous when raw. The herb, sold as a medicinal herb, is processed in a way that detoxifies it. Processing involves soaking the herb in water for 1 week, mixing it with 4% Zingiberis *Sheng Jiang* and 2% Glycyrrhiza *Gan Cao*. The herb is again soaked in water for 2 days, and then steamed, sliced, and dried.
5. Good quality Aconite *Fu Zi* is large and solid with a salty-white surface.
6. Aconite *Wu Tou* is related to Aconite *Fu Zi*. Both herbs come from the aconite plant, but *Wu Tou* is the main root while *Fu Zi* consists of the branches from the main root. There are two subtypes of *Wu Tou*: Aconiti Carmichaeli Radix (*Chuan Wu*) and Aconiti Kusnezoffii Radix (*Cao Wu*). Aconite *Chuan Wu* is hotter, more toxic, and stronger for clearing Wind-Cold Damp Bi than *Fu Zi*. Even though *Chuan Wu* and *Cao Wu* come from different plant species, they have similar actions and properties. *Cao Wu* is usually wild rather than cultivated and is even more toxic and potent than *Chuan Wu*. *Cao Wu* is rarely used.

Pharmaceutical Ingredients:[1–4]

1. Alkaloids (aconite, hypaconite, mesaconite, isodelphinine, benzoylmesaconitine)
2. Talatisamine, *chuan-wu*-base A, *chuan-wu*-base B
3. Higenamine, salsolinol, coryneine, atisines, aminophenols, neoline, 15-α-hydroxyneoline, higenamine, dl-demethyl coclaurine, salsolinol

Cinnamomum *Rou Gui* 肉桂

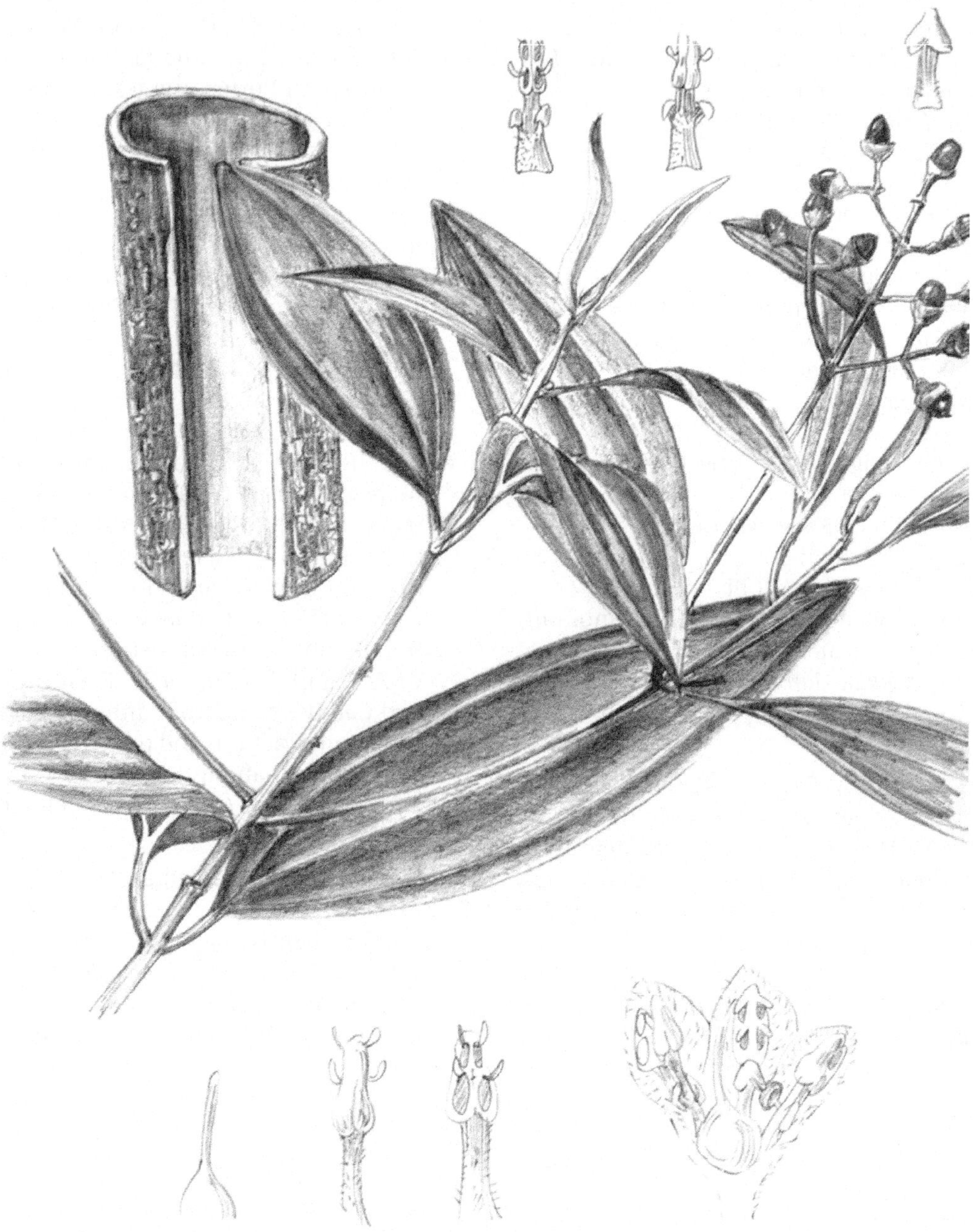

Original Reference: *Shen Nong Ben Cao Jing* (*Shen Nong's Materia Medica*, 1st century BCE) 神农本草经

Part Used: Bark

Name:
Pharmaceutical: Cinnamomum Cassiae, Cortex
Botanical: Cinnamomum cassia
Common: Cinnamon bark
Wade-Giles: *Jou-Kuei*
Translation: Meat bark

Energy/Taste: Hot, pungent, sweet

Channel-Organ: Kidney, Spleen, Heart, Liver

Actions:
1. Warm the Middle and Lower Burners
2. Dispel Coldness and stop pain
3. Warm Channels to promote circulation
4. Lead Fire back to source and treat upward floating of Deficient *Yang*

Form and Preparation: Powder or decoction

Dosage:
Horses and Cattle: 25–30g
Llamas, Alpacas, Goats, and Pigs: 5–10g
Dogs: 2–5g
Cats and Rabbits: 0.5–1g
Birds: 0.1–2g

Cautions and Contraindications:
1. Contraindicated during pregnancy
2. Caution during hot conditions such as *Yin* Deficiency

Side Effects: This herb is pungent and hot and may induce bleeding.

Clinical Applications:
1. Kidney *Yang* Deficiency
   Clinical signs: Sore and cold lumbar region, hind limb weakness, impotence or infertility, frequent urination
   Combine with: Rehmannia *Shu Di Huang*, Cornus *Shan Zhu Yu*, Aconite *Fu Zi*
   Classical herbal formula: *Shen Qi Wan (Jin Gui Shen Qi Wan)*
2. Deficiency of Kidney *Yang* and Lung *Qi*
   Clinical signs: Difficult breathing (especially inhalation), asthma
   Combine with: Ginkgo *Bai Guo*
3. Spleen and Kidney *Yang* Deficiency
   Clinical signs: Cold or pain in abdomen, edema, water accumulation, diarrhea, poor appetite
   Combine with: Aconite *Fu Zi*, Zingiberis *Gan Jiang* and Atractylodes *Bai Zhu*
   Classical herbal formula: *Gui Fu Li Zhong Wan*
4. Kidney and Heart *Yang* Deficiency
   Clinical signs: Congestive heart failure, edema, shortness of breath
   Combine with: Ginseng *Ren Shen* and Rehmannia *Shu Di Huang*
5. Cold Bi in the Channels or uterus
   Clinical signs: Painful joints and extremities, cold abdomen, dysmenorrhea, back pain
   Combine with: Zingiberis *Gan Jiang*, Evodia *Wu Zhu Yu*, Angelica *Dang Gui*, Ligusticum *Chuan Xiong*, and Carthamus *Hong Hua*

History and Comments:
1. Cinnamomum *Rou Gui* varies in strength depending on its grade. Thicker, older, and more expensive bark requires smaller doses due to its greater strength.
2. Adding a small amount of Cinnamomum *Rou Gui* to *Qi* and Blood tonic formulas can help generate *Qi* and Blood.
3. It can be used for hernia due to Cold.

Pharmaceutical Ingredients:[1–4]
1. Cinnamon oil
2. Cinnamic aldehyde, cinnamic acid, cinnamyl acetate, phenylpropyl acetate
3. Cinncassiol-A, -B, -C1, -C2, C3
4. Alkaloids, coumarin, tannin, cinnzeylanine, cinnzeylanol

Zingiberis *Gan Jiang* 干姜

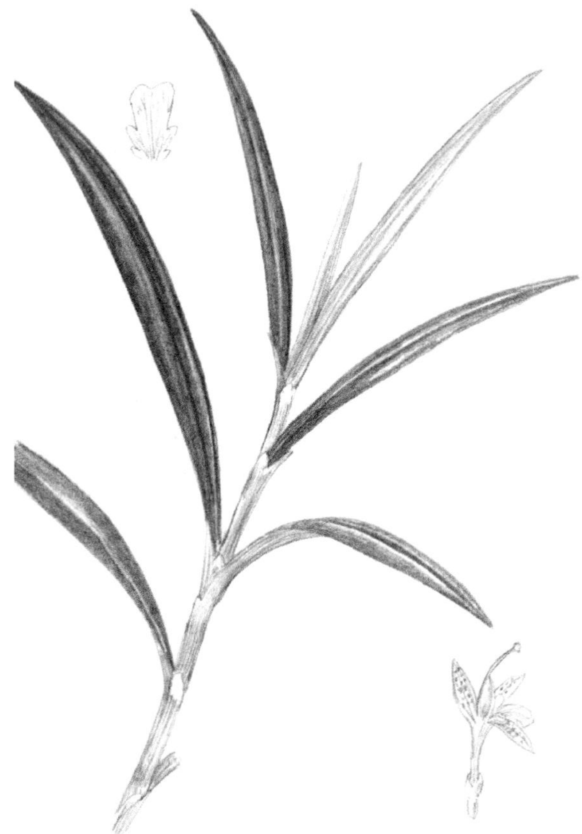

Original Reference: *Shen Nong Ben Cao Jing* (*Shen Nong's Materia Medica*, 1st century BCE) 神农本草经

Part Used: Rhizome and root

Name:
Pharmaceutical: Zingiberis Officinalis, Rhizoma
Botanical: Zingiber officinale
Common: Dried ginger
Wade-Giles: *Kan-Chiang*
Translation: Dry ginger

Energy/Taste: Hot, pungent

Channel-Organ: Spleen, Stomach, Lung, Heart, Kidney

Actions:
1. Warm the Middle Burner and dispel Cold
2. Warm the Lung to remove Phlegm
3. Restore *Yang* after collapse
4. Warm Channels and stop bleeding

Form and Preparation: Powder or decoction; roast before decoction

Dosage:
Horses and Cattle: 15–30g
Camels: 35–65g
Llamas, Alpacas, Goats, and Pigs: 3–10g
Dogs: 1–3g
Cats and Rabbits: 0.5–1g
Birds: 0.3–1g

Cautions and Contraindications:
1. Caution during pregnancy
2. Bleeding due to Heat or Excess
3. *Yin* Deficiency with Heat

Side Effects: None known

Clinical Applications:
1. Invasion of Cold to the Spleen and Stomach
   Clinical signs: Colic, vomiting, diarrhea
   Combine with: Evodia *Wu Zhu Yu* or Alpinia *Gao Liang Jiang*, and Pinellia *Ban Xia*
   Classical herbal formula: *Ban Xia Gan Jiang San*
2. Interior False Cold due to Spleen *Yang* Deficiency
   Clinical signs: Chronic intermittent colic, distended abdomen, vomiting, nausea, diarrhea, poor appetite, lassitude, weak pulse
   Combine with: Glycyrrhiza *Gan Cao*, Atractylodes *Bai Zhu*, Jujube *Da Zao*, Poria *Fu Ling*, and Ginseng *Ren Shen*
   Classical herbal formula: *Li Zhong Wan*
3. Collapsing of *Yang*
   Clinical signs: Cold profuse sweating, cold limbs, listless, minute pulse
   Combine with: Aconite *Fu Zi*
   Classical herbal formula: *Si Ni Tang*
4. Cold Phlegm or Phlegm-fluid in the Lung
   Clinical signs: Chills, difficult breathing, cough with profuse watery sputum, cold upper back, chronic lingering Phlegm
   Combine with: Ephedra *Ma Huang*, Asarum *Xi Xin*, and Pinellia *Ban Xia*, Schisandra *Wu Wei Zi*
   Classical herbal formula: *Xiao Qing Long Tang* (Small Blue Dragon Decoction)
5. Hemorrhaging due to Deficiency Cold
   Clinical signs: Uterine bleeding, bleeding in stool or in vomit
   Combine with: Codonopsis *Dang Shen* and Jujube *Da Zao*, Atractylodes *Bai Zhu*

History and Comments:
1. Zingiberis *Gan Jiang* (dried Ginger) has a similar effect as Zingiberis *Sheng Jiang* (fresh Ginger). These two herbs are often substituted for each other. Zingiberis *Sheng Jiang* is preferred for Wind invasions and nausea, while Zingiberis *Gan Jiang* is preferred for Internal Cold.
2. *Gan Jiang* is used when there is Dampness and Cold. *Sheng Jiang* is used when there is Dryness and Heat.
3. *Gan Jiang* is said to enter the Heart and Kidney Channels while *Sheng Jiang* enters the Lung and Spleen.
4. Ginger also detoxifies other herbs, such as Pinellia *Ban Xia*.
5. Good quality Ginger is solid with a grayish yellow exterior and a powdery grayish-white appearance on cross section.

Pharmaceutical Ingredients:[1–4]
1. Essential oils (zingiberol, zingiberene, phellandrene, camphene, borneol, bisabolene, α-curcumene, α-farnesene, β-farnesene, linalool, cineole, β-sesouiphellandrene)
2. 6-gingerol, 6-shogaol, zingiberone, gingerol, zingerone, dihydroginerol, hexyhydrocurcumin, L-pipecolic acid
3. Asparagine, pipeolic acid, glutamate, aspartic acid, serine, glycine

Foeniculum *Xiao Hui Xiang* 小茴香

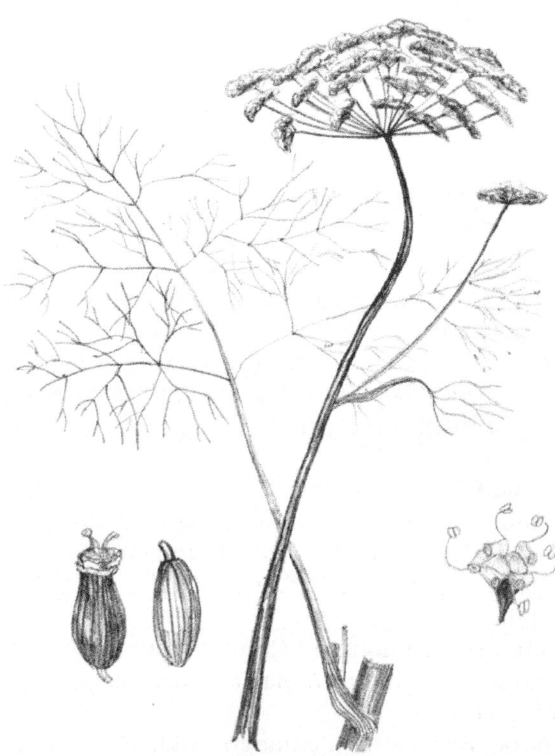

Original Reference: *Tang Ben Cao* (*Tang Materia Medica*) by *Su Jing* et al., *Tang* Dynasty 唐本草

Part Used: Fruit

Name:
Pharmaceutical: Foeniculi Vulgaris, Fructus
Botanical: Foeniculum vulgare
Common: Fennel
Wade-Giles: *Hsiao-Hui-Hsiang*
Translation: Fennel Fragrant

Energy/Taste: Warm, pungent

Channel-Organ: Liver, Kidney, Spleen, Stomach

Actions:
1. Dispel Cold and stop pain
2. Regulate *Qi* and harmonize the Stomach

Form and Preparation: Powder or decoction

Dosage:
Horses and cattle: 15–60 g
Llamas, Alpacas, Goats, and Pigs: 10–15 g
Dogs: 1–3 g
Cats and Rabbits: 0.5–1 g
Bird and Rabbit: 0.5–2 g

Cautions and Contraindications: Caution if False Heat due to *Yin* Deficiency

Side Effects: None known

Clinical Applications:
1. Cold Stagnation in the Liver Channel
   Clinical signs: Hernia, swollen or painful testicles, sharp localized pain in lower abdomen, aggravated by Cold
   Combine with: Cinnamomum *Rou Gui* and Lindera *Wu Yao*, Litchi *Li Zhi He*
2. Cold in the Stomach
   Clinical signs: Vomiting, epigastric distension, epigastric pain
   Combine with: Zingiberis *Gan Jiang* and Saussurea *Mu Xiang*
   Clinical signs: Vomiting and reduced appetite
   Combine with: Zingiberis *Sheng Jiang* and Magnolia *Hou Po*

History and Comments:
1. Foeniculum *Xiao Hui Xiang* is also called *Hui Xiang*.
2. It induces milk secretion in cows and mares.
3. It is also used for infertility.
4. It regulates the peristaltic functions of the gastrointestinal tract and thereby reduces emptying time and increasing the passage of gas.

Pharmaceutical Ingredients: [1–4]
1. Essential oil (trans-anethole, limonene, fenchone, estragole, r-terpinene, α-pinene, mycene, β-pinene, camphor, camphene, methoxyphenyl acetone, sabinene, α-phellandrene, p-cymene, cineole, 4-terpineol, transfenchol acetate, anethole, anisaldenyle)
2. Petroselinic acid

Evodia *Wu Zhu Yu* 吴茱萸

Original Reference: *Shen Nong Ben Cao Jing* (*Shen Nong's Materia Medica*, 1st century BCE) 神农本草经

Part Used: Fruit

Name:
Pharmaceutical: Evodiae Rutaecarpae, Fructus
Botanical: Evodia rutaecarpa
Common: Evodia fruit
Wade-Giles: *Wu-Chu-Yu*

Energy/Taste: Hot, pungent, bitter, slightly toxic

Channel-Organ: Liver, Spleen, Stomach, Kidney

Actions:
1. Dispel Cold and stop pain
2. Pacify the Liver and lead Fire downward
3. Descend *Qi* and stop vomiting

Form and Preparation: Powder or decoction

Dosage:
Horses and Cattle: 10–30 g
Llamas, Alpacas, Goats, and Pigs: 3–10 g
Dogs: 1–5 g
Cats and Rabbits: 0.5–1 g

Cautions and Contraindications:
1. Caution during pregnancy
2. Avoid prolonged usage, especially in *Yin* Deficiency; *Yin* Deficiency with Heat
3. May antagonize Salvia *Dan Shen*

Side Effects:
1. Slightly toxic
2. Overdosing can cause very dry throat.
3. Unpleasant taste—too Pungent, too bitter
4. Very drying and can injure *Yin*

Caryophyllum *Ding Xiang* 丁香

Original Reference: *Lei Gong Pao Zhi Lun* (*Lei's Method of Preparing Drugs*) by *Lei Xiao* in 5th century 雷公炮炙论

Part Used: Flower-bud

Name:
Pharmaceutical: Caryophylli, Flos
Botanical: Eugenia caryophyllata; Syzygym aromaticum
Common: Clove
Wade-Giles: *Ting-Hsiang*
Translation: Spike Fragrance

Energy/Taste: Warm, pungent

Channel-Organ: Spleen, Stomach, Lung, Kidney

Actions:
1. Warm Spleen and Stomach
2. Descend Stomach *Qi*
3. Warm Kidney and Tonify *Yang*

Form and Preparation: Powder or decoction

Dosage:
Horses and Cattle: 9–30 g
Llamas, Alpacas, Goats, and Pigs: 3–6 g
Dogs: 1–2 g
Cats and Rabbits: 0.5–1 g
Birds: 0.1–1 g

Cautions and Contraindications:
1. Do not combine with Curcuma *Yu Jin*.
2. Caution for febrile diseases and *Yin* Deficiency

Side Effects: None known

Zanthoxylum *Chuan Jiao* 川椒

Original Reference: *Shen Nong Ben Cao Jing* (*Shen Nong's Materia Medica*, 1st century BCE) 神农本草经

Part Used: Fruit

Name:
Pharmaceutical: Zanthoxyli, Pericarpium (Prickly-ash)
Botanical: Zanthoxylum bungeanum; Z. schinifolium; Z. simulans
Common: *Sichuan* pepper
Wade-Giles: *Ch'uan-Chiao*
Translation: *Sichuan* pepper
Alternative: Flower Pepper (*Hua Jiao*)

Energy/Taste: Hot, pungent, slightly toxic

Channel-Organ: Spleen, Stomach, Kidney

Actions:
1. Warm the Stomach and Spleen
2. Stop pain
3. Kill parasites

Form and Preparation: Powder or decoction

Dosage:
Horses and Cattle: 10–20 g
Llamas, Alpacas, Goats, and Pigs: 5–10 g

Cautions and Contraindications:
1. Contraindicated for *Yin* Deficiency with Heat or Pregnancy
2. May counteract Tussilago *Kuan Dong Hua*, Aconite *Fu Zi*, and Ledebouriella *Fang Feng*, and antagonize Trichosanthes *Gua Lou*

Side Effects: May cause diarrhea

Piper *Hu Jiao* 胡椒

Original Reference: *Tang Ben Cao* (*Tang Materia Medica*) by Su Jing et al., *Tang* Dynasty 唐本草

Part Used: Fruit

Name:
Pharmaceutical: Piperis Nigri, Fructus
Botanical: Piper nigrum L.
Common: Black pepper
Wade-Giles: *Hu-Chiao*
Translation: Foreign pepper

Energy/Taste: Warm, pungent

Channel-Organ: Stomach, Large intestine

Actions: Warm Spleen and Stomach and dispel Cold

Form and Preparation: Powder or decoction

Dosage:
Horses and Cattle: 9–27 g
Llamas, Alpacas, Goats, and Pigs: 3–7 g

Cautions and Contraindications: Heat due to *Yin* Deficiency

Side Effects: None known

Alpinia *Gao Liang Jiang* 高良姜

Original Reference: *Ming Yi Bie Lu* (*Miscellaneous Records of Famous Physicians*) by *Tao Hong-Jing*, North and South Kingdoms (5th century) 名医别录

Part Used: Rhizome

Name:
Pharmaceutical: Alpiniae officinari, Rhizoma
Botanical: Alpinia officinarum
Common: Galanga
Wade-Giles: *Kao-Liang-Chiang*
Translation: Tall, Good Ginger

Table 6.2. Herbs to Warm the Interior: A quick overview and comparison.

Herbs	Special Actions	Common Characteristics
Tonify *Yang* and resuscitate collapsed *Yang Qi*		Energy: Hot or warm Taste: Pungent Action: Warm the interior to expel coldness Indication: Interior Cold or *Yang* Deficiency Signs: Cold extremities, warm-seeking behavior, lack of thirst or attraction to warm water, loose stools, clear and prolonged urination, pale tongue with white thin coating, deep and slow pulse
Fu Zi	#1 herb to Warm and strengthen Kidney/Heart *Yang*	
	Dispel water and dampness	
	Toxic	
Rou Gui	Warm the Middle and channels to move Blood	
	Lead fire back to the source	
Gan Jiang	Warm the Middle to dispel Cold	
	Warm the Lung to remove Phlegm	
Warm the Middle Burner to dispel Coldness		
Xiao Hui Xiang	Warm the Kidney to dispel Coldness in lumbar region	
	Regulate *Qi* and harmonize the stomach	
Wu Zhu Yu	Pacify the Liver and lead fire downward	
	Descend *Qi* and stop vomiting	
	Slightly Toxic	
Ding Xiang	Descend Stomach *Qi*, Warm Kidney	
Chuan Jiao	Stop pain, kill parasites	
Hu Jiao	Dispel Cold to stop pain	
Gao Liang Jiang	Stop pain and stop vomiting	

Energy/Taste: Hot, pungent

Channel-Organ: Spleen, Stomach

Actions:

1. Warm Spleen and Stomach
2. Stop pain

Form and Preparation: Powder or decoction

Dosage:

Horses and Cattle: 15–30 g
Llamas, Alpacas, Goats, and Pigs: 3–10 g
Dogs: 1–3 g
Cats and Rabbits: 0.3–0.5 g
Birds: 0.2–1 g

Cautions and Contraindications:

1. Contraindication for *Yin* Deficiency with Heat signs
2. In patients with weak constitutions, Alpinia *Gao Liang Jiang* should not be used alone. Instead, combine with Codonopsis *Dang Shen* and Atractylodes *Bai Zhu* to moderate its potential irritating side effects.

Side Effects: None known

SUMMARY OF HERBS THAT WARM THE INTERIOR

Table 6.2 summarizes and compares the herbs that warm The Interior.

REFERENCES

1. Chen JK, Chen TT. Chinese Medical Herbology and Pharmacology. City of Industry, CA: Art of Medicine Press, 2004.
2. Brinker FJ. The Toxicology of Botanical Medicines. Sandy, OR: Eclectic Medical Publications, 2000.
3. Duke JA. Handbook of Medicinal Herbs. New York: Chemical and Rubber Company Press, 2001.
4. Huang KC. The Pharmacology of Chinese Herbs, 2nd Edition. New York: Chemical and Rubber Company Press, 1999.

7 Herbs to Dispel Damp 祛湿药

Huisheng Xie, Min Su Kim, Cheryl Chrisman

Damp, which is one of Six Pathogenic *Qi*, is characterized as a thick, heavy, greasy, sticky, mucoid pathogen. Damp can be divided into Interior Damp, which is generated from the internal organs, and Exterior Damp, which enters from the external environment. External Damp combines with pathogenic Wind, Cold, Summer Heat and Heat, when it invades the body. Therefore, the pathogens related to Damp include Wind-Damp, Cold-Damp, and Damp-Heat.

As their name suggests Herbs to Dispel Damp treat Damp. These herbs are divided into three categories: 1) Herbs to Dispel Wind-Damp, 2) Aromatic Herbs to Transform Damp, and 3) Herbs to Benefit Urination and Drain Damp.

HERBS TO DISPEL WIND-DAMP

Herbs to dispel Wind-Damp are often used to treat *Bi* Syndrome. *Bi* Syndrome refers to *Qi*-Blood Stagnation in the muscles, sinews, joints, bones, and Channels. There are four types of *Bi* Syndrome (Table 7.1).

Herbs to dispel Wind-Damp can relieve pain; relax tendons; promote *Qi* circulation in Channels; and strengthen tendons, joints, and bones. These herbs have analgesic, antiinflammatory, and antipyretic effects, and promote circulation. They are indicated for the following conditions: soft tissue pain, muscle spasms, muscle numbness, hemiplegia, degenerative joint diseases, arthritis, soreness, and pain and weakness in the back and limbs.

Because alcohol can enhance the herbs' ability to expel Wind-Damp, herbs are commonly used as tinctures or in other prepared forms. The herbs are generally aromatic and warm, which makes them drying in nature. Because this drying effect may injure the *Yin* and Blood, these herbs are contraindicated for Blood or *Yin* Deficiency. Herbs to dispel Wind-Damp may be combined with Wind dispersing herbs, *Qi* and Blood invigorating herbs, or warming or cooling Herbs.

Angelica *Du Huo* 独活

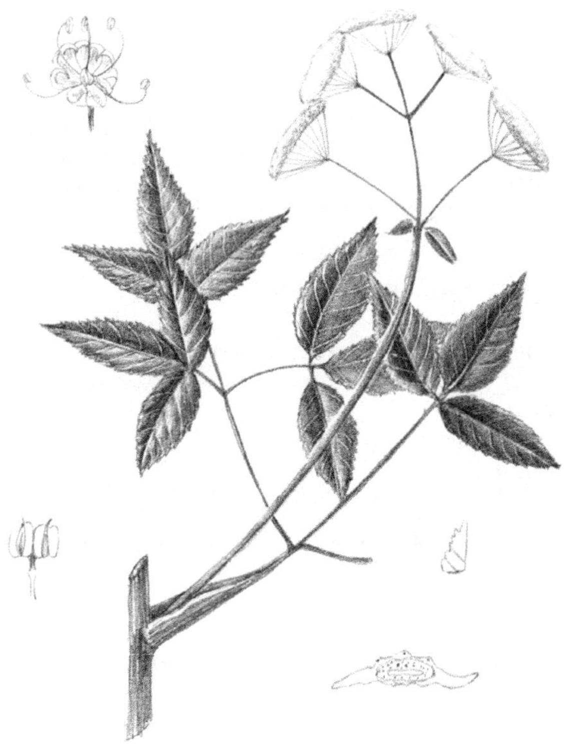

a

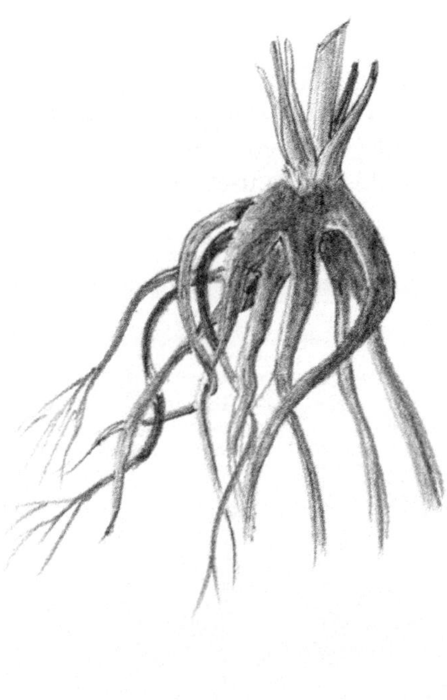

b

Table 7.1. Differentiation of *Bi* syndrome.

Types of *Bi* Syndrome	Clinical Signs	Treatment Principles and Examples of Herbs
Wind *Bi* (*Xing-Bi*)	Pain migrates from joint to joint. More acute onset	Dispel *Wind*-Damp and invigorate Blood Angelica *Du Huo*
Cold-*Bi* (*Tong-Bi*)	Fixed, severe pain Aggravated by exposure to cold Decrease in joint mobility Cold-extremities	Strong warming, dispel Wind, and regulate *Yang* Aconite *Chuan Wu*
Damp *Bi* (*Zuo-Bi*)	Fixed, lingering pain Swelling of extremities and joints Stiffness worse than pain Worse when weather changes	Warming expel *Wind* and Dampness, tonify the *Spleen*, leach out the Damp Chaenomeles *Mu Gua*
Heat *Bi* (*Re-Bi*)	Acute pain Swelling, heat, redness, and pain	Cool dispel *Wind*-damp + clear heat Gentiana *Qin Jiao*

Original Reference: *Shen Nong Ben Cao Jing* (*Shen Nong's Materia Medica*, 1st century BCE) 神农本草经

Part Used: Root

Name:
Pharmaceutical: Angelicae Pubescentis, Radix
Botanical: Angelica Pubescens; A. Laxiflora
Wade-Giles: *Tu-Huo*
Translation: Self-reliant Existence

Energy/Taste: Slightly warm, pungent, bitter

Channel-Organ: Kidney, Bladder

Actions:
1. Dispel Wind-Damp and Cold
2. Unblock *Bi* to stop pain
3. Release Exterior Patterns

Form and Preparation: Powder, decoction, or pill

Dosage:
Horses and Cattle: 15–45 g
Llamas, Alpacas, Goats, and Pigs: 3–10 g
Dogs: 2–5 g
Cats: 0.5–1 g
Birds and Rabbits: 0.5–1.5 g

Cautions and Contraindications: Caution for Deficiency of *Yin* or Blood with Heat

Side Effects: May cause dizziness, headache, nausea, vomiting

Clinical Applications:
1. Wind-Damp *Bi* Syndrome and joint pain
   Clinical signs: Pain in the lower back and limbs, soreness, pain, numbness of joints, and motor impairment
   Combine with: Gentiana *Qin Jiao*, Ledebouriella *Fang Feng*, Loranthus *Sang Ji Sheng*
   Classical herbal formula: *Du Huo Ji Sheng Tang*
2. Wind-Cold Exogenous invasion
   Clinical signs: Cold, chills and fever, stiff neck and shoulders
   Combine with: Notopterygium *Qiang Huo*, Ligusticum *Chuan Xiong*, Vitex *Man Jing Zi*, and Ligusticum *Gao Ben*

History and Comments:
1. Combining Notopterygium *Qiang Huo* with Angelica *Du Huo* will reinforce Angelica's effect. Angelica *Du Huo* is best for *Bi* Syndrome or pain in the lower back and pelvic limbs. Notopterygium *Qiang Huo* is good for *Bi* Syndrome in the neck, shoulders, and thoracic limbs.
2. Good quality *Du Huo* is thick, glistening, and aromatic.

Pharmaceutical Ingredients:[1–4]
1. Coumarine (othol, columbiamotin, columbianetin acetate, bergapten, columbianadin, xanthotoxin, isoimperotorin, angelol, isoangelol, anpubesol, angelol B, umbelliferone, columbianetin-d-glucopyranoside)
2. Anpubesol
3. Sylvestreene, α-pinene, 3-methylnonane, eremophilene, thymol, α-cedrene, humulene

Gentiana *Qin Jiao* 秦艽

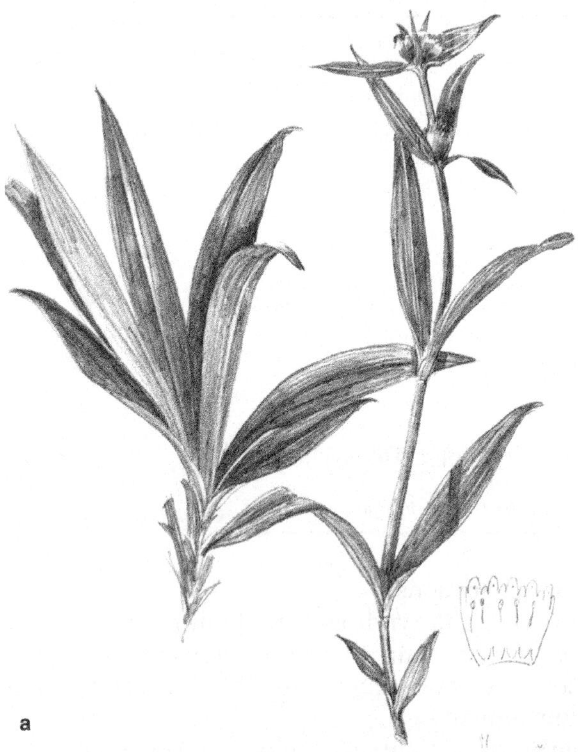

a

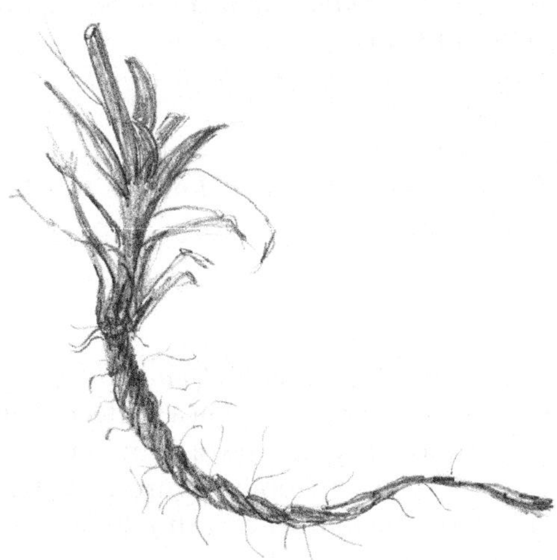

b

Original Reference: *Shen Nong Ben Cao Jing* (*Shen Nong*'s *Materia Medica*, 1st century BCE) 神农本草经

Part Used: Root

Name:
Pharmaceutical: Gentianae *Qinjiao*, Radix
Botanical: Gentiana Macrophylla; G. Straminea; G. Crassicaulis; G. Dahurica
Common: Large-leaf Gentian root
Wade-Giles: *Chin-Chiu*

Energy/Taste: Neutral, bitter, pungent

Channel-Organ: Stomach, Liver, Gallbladder

Actions:
1. Dispel Wind-Damp
2. Clear False Heat due to *Yin* Deficiency
3. Clear Damp-Heat or Fire from Liver/Gallbladder
4. Relax *Jin* (the sinews)

Form and Preparation: Powder, decoction, or pill

Dosage:
Horses and Cattle: 30–45 g
Llamas, Alpacas, Goats, and Pigs: 3–10 g
Dogs: 2–5 g
Cats: 0.5–1 g
Birds and Rabbits: 0.5–1.5 g

Cautions and Contraindications: Caution for diarrhea, frequent urination, or chronic pain with emaciation

Side Effects: Overdose will cause diarrhea, nausea, vomiting, and palpitations.

Clinical Applications:
1. Joint pain due to Wind-Damp *Bi* Syndrome with Heat signs
   Combine with: Stephania *Han Fang Ji*, Ledebouriella *Fang Feng*, and Anemarrhena *Zhi Mu*.
   Classical herbal formula: *Qin Jiao San*
2. False Heat from *Yin* Deficiency
   Clinical signs: "Bone-steaming" fever, low-grade fever due to *Yin* Deficiency
   Combine with: Artemisia *Qing Hao*, Testudinis *Gui Ban*, Anemarrhena *Zhi Mu*, Lycium *Di Gu Pi*
3. Hemiplegia with Deficiency of Blood
   Combine with: Angelica *Dang Gui*, Paeonia *Bai Shao*
4. Jaundice due to Liver Damp Heat with Jaundice
   Combine with: Artemisia *Yin Chen Hao*, Gardenia *Zhi Zi* and Scuttellaria *Huang Qin*

History and Comments: This herb is good for treating *Bi* Syndromes with *Yin* Deficiency.

Pharmaceutical Ingredients:[1–4]
1. Gentianine, gentianidine, gentiopieroside, gentianel, homoorientin
2. Sapoknaretin

Loranthus *Sang Ji Sheng* 桑寄生

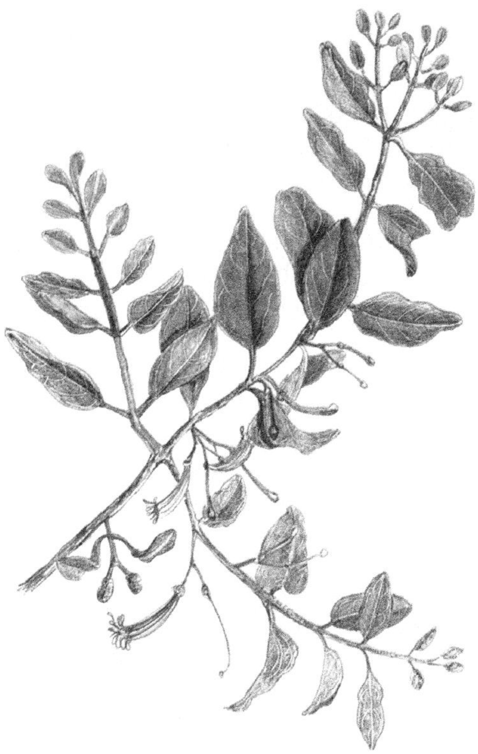

Original Reference: *Shen Nong Ben Cao Jing* (*Shen Nong*'s *Materia Medica*, 1st century BCE) 神农本草经

Part Used: Stem and branch with leaves

Name:
Pharmaceutical: Ramulus Loranthi
Botanical: Loranthus parasiticus; L. gracilifolius
Common: Mistletoe stems
Wade-Giles: *Sang-Chi-Sheng*
Translation: Mulberry Parasite

Energy/Taste: Neutral, bitter

Channel-Organ: Liver, Kidney

Actions:
1. Dispel Wind-Damp and Cold
2. Strengthen tendons and bones
3. Tonify Liver and Kidney *Yin*
4. Nourish Blood to calm fetus and prevent abortion

Form and Preparation: Powder, decoction, or pill

Dosage:
Horses and Cattle: 30–60 g
Llamas, Alpacas, Goats, and Pigs: 5–15 g
Dogs: 2–3 g
Cats: 1–2 g

Cautions and Contraindications: Caution for Damp-Heat

Side Effects: None known

Clinical Applications:
1. Wind-Damp *Bi* Syndrome due to Kidney *Yang/Qi* Deficiency
   Clinical signs: Pain and soreness in lower back and stifles, stiffness
   Combine with: Angelica *Du Huo*, Achyranthes *Niu Xi*, Eucommia *Du Zhong*, Cibotium *Gou Ji*
2. Restless fetus due to Deficiency of Liver and Kidney, and *Ren* and *Chong* Channels
   Combine with: Dipsacus *Xu Duan*, Eucommia *Du Zhong*, Artemisia *Ai Ye*, and Asinum Gelatinum *E Jiao*
3. Hypertension due to Liver/Kidney *Yin* Deficiency
   Combine with: Gastrodia *Tian Ma*, Chrysanthemum *Ju Hua*, and Lycium *Gou Qi Zi*
4. Dry and scaly skin due to Blood Deficiency
   Combine with: Chicken eggs and brown sugar

History and Comments:
1. Frying Loranthus *Sang Ji Sheng* in wine strengthens its ability to expel Wind-Damp.
2. Loranthus *Sang Ji Sheng* is effective for hypertension.

Pharmaceutical Ingredients:[1–4] Avicullarin, quercetin, coriamyrtin, tutin, coratin, d-catechin, quercitrin, hyoerin, hyperoside

Clematis *Wei Ling Xian* 威灵仙

Original Reference: *Tang Ben Cao* (*Tang Materia Medica*) by *Su Jing* et al., *Tang* Dynasty 唐本草

Part Used: Root

Name:
Pharmaceutical: Clematidis, Radix
Botanical: Clematis Chinensis; C. Hexapetala; C. Manchurica
Common: Chinese Clematis Root
Wade-Giles: *Wei-Ling-Hsien*
Translation: Awesome Spiritual Immortal

Energy/Taste: Warm, pungent, salty

Channel-Organ: Bladder

Actions:
1. Dispel Wind and Damp
2. Invigorate *Qi* in the Channels, stop pain

Form and Preparation: Powder, decoction, or pill

Dosage:
Horses and Cattle: 15–60g
Llamas, Alpacas, Goats, and Pigs: 3–10g
Dogs: 2–5g
Cats: 0.5–2g
Birds and Rabbits: 0.5–1.5g

Cautions and Contraindications:
1. Contraindicated for weak patients with *Qi*-Blood Deficiency
2. Caution during pregnancy

Side Effects:
1. Scatters *Qi* and Blood
2. May be adulterated with aristolochic acid

History and Comments: During the *Tang* Dynasty (785–805 CE), a man had suffered from severe paralysis for over 10 years. He had tried many therapies without success. He was about to give up, but a friend advised him to try a new therapy from a visiting monk. After examining the paralyzed man, the monk said he believed the herb *Wei Ling Xian* could help. The monk made a special trip to the mountains and collected the herb. After using this herbal medication for several days, the man could walk again.

Aconite *Chuan Wu* 川乌

Original Reference: *Shen Nong Ben Cao Jing* (*Shen Nong's Materia Medica*, 1st century BCE) 神农本草经

Part Used: Main root

Name:
Pharmaceutical: Aconiti Carmichaeli Radix
Botanical: Aconitum carmichaeli Debx
Common: Aconiti Carmichaeli
Wade-Giles: *Ch'uan-Wu*
Translation: *Sichuan* Aconite

Energy/Taste: Hot, pungent, bitter, very toxic

Channel-Organ: Heart, Liver, Kidney, Spleen

Actions:
1. Clear Wind-Damp
2. Warm the Channel to stop pain

Form and Preparation: Powder, decoction, or pill; long decoction for oral use, or raw for topical application

Dosage:
Horses and Cattle: 9–18g
Llamas, Alpacas, Goats, and Pigs: 1.5–3g
Dogs: 0.5–1g

Cautions and Contraindications:
1. Contraindicated during pregnancy
2. Prohibited for young pediatric patients (too *Yang*)
3. Contraindicated for *Yang* Excess or *Yin* Deficiency
4. May antagonize Fritillaria *Bei Mu*, Trichosanthes *Gua Lou*, Trichosanthes *Tian Hua Fen*, Pinellia *Ban Xia*, Bletilla *Bai Ji*, Cynanchum *Bai Wei*, and Scolopendra *Wu Gong*, and counteract Rhinoceros *Xi Jiao*.

Side Effects:
1. It is very toxic.
2. It may cause numb lips, paralysis, excessive salivation, nausea, vomiting, diarrhea, dizziness, dyspnea, convulsions, fecal or urinary incontinence, arrhythmia, or coma.

Aconite *Cao Wu* 草乌

Original Reference: *Shen Nong Ben Cao Jing* (*Shen Nong's Materia Medica*, 1st century BCE) 神农本草经

Part Used: Main root

Name:
Pharmaceutical: Aconiti Kusnezoffii Radix
Botanical: Aconitum kusnezoffii Reichb
Common: Aconiti Kusnezoffii
Wade-Giles: *Cao-Wu*
Translation: Grass Aconite

Energy/Taste: Hot, pungent, bitter, very toxic

Channel-Organ: Heart, Liver, Kidney, Spleen

Actions:
1. Clear Wind-Damp
2. Warm the Channels to stop pain
3. More potent than *Chuan Wu*

Form and Preparation: Powder, decoction, or pill; prepared form for oral use only; raw form for topical application

Dosage:
Horses and Cattle: 5–10g
Llamas, Alpacas, Goats, and Pigs: 1–2g
Dogs: 0.5–1g

Cautions and Contraindications:
1. Contraindicated during pregnancy
2. Prohibited for young patients (too *Yang*)
3. Contraindicated for *Yang* Excess or *Yin* Deficiency

4. May antagonize Fritillaria *Bei Mu*, Trichosanthes *Gua Lou*, Trichosanthes *Tian Hua Fen*, Pinellia *Ban Xia*, Bletilla *Bai Ji*, Cynanchum *Bai Wei*, Scolopendra *Wu Gong* and counteracts Rhinoceros *Xi Jiao*.

Side Effects:
1. It is more toxic and potent than *Chuan Wu*.
2. It may cause numb lips, paralysis, excessive salivation, nausea, vomiting, diarrhea, dizziness, dyspnea, convulsions, fecal or urinary incontinence, arrhythmia, or coma.

Chaenomeles *Mu Gua* 木瓜

Original Reference: *Ming Yi Bie Lu* (*Miscellaneous Records of Famous Physicians*) by *Tao Hong-Jing*, North and South Kingdoms (5th century) 名医别录

Part Used: Fruit

Name:
Pharmaceutical: Chaenomelis, Fructus
Botanical: Chaenomeles Speciosa; C. Lagenaria (Chinese Quince)
Common: Chinese Quince
Wade-Giles: *Mu-Kua*
Translation: Wood Melon

Energy/Taste: Warm, sour

Channel-Organ: Liver, Spleen

Actions:
1. Invigorate *Qi* and Blood Circulation in the Channels
2. Relax muscles and tendons
3. Transform Damp and Harmonize the Stomach
4. Reduce Food Stagnation

Form and Preparation: Powder, decoction, or pill; do not cook in iron.

Dosage:
Horses and Cattle: 15–30 g
Llamas, Alpacas, Goats, and Pigs: 5–12 g
Dogs: 2–5 g
Cats: 0.5–2 g
Birds and Rabbits: 0.2–2 g

Cautions and Contraindications:
1. Caution for *Yin* Deficiency
2. Contraindicated for Interior Excess Heat

Side Effects: Excessive use can harm the teeth and bones.

Lycopodium *Shen Jin Cao* 伸筋草

Original Reference: *Ben Cao Shi Yi* (*Supplement to Materia Medica*) by *Chen Cang-Qi* in 8th century 本草拾遗

Part Used: Whole plant

Name:
Pharmaceutical: Lycopodium, Herb
Botanical: Lycopodium japonicum Thunb.
Common: Lycopodium
Wade-Giles: *Shen-Chin-Ts'ao*
Translation: Stretch Tendon Herb

Energy/Taste: Warm, slightly bitter, pungent

Channel-Organ: Kidney, Spleen

Actions:
1. Clear Wind-Damp
2. Invigorate *Qi* and Blood Circulation in the Channels
3. Relax muscles and tendons

Form and Preparation: Powder, decoction, or pill

Dosage:
Horses and Cattle: 15–45 g
Llamas, Alpacas, Goats, and Pigs: 3–12 g
Dogs: 1–5 g
Cats: 0.5–1 g
Birds and Rabbits: 0.3–2 g

Cautions and Contraindications: Contraindicated during pregnancy

Side Effects: May cause a skin allergy

Bombyx *Can Sha* 蚕沙

Original Reference: *Ming Yi Bie Lu* (*Miscellaneous Records of Famous Physicians*) by *Tao Hong-Jing*, North and South Kingdoms (5th century) 名医别录

Part Used: Silkworm Droppings

Name:
Pharmaceutical: Bombycis Mori, Excrementum
Zoological: Bombyx Mori
Common: Silkworm Feces
Wade-Giles: *Ts'an-Sha*
Translation: Silkworm Sand

Energy/Taste: Warm, sweet, pungent

Channel-Organ: Liver, Spleen, Stomach

Actions:
1. Dispel Wind and Damp
2. Harmonize Stomach and transform Damp

Form and Preparation: Powder or pill

Dosage:
Horses and Cattle: 20–90 g
Llamas, Alpacas, Goats, and Pigs: 5–12 g
Dogs: 2–5 g
Cats: 0.5–1 g
Birds and Rabbits: 0.3–5 g

Cautions and Contraindications: Contraindicated for External application

Side Effects: None known

Agkistrodon *Bai Hua She* 白花蛇

Original Reference: *Lei Gong Pao Zhi Lun* (*Lei's Method of Preparing Drugs*) by *Lei Xiao*, 5th century 雷公炮炙论

Part Used: Whole Body

Name:
Pharmaceutical: Agkistrodon Seu Bungarus
Zoological: Agkistrodon Acutus or Bungarus Multicinctus
Common: White Banded Krait; Agkistrodon
Wade-Giles: *Pai-Hua-She*
Translation: White-patterned Snake

Energy/Taste: Warm, sweet, salty, toxic

Channel-Organ: Liver, Spleen

Actions:
1. Unblock the Channels and Extinguish Wind
2. Dispel Wind from the skin to stop itching
3. Dispel Internal Wind to stop convulsions

Form and Preparation: Decoction or used in wine for *Bi* Syndrome or arthritis

Dosage:
Horses and Cattle: 30–60 g
Llamas, Alpacas, Goats, and Pigs: 5–10 g
Dogs: 2–5 g
Cats: 1–2 g

Cautions and Contraindications:
1. Contraindicated for pregnancy
2. Caution for *Yin* Deficiency with Heat or Blood Deficiency

Side Effects:
1. **It is toxic.**
2. May cause a skin allergy

Zaocys *Wu Shao She* 乌梢蛇

Original Reference: *Yao Xing Lun* (*Discussion of Medicinal Properties*) by *Chen Zhou* in 19th century 药性论

Part Used: Whole Body

Name:
Pharmaceutical: Zaocys Dhumnades
Zoological: Zaocys Dhumnades
Common: Black-striped Snake
Wade-Giles: *Wu-Shao-She*
Translation: Black-striped Snake

Energy/Taste: Neutral, sweet, salty

Channel-Organ: Liver, Spleen

Actions:
1. Dispel Wind and Damp
2. Clear External Wind to stop itching
3. Clear Internal Wind to stop seizures

Form and Preparation: Decoction, or used in wine for joint pain and severe *Bi* syndrome

Dosage:
Horses and Cattle: 15–30 g
Llamas, Alpacas, Goats, and Pigs: 2–6 g
Dogs: 1–3 g
Cats: 0.5–1 g

Cautions and Contraindications: Caution for *Yin* Deficiency with Heat or Blood Deficiency

Side Effects: None known

Piper *Hai Feng Teng* 海风藤

Original Reference: *Ben Cao Cong Xin* (*Thoroughly Revised Materia Medica*) by *Wu Yi-luo* and *Wu Zun-cheng*) in 1751 CE 本草从新

Part Used: Stems

Name:
Pharmaceutical: Caulis Piperis Futokadsurae, Caulis
Botanical: Piper Futokadsura Sieb. Et Zucc.
Common: Kadsura; Kadsura Stem; Futokadsura Stem
Wade-Giles: *Hai-Feng-T'eng*
Translation: Sea Wind Vine

Energy/Taste: Warm, pungent, bitter

Channel-Organ: Liver

Actions:
1. Dispel Wind and Damp
2. Clear Channels and Collaterals
3. Disperse Cold and alleviate pain

Form and Preparation: Powder, decoction, or pill

Dosage:
Horses and Cattle: 30–60 g
Llamas, Alpacas, Goats, and Pigs: 3–9 g
Dogs: 1–3 g

Cautions and Contraindications: Caution during pregnancy

Side Effects: May cause a skin allergy

Aconite *Xue Shang Yi Zhi Hao* 雪上一枝蒿

Original Reference: *Ke Xue De Min Jian Yao Cao* (*Scientific Folk Materia Medica*) by *Zhongde Zhu* in 1951 科学的民间药草

Part Used: Root

Name:
Pharmaceutical: Aconiti Brachypodum Radix
Botanical: Aconitum Brachypodum Diels.
Common: Aconiti Brachypodum
Wade-Giles: *Hsueh-Shang-I-Chih-Hao*
Translation: One Plant Above Snow

Energy/Taste: Warm, pungent, bitter, very toxic

Channel-Organ: Liver

Actions:
1. Clear Wind-Damp
2. Invigorate Blood to stop pain

Form and Preparation: Powder, decoction, or pill

Dosage: Horses and Cattle: 0.3–1 g

Cautions and Contraindications:
1. Contraindicated during pregnancy
2. Contraindicated for weak, geriatric and pediatric patients
3. Contraindicated for any ulceration

Side Effects:
1. **It is very toxic.**
2. It may cause colic, vomiting, diarrhea, paralysis, dizziness, dyspnea, convulsions, fecal or urinary incontinence, arrhythmia, or coma

Liquidambar *Lu Lu Tong* 路路通

Original Reference: *Ben Cao Gang Mu Shi Yi* (*Omissions for the Materia Medica Compendium*) by *Zhao Xue-min* et al., in 1765 CE. 本草纲目拾遗

Part Used: Fruit

Name:
Pharmaceutical: Fructus Liquidambaris Taiwanianae
Botanical: Liquidambar taiwaniana
Common: Sweetgum fruit
Wade-Giles: *Lu-Lu-T'ung*
Translation: All Roads Open

Energy/Taste: Neutral, bitter

Channel-Organ: Liver, Stomach, All Twelve Channels

Actions:
1. Promote movement of *Qi* and Blood to stop pain
2. Clear Wind-Damp, promote urination
3. Open Channels to promote milk production

Form and Preparation: Powder, decoction, or pill

Dosage:
Horses and Cattle: 20–40 g
Llamas, Alpacas, Goats, and Pigs: 3–9 g
Dogs: 1–3 g

Cautions and Contraindications: Contraindicated during pregnancy

Side Effects: May induce palpitations

Siegesbeckia *Xi Xian Cao* 豨莶草

Original Reference: *Tang Ben Cao* (*Tang Materia Medica*) by *Su Jing* et al., *Tang* Dynasty 唐本草

Part Used: Leaf and Stem

Name:
Pharmaceutical: Siegesbeckiae, Herba
Botanical: Siegesbeckia Orientalis; S. Pubsescens
Common: St. Paul's Wort; Siegesbeckia
Wade-Giles: *Hsi-Hsien-Ts'ao*

Energy/Taste: Cold, bitter

Channel-Organ: Liver, Kidney

Actions:
1. Dispel Wind and Damp
2. Clear the Channels and Collaterals
3. Dispel Toxic Heat

Form and Preparation: Powder, decoction, or pill

Dosage:
Horses and Cattle: 20–60 g
Llamas, Alpacas, Goats, and Pigs: 5–15 g
Dogs: 3–8 g
Cats: 1–3 g
Birds and Rabbits: 1–5 g

Cautions and Contraindications: Contraindicated for Deficiency of Blood or *Yin*

Side Effects: None known

Morus *Sang Zhi* 桑枝

Original Reference: *Ben Cao Tu Jing* (*Illustrated Classic of Materia Medica*) by *Su Song* and *Su Zi-rong* in 1061 本草图经

Part Used: Twig

Name:
Pharmaceutical: Mori Albae, Ramulus
Botanical: Morus Alba
Common: Mulberry Twig
Wade-Giles: *Sang-Chih*
Translation: Mulberry Twig

Energy/Taste: Neutral, slightly bitter, sweet

Channel-Organ: Liver

Actions:
1. Dispel Wind and Damp
2. Clear the Channels and Collaterals
3. Serve as a transporter to the limbs (especially for the thoracic limbs)

Form and Preparation: Powder, decoction, or pill; the twigs are collected in the spring, when they are tender.

Dosage:
Horses and Cattle: 30–45 g
Llamas, Alpacas, Goats, and Pigs: 3–12 g
Dogs: 1–5 g
Cats: 0.5–1 g
Birds and Rabbits: 0.2–1 g

Cautions and Contraindications: Caution for *Yin* Deficiency with Heat

Side Effects: None known

Erythrinia *Hai Tong Pi* 海桐皮

Original Reference: *Ben Cao Gang Mu* (*Materia Medica Compendium*) by *Li Shi-Zhen* in 1590 本草纲目

Part Used: Bark

Name:
Pharmaceutical: Erythriniae, Cortex
Botanical: Erythrinia Variegata L. Var. Orientalis
Common: Erythrinia Bark
Wade-Giles: *Hai-T'ung-P'i*

Energy/Taste: Neutral, bitter, pungent

Channel-Organ: Liver

Actions:
1. Dispel Wind and Damp
2. Clear the Channels/unblock the Channels in the pelvic limbs
3. Kill parasites, stop itching

Form and Preparation: Powder, decoction, or pill

Dosage:
Horses and Cattle: 20–60 g
Llamas, Alpacas, Goats, and Pigs: 3–10 g
Dogs: 2–5 g
Cats: 0.5–1 g
Birds and Rabbits: 0.3–2 g

Cautions and Contraindications: Contraindicated for Blood Deficiency

Side Effects: None known

Clerodentrum *Chou Wu Tong* 臭梧桐

Original Reference: *Ben Cao Tu Jing* (*Illustrated Classic of Materia Medica*) by *Su Song* and *Su Zi-rong* in 1061 本草图经

Part Used: Leaf

Name:
Pharmaceutical: Clerodendri Trichotomi, Folium
Botanical: Clerodendrum Trichotomum
Common: Hairy Clerodendron
Wade-Giles: *Ch'ou-Wu-T'ung*

Energy/Taste: Cool, pungent, bitter, sweet

Channel-Organ: Liver

Actions:
1. Dispel Wind and Damp
2. Reduce hypertension

Form and Preparation: Powder, decoction, or pill

Dosage:
Horses and Cattle: 20–40 g
Llamas, Alpacas, Goats, and Pigs: 3–10 g
Dogs: 1–5 g
Cats: 0.5–1 g
Birds and Rabbits: 0.3–2 g

Cautions and Contraindications: None known

Side Effects: None known

Stephania *Han Fang Ji* 防己

Original Reference: *Shen Nong Ben Cao Jing* (*Shen Nong's Materia Medica*, 1st century BCE) 神农本草经

Part Used: Root

Name:
Pharmaceutical: Stephaniae Tetrandrae, Radix
Botanical: Stephania tetranda
Common: Stephania root
Wade-Giles: *Han-Fang-Chi*
Translation: Defense self
Alternate: It is also called *Han Fang Ji* to distinguish it from Aristolochia *Guang Fang Ji*

Energy/Taste: Cold, bitter, pungent

Channel-Organ: Lung, Spleen, Bladder, Kidney

Actions:
1. Dispel Wind-Damp, stop pain
2. Reduce edema

Form and Preparation: Powder, decoction, or pill

Dosage:
Horses and Cattle: 14–45 g
Llamas, Alpacas, Goats, and Pigs: 3–10 g
Dogs: 2–6 g
Cats: 0.5–1 g
Birds and Rabbits: 0.1–1 g

Cautions and Contraindications:
1. Caution for *Yin* Deficiency.
2. Caution with a weak Spleen and Stomach

Side Effects:
1. *Fang Ji* or *Han Fang Ji* is suspected of containing aristolochic acid or of being adulterated with aristolochic acid.
2. Aristolochia *Guang Fang Ji* has aristolochic acid, which can damage Kidneys.

Luffa *Si Gua Luo* 丝瓜络

Original Reference: *Ben Cao Gang Mu* (*Materia Medica Compendium*) by *Li Shi-Zhen* in 1590 本草纲目

Part Used: Skeleton of the vegetable sponge of the fruit

Name:
Pharmaceutical: Fasciculus Vascularis Luffae
Botanical: Luffa cylindrical Roem
Common: String Melon's dry skeleton
Wade-Giles: *Ssu-Kua-Luo*
Translation: String melon's Net

Energy/Taste: Neutral, sweet

Channel-Organ: Lung, Spleen, Bladder, Kidney

Actions:
1. Dispel Wind-Damp
2. Invigorate Blood to stop pain
3. Open the Channel to promote milk production

Form and Preparation: Powder, decoction, or pill

Dosage:
Horses and Cattle: 50–100 g
Llamas, Alpacas, Goats, and Pigs: 5–30 g
Dogs: 2–5 g
Cats: 1–2 g
Birds and Rabbits: 0.1–1 g

Cautions and Contraindications: None known

Side Effects: None known

Tripterygium *Lei Gong Teng* 雷公藤

Original Reference: *Ben Cao Gang Mu Shi Yi* (*Omissions for the Materia Medica Compendium*) by *Zhao Xue-min* et al., in 1765 CE 本草纲目拾遗

Part Used: Root

Name:
Pharmaceutical: Tripterygium, Radix
Botanical: Tripterygium wilfordii Hook
Common: Tripterygium
Wade-Giles: *Lei-Kung-T'eng*
Translation: Thunder God's Cane

Energy/Taste: Cold, bitter, pungent, very toxic

Channel-Organ: Liver, Kidney

Actions:
1. Dispel Wind-Damp to stop pain
2. Move Blood and invigorate Channels
3. Reduce edema, kill parasites

Form and Preparation: Powder, decoction, or pill

Dosage:
Horses and Cattle: 10–20 g
Llamas, Alpacas, Goats, and Pigs: 2–5 g
Dogs: 1–2 g

Cautions and Contraindications: Contraindicated during pregnancy

Side Effects:
1. **It is very toxic.**
2. It may cause skin allergy, nausea, vomiting, poor appetite, colic, bloody diarrhea, dizziness, infertility, ulceration, arrhythmia, convulsions, and coma.

Acanthopanax *Wu Jia Pi* 五加皮

Original Reference: *Shen Nong Ben Cao Jing* (*Shen Nong's Materia Medica*, 1st century BCE) 神农本草经

Part Used: Root bark

Name:
Pharmaceutical: Acanthopanacis Gracilistyli Radicis, Cortex
Botanical: Acanthopanax Gracilistylus
Common: Acanthopanax Root Bark
Wade-Giles: *Wu-Chia-P'i*
Translation: Five Additions Bark

Energy/Taste: Warm, pungent, bitter

Channel-Organ: Liver, Kidney

Actions:
1. Dispel Wind-Damp
2. Strengthen tendons and bones
3. Benefit urination
4. Transform Damp and reduce swelling

Form and Preparation: Powder, decoction, or pill; can be soaked in wine for rear or back weakness

Dosage:
Horses and Cattle: 15–45 g
Llamas, Alpacas, Goats, and Pigs: 5–12 g
Dogs: 2–5 g
Cats: 1–2 g
Birds and Rabbits: 0.1–1 g

Cautions and Contraindications: Caution for *Yin* Deficiency with Heat

Side Effects: None known

Cibotium *Gou Ji* 狗脊

Original Reference: *Shen Nong Ben Cao Jing* (*Shen Nong's Materia Medica*, 1st century BCE) 神农本草经

Part Used: Rhizome

Name:
Pharmaceutical: Cibotii Barometz, Rhizoma
Botanical: Cibotium barometz
Wade-Giles: *Kou-Chi*
Translation: Dog's Spine

Energy/Taste: Warm, bitter, sweet

Channel-Organ: Liver, Kidney

Actions:
1. Tonify Liver and Kidney and strengthen bones and tendons
2. Dispel Wind-Damp
3. Stabilize Kidney to stop urinary incontinence and vaginal discharge

Form and Preparation: Powder, decoction, or pill

Dosage:
Horses and Cattle: 15–45 g
Llamas, Alpacas, Goats, and Pigs: 5–12 g
Dogs: 2–5 g
Cats: 1–3 g
Birds and Rabbits: 0.1–1 g

Cautions and Contraindications:
1. Caution for dysuria or urinary dysfunction or *Yin* Deficiency with Heat
2. May antagonize Patrinia *Bai Jiang Cao*

Side Effects: None known

Saussurea *Xue Lian Hua* 雪莲花

Original Reference: *Ben Cao Gang Mu Shi Yi* (*Omissions for the Materia Medica Compendium*) by *Zhao Xue-min* et al., in 1765 CE 本草纲目拾遗

Part Used: Whole plant with flower

Name:
Pharmaceutical: Saussurea Laniceps Herba
Botanical: Saussurea laniceps Hand

Common: Saussurea Laniceps
Wade-Giles: *Hsueh-Lien-Hua*
Translation: Snow Flower

Energy/Taste: Warm, sweet, slightly bitter

Channel-Organ: Liver, Kidney

Actions:
1. Clear Wind-Damp and strengthen bones and tendons
2. Tonify Kidney *Yang*
3. Regulate Liver and stop bleeding

Form and Preparation: Powder, decoction, or pill

Dosage:
Horses and Cattle: 15–45 g
Llamas, Alpacas, Goats, and Pigs: 5–12 g
Dogs: 2–5 g
Cats: 0.5–1 g
Birds and Rabbits: 0.1–1 g

Cautions and Contraindications: Contraindicated during pregnancy

Side Effects: None known

AROMATIC HERBS TO TRANSFORM DAMP

Herbs to transform Damp are warm, aromatic, fragrant, pungent, and drying. They can expel the pathogenic Damp, which stagnates in the Middle Burner (*Zhong Jiao*), mainly the Spleen and Stomach. The primary clinical signs include bloated abdomen (or abdominal distension), vomiting, nausea, acid regurgitation, poor appetite, lack of thirst, diarrhea, lassitude, a pale or yellow tongue with white and greasy coating, and a slippery pulse or soft pulse.

According to an old TCVM saying the "Spleen dislikes Damp but enjoys fragrance." Excessive Damp stagnates in the Middle Burner (*Zhong Jiao*) and limits the Spleen's ability to transform and transport water and Body Fluids, which allows Damp to build up. On the other hand, fragrant herbs can revive the Spleen's ability to transform and transport Damp, which subsequently decreases the Damp. Thus, these aromatic herbs combat Damp by strengthening the Spleen, transforming turbid Damp, and promoting *Qi* flow in the Spleen and Stomach. The herbs can treat Damp due to Spleen *Qi* or *Yang* Deficiency, Summer Damp-Heat, Damp *Bi* Syndromes, and diarrhea. They are often combined with other herbs to treat specific conditions. For example, combine aromatic herbs with 1) herbs to warm the Interior for Cold-Damp conditions, 2) herbs to clear Heat for Damp-Heat conditions, 3) herbs to invigorate *Qi* flow for Damp Stagnation, or 4) herbs to tonify Spleen *Qi* for Damp due to Spleen *Qi* Deficiency.

The pungent, warm, aromatic, and dry nature of aromatic herbs can exhaust the *Yin*; thus, these herbs should be used cautiously in patients with *Yin* Deficiency. However, the herbs' effectiveness can be affected by their processing. Overcooking can damage the aromatic and fragrant properties, so these herbs should be cooked quickly or added near the end of the preparation process.

Atractylodes *Cang Zhu* 苍术

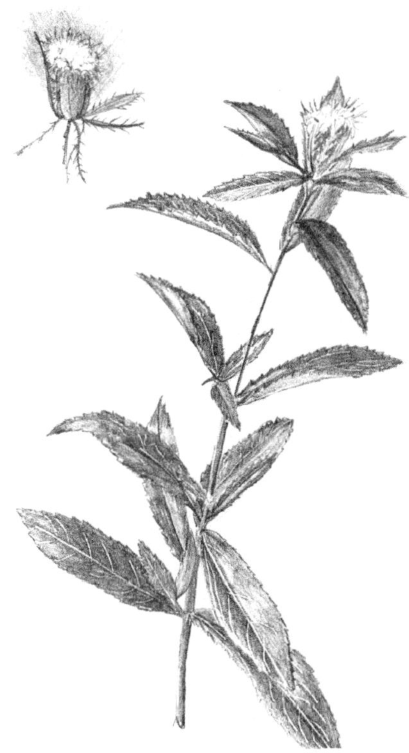

a

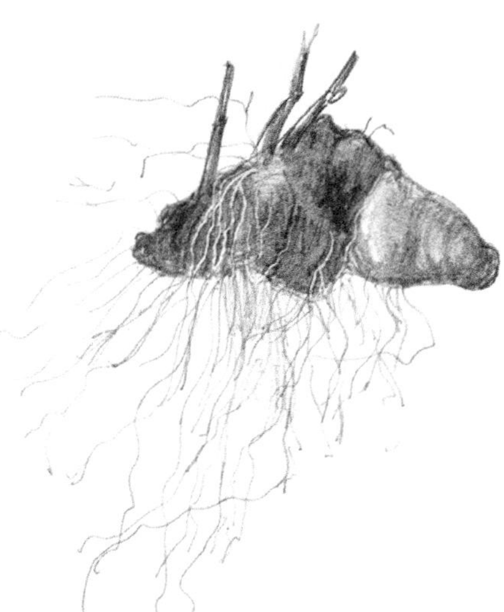

b

Original Reference: *Shen Nong Ben Cao Jing* (*Shen Nong's Materia Medica*, 1st century BCE) 神农本草经

Part Used: Root and Rhizome

Name:
Pharmaceutical: Atractylodis, Rhizoma
Botanical: Atractylodes Lancea; A. Chinensis; A. Japonica
Common: Atractylodes
Wade-Giles: *Ts'ang-Shu*
Translation: Dark Bundle

Energy/Taste: Warm, pungent, bitter

Channel-Organ: Spleen, Stomach

Actions:
1. Dry Damp and strengthen the Spleen
2. Expel Wind-Damp
3. Induce sweating
4. Improve vision

Form and Preparation: Powder, decoction, or pill

Dosage:
Horses and Cattle: 15–60 g
Camels: 35–65 g
Llamas, Alpacas, Goats, and Pigs: 5–15 g
Dogs: 3–8 g
Cats: 1–2 g
Birds and Rabbits: 0.3–3 g

Cautions and Contraindications:
1. Because it is very drying, caution in *Yin* Deficiency.
2. Contraindicated with sweating due to *Qi* Deficiency

Side Effects: None known

Clinical Applications:
1. Damp accumulating and Stagnant in the Spleen and Stomach
   Clinical signs: Abdominal fullness or distension, poor appetite, nausea, vomiting, diarrhea, greasy tongue/coat
   Combine with: Pogostemon *Huo Xiang*, Magnolia *Hou Po*, and Citrus *Chen Pi*
   Classical herbal formula: *Ping Wei San*
2. Wind-Cold-Damp in the Channels and Collaterals
   Clinical signs: Swollen and painful joints, weakness of the lower limbs, headache, arthritis, muscle pain
   Combine with: Chaenomeles *Mu Gua*, Morus *Sang Zhi*, and Angelica *Du Huo*
3. Exterior Pattern due to the invasion of Wind-Cold with Damp
   Clinical signs: Soreness of limbs, chills, fever
   Combine with: Ledebouriella *Fang Feng*, Asarum *Xi Xin*, and Notopterygium *Qiang Huo*
4. Downward flowing Of Damp-Heat
   Clinical signs: Swollen, painful and weak stifles and pelvic limbs, or skin lesions
   Combine with: Phellodendron *Huang Bai*, Achyranthes *Niu Xi*
   Classical herbal formula: *San Miao Wan*
5. Summer Heat with Damp
   Combine with: Lonicera *Jin Yin Hua*
6. Cataracts, glaucoma, night blindness
   Combine with: Sesame *Hei Zhi Ma*

History and Comments:
1. Atractylodes *Cang Zhu* acts internally by drying Damp to strengthen the Spleen, and it acts externally by expelling Wind-Cold to relieve an Exterior Pattern.
2. Atractylodes *Cang Zhu* and *Bai Zhu* are very similar plants, which can substitute for each other in a formula, but they are not the same species. Atractylodes *Cang Zhu* is preferred for Damp conditions, whereas Atractylodes *Bai Zhu* is preferred as a Spleen *Qi* tonic. Also, Atractylodes *Bai Zhu* is more expensive.
3. Atractylodes *Cang Zhu* is combined with Poria *Fu Ling* or Magnolia *Hou Po* to synergize and enhance its effect.
4. Good quality *Cang Zhu* is large and solid, lacks small hairs, has a cinnabar-colored cross section, and is aromatic.
5. *Cang Zhu* can promote sweating, improve night vision, and also reduce blood sugar levels.

Pharmaceutical Ingredients:[1–4]
1. Essential oils (β-eudesmol, hinesol, atractylodin, atractylone, atractyloside, atractylol, eudesmol)
2. β-eudesmol, atractyloain
3. Vitamin A

Magnolia *Hou Po* 厚朴

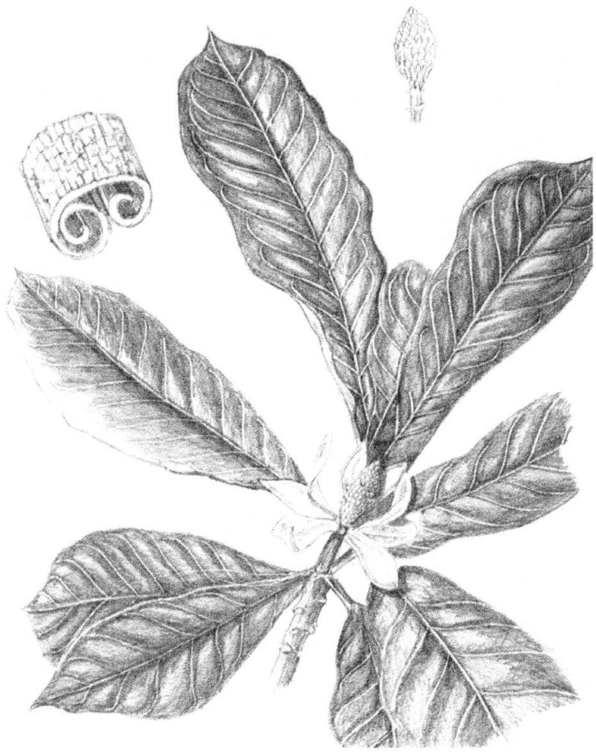

Original Reference: *Shen Nong Ben Cao Jing* (*Shen Nong's Materia Medica*, 1st century BCE) 神农本草经

Part Used: Bark

Name:
Pharmaceutical: Magnoliae Officinalis, Cortex
Botanical: Magnolia Officinales; M. Biloba
Common: Magnolia Bark
Wade-Giles: *Hou-Pu*
Translation: Thick bark

Energy/Taste: Slightly cold, bitter, sour

Channel-Organ: Spleen, Stomach, Lung, Large Intestine

Actions:
1. Dry Damp and transform Phlegm
2. Regulate *Qi* and relieve Food Stagnation
3. Direct rebellious *Qi* downward to stop asthma

Form and Preparation: Powder, decoction, or pill

Dosage:
Horses and Cattle: 15–45 g
Camels: 30–60 g
Llamas, Alpacas, Goats, and Pigs: 5–15 g
Dogs: 2–5 g
Cats: 0.5–1 g
Birds and Rabbits: 0.2–1 g

Cautions and Contraindications:
1. Caution during pregnancy
2. May antagonize Alisma *Ze Xie*

Side Effects: Overdosage may damage *Qi* and Body Fluids.

Clinical Applications:
1. Disharmony of the Spleen and Stomach due to Stagnation of Damp
   Clinical signs: Abdominal distension and fullness, regurgitation, nausea, vomiting
   Combine with: Atractylodes *Cang Zhu* and Citrus *Chen Pi*
   Classical herbal formula: *Ping Wei San*
2. Food retention or constipation
   Clinical signs: Abdominal distension, colic, nausea, poor appetite, constipation
   Combine with: Rheum *Da Huang* and Aurantium *Zhi Shi*
   Classical herbal formula: *Da Xiao Cheng Qi Tang*
3. Cough or asthma
   Combine with: Perilla *Zi Su Zi*, Peucedanum *Qian Hu*, and Cinnamomum *Gui Zhi*
   Classical herbal formula: *Su Zi Jiang Qi Tang*

History and Comments:
1. Magnolia *Hou Po* is an important herb that relieves bloating or distention due to Damp, Food Stagnation, or *Qi* Stagnation in the gastrointestinal system. It is often combined with Poria *Fu Ling* and Citrus *Chen Pi*.
2. Its energy goes downward; thus, it can treat asthma or cough.
3. Good quality Magnolia *Hou Po* is thick, finely textured, oily, and aromatic.
4. Magnolia *Hou Po* is effective for the prevention of postoperative intestinal adhesions.

Pharmaceutical Ingredients:[1–4]
1. Essential oils (β-eudesmol, magnolol, honokiol, tetrahydromagnolol, isomagnolol)
2. Magnocurarine, magnoloside, alkaloids, saponin

Pogostemon *Huo Xiang* 藿香

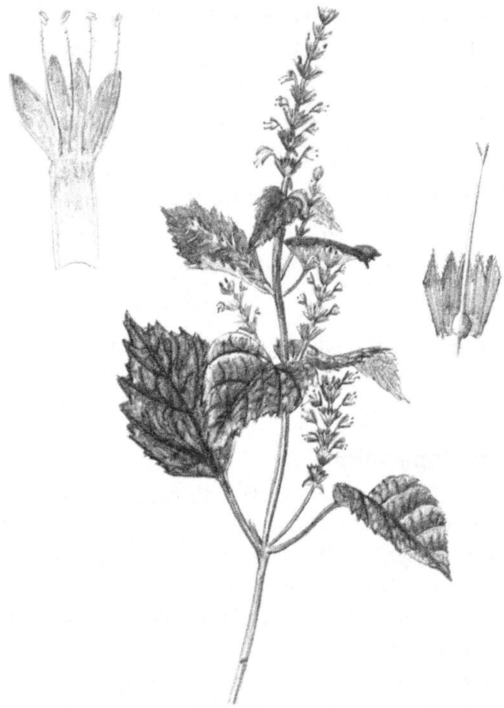

Original Reference: *Ming Yi Bie Lu* (*Miscellaneous Records of Famous Physicians*) by *Tao Hong-Jing*, North and South Kingdoms (5th century) 名医别录

Part Used: Aboveground parts of the plant

Name:
Pharmaceutical: Pogostemi, Herba
Botanical: Pogostemon Cablin or Agastache Rugosa
Common: Pogostemon
Wade-Giles: *Huo-Hsiang*
Translation: Leaf Fragrant

Energy/Taste: Slightly warm, pungent

Channel-Organ: Spleen, Stomach, Lung

Actions:
1. Transform Damp
2. Harmonize the Stomach and stop vomiting
3. Clear Summer Heat and relieve the Exterior

Form and Preparation: Powder, decoction, or pill

Dosage:
Horses and Cattle: 20–45 g
Llamas, Alpacas, Goats, and Pigs: 5–10 g
Dogs: 2–5 g
Cats: 0.5–1 g
Birds and Rabbits: 0.1–2 g

Cautions and Contraindications: Contraindicated for *Yin* Deficiency and Blood Deficiency

Side Effects: None known

Clinical Applications:
1. Damp blocking Middle Burner (*Zhong Jiao*, Spleen, and Stomach)
   Clinical signs: Abdominal distension, nausea, vomiting, poor appetite, diarrhea
   Combine with: Atractylodes *Cang Zhu*, Magnolia *Hou Po*, Pinellia *Ban Xia*
   Classical herbal formula: *Wei Cang He*
2. Internal injury by raw and Cold Food with Exogenous invasion of Wind-Cold
   Clinical signs: Chills and fever, headache, nausea, vomiting, abdominal fullness, diarrhea
   Combine with: Perilla *Zi Su Ye*, Pinellia *Ban Xia*, Magnolia *Hou Po*, Eupatorium *Pei Lan*, and Citrus *Chen Pi*
   Classical herbal formula: *Hou Xiang Zheng Qi San*

History and Comments:
1. Pogostemon *Huo Xiang* is also called Agastache.
2. Pogostemon *Huo Xiang* is an important herb for transforming Damp and removing turbidity. Damp obstructs the Middle Burner (*Zhong Jiao*) and interferes with the Spleen's transporting function.
3. Pogostemon *Huo Xiang*, Perilla *Zi Su Ye*, and Phragmites *Lu Gen* are all effective in controlling vomiting. However, *Huo Xiang* is better for transforming Damp, *Zi Su Ye* is better for releasing the Exterior, and *Lu Gen* is better for clearing Stomach Heat.
4. Good quality *Huo Xiang* has many leaves, with blue-green stems and branches, and is aromatic (Agastache). It also is good quality if it has a coarse stem, has soft and thick leaves, and is green and aromatic (Pogostemon). In general, Pogostemon *Huo Xiang* is considered to be of higher quality than Agastache.
5. *Huo Xiang* has significant inhibitory effects on many pathogenic fungi in vitro.

Pharmaceutical Ingredients:[1–4]
1. Patchoulialcohol
2. Cinnamic aldehyde, benzaldehyde, eugenol, patchoulipyridine, epiguaipyridine
3. β-elemene, caryophyllen, alloaromadendrene, r-patchoulene, α-guaiene, δ-guaiene, α-patchoulene

4. Methylchavicol, anethole, anisaldehyde, d-limonene, α-pinene, β-pinene, p-methoxy cinnamaldehyde, linalool, 1-octen-3-ol, β-humulene, α-xylangene, β-farnesene

Amomum *Sha Ren* 砂仁

Original Reference: *Yao Xing Lun* (*Discussion of Medicinal Properties*) by *Chen Zhou* in 19th century 药性论

Part Used: Fruit

Name:
Pharmaceutical: Amomi, Fructus
Botanical: Amomum Vilosum; A. Longiligulare; A. Xanthioides
Common: Cardamon
Wade-Giles: *Sha-Jen*
Translation: Sand Seeds

Energy/Taste: Warm, pungent

Channel-Organ: Spleen, Stomach

Actions:
1. Transform Damp, promote *Qi* flow
2. Warm the Middle Burner (*Zhong Jiao*), stop diarrhea
3. Calm the fetus to prevent abortion

Form and Preparation: Powder, decoction, or pill

Dosage:
Horses and Cattle: 15–30 g
Llamas, Alpacas, Goats, and Pigs: 3–9 g
Dogs: 1–3 g
Cats: 0.3–1 g
Birds and Rabbits: 0.5–1.5 g

Cautions and Contraindications: Caution for *Yin* Deficiency and Blood Deficiency

Side Effects: None known

Amomum *Bai Dou Kou* 白豆蔻

Original Reference: *Ming Yi Bie Lu* (*Miscellaneous Records of Famous Physicians*) by *Tao Hong-Jing*, North and South Kingdoms (5th century) 名医别录

Part Used: Fruit

Name:
Pharmaceutical: Amomi Kravanh, Fructus
Botanical: Amomum Kravanh Pierre
Common: Round Cardamon fruit
Wade-Giles: *Pai-Tou-K'ou*
Translation: White Bean

Energy/Taste: Warm, pungent

Channel-Organ: Lung, Spleen, Stomach

Actions:
1. Transform Damp and promote *Qi* flow
2. Warm Spleen and Stomach and stop vomiting
3. Transform Phlegm and resolve Stagnation
4. Promote gastrointestinal functions in chronic renal failure patients

Form and Preparation: Powder, decoction, or pill

Dosage:
Horses and Cattle: 15–30 g
Llamas, Alpacas, Goats, and Pigs: 3–10 g
Dogs: 2–5 g
Cats: 0.5–1 g
Birds and Rabbits: 0.5–1.5 g

Cautions and Contraindications: Caution for Blood and *Yin* Deficiency

Side Effects: None known

Alpinia Cao Dou Kou 草豆蔻

Original Reference: *Lei Gong Pao Zhi Lun* (*Lei's Method of Preparing Drugs*) by *Lei Xiao* (5th century) 雷公炮炙论

Part Used: Seed

Name:
Pharmaceutical: Alpinia Katsumadai, Semen
Botanical: Alpinia katsumadai Hayata
Common: Katsumada's galangal seeds
Wade-Giles: *Pai-Tou-K'ou*
Translation: Grass Bean

Energy/Taste: Warm, pungent

Channel-Organ: Spleen, Stomach

Actions:
1. Dry Damp and promote *Qi* flow
2. Warm the Middle Burner (*Zhong Jiao*) and stop vomiting

Form and Preparation: Powder, decoction, or pill

Dosage:
Horses and Cattle: 15–30 g
Camels: 35–65 g
Llamas, Alpacas, Goats, and Pigs: 3–10 g

Dogs: 2–5 g
Cats: 0.5–1 g
Birds and Rabbits: 0.1–2 g

Cautions and Contraindications: Caution for Blood and *Yin* Deficiency

Side Effects: None known

Eupatorium *Pei Lan* 佩兰

Original Reference: *Shen Nong Ben Cao Jing* (*Shen Nong's Materia Medica*, 1st century BCE) 神农本草经

Part Used: Aboveground part of the plant

Name:
Pharmaceutical: Eupatorii Fortunei, Herba
Botanical: Eupatorium Forunei
Common: Eupatorium
Wade-Giles: *P'ei-Lan*
Translation: Ornamental Orchid

Energy/Taste: Neutral, pungent

Channel-Organ: Spleen, Stomach

Actions:
1. Transform Damp
2. Clear Summer Heat

Form and Preparation: Powder, decoction, or pill

Dosage:
Horses and Cattle: 15–45 g
Llamas, Alpacas, Goats, and Pigs: 5–15 g
Dogs: 1–4 g
Cats: 0.5–1 g
Birds and Rabbits: 0.1–2 g

Cautions and Contraindications: None known

Side Effects: None known

Amomum *Cao Guo* 草果

Original Reference: *Ben Cao Gang Mu* (*Materia Medica Compendium*) by *Li Shi-Zhen* in 1590 本草纲目

Part Used: Fruit

Name:
Pharmaceutical: Amomi Tsao-Ko, Fructus
Botanical: Amomum Tsao-Ko
Common: Tsao-Ko fruit
Wade-Giles: *Ts'ao-Kuo*
Translation: Grass Fruit

Energy/Taste: Warm, pungent

Channel-Organ: Spleen, Stomach

Actions: Dry Damp and warm the Middle Burner (*Zhong Jiao*)

Form and Preparation: Powder, decoction, or pill

Dosage: Horses and Cattle: 15–45 g
Llamas, Alpacas, Goats, and Pigs: 3–9 g
Dogs: 1–4 g
Cats: 0.3–1 g
Birds and Rabbits: 0.1–2 g

Cautions and Contraindications: Caution for Blood and *Yin* Deficiency

Side Effects: None known

HERBS TO BENEFIT URINATION AND DRAIN DAMP

The herbs in this section are used in treating two types of Damp: Water-Damp and Damp-Heat (Table 7.2). These herbs eliminate Damp accumulation by increasing urine volume to facilitate water excretion. They are either sweet or bland with neutral, cool or cold energy. They can be used for dysuria, *Lin* Syndrome, diarrhea, edema, urinary tract infections, Phlegm-Fluid, jaundice and eczema. These herbs are often combined with other herbs, depending on the kind of Damp. They are combined with aromatic herbs to transform Damp for

Table 7.2. Differentiation of Damp Patterns.

Pattern	Clinical Signs	Examples of Herbs
Water-Damp or Fluid Accumulation	Edema in limbs Ascites Wet cough due to Damp-Phlegm	Poria *Fu Ling*
Damp-Heat	Lower Burner: UTI, cystitis, bladder/kidney crystal, or stone Pyometra, endometritis Middle Jiao: Liver Damp-Heat, jaundice, GB stones GI Damp-Heat, or IBD Skin: Moisture dermatitis, open and oozing sore, hot spot	Plantago *Che Qian Zi*

Damp accumulation in Stomach or Spleen and herbs to clear Damp-Heat (Chapter 4) in the Middle Burner (*Zhong Jiao*). In general, these herbs should be used cautiously in *Yin* Deficiency or internal dryness.

Poria *Fu Ling* 茯苓

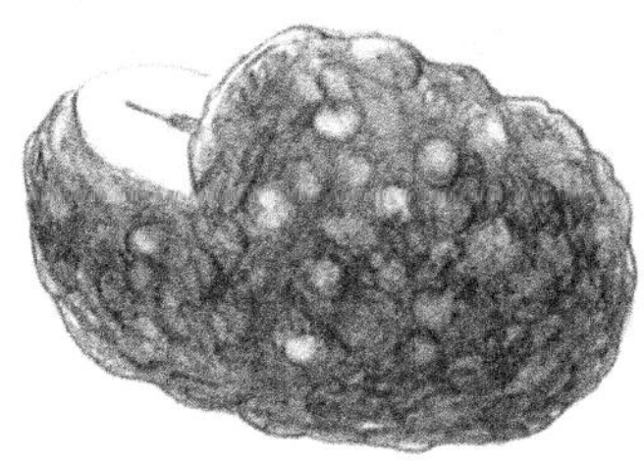

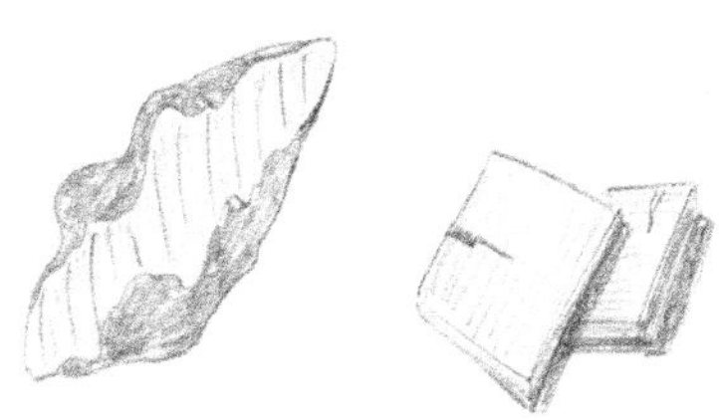

Original Reference: *Shen Nong Ben Cao Jing* (*Shen Nong's Materia Medica*, 1st century BCE) 神农本草经

Part Used: Fungus

Name:
Pharmaceutical: Poriae Cocos, Sclerotium
Botanical: Poria Cocus
Common: Poria
Wade-Giles: *Fu-Ling*
Translation: Hidden root

Energy/Taste: Neutral, sweet, bland

Channel-Organ: Heart, Spleen, Bladder, Kidney

Actions:
1. Promote urination and drain Damp
2. Strengthen the Spleen and tonify the Middle Burner (*Zhong Jiao*)
3. Calm the *Shen*
4. Transform Phlegm

Form and Preparation: Powder, decoction, or pill

Dosage:
Horses and Cattle: 20–60 g
Camels: 45–90 g
Llamas, Alpacas, Goats, and Pigs: 5–10 g
Dogs: 2–6 g
Cats: 1–2 g
Birds and Rabbits: 0.3–2 g

Cautions and Contraindications:
1. Contraindicated for polyuria or spermatorrhea
2. May counteract Sanguisorba *Di Yu*, Gentiana *Qin Jiao*, and Amyda *Bie Jia*

Side Effects: Avoid overdosing because it can be too drying

Clinical Applications:
1. Damp, water retention, or fluid accumulation
   Clinical signs: Edema, ascites, pleural effusion, painful or scanty urination, diarrhea
   Combine with: Polyporus *Zhu Ling*, Alisma *Ze Xie*, Atractylodes *Bai Zhu*, and Cinnamomum *Gui Zhi*
   Classical herbal formula: *Wu Ling San* or *Wu Pi Yin*
2. Retention of Phlegm-fluid in the Lung or Heart
   Clinical signs: Dizziness, palpitations, cough
   Combine with: Cinnamomum *Gui Zhi*, Atractylodes *Bai Zhu*
   Classical herbal formula: *Ling Gui Zhu Gan Tang*
3. Excess Damp due to Spleen *Qi* Deficiency
   Clinical signs: Poor appetite, poor digestion, diarrhea, nausea, lassitude
   Combine with: Codonopsis *Dang Shen*, Atractylodes *Bai Zhu*, and Glycyrrhiza *Gan Cao*
   Classical herbal formula: Si Jun Zi Tang
4. Nausea due to Phlegm accumulation
   Combine with: Pinellia *Ban Xia*, Citrus *Chen Pi* and Glycyrrhiza *Gan Cao*
   Classical herbal formula: *Er Chen Tang*
5. Palpitations and insomnia
   Combine with: Codonopsis *Dang Shen*, Longan *Long Yan Rou*, Ziziphus *Suan Zao Ren*
   Classical herbal formula: *Gui Pi Tang*

History and Comments:
1. Poria *Fu Ling* is a fungus that grows around the roots of various pine trees. The center of the fungus (*Fu Shen*) is used to Calm *Shen* and benefit the Heart. The dark skin of the fungus (*Fu Ling Pi*) is a strong diuretic.
2. Poria *Fu Ling* is often combined with Atractylodes (*Bai Zhu* or *Cang Zhu*) to reinforce its effects.
3. Poria *Fu Ling* comes in flat, cubed, or shaven curled pieces, but the latter is preferred.
4. Lui-zhong Yuan, a famous novelist from the *Tong* Dynasty (773–819 CE) suffered from acute heart palpitations and a bloating sensation in his upper

abdomen area. When a doctor said that *Fu Ling* could treat his illness, Lui-zhong purchased the herb, made a soup from it, and drank it. His condition did not improve; rather, it worsened. Lui-zhong called this doctor to his house. When the doctor arrived, he listened to Lui-zhong complain about the treatment, then he examined the herb. The doctor said, "That is not *Fu Ling*. It is an old sweet potato. The herbal salesman cheated you. You should not blame me." The novelist got some real *Fu Ling*, and he was completely healed after taking a couple of doses. Afterward, this novelist wrote an article explaining how to differentiate *Fu Ling* from imitations and warning others to be wary of unscrupulous herbalists.

Pharmaceutical Ingredients:[1–4]

1. β-pachyman, pachymose, pachyman, pachymaran, poriaic acid A, B, C
2. Terpene (pachymic acid, tumulosic acid, 3β-hydroxylanosta-7, 9(11), 24-trien-21 acid)
3. Sylvite sterol, lecithin, choline, histidine

Alisma *Ze Xie* 泽泻

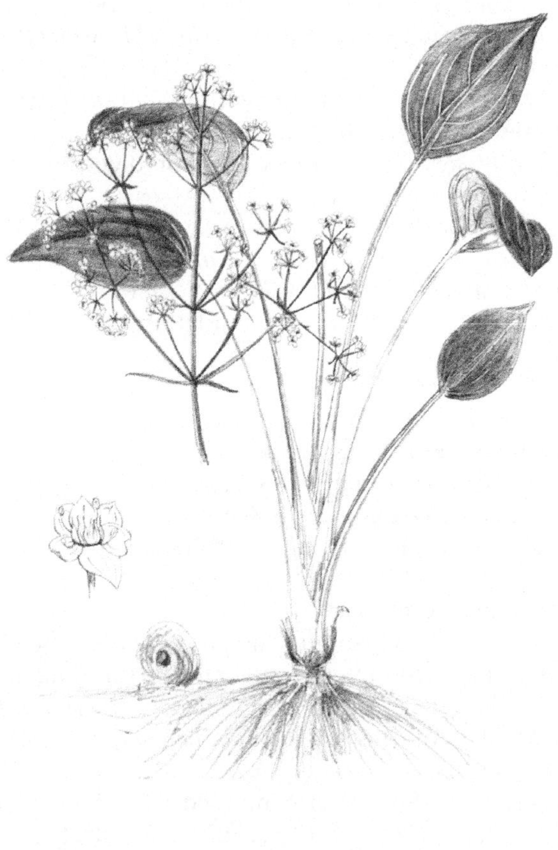

Original Reference: *Shen Nong Ben Cao Jing* (*Shen Nong's Materia Medica*, 1st century BCE) 神农本草经

Part Used: Rhizome

Name:
Pharmaceutical: Alismatis Orientalitis, Rhizoma
Botanical: Alsima orientalis; Alisma plantago-aquatica L.
Common: Alisma
Wade-Giles: *Tse-Hsieh*
Translation: Marsh Drain

Energy/Taste: Cold, sweet, bland

Channel-Organ: Kidney, Bladder

Actions:

1. Promote urination, drain Damp
2. Clear Kidney Fire

Form and Preparation: Powder, decoction, or pill

Dosage:
Horses and Cattle: 20–45 g
Camels: 35–65 g
Llamas, Alpacas, Goats, and Pigs: 5–15 g
Dogs: 3–8 g
Cats: 0.5–1 g
Birds and Rabbits: 0.5–1 g

Cautions and Contraindications:

1. Glycyrrhiza *Gan Cao* inhibits its diuretic effect.
2. Caution for Cold-Damp conditions

Side Effects: Overdose may damage sperm.

Clinical Applications:

1. Water retention and urination disorders
   Clinical signs: Dysuria, turbid urine, painful urination, edema, diarrhea, leukorrhea, urinary tract infections
   Combine with: Poria *Fu Ling*, Polyporus *Zhu Ling*, Atractylodes *Bai Zhu*; avoid using Glycyrrhiza *Gan Cao*
   Classical herbal formula: *Wu Ling San*
2. False Fire/Heat due to Kidney *Yin* Deficiency
   Combine with: Anemarrhena *Zhi Mu* and Phellodendron *Huang Bai*
   Classical herbal formula: *Zhi Bai Di Huang Wan*
3. Organ transporter for the Kidney
   Classical herbal formula: *Liu Wei Di Huang Wan*

History and Comments:

1. Alisma *Ze Xie* is a safe herb for removing Damp from the Lower Burner. It does not injure *Yin*. Its ability to attract Damp to the Kidney facilitates the nourishing of Kidney *Yin*.
2. Alisma *Ze Xie* is a mild herb and should be used in large quantities in most formulas.

3. Good quality *Ze Xie* is large, yellowish white, lustrous, and powdery.
4. *Ze Xie* can reduce serum cholesterol and fat in the liver. It is also effective for hypertension.

Pharmaceutical Ingredients:[1–4]
1. Alkaloids, glycosides
2. Terpenoids (alisol A, B, alisol A monoacetate, alisol B monoacetate, alisol C monoacetate, epialisol A, alismol, alismoxide, alismin)
3. Starch, protein, fatty acids, amino acids, essential oils, choline, phytosterols
4. K, Na, Mg, Ca, Fe, Mn, Cu, Zn

Polyporous *Zhu Ling* 猪苓

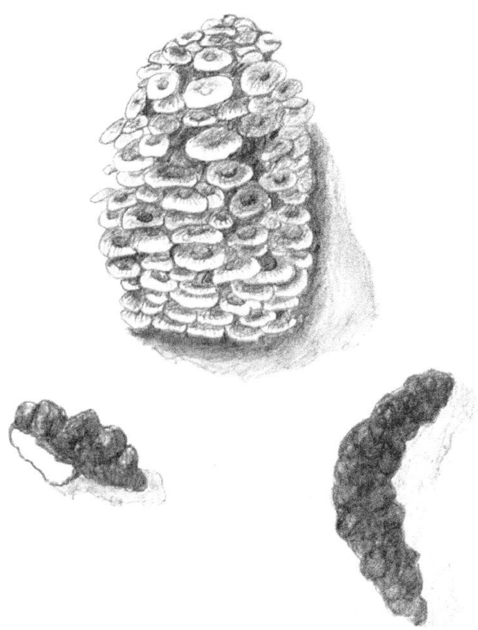

Original Reference: *Shen Nong Ben Cao Jing* (*Shen Nong*'s *Materia Medica*, 1st century BCE) 神农本草经

Part Used: Fungus

Name:
Pharmaceutical: Polypori Umbellati, Sclerotium
Botanical: Polyporous umbellatus; Grifolia umbellata
Common: Polyporus
Wade-Giles: *Chu-Ling*
Translation: Pig root

Energy/Taste: Neutral, sweet, bland

Channel-Organ: Kidney, Bladder

Actions:
1. Promote urination and drain Damp
2. Promote water metabolism and relieve edema

Form and Preparation: Powder, decoction, or pill

Dosage:
Horses and Cattle: 20–60 g
Camels: 35–65 g
Llamas, Alpacas, Goats, and Pigs: 5–20 g
Dogs: 2–6 g
Cats: 1–2 g
Birds and Rabbits: 0.3–3 g

Cautions and Contraindications: Caution for absence of Damp

Side Effects: Long-term use is discouraged, because it may injure the *Yin*. However, it is the most neutral and safe herb in this category.

Clinical Applications:
1. Urination disorders and water retention
   Clinical signs: Dysuria, turbid urine, painful urination, edema, diarrhea, leukorrhea, urinary tract infections, thirst unrelated to Heat, scanty urine
   Combine with: Poria *Fu Ling* and Alisma *Ze Xie*
   Classical herbal formula: *Wu Ling San*
2. Organ transporter for Bladder and Kidney

History and Comments:
1. Polyporus *Zhu Ling* is excellent for treating abdominal water retention due to Kidney *Qi* or *Yang* Deficiency.
2. During times of reduced availability, it is all right to substitute Polyporus *Zhu Ling* for Poria *Fu Ling*. Polyporus is a stronger diuretic than Poria *Fu Ling*, but does not strengthen Spleen or calm *Shen*.
3. When used alone, Polyporus *Zhu Ling* can treat mild cases of water retention and urinary disorders such as difficult urination and edema.
4. Polyporus *Zhu Ling* is routinely combined with Alisma *Ze Xie*.
5. Good quality *Zhu Ling* is large and lustrous, has a very dark red outer skin, and is powdery and white on the inside.
6. *Zhu Ling* contains immune-enhancing polysaccharides. It can also lower blood sugar levels.

Pharmaceutical Ingredients:[1–4]
1. Glucan, ergosterol, biotin, polyporenic acid A, C, polyporusterone
2. Protein, sylvite

Plantago *Che Qian Zi* 车前子

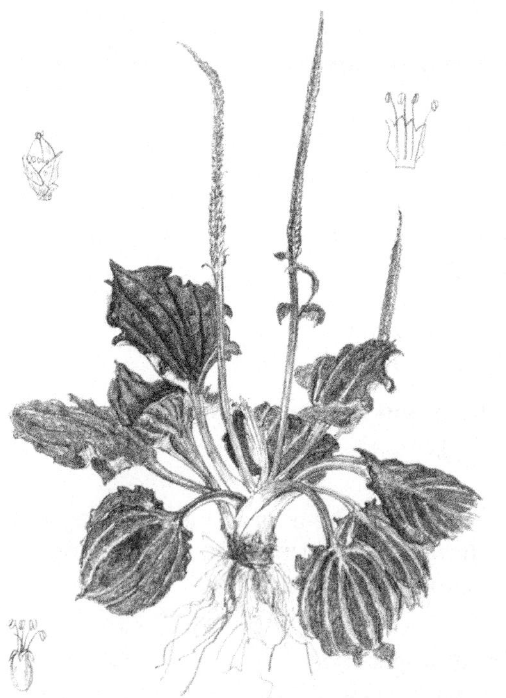

Original Reference: *Shen Nong Ben Cao Jing* (*Shen Nong's Materia Medica*, 1st century BCE) 神农本草经

Part Used: Seed

Name:
Pharmaceutical: Plantagaginis, Semen
Botanical: Plantago asiatica; P. depressa
Common: Plantago seed
Wade-Giles: *Ch'e-Ch'ien-Tzu*
Translation: Cart Front Seed

Energy/Taste: Slightly cold, sweet

Channel-Organ: Kidney, Lung, Bladder, Liver

Actions:
1. Promote urination and relieve abnormal urination
2. Clear Heat and improve vision
3. Clear the Lung and resolve Phlegm

Form and Preparation: Powder, decoction, or pill

Dosage:
Horses and Cattle: 20–30 g
Camels: 30–50 g
Llamas, Alpacas, Goats, and Pigs: 5–15 g
Dogs: 2–5 g
Cats: 1–2 g
Birds and Rabbits: 0.3–3 g

Cautions and Contraindications:
1. Caution for polyuria, constipation, or pregnancy
2. Contraindicated for *Yang* Deficiency

Side Effects: None known

Clinical Applications:
1. Damp-Heat in the Bladder and Lower Burner (*Xiao Jiao*)
   Clinical signs: Dysuria, painful urination, frequent urination, distension in lower abdomen, edema
   Combine with: Akebia *Mu Tong*, Gardenia *Zhi Zi*, Talcum, *Hua Shi*, Alisma *Ze Xie*
   Classical herbal formula: *Ba Zheng San*
2. Urinary crystals or calculi due to Damp-Heat
   Combine with: Lygodium *Hai Jin Sha*, Gardenia *Zhi Zi*
3. Liver Heat affecting the eyes
   Clinical signs: Painful eyes, red eyes, photophobia
   Combine with: Chrysanthemum *Ju Hua*, Gentiana *Long Dan Cao*, and Scutellaria *Huang Qin*
4. Profuse Lung Phlegm-Heat with cough
   Combine with: Trichosanthes *Gua Lou*, Scutellaria *Huang Qin*, and Fritillaria *Chuan Bei Mu* or combine with Platycodon *Jie Geng*, and Armeniaca *Xing Ren*

History and Comments:
1. During the *Han* Dynasty (206 BC–220 CE), General Wu Ma and his troops were trapped in a barren area by an enemy army. It was summer, which is the most Hot and Damp time of the year. The food and water supplies were nearly gone, and both the soldiers and their horses became ill. Their abdomens swelled like large drums and they developed hematuria and dysuria. One day, a horseman found that his horse's urine was no longer bloody, so he carefully observed the horse's actions. The horseman saw the horse eating a cow-ear–shaped herb. He collected this herb, cooked it, and ate it himself. His urine became normal too. The horseman reported his finding to the General. When the General asked how he found this herb, the horseman pointed to the horse saying, "front of the cart." The General ordered all troops to eat the herb and to feed it to their horses. Several days later, all soldiers and their horses were almost healed. Then General Wu Ma decided to call this herb the "Cart Front Herb" (*Ce Qian Cao*).
2. During the *Ming* Dynasty (1368–1644 CE), a famous writer, Ou *Yang* Shou, suffered from acute diarrhea so terrible that his stool was like water. He did not improve even after following several famous doctors'

prescribed treatments. One day, his wife suggested he buy the 30-cent bag of herbs sold by a street vendor for diarrhea. Because Ou *Yang* Shou did not trust that this street vendor's classical herbal formula was safe, he rejected her idea. Seeing no other available option, Ou *Yang* Shou's wife asked her family members to purchase the herb and pretend that they had received a new herbal recipe from a famous doctor. Believing their story, the writer accepted the new herbs and made an herbal soup. One dose of the soup cured Ou *Yang* Shou's illness.
3. Plantago *Che Qian Zi* is often dry-fried or fried in salt water prior to decoction. It is a transporter to the Lower Burner *(Xia Jiao)*. It can be used in formulas for endometritis, prostate problems, and urinary tract infections. It has also been used for malposition of the fetus.
4. The seed contains mucilage, which soothes an irritated urinary tract, vagina, and colon.
5. Plantago *Che Qian Cao* is the entire plant, which is sweet and cold. It is more effective at clearing Heat and relieving toxicity than the seed alone.
6. Good quality *Che Qian Zi* is large, black, round, and full.

Pharmaceutical Ingredients:[1–4]
1. Planteroic acid
2. Flavonoids (plantagin, plantenolic acid, plantasan), D-xylose, D-galacturonic acid, L-rhamnose, D-galactose, L-arabinose
3. Protein, succinic acid, adenine, choline, catalpol, palmitic acid, stearic acid, arachidonic acid, linoleic acid, oleic acid

Talcum *Hua Shi* 滑石

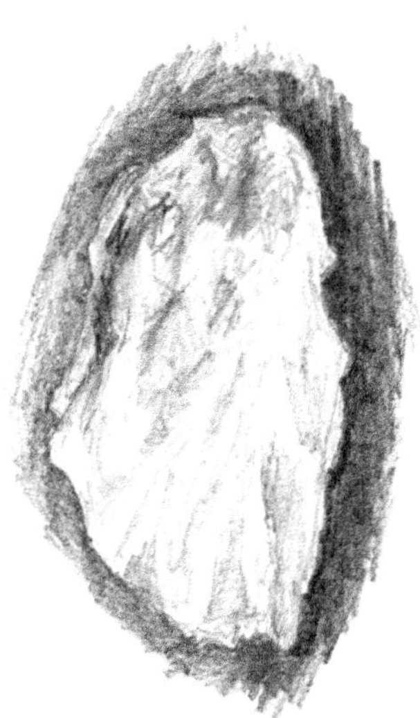

Original Reference: *Shen Nong Ben Cao Jing* (*Shen Nong's Materia Medica*, 1st century BCE) 神农本草经

Part Used: Rock–mineral $Mg_3(Si_4O_{10})(OH)_2$

Name:
Pharmaceutical: Talcum
Chemical: Magnesium silicate, hydrated
Common: Talcum
Wade-Giles: *Hua-Shih*
Translation: Slippery Rock

Energy/Taste: Cold, pungent, bland, sweet

Channel-Organ: Stomach, Bladder

Actions:
1. Promote water metabolism and relieve abnormal urination
2. Clear Heat and release Summer Heat
3. Aid movement of urinary crystals and calculi

Form and Preparation: Powder, decoction, or pill

Dosage:
Horses and Cattle: 25–45 g
Camels: 30–60 g
Llamas, Alpacas, Goats, and Pigs: 5–20 g
Dogs: 2–9 g
Cats: 1–3 g
Birds and Rabbits: 0.3–3 g

Cautions and Contraindications:
1. Caution during pregnancy
2. Caution for chronic diarrhea due to Spleen *Qi* or *Yang* Deficiency
3. Caution for depleted Body Fluids due to a warm-febrile disease and for excessive urination

Side Effects: Long-term use may cause ovarian cancer.

Clinical Applications:
1. Damp-Heat in the Bladder and Kidney
   Clinical signs: Painful, urgent, or frequent urination; hematuria; lower abdominal distension; occasional fever
   Combine with: Akebia *Mu Tong*, Plantago *Che Qian Zi*, Polygonum *Bian Xu*, Gardenia *Zhi Zi*
   Classical herbal formula: *Ba Zheng San*
2. Urinary crystals or calculi
   Combine with: Alisma *Ze Xie*, Polyporous *Zhu Ling*, Lygodium *Hai Jin Sha*
3. Summer Heat Pattern
   Clinical signs: Thirst, anhidrosis, profuse sweating, vomiting, nausea, diarrhea
   Combine with: Glycyrrhiza *Gan Cao* (6:1 ratio)
4. Skin diseases, boils, Heat rash (prickly Heat), eczema, wounds
   Combine with: Gypsum *Shi Gao* and Calamina *Lu Gan Shi*, Phellodendron *Huang Bai* and Alum *Ming Fan*
   Apply topically

5. Edema accompanying dysentery
   Combine with: Alisma *Ze Xie*, Plantago *Che Qian Zi*, and Poria *Fu Ling*

History and Comments:
1. Talcum *Hua Shi* comes as an easily crushed rock or as a fine powder. The latter is preferred. Use caution not to inhale the dust. Inhaled talc is carcinogenic, but ingested talc is not.
2. Talcum *Hua Shi* is similar to Gypsum *Shi Gao*. Both are very cooling minerals.
3. Talcum *Hua Shi* is soothing to the urinary tract and is useful to treat urinary irritation and burning due to Heat or infection. The herb is also recommended for hematuria.
4. Good quality Talcum *Hua Shi* is soft, smooth, bluish white, and without dust.
5. Talcum *Hua Shi* has antibacterial effects and is soothing to the skin and mucus membranes. It is useful not only for the urinary tract and intestines, but also for skin lesions, including traumatic wounds and infections.

Pharmaceutical Ingredients:[5]
1. $Mg_3(Si_4O_{10})(OH)_2$
2. $Al_4(Si_4O_{10})(OH)_8$

Akebia *Mu Tong* 木通

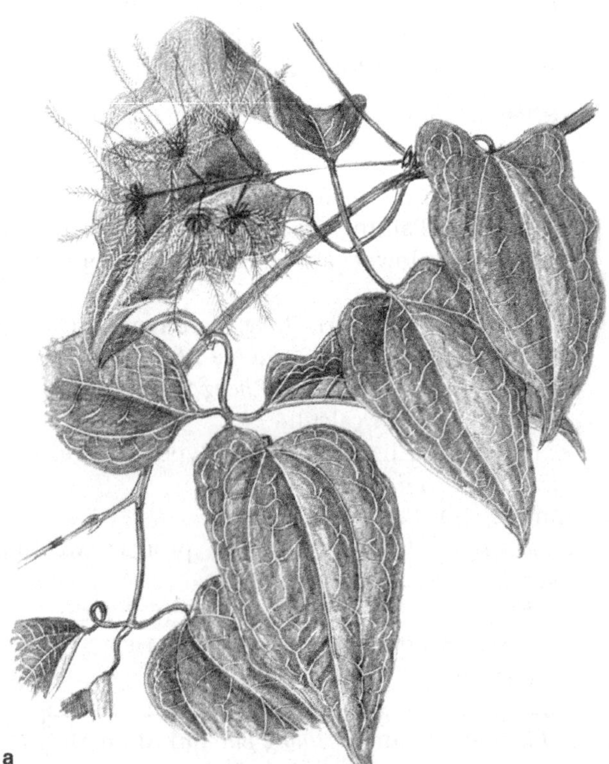

a

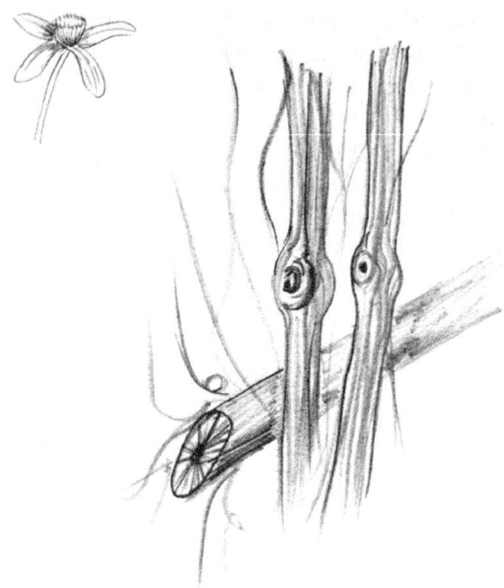

b

Original Reference: *Shen Nong Ben Cao Jing* (*Shen Nong*'s *Materia Medica*, 1st century BCE) 神农本草经

Part Used: Stem

Name:
Pharmaceutical: Mutong, Caulis (Formerly: Caulis Akebiae)
Botanical: Akebia quinata; Aristolochia manshuriensis
Common: Akebia
Wade-Giles: *Mu-T'ung*
Translation: Wood (with) Holes

Energy/Taste: Cold, bitter

Channel-Organ: Heart, Small Intestine, Bladder, Lung

Actions:
1. Clear Heat and relieve abnormal urination
2. Improve circulation of Blood and promote lactation
3. Clear Heart Fire and calm *Shen*

Form and Preparation: Powder, decoction, or pill

Dosage:
Horses and Cattle: 25–40 g
Llamas, Alpacas, Goats, and Pigs: 2–6 g
Dogs: 2–4 g
Cats: 0.5–1 g
Birds and Rabbits: 0.1–1.5 g

Cautions and Contraindications:
1. Contraindicated during pregnancy
2. Contraindicated with Deficiency of *Yin* or *Qi*

Side Effects:
1. Overdosing (60 g/day) in people can cause acute renal failure.
2. It is suspected of containing aristolochic acid.

Clinical Applications:

1. Damp-Heat in the Bladder
   Clinical signs: Painful, frequent, difficult, or urgent urination; dysuria; full lower abdomen; edema
   Combine with: Plantago *Che Chian Zi*, Alisma *Ze Xie*, Talcum *Hua Shi*, or Coix *Yi Yi Ren*
2. Hematuria due to Heart Fire affecting the Small Intestine
   Clinical signs: Mouth or tongue ulcers, sore throat, irritability, insomnia, painful urination, bloody urine
   Combine with: Bambusa *Zhu Ye*, Lophatherum *Dan Zhu Ye*, Rehmannia *Sheng Di Huang*, and Glycyrrhiza *Gan Cao*
   Classical herbal formula: *Dao Che San* (Red Front Door)
3. Insufficient lactation or failure to start lactation
   Combine with: Vaccaria *Wang Bu Liu Xing*, Astragalus *Huang Qi*, Angelica *Dang Gui*, and Pig's feet
4. Joint pain and obstruction due to Wind-Damp
   Combine with: Atractylodes *Cang Zhu*

History and Comments:

1. Akebia *Mu Tong* has antibacterial and antiinfectious effects.
2. Tetrapanax *Tong Cao* and Akebia *Mu Tong* have similar actions, and can be substituted for each other.

Pharmaceutical Ingredients:[1–4]

1. Akebin
2. Hederagerin, oleanolic acid
3. Na, akebic acid B, D, debilicacid, aristoloside

Tetrapanax *Tong Cao* 通草

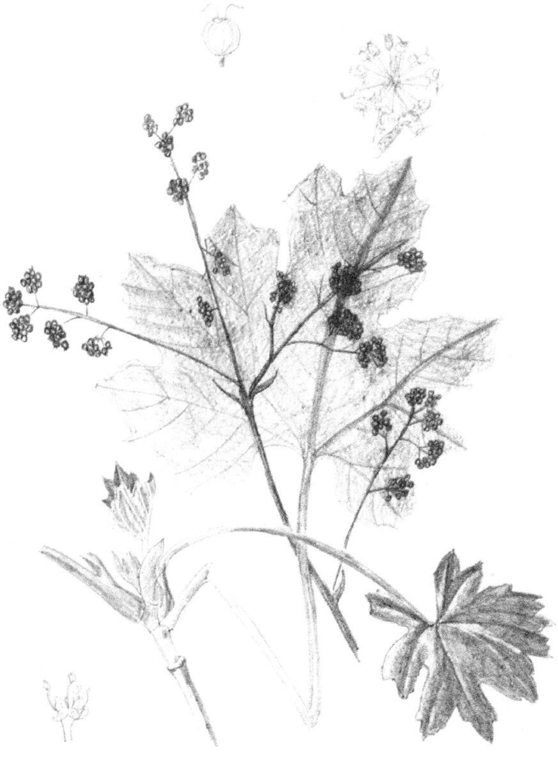

Original Reference: *Ben Cao Shi Yi* (*Supplement to Materia Medica*) by *Chen Cang-Qi* (8th century) 本草拾遺

Part Used: Rice paper pith

Name:
Pharmaceutical: Tetrapanacis Papyriferi, Medulla
Botanical: Tetrapanax papyriferus
Common: Rice paper pith, tetrapanax
Wade-Giles: *T'ung-Ts'ao*
Translation: Unblocking Herb

Energy/Taste: Cool, sweet, bland

Channel-Organ: Lung, Stomach

Actions:

1. Clear Heat and promote urination
2. Promote lactation

Form and Preparation: Powder, decoction, or pill

Dosage:
Horses and Cattle: 15–30 g
Camels: 30–60 g
Llamas, Alpacas, Goats, and Pigs: 3–10 g
Dogs: 2–5 g
Cats: 0.5–1 g
Birds and Rabbits: 0.5–2 g

Cautions and Contraindications:

1. Caution for Deficient *Qi* or *Yin*
2. Caution during pregnancy

Side Effects: None known

Clinical Applications:

1. Damp-Heat in the Bladder
   Clinical signs: Dysuria; painful, frequent, urgent urination
   Combine with: Talcum *Hua Shi* and Plantago *Che Qian Zi*
2. Edema and distention due to obstruction from Damp Heat
   Combine with: Areca *Da Fu Pi*
3. Bloody urination
   Combine with: Dianthus *Qu Mai*
4. Insufficient lactation after parturition
   Combine with: Vaccaria *Wang Bu Liu Xing*, Angelica *Dang Gui*, Astragalus *Huang Qi*, and Ligusticum *Chuang Xiong*

History and Comments: Tetrapanax *Tong Cao* may be substituted for Akebia *Mu Tong*.

Pharmaceutical Ingredients:[1–4]
1. Uronic acid, galactose, galacturonic acid
2. Glucose, xylose, lipids, protein, fiber, ash

Artemisia *Yin Chen Hao* 茵陈蒿

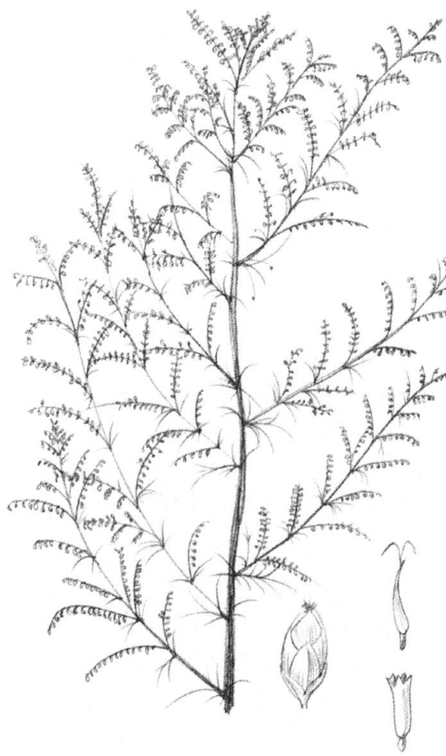

Original Reference: *Shen Nong Ben Cao Jing* (*Shen Nong's Materia Medica*, 1st century BCE) 神农本草经

Part Used: The whole aboveground plant

Name:
Pharmaceutical: Artemisiae Yinchenhao, Herba
Botanical: Artemisia capillaris; A. scoparia
Common: Capillaris
Wade-Giles: *Yin-Ch'en-Hao*

Energy/Taste: Slightly cold, bitter, pungent

Channel-Organ: Spleen, Stomach, Liver, Gallbladder

Actions:
1. Drain Damp, relieve jaundice
2. Detoxify and heal wounds

Form and Preparation: Powder, decoction, or pill

Dosage:
Horses and Cattle: 20–45 g
Camels: 35–65 g
Llamas, Alpacas, Goats, and Pigs: 5–15 g
Dogs: 2–6 g
Cats: 1–2 g
Birds and Rabbits: 0.1–2 g

Cautions and Contraindications: Caution for *Yin* jaundice with pale yellow skin and Blood Deficiency

Side Effects: None known

Clinical Applications:
1. Damp-Heat *Yang* Jaundice
   Clinical signs: Fever, bright yellow mucous membranes and conjunctiva, explosive diarrhea, constipation
   Combine with: Gardenia *Zhi Zi* and Rheum *Da Huang*
   Classical herbal formula: *Yin Chen Hao Tang* (Artemisia Combination)
2. Cold-Damp *Yin* jaundice
   Clinical signs: Fatigue, cold limbs, no appetite, chronic jaundice, diarrhea
   Combine with: Aconite *Fu Zi*, Atractylodes *Bai Zhu*, Poria *Fu Ling*, and Zingiberis *Gan Jiang*
   Classical herbal formula: *Yin Chen Zhu Fu Tang*
3. Gallstones
   Combine with: Lysimachia *Jin Qian Cao*, Rheum *Da Huang*, and Gardenia *Zhi Zi*
4. Skin diseases with itching and erosion
   Combine with: Phellodendron *Huang Bai*, Sophora *Ku Shen* and Kochia *Di Fu Zi* if taken orally, or may be used alone topically on the skin

History and Comments:
1. Artemisia *Yin Chen Hao* is the primary herb used for hepatitis and jaundice.
2. Artemisia *Yin Chen Hao* and Bupleurum *Chai Hu* both enter the Liver and Gallbladder Channels. They both drain Fire from the Liver and Gallbladder, but the former is less drying and softer than the latter. Artemisia *Yin Chen Hao* is especially useful when a patient with a *Yin*-Deficient or Excessive constitution needs the Heat clearing action of Bupleurum *Chai Hu*, but is unable to tolerate its drying nature.
3. Good quality *Yin Chen Hao* is young, soft, gray-green, and aromatic.
4. *Yin Chen Hao* has both antibacterial and antiviral properties. It can also reduce serum cholesterol and is useful for the treatment of gallstones.
5. *Yin Chen Hao* is effective for ulceration of the tongue and mouth.

Pharmaceutical Ingredients:[1–4]
1. Chlorogenic acid, caffeic acid, p-hydroxyacetophenone, 6,7-dimethoxycoumarin, capillarisin, salicylic acid, phydroxya cetophenone

2. β-pinene; capilline; capillone; capillene; capillarin; stearic acid; palmitic acid; oleic acid; linoleic acid; arachidic acid; montanic acid; 6,7-dimethoxycoumarine; 1-(2″-methoxyphenil)-2, 4-hexadiene; capillanol
3. Scoparone, folic acid

Phaseolus *Chi Xiao Dou* 赤小豆

Original Reference: *Shen Nong Ben Cao Jing* (*Shen Nong's Materia Medica*, 1st century BCE) 神农本草经

Part Used: Seeds

Name:
Pharmaceutical: Phaseoli Calcarati, Semen
Botanical: Phaseolus calcaratus
Common: Aduki bean
Wade-Giles: *Ch'ih-Hsiao-Tou*
Translation: Dark red little bean

Energy/Taste: Neutral, sweet, sour

Channel-Organ: Heart, Small Intestine

Actions:
1. Promote water metabolism and reduce edema
2. Relieve jaundice, clear Heat
3. Dispel toxins and eliminate pus

Form and Preparation: Powder, decoction, or pill

Dosage:
Horses and Cattle: 50–100 g
Llamas, Alpacas, Goats, and Pigs: 10–60 g
Dogs: 2–10 g
Cats: 1–3 g
Birds and Rabbits: 0.5–5 g

Cautions and Contraindications: Caution with Internal Dryness

Side Effects: Frequent ingestion of this bean can cause dryness.

Coix *Yi Yi Ren* 薏苡仁

Original Reference: *Shen Nong Ben Cao Jing* (*Shen Nong's Materia Medica*, 1st century BCE) 神农本草经

Part Used: Seed

Name:
Pharmaceutical: Coicis Lachryma-jobi, Semen
Botanical: Coix lacryma-jobi
Common: Job's tears
Wade-Giles: *I-I-Jen*
Translation: Coix seed

Energy/Taste: Cool, sweet, bland

Channel-Organ: Spleen, Stomach, Lung

Actions:
1. Drain Damp and promote urination
2. Strengthen Spleen and reduce edema
3. Clear Heat and eliminate pus
4. Relieve spasms and stop pain

Form and Preparation: Powder, decoction, or pill

Dosage:
Horses and Cattle: 30–60 g
Llamas, Alpacas, Goats, and Pigs: 5–20 g
Dogs: 2–10 g
Cats: 1–3 g
Birds and Rabbits: 0.3–3 g

Cautions and Contraindications: Caution if Deficient of Body Fluids and dehydrated

Side Effects: None known

Benincasa *Dong Gua Ren* 冬瓜仁

Original Reference: *Kai Bao Ben Cao* (*Materia Medica of the Kai Bao Era*) by *Ma Zhi* in 973 开宝本草

Part Used: Seed

Name:
Pharmaceutical: Exocarpium Benincasae
Botanical: Benincasa hispida
Common: Benincasa peel, Chinese wax gourd
Wade-Giles: *Tung-Kua-Jen*
Translation: Winter Melon Seed
Alternate: *Dong Gua Zi*

Energy/Taste: Cool, sweet

Channel-Organ: Lung, Small Intestine

Actions:
1. Clear Lung and transform Phlegm
2. Drain Damp and dispel pus

Form and Preparation: Powder, decoction, or pill

Dosage:
Horses and Cattle: 20–60 g
Llamas, Alpacas, Goats, and Pigs: 5–12 g
Dogs: 2–5 g
Cats: 1–2 g
Birds and Rabbits: 0.3–3 g

Cautions and Contraindications: None known

Side Effects: None known

Benincasa *Dong Gua Pi* 冬瓜皮

Original Reference: *Kai Bao Ben Cao* (*Materia Medica of the Kai Bao Era*) by *Ma Zhi* in 973 开宝本草

Part Used: Peel

Name:
Pharmaceutical: Exocarpium Benincasae
Botanical: Benincasa hispida
Common: Chinese wax gourd
Wade-Giles: Tung-Kua-P'i
Translation: Winter Melon Peel

Energy/Taste: Cool, sweet

Channel-Organ: Spleen, Small Intestine

Actions:
1. Promote water metabolism and reduce edema
2. Clear Heat and Summer Heat
3. Promote milk production

Form and Preparation: Powder, decoction, or pill, or used as Food Therapy

Dosage:
Horses and Cattle: 20–45 g
Llamas, Alpacas, Goats, and Pigs: 5–10 g
Dogs: 2–5 g
Cats: 1–1.5 g
Birds and Rabbits: 0.3–3 g

Cautions and Contraindications: None known

Side Effects: None known

Zea Yu Mi Xu 玉米须

Original Reference: *Lingnan Cai Yao Lu* (*Records of Picking Herbs in Lingnan*) by *Xiao Bu-dan* in 1936

Part Used: Whiskers of the flower

Name:
Pharmaceutical: Stylus Zeae Mays
Botanical: Zea Mays L.
Common: Cornsilk
Wade-Giles: *Yu-Mi-Hsu*
Translation: Jade Rice whiskers

Energy/Taste: Neutral, sweet

Channel-Organ: Bladder, Liver, Gallbladder

Actions:
1. Promote Water metabolism and reduce edema
2. Drain Damp and relieve jaundice
3. Has been used for chronic edema, renal failure, diabetes, cystitis, and jaundice

Form and Preparation: Use fresh or in a decoction

Dosage:
Horses and Cattle: 20–45 g
Llamas, Alpacas, Goats, and Pigs: 5–12 g
Dogs: 2–5 g
Cats: 1–2 g
Birds and Rabbits: 0.3–3 g

Cautions and Contraindications: None known

Side Effects: None known

Lagenaria Hu Lu 葫芦

Original Reference: *Ri Hua-Zi Ben Cao* (*Materia Medica of Ri Hua-Zi*) *Ri Hua-Zi* in 713 日华子本草

Part Used: Fruit

Name:
Pharmaceutical: Fructus Lagenaria
Botanical: Lagenaria siceraria
Common: Mini gourd
Wade-Giles: *Hu-Lu*
Translation: Bottle Gourd

Energy/Taste: Neutral, sweet

Channel-Organ: Lung, Kidney

Actions:
1. Promote water metabolism and reduce edema
2. Has been used for edema, jaundice, and diabetes

Form and Preparation: Powder, decoction, pill, or use as Food Therapy

Dosage:
Horses and Cattle: 60–120 g
Llamas, Alpacas, Goats, and Pigs: 10–60 g
Dogs: 2–15 g
Cats: 1–3 g
Birds and Rabbits: 0.3–3 g

Cautions and Contraindications: None known

Side Effects: None known

Capsella *Ji Cai* 荠菜

Original Reference: *Qian Jin Yao Fang* (*Thousand Ducat Formulas*) by *Sun Si-Miao* in 652 千金要方

Part Used: Whole plant

Name:
Pharmaceutical: Herba Capsella bursa
Botanical: Capsella bursa Medle
Common: Shepherd's purse
Wade-Giles: *Chi-Ts'ai*
Translation: Wild Vegetable

Energy/Taste: Cool, sweet

Channel-Organ: Liver, Stomach

Actions:
1. Promote water metabolism and reduce edema
2. Brighten eyes and stop bleeding
3. Has been used for inflammatory bowel disease and uveitis

Form and Preparation: Decoction or Food Therapy

Dosage:
Horses and Cattle: 30–100 g
Llamas, Alpacas, Goats, and Pigs: 5–30 g
Dogs: 2–8 g
Cats: 1–3 g
Birds and Rabbits: 0.3–3 g

Cautions and Contraindications: None known

Side Effects: None known

Dianthus *Qu Mai* 瞿麦

Original Reference: *Shen Nong Ben Cao Jing* (*Shen Nong's Materia Medica*, 1st century BCE) 神农本草经

Part Used: Whole plant

Name:
Pharmaceutical: Dianthi, Herba
Botanical: Dianthus superbus
Common: Chinese pink, fringed pink, dianthus
Wade-Giles: *Chu-Mai*
Translation: *Qu* wheat

Energy/Taste: Cold, bitter

Channel-Organ: Heart, Small Intestine

Actions:
1. Promote urination and treat *Lin* Syndrome
2. Invigorate blood circulation and unblock the Channels

Form and Preparation: Powder, decoction, or pill

Dosage:
Horses and Cattle: 20–45 g
Llamas, Alpacas, Goats, and Pigs: 5–15 g
Dogs: 2–6 g
Cats: 0.5–1 g
Birds and Rabbits: 0.5–1.5 g

Cautions and Contraindications: Contraindicated during pregnancy

Side Effects: None known

Kochia *Di Fu Zi* 地肤子

Original Reference: *Shen Nong Ben Cao Jing* (*Shen Nong's Materia Medica*, 1st century BCE) 神农本草经

Part Used: Fruit

Name:
Pharmaceutical: Kochiae Scopariae, Fructus
Botanical: Kochia Scoparia
Common: Broom Cypress, Kochia fruit
Wade Giles: *Ti Fu Tzu*
Translation: Earth Skin Seeds

Energy/Taste: Cold, bitter, pungent

Channel-Organ: Kidney, Bladder

Actions:
1. Promote urination and treat *Lin* Syndrome
2. Clear Heat and transform Damp
3. Stop itching

Form and Preparation: Powder, decoction, or pill

Dosage:
Horses and Cattle: 15–45 g
Llamas, Alpacas, Goats, and Pigs: 3–10 g
Dogs: 1–3 g
Cats: 0.5–1 g
Birds and Rabbits: 0.3–3 g

Cautions and Contraindications: Do not use in combination with Sepia *Hai Piao Xiao*.

Side Effects: None known

Lygodium *Hai Jin Sha* 海金沙

Original Reference: *Jia You Ben Cao* (*Materia Medica of the Jia You Era*) by *Zhang Yu-xi* and *Su Song* in 1061 CE 嘉佑本草

Part Used: Spores

Name:
Pharmaceutical: Lygodii Japonici, Spora
Botanical: Lygodium Japonicum
Common: Japanese Fern, Lygodium
Wade-Giles: *Hai-Chin-Sha*
Translation: Sea Golden Sand

Energy/Taste: Cold, sweet, salty

Channel-Organ: Bladder, Small Intestine

Actions:
1. Promote urination and clear *Lin* Syndrome
2. Clear Damp Heat and stop pain

Form and Preparation: Powder, decoction, or pill

Dosage:
Horses and Cattle: 30–45 g
Camels: 35–65 g
Llamas, Alpacas, Goats, and Pigs: 5–20 g
Dogs: 2–5 g
Cats: 0.5–1 g
Birds and Rabbits: 1–2 g

Cautions and Contraindications: Caution for Kidney *Yin* Deficiency

Side Effects: None known

Juncus *Deng Xin Cao* 灯心草

Original Reference: *Kai Bao Ben Cao* (*Materia Medica of the Kai Bao Era*) by *Ma Zhi* in 973 开宝本草

Part Used: Pith

Name:
Pharmaceutical: Junci Effusi, Medulla
Botanical: Juncus effusus
Common: Bulrush pith
Wade-Giles: *Teng-Hsin-T'sao*
Translation: Lamp Wick Herb

Energy/Taste: Slightly cold, sweet, bland

Channel-Organ: Heart, Lung, Small Intestine

Actions:
1. Promote urination and clear *Lin* Syndrome
2. Drain Heat from the Heart, calm *Shen*

Form and Preparation: Powder, decoction, or pill

Dosage:
Horses and Cattle: 10–25 g
Llamas, Alpacas, Goats, and Pigs: 3–9 g
Dogs: 1–3 g
Cats: 0.5–1 g
Birds and Rabbits: 0.1–1.5 g

Cautions and Contraindications: Caution for Cold due to *Yang* Deficiency

Side Effects: None known

Polygonum *Bian Xu* 扁蓄

Original Reference: *Shen Nong Ben Cao Jing* (*Shen Nong's Materia Medica*, 1st century BCE) 神农本草经

Part Used: Aboveground parts of the plant

Name:
Pharmaceutical: Polygoni Avicularis, Herba
Botanical: Polygonum aviculare L.
Common: Polygonum

Energy/Taste: Slightly cold, bitter

Channel-Organ: Bladder

Actions:
1. Promote water metabolism and regulate abnormal urination
2. Expel parasites and stop itching

Form and Preparation: Powder, decoction, or pill

Dosage:
Horses and Cattle: 20–60 g
Camels: 30–80 g
Llamas, Alpacas, Goats, and Pigs: 5–10 g
Dogs: 1–5 g
Cats: 0.5–1 g
Birds and Rabbits: 0.3–3 g

Cautions and Contraindications: Caution for Spleen *Qi* Deficiency

Side Effects: Overdose can cause drainage of the Essential *Qi*.

Pyrrosia *Shi Wei* 石韦

Original Reference: *Shen Nong Ben Cao Jing* (*Shen Nong's Materia Medica*, 1st century BCE) 神农本草经

Part Used: Leaf

Name:
Pharmaceutical: Pyrossiae, Herba
Botanical: Pyrossia sheareri; P. lingua; P. petiolosa
Common: Pyrrosia leaves
Wade-Giles: *Shih-Wei*
Translation: Stone Reed

Energy/Taste: Slightly cold, bitter, sweet

Channel-Organ: Bladder, Lung

Actions:
1. Promote urination and clear *Lin* Syndrome
2. Cool Blood and stop bleeding
3. Cool Lung Heat and stop cough

Form and Preparation: Powder, decoction, or pill

Dosage:
Horses and Cattle: 15–45 g
Camels: 30–60 g
Llamas, Alpacas, Goats, and Pigs: 5–10 g
Dogs: 2–5 g
Cats: 0.5–1 g
Birds and Rabbits: 0.3–2 g

Cautions and Contraindications: Caution for *Yin* Deficiency

Side Effects: None known

Malva *Dong Kui Zi* 冬葵子

Original Reference: *Shen Nong Ben Cao Jing* (*Shen Nong's Materia Medica*, 1st century BCE) 神农本草经

Part Used: Seed

Name:
Pharmaceutical: Semen Malva
Botanical: Malva verticillata L.
Common: Musk mallow seeds, or abutilon seeds
Wade-Giles: *Tung-K'uei-Tzu*
Translation: Winter Seed

Energy/Taste: Cool, sweet

Channel-Organ: Large Intestine, Small Intestine, Bladder

Actions:
1. Promote urination to resolve *Lin* Syndrome
2. Promote milk production
3. Moisten intestines to promote bowel movements

Form and Preparation: Powder, decoction, or pill

Dosage:
Horses and Cattle: 30–45 g
Llamas, Alpacas, Goats, and Pigs: 5–20 g
Dogs: 2–5 g
Cats: 0.5–1 g
Birds and Rabbits: 0.1–1.5 g

Cautions and Contraindications:
1. Caution for diarrhea due to Spleen *Qi* Deficiency
2. Caution during pregnancy

Side Effects: Overdosage may cause diarrhea.

Dioscorea *Bi Xie* 卑解

Original Reference: *Shen Nong Ben Cao Jing* (*Shen Nong's Materia Medica*, 1st century BCE) 神农本草经

Part Used: Rhizome

Name:
Pharmaceutical: Dioscoreae Hypoglaucae, Rhizoma
Botanical: Dioscorea hypoglauca Palib, Dioscorea tokoro, Dioscorea septemloba, Dioscorea futschauensis
Common: Hypoglauca Yam

Energy/Taste: Neutral, bitter

Channel-Organ: Kidney, Bladder, Stomach

Actions:
1. Drain Damp, resolve turbid urine
2. Expel Wind-Damp and relieve *Bi* Syndrome
3. Clear Damp Heat from the skin

Form and Preparation: Powder, decoction, or pill

Dosage:
Horses and Cattle: 25–45 g
Llamas, Alpacas, Goats, and Pigs: 5–15 g
Dogs: 2–8 g
Cats: 0.5–1 g
Birds and Rabbits: 0.5–1.5 g

Cautions and Contraindications: Caution for Kidney *Yin* Deficiency

Side Effects: None known

Lysimachia *Jin Qian Cao* 金钱草

Original Reference: *Ben Cao Gang Mu Shi Yi* (*Omissions for the Materia Medica Compendium*) by *Zhao Xue-min* et al., in 1765 本草纲目拾遗

Part Used: Whole plant

Name:
Pharmaceutical: Lysimachiae au Desmodii, Herba
Botanical: Lysimachia christiniae; Desmodium styracifolium
Common: Desmodium
Wade-Giles: *Chin-Ch'ien-Ts'ao*
Translation: Golden Money Herb

Energy/Taste: Slightly cold, sweet, salty

Channel-Organ: Liver, Kidney, Gallbladder, Bladder

Actions:
1. Promote urination and resolve *Lin* Syndrome
2. Clear calculi from the Kidney and Bladder
3. Drain Damp and clear jaundice

Form and Preparation: Powder, decoction, or pill

Dosage:
Horses and Cattle: 30–120 g
Llamas, Alpacas, Goats, and Pigs: 5–25 g
Dogs: 2–10 g
Cats: 1–3 g
Birds and Rabbits: 0.3–3 g

Cautions and Contraindications: Prolonged use can lead to dizziness or palpitations associated with depletion of potassium from the body owing to the herb's diuretic effect.

Side Effects: May cause a skin allergy

Polygonum *Hu Zhang* 虎杖

Original Reference: *Ming Yi Bie Lu* (*Miscellaneous Records of Famous Physicians*) by *Tao Hong-Jing*, North and South Kingdoms (5th century) 名医别录

Part Used: Stem and root

Name:
Pharmaceutical: Cuspidati, Radix Et Rhizoma
Botanical: Polygonum Cuspidatum Sieb. Et Zucc.
Common: Bushy Knotweed Root and stem
Wade-Giles: *Hu-Chang*
Translation: Tiger's Cane

Energy/Taste: Slightly cold, bitter

Channel-Organ: Liver, Gallbladder, Lung

Actions:
1. Clear Heat, resolve Damp, and clear jaundice
2. Invigorate Blood, dispel Stasis, and stop pain
3. Transform Phlegm, stop cough

Form and Preparation: Powder, decoction, or topical application

Dosage:
Horses and Cattle: 20–45 g
Llamas, Alpacas, Goats, and Pigs: 5–10 g
Dogs: 2–5 g
Cats: 0.5–1 g
Birds and Rabbits: 0.5–1.5 g

Cautions and Contraindications: Contraindicated during pregnancy

Side Effects: Overdosage or long-term use may cause nausea, vomiting, anorexia, diarrhea, and palpitations.

Abrus *Ji Gu Cao* 鸡骨草

Original Reference: *Lingnan Cai Yao Lu* (*Records of Picking Herbs in Lingnan*) by *Xiao Bu-dan* in 1936

Part Used: Whole plant

Name:
Pharmaceutical: Herba Abrus
Botanical: Abrus cantoniensis Hance
Common: Abrus
Wade-Giles: *Chi-Ku-Ts'ao*
Translation: Chicken Bone Herb

Energy/Taste: Cool, sweet, slightly bitter

Channel-Organ: Liver, Stomach

Actions:
1. Drain Damp and clear jaundice
2. Clear Heat and detoxify
3. Move Liver *Qi* to stop pain

Form and Preparation: Powder, decoction, or pill

Dosage:

Horses and Cattle: 20–40 g
Camels: 35–65 g
Llamas, Alpacas, Goats, and Pigs: 3–10 g
Dogs: 2–5 g

Cautions and Contraindications: None known

Side Effects: None known

SUMMARY

Table 7.3 summarizes and compares the herbs that dispel Damp.

REFERENCES

1. Chen JK, Chen TT. Chinese Medical Herbology and Pharmacology. City of Industry, CA: Art of Medicine Press, 2004.
2. Brinker FJ. The Toxicology of Botanical Medicines. Sandy, OR: Eclectic Medical Publications, 2000.
3. Duke JA. Handbook of Medicinal Herbs. New York: Chemical and Rubber Company Press, 2001.
4. Huang KC. The Pharmacology of Chinese Herbs, 2nd Edition. New York: Chemical and Rubber Company Press, 1999.
5. Bensky D, Clavey S, Stoger E. Chinese Herbal Medicine Materia Medica (3rd Edition). Seattle, WA: Eastland Press, Inc., 2004.

Table 7.3. Herbs to Dispel Dampness: A quick overview and comparison.

Herbs	Special Actions	Common Characteristics
Herbs to dispel Wind-Damp		
Herbs to dispel Wind-Cold-Damp		Taste: Pungent
(Wind/Cold/Damp *Bi*)		Action: Promote *Qi* flow
Du Huo	Clear *Bi* in the rear limb, clear Wind *Bi*	Relieve pain
Wei Ling Xian	Invigorate Channels, soften hardness	Indication: *Bi* Syndrome
Chuan Wu	Clear Cold *Bi*, topically relieve pain, **very toxic**	*Modern Study*
Cao Wu	Clear Cold *Bi*, topically relieve pain, **very toxic**	These herbs have
Mu Gua	Clear Damp *Bi*, harmonize Stomach, stop vomiting	analgesic,
Shen Jin Cao	Invigorate Channels	antiinflammatory,
Can Sha	Harmonize Stomach, transform Damp	antipyretic, and
Bai Hua She	Clear Wind to stop itching and convulsions, **toxic**	circulation-promoting
Wu Shao She	Clear Wind to stop itching and convulsions	properties. Their
Hai Feng Teng	Invigorate Channels, clear Cold *Bi*	indication includes
Xue Shang Yi Zhi Hao	Invigorate Blood, clear Cold *Bi*, **very toxic**	soft tissue pain, spasm
Lu Lu Tong	Open Channels, promote milk production	and convulsion of
Herbs to dispel Wind-Damp-Heat (Hot		tendons and muscles,
Bi)		numbness of muscle
Qin Jiao	Clear False Heat, clear Damp-Heat	and skin, hemiplegia
Xi Xian Cao	Clear Channels, dispel Toxic Heat	and flaccid limbs,
Sang Zhi	Clear Channels, be the transporter to limbs	degenerative joint
Hai Tong Pi	Clear *Bi* in rear limbs, kill scabies	diseases, rheumatism
Chou Wu Tong	Cool Liver to decrease hypertension	and arthritis, soreness,
Fang Ji	Reduce edema. **May be adulterated with aristolochic acid**	pain and weakness in
Si Gua Luo	Open Channel to promote milk production	back and limbs.
Lei Gong Teng	Reduce edema, kill parasites, **very toxic**	
Herbs to strengthen bones and Clear Wind-Damp (Deficiency Bi)		
Sang Ji Sheng	Tonify Liver and Kidney, calm fetus	
Wu Jia Pi	Tonify Liver and Kidney, transform Damp to reduce swelling	
Gou Ji	Tonify Liver and Kidney, stop urinary incontinence	
Xue Lian Hua	Tonify Kidney *Yang*, stop bleeding	
Aromatic Herbs o transform Dampness		
Cang Zhu	#1 herb to dry up Dampness for Spleen	Taste: Pungent, aromatic
	Clear Wind-Cold-Damp	Energy: Warm and dry
	Good for Vitamin A deficiency	Action: Transform Damp
Hou Po	Transform Phlegm to stop asthma or cough	Promote *Qi* flow
	Direct *Qi* downward to treat constipation	Strengthen Spleen
Huo Xiang	Clear Exterior Wind Cold	Indications:
	Clear Summer Heat with Damp	Dampness Stagnation
Sha Ren	Wake up Spleen, stop diarrhea	Stomach *Qi* Stagnation
	Calm fetus to prevent abortion	Spleen *Qi* Deficiency
Bai Dou Kou	Transform Phlegm, stop vomiting	**Cautions:** May damage
	Promote GI functions in chronic renal failure	*Yin*
Cao Dou Kou	Warm the Middle *Jiao*, stop vomiting	
Pei Lan	The only neutral one to transform Damp	
	Wake up Spleen	
	Clear Summer Heat, promote body fluids	
Cao Guo	Clear malaria	

Table 7.3. *(Continued)*

Herbs	Special Actions	Common Characteristics
Herbs to benefit urination and drain Dampness		
Herbs to drain Dampness and eliminate edema		
Fu Ling	Strengthen Spleen, calm *Shen*, potent diuretic	Taste: Sweet or bland Energy: Neutral, cool, or cold Action: Promote urination, a drain Dampness Indications: Dysuria, or *Lin* Syndrome Edema Diarrhea Phlegm–fluid Jaundice Eczema **Cautions:** May consume *Yin* and body fluids *Modern Study* These herbs have a diuretic effect. They clear Dampness via increase in urine volume and frequency.
Ze Xie	Clear Kidney False Fire to be a transporter to the Kidney, mild diuretic	
Zhu Ling	The most potent diuretic, to be a transporter to Kidney and Bladder	
Chi Xiao Dou	Relieve jaundice, clear heat	
Yi Yi Ren	Strengthen Spleen, clear *Bi* syndrome, clear pus	
Dong Gua Ren	Clear Lung Heat and transform Phlegm	
Dong Gua Pi	Clear Summer Heat, promote milk production	
Yu Mi Xu	Relieve jaundice, reduce edema	
Hu Lu	Reduce edema, clear jaundice	
Ji Cai	Brighten eyes and stop bleeding	
Diuretic herbs to resolve Lin syndrome		
Che Qian Zi	Clear Liver Heat and brighten eyes	
Hua Shi	Clear Heat and Summer Heat	
Mu Tong	Clear Heat from Heart and Small Intestine	
Tong Cao	Promote milk production	
Qu Mai	Invigorate Blood, potent to clear *Lin* syndrome	
Di Fu Zi	Clear skin Damp-Heat and stop itching	
Hai Jin Sha	Clear stone and crystal, stop pain	
Deng Xin Cao	Clear Heart Heat	
Bian Xu	Clear Heat, kill parasites, stop itching	
Shi Wei	Clear Heat, cool Blood	
Dong Kui Zi	Promote milk production, moisten intestines	
Bi Xie	Clear Wind-Damp, clear skin Damp-Heat	
Herbs to drain Dampness to resolve jaundice		
Yin Chen Hao	Detoxify and heal sores	
Jin Qian Cao	Clear crystal and stone from Kidney and Bladder	
Hu Zhang	Invigorate Blood, dispel Stasis, and stop pain	
Ji Gu Cao	Clear Heat and detoxify, move Liver *Qi*	

8 Herbs to Regulate (Stagnant) *Qi* 理气药

Huisheng Xie, Cheryl Chrisman, Min Su Kim

Qi is the most essential substance for forming an animal's body and maintaining its life activities. When the body is functioning properly, the *Qi* flows smoothly and freely. This *Qi* flow is known as *Qi Ji*. Disturbances of *Qi* flow result in disease. *Qi* flow disorders occur in one of two forms: Stagnation (blockage) or rebellion.

Qi Stagnation in the Exterior, which includes the Channels, muscles, joints, and connective tissues, leads to pain (*Bi* Syndrome). *Qi* Stagnation in the blood circulation leads to Blood Stagnation. *Qi* Stagnation in the Interior can lead to internal organ dysfunction. There are three primary categories of Internal *Qi* Stagnation: Stomach *Qi* Stagnation, Liver *Qi* Stagnation, and Lung *Qi* Stagnation (Table 8.1).

The herbs to regulate *Qi* support *Qi* functions by promoting free *Qi* flow and eliminating *Qi* Stagnation or rebellious *Qi*. These herbs are mostly warm, aromatic, drying, invigorating, pungent, or bitter in nature. They are used to treat gastrointestinal disorders, asthma, and emotional and behavioral disorders. Because these herbs are drying, prolonged use can damage stomach *Yin*. Their pungent and invigorating qualities can scatter and disperse *Qi*. Thus, use them cautiously in patients with *Qi* Deficiency. During preparation, cook the herbs for only a short time (15 minutes) to preserve their aromatic aspects and rich volatile oils.

To understand *Qi* from a modern biomedical perspective, one can imagine *Qi* as the physiological activities of the tissues. *Qi* Stagnation is an impediment or malfunction in the activity of the tissues. Herbs that regulate *Qi* primarily act to optimize the physiological functions of the gastrointestinal tract and Liver.

Citrus *Chen Pi* 陈皮

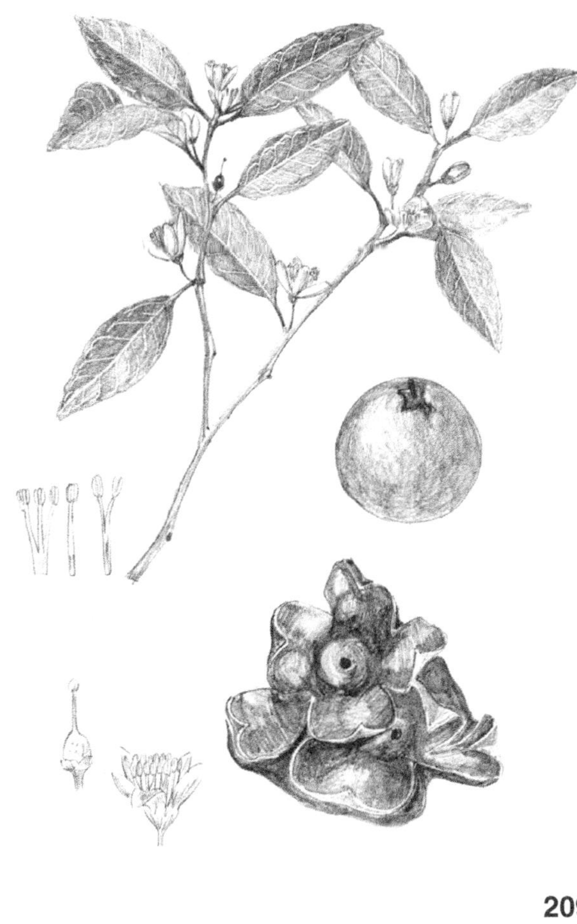

Table 8.1. Comparison between different Patterns of *Qi* Stagnation.

Patterns	Main Clinical Signs	Examples of Herbs
Stomach *Qi* Stagnation (including Large Intestine *Qi* Stagnation)	Abdominal distension, or colic Belching or flatulence Acid or sour regurgitation Nausea and vomiting Diarrhea or constipation	Citrus *Chen Pi* Saussurea *Mu Xiang*
Liver *Qi* Stagnation	Sensitive in chest or flanks (hypochondriac region) Loss of appetite Hiccups, belching, acid regurgitation Depression or irritability Irregular estrous cycle Red eyes Breast nodules or lumps Hernia or testicular pain Complications 1) Stagnant Liver *Qi* can lead to Heat 2) Can affect Stomach or Lungs	Cyperus *Xiang Fu*
Lung *Qi* Stagnation	Wheezing and cough Labored breathing or asthma Sensitive in the chest region on palpation	Aquilaria *Chen Xiang*

Original Reference: *Shen Nong Ben Cao Jing* (*Shen Nong's Materia Medica*, 1st century BCE) 神农本草经

Part Used: Peel or skin

Name:
Pharmaceutical: Citri Reticulatae, Pericarpium
Botanical: Citrus Reticulata; C. Tangerina; C. Erythrosa
Common: Tangerine Peel
Wade-Giles: *Ch'en P'i*
Translation: Aged Peel

Energy/Taste: Warm, pungent, bitter

Channel-Organ: Spleen, Lung

Actions:
1. Regulate *Qi* and strengthen the Spleen
2. Dry *Dampness* and transform Phlegm

Form and Preparation: Powder, decoction, pill, or Food Therapy

Dosage:
Horses and Cattle: 30–60 g
Llamas, Alpacas, Goats, and Pigs: 3–10 g
Dogs: 1–5 g
Cats and Rabbits: 0.5–1 g
Birds: 0.3–3 g

Cautions and Contraindications: Caution in *Yin* Deficiency with a dry cough

Side Effects: None known

Clinical Applications:
1. *Qi* Stagnation in the Spleen and Stomach
   Clinical signs: Abdominal distension, belching, hiccups, nausea, vomiting, colic, poor appetite, diarrhea
   Combine with: Aurantium *Zhi Ke* and Saussurea *Mu Xiang*, Zingiberis *Sheng Jiang*
   Herbal formula: *Wei Cang He* (Happy Earth)
2. Cold-Damp obstructed in the Spleen and Stomach
   Clinical signs: Abdominal fullness, poor appetite, fatigue, diarrhea, white and sticky tongue coating
   Combine with: Atractylodes Cang *Zhu* and Magnolia *Hou Po*
   Classical herbal formula: *Wei Lin San*
3. Damp-Phlegm obstructing the Lung
   Clinical signs: Cough with profuse watery Phlegm
   Combine with: Pinellia *Ban Xia* and Poria *Fu Ling*
   Classical herbal formula: *Er Chen Tang*

History and Comments:
1. Citrus *Chen Pi* is pungent, bitter, fragrant, and warm. The pungent taste moves *Qi* for treating *Qi* Stagnation. The bitter taste causes *Qi* to descend, which helps treat vomiting and cough. The warm temperature and fragrant smell helps to regulate *Qi* and normalize Spleen *Qi's* actions, namely to dry Damp and transform Phlegm. Citrus *Chen Pi* is a *Qi* herb for both the Spleen and Lung Channels.
2. Citrus *Chen Pi* is aged and has a dark appearance. The older the peel, while retaining aroma, the better the quality.
3. Citrus *Chen Pi* is often added to *Qi* tonic herbal formulas to prevent clotting and *Qi* Stagnation. It is also combined with Zingiberis *Sheng Jiang* for nausea and vomiting.

Pharmaceutical Ingredients: [1–4]
1. Essential oils (nobiletin, limonene, α-pinene, β-pinene, β-phellandrene)
2. Flavonoids (hesperidin, neohesperidin, tangeretin, citromitin, 5-o-desmethyl citromitin)
3. Inositol, Vitamin B1

Citrus *Ju Hong* 桔红, *Ju He* 桔核, and *Ju Ye* 桔叶

These three herbs are related to Citrus *Chen Pi*. They all come from the same plant.

Citrus *Ju Hong* is red tangerine peel. It is milder and used to strengthen the Spleen and has a more drying effect for the treatment of vomiting and wet cough. It can often substitute for *Chen Pi*.

Citrus *Ju He* is the tangerine seed. It can regulate *Qi*, dissipate masses and relieve pain. It is used to treat testicular pain and hernia with swollen testicles.

Citrus *Ju Ye* is the tangerine leaf. It can regulate liver *Qi*, eliminate masses and nodules. It can be used to treat breast masses.

Saussurea *Mu Xiang* 木香

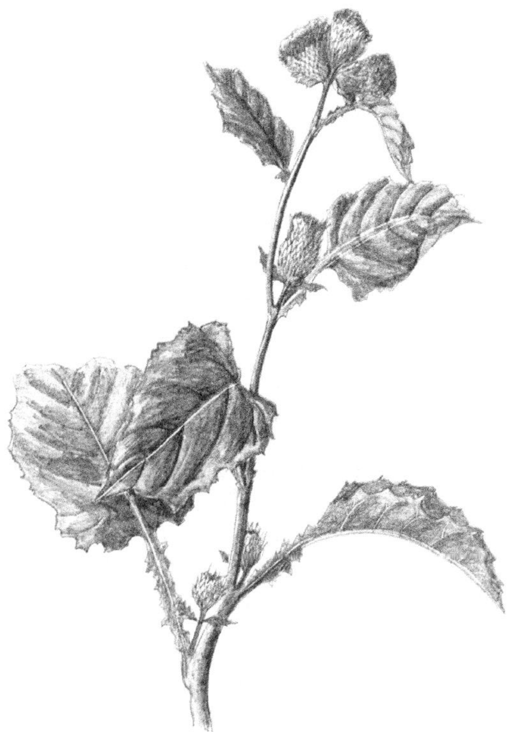

a

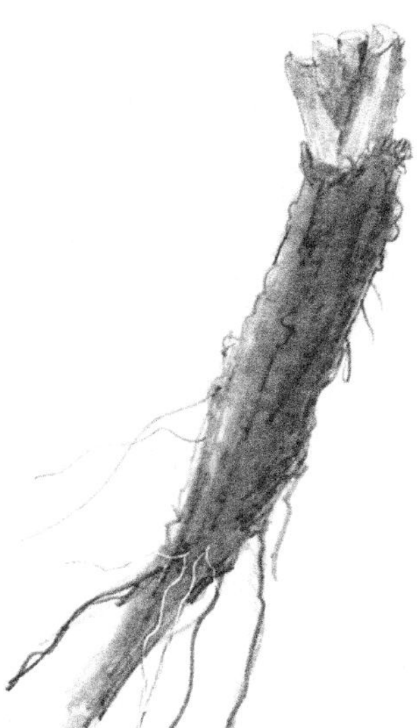

b

Original Reference: *Shen Nong Ben Cao Jing* (*Shen Nong's Materia Medica*, 1st century BCE) 神农本草经

Part Used: Root

Name:
Pharmaceutical: Saussureae, Radix
Botanical: Saussurea Lappa
Common: Auklandia
Wade-Giles: *Mu-Hsiang*
Translation: Wood Fragrance

Energy/Taste: Warm, pungent, bitter

Channel-Organ: Spleen, Stomach, Large Intestine, Gallbladder

Actions:
1. Regulate *Qi* and stop pain
2. Strengthen Spleen and stop diarrhea

Form and Preparation: Powder, decoction, or pill

Dosage:
Horses and Cattle: 30–60 g
Llamas, Alpacas, Goats, and Pigs: 5–15 g
Dogs: 2–5 g
Cats and Rabbits: 0.5–2 g
Birds: 0.1–1 g

Cautions and Contraindications: Caution for *Yin* Deficiency with Fire

Side Effects: None known

Clinical Applications:
1. Stomach and Spleen *Qi* Stagnation
   Clinical signs: Abdominal pain or distension, belching, hiccups, nausea, vomiting, poor appetite, diarrhea
   Combine with: Poria *Fu Ling*, Amomum *Sha Ren*, and Citrus *Chen Pi*
   Classical herbal formula: *Xiang Sha Liu Jun Zi Tang* (Eight Gentlemen)
2. Damp Heat dysentery
   Clinical signs: Abdominal pain, tenesmus, diarrhea
   Combine with: Coptis *Huang Lian* and Areca *Bing Lang*
   Classical herbal formula: *Da Xiang Lian Wan*
3. Liver *Qi* Stagnation
   Clinical signs: flank pain, distension, soreness

History and Comments:
1. Saussurea *Mu Xiang* is quite warm and is a strong *Qi* mover. In addition to regulating *Qi* in the Upper, Middle, and Lower Burners (*Shang, Zhong, and Xia*

Jiaos), this herb is very good for pain due to *Qi* Stagnation of the Spleen and Stomach. Stir-fried *Mu Xiang* is good to stop diarrhea.
2. *Mu Xiang* dilates the biliary duct to assist the discharge of gallstones.
3. Alkaloids from this herb have a strong inhibitory effect on histamine-induced bronchospasms and intestinal spasms. Water herbal extracts have antispasmodic and bronchodilatory effects and will lower blood pressure.

Pharmaceutical Ingredients:[1–4]
1. Essential oils (aplotaxene, α-costene, β-costene, costunolide, dehydrocostus lactone, 12-methoxydihydrocostus lactone, costic acid, costol, costus lactone, dihydrocostunolide, α-costol, α-costic acid)
2. Saussurine, synanthrin, stigmasterol

Aurantium *Zhi Shi* 枳实

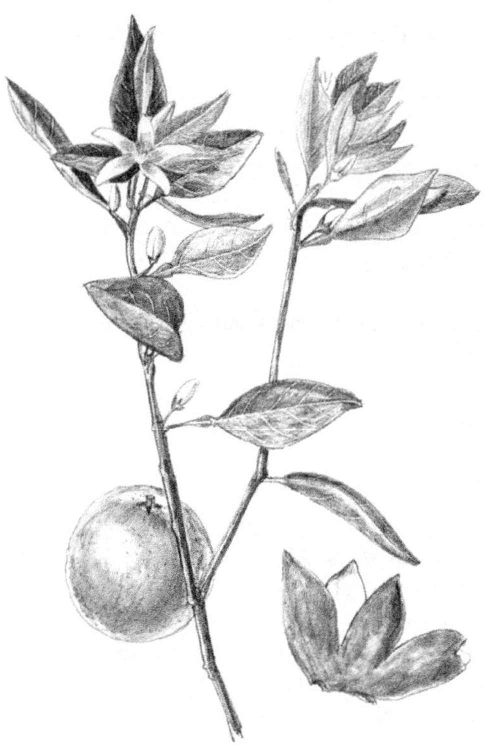

Original Reference: *Shen Nong Ben Cao Jing* (*Shen Nong's Materia Medica*, 1st century BCE) 神农本草经

Part Used: Immature fruit

Name:
Pharmaceutical: Citri Aurantii, Fructus Immaturus
Botanical: Citrus Aurantium; C. Wilsonii; Poncirus Trifoliata
Common: Bitter Orange
Wade-Giles: *Chih-Shih*
Translation: Orange solid

Energy/Taste: Slightly cold, bitter, pungent

Channel-Organ: Spleen, Stomach, Large Intestine

Actions:
1. Break up *Qi* Stagnation to remove Stasis
2. Direct *Qi* downward to unblock the bowels

Form and Preparation: Powder, decoction, or pill

Dosage:
Horses and Cattle: 30–60 g
Llamas, Alpacas, Goats, and Pigs: 3–10 g
Dogs: 2–6 g
Cats and Rabbits: 0.3–0.5 g
Birds: 0.2–3 g

Cautions and Contraindications:
1. Caution during Pregnancy
2. Caution in Spleen *Qi* Deficiency or Stomach False Cold due to *Yang* Deficiency

Side Effects: May cause diarrhea

Clinical Applications:
1. Constipation or Food Stasis
   Clinical signs: Food retention, abdominal distension, colic, belching with foul odor, nausea or vomiting
   Combine with: Rheum *Da Huang*, Magnolia *Hou Po*, Crataegus *Sha Zha*, Hordeum *Mai Ya*, and Massa Fermentata *Shen Qu*
   Classical herbal formula: *Da Cheng Qi Tang*
2. Damp-Heat Stagnation in the Intestines
   Clinical signs: Dysentery with tenesmus and abdominal pain
   Combine with: Rheum *Da Huang*, Coptis *Huang Lian*, Scutellaria *Huang Qin*
3. Prolapse of the uterus, rectum, or stomach due to Spleen *Qi* Deficiency
   Combine with: Atractylodes *Bai Zhu* and Astragalus *Huang Qi*
4. Turbid Phlegm Obstructing the Chest
   Clinical signs: Pain in the chest, sensitive on palpation
   Combine with: Allium *Xie Bai*, Cinnamomum *Gui Zhi*, Trichosanthes *Gua Lou*
   Classical herbal formula: *Zhi Shi Xia Bai Hui Zhi Tang*

History and Comments:

1. Auratium *Zhi Shi* is excellent for treating nausea. It is also effective for breaking up Phlegm and descending Stomach *Qi*.
2. Aurantium *Zhi Shi* is the immature fruit. The mature fruit is called Aurantium *Zhi Ke* or Aurantium *Zhi Qiao*. Although their properties are slightly different, one can be substituted for the other.
3. Aurantium *Zhi Ke* is milder than Aurantium *Zhi Shi* and thus is preferred for chronic or less serious diseases. Aurantium *Zhi Ke* has a more ascending direction, and Aurantium *Zhi Shi* has a more descending direction. If there is constipation, Aurantium *Zhi Shi* is more appropriate.
4. Auratium *Zhi Shi* is used especially when the formula contains purgative and diuretic therapies. It is combined with Citrus *Chen Pi* to strengthen the Middle Burner (*Zhong Jiao*).

Pharmaceutical Ingredients:[1–4]

1. Flavonoids (synephrine, N-methyltyramine, nobiletin, quinoline, narcotine, noradrenaline, tryptamine, tyramine, naringin, tergeretin, lonicerin, poncirin, hesperidin, rhoifolin, naringin, neohesperidin)
2. Skimmianine, α-pinene, β-pinene, myrcene, limonene, camphene, r-terpinene, p-cymene, caryophyllene

Cyperus *Xiang Fu* 香附

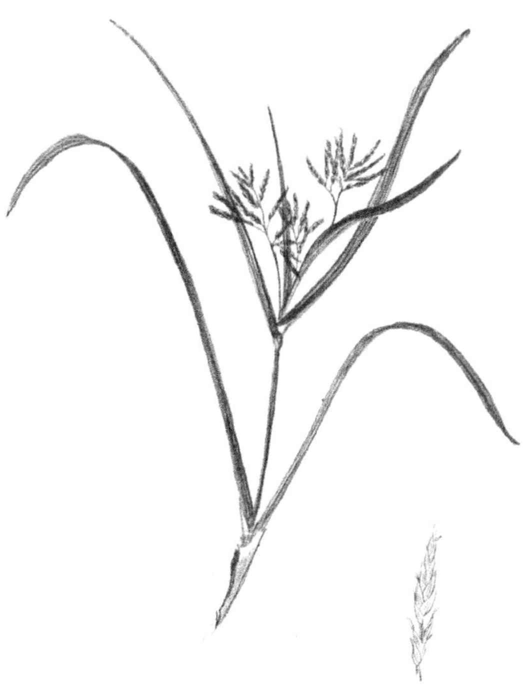

a

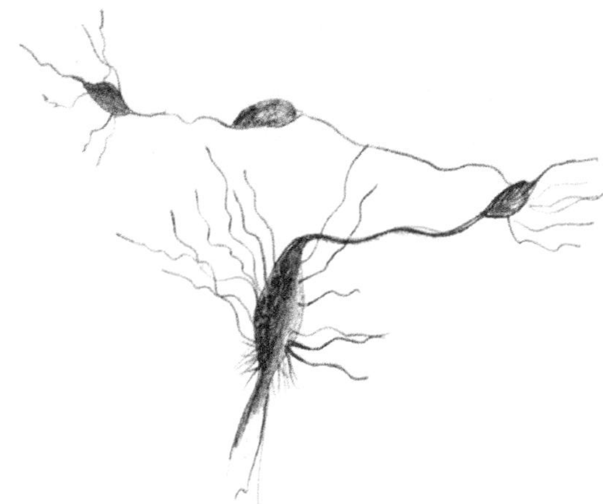

b

Original Reference: *Ming Yi Bie Lu* (*Miscellaneous Records of Famous Physicians*) by *Tao Hong-Jing*, North and South Kingdoms (5th century) 名医别录

Part Used: Root and rhizome

Name:
Pharmaceutical: Cyperi Rotunda, Rhizoma
Botanical: Cyperus Rotundus
Common: Cyperus
Wade-Giles: *Hsiang-Fu*
Translation: Fragrant Attachment

Energy/Taste: Neutral, pungent, bitter, slightly sweet

Channel-Organ: Liver, Triple Burners (*San Jiao*)

Actions:

1. Smooth Liver *Qi* to resolve Stagnation
2. Disperse Stasis to stop pain

Form and Preparation: Powder, decoction, or pill

Dosage:
Horses and Cattle: 30–60 g
Llamas, Alpacas, Goats, and Pigs: 5–15 g
Dogs: 3–8 g
Cats and Rabbits: 0.5–1 g
Birds: 0.3–3 g

Cautions and Contraindications:

1. Caution during pregnancy
2. Caution in *Qi* Deficiency without Stagnation

Side Effects: None known

Clinical Applications:

1. Liver *Qi* Stagnation

Clinical signs: Sensitive in the flank area on palpation, irritability, aggression, abdominal distension and pain, hiccups, belching, nausea, vomiting, acid regurgitation

Combine with: Bupleurum *Chai Hu*, Paeonia *Bai Shao*, Angelica *Dang Gui*, Ligusticum *Chuan Xiong*

Classical herbal formula: *Chai Hu Shu Gan Wan*

2. Cold Stagnation in the Liver Channel

   Clinical signs: Hernia, testicular or scrotal swelling and pain

   Combine with: Foeniculum *Xiao Hui Xiang* and Lindera *Wu Yao*

3. Food Stagnation in the Stomach

   Combine with: Atractylodes *Cang Zhu*

History and Comments:

1. Cyperus *Xiang Fu* is excellent for Liver *Qi* Stagnation. It is also considered the best herb for gynecological conditions.
2. Cyperus *Xiang Fu* is used in combination with either Bupleurum *Chai Hu* or Lindera *Wu Yao*, but not both.
3. *Xiang Fu* has an inhibitory effect on the uterus, similar to but weaker than that of Angelica *Dang Gui*. Its volatile oils contain an estrogenlike substance.

Pharmaceutical Ingredients:[1–4]

1. Essential oils (cyperene β, cyperene β, cyperol, isocyperol, α-cyperone, β-cyperone, β-selinene, patchoulenone, limonene, β-pinene, pcymene, camphene, sugenolacetate, α-rotunol, β-rotunol, cyperolone, cyperotundone)
2. Triterpenoids, flavonoids, alkaloids

Lindera *Wu Yao* 乌药

Original Reference: *Ben Cao Shi Yi* (*Supplement to Materia Medica*) by *Chen Cang-Qi* in 8th century 本草拾遗

Part Used: Root

Name:

Pharmaceutical: Linderae Strychnifoliae, Radix
Botanical: Lindera Strychnifolia
Common: Lindera
Wade-Giles: *Wu-Yao*
Translation: Dark Medicine

Energy/Taste: Warm, pungent

Channel-Organ: Spleen, Stomach, Lung, Kidney

Actions:

1. Regulate *Qi*, stop pain
2. Warm Kidney to dispel Cold

Form and Preparation: Powder, decoction, or pill; Lindera *Wu Yao* is better if decocted only briefly because many constituents are volatile oils.

Dosage:

Horses and Cattle: 30–60 g
Llamas, Alpacas, Goats, and Pigs: 5–15 g
Dogs: 1–6 g
Cats and Rabbits: 0.5–3 g
Birds: 0.3–3 g

Cautions and Contraindications: Caution in Blood Deficiency or Internal Heat Pattern

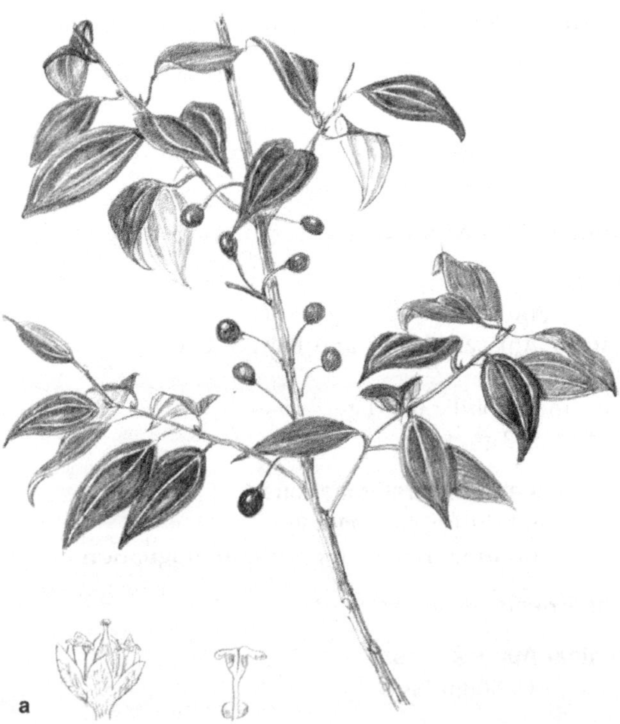

a

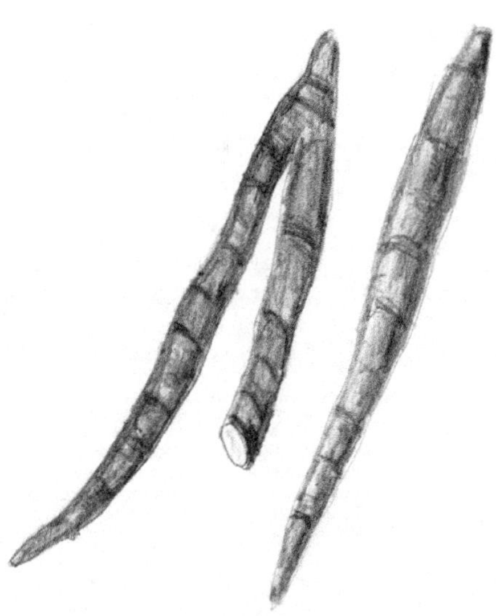

b

Side Effects: None known

Clinical Applications:
1. *Qi* Stagnation with Cold and chest pain
   Clinical signs: Chest pain on palpation
   Combine with: Trichosanthes *Gua Lou*, Curcuma *Yu Jin*, Aurantium *Zhi Ke*
2. *Qi* Stagnation with Cold and colic
   Clinical signs: Abdominal pain, bloating, belching, borborygmus, hiccups
   Combine with: Saussurea *Mu Xiang*
3. *Qi* Stagnation with Cold and testicular pain and hernia
   Clinical signs: Pain on palpation of testicles or hernia
   Combine with: Foeniculum *Xiao Hui Xiang*, Evodia *Wu Zhu Yu*, and Citrus *Qing Pi*
   Classical herbal formula: *Tian Tai Wu Yao San*
4. Urinary leakage due to Kidney *Qi* or *Yang* Deficiency
   Clinical signs: Urinary dribbling or incontinence, frequent urination, lower back pain, pain or weakness in the pelvic limbs
   Combine with: Alpinia *Yi Zhi Ren* and Dioscorea *Shan Yao*
   Classical herbal formula: Suo Quan Wan

History and Comments:
1. Lindera *Wu Yao* is a warming and invigorating herb. It is considered a master herb for the canine species.
2. Lindera *Wu Yao* can be reinforced by combining it with Evodia *Wu Zhu Yu*.
3. Good quality Lindera *Wu Yao* is powdery, lacks black spots, and is light brown.

Pharmaceutical Ingredients:[1–4]
1. Essential oils (lindenenol, lindenene, linderoxide, isolinderoxide, isofuranogermacrene, lindestrene, lindestrenolide, linderalactone, isolinderalactone, linderane, neolinderalactone)
2. Laurolitsine, linderol, linderic acid, sitosterol

Aurantium *Zhi Ke* (*Zhi Qiao*) 枳壳

Original Reference: *Shen Nong Ben Cao Jing* (*Shen Nong's Materia Medica*, 1st century BCE) 神农本草经

Part Used: Fruit

Name:
Pharmaceutical: Citri Aurantii, Fructus
Botanical: Citrus Aurantium; C. Wilsonii; Poncirus Trifoliata
Common: Bitter Orange
Wade-Giles: *Ch'ih-K'e*
Translation: Orange skin

Energy/Taste: Cold, pungent, bitter

Channel-Organ: Spleen, Stomach, Liver

Actions:
1. Move *Qi* and disperse chest *Qi*
2. Widen the Middle Burner to relieve fullness

Form and Preparation: Powder, decoction, or pill

Dosage:
Horses and Cattle: 30–60 g
Llamas, Alpacas, Goats, and Pigs: 3–10 g
Dogs: 1–6 g
Cats and Rabbits: 0.5–1 g
Birds: 0.3–3 g

Cautions and Contraindications: Caution during pregnancy

Side Effects: May cause diarrhea

Citrus *Qing Pi* 青皮

Original Reference: *Ben Cao Gang Mu* (*Materia Medica* Compendium) by *Li Shi-Zhen* in 1590 本草纲目

Part Used: Skin of the green unripe fruit

Name:
Pharmaceutical: Citri Reticulatae Viride, Pericarpium
Botanical: Citrus Reticulata; C. Tangerina; C. Erythrosa
Common: Immature Tangerine Peel
Wade-Giles: *Ch'ih-K'e*
Translation: Green Skin

Energy/Taste: Warm, bitter, pungent

Channel-Organ: Liver, Gallbladder, Stomach

Actions:
1. Soothe Liver *Qi* and break up Stasis
2. Dissipate masses and reduce Stagnation

Form and Preparation: Powder, decoction, or pill

Dosage:
Horses and Cattle: 15–30 g
Llamas, Alpacas, Goats, and Pigs: 3–10 g
Dogs: 1–5 g
Cats and Rabbits: 0.5–1 g
Birds: 0.3–5 g

Cautions and Contraindications: Caution in *Yin* Deficiency with Excess Heat

Side Effects: None known

Aquilaria *Chen Xiang* 沉香

Original Reference: *Ming Yi Bie Lu* (*Miscellaneous Records of Famous Physicians*) by *Tao Hong-Jing*, North and South Kingdoms (5th century) 名医别录

Part Used: The resinous heartwood

Name:
Pharmaceutical: Aquilariae, Lignum
Botanical: Aquilaris Sinensis; A. Agallocha
Common: Aquilaria
Wade-Giles: *Ch'en-Hsiang*
Translation: Sinking Fragrance

Energy/Taste: Warm, pungent, aromatic, bitter

Channel-Organ: Spleen, Liver, Kidney

Actions:
1. Regulate *Qi* to stop pain
2. Descend rebellious *Qi* to stop vomiting
3. Strengthen Kidney to stop asthma

Form and Preparation: Powder, decoction, or pill

Dosage:
Horses and Cattle: 6–16 g
Llamas, Alpacas, Goats, and Pigs: 1–5 g
Dogs: 0.5–2 g
Cats and Rabbits: 0.2–0.5 g
Birds: 0.1–0.5 g

Cautions and Contraindications:
1. Caution in Deficiency of *Yin* with Heat
2. Caution for prolapse of organs due to *Qi* Deficiency

Side Effects: May cause a skin allergy

Areca *Da Fu Pi* 大腹皮

Original Reference: *Kai Bao Ben Cao* (*Materia Medica* of the *Kai Bao Era*) by *Ma Zhi* in 973 开宝本草

Part Used: Husk

Name:
Pharmaceutical: Arecae Catechu, Pericarpium
Botanical: Areca Catechu
Common: Areca Peel
Wade-Giles: *Ta-Fu-P'i*
Translation: Big Abdomen Skin

Energy/Taste: Warm, pungent

Channel-Organ: Spleen, Stomach, Large Intestine

Actions:
1. Invigorate Stomach *Qi* and dispel Food Stagnation
2. Dispel Stagnation of Damp
3. Promote urination and reduce edema

Form and Preparation: Powder, decoction, or pill

Dosage:
Horses and Cattle: 15–45 g
Llamas, Alpacas, Goats, and Pigs: 5–12 g
Dogs: 1–2 g
Cats and Rabbits: 0.5–1 g
Birds: 0.1–1.5 g

Cautions and Contraindications: Caution in *Qi* Deficiency

Side Effects: Overdosing may cause diarrhea.

Kaki *Shi Di* 柿蒂

Original Reference: *Ben Cao Shi Yi* (*Supplement to Materia Medica*) by *Chen Cang-Qi* in 8th century 本草拾遗

Part Used: Whole and broken pieces of calyx

Name:
Pharmaceutical: Diospyri Kaki, Calyx
Botanical: Diospyros Kaki L.
Common: Persimmon Calyx
Wade-Giles: *Shih-Ti*
Translation: Persimmon calyx

Energy/Taste: Neutral, bitter, astringent

Channel-Organ: Lung, Stomach

Actions:
1. Direct *Qi* downward, stop nausea or vomiting
2. Consolidate the intestines to stop diarrhea

Form and Preparation: Powder, decoction, or pill

Dosage:
Horses and Cattle: 60–120 g
Llamas, Alpacas, Goats, and Pigs: 20–60 g
Dogs: 5–10 g
Cats and Rabbits: 1–5 g

Cautions and Contraindications: None known

Side effects: None known

Melia *Chuan Lian Zi* 川楝子

Original Reference: *Shen Nong Ben Cao Jing* (*Shen Nong's Materia Medica*, 1st century BCE) 神农本草经

Part Used: Fruit

Name:
Pharmaceutical: Melia Toosendan, Fructus
Botanical: Melia Toosendan
Common: Sichuan Chinaberry
Wade-Giles: *Ch'uan-Lien-Tzu*
Translation: Sichuan Chinaberry Seed

Energy/Taste: Cold, bitter, sour, slightly toxic

Channel-Organ: Liver, Stomach, Small Intestine, Bladder

Actions:
1. Regulate *Qi* stop pain
2. Dispel Damp, kill parasites

Form and Preparation: Powder, decoction, or pill

Dosage:
Horses and Cattle: 15–45 g
Camels: 40–70 g
Llamas, Alpacas, Goats, and Pigs: 3–10 g
Dogs: 1–5 g

Cautions and Contraindications:
1. Contraindicated for long-term use
2. Do not overdose.
3. Caution in Deficiency and Cold in the Spleen and Stomach

Side Effects: Overdosing leads to diarrhea or nausea.

Rosa *Mei Gui Hua* 玫瑰花

Original Reference: *Ben Cao Gang Mu Shi Yi* (*Omissions for the Materia Medica Compendium*) by *Zhao Xue-min* et al., in 1765. 本草纲目拾遗

Part Used: Flower bud

Name:
Pharmaceutical: Rosae Rugosae, Flos
Botanical: Rosa Rugosa Thunb.
Common: Chinese Rose (previously: Rose)
Wade-Giles: *Mei-Kuei-Hua*
Translation: Rose Flower

Energy/Taste: Warm, sweet, slightly bitter

Channel-Organ: Liver, Spleen

Actions:
1. Regulate *Qi* to resolve Stagnation
2. Removes Blood Stagnation

Form and Preparation: Powder, decoction, or pill

Dosage:
Horses and Cattle: 15–30 g
Llamas, Alpacas, Goats, and Pigs: 3–10 g
Dogs: 1–5 g
Cats and Rabbits: 0.5–1 g
Birds: 0.1–1 g

Cautions and Contraindications: None known

Side Effects: None known

Litchi *Li Zhi He* 荔枝核

Original Reference: *Ben Cao Yan Yi* (*Extension of the Materia Medica*) by *Kou Zong-Shi* in 1116 本草衍义

Part Used: Nut and seed

Name:
Pharmaceutical: Semen Litchi Chinensis
Botanical: Litchi chinensis Sonn.
Common: Leechee nut
Wade-Giles: *Li-Chih-He*
Translation: Leechee nut

Energy/Taste: Warm, sweet, pungent

Channel-Organ: Liver, Stomach

Actions:
1. Move *Qi* and disperse masses
2. Dispel Cold to stop pain in hernias and testicles

Form and Preparation: Powder, decoction, or Food Therapy

Dosage:
Horses and Cattle: 30–60 g
Llamas, Alpacas, Goats, and Pigs: 3–10 g
Dogs: 1–5 g
Cats and Rabbits: 0.5–1 g
Birds: 0.3–3 g

Cautions and Contraindications: None known

Side Effects: None known

Allium *Xie Bai* 薤白

Original Reference: *Shen Nong Ben Cao Jing* (*Shen Nong's Materia Medica*, 1st century BCE) 神农本草经

Part Used: Bulb

Name:
Pharmaceutical: Allii, Bulbus
Botanical: Allium Macrostemon; A. Chinensis; A. Bakeri
Common: Chinese Chive
Wade-Giles: *Hsieh-Pai*
Translation: Chive White

Energy/Taste: Warm, pungent, bitter

Channel-Organ: Lung, Heart, Stomach, Large Intestine

Actions:
1. Invigorate *Yang* and disperse masses
2. Regulate *Qi* and resolve Stagnation

Form and Preparation: Powder, decoction, or Food Therapy

Dosage:
Horses and Cattle: 50–100g
Llamas, Alpacas, Goats, and Pigs: 10–50g

Cautions and Contraindications: Caution in *Qi* Deficiency without Stagnation

Side Effects: None known

Santalum *Tan Xiang* 檀香

Original Reference: *Ming Yi Bie Lu* (*Miscellaneous Records of Famous Physicians*) by *Tao Hong-Jing*, North and South Kingdoms (5th century) 名医别录

Part Used: Heart of Sandalwood

Name:
Pharmaceutical: Santali Albi, Lignum
Botanical: Santatum Album L.
Common: Sandalwood
Wade-Giles: *T'an-Hsiang*
Translation: Sandalwood Fragrance

Energy/Taste: Warm, pungent, aromatic

Channel-Organ: Spleen, Stomach, Lung, Heart

Actions:
1. Regulate *Qi* in Spleen and Stomach, stop colic
2. Dispel Cold and Stagnation in the chest

Form and Preparation: Powder, decoction, or pill

Dosage:
Horses and Cattle: 30–60g
Llamas, Alpacas, Goats, and Pigs: 5–20g
Dogs: 1–5g
Cats and Rabbits: 0.5–1g
Birds: 0.3–3g

Cautions and Contraindications: Caution in *Yin* Deficiency with Heat

Side Effects: None known

Citrus *Fo Shou* 佛手

Original Reference: *Ben Cao Gang Mu* (*Materia Medica Compendium*) by *Li Shi-Zhen* in 1590 本草纲目

Part Used: Ripe fruit

Name:
Pharmaceutical: Citri Sarcodctylis, Fructus
Botanical: Citrus Medica L Var Sarcodactylis (Noot.) Swingle
Common: Finger Citron Fruit
Wade-Giles: *Fo-Shou*
Translation: Buddha Hand

Energy/Taste: Warm, pungent, bitter

Channel-Organ: Liver, Lung, Stomach, Spleen

Actions:
1. Soothe Liver *Qi* to resolve Stagnation
2. Regulate *Qi* to harmonize the Middle Burner
3. Dry Dampness and transform Phlegm

Form and Preparation:
Powder, decoction, or pill

Dosage:
Horses and Cattle: 30–60g
Llamas, Alpacas, Goats, and Pigs: 3–10g
Dogs: 1–5g
Cats and Rabbits: 0.5–1g
Birds: 0.3–3g

Cautions and Contraindications:
1. Caution in *Yin* Deficiency with Heat
2. Caution in *Qi* Deficiency without Stagnation

Side Effects: None known

SUMMARY OF HERBS THAT REGULATE (STAGNANT) *QI*

Table 8.2 summarizes and compares the herbs that Regulate (Stagnant) *Qi*.

REFERENCES

1. Chen JK, Chen TT. Chinese Medical Herbology and Pharmacology. City of Industry, CA: Art of Medicine Press, 2004.
2. Brinker FJ. The Toxicology of Botanical Medicines. Sandy, OR: Eclectic Medical Publications, 2000.
3. Duke JA. Handbook of Medicinal Herbs. New York: Chemical and Rubber Company Press, 2001.
4. Huang KC. The Pharmacology of Chinese Herbs, 2nd Edition. New York: Chemical and Rubber Company Press, 1999.

Table 8.2. Herbs to regulate *Qi*: A quick overview and comparison.

Herbs	Special Actions	Common Characteristics
Herbs to regulate *Qi* in the Spleen and Stomach (GI)		Taste: Aromatic, pungent, bitter Energy: Warm and drying Action: Promote the free flow of *Qi* Indications: Nausea or vomiting due to Stomach *Qi* Rebellion Colic due to GI *Qi* Stagnation Bloat due to GI *Qi* Stagnation Liver *Qi* Stagnation Lung *Qi* Stagnation and cough or asthma *Qi* Stagnation and pain Cautions: Long-term use can damage Stomach *Yin* because of dryness. Use caution in *Qi* Deficiency because they scatter *Qi*. Decoction times are often short (15 min) to preserve aromatic aspect.
Chen Pi	Strengthen Spleen and transform Phlegm	
Ju Hong	Dry up Dampness, stop vomiting and cough	
Ju He	Dissipate mass and relieve testicle pain	
Mu Xiang	Strengthen Spleen and stop diarrhea	
Zhe Shi	Direct *Qi* downward to promote bowel movement	
Zhi Ke	Widen the GI to relieve fullness and bloat	
Da Fu Pi	Promote urination and reduce edema	
Shi Di	Direct *Qi* downward, stop nausea or GI reflux	
Herbs to regulate Liver *Qi*		
Xiang Fu	Disperse stasis to stop pain	
Qing Pi	Break up stasis and dissipate lumps	
Chuan Lian Zi	Dispel Damp, expel parasites, slightly toxic	
Mei Gui Hua	Remove Blood Stagnation	
Li Zhi He	Dispel Cold to stop pain in hernia and testicle	
Fo Shou	Dry up Dampness and transform Phlegm	
Herbs to regulate mixed *Qi* Stagnation		
Wu Yao	Warm Kidney to dispel Coldness, relieve Bi	
Chen Xiang	Descend rebellious *Qi* to stop vomiting and asthma	
Xie Bai	Invigorate *Yang* and disperse Stagnation in chest and abdomen	
Tan Xiang	Dispel Coldness and Stagnation in the chest	

9 Herbs to Relieve Food Stagnation 消食药

Huisheng Xie, Min Su Kim, Cheryl Chrisman

Herbs to relieve Food Stagnation primarily act to promote appetite, improve digestion, and remove accumulated Food (Food Stagnation). The causes of Food Stagnation include Spleen *Qi* Deficiency, excessive consumption of cold or raw food, and too much food and drink.

These herbs are sweet, pungent, and warm. They primarily enter the Spleen and Stomach Channels and organs, where they act to improve appetite, promote digestion and absorption, and relieve Food Stagnation. In general, these herbs are often combined with herbs to invigorate *Qi*; however, they are also combined with other herbs, depending on the disease. A combination of herbs may be used to relieve Food Stagnation including 1) cool bitter herbs for Accumulation of Interior Heat, 2) warming herbs for Cold conditions, 3) aromatic herbs to dispel Damp in turbid Damp conditions, and 4) *Qi* tonic herbs for Spleen *Qi* Deficiency.

Crataegus *Shan Zha* 山楂

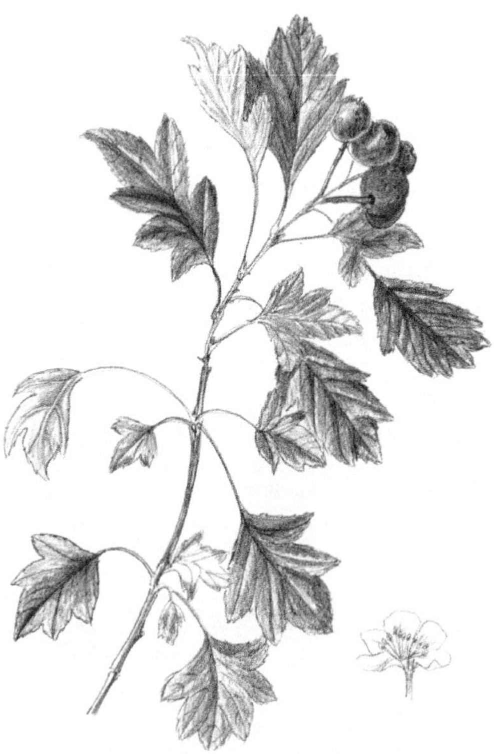

Original Reference: *Tang Ben Cao* (*Tang Materia Medica*) by *Su Jing* et al., *Tang* Dynasty 唐本草

Part Used: Fruit

Name:
Pharmaceutical: Fructus Crataegi, Fructus
Botanical: Crataegus pinnatifida; C. cuneata
Common: Hawthorn Berry
Wade-Giles: *Shan-Cha*
Translation: Mountain Berry

Energy/Taste: Slightly warm, sour, sweet

Channel-Organ: Spleen, Stomach, Liver

Actions:
1. Eliminate Food Stagnation, stop diarrhea
2. Invigorate Blood to disperse Stagnation

Form and Preparation: Powder, decoction, pill, or Food Therapy; stir-frying enhances its actions

Dosage:
Horses and Cattle: 15–45 g
Llamas, Alpacas, Goats, and Pigs: 5–15 g
Dogs: 2–6 g
Cats: 0.5–1.5 g
Birds and Rabbits: 0.5–2 g

Cautions and Contraindications: Caution in acid regurgitation

Side Effects: Overdose and long-term use may increase the gastric acidity and cause constipation.

Clinical Applications:
1. Food Stagnation and retention of Food, especially fats and meat
   Clinical signs: Abdominal distension, colic, retention of food, belching with foul odor, nausea, flatulence, diarrhea

Combine with: Saussurea *Mu Xiang*, Hordeum *Mai Ya*, Massa Fermentata *Shen Qu*, Aurantium *Zhi Ke*
Classical herbal formula: *Bao He Wan*
2. Postpartum abdominal pain due to Blood Stagnation
Combine with: Angelica *Dang Gui*, Ligusticum *Chuan Xiong*, Leonurus *Yi Mu Cao*
3. Chest pain due to Blood Stagnation
Combine with: Salvia *Dan Shen*
4. Hernia and swollen testicles
Combine with: Foeniculum *Xiao Hui Xiang*

History and Comments:
1. During the *Ming* Dynasty (1368–1644 CE), a mother following the advice of a village doctor, fed her skinny, jaundiced child too much meat. The child was unable to digest such big, rich meals, so his abdomen became painful and looked like a very big drum. Seeking relief, this child wandered into the mountains. He was attracted to a wild, red berry on a nearby plant. He picked off a berry and ate it. He loved the sour and sweet taste so much that he then ate many berries until he was full. After returning home, he vomited a large amount of Phlegm. To everyone's surprise, his belly immediately shrunk. With time, he gradually gained weight and his face became a healthy color. The village decided to call this wild mountain berry, *Shan* (Mountain) *Zha* (Berry).
2. Crataegus *Shan Zha* is often combined with Massa Fermentata *Shen Qu* and Hordeum *Mai Ya*. Together these three herbs are referred to as the "3 Immortals."
3. *Shan Zha* is clinically effective for lowering elevated cholesterol and high blood pressure. It is often used as a heart tonic in Western herbal medicine.

Pharmaceutical Ingredients:[1,2]
1. Crataegolic acid, citric acid, succinic acid, chlorogenic acid, caffeic acid, oleanolic acid, ursolic acid, maslinic acid, tartaric acid
2. Flavonoids (quercetin, vitexin, hyperin, amygdalin, quercitin, epicatechin, rutin)
3. Lipase, vitamin B2, vitamin C, pectin, carotene, Na, Fe

Massa Fermentata *Shen Qu* 神曲

Original Reference: *Yao Xing Lun* (*Discussion of Medicinal Properties*) by *Chen Zhou* in the 19th century 药性论

Part Used: Dried fermented mass of wheat flour, bran, Artemisia *Qing Hao*, Armeniaca *Xing Ren*, Xanthium *Cang Er Zi*, Phaseolus *Chi Xiao*, and other herbs

Name:
Pharmaceutical name: Medicata Fermentata, Massa
Common: Medicated Leaven, *shen-chu*
Wade-Giles: *Shen-Chu*
Translation: Divine Fermented Mass

Energy/Taste: Warm, sweet, pungent

Channel-Organ: Spleen, Stomach

Actions:
1. Eliminate Food Stagnation, especially grain or hay retention
2. Strengthen Stomach and harmonize the Middle Burner (*Zhong Jiao*)

Form and Preparation: Powder, decoction, or pill

Dosage:
Horses and Cattle: 20–60 g
Llamas, Alpacas, Goats, and Pigs: 5–15 g
Dogs: 2–8 g
Cats: 0.5–1.5 g
Birds and Rabbits: 0.5–2 g

Cautions and Contraindications: None known

Side Effects: None known

Hordeum *Mai Ya* 麦芽

Original Reference: *Yao Xing Lun* (*Discussion of Medicinal Properties*) by *Chen Zhou* in the 19th century 药性论

Part Used: Germinated seed

Name:
Pharmaceutical: Hordei Vularis Germinatus, Fructus
Botanical: Hordeum vulgare
Common: Sprouted Barley
Wade-Giles: *Mai-Ya*
Translation: Barley Sprout

Energy/Taste: Neutral, sweet

Channel-Organ: Spleen, Stomach, Liver

Actions:
1. Eliminate Food Stagnation and harmonize the Stomach
2. Stop lactation, smooth Liver *Qi*

Form and Preparation: Powder, decoction, pill, or Food Therapy

Dosage:
Horses and Cattle: 15–45 g
Llamas, Alpacas, Goats, and Pigs: 5–15 g
Dogs: 2–8 g
Cats: 0.5–1.5 g
Birds and Rabbits: 0.1–1.5 g

Cautions and Contraindications: Prohibited for use in lactating animals

Side Effects: Overdose or long-term use may damage the Liver.

Oryza *Gu Ya* 谷牙

Original Reference: *Ming Yi Bie Lu* (*Miscellaneous Records of Famous Physicians*) by *Tao Hong-Jing*, North and South Kingdoms (5th century) 名医别录

Part Used: Germinated seed

Name:
Pharmaceutical: Oryzae Sativae Germinatus, Fructus
Botanical: Oryza sativa, L.
Common: Sprouted rice
Wade-Giles: *Ku-ya*
Translation: Rice Sprout

Energy/Taste: Warm, sweet

Channel-Organ: Spleen, Stomach

Actions:
1. Eliminate Food Stagnation and harmonize the Stomach
2. Improve appetite

Form and Preparation: Powder, decoction, pill, or Food Therapy

Dosage:
Horses and Cattle: 15–45 g
Llamas, Alpacas, Goats, and Pigs: 5–15 g
Dogs: 2–6 g
Cats: 0.5–1 g
Birds and Rabbits: 0.5–2 g

Cautions and Contraindications: Contraindicated for lactating animals

Side Effects: Long-term use may injure the Kidneys.

Raphanus *Lai Fu Zi* 莱菔子

Original Reference: *Ri Hua-Zi Ben Cao* (*Materia Medica of Ri Hua-Zi*) by *Ri Hua-Zi* in 713 日华子本草

Part Used: Seed

Name:
Pharmaceutical: Raphani Sativi, Semen
Botanical: Raphanus sativus L.
Common: Radish Seed
Wade-Giles: *Lai-Fu-Tzu*

Energy/Taste: Neutral, pungent, sweet

Channel-Organ: Spleen, Stomach, Lung

Actions:
1. Eliminate Food Stagnation
2. Descend *Qi* and transform Phlegm

Form and Preparation: Powder, decoction, or pill

Dosage:
Horses and Cattle: 20–60 g
Camel: 45–100 g
Llamas, Alpacas, Goats, and Pigs: 5–15 g
Dogs: 2–6 g
Cats: 0.5–1 g
Birds and Rabbits: 0.2–2 g

Cautions and Contraindications:
1. Caution in *Qi* Deficiency
2. May decrease the energetic actions of Ginseng *Ren Shen*

Side Effects: Overdose or long-term use may damage the Liver.

Corneum Gigeria *Ji Nei Jin* 鸡内金

Original Reference: *Shen Nong Ben Cao Jing* (*Shen Nong's Materia Medica*, 1st century BCE) 神农本草经

Part Used: Dried membrane of chicken gizzards

Name:
Pharmaceutical: Gigeriae Galli, Endothelium Corneum
Zoological: Gallus gallus domesticus
Common: Chicken gizzard lining
Wade-Giles: *Chi-Nei-Chin*
Translation: Chicken's Interior Gold

Energy/Taste: Neutral, sweet, salty

Channel-Organ: Spleen, Stomach, Small Intestine, Bladder

Actions:
1. Eliminate Food Stagnation and strengthen Spleen *Qi*
2. Dissolve cystic calculi
3. Secure Essence and stop incontinence

Form and Preparation: Powder, decoction, pill, or Food Therapy

Dosage:
Horses and Cattle: 15–30 g
Llamas, Alpacas, Goats, and Pigs: 3–9 g
Dogs: 2–4 g

Table 9.1. Herbs to relieve Food Stagnation: A quick overview and comparison.

Herbs	Special Actions	Common Characteristics
Shan Zha	Eliminate fat and meat food retention Stop diarrhea, invigorate Blood	Taste: Sweet, pungent Energy: Warm or neutral Channel-Organ: Spleen, Stomach Action: Remove food retention Indication: Food Stagnation
Shen Qu	Eliminate grain food retention Strengthen Stomach	
Mai Ya	Stop lactation, reduce mammary swelling Soothe Liver *Qi*	
Gu Ya	Mildly strengthen Spleen *Qi* Improve appetite	
Lai Fu Zi	Descend *Qi* and transform Phlegm	
Ji Nei Jin	Strengthen Spleen *Qi* Stop urinary leakage, resolve stones	

Cats: 0.5–1 g
Birds and Rabbits: 0.5–1.5 g

Cautions and Contraindications: Caution in *Qi* Deficiency

Side Effects: None known

SUMMARY OF HERBS THAT RELIEVE FOOD STAGNATION

Table 9.1 summarizes and compares the herbs that relieve Food Stagnation.

REFERENCES

1. Chen JK, Chen TT. Chinese Medical Herbology and Pharmacology. City of Industry, CA: Art of Medicine Press, 2004.
2. Bensky D, Clavey S, Stoger E. Chinese Herbal Medicine Materia Medica, 3rd Edition. Seattle, WA: Eastland Press, Inc., 2004.

10 Herbs to Stop Bleeding 止血药

Huisheng Xie, Min Su Kim, Cheryl Chrisman

Herbs to stop bleeding are used to stop many types of hemorrhage. They may be used to treat traumatic bleeding, hematemesis, epistaxis (nosebleed), hemoptysis (coughing up blood), hematochezia (blood in feces), hematuria (blood in urine), uterine bleeding, and bleeding from gastrointestinal ulcers. The energy of these herbs goes to the Blood Level (*Xue* stage). Herbs to stop bleeding are associated with Liver, Heart, and Spleen because the Liver stores Blood, the Heart governs Blood, and the Spleen holds Blood inside the blood vessels. In addition to hemostasis, some of these herbs cool Blood Heat, invigorate the Blood to stop Blood Stasis, warm the Channels, or are astringents.

Bleeding can be caused by systemic Heat, Blood Heat, Liver *Yang* Rising, False Heat due to *Yin* Deficiency, Spleen *Qi* Deficiency, and Spleen *Yang* Deficiency. Bleeding then leads to other secondary conditions, including Blood Stagnation. The herbs to stop bleeding are for symptomatic treatment only. They stop the hemorrhage, but they do not treat the underlying "root" cause of the hemorrhage. Therefore, these herbs should be combined with other herbs to treat the patient's underlying condition. Herbs to stop bleeding are combined with herbs that 1) dispel systemic Heat, 2) cool Blood Heat, 3) subdue the Liver *Yang*, 4) nourish the *Yin*, 5) tonify Spleen *Qi*, 6) tonify *Yang Qi* to prevent collapse, or 7) invigorate Blood.

Sanguisorba *Di Yu* 地榆

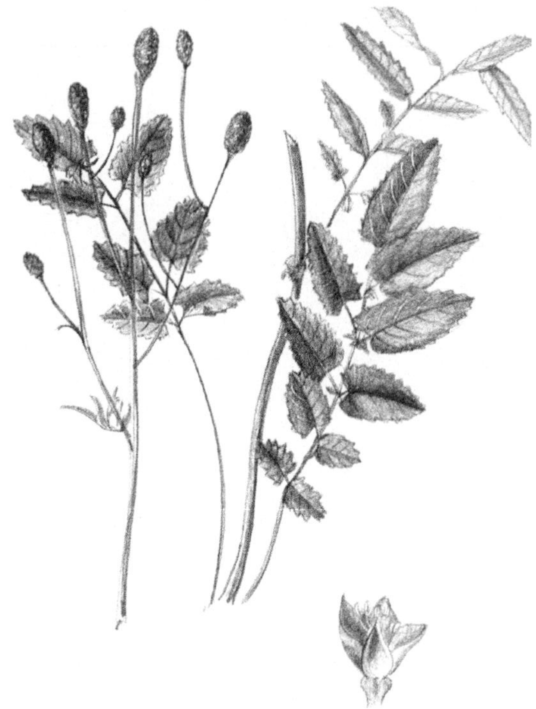

a

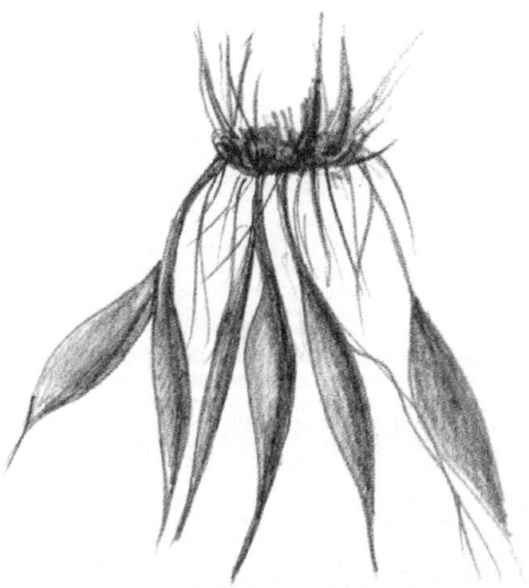

b

Original Reference: *Shen Nong Ben Cao Jing* (*Shen Nong's Materia Medica*, 1st century BCE) 神农本草经

Part Used: Root

Name:
Pharmaceutical: Sanguisorbae Officinalis, Radix
Botanical: Sanguisorba Officinalis
Common: Sanguisorba
Wade-Giles: *Ti-Yu*
Translation: Earth Elm

Energy/Taste: Slightly cold, bitter, sour

Channel-Organ: Liver, Stomach, Large Intestine

Actions:
1. Cool Blood and stop bleeding
2. Relieve toxicity and heal ulcers

Form and Preparation: Powder, decoction, or pill

Dosage:
Horses and Cattle: 15–60 g
Llamas, Alpacas, Goats, and Pigs: 5–12 g
Dogs: 2–5 g
Cats: 0.5–1 g
Birds and Rabbits: 0.5–2 g

Cautions and Contraindications:
1. Do not apply topically to large burns.
2. Caution in patients with uterine bleeding due to Spleen *Qi* Deficiency

Side Effects: None known

Clinical Applications:
1. Bleeding due to Blood Heat
   Clinical signs: Ulcers and bleeding gums, hematochezia, hematuria, hemorrhoids, uterine bleeding
   Combine with: Sophora *Huai Hua*, Scutellaria *Huang Qin* and Rehmannia *Sheng Di Huang*
2. Burns, skin ulcers, eczema, infected and open wounds
   Combine with: Coptis *Huang Lian* or Phellodendron *Huang Bai*
   Apply topically

History and Comments:
1. Sanguisorba *Di Yu* is used for bleeding disorders due to Blood Heat, usually in the Lower Burner (*Xia Jiao*). The herb is often stir-fried until brown or charred to enhance its astringent and hemostatic effects.
2. Good quality Sanguisorba *Di Yu* is coarse, hard, and reddish in color.
3. Sanguisorba *Di Yu* has strong antibiotic effects and can heal second- and third-degree burns.

Pharmaceutical Ingredients:[1–4]
1. Tannin, triterpenoidal saponin, pomolic acid, arabinose, glucose
2. Ziyuglycoside I, ziyuglycoside II, sanguiin, sanguisorbin, sanguisorbigenin tannins, saurissimoside R1, quercetin, kaempferol

Notoginseng *Tian Qi* or *San Qi* 田七 or 三七

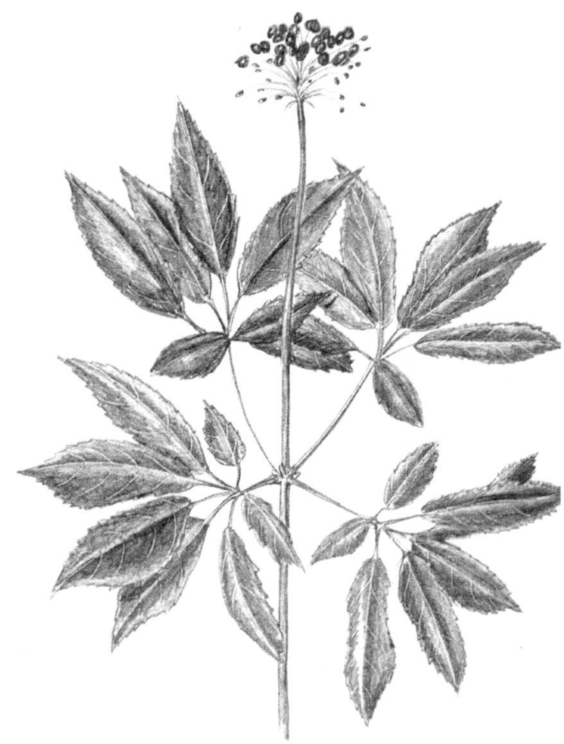

a

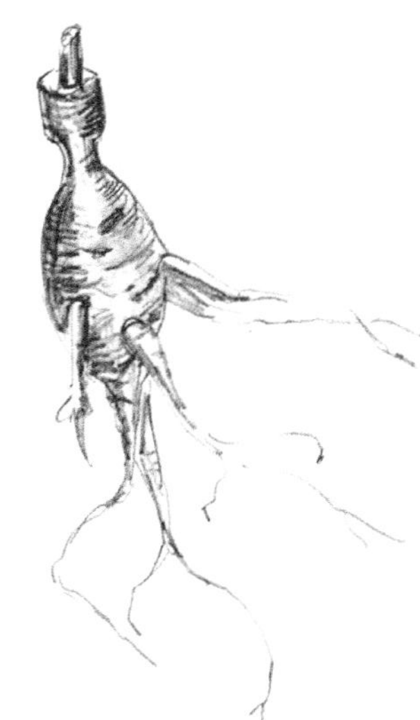

b

Original Reference: *Ben Cao Gang Mu* (*Materia Medica Compendium*) by *Li Shi-Zhen* in 1590 本草纲目

Part Used: Root

Name:
Pharmaceutical: Notoginseng, Radix
Botanical: Panax Pseudoginseng; Panax Notoginseng
Common: Raw Pseudoginseng, *San Qi*
Wade-Giles: *San Ch'i* or *Tien-Ch'i*
Translation: "Field Seven"
Alternative: *San Qi* (Three Seven)

Energy/Taste: Warm, sweet, slightly bitter

Channel-Organ: Liver, Stomach, Large Intestine

Actions:
Stop Bleeding and relieve Stagnation
Invigorate Blood, stop pain, and reduce swelling

Form and Preparation: Powder, decoction, or pill

Dosage:
Horses and Cattle: 10–30 g
Camels: 15–45 g
Llamas, Alpacas, Goats, and Pigs: 3–6 g
Dogs: 1–3 g
Cats: 0.5–1 g
Birds and Rabbits: 0.5–2 g

Cautions and Contraindications:
1. Caution during pregnancy
2. Caution with *Yin* Deficiency (in *Yin*-Deficient patients; always combine with *Yin* tonic herbs)

Side Effects: None known

Clinical Applications:
1. Internal or *External* hemorrhaging
   Clinical signs: Traumatic bleeding, hematemesis, epistaxis, hemoptysis, hematochezia, hematuria, menorrhagia, uterine bleeding, or bleeding due to ulcers
   Use alone or combine with: Hominis *Xue Yu Tan*
2. Hemorrhage and swelling due to trauma
   Single herb: Apply externally or take internally
   Combine with: (Roasted) Draconis *Duan Long Gu* and Rhus *Wu Bei Zi* for topical use
3. Chest pain due to Heart Blood Stagnation or congestive heart failure
   Combine with: Salvia *Dan Shen*

History and Comments:
1. Notoginseng *Tian Qi* is a highly valuable hemostasis herb. The herb will stop bleeding, while simultaneously dispersing blood clots.
2. Notoginseng *Tian Qi* is usually taken in its raw form. It may be used in patients undergoing surgery to prevent or treat postoperative hemorrhage.
3. Steamed or stir-fried Notoginseng *Tian Qi* acts as a *Blood* tonic following traumatic (or surgical) blood loss.
4. Notoginseng *Tian Qi*, or *San Qi*, refers to its characteristic seven leaves (*Qi*). Good quality Notoginseng is large, solid, and heavy with a thin cortex and dark color.
5. Notoginseng *Tian Qi* is the primary hemostatic herb in the patented medicine, *Yunnan Bai Yao*.

Pharmaceutical Ingredients:[1–4]
1. Triterpenoid, dencichine
2. Sapnin (notoginsenoside R1, R2, R3, R4, R6, Rh2panaxosides Rb1, Rb2, Rc, Rd, Re, Rf, Rg1, Rg2, Rh, D1, D2, E2, 20-glucoginsenoside Rf, gypenoside XVII)
3. Sapogenin (panaxadiol, panaxatriol)
4. Essential oils (α-copaene, β-cubebene, caryophyllene, guaiene, α-cedrene)

Bletilla *Bai Ji* 白及

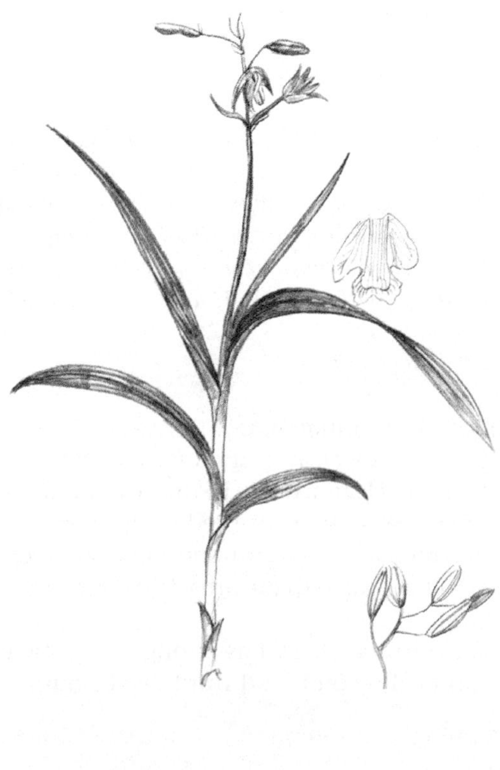

a

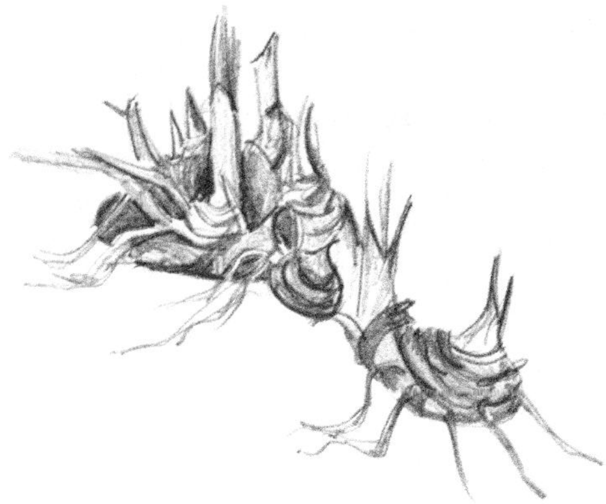

b

Original Reference: *Shen Nong Ben Cao Jing* (*Shen Nong's Materia Medica*, 1st century BCE) 神农本草经

Part Used: Rhizome

Name:
Pharmaceutical: Bletillae Striatae, Rhizoma
Botanical: Bletilla Striata (Thunb.) Reichb.
Common: Bletilla
Wade-Giles: *Pai-Chi*
Translation: White Arrival

Energy/Taste: Slightly cold, bitter, sweet, astringent

Channel-Organ: Lung, Stomach, Liver

Actions:
1. Stop bleeding with astringent actions
2. Reduce swelling and promote healing

Form and Preparation: Powder, decoction, or pill

Dosage:
Horses and Cattle: 20–60 g
Camels: 30–80 g
Llamas, Alpacas, Goats, and Pigs: 5–12 g
Dogs: 2–5 g
Cats: 0.5–2 g
Birds and Rabbits: 0.5–1.5 g

Cautions and Contraindications: Incompatible with Aconite *Wu Tou* and Aconite *Fu Zi*

Side Effects: None known

Clinical Applications:
1. Hemorrhage
   Clinical signs: Bleeding from the Lung, Stomach, or a traumatic injury
   Combine with: Asinum Gelatinum *E Jiao*, Nelumbo *Ou Jie*, or Stemona *Bai Bu*
2. Boils, carbuncles, and swellings
   Clinical signs: Affected areas exhibit redness, swelling, heat, and pain
   Combine with: Lonicera *Jin Yin Hua*, Fritillaria *Chuan Bei Mu*, Trichosanthes *Tian Hua Fen*, Gleditsia *Zao Jiao Ci*
   Classical herbal formula: *Nei Xiao San*
3. Chronic nonhealing ulcers
   Single use: Apply powder directly to wounds
4. Chapped skin on feet and cracked paws or hooves
   Combine with: sesame oil for *External* use

History and Comments: Good quality Bletilla *Bai Ji* is thick, solid, and without any particular color

Pharmaceutical Ingredients:[1–4]
Starch, glucose, acacia gum, tragacanth
Bletilla mannan, bletilla-gluco mannan, physcion, batatasin III

Artemisia *Ai Ye* 艾叶

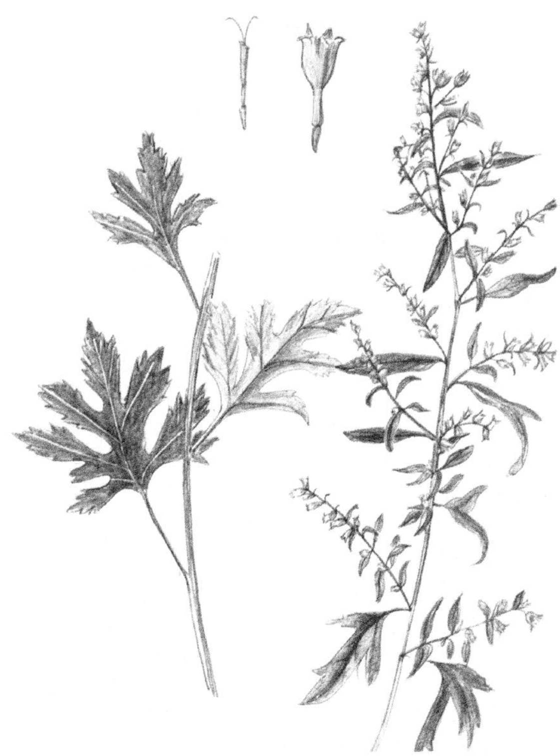

Original Reference: *Ming Yi Bie Lu* (*Miscellaneous Records of Famous Physicians*) by *Tao Hong-Jing*, North and South Kingdoms (5th century) 名医别录

Part Used: Leaf

Name:
Pharmaceutical: Artemisia Argyi, Folium
Botanical: Artemisia Argyi; A. Vulgaris
Common: Mugwort, Artemisia
Wade-Giles: *Ai-Yeh*
Translation: Artemisia Leaf

Energy/Taste: Warm, pungent, bitter

Channel-Organ: Liver, Spleen, Kidney

Actions:
1. Warm the Channels and stop bleeding
2. Dispel Cold and stop pain
3. Calm the fetus and warm the womb

Form and Preparation: Powder, decoction, or pill for oral use; Moxibustion for *External* use

Dosage:
Horses and Cattle: 15–45 g
Camels: 30–60 g
Llamas, Alpacas, Goats, and Pigs: 5–12 g
Dogs: 1–3 g
Cats: 0.5–1 g
Birds and Rabbits: 0.5–1.5 g

Cautions and Contraindications: Caution during pregnancy

Side Effects: Overdosing may cause nausea.

Clinical Applications:
1. Uterine bleeding due to *Yang Qi* Deficiency, parturition, and abortion
   Combine with: Asinum Gelatinum *E Jiao*
2. Coldness due to *Yang* Deficiency in the Lower Burner (*Xia Jiao*)
   Clinical signs: Colic, irregular estrous cycle, infertility, risk of miscarriage, diarrhea
   Combine with: Angelica *Dang Gui*, Cyperus *Xiang Fu*, Ligusticum *Chuan Xiong*, and Lindera *Wu Yao*
3. Fungal infections and warts
   Use alone: apply topically
4. Skin lesions due to Damp/Cold with itching
   Combine with: Kochia *Di Fu Zi*

History and Comments:
1. Good quality Artemisia *Ai Ye* is gray-white in color, aromatic, and has a thick, hairy texture. It disperses the Lung, transforms Phlegm, and benefits asthma.
2. Artemisia *Ai Ye* is often used for moxibustion and it warms the Channels and promotes *Qi* and Blood circulation.

Pharmaceutical Ingredients:[1–4]
1. Essential oils (D-α-phellandrene, α-cadinene, 1,8-cineole, camphene, trans-carveol, cineole, limonene, α-thujone, β-pinene, α-terpineneol, borneol acetate, elemol, isoborneol, carvone)
2. Adenine; choline; vitamins A, B, C, D; amylase; thujone; cadinene

Cephalanoplos *Xiao Ji* 小蓟

Original Reference: *Ming Yi Bie Lu* (*Miscellaneous Records of Famous Physicians*) by *Tao Hong-Jing*, North and South Kingdoms (5th century) 名医别录

Part Used: Aboveground part of the plant and the root

Name:
Pharmaceutical: Cephanoplos Setosum, Herba Seu Radix
Botanical: Cephanoplos setosum Kitarn
Common: Cephalanoplos
Wade-Giles: *Shiao-Chi*
Translation: Small Thistle

Energy/Taste: Cool, sweet, bitter

Channel-Organ: Liver, Heart

Actions:
1. Cool Blood and stop bleeding
2. Reduce swelling and clear Heat toxin
3. Promote urination and clear *Lin* Syndrome

Form and Preparation: Powder, decoction, or pill

Dosage:
Horses and Cattle: 30–90 g
Llamas, Alpacas, Goats, and Pigs: 10–40 g
Dogs: 2–10 g
Cats: 0.5–2 g
Birds and Rabbits: 0.5–3 g

Cautions and Contraindications: Caution during pregnancy or with Spleen *Qi* Deficiency. Do not combine with Glycerrhiza *Gan Cao*.

Side Effects: May cause diarrhea

Cirsium *Da Ji* 大蓟

Original Reference: *Ming Yi Bie Lu* (*Miscellaneous Records of Famous Physicians*) by *Tao Hong-Jing*, North and South Kingdoms (5th century) 名医别录

Part Used: Aboveground part of the plant and the root

Name:
Pharmaceutical: Herba Cirsii Japonici, Herba Seu Radix
Botanical: Cirsium Japonica
Common: Japanese Thistle
Wade-Giles: *Ta-Chi*
Translation: Big Thistle

Energy/Taste: Cool, sweet, bitter

Channel-Organ: Spleen, Liver, Heart

Actions:
1. Cool Blood and stop bleeding
2. Reduce swelling and resolve Stagnation
3. Promote healing and generate new tissue at wound sites

Form and Preparation: Powder, decoction, or pill

Dosage:
Horses and Cattle: 30–60 g
Llamas, Alpacas, Goats, and Pigs: 5–20 g
Dogs: 2–5 g
Cats: 0.5–1 g
Birds and Rabbits: 0.5–1.5 g

Cautions and Contraindications:
1. Caution during pregnancy or with Spleen *Qi* Deficiency
2. Do not combine with Glycyrrhiza *Gan Cao*.

Side Effects: May cause diarrhea

Sophora *Huai Hua* 槐花

Original Reference: *Ri Hua-Zi Ben Cao* (*Materia Medica of Ri Hua-Zi*) by *Ri Hua-Zi* in 713 CE 日华子本草

Part Used: Flower and flower bud

Name:
Pharmaceutical: Sophorae Japonicae, Flos
Botanical: Sophora Japonica
Common: Scholar Tree
Wade-Giles: *Huai-Hua*
Translation: Sophora Flower

Energy/Taste: Cold, bitter

Channel-Organ: Liver, Large Intestine

Actions:
1. Cool Blood and stop bleeding
2. Cool Liver and clear Fire

Form and Preparation: Powder, decoction, or pill

Dosage:
Horses and Cattle: 20–45 g
Camels: 40–80 g
Llamas, Alpacas, Goats, and Pigs: 5–15 g
Dogs: 2–8 g
Cats: 0.5–1 g
Birds and Rabbits: 0.5–1.5 g

Cautions and Contraindications: Caution in patients with False Heat due to *Yin* Deficiency or Spleen *Qi* Deficiency

Side Effects: None known

Biota *Ce Bai Ye* 侧柏叶

Original Reference: *Ming Yi Bie Lu* (*Miscellaneous Records of Famous Physicians*) by *Tao Hong-Jing*, North and South Kingdoms (5th century) 名医别录

Part Used: Leafy twig tops

Name:
Pharmaceutical: Biotae Orientalis, Folium
Botanical: Biota Orientalis
Common: Thuja Leaf
Wade-Giles: *Ts'e Pai Yeh*
Translation: Flat Fir Leaves

Energy/Taste: Slightly cold, bitter, astringent

Channel-Organ: Lung, Liver, Large Intestine

Actions:
1. Cool Blood and stop bleeding
2. Transform Phlegm to stop coughing
3. Promote hair growth and darken the hair

Form and Preparation: Powder, decoction, or pill

Dosage:
Horses and Cattle: 15–60 g
Llamas, Alpacas, Goats, and Pigs: 5–12 g
Dogs: 2–5 g
Cats: 0.5–1 g
Birds and Rabbits: 0.2–2 g

Cautions and Contraindications: Caution with *Yang* Deficiency

Side Effects: A large dose or long-term ingestion may cause dizziness, nausea, and vomiting.

Imperata *Bai Mao Gen* 白茅根

Original Reference: *Shen Nong Ben Cao Jing* (*Shen Nong's Materia Medica*, 1st century BCE) 神农本草经

Part Used: Rhizome

Name:
Pharmaceutical: Imperatae Cyclindricae, Rhizoma
Botanical: Imperata Cyclindrica
Common: Imperata rhizome
Wade-Giles: *Pai-Mao-Ken*
Translation: White Grass Root

Energy/Taste: Cold, sweet

Channel-Organ: Lung, Stomach, Bladder, Small Intestine

Actions:
1. Cool Blood and stop bleeding
2. Clear Heat to promote urination
3. Clear Heat from the Stomach and Lung

Form and Preparation: Powder, decoction, or pill

Dosage:
Horses and Cattle: 20–45 g
Llamas, Alpacas, Goats, and Pigs: 5–10 g
Dogs: 2–5 g
Cats: 0.5–1 g
Birds and Rabbits: 0.5–1.5 g

Cautions and Contraindications: Caution during pregnancy if there is a history of spontaneous abortion

Side Effects: Overdosing may cause diarrhea.

Rubia *Qian Cao* 茜草

Original Reference: *Shen Nong Ben Cao Jing* (*Shen Nong*'s *Materia Medica*, 1st century BCE) 神农本草经

Part Used: Root

Name:
Pharmaceutical: Rubiae Cordifoliae, Radix
Botanical: Rubia Cordifolia
Common: Madder
Wade-Giles: *Ch'ien-Ts'ao*
Translation: Red Plant
Alternative: *Qian Cao Gen* (Red Plant Root)

Energy/Taste: Cold, bitter

Channel-Organ: Liver

Actions:
1. Cool Blood and stop bleeding
2. Invigorate Blood and disperse Stagnation from traumatic injuries

Form and Preparation: Powder, decoction, or pill

Dosage:
Horses and Cattle: 30–60 g
Llamas, Alpacas, Goats, and Pigs: 5–20 g
Dogs: 2–5 g
Cats: 0.5–1 g
Birds and Rabbits: 0.5–1.5 g

Cautions and Contraindications: Caution during pregnancy or with Cold due to Spleen *Yang* Deficiency

Side Effects: None known

Typha *Pu Huang* 蒲黄

Original Reference: *Shen Nong Ben Cao Jing* (*Shen Nong*'s *Materia Medica*, 1st century BCE) 神农本草经

Part Used: Pollen

Name:
Pharmaceutical: Typha, Pollen
Botanical: Typha Orientalis; T. Angustifolia; T. Latifolia
Common: Cats-Tail Bullrush Pollen
Wade-Giles: *P'u-Huang*
Translation: Typha Yellow

Energy/Taste: Neutral, sweet

Channel-Organ: Liver, Heart, Spleen, Pericardium

Actions:
1. Stop bleeding, promote urination
2. Disperse Stagnation and stop pain

Form and Preparation: Powder, decoction, or pill

Dosage:
Horses and Cattle: 15–45 g
Camels: 30–60 g
Llamas, Alpacas, Goats, and Pigs: 5–10 g
Dogs: 2–5 g
Cats: 0.5–1 g
Birds and Rabbits: 0.5–1.5 g

Cautions and Contraindications: Caution during pregnancy

Side Effects: None known

Dalbergia *Jiang Xiang* 降香

Original Reference: *Ben Cao Gang Mu* (*Materia Medica Compendium*) by *Li Shi-Zhen* in 1590 CE 本草纲目

Part Used: Wood

Pharmaceutical: Dalergiae Odoriferae, Lignum
Botanical: Dalbergia odorifera T. Chen

Common: Dalbergia Wood
Wade-Giles: *Chiang-Hsiang*
Translation: Sinking Fragrance

Energy/Taste: Warm, pungent

Channel-Organ: Heart, Liver

Actions:
1. Invigorate Blood and remove Stagnation
2. Stop bleeding and pain
3. Conduct *Qi* downward and stop vomiting

Form and Preparation: Decoction, powder, or topical application

Dosage:
Horses and Cattle: 10–30 g
Llamas, Alpacas, Goats, and Pigs: 3–9 g
Dogs: 1–3 g

Cautions and Contraindications: None known

Side Effects: None known

Agrimony *Xian He Cao* 仙鶴草
Original Reference: *Shen Nong Ben Cao Jing* (*Shen Nong's Materia Medica*, 1st century BCE) 神农本草经

Part Used: Whole plant

Name:
Pharmaceutical: Agrimoniae Pilosae, Herba
Botanical: Agrimonia Pilosia
Common: Agrimony
Wade-Giles: *Hsien-He-Ts'ao*
Translation: Immortal Crane Herb

Energy/Taste: Neutral, bitter, astringent

Channel-Organ: Lung, Liver, Spleen

Actions:
1. Stop Bleeding with astringent actions
2. Relieve dysentery

Form and Preparation: Powder, decoction, or pill

Dosage:
Horses and Cattle: 15–60 g
Camels: 30–100 g
Llamas, Alpacas, Goats, and Pigs: 5–15 g
Dogs: 2–5 g
Cats: 0.5–2 g
Birds and Rabbits: 0.1–1.5 g

Cautions and Contraindications: Caution in patients with Excess Fire

Side Effects: None known

Nelumbo (Lotus) *Ou Jie* 藕节
Original Reference: *Yao Xing Lun* (*Discussion of Medicinal Properties*) by *Chen Zhou* in 19th century 药性论

Part Used: Node of the rhizome

Name:
Pharmaceutical: Nelumbinis Nuciferae Rhizomatis, Nodus
Botanical: Nelumbo Nucifera Gaertn
Common: Lotus Node
Wade-Giles: *Ou-Chieh*
Translation: Lotus Node

Energy/Taste: Neutral, sweet, astringent

Channel-Organ: Liver, Lung, Stomach

Actions:
1. Stop Bleeding with astringent actions
2. Resolve Stagnation

Form and Preparation: Powder, decoction, or Food Therapy

Dosage:
Horses and Cattle: 30–90 g
Llamas, Alpacas, Goats, and Pigs: 9–30 g
Dogs: 2–8 g
Cats: 0.5–1 g
Birds and Rabbits: 0.5–3 g

Cautions and Contraindications: None known

Side Effects: None known

Trachycarpus *Zong Lu* 棕榈
Original Reference: *Ben Cao Shi Yi* (*Supplement to Materia Medica*) by *Chen Cang-Qi* in 8th century 本草拾遗

Part Used: Stipule fiber

Name:
Pharmaceutical: Fibra Stipulae Trachycarpi
Botanical: Trachycarpus fortunei Wendl
Common: Trachycarpus stiple fiber
Wade-Giles: *Tsung-Lu*
Translation: Palm Stipule

Energy/Taste: Neutral, bitter, astringent

Channel-Organ: Liver, Lung, Large Intestine

Actions:
1. Stop bleeding with astringent actions
2. Stop diarrhea and uterine discharge

Form and Preparation: Powder, decoction, or pill

Dosage:
Horses and Cattle: 15–45 g
Camels: 20–60 g
Llamas, Alpacas, Goats, and Pigs: 5–15 g
Dogs: 2–5 g
Cats: 0.5–1 g
Birds and Rabbits: 0.5–1.5 g

Cautions and Contraindications: Caution in patients suffering from bleeding with Stagnation

Side Effects: None known

Hominis *Xue Yu Tan* 血余炭

Original Reference: *Shen Nong Ben Cao Jing* (*Shen Nong's Materia Medica*, 1st century BCE) 神农本草经

Part Used: Charred human hair

Name:
Pharmaceutical: Crinis Carbonisatus Hominis
Zoological: Homo sapiens L.
Common: Charred human hair
Wade-Giles: *Hsueh-Chieh*
Translation: Blood Residue Char

Energy/Taste: Neutral, bitter

Channel-Organ: Liver, Stomach

Actions:
1. Stop bleeding with astringent actions
2. Promote urination to stop dribbling

Form and Preparation: Powder, decoction, or pill

Dosage:
Horses and Cattle: 15–30 g
Camels: 25–50 g
Llamas, Alpacas, Goats, and Pigs: 5–12 g
Dogs: 2–5 g
Cats: 0.5–1 g
Birds and Rabbits: 0.5–1.5 g

Cautions and Contraindications: None known

Side Effects: None known

Terra Flava *Fu Long Gan* 伏龙肝 (灶心土)

Original Reference: *Ming Yi Bie Lu* (*Miscellaneous Records of Famous Physicians*) by *Tao Hong-Jing*, North and South Kingdoms (5th century) 名医别录

Part Used: Ignited yellow earth

Name:
Pharmaceutical: Terra Flava Usta
Common: Furnace Soil; Ignited Yellow Earth
Wade-Giles: *Fu-Lung-Ken*
Translation: Hidden Dragon Liver
Alternative: *Zao Xin Tu* (Furnace soil)

Energy/Taste: Warm, pungent

Channel-Organ: Spleen, Stomach

Actions:
1. Warm the Middle Burner (*Zhong Jiao*) and stop bleeding
2. Stop vomiting and diarrhea

Form and Preparation: Powder, decoction, or pill

Dosage:
Horses and Cattle: 100–240 g
Llamas, Alpacas, Goats, and Pigs: 10–60 g
Dogs: 2–10 g
Cats: 0.5–3 g
Birds and Rabbits: 0.5–5 g

Cautions and Contraindications: None known

Side Effects: None known

SUMMARY OF HERBS THAT STOP BLEEDING

Table 10.1 summarizes and compares the herbs that stop Bleeding.

REFERENCES

1. Chen JK, Chen TT. Chinese Medical Herbology and Pharmacology. City of Industry, CA: Art of Medicine Press, 2004.
2. Brinker FJ. The Toxicology of Botanical Medicines. Sandy, OR: Eclectic Medical Publications, 2000.
3. Duke JA. Handbook of Medicinal Herbs. New York: Chemical and Rubber Company Press, 2001.
4. Huang KC. The Pharmacology of Chinese Herbs, 2nd Edition. New York: Chemical and Rubber Company Press, 1999.

Table 10.1. Herbs to stop Bleeding: A quick overview and comparison.

Herbs	Special Actions	Common Characteristics
Herbs to cool Blood and stop Bleeding		Taste: Sweet or bitter
Di Yu	Relieve Heat toxin and heal ulcers	Energy: Cool or cold
Xiao Ji	Promote urination Clear Heat Lin and Bleeding Lin syndromes	Action: Cool Blood and stop Bleeding
Da Ji	Reduce swelling and resolve Stagnation Promote healing and generate new flesh at sores	Indication: Hemorrhage due to Excess Heat or Blood Heat
Huai Hua	Clear Large Intestine Damp-Heat for any bleeding of anus and colon; clear Liver Fire to brighten eyes	Cautions: May consume *Yang Qi*
Ce Bai Ye	Transform Phlegm to stop cough Promote hair growth and blacken hair	
Bai Mao Gen	Clear Heat to promote urination Clear Stomach Heat to stop bleeding gums	
Herbs to resolve Stagnation and stop Bleeding		Taste: Invigorating
Tian Qi	Warm, very potent Stop pain, reduce swelling	Action: Move Blood, resolve Stagnation and stop bleeding
Qian Cao	Cold, Cool Blood, and clear Heat Invigorate Blood for traumatic injuries	Indication: Hemorrhage with secondary Stagnation
Pu Huang	Neutral Stop pain and promote urination	Cautions: Caution with Stagnation
Jiang Xiang	Warm, conduct *Qi* downward, and stop vomiting	
Herbs to stop Bleeding with astringent actions		Taste: Astringent
Bai Ji	Cold; Reduce Swelling and promote healing	Action: Astringently stop bleeding
Xian He Cao	Neutral; relieve Dysentery	Indication: Any hemorrhage
Ou Jie	Neutral; resolve Stagnation	Cautions: in pregnancy
Zong Lu	Neutral; stop diarrhea and uterine discharge	
Xue Yu Tan	Neutral; promote urination to stop dribbling	
Herbs to warm Channels and stop Bleeding		Energy: Warm
Ai Ye	Dispel Cold and stop pain Calm fetus and warm the womb	Indication: Hemorrhage due to Spleen *Qi* Deficiency or *Yang* Deficiency
Fu Long Gan	Warm the Middle Jiao and stop bleeding Stop vomiting and diarrhea	Cautions: Caution in Excess Heat

11 Herbs to Invigorate Blood and Break Blood Stasis 活血化瘀药

Huisheng Xie, Vanessa Preast, Min Su Kim

According to Traditional Chinese Veterinary Medicine (TCVM), pain arises due to *Qi* Stagnation, Blood Stagnation, or both. This principle is based on ancient TCVM maxims stating, "where there is pain, there must be Stagnation" and "where there is free flow (of *Qi* and/or Blood), there must be no pain." Stagnation is essentially the result when *Qi* or Blood does not flow freely. Blood Stagnation in particular occurs when the Blood flow slows down, becomes blocked, or is otherwise static.

TCVM practitioners, working from this understanding that pain is caused by Stagnation, realized that removing Stagnation could resolve the pain. For this reason, effective pain relief often involves using herbs that encourage *Qi* and Blood flow. The herbs to regulate *Qi*, as discussed in Chapter 8, are primarily used to treat *Qi* Stagnation, and the herbs discussed in this chapter primarily treat Blood Stagnation or Blood Stasis. Blood Stagnation is associated with bruising, swelling, and pain; Blood Stasis is associated with larger, more solid masses (Table 11.1).

Herbs to invigorate Blood and break Blood Stasis are mostly pungent and fragrant herbs that associate with the Heart and Liver Meridians. These herbs harmonize blood vessels, promote Blood circulation, resolve Blood Stagnation, reduce swelling, and stop pain. Depending on their strength category, the herbs are used for different conditions. "Blood-invigorators" are the milder Blood-moving herbs often used for Blood Stagnation. "Stasis-breakers" are the stronger Blood-moving herbs used to treat Blood Stasis.

Blood Stagnation or Stasis can be caused by Cold, *Qi* Stagnation, trauma or surgery, Heat accumulation, Wind-Damp invasion, or any chronic illness. Regarding the last cause, an ancient TCVM maxim states, "Any long-term disease must have Blood Stagnation."

Herbs to invigorate Blood and break Blood Stasis are often combined with other herbs in order to treat the underlying causes of disease. For example, these herbs may be combined with 1) herbs to warm Interior and dispel Cold, 2) herbs to invigorate *Qi*, 3) herbs to clear Heat and cool Blood, and 4) herbs to dispel Wind-Damp. Generally, *Qi*-invigorating herbs accompany Blood-invigorating herbs within formulas because the *Qi* is the force that causes Blood to circulate through the whole body. Herbs to invigorate Blood and break Stasis should be used cautiously for a weak Spleen or Stomach because they sedate the Stomach and decrease the appetite; In addition, these herbs should be used cautiously during pregnancy.

Table 11.1. Comparison between Blood Stagnation and Blood Stasis.

Patterns	Clinical Signs	Examples of Herbs
Blood Stagnation	Pain due to lack of flow of *Qi* and Blood Location of pain is fixed Visible bruise Deep, sharp, stabbing pain Common locations: Sites due to trauma or surgery to chest, including Heart and Lung, Spine and disc, Abdomen, Liver, Spleen, Uterus, Large Intestine	Ligusticum *Chuan Xiong* Corydalis *Yan Hu Suo*
Blood Stasis	Tumors and swollen masses of internal organs (palpable but mobile) 1) Spleen 2) Liver Fixed tumors (hard, palpable, immobile) 1) Skin tumors and cancer 2) Lymphoma 3) Osteosarcoma 4) Fibroid cysts in uterus or ovaries 5) Other various cancers	Sparganium *San Leng* Zedoaria *E Zhu*

Ligusticum *Chuan Xiong* 川芎

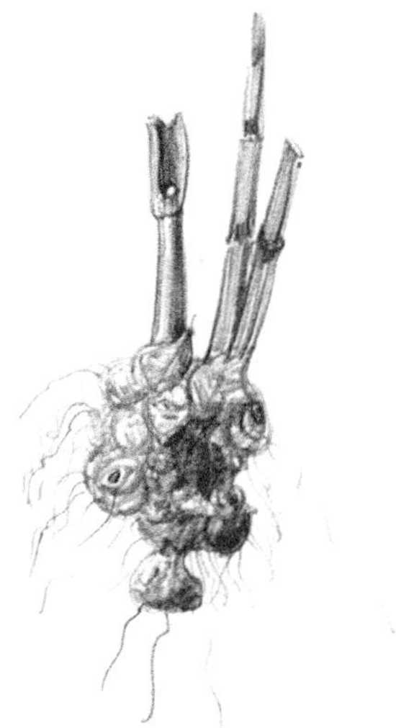

Original Reference: *Shen Nong Ben Cao Jing* (*Shen Nong*'s *Materia Medica*, 1st century BCE) 神农本草经

Part Used: Rhizome

Name:
Pharmaceutical: Ligustici Chuanxiong, Rhizoma
Botanical: Ligusticum wallichi
Common: Ligusticum
Wade-Giles: *Ch'uan-Hsiung*
Translation: Sichuan Ligusticum

Energy/Taste: Warm, pungent

Channel-Organ: Liver, Gallbladder, Pericardium

Actions:
1. Invigorate Blood and move *Qi*
2. Expel Wind and stop pain

Form and Preparation: Powder, decoction, or pill

Dosage:
Horses and Cattle: 15–45 g
Camels: 30–60 g
Llamas, Alpacas, Goats, Sheep, and Pigs: 3–10 g
Dogs: 2–5 g
Cats and Rabbits: 0.5–2 g
Birds: 0.1–1.5 g

Cautions and Contraindications:
1. Caution during pregnancy
2. If used together in a formula, this herb may counteract the effects of Cornus *Shan Zhu Yu*, Astragalus *Huang Qi*, Talcum *Hua Shi*, *or* Coptis *Huang Lian*

Side Effects: Overdosage may cause nausea and vomiting.

Clinical Application:
1. Postpartum abdominal pain or retained placenta due to *Qi*-Blood Stagnation
   Combine with: Leonurus *Yi Mu Cao*, Persica *Tao Ren* and Carthamus *Hong Hua*
   Classical herbal formula: *Tao Hong Si Wu Tang*
2. Hypochondriac pain due to *Qi*-Blood Stagnation
   Combine with: Bupleurum *Chai Hu*, Cyperus *Xiang Fu* and Curcuma *Yu Jin*
3. Weakness and numbness of limbs due to *Qi*-Blood Stagnation
   Combine with: Paeonia *Chi Shao*, Lumbricus *Di Long* and Millettia *Ji Xue Teng*
   Classical herbal formula: *Bu Yang Huan Wu Tang*
4. *Bi* syndrome due to obstruction of Wind Damp in the Channels
   Combine with: Notopterygium *Qiang Huo*, Angelica *Du Huo*, Ledebouriella *Fang Feng*, and Morus *Sang Zhi*
   Classical herbal formula: *Du Huo Ji Sheng Tang*
5. Itchy skin
   Combine with: Paeonia *Bai Shao*, Schizonepeta *Jing Jie*
   Classical herbal formula: *Si Wu Xiao Feng San*

History and Comments:
1. Ligusticum *Chuan Xiong* is a strong Blood invigorator. Preparing the herb in sugar is preferred for its taste and reddish color. When it is prepared in wine, the herb is more invigorating, but it turns more white or brown.
2. *Chuan Xiong* is useful for stroke, embolism, heart attack, and severe congestive heart disease.

Pharmaceutical Ingredients:[1–4]
1. Alkaloids (chuanxiongzine, etramethylpyrazine, L-isoleucine-L-valine anhydride, L-valine-L-valine anhydride, trimethylamine, choline, perlolyrine, cnidiumlactone, chuanxingol, hydroxy-3-butylphathalide, ligustilide, ligustilide, wallichilide, neocnidilide, senkyunolide
2. Organic acid (caffeic acid, varillic acid, ferulic acid, sedanonic acid, folic acid, vanillic, protocatechuic acid, palmitic acid, linolenic acid, chrysophanol, methyl phenylacetate, sedanoic acid lactone, perlolyrine)
3. Essential olis (ethyl pentadecanoate, ethyl palmitate, ethyl heptadecanoate, ethyl isoheptadecanoate, ethyl octadecanoate, ethyl isoctadecanoate, methyl palmitate, methyl linolenate)

Corydalis *Yan Hu Suo* 延胡索

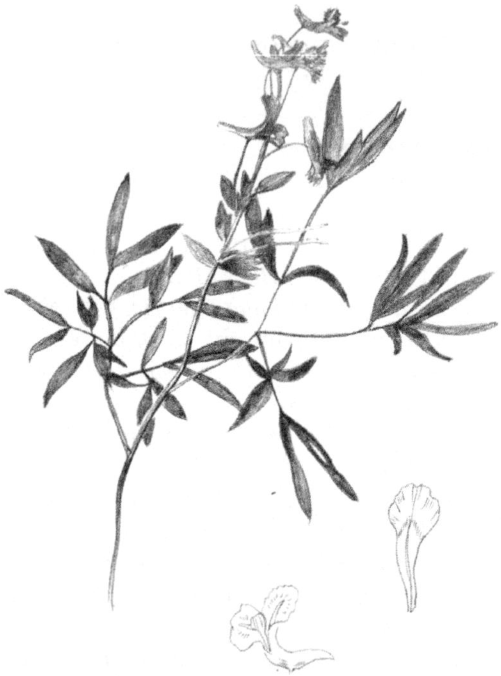

a

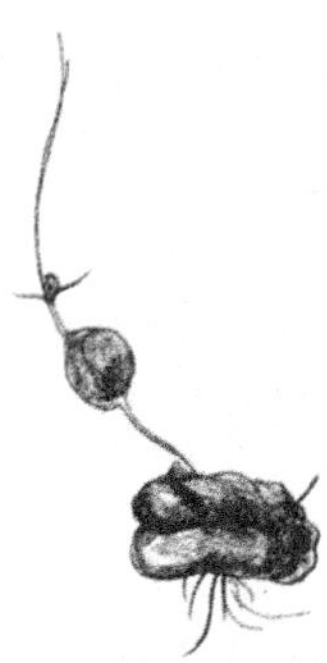

b

Original Reference: *Lei Gong Pao Zhi Lun* (*Lei's Method of Preparing Drugs*) by *Lei Xiao*, 5th century CE 雷公炮炙论

Part Used: Rhizome

Name:
Pharmaceutical: Corydalis Yanhusuo, Rhizoma
Botanical: Corydalis yanhusuo; C. turtschaninovii
Common: Corydalis
Wade-Giles: *Yan-Hu-So*
Translation: Extended Northern Rope
Alternative: *Xuan Hu*

Energy/Taste: Warm, pungent, bitter

Channel-Organ: Heart, Liver, Spleen

Actions:
1. Invigorate Blood and move *Qi*
2. Resolve Stagnation and stop pain

Form and Preparation: Powder, decoction, or pill

Dosage:
Horses and Cattle: 15–30 g
Camels: 30–75 g
Llamas, Alpacas, Goats, Sheep, and Pigs: 3–10 g
Dogs: 1–5 g
Cats and Rabbits: 0.5–1 g
Birds: 0.1–1.5 g

Cautions and Contraindications: Caution during pregnancy

Side Effects: None known

Clinical Application
1. Pain due to *Qi* Stagnation
   Clinical signs: Pain in stomach, heart, chest, abdomen, uterus, hernia
   Combine with: Melia *Chuan Lian Zi* and Angelica *Dang Gui*
2. Pain due to Blood Stagnation
   Clinical signs: Traumatic pain, postoperative pain, soreness in lower back, pain in limbs
   Combine with: Olibanum *Ru Xiang*, Myrrh *Mo Yao*, and Ligusticum *Chuan Xiong*
3. Headache due to *Qi*-Blood Stagnation or Wind-Damp in Channels
   Combine with: Angelica *Bai Zhi* and Ligusticum *Chuan Xiong*

History and Comments:
1. Corydalis *Yan Hu Suo* is excellent for pain control and may have pain management effects similar to morphine and codeine. Frying with vinegar enhances this herb's ability to stop pain.
2. *Yan Hu Suo* is effective for healing stomach and intestinal ulcers and for suppressing stomach acidity.

Pharmaceutical Ingredients:[1–4] Alkaloids (dl-tetrahydropalmatine, d-corydaline, corydalis, protopine, 1-tetrahydrocoptisine, 1-tetrahydrocolumbamine, corydalis H, corydalis I, corybulbine, B-homochelidonine, coptisine, dehydrocorydaline, corydalmine, dehydrocorydalmine, columbamine

Curcuma *Yu Jin* 郁金

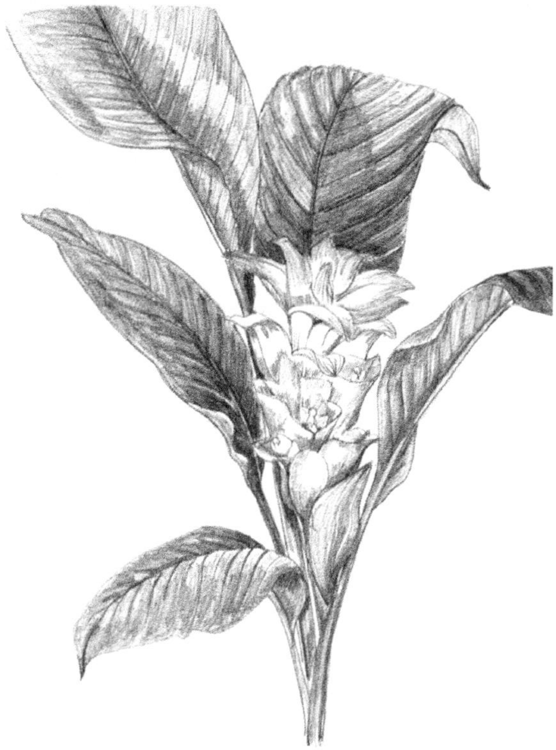

a

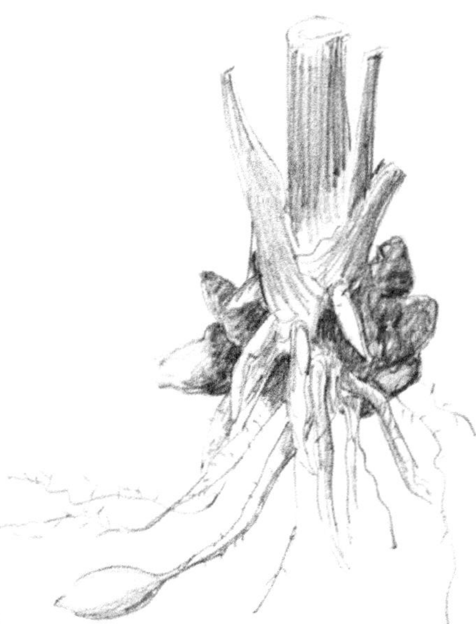

b

Original Reference: *Yao Xing Lun* (*Discussion of Medicinal Properties*) by *Chen Zhou* in 19th century 药性论

Part Used: Root

Name:
Pharmaceutical: Curcumae, Tuber
Botanical: Curcuma aromatica; C. zedoaria; C. longa
Common: Turmeric tuber
Wade-Giles: *Yu-Chin*
Translation: Jade Gold

Energy/Taste: Cold, pungent, bitter

Channel-Organ: Heart, Liver, Gallbladder

Actions:
1. Invigorate Blood and relieve pain
2. Regulate *Qi* and dispel Stagnation
3. Cool Blood and clear Heat in the Heart
4. Relieve jaundice and benefit the Gallbladder

Form and Preparation: Powder, decoction, or pill

Dosage:
Horses and Cattle: 15–45 g
Camels: 30–60 g
Llamas, Alpacas, Goats, Sheep, and Pigs: 3–10 g
Dogs: 2–6 g
Cats and Rabbits: 0.5–1 g
Birds: 0.2–1.5 g

Cautions and Contraindications:
1. Caution during pregnancy
2. Do not combine with Caryophyllum *Ding Xiang*.

Side Effects: None known

Clinical Application
1. Pain due to *Qi* and Blood Stagnation
   Clinical signs: Pain in the chest, abdomen, or hypochondrium; trauma
   Combine with: Salvia *Dan Shen*, Cyperus *Xiang Fu*, Bupleurum *Chai Hu*, and Aurantium *Zhi Ke*
2. Shen disturbance due to Heat-Phlegm and Interior Damp and Phlegm
   Clinical signs: Mental agitation, mania, restlessness, insomnia, epilepsy
   Combine with: Acorus *Shi Chang Pu* or Alum *Ming Fan*
3. Jaundice due to Liver Damp-Heat
   Clinical signs: *Yang* jaundice, flank pain, reduced urine output, loss of appetite
   Combine with: Bupleurum *Chai Hu*, Cyperus *Xiang Fu*, Artemisia *Yin Chen Hao*, Gardenia *Zhi Zi*
4. Hemorrhage due to Blood Heat with Blood Stasis
   Clinical signs: Purplish blotches on skin, bloody diarrhea, epistaxis
   Combine with: Mouton *Mu Dan Pi*, Cyathula *Niu Xi*
5. Pain associated with urinary dysfunction and uroliths
   Combine with: Lysimachia *Jin Qian Cao*

History and Comments:
1. Curcuma *Yu Jin* cools Blood and clears Heat from the Heart, Small Intestine, and Large Intestine. It is used to treat colitis and bloody diarrhea in horses. It also

effectively treats Heat-Phlegm misting in the Heart, which can cause mania and epilepsy.
2. Curcuma *Yu Jin* can invigorate Liver Blood Stagnation and is usually combined with herbs to soothe Liver *Qi*.
3. Stir-fry Curcuma *Yu Jin* with wine or vinegar to reduce its cold nature while enhancing its ability to circulate *Qi*.

Pharmaceutical Ingredients:[1–4]
1. Curcumin, demethoxy curcumin, bisdemethoxy curcumin, d-camphene, d-camphor, 1-α-curcumene, 1-β-curcumene, curcumin, turmerone
2. Essential oils (turmerone, zingiberene, phellandrene, 1,8-cineole, sabinene, borneol)
3. Ar-turmerone, caryophyllene, glucose, starch, bisabolane, curlone, lipids, carvone

Salvia *Dan Shen* 丹参

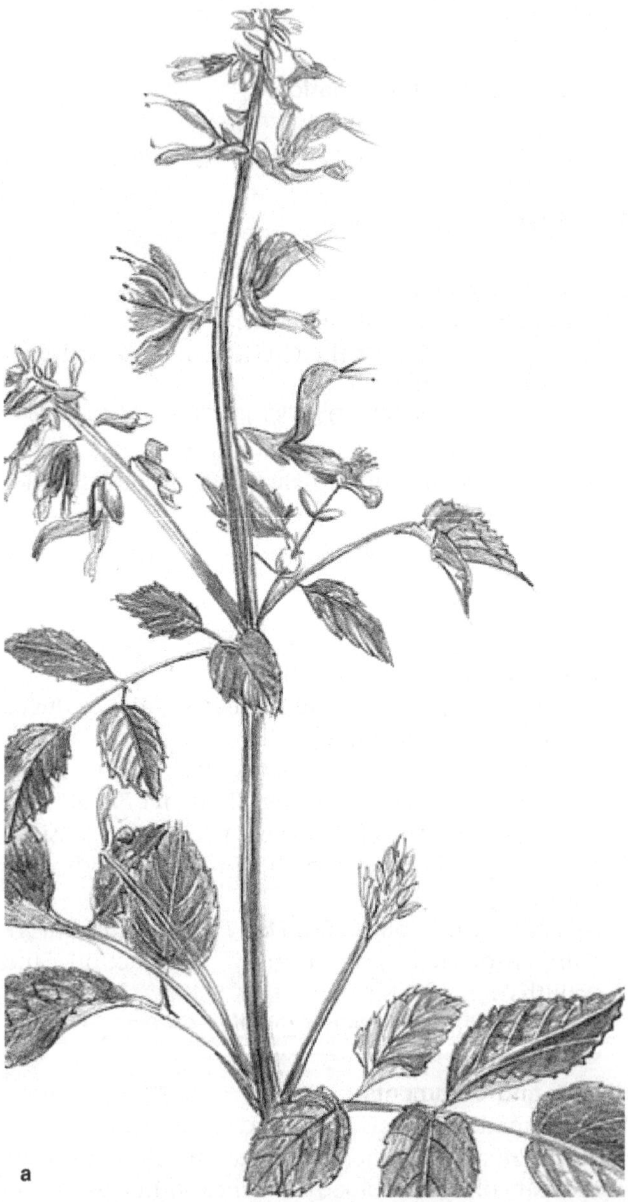

a

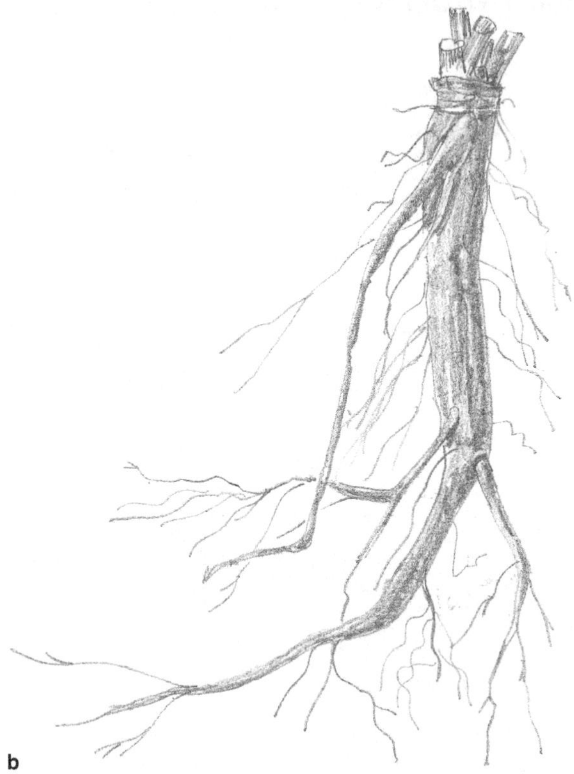

b

Original Reference: *Shen Nong Ben Cao Jing* (*Shen Nong*'s *Materia Medica*, 1st century BCE) 神农本草经

Part Used: Root

Name:
Pharmaceutical: Salviae Miltiorrhizae, Radix
Botanical: Salvia miltiorrhiza
Common: Sage
Wade-Giles: *Tan-Shen*
Translation: Red Sage Root

Energy/Taste: Slightly cold, bitter

Channel-Organ: Heart, Pericardium, Liver

Actions:
1. Invigorate Blood and resolve Stagnation
2. Cool Blood and eliminate abscess
3. Nourish Blood and calm Shen

Form and Preparation: Powder, decoction, or pill

Dosage: Preparing Salvia *Dan Shen* with wine can enhance its Blood-invigorating actions.
Horses and Cattle: 15–45 g

Camels: 30–60 g
Llamas, Alpacas, Goats, Sheep, and Pigs: 3–10 g
Dogs: 2–5 g
Cats and Rabbits: 0.5–2 g
Birds: 0.1–1.5 g

Cautions and Contraindications:

1. This herb may be incompatible with Veratrum *Li Lu*. If they combine, effectiveness of one or both of the herbs decreases. Therefore, avoid using it with *Li Lu*.
2. Do not prescribe large doses for patients with congenital bleeding disorders.

Side Effects: None known

Clinical Application:

1. Blood Stagnation in and around the uterus
   Clinical signs: Uterine cysts, fibroid tumors, postpartum pain, retained placenta, false pregnancy, endometriosis, irregular estrus cycles
   Combine with: Leonurus *Yi Mu Cao*, Persica *Tao Ren*, Carthamus *Hong Hua*, Angelica *Dang Gui*
2. Chest pain and cardiomyopathy due to Blood Stagnation
   Use alone or combine with: Notoginseng *Tian Qi*
   Classical herbal formula: *Fu Fang Dan Shen Pian* (Compound *Dan Shen*)
3. *Qi* and Blood Stagnation in the Channels and limbs
   Clinical signs: Joint or muscle pain, or traumatic pain
   Combine with: Angelica *Dang Gui*, Carthamus *Hong Hua*, Ligusticum *Chuan Xiong*, Olibanum *Ru Xiang* and Myrrh *Mo Yao*
4. Blood Heat with ulcerations, sores, abscess, carbuncles, furuncles, swellings
   Combine with: Lonicera *Jin Yin Hua*, Forsythia *Lian Qiao*, and Olibanum *Ru Xiang*
5. Heat in the *Ying* level
   Clinical signs: High fever, irritability, behavioral changes or Shen disturbance, skin rash, epistaxis, dark-red tongue
   Combine with: Rehmannia *Sheng Di Huang*, Scrophularia *Xuan Shen*, Mouton *Mu Dan Pi*
   Classical herbal formula: *Qing Ying Tang*
6. Blood Deficiency with internal Heat
   Combine with: Ziziphus *Suan Zao Ren*, Polygonum *Ye Jiao Teng*

History and Comments:

1. Be careful: Do not confuse *Dan Shen* with Codonopsis *Dang Shen* (*Qi* Tonic).
2. The inside of good quality *Dan Shen* is coarse and purplish black with small white spots. Depending on its preparation, the herb has different effects. Stir-fry in wine to invigorate Blood; stir-fry until brown to stop bleeding.
3. When used alone, Salvia *Dan Shen* is also known to have the same actions as the formula *Si Wu Tang* (Four Substances) to tonify and move Blood.
4. In China, Salvia *Dan Shen* is administered via an intravenous drip for embolic stroke, heart attack, and severe heart congestion.
5. In China, Salvia *Dan Shen* has recently been used to treat patients with an enlarged liver, spleen disorders, and coronary heart disease.

Pharmaceutical Ingredients:[1–4]

1. Terpenoids (tanshinone, cryptotanshinone, dihydrotanshinone, hydroxytanshinone, miltionone, salvilenone, methyltanshinonate, methylenetanshinquinone, przewatanshinquinone A, miltirone, dihydrotanshinone, tanshinol A, tanshinol B, tanshinol C, nortanshinone, 1,2,15,16-tetrahydrotanshiquinone, isotanshinone), isocryptotanshinone, tanshiquinone A, B, C
2. Flavonoids, steroids

Carthamus *Hong Hua* 红花

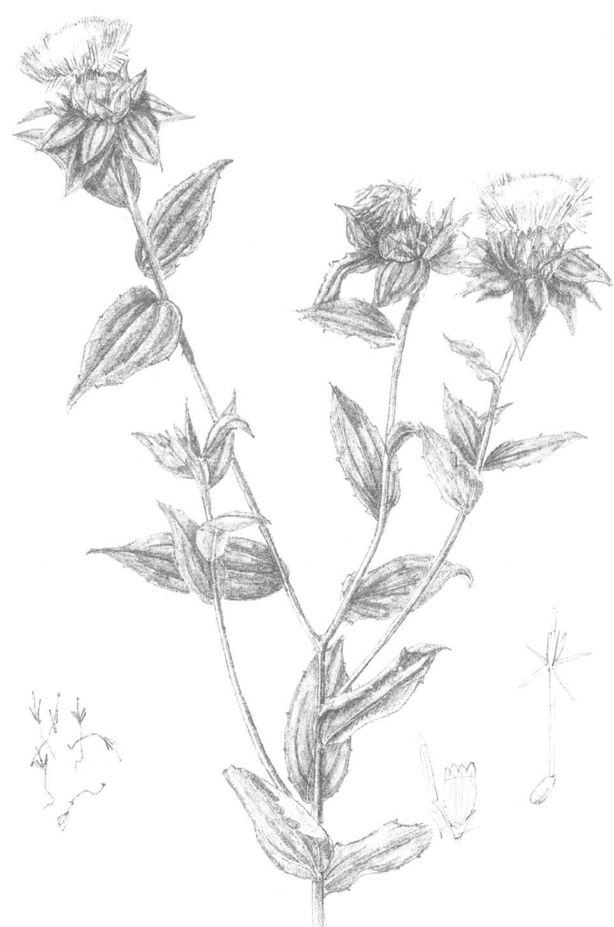

Original Reference: *Tang Ben Cao* (*Tang Materia Medica*) by *Su Jing* et al., *Tang* Dynasty 唐本草

Part Used: Flower

Name:
Pharmaceutical: Carthami Tictori, Flos
Botanical: Carthamus tinctorius
Common: Safflower
Wade-Giles: *Hung-Hua*
Translation: Red Flower

Energy/Taste: Warm, pungent, bitter

Channel-Organ: Heart, Liver

Actions:
1. Invigorate Blood and remove Stasis
2. Unblock the Channels and stop pain

Form and Preparation: Powder, decoction, or pill

Dosage:
Horses and Cattle: 15–30 g
Llamas, Alpacas, Goats, Sheep, and Pigs: 3–10 g
Dogs: 2–5 g
Cats and Rabbits: 0.5–1 g
Birds: 0.1–1 g

Cautions and Contraindications:
1. Contraindicated during pregnancy
2. Caution in bleeding patients

Side Effects: Overdose may cause abdominal pain, colic, diarrhea, or gastrointestinal bleeding.

Clinical Application
1. Blood Stagnation in and around the uterus
   Clinical signs: Ovarian or uterine cysts, fibroid masses, postpartum pain, false pregnancy, retained placenta
   Combine with: Persica *Tao Ren*, Angelica *Dang Gui*, Ligusticum *Chuan Xiong*, Paeonia *Chi Shao Yao*
   Classical herbal formula: *Tao Hong Si Wu Tang*
2. Blood Stagnation due to trauma or postsurgery
   Combine with: Persica *Tao Ren*
   Classical herbal formula: *Fu Yuan Huo Xue Tang*
3. Masses and Liver or Spleen enlargement due to Blood Stagnation
   Combine with: Salvia *Dan Shen* and Persica *Tao Ren*
4. Pain and numbness due to Blood Stagnation in the Channels
   Combine with: Chaenomeles *Mu Gua*
5. Skin rash with dark color due to Heat and Blood Stagnation
   Combine with: Paeonia *Chi Shao Yao* and Ledebouriella *Fang Feng*

History and Comments
1. Carthamus *Hong Hua* is usually combined with Persica *Tao Ren* to treat masses and lumps due to Blood Stasis. It is also effective for dispersing bruises due to trauma.
2. A good quality *Hong Hua* feels greasy.

Pharmaceutical Ingredients:[1–4]
1. Carthamin, neocarthamin, carthamone, carthamidin, precarthamin, saffloryellow A, B, safflomin A
2. Chlorogenic acid, caffeic acid

Persica *Tao Ren* 桃仁

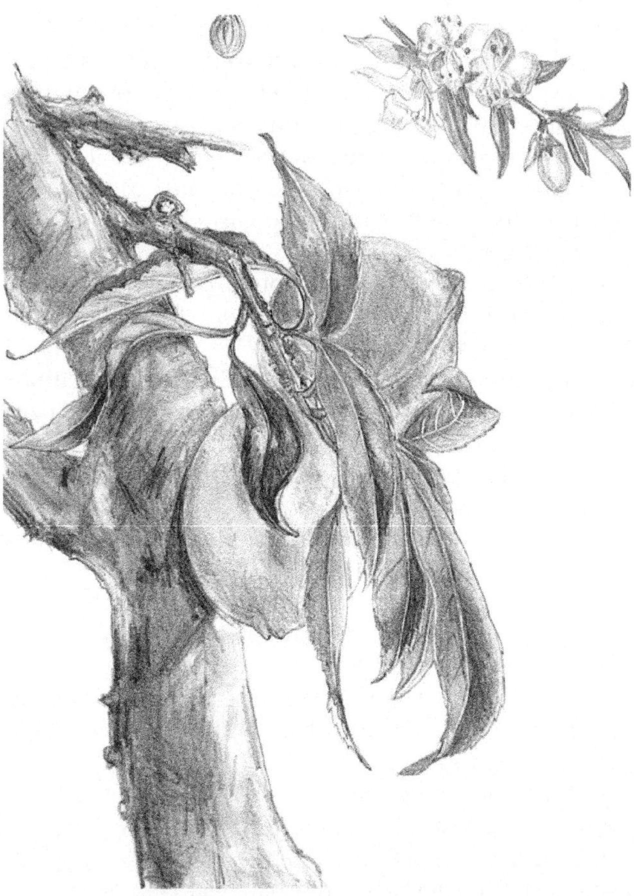

Original Reference: *Shen Nong Ben Cao Jing* (*Shen Nong's Materia Medica*, 1st century BCE) 神农本草经

Part Used: Seed

Name:
Pharmaceutical: Persicae, Semen
Botanical: Prunus Persica; P. davidiana

Common: Peach kernel
Wade-Giles: *T'ao-Jen*
Translation: Peach Kernel

Energy/Taste: Neutral, bitter, sweet, mild toxic

Channel-Organ: Heart, Liver, Large Intestine, Lung

Actions:
1. Invigorate Blood and dispel Stagnation
2. Moisten the intestines and purge stool
3. Stop asthma and cough

Form and Preparation: Powder, decoction, or pill

Dosage:
Horses and Cattle: 15–30g
Llamas, Alpacas, Goats, Sheep, and Pigs: 3–10g
Dogs: 2–5g
Cats and Rabbits: 0.5–1g
Birds: 0.1–1g

Cautions and Contraindications:
1. Contraindicated during pregnancy
2. Caution in patients with diarrhea

Side Effects: Overdosage may damage the nervous system and cause nausea, vomiting, headache, palpitations, restlessness, convulsions, and coma.

Clinical Application
1. Blood Stagnation in and around the uterus
   Clinical signs: Uterine or ovarian cysts, fibroid masses, postpartum pain, expelling a dead fetus or placenta, scanty flow, abdominal pain
   Combine with: Carthamus *Hong Hua*, Angelica *Dang Gui*, Ligusticum *Chuan Xiong*, Paeonia *Chi Shao Yao*
   Classical herbal formula: *Tao Hong Si Wu Tang*
2. Blood Stagnation due to trauma or postsurgery
   Combine with: Carthamus *Hong Hua*
   Classical herbal formula: *Fu Yuan Huo Xue Tang*
3. Constipation due to dryness in the intestines
   Combine with: Angelica *Dang Gui*, Cannabis *Huo Ma Ren*, and Armeniaca *Xing Ren*
4. Intestinal abscess; also used for trauma accompanied by constipation
   Combine with: Rheum *Da Huang*, Mirabilite *Mang Xiao*, Moutan *Mu Dan Pi*
5. Lung abscess
   Combine with: Coix *Yi Yi Ren*, Benincasa *Dong Gua Ren*

History and Comments:
1. Persica *Tao Ren* is often combined with Carthamus *Hong Hua* to reinforce its effect.
2. *Tao Ren* can cause abortion; thus, it is prohibited during pregnancy.

Pharmaceutical Ingredients:[1–4]
1. Amygdalin, emulsion, lactase, allontoinase, allantoinase, lipids, vitamin B1, fatty acid
2. Essential oils (oleic acid, glyceric acid, palmitic acid, gibberellin A_5, A_{33}), emulsin

Sanguis Draconis *Xue Jie* 血竭

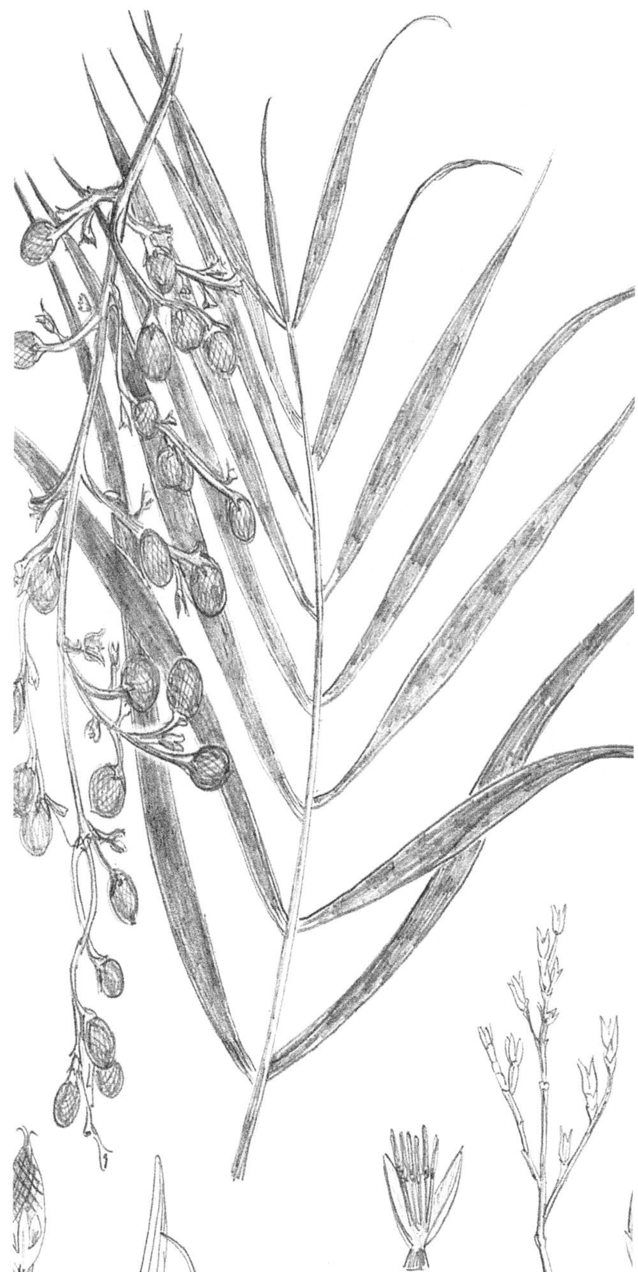

Original Reference: *Lei Gong Pao Zhi Lun* (*Lei's Method of Preparing Drugs*) by *Lei Xiao* in 5th century 雷公炮炙论

Part Used: Resin from the fruit and stem

Name:
Pharmaceutical: Draconis, Sanguis
Botanical: Daemonorops draco. Bl
Common: Dragon's Blood (a resin)
Wade-Giles: *Hsueh-Yu-T'an*
Translation: Exhausted Blood

Energy/Taste: Neutral, sweet, salty

Channel-Organ: Heart, Liver

Actions:
1. Invigorate Blood and dispel Stagnation
2. Stop pain and bleeding
3. Promote wound healing

Form and Preparation: Powder, decoction, or pill

Dosage:
Horses and Cattle: 15–25 g
Llamas, Alpacas, Goats, Sheep, and Pigs: 3–6 g
Dogs: 1–3 g
Cats and Rabbits: 0.2–0.5 g

Cautions and Contraindications:
1. Contraindicated during pregnancy
2. Caution when Blood Stagnation is not present

Side Effects: May cause abortion

Clinical Application
1. Swelling and pain due to Blood Stagnation caused by external injuries, especially of the chest and abdomen
   Combine with: Olibanum *Ru Xiang*, Myrrh *Mo Yao*
   Classical herbal formula: *Qi Li San*
2. Chronic, nonhealing ulcers
   Single topical use, or *combine with*: Olibanum *Ru Xiang*, Myrrh *Mo Yao*
3. Hemorrhages due to external injuries
   Single topical use, or *combine with*: Acacia *Er Cha*, Olibanum *Ru Xiang*, Myrrh *Mo Yao*, Typha *Pu Huang*

History and Comments:
1. Good quality Draconis *Xue Jie* has an iron black color. When it is powdered, it turns blood-red.
2. Draconis *Xue Jie* is effective for treating gastrointestinal bleeding. It is also topically used to treat anal bleeding.

Pharmaceutical Ingredients:[1–4]
1. Dracorubin, dracorhodin, nordracorhodin, nordracorubin, dracoresene
2. Pimaric acid, sandaracopimaric acid

Sparganium *San Leng* 三棱

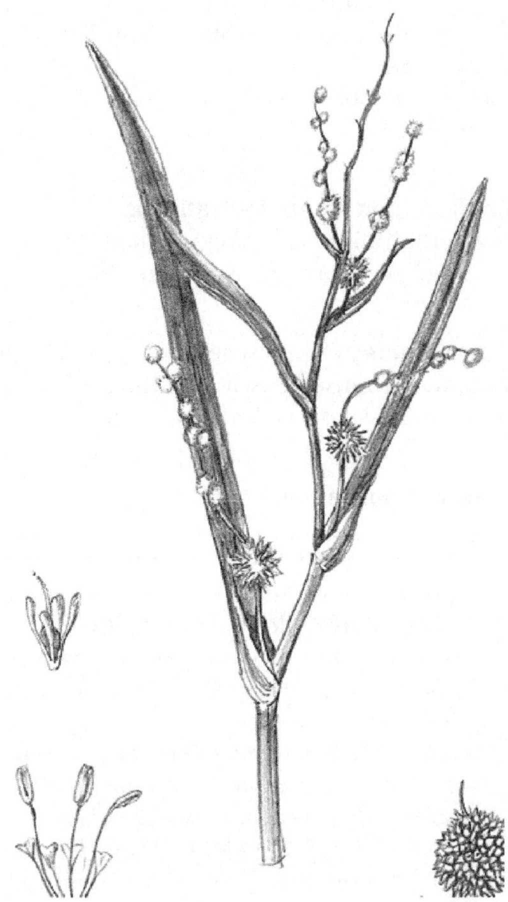

a

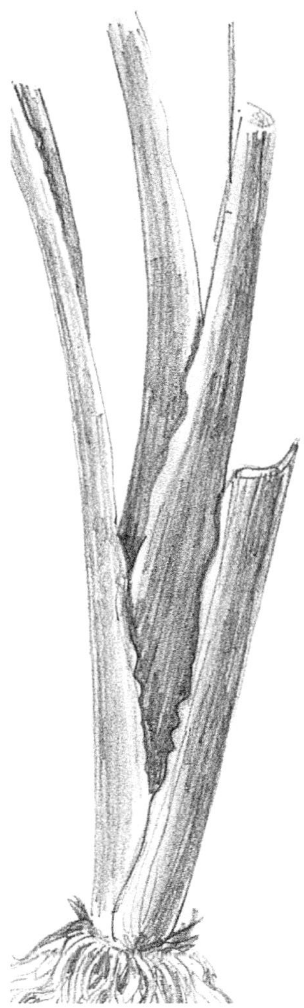

b

Original Reference: *Ben Cao Shi Yi* (*Supplement to Materia Medica*) by *Chen Cang-Qi* in 8th century 本草拾遗

Part Used: Rhizome

Name:
Pharmaceutical: Sparganii Stoloniferi, Rhizoma
Botanical: Sparganium stoloniferum
Common: Sparganium rhizome
Wade-Giles: *San-Leng*
Translation: Three Edged

Energy/Taste: Neutral, bitter, pungent

Channel-Organ: Liver, Spleen

Actions:
1. Break up and drive out Blood Stasis
2. Promote *Qi* circulation and stop pain

Form and Preparation: Powder, decoction, or pill

Dosage:
Horses and Cattle: 15–60 g
Llamas, Alpacas, Goats, Sheep, and Pigs: 3–10 g
Dogs: 1–3 g
Cats and Rabbits: 0.2–0.5 g

Cautions and Contraindications:
1. Prohibited during pregnancy
2. Contraindicated in patients with profuse bleeding
3. Caution in patients with Deficiency

Side Effects: May cause diarrhea

Clinical Application
1. Masses, lumps, and nodules due to Blood Stasis
   Combine with: Zedoaria *E Zhu*, Fritillaria *Zhe Bei Mu*
   Classical herbal formula: *Nei Xiao Wan* (Stasis Breaker)
2. Retention of food with *Qi* Stagnation
   Clinical signs: Food retention, abdominal distension with pain
   Combine with: Zedoaria *E Zhu*, Citrus *Qing Pi*, and Hordeum *Mai Ya*; or Saussurea *Mu Xiang*, Areca *Da Fu Pi*, and Massa Fermentata *Shen Qu*

History and Comments:
1. Sparganium *San Leng* and Zedoaria *E Zhu* are the top two herbs for breaking down Deficiency and invigorating Blood. They are often used to treat tumors and growths.
2. Stir-frying the herb with vinegar enhances its ability to stop pain.
3. Good quality Sparganium *San Leng* is heavy and solid with a yellowish white color.

Pharmaceutical Ingredients:[1–4]
1. Essential oils (benzene ethanol, 1, 4-benzenediol, hexadecanoic acid, dehydrocostuslactone, βelemene, 2-furan-methanol, 2-cetylpyrrole
2. Formonetin, stigmasterol, β-sitosterol, daucosterol, starch

Zedoaria *E Zhu* 莪术

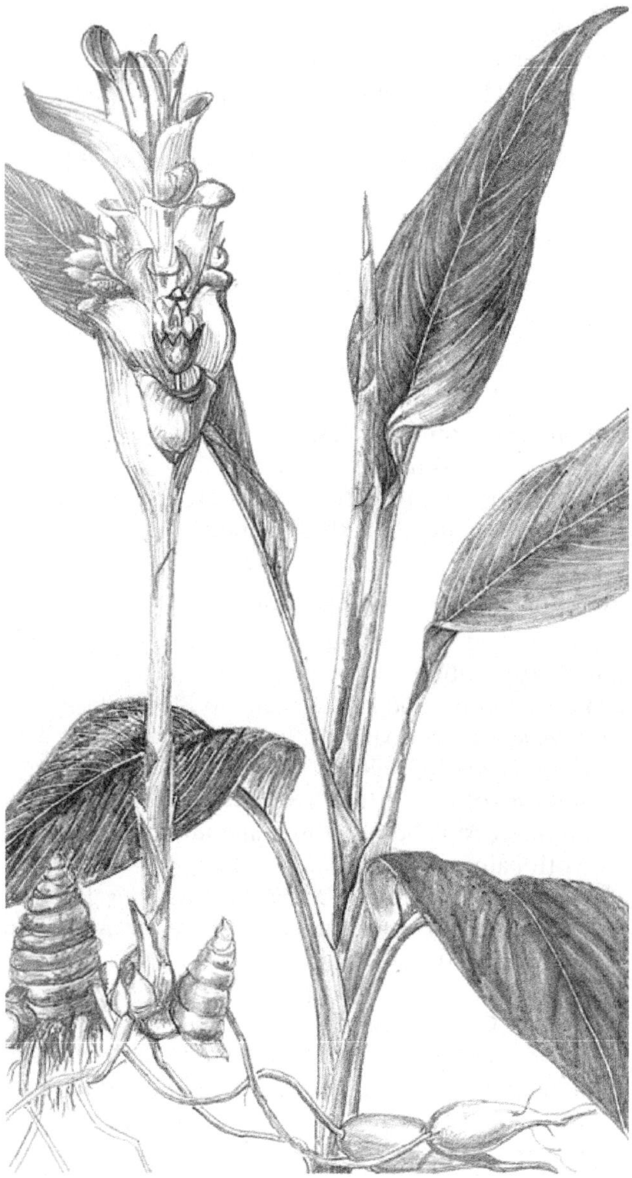

Original Reference: *Yao Xing Lun (Discussion of Medicinal Properties)* by *Chen Zhou* in 19th century 药性论

Part Used: Rhizome

Name:
Pharmaceutical: Zedoariae, Rhizoma
Botanical: Curcuma zedoaria; C. aromatica; C. kwangsiensis
Common: Zedoary rhizome
Wade-Giles: *E-Chu*
Translation: Zedoary Bundle

Energy/Taste: Warm, pungent, bitter

Channel-Organ: Liver, Spleen

Actions:
1. Break up Blood and drive out Stasis
2. Promote *Qi* circulation and stop pain
3. Dissolve accumulations

Form and Preparation: Powder, decoction, or pill

Dosage:
Horses and Cattle: 15–60 g
Llamas, Alpacas, Goats, Sheep, and Pigs: 3–10 g
Dogs: 1–3 g
Cats and Rabbits: 0.2–0.5 g
Birds: 0.1–1 g

Cautions and Contraindications:
1. Contraindicated during pregnancy
2. Caution in patients with Deficiency

Side Effects: May cause dizziness, nausea, dyspnea, fever, or an increase in liver enzymes

Clinical Application
1. *Qi* and Blood Stagnation affecting the uterus
   Clinical signs: Dysmenorrhea, amenorrhea, fibroid masses, abdominal masses, postpartum retention of placenta, emotional depression, and wiry pulse
   Combine with: Sparganium *San Leng*; or with Angelica *Dang Gui* and Carthamus *Hong Hua*
   Combine with: Angelica *Dang Gui*, Paeonia *Chi Shao*, and Ligusticum *Chuan Xiong*
   Classical herbal formula: *E Zhu Wan*
2. Retention of food with Stagnation of *Qi*
   Clinical signs: Epigastric and abdominal distension with pain
   Combine with: Sparganium *San Leng*, Saussurea *Mu Xiang*, Crataegus *Shan Zha*, and Aurantium *Zhi Shi*
3. Pain and fullness in the chest and abdomen due to *Qi* Stagnation
   Combine with: Citrus *Qing Pi*
4. Immobile palpable masses of the epigastrium, abdomen, and subcostal areas, usually accompanied by pain and distention (as in cases of liver and spleen enlargement); indicated in robust patients (constitutionally)
   Combine with: Sparganium *San Leng*
   If concurrent heat signs: combine with Gardenia *Zhi Zi*, Rehmannia *Sheng Di Huang*

History and Comments
1. The combination of Sparganium *San Leng* and Zedoaria *E Zhu* forcefully breaks up any Stasis and Stagnation and is commonly used for cancerous masses.
2. Sparganium *San Leng* and Zedoaria *E Zhu* have similar energetic actions. However, *Sang Leng* is

stronger for breaking down Stasis, and *E Zhu* more strongly moves *Qi* and stops pain.
3. Stir-fry Zedoaria *E Zhu* with vinegar to enhance its function to move Blood and stop pain.

Pharmaceutical Ingredients:[1–4] Zingiberene, zedoarone, furanodine, furanodienone, isofuranodienone, curcumol, curdione, isocurcumol, curzerene, curzerenone, epicurzerenone, curcumenol, procurcumenol, isocurcumenol, curcumadiol, curcumin, turmerol

Olibanum *Ru Xiang* 乳香

Original Reference: *Ming Yi Bie Lu (Miscellaneous Records of Famous Physicians)* by *Tao Hong-Jing*, North and South Kingdoms (5th century) 名医别录

Part Used: Gummy resin

Name:
Pharmaceutical: Resina Olibani, Olibanum
Botanical: Boswellia carterri
Common: Mastic
Wade-Giles: *Ju-Hsiang*
Translation: Milk Fragrant

Energy/Taste: Warm, pungent, bitter

Channel-Organ: Heart, Liver, Spleen

Actions:
1. Invigorate Blood and stop pain
2. Reduce swelling and regenerate tissue
3. Promote *Qi* flow to relax sinews and the Channels

Form and Preparation: Powder, decoction, or pill

Dosage:
Horses and Cattle: 15–30 g
Llamas, Alpacas, Goats, Sheep, and Pigs: 3–6 g
Dogs: 1–3 g
Cats and Rabbits: 0.2–0.5 g
Birds: 0.2–1 g

Cautions and Contraindications:
1. Prohibited during pregnancy
2. Caution in patients with Spleen Deficiency

Side Effects: May cause vomiting, colic, diarrhea, and allergic skin reactions

Myrrh *Mo Yao* 没药

Original Reference: *Kai Bao Ben Cao (Materia Medica of the Kai Bao* Era) by *Ma Zhi* in 973 开宝本草

Part Used: Gummy resin

Name:
Pharmaceutical: Resina Myrrha; Myrrha
Botanical: Commiphora molmol; C. myrrh
Common: Myrrh
Wade-Giles: *Mo-Yao*
Translation: Hidden Medicine

Energy/Taste: Neutral, bitter

Channel-Organ: Heart, Liver, Spleen

Actions:
1. Invigorate Blood and stop pain
2. Reduce swelling and regenerate tissues

Form and Preparation: Powder, decoction, or pill

Dosage:
Horses and Cattle: 25–45 g
Llamas, Alpacas, Goats, Sheep, and Pigs: 5–10 g
Dogs: 1–3 g
Cats and Rabbits: 0.2–0.5 g
Birds: 0.1–1 g

Cautions and Contraindications:
1. Prohibited during pregnancy
2. Caution in patients with Spleen Deficiency

Side Effects: Excessive dosage can cause nausea

Curcuma *Jiang Huang* 姜黄

Original Reference: *Tang Ben Cao (Tang Materia Medica)* by *Su Jing* et al., *Tang* Dynasty 唐本草

Part Used: Rhizome

Name:
Pharmaceutical: Curcumae Longae, Rhizoma
Botanical: Curcuma longa L.
Common: Turmeric
Wade-Giles: *Chiang-Huang*
Translation: Ginger Yellow

Energy/Taste: Warm, pungent, bitter

Channel-Organ: Spleen, Stomach, Liver

Actions:
1. Invigorate Blood and promote *Qi* flow
2. Expel Wind-Damp in the Channel and stop pain

Form and Preparation: Powder, decoction, or pill

Dosage:
Horses and Cattle: 25–45 g
Llamas, Alpacas, Goats, Sheep, and Pigs: 5–10 g
Dogs: 1–3 g

Cats and Rabbits: 0.2–0.5 g
Birds: 0.1–1 g

Cautions and Contraindications:
1. Caution during pregnancy
2. Caution in patients with Blood Deficiency without Blood Stagnation

Side Effects: None known

Trogopterus *Wu Ling Zhi* 五灵脂

Original Reference: *Kai Bao Ben Cao* (*Materia Medica of the Kai Bao Era*) by *Ma Zhi* in 973 开宝本草

Part Used: Stool of the flying squirrel

Name:
Pharmaceutical: Trogopterori seu Pteromi, Excrementum
Zoological: Trogopterus xanthipes; Pteromys volans; P. pselaphon
Common: Flying squirrel feces
Wade-Giles: *Wu-Ling-Chih*
Translation: Five Effective Fats

Energy/Taste: Warm, salty, bitter, sweet

Channel-Organ: Liver

Actions:
1. Invigorate Blood and stop pain
2. Resolve Stagnation and stop bleeding

Form and Preparation: Powder or pill

Dosage:
Horses and Cattle: 15–30 g
Llamas, Alpacas, Goats, Sheep, and Pigs: 5–10 g
Dogs: 2–5 g
Cats and Rabbits: 0.5–1 g
Birds: 0.1–1 g

Cautions and Contraindications:
1. Caution during pregnancy
2. Do not combine with Ginseng *Ren Shen*.

Side Effects: May weaken Spleen *Qi*

Corydalis *Xia Tian Wu* 夏天无

Original Reference: *Zhen Jiang Min Jian Chang Yong Cao Yao* (*Zhe Jiang Folk Materia Medica*) by Public Health Department of *Zhejiang* Province in 1969 浙江民间常用草药

Part Used: Rhizome

Name:
Pharmaceutical: Corydalis decumbens, Rhizoma
Botanical: Corydalis decumbens Pres.
Common: Corydalis decumbens
Wade-Giles: *Hsia-T'ien-Wu*
Translation: Summer Time Disappearance

Energy/Taste: Warm, pungent, pitter

Channel-Organ: Liver

Actions:
1. Invigorate Blood to stop pain
2. Relax sinews and eliminate Wind-Damp

Form and Preparation: Powder, decoction, or pill

Dosage:
Horses and Cattle: 15–60 g
Llamas, Alpacas, Goats, Sheep, and Pigs: 3–10 g
Dogs: 2–5 g
Cats and Rabbits: 0.5–1 g
Birds: 0.1–1.5 g

Cautions and Contraindications: None known

Side Effects: None known

Vaccaria *Wang Bu Liu Xing* 王不留行

Original Reference: *Shen Nong Ben Cao Jing* (*Shen Nong's Materia Medica*, 1st century BCE) 神农本草经

Part Used: Seed

Name:
Pharmaceutical: Vaccariae Segetalis, Semen
Botanical: Vaccara segetalis (Neck.) Garcke
Common: Vaccaria
Wade-Giles: *Wang-Pu-Liu-Hsing*
Translation: King who does not stay but departs

Energy/Taste: Neutral, bitter

Channel-Organ: Liver, Stomach

Actions:
1. Move Blood and invigorate Channels
2. Reduce swelling and promote lactation

Form and Preparation: Powder, decoction, or pill

Dosage: Because the herb is an irritant, pellets have been implanted in ear acupuncture points to treat various conditions.

Horses and Cattle: 30–100 g
Llamas, Alpacas, Goats, Sheep, and Pigs: 10–30 g
Dogs: 2–5 g
Cats and Rabbits: 0.5–2 g
Birds: 0.1–1.5 g

Cautions and Contraindications: Caution during pregnancy

Side Effects: May cause skin photosensitivity

Cyathula *Chuan Niu Xi* 川牛膝

Original Reference: *Shen Nong Ben Cao Jing* (*Shen Nong's Materia Medica*, 1st century BCE) 神农本草经

Part Used: Root

Name:
Pharmaceutical: Cyathulae, Radix
Botanical: Achyranthes bidentatae; Cyathula capitata; C. officinalis
Common: Cyathula or Achyranthes root
Wade-Giles: *Niu-Hsi*
Translation: Ox's Knee

Energy/Taste: Neutral, bitter, sour

Channel-Organ: Liver, Kidney

Actions:
1. Invigorate Blood and dispel Stagnation
2. Tonify Liver and Kidney and strengthen tendons and bones
3. Promote urination and direct *Qi*-Blood down to rear limbs and stifle

Form and Preparation: Powder, decoction, or pill

Dosage:
Horses and Cattle: 20–60 g
Llamas, Alpacas, Goats, Sheep, and Pigs: 5–12 g
Dogs: 2–5 g
Cats and Rabbits: 0.5–2 g
Birds: 0.1–1.5 g

Cautions and Contraindications:
1. Prohibited during pregnancy
2. Caution during diarrhea due to Spleen *Qi* Deficiency
3. Do not use with Cynanchum *Bai Qian.*

Side Effects: None known

Leonurus *Yi Mu Cao* 益母草

Original Reference: *Shen Nong Ben Cao Jing* (*Shen Nong's Materia Medica*, 1st century BCE) 神农本草经

Part Used: Entire plant

Name:
Pharmaceutical: Leonuri Heterophylii, Herba
Botanical: Leonurus heterophyllus
Common: Motherwort
Wade-Giles: *I-Mu-Ts'ao*
Translation: Benefit Mother Herb

Energy/Taste: Cold, bitter, pungent

Channel-Organ: Liver, Heart, Bladder

Actions:
1. Invigorate Blood and resolve Stagnation
2. Promote urination and reduce edema
3. Clear Heat and detoxify

Form and Preparation: Powder, decoction, or pill

Dosage:
Horses and Cattle: 30–60 g
Llamas, Alpacas, Goats, Sheep, and Pigs: 5–30 g
Dogs: 2–10 g
Cats and Rabbits: 0.5–2 g
Birds: 0.1–1.5 g

Cautions and Contraindications: Caution during pregnancy

Side Effects:
1. Overdose may damage the central nerve system; it first causes excitement, and then paralysis.
2. Overdosage may also cause hematuria and abortion.

Millettia *Ji Xue Teng* 鸡血藤

Original Reference: *Ben Cao Gang Mu Shi Yi* (*Omissions for the Materia Medica Compendium*) by *Zhao Xue-min* et al., in 1765 本草纲目拾遗

Part Used: Vine, or vine and root

Name:
Pharmaceutical: Millettiae, Radix et Caulis
Botanical: Millettia dielsiana
Common: Millettia root and vine
Wade-Giles: *Chi-Hsue–tang*
Translation: Chicken Blood Vine

Energy/Taste: Warm, bitter, sweet

Channel-Organ: Liver, Heart, Spleen, Kidney

Actions:
1. Invigorate Blood and tonify Blood
2. Relax the tendons and invigorate the Channels

Form and Preparation: Powder, decoction, or pill

Dosage:
Horses and Cattle: 15–60 g
Llamas, Alpacas, Goats, Sheep, and Pigs: 3–10 g
Dogs: 2–5 g
Cats and Rabbits: 0.5–2 g
Birds: 0.1–1.5 g

Cautions and Contraindications: None known

Side Effects: None known

Lycopus *Ze Lan* 泽兰

Original Reference: *Shen Nong Ben Cao Jing* (*Shen Nong's Materia Medica*, 1st century BCE) 神农本草经

Part Used: Aboveground part

Name:
Pharmaceutical: Lycopi Lucidi, Herba
Botanical: Lycopus lucidus Turcz. var. hirtus Regel
Common: Bugleweed
Wade-Giles: *Tse-Lan*
Translation: Marsh Orchid

Energy/Taste: Slightly warm, bitter, pungent, aromatic

Channel-Organ: Liver, Spleen

Actions:
1. Invigorate Blood and regulate the estrous cycle
2. Promote urination and reduce edema

Form and Preparation: Powder, decoction, or pill

Dosage:
Horses and Cattle: 15–60g
Llamas, Alpacas, Goats, Sheep, and Pigs: 3–10g
Dogs: 2–5g
Cats and Rabbits: 0.5–2g
Birds: 0.1–1.5g

Cautions and Contraindications:
1. Caution during pregnancy
2. Caution in patients without Blood Stasis

Side Effects: None known

Rosa *Yue Ji Hua* 月季花

Original Reference: *Ben Cao Gang Mu* (*Materia Medica Compendium*) by *Li Shi-Zhen* in 1590 本草纲目

Part Used: Flower

Name:
Pharmaceutical: Rosae chinensis Flos
Botanical: Rosa chinesis Jacq.
Common: Chinese tea rose flower
Wade-Giles: *Yueh-Chi-Hua*
Translation: Moon Seasonal Flower

Energy/Taste: Neutral, sweet, slightly bitter

Channel-Organ: Liver

Actions:
1. Invigorate Blood and regulate the estrous cycle
2. Soothe Liver *Qi* and reduce swelling

Form and Preparation: Powder, decoction, or pill

Dosage:
Horses and Cattle: 15–60g
Llamas, Alpacas, Goats, Sheep, and Pigs: 3–10g
Dogs: 2–5g
Cats and Rabbits: 0.5–2g
Birds: 0.1–1.5g

Cautions and Contraindications:
1. Caution during pregnancy
2. Caution in patients without Blood Stasis

Side Effects: None known

Eupolyphaga *Tu Bie Chong* 土鳖虫

Original Reference: *Shen Nong Ben Cao Jing* (*Shen Nong's Materia Medica*, 1st century BCE) 神农本草经

Part Used: Whole dried insect

Name:
Pharmaceutical: Eupolyphaga seu Opisthoplatia
Zoological: Eupolyphaga sinensis Walker
Common: Wingless Cockroach
Wade-Giles: *T'u-Pieh-Ch'ung*
Translation: Land Soft-Shelled Turtle Bug

Energy/Taste: Cold, salty, toxic

Channel-Organ: Liver

Actions:
1. Break up and drive out Blood Stasis
2. Renew sinews and heal bones

Form and Preparation: Powder, decoction, or pill

Dosage:
Horses and Cattle: 10–15g
Llamas, Alpacas, Goats, Sheep, and Pigs: 3–6g
Dogs: 1–3g
Cats and Rabbits: 0.2–0.5g
Birds: 0.1–1g

Cautions and Contraindications: Caution during pregnancy

Side Effects: May cause diarrhea

Strychnos *Ma Qian Zi* 马钱子

Original Reference: *Ben Cao Gang Mu* (*Materia Medica Compendium*) by *Li Shi-Zhen* in 1590 本草纲目

Part Used: Seed

Name:
Pharmaceutical: Strychni Semen
Botanical: Strychnos nux-vomica L.

Common: Nux-vomica
Wade-Giles: *Ma-Ch'ien-Tzu*
Translation: Equine Money Seed

Energy/Taste: Cold, bitter, extremely toxic

Channel-Organ: Liver, Spleen

Actions:
1. Disperse lumps and reduce swelling to promote healing
2. Unblock the Channels to stop pain
3. Resolve stubborn Wind-Damp

Form and Preparation: Powder, decoction, or pill

Dosage:
Horses and Cattle: 1.5–6 g
Llamas, Alpacas, Goats, Sheep, and Pigs: 0.2–1 g
Dogs: 0.1–0.3 g

Cautions and Contraindications:
1. Contraindicated during pregnancy or in weak patients
2. Extremely toxic
3. Use only when no other choices are available

Side Effects: May damage the central nervous system and cause dry mouth, dizziness, headache, restlessness, ataxia, convulsions, coma, or even death

Pyritum *Zi Ran Tong* 自然铜

Original Reference: *Lei Gong Pao Zhi Lun* (*Lei's Method of Preparing Drugs*) by *Lei Xiao*, 5th century 雷公炮炙论

Part Used: Mineral

Name:
Pharmaceutical: Pyritum
Common: Pyrite
Wade-Giles: *Tzu-Jan-T'ung*
Translation: Natural Copper

Energy/Taste: Neutral, pungent, bitter

Channel-Organ: Liver, Kidney

Actions:
1. Dispel Blood Stasis and stop pain
2. Join bones and sinews and promote healing

Form and Preparation: Powder, decoction, or pill

Dosage:
Horses and Cattle: 15–45 g
Llamas, Alpacas, Goats, Sheep, and Pigs: 3–10 g
Dogs: 2–5 g
Cats and Rabbits: 0.2–0.5 g
Birds: 0.2–1 g

Cautions and Contraindications:
1. Caution in *Yin* Deficiency with Heat or in Blood Deficiency

Side Effects: Like any mineral, long-term use is hard on the digestive system.

Sappan *Su Mu* 苏木

Original Reference: *Tang Ben Cao* (*Tang Materia Medica*) by *Su Jing* et al., *Tang* Dynasty 唐本草

Part Used: Central wood

Name:
Pharmaceutical: Sappan Lignum
Botanical: Caesalpinia sappan L.
Common: Sappan wood
Wade-Giles: *Su-Mu*
Translation: Sumatra Wood

Energy/Taste: Neutral, sweet, salty, pungent

Channel-Organ: Heart, Liver

Actions:
1. Invigorate Blood and promote healing
2. Dispel Stagnation and regulate the estrous cycle

Form and Preparation: Powder, decoction, or pill

Dosage:
Horses and Cattle: 15–30 g
Llamas, Alpacas, Goats, Sheep, and Pigs: 3–9 g
Dogs: 1–3 g
Cats and Rabbits: 0.2–0.5 g
Birds: 0.1–1 g

Cautions and Contraindications: Caution during pregnancy

Side Effects: None known

Artemisia *Liu Ji Nu* 刘寄奴

Original Reference: *Tang Ben Cao* (*Tang Materia Medica*) by *Su Jing* et al., *Tang* Dynasty 唐本草; also known as *Xin Xiu Ben Cao* (*Newly Revised Materia Medica*)

Part Used: Whole plant

Name:
Pharmaceutical: Artemisiae anomalae Herba
Botanical: Artemisia anomala S. Moore
Common: Anomala
Wade-Giles: *Liu-Chi-Nu*

Energy/Taste: Warm, bitter

Channel-Organ: Heart, Liver, Spleen

Actions:
1. Invigorate Blood and promote healing
2. Dispel Stagnation and stop bleeding
3. Promote digestion to resolve Food Stasis

Form and Preparation: Powder, decoction, or pill

Dosage:
Horses and Cattle: 15–60 g
Llamas, Alpacas, Goats, Sheep, and Pigs: 2–10 g
Dogs: 1–3 g

Cautions and Contraindications: Caution during pregnancy

Side Effects: None known

Hirudo *Shui Zhi* 水蛭

Original Reference: *Shen Nong Ben Cao Jing* (*Shen Nong's Materia Medica*, 1st century BCE) 神农本草经

Part Used: Whole leech; dried, pounded, or carbonized

Name:
Pharmaceutical: Hirudo seu Whitmania
Zoological: Hirudo nipponia Whitman, Whitmania pigra, W. aeranulata
Common: Leech
Wade-Giles: *Shui-Chih*
Translation: Water Bug

Energy/Taste: Neutral, salty, bitter, slightly toxic

Channel-Organ: Liver, Bladder

Actions:
1. Break up and drive out Deficiency and reduce immobile masses
2. Dissolve accumulations

Form and Preparation: Powder, decoction, or pill

Dosage:
Horses and Cattle: 15–30 g
Llamas, Alpacas, Goats, Sheep, and Pigs: 2–9 g
Dogs: 1–3 g
Cats and Rabbits: 0.2–1 g

Cautions and Contraindications:
1. Contraindicated during pregnancy
2. Contraindicated in patients with weakness without Deficiency

Side Effects: May cause fetal injury and abortion

Tabanus *Meng Chong* 虻虫

Original Reference: *Shen Nong Ben Cao Jing* (*Shen Nong's Materia Medica*, 1st century BCE) 神农本草经

Part Used: Dried female insect's body

Name:
Pharmaceutical: Tabanus
Zoological: Tabanus bivittatus Mats.
Common: Gadfly
Wade-Giles: *Meng-Ch'ung*
Translation: Gadfly Bug

Energy/Taste: Slightly cold, bitter, slightly toxic

Channel-Organ: Liver

Actions:
1. Break up and drive out Deficiency and reduce immobile masses
2. Dissolve accumulations

Form and Preparation: Powder, decoction, or pill

Dosage:
Horses and Cattle: 9–30 g
Llamas, Alpacas, Goats, Sheep, and Pigs: 2–9 g
Dogs: 0.5–3 g

Cautions and Contraindications: Caution during pregnancy

Side Effects: May cause abortion

Manitis *Chuan Shan Jia* 穿山甲

This substance is prohibited as is from an endangered species. The following information is just for educational purposes

Original Reference: *Ming Yi Bie Lu* (*Miscellaneous Records of Famous Physicians*) by *Tao Hong-Jing*, North and South Kingdoms (5th century) 名医别录

Part Used: Scales of the Pangolin scaly anteater

Name:
Pharmaceutical: Manitis Pentadectylae, Squama
Zoological: Manis pentadactyla
Common: Pangolin anteater scales
Wade-Giles: *Ch'uan-Shan-Chia*
Translation: Penetrate Mountain Scales

Energy/Taste: Cold, salty

Channel-Organ: Liver, Stomach

Actions:
1. Invigorate Blood and clear the Channels
2. Promote lactation
3. Reduce swelling and dispel pus

Form and Preparation: Powder, decoction, or pill

Dosage:
Horses and Cattle: 25–45 g
Llamas, Alpacas, Goats, Sheep, and Pigs: 3–10 g
Dogs: 2–5 g

Table 11.2. Herbs to invigorate Blood and Break Stasis: A quick overview and comparison.

Herbs	Special Actions	Common Characteristics
Herbs to invigorate Blood to relieve pain		
Chuan Xiong	Move *Qi*, expel Wind	Taste: Pungent
Yan Hu Suo	Move *Qi*, resolve Stagnation	Action: Move *Qi* and Blood, relieve pain
Yu Jin	Cool Blood and clear Heat in the Heart Relieve Jaundice and benefit Gallbladder	Indications:
Ru Xiang	Reduce swelling and regenerate tissue Move *Qi* to relax sinews and the Channels	*Qi*-Blood Stagnation Various pain conditions
Mo Yao	Reduce swelling and regenerate tissue	*Bi* syndrome
Jiang Huang	Promote *Qi* flow and eliminate Wind-Damp	
Wu Ling Zhi	Stop bleeding	
Xia Tian Wu	Relax sinews and eliminate Wind-Damp	
Herbs to invigorate Blood to regulate estrous cycle		
Dan Shen	Cool Blood and eliminate abscess	Taste: Pungent and bitter
Hong Hua	Remove stasis, unblock the Channels	Channels/Organs: Liver
Tao Ren	Moisten the intestines, purge stool, stop asthma	Action: Invigorate Blood, resolve Stagnation, Regulate estrous cycle
Wang Bu Liu Xing	Reduce swelling and promote lactation	Indications:
Chuan Niu Xi	Tonify Liver/Kidney to strengthen tendons/bones Promote urination, direct *Qi*-Blood down to stifle/rear limbs	Parturition *Qi*-Blood Stagnation Irregular cycle Lower *Jiao* Stagnation
Yi Mu Cao	Promote urination to reduce edema, clear Heat	
Ji Xue Teng	Tonify Blood, relax the tendons	
Ze Lan	Promote urination to reduce swelling	
Yue Ji Hua	Soothe Liver *Qi* and reduce swelling	
Herbs to invigorate Blood to promote healing		
Xue Jie	Stop pain and bleeding	Taste: Pungent, bitter, salty
Tu Bie Chong	Break up Stasis, renew sinews and join bones	Channels/organs: Liver, Kidney
Ma Qian Zi	Disperse lumps, resolve stubborn Wind-Damp	Action: Move Blood, promote healing, join bones, regenerate flesh
Zi Ran Tong	Dispel Blood Stasis, join bones and sinews	Indications:
Su Mu	Regulate the estrous cycle	Traumatic injuries
Liu Ji Nu	Stop bleeding, resolve Food Stasis	Fracture Soft tissue damage
Herbs to break up Stasis to shrink masses		
San Leng	Promote *Qi* circulation and stop pain	Taste: Pungent, potent, **toxic**
E Zhu	Move *Qi*, stop pain, dissolve accumulations	Action: Break up and drive out Blood Stasis, shrink masses
Shui Zhi	Dissolve accumulations	Indications:
Meng Chong	Dissolve accumulations	Any masses and growth
Chuan Shan Jia	Promote lactation, dispel pus	Accumulations

Cautions and Contraindications:

1. Prohibited during pregnancy
2. Caution in patients with *Qi* and Blood Deficiency
3. Caution in patients with skin ulcers

Side Effects: May cause abdominal fullness, indigestion, and damage to liver functions

SUMMARY OF HERBS THAT INVIGORATE BLOOD AND BREAK BLOOD STASIS

Table 11.2 summarizes and compares the herbs that invigorate Blood and break Blood Stasis.

REFERENCES

1. Chen JK, Chen TT. Chinese Medical Herbology and Pharmacology. City of Industry, CA: Art of Medicine Press, 2004.
2. Brinker FJ. The Toxicology of Botanical Medicines. Sandy, OR: Eclectic Medical Publications, 2000.
3. Duke JA. Handbook of Medicinal Herbs. New York: Chemical and Rubber Company Press, 2001.
4. Huang KC. The Pharmacology of Chinese Herbs, 2nd Edition. New York: Chemical and Rubber Company Press, 1999.

12 Herbs to Calm *Shen* 安神药

Huisheng Xie, Vanessa Preast, Min Su Kim

The *Shen* (Spirit or Mind) describes the external manifestation of the body's consciousness and psychological activities. The *Shen* rules the mind, mental activities, memory and sleep. It provides awareness, clarity, and inner peace. Animals with normal *Shen* express a calm outward appearance, mental alertness, inner peace, normal behavior, good memory, and normal sleeping Patterns. The Heart stores the *Shen* and the Liver hosts the *Hun* (*Yang* Soul or Ethereal Soul). *Hun* represents the psychological faculty of vision, imagination, clear direction, and capacity for justice. *Hun* is energized by the coming and going of the *Shen*. The *Hun* is a slightly more materialized psychospiritual substance than the *Shen*. Mental disorders occur when the *Hun* leaks (or escapes) out of the body.

A disorder of *Shen* is called *Shen* Disturbance or Disturbed *Shen*. *Shen* Disturbance includes signs such as irritability, palpitations, separation anxiety, restlessness, hyperactivity or mania, thunderstorm phobia, stall anxiety (horses), inability to concentrate, timidity, skittishness, excessive verbalization, insomnia, and nightmares accompanied by movement and vocalizations. Due to the link between the *Shen*, the Heart, and the Liver, an imbalance in one system can adversely affect the other. Thus, *Shen* Disturbance may result in Heart and Liver disorders just as Heart *Yin* and/or Blood Deficiency, Heart Excess Fire, Liver *Yang* Rising, and Phlegm can cause *Shen* Disturbance.

The Herbs to Calm the *Shen* are useful for treating *Shen* Disturbance. These herbs are divided into two categories based on their nature and actions: 1) Light Herbs to Nourish the Heart and Calm *Shen* and 2) Heavy Substances to Anchor and Settle *Shen*. Light Herbs to Nourish the Heart and Calm the *Shen* are very light herbs that calm *Shen* by nourishing *Yin* and Blood. Heavy Substances to Anchor and Settle the *Shen* are heavy because they contain mostly minerals and shells. In addition to settling the *Shen* disturbance, they sedate Liver *Yang* Rising (dizziness, anger, irritability), astringe leaky Lung *Qi* (cough and wheezing, difficult breathing), and redirect rebellious Stomach *Qi* (vomiting and nausea, hiccups and belching) downward.

Depending on the cause of the *Shen* Disturbance, the treatment involves different herbal combinations. For *Shen* Disturbance due to Heart *Yin* or/and Blood Deficiency, combine the Light Herbs with herbs to nourish *Yin* or Blood. To treat *Shen* Disturbance due to Liver *Yang* Rising or Fire, combine the Heavy Substances with herbs to pacify Liver *Yang*. When *Shen* Disturbance is due to Heart Excess Heat, combine either Light Herbs or Heavy Substances with herbs to clear Heart Fire. Combine either Light Herbs or Heavy Substances with herbs to transform Phlegm to treat *Shen* Disturbance due to Phlegm misting the Mind.

There are some cautions to consider when using these herbs. Heavy minerals tend to injure the Stomach and Spleen. Thus, the Heavy Substances should be used cautiously in patients with diarrhea or inappetence when they are used alone. Alternatively, the heavy minerals could be combined with herbs to tonify Stomach and Spleen *Qi*. Another concern is that some Heavy Substances may contain heavy metals. For example, Cinnabar contains mercury. For this reason, these herbs should not be used for a prolonged period of time.

LIGHT HERBS TO NOURISH THE HEART AND CALM *SHEN*

Ziziphus *Suan Zao Ren* 酸枣仁

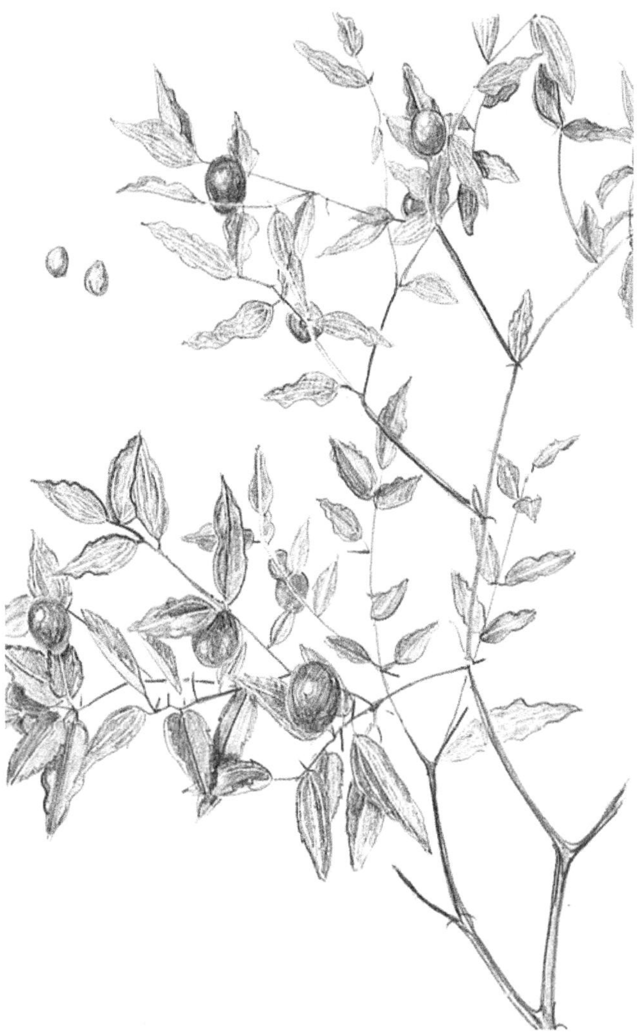

Original Reference: *Shen Nong Ben Cao Jing* (*Shen Nong's Materia Medica*, 1st century BCE) 神农本草经

Part Used: Seed

Name:
Pharmaceutical: Ziziphi Spinosae, Semen
Botanical: Ziziphus Spinosa
Common: Wild Jujube Seed
Wade-Giles: *Suan-Tsao-Jen*
Translation: Sour Date Seed

Energy/Taste: Neutral, sweet, sour

Channel-Organ: Heart, Liver, Spleen

Actions:
1. Nourish Heart *Yin* and Blood and calm *Shen*
2. Stop sweating
3. Tonify Liver

Form and Preparation: Powder, decoction, or pill

Dosage:
Horses and Cattle: 20–60 g
Llamas, Alpacas, Goats, Sheep, and Pigs: 3–10 g
Dogs: 2–5 g
Cats and Rabbits: 0.5–1 g
Birds: 0.2–2 g

Cautions and Contraindications: Caution in patients with Excess Fire conditions

Side Effects: May cause allergic skin reactions, chills, fever, or aching joints

Clinical Applications:
1. *Shen* Disturbance due to Heart Blood Deficiency
   Clinical signs: anxiety, barking at night or other abnormal behavior, palpitations, vivid dreaming, frightened or distracted easily
   Combine with: Angelica *Dang Gui*, Polygala *Yuan Zhi*, Schisandra *Wu Wei Zi*, Paeonia *Bai Shao*, Polygonum *He Shou Wu*, Longan *Long Yan Rou*
   Classical herbal formula: *Tian Wang Bu Xin Tang*
2. Liver and Heart Blood Deficiency
   Clinical signs: Anxiety, irritability or aggression, poor vision, palpitations, vivid dreaming
   Combine with: Angelica *Dang Gui*, Polygonum *He Shou Wu*, Longan *Long Yan Rou*, Lycium *Gou Qi Zi*, and Rehmannia *Shu Di*
   Classical herbal formula: *Suan Zao Ren Tang*
3. *Shen* Disturbance due to Heart and Liver *Yin* Deficiency with Heat
   Combine with: Anemarrhena *Zhi Mu* and Poria *Fu Shen*
4. Spontaneous day or night sweating due to *Qi* Deficiency
   Combine with: Ginseng *Ren Shen*, Ostrea *Mu Li*, Astragalus *Huang Qi*, and Schisandra *Wu Wei Zi*

History and Comments:
1. Ziziphus *Suan Zao Ren* is recommended for all cases of *Shen* Disturbance that also have *Yin* or Blood Deficiency, because the herb has both sedating and tonifying effects.
2. The effects of Ziziphus *Suan Zao Ren* are reinforced when combined with Polygala *Yuan Zhi* and Biota *Bai Zi Ren*.
3. The raw herb has a stronger calming effect than the prepared forms. Use the raw herb for restlessness due to Fire from Deficiency. Use the dry fried herb for Stomach and Spleen Deficiency or excessive sweating.
4. Good quality Ziziphus *Suan Zao Ren* is large, full, and purplish red.

5. *Suan Zao Ren* reduces renal hypertension and also reduces edema due to severe burns when combined with Schisandra *Wu Wei Zi* and taken internally.

Pharmaceutical Ingredients:[1–4]

1. Protein, saponin, flavonoids glycosides, vitamin C
2. Betulin, betulinic acid, jujuboside, jujubogenin, ebetinlaetone, ceanothic acid, alphitolic acid
3. Flavonoid glycosides (zivulgarin, spinosin, swertisin), sterol, vitamin

Biota *Bai Zi Ren* 柏子仁

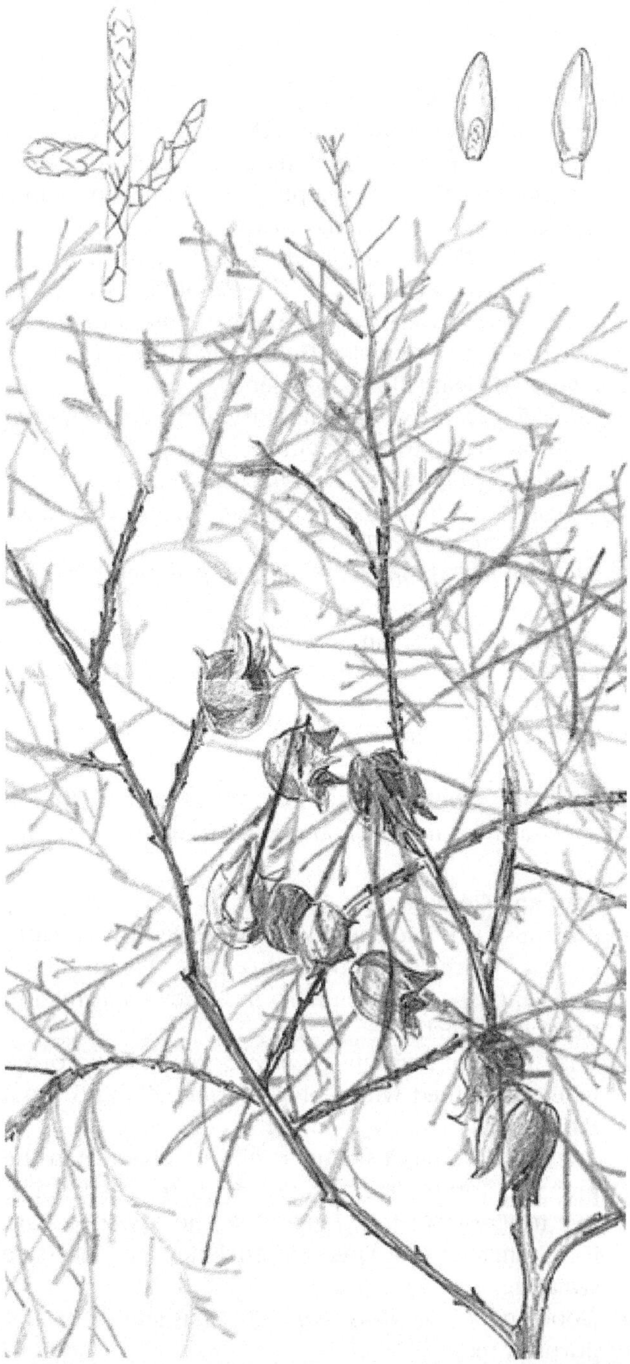

Original Reference: *Shen Nong Ben Cao Jing* (*Shen Nong's Materia Medica*, 1st century BCE) 神农本草经

Part Used: Seed

Name:
Pharmaceutical: Biotae Orientalis, Semen
Botanical: Biota Orientalis
Common: Biota seed
Wade-Giles: *Pai-Tzu-Jen*
Translation: Biota Seed

Energy/Taste: Neutral, sweet

Channel-Organ: Heart, Liver, Kidney, Large Intestine

Actions:

1. Nourish the Heart and calm the *Shen*
2. Moisten the Intestines to move stool

Form and Preparation: Powder, decoction, or pill

Dosage:
Horses and Cattle: 30–60 g
Camels: 40–80 g
Llamas, Alpacas, Goats, Sheep, and Pigs: 5–20 g
Dogs: 2–10 g
Cats and Rabbits: 1–2 g
Birds: 0.2–5 g

Cautions and Contraindications:

1. Caution in patients with excessive Phlegm Damp in the chest
2. May antagonize Chrysanthemum *Ju Hua*

Side Effects: May cause diarrhea

Clinical Applications:

1. Heart-Blood or *Yin* Deficiency
   Clinical signs: Restlessness, palpitations, anxiety
   Combine with: Ziziphus *Suan Zao Ren*, Polygala *Yuan Zhi*, and Schisandra *Wu Wei Zi*
   Classical herbal formula: *Tian Wang Bu Xin Tang*
2. Constipation due to Dryness in the Intestines
   Combine with: Armeniaca *Xing Ren*, Prunus *Yu Li Ren*, and Persica *Tao Ren*

History and Comments:

1. The effects of Biota *Bai Zi Ren* are reinforced when combined with Ziziphus *Suan Zao Ren* and Polygala *Yuan Zhi*.
2. To prepare Biota *Bai Zi Ren* for topical use, it is dry-fried until the oil seeps out.
3. Good quality Biota *Bai Zi Ren* is full, oily, and yellowish white.

Pharmaceutical Ingredients:[1–4]
1. Lipids, saponins
2. Essential oils (α-thujone, thujene, fenchone, pinene)
3. Fatty oils (palmitic acid, stearic acid, linoleic acid)
4. Flavonoids (cupressuflavone, apigenin)
5. β-sitosterol, tannin

Polygala *Yuan Zhi* 远志

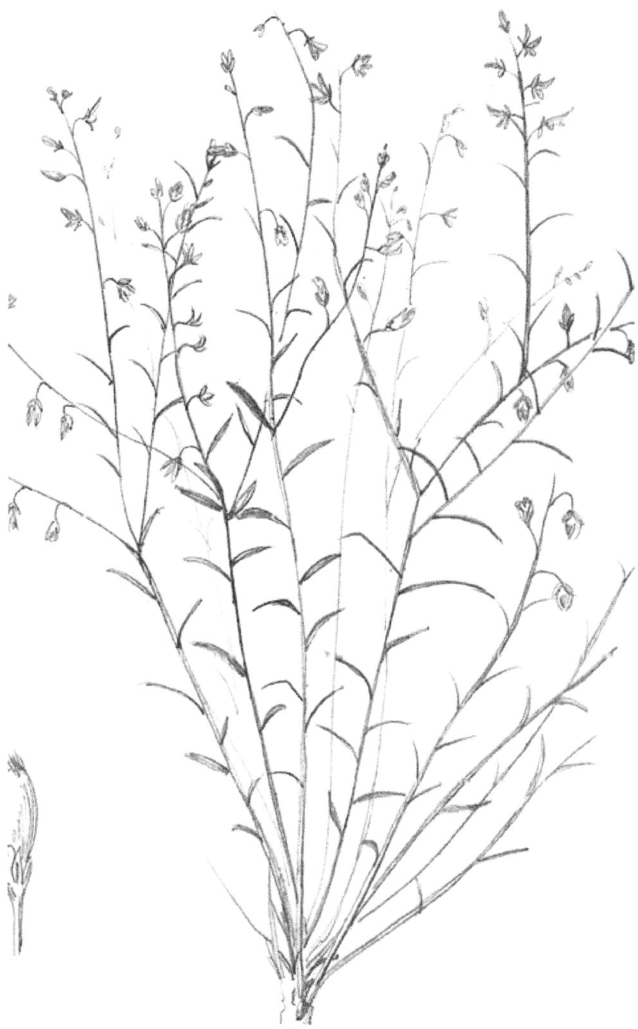

Original Reference: *Shen Nong Ben Cao Jing* (*Shen Nong's Materia Medica*, 1st century BCE) 神农本草经

Part Used: Root

Name:
Pharmaceutical: Polygalae Tenuifoliae, Radix
Botanical: Polygala Tenuifolia; P. Siberica
Common: Polygala root
Wade-Giles: *Yuan-Chih*
Translation: Profound Will

Energy/Taste: Slightly warm, bitter, pungent

Channel-Organ: Heart, Kidney, Lung

Actions:
1. Pacify the Heart and calm the *Shen*
2. Remove Phlegm and open orifices
3. Reduce abscesses and dissipate swelling

Form and Preparation: Powder, decoction, or pill

Dosage:
Horses and Cattle: 10–30 g
Camels: 45–90 g
Llamas, Alpacas, Goats, Sheep, and Pigs: 5–10 g
Dogs: 2–6 g
Cats and Rabbits: 0.5–1 g
Birds: 0.1–1.5 g

Cautions and Contraindications:
1. Caution during pregnancy or in patients with a gastric ulcer
2. May counteract Margarita *Zhen Zhu*

Side Effects: May cause allergic skin reactions, asthma, or numbness in the tongue and lower jaw

Clinical Applications
1. *Shen* Disturbance due to Heart *Yin* or Blood Deficiency
   Clinical signs: Anxiety, restlessness, palpitation, insomnia, poor memory
   Combine with: Poria *Fu Shen* and Ziziphus *Suan Zao Ren*
   Classical herbal formula: *Gui Pi Tang*
2. Turbid Phlegm obstructing the Heart
   Clinical signs: Mental disorder, epilepsy, unconsciousness
   Combine with: Buthus *Quan Xie*, Gastrodia *Tian Ma*
3. Cough with sticky thick Phlegm
   Combine with: Armeniaca *Xing Ren*, Platycodon *Jie Geng*, Fritillaria *Chuan Bei Mu*, and Glycerrhiza *Gan Cao*
4. Abscesses, boils, furuncles
   Combine with: Chrysanthemum *Ju Hua*, Taraxacum *Pu Gong Ying*, and Forsythia *Lian Qiao*

History and Comments:
1. To prepare a topical application for early-stage skin lesions, mix a decoction of Polygala *Yuan Zhi* with a little rice wine.
2. Good quality Polygala *Yuan Zhi* is thick and has a thick cortex.

Pharmaceutical Ingredients:[1–4]
1. Onjisaponin A, B, C, D, E, F, G; tenuigenin A, B; tenuifolin
2. Prosaponins, presenegenin, tenuidine, polygalitol, xanthones, cinnamic acid
3. 3, 4, 5-trimethoxycinnamic acid, 6-hydroxy-1, 2, 3, 7-tetramethoxyxanthone, 1, 2, 3, 7-pentamethoxyxanthone

HEAVY SUBSTANCES TO ANCHOR, SETTLE, AND CALM *SHEN*

Ostrea *Mu Li* 牡蛎

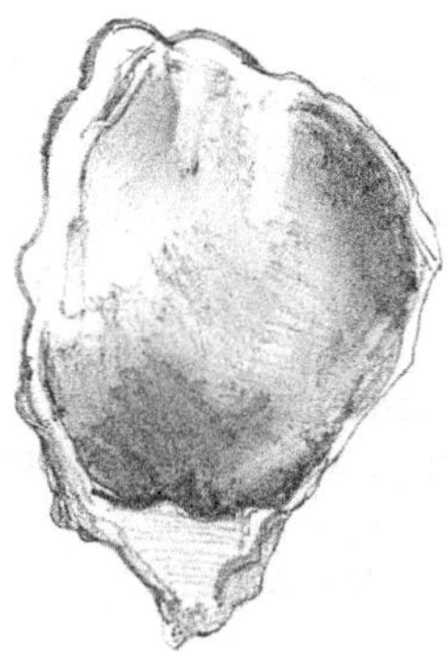

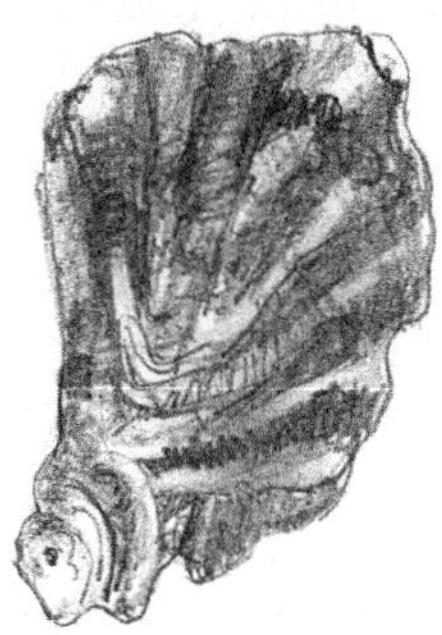

Original Reference: *Shen Nong Ben Cao Jing* (*Shen Nong's Materia Medica*, 1st century BCE) 神农本草经

Part Used: Oyster shell

Name:
Pharmaceutical: Ostreae, Concha
Zoological: Ostrea Gigas; O. Talienwhanensis
Common: Oyster Shell
Wade-Giles: *Mu-Li*
Translation: Oyster Shell

Energy/Taste: Slightly cold, salty

Channel-Organ: Liver, Kidney

Actions:
1. Pacify the Liver and Subdue *Yang*
2. Soften the hardness and dissipate nodules
3. Act as an astringent to bind the leakage

Form and Preparation: Powder, decoction, or pill

Dosage:
Horses and Cattle: 30–90 g
Llamas, Alpacas, Goats, Sheep, and Pigs: 5–30 g
Dogs: 2–10 g
Cats and Rabbits: 0.5–2 g
Birds: 0.2–3 g

Cautions and Contraindications:
1. Prohibited in patients who have high fevers without sweating
2. Adverse reactions occur when combined with Ephedra *Ma Huang*, Evodia *Wu Zhi Yu*, and Asarum *Xi Xin*.

Side Effects: Prolonged use injures the Stomach.

Clinical Applications:
1. Liver and Kidney *Yin* Deficiency with upward flaring *Yang*
   Clinical signs: Dizziness, vertigo, blurred vision, tinnitus, palpitation, hypertension, headache, irritability, insomnia
   Combine with: Draconis *Long Gu*, Testudinus *Gui Ban*, Paeonia *Bai Shao*
2. Hardness and masses due to Fire-Phlegm
   Clinical signs: Tumor masses, enlarged Liver and Spleen, scrofula nodules, swollen lymph nodes and goiter
   Combine with: Fritillaria *Zhe Bei Mu*, Scrophularia *Xuan Shen*, and Prunella *Xia Ku Cao*
   Classical herbal formula: *Xiao Lei Wan*
3. Spontaneous day or night sweating due to *Qi* Deficiency
   Combine with: Astragalus *Huang Qi*, Ephedra *Ma Huang Gen*, and Triticum *Fu Xiao Mai*
   Classical herbal formula: *Mu Li San*
4. Urinary leakage due to Kidney *Qi* Deficiency
   Combine with: Astraglaus *Sha Yuan Zi*, Euryale *Qian Shi*, Rosa *Jin Ying Zi*, and Nelumbo *Lian Xu*
   Classical herbal formula: *Jin Suo Gu Jing Wan*
5. Gastric ulceration with acid regurgitation
   Combine with: Haliotis *Shi Jue Ming*

History and Comments:
1. Ostrea *Mu Li* is available as a white shell that is crushed into a powder. Boil the powder for 20 minutes before adding the remaining herbs in the prescription.

2. The effects of Ostrea *Mu Li* are enhanced when combined with Draconis *Long Gu*.
3. Ostrea *Mu Li*, like most shells, has astringent qualities. It also has the ability to moisten Kidney *Yin*.
4. Charring Ostrea *Mu Li* enhances its astringency and hemostatic effects.
5. Good quality Ostrea *Mu Li* is large, white, and has a clean and shiny inner surface.
6. Ostrea *Mu Li* is used to treat excessive Stomach acid and ulcer. Dry-roasting enhances its effectiveness for this purpose.

Pharmaceutical Ingredients:[1–4]
1. Calcium carbonate, calcium phosphate, calcium sulfate, amino acid
2. Mg, Fe, Al, Na

Draconis *Long Gu* 龙骨

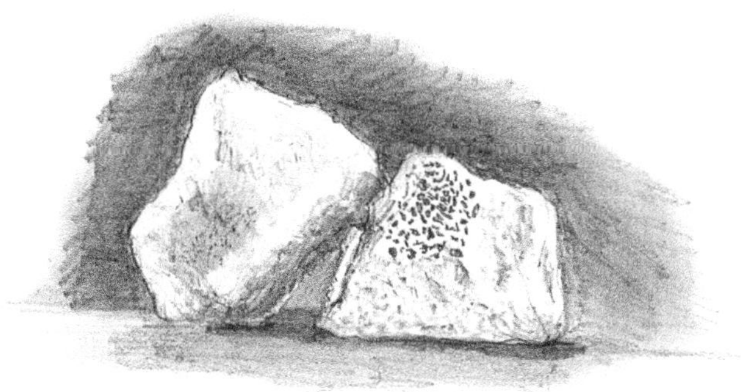

Original Reference: *Shen Nong Ben Cao Jing* (*Shen Nong's Materia Medica*, 1st century BCE) 神农本草经

Part Used: Fossilized bone

Name:
Pharmaceutical: Draconis, Os
Zoological: Stegodon Orientalis; Rhinoceros Sinensis
Common: Dragon Bone
Wade-Giles: *Lung-Ku*
Translation: Dragon Bone

Energy/Taste: Neutral, sweet, astringent

Channel-Organ: Heart, Liver, Kidney

Actions:
1. Settle *Shen* and pacify Spirit
2. Tranquilize the Liver and Subdue raised *Yang*
3. Act as an astringent to stabilize leakage

Form and Preparation: Powder, decoction, or pill

Dosage:
Horses and Cattle: 30–60 g
Llamas, Alpacas, Goats, Sheep, and Pigs: 3–8 g
Dogs: 2–5 g
Cats and Rabbits: 0.5–1 g
Birds: 0.2–2 g

Cautions and Contraindications:
1. Prohibited in Damp-Heat conditions
2. May counteract Gypsum *Shi Gao* and should not be mixed with fish

Side Effects: May cause allergic skin reactions or arrhythmia

Clinical Applications:
1. Liver and Kidney *Yin* Deficiency with upward flaring *Yang*
   Clinical signs: Dizziness, vertigo, blurred vision, tinnitus, palpitation, hypertension, headache, irritability, anxiety, insomnia
   Combine with: Ostrea *Mu Li*, Hematite *Dai Zhe Shi*, Paeonia *Bai Shao*, and Achyranthes *Niu Xi*
2. Urinary leakage due to Kidney *Qi* Deficiency
   Combine with: Ostrea *Mu Li*, Astragalus *Sha Yuan Zi*, and Euryale *Qian Shi*
   Classical herbal formula: *Jin Suo Gu Jing*
3. Palpitations, fright, anxiety, and insomnia
   Combine with: Ostrea *Mu Li*, Polygala *Yuan Zhi*, Ziziphus *Suan Zao Ren*, and Testudinis *Gui Ban*
4. Spontaneous day or night sweating due to *Qi* Deficiency
   Combine with: Astragalus *Huang Qi*, Ostrea *Mu Li* and Schisandra *Wu Wei Zi*
5. Topically as a powder for chronic, nonhealing sores and ulcerations
   Combine with: Alum *Ming Fan*

History and Comments:
1. Draconis *Long Gu* traditionally comes from the fossilized extremities and vertebrae of the prehistoric rhinoceros, which is found in the large burial grounds in central China. The traditional supply has diminished, so most Draconis available today comes from ox bones that have been synthetically treated to duplicate the effect of Draconis *Long Gu*.
2. Draconis and Ostrea are often combined to take advantage of their complementary effects. Ostrea

Mu Li has *Yin* nourishing effects, but Draconis *Long Gu* supports the *Yang*.
3. *Duan Long Gu* is burnt Draconis. It acts as an astringent for bleeding problems.
4. Stir-frying or baking Draconis *Long Gu* enhances its astringent effect.
5. Good quality Draconis *Long Gu* is hard and white with a strong, moisture-absorbing quality.
6. The sedating effect of *Long Gu* and *Mu Li* is due largely to their heavy calcium content.

Pharmaceutical Ingredients:[1–4]
1. Calcium carbonate, calcium phosphate, oxides of silicone
2. Fe, Al, Mg, uranium, Ca, titanium, P, Na, K, Zn

Polygonum *Ye Jiao Teng* 夜交藤

Original Reference: *Ben Cao Gang Mu* (*Materia Medica Compendium*) by *Li Shi-Zhen* in 1590 本草纲目

Part Used: Stem

Name:
Pharmaceutical: Caulis Polygoni Multiflori
Botanical: Polygonum Multiflorum
Common: Fleece flower
Wade-Giles: *Yeh-Chiao-T'eng*
Translation: Evening Friends Vine

Energy/Taste: Neutral, sweet

Channel-Organ: Heart, Liver

Actions:
1. Nourish the Heart and calm *Shen*
2. Dispel Wind and activate the Channels
3. Alleviate itching

Form and Preparation: Powder, decoction, or pill

Dosage:
Horses and Cattle: 20–60 g
Llamas, Alpacas, Goats, Sheep, and Pigs: 5–20 g
Dogs: 2–8 g
Cats and Rabbits: 0.5–1 g
Birds: 0.2–2 g

Cautions and Contraindications: None known

Side Effects: May cause allergic skin reactions, chills and fever

Poria *Fu Shen* 伏神

Original Reference: *Shen Nong Ben Cao Jing* (*Shen Nong*'s *Materia Medica*, 1st century BCE) 神农本草经

Part Used: Central part of the fungus

Name:
Pharmaceutical: Poriae Cocos, Sclerotium
Botanical: Poria Cocos
Common: Tuckahoe, Hoelen, Indian Bread
Wade-Giles: *Fu-Shen*
Translation: Poria Spirit

Energy/Taste: Neutral, sweet, bland

Channel-Organ: Heart, Spleen

Actions:
1. Pacify the Heart and calm *Shen*
2. Tonify the Spleen and benefit urination

Form and Preparation: Powder, decoction, or pill

Dosage:
Horses and Cattle: 20–60 g
Llamas, Alpacas, Goats, Sheep, and Pigs: 5–15 g
Dogs: 2–5 g
Cats and Rabbits: 0.5–1 g
Birds: 0.2–2 g

Cautions and Contraindications: None known

Side Effects: May cause polyuria

Albizzia *He Huan Pi* 合欢皮

Original Reference: *Shen Nong Ben Cao Jing* (*Shen Nong*'s *Materia Medica*, 1st century BCE) 神农本草经

Part Used: Bark

Name:
Pharmaceutical: Albizziae Julibrissin, Cortex
Botanical: Albizzia Julibrissin; A. Kalkora
Common: Albizzia Bark
Wade-Giles: *Ho-Huan-Pi*
Translation: Collective Happiness Bark

Energy/Taste: Neutral, sweet

Channel-Organ: Heart, Liver, Lung

Actions:
1. Calm *Shen* and relieve depression
2. Invigorate Blood and eliminate swelling

Form and Preparation: Powder, decoction, or pill

Dosage:
Horses and Cattle: 20–60 g
Llamas, Alpacas, Goats, Sheep, and Pigs: 5–15 g

Dogs: 2–5 g
Cats and Rabbits: 0.5–1 g
Birds: 0.2–2 g

Cautions and Contraindications: None known

Side Effects: None known

Succinum *Hu Po* 琥珀

Original Reference: *Ming Yi Bie Lu* (*Miscellaneous Records of Famous Physicians*) by *Tao Hong-Jing*, North and South Kingdoms (5th century) 名医别录

Part Used: Resin

Name:
Pharmaceutical: Succinum
Botanical: Pinus Spp.
Common: Amber
Wade-Giles: *Hu-P'o*
Translation: Amber

Energy/Taste: Neutral, sweet

Channel-Organ: Bladder, Heart, Liver

Actions:
1. Tranquilize and settle *Shen*
2. Invigorate Blood and release Stagnation
3. Promote urination and reduce swelling

Form and Preparation: Powder, decoction, or pill

Dosage:
Horses and Cattle: 10–15 g
Llamas, Alpacas, Goats, Sheep, and Pigs: 1–3 g
Dogs: 0.5–2 g

Cautions and Contraindications: Contraindicated in *Yin*-Deficient patients with heat signs

Side Effects: None known

Magnetite *Ci Shi* 磁石

Original Reference: *Shen Nong Ben Cao Jing* (*Shen Nong's Materia Medica*, 1st century BCE) 神农本草经

Part Used: Rock

Name:
Pharmaceutical: Magnetitum
Common: Magnetite
Wade-Giles: *Tz'u-Shih*
Translation: Magnetic Stone

Energy/Taste: Cold, salty

Channel-Organ: Heart, Kidney, Liver

Actions:
1. Tranquilize and settle *Shen*
2. Anchor ascendant Liver *Yang*, improve hearing and vision
3. Aid Kidney in grasping *Qi* to stop asthma

Form and Preparation: Powder, decoction, pill, or topical application

Dosage:
Horses and Cattle: 30–60 g
Llamas, Alpacas, Goats, Sheep, and Pigs: 5–24 g
Dogs: 1–3 g
Cats and Rabbits: 0.5–1 g
Birds: 0.2–2 g

Cautions and Contraindications: Caution in patients with Spleen *Qi* Deficiency

Side Effects: Long-term use or overdose causes indigestion.

Cinnabaris *Zhu Sha* 朱砂

Original Reference: *Shen Nong Ben Cao Jing* (*Shen Nong's Materia Medica*, 1st century BCE) 神农本草经

Part Used: Minera

Name:
Pharmaceutical: Cinnabaris
Common: Cinnabar Mineral
Wade-Giles: *Chu-Sha*
Translation: Vermillion Seed

Energy/Taste: Slightly cold, sweet, toxic

Channel-Organ: Heart

Actions:
1. Calm down the Spirit and *Shen*
2. Clear Heat from the Heart

Form and Preparation: Powder, decoction, pill, or topical application

Dosage:
Horses and Cattle: 3–6 g
Llamas, Alpacas, Goats, Sheep, and Pigs: 0.2–1.5 g
Dogs: 0.05–0.45 g

Cautions and Contraindications:
1. Do not overdose when administering orally.
2. Avoid long-term use to prevent mercury poisoning.

Table 12.1. Herbs to calm *Shen*: A quick overview and comparison.

Herbs	Special Actions	Common Characteristics
Light Herbs to Nourish Heart and Calm *Shen*		
Suan Zao Ren	Stop sweating, tonify Liver	Action: Moisten Heart and Liver, nourish *Yin* and Blood and calm *Shen*
Bai Zi Ren	Moisten the Intestines to move stool	
Yuan Zhi	Remove Phlegm and open orifices, reduce abscesses and dissipate swelling	Indication: *Shen* Disturbance due to *Yin* or/and Blood Deficiency, Heart and Spleen Deficiency, Heart-Kidney disharmony
Ye Jiao Teng	Dispel Wind, alleviate itching	
Fu Shen	Tonify Spleen, benefit urination	
He Huan Pi	Invigorate Blood and eliminate swelling	
Heavy Substances to Anchor and Settle *Shen*		
Mu Li	Pacify the Liver and subdue *Yang*, soften hardness and dissipate nodules, act as an astringent to bind the leakage	Parts used: Minerals or rocks Action: Tranquilize and settle Heart and *Shen* Indication: *Shen* Disturbance due to Phlegm-Fire, Liver *Qi* Stagnation with Heat, Excessive Heart Heat
Long Gu	Tranquilize the Liver and subdue raised *Yang*, act as an astringent to stabilize leakage	
Hu Po	Invigorate Blood and release Stagnation, promote urination and reduce swelling	
Ci Shi	Improve hearing and vision, aid kidney in grasping *Qi* to stop asthma	
Zhu Sha	Clear Heat from the Heart	

3. Contraindicated in patients with poor Liver and Kidney functions

Side Effects: May damage the nervous system and cause mercury poisoning, which may result in urine retention, edema, coma, convulsions, hypotension, renal failure, or death

SUMMARY OF HERBS THAT CALM *SHEN*

Table 12.1 summarizes and compares the herbs that Calm *Shen*.

REFERENCES

1. Chen JK, Chen TT. Chinese Medical Herbology and Pharmacology. City of Industry, CA: Art of Medicine Press, 2004.
2. Brinker FJ. The Toxicology of Botanical Medicines. Sandy, OR: Eclectic Medical Publications, 2000.
3. Duke JA. Handbook of Medicinal Herbs. New York: Chemical and Rubber Company Press, 2001.
4. Huang KC. The Pharmacology of Chinese Herbs, 2nd Edition. New York: Chemical and Rubber Company Press, 1999.

13 Herbs to Pacify the Liver and Extinguish Endogenous Wind 平肝熄风药

Huisheng Xie, Vanessa Preast, Min Su Kim

Herbs that pacify the Liver and extinguish Endogenous Wind primarily consist of animal by-products, shells, or bugs. Shells are believed to anchor the *Yang*, and worms (including insects and bugs) are said to gather and subdue Wind. These herbs are divided into three subcategories: 1) herbs to pacify the Liver and tranquilize *Yang*, 2) herbs to pacify the Liver and brighten the eyes, and 3) herbs to extinguish Internal Wind and stop spasm. All these herbs exhibit their effects by entering the Liver Channel (see Table 13.1, later in this chapter). The herbs that pacify the Liver and tranquilize *Yang* are cold or cool herbs that treat Liver *Yang* Rising and clinical signs, including dizziness or vertigo, hyperactivity, hypertension, red eyes, and otitis. *Huang Di Nei Jing* explains that "all Wind-related, dizziness-like clinical signs are from the Liver." Thus, treating the Liver will help clear the clinical signs.

The herbs that pacify the Liver and brighten the eyes are very similar to the herbs that pacify the Liver and tranquilize *Yang*. These herbs, however, have greater effect on eye disorders.

The herbs to extinguish the Internal Wind and stop spasm may be cold or warm. They are used to treat tremors, convulsions, spasm, and seizures. Internal Wind can be caused by 1) extreme Heat or excessive Heat, 2) *Yin* and/or Blood Deficiency, 3) Liver *Yang* Rising, and 4) Phlegm. Depending on the patient's additional clinical signs, these herbs may be combined with 1) herbs to tonify Blood and *Yin*, 2) herbs to clear Heat, 3) herbs to clear Phlegm, or 4) herbs to calm *Shen*.

Haliotis *Shi Jue Ming* 石决明

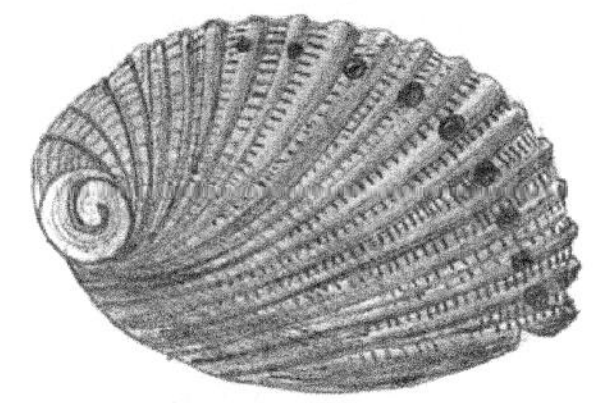

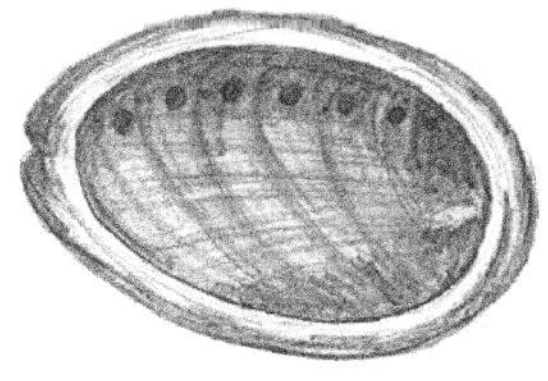

Original Reference: *Ming Yi Bie Lu* (*Miscellaneous Records of Famous Physicians*) by *Tao Hong-Jing*, North and South Kingdoms (5th century) 名医别录

Part Used: Shell

Name:
Pharmaceutical: Haliotidis, Concha
Zoological: Haliotis Diversicolor
Common: Haliotis Shell
Wade-Giles: *Shih-Chueh-Ming*
Translation: Stone Decisive Brightness

Table 13.1. Herbs to pacify the Liver and Extinguish Wind: A quick overview and comparison.

Herbs	Special Actions	Common Characteristics
Herbs to pacify the Liver and tranquilize *Yang*		
Shi Jue Ming	Clear Heat from the Liver and brighten the eyes	Energy: Cool or Cold
Bai Ji Li	Brighten the eyes, expel Wind and stop itching	Action: Pacify the Liver, subdue the rising Liver *Yang*
Zhen Zhu Mu	Calm the *Shen* and brighten the eyes	
Zhen Zhu	Calm the *Shen* and brighten the eyes Promote healing and generate flesh	Indications: Liver *Yang* Rising, dizziness or vertigo, irritability, hyperactivity, hypertension, blurred vision
Dai Zhe Shi	Conduct rebellious *Qi* downward Cool Blood and stop bleeding	
Luo Bu Ma	Clear Heat and benefit urination	
Herbs to pacify the Liver and brighten the eyes		
Jue Ming Zi	Moisten intestines and move stool	Action: Pacify Liver, brighten the eyes, eliminate superficial visual obstruction
Qing Xiang Zi	Reduce corneal opacity, clear Wind-Heat	
Mi Meng Hua	Brighten eyes and reduce corneal opacity	Indications: Eye problems due to Liver Wind Heat or Liver Fire flaring up, ocular opacity
Mu Zei	Disperse Wind-Heat, stop bleeding	
Gu Jing Cao	Disperse Wind-Heat, eliminate visual opacity	
Ye Ming Sha	Disperse Blood Stasis and reduce accumulations	
Herbs to extinguish Endogenous Wind and stop spasm and seizure		
Tian Ma	Pacify the Liver and subdue the raised *Yang* Invigorate the Channels and stop pain	Action: Extinguish Internal Wind and stop spasm and seizure
Gou Teng	Clear Heat and pacify the Liver	Indications: Tremors, convulsions, spasm, seizures
Di Long	Stop asthma and promote urination Activate the Channels	
Jiang Can	Expel Wind and stop pain Dispel toxin and disperse nodules	
Man Jing Zi	Benefit eyes and act as a transporter to the head	
Quan Xie	Dissipate nodules, activate the Channels	
Wu Gong	Dispel toxin and dissipate Nodules Activate the Channels and relieve pain	
Ling Yang Jiao	Pacify the Liver and anchor *Yang* Clear Heat, brighten eyes, release toxins	

Energy/Taste: Cold, salty

Channel-Organ: Liver

Actions:
1. Pacify the Liver and subdue *Yang*
2. Clear Heat from the Liver and brighten the eye

Form and Preparation: Powder, decoction, or pill

Dosage:
Horses and Cattle: 30–60 g
Camels: 45–100 g
Llamas, Alpacas, Goats, Sheep, and Pigs: 10–25 g
Dogs: 2–5 g
Cats and Rabbits: 0.5–2 g
Birds: 0.2–2 g

Cautions and Contraindications: May counteract Inula *Xuan Fu Hua*

Side Effects: May cause diarrhea

Clinical Application
1. Liver *Yang* Rising due to Liver and Kidney *Yin* Deficiency
   Clinical signs: Headache, hypertension, dizziness, vertigo, blurred vision, hyperactivity, Shen disturbance
   Combine with: Ostrea *Mu Li*, Paeonia *Bai Shao*, Testudinus *Gui Ban Jiao*, Uncaria *Gou Teng*, Chrysanthemum *Ju Hua*, and Prunella *Xia Ku Cao*

2. Uveitis due to Liver Fire Flaring Up
   Clinical signs: Blurred Vision; red, swollen, and painful eyes
   Combine with: Chrysanthemum *Ju Hua* and Cassia *Jue Ming Zi*
   Classical herbal formula: *Jue Ming San* (Haliotis Powder)

History and Comments:
1. Cook Haliotis *Shi Jue Ming* for 30 minutes before adding other herbs.
2. Commonly used for treatment of headaches behind the eyes, cataracts, and glaucoma

Pharmaceutical Ingredients:[1–4] Calcium carbonate, Magnesium (Mg), Iron (Fe), Silica, Phosphate, 20 different amino acids

Tribulus *Bai Ji Li* 白蒺藜 (刺蒺藜)

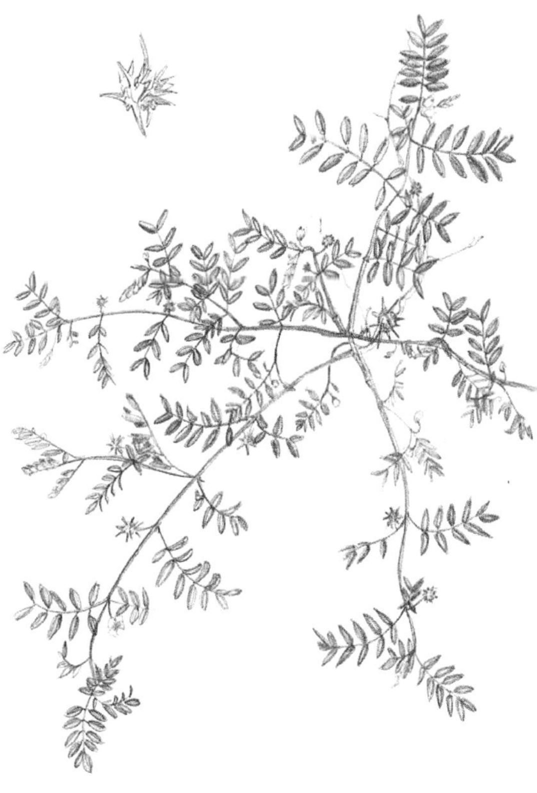

Original Reference: *Shen Nong Ben Cao Jing* (*Shen Nong's Materia Medica*, 1st century BCE) 神农本草经

Part Used: Ripe fruit

Name:
Pharmaceutical: Tribuli Terrestris, Fructus
Botanical: Tribulus Terrestis
Common: Tribulus Fruit
Wade-Giles: *Pai-Chi-Li*
Translation: White Tribulus
Alternative: *Ci Ji Li*

Energy/Taste: Slightly warm, bitter, pungent

Channel-Organ: Liver

Actions:
1. Pacify the Liver and smooth the Liver
2. Subdue the raised Liver *Yang*, brighten the eyes
3. Expel Wind and stop itching

Form and Preparation: Powder, decoction, or pill

Dosage:
Horses and Cattle: 20–45 g
Llamas, Alpacas, Goats, Sheep, and Pigs: 5–18 g
Dogs: 2–5 g
Cats and Rabbits: 0.5–1 g
Birds: 0.1–1.5 g

Cautions and Contraindications: Caution during pregnancy

Side Effects: May cause fatigue, narcolepsy, dizziness, nausea, vomiting, palpitation, pulmonary edema, and dyspnea

Clinical Application
1. Liver *Yang* Rising
   Clinical signs: Inflamed eyes, hypertension, irritability, dizziness, vertigo, distention and pain in the head
   Combine with: Uncaria *Gou Teng*, Chrysanthemum *Ju Hua*, and Paeonia *Bai Shao*
2. Liver *Qi* Stagnation
   Clinical signs: Aggression, sensitivity on chest and hypochondria area, and obstructed lactation
   Combine with: Bupleurum *Chai Hu*, Chrysanthemum *Ju Hua*, Citrus *Qing Pi*, and Cyperus *Xiang Fu*
3. Hives or itching due to Wind-Heat
   Combine with: Schizonopeta *Jing Jie*, Cicada *Chuan Tui*, and Ledebouriella *Fang Feng*

History and Comments: Tribulus *Bai Ji Li* is effective for genital inflammation.

Pharmaceutical Ingredients:[1–4]

1. Kaempferol, kaempferol-3-glycosides, kaempferol-3-rutinose, tribuloside, furostanol bisglycoside
2. Alkaloids (harmane, harmine)

Cassia *Jue Ming Zi* 决明子

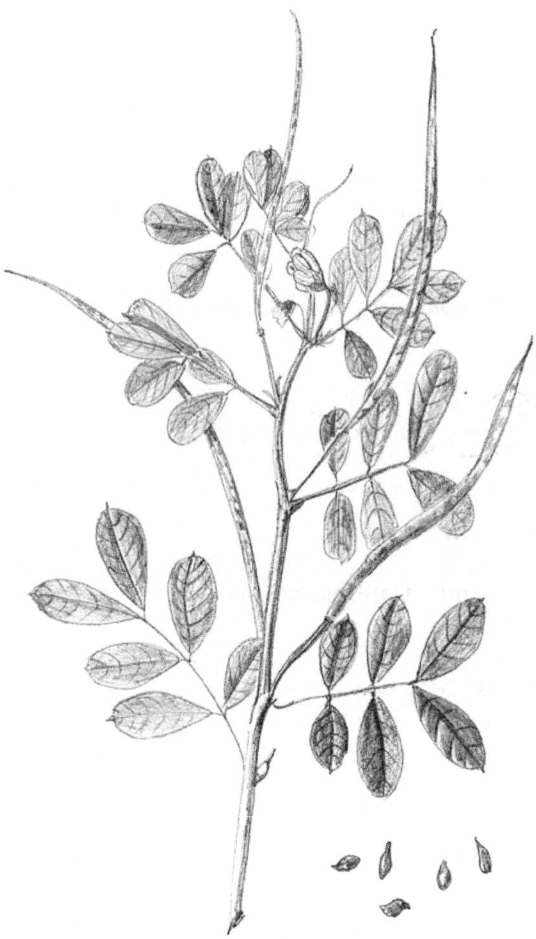

Original Reference: *Shen Nong Ben Cao Jing* (*Shen Nong's Materia Medica*, 1st century BCE) 神农本草经

Part Used: Seed

Name:
Pharmaceutical: Cassiae, Semen
Botanical name: Cassia tora; C. obtusifolia
Common: Cassia seed
Wade-Giles: *Chueh-Ming-Tzu*
Translation: Decisive Bright Seed

Energy/Taste: Slightly cold, sweet, bitter, salty

Channel-Organ: Liver, Large Intestine

Actions:

1. Clear Liver Heat and brighten the eyes
2. Moisten intestines and move stool

Form and Preparation: Powder, decoction, or pill

Dosage:
Horses and Cattle: 20–60 g
Llamas, Alpacas, Goats, Sheep, and Pigs: 5–15 g
Dogs: 3–8 g
Cats and Rabbits: 0.5–2 g
Birds: 0.2–5 g

Cautions and Contraindications: Do not combine with Cannabis *Huo Ma Ren*

Side Effects: May cause diarrhea

Clinical Application

1. Acute eye problems due to Liver Fire Flaring Upward or Liver *Yang* Rising
   Clinical signs: Red, swollen, painful eyes, photophobia, dizziness, vertigo, blurred vision, glaucoma, headache
   Combine with: Chrysanthemum *Ju Hua*, Morus *Sang Ye*, Gardenia *Zhi Zi*, Vitex *Man Jing Zi* and Prunella *Xia Ku Cao*
2. Constipation:
   Use alone, or combine with: Angelica *Dang Gui*, Lophatherum *Dan Zhu Ye* and Trichosanthes *Gua Lou Ren*
3. Chronic eye problems due to Kidney and Liver *Yin* Deficiency
   Clinical signs: Blurred vision, glaucoma, and cataract
   Combine with: Ligustrum *Nü Zhen Zi*, Prunella *Xia Ku Cao*, and Lycium *Gou Qi Zi*

History and Comments:

1. Cassia *Jue Ming Zi* is used both as a general eye and vision tonic and as a treatment for various eye and vision problems.
2. *Jue Ming Zi* more effectively clears Liver Fire and benefits the Kidneys than does Chrysanthemum *Ju Hua*; however, Chrysanthemum *Ju Hua* more effectively clears the Liver and disperses Wind Heat.
3. *Jue Ming Zi* is beneficial for lowering blood cholesterol and blood pressure.

Pharmaceutical Ingredients:[1–4]

1. Chrysophanol, emodin, aloe-emodin, rhein, modinan, physcion, obtusin, aurantio-obtusin, chrysobtusin, torachrsone, rubrofusarin, norrubrofusarin, toralactone
2. Palmitic acid, stearic acid, oleic acid
3. Fe, Mn, Cu, Zn, Ni, Co, Vitamin A

Gastrodia *Tian Ma* 天麻

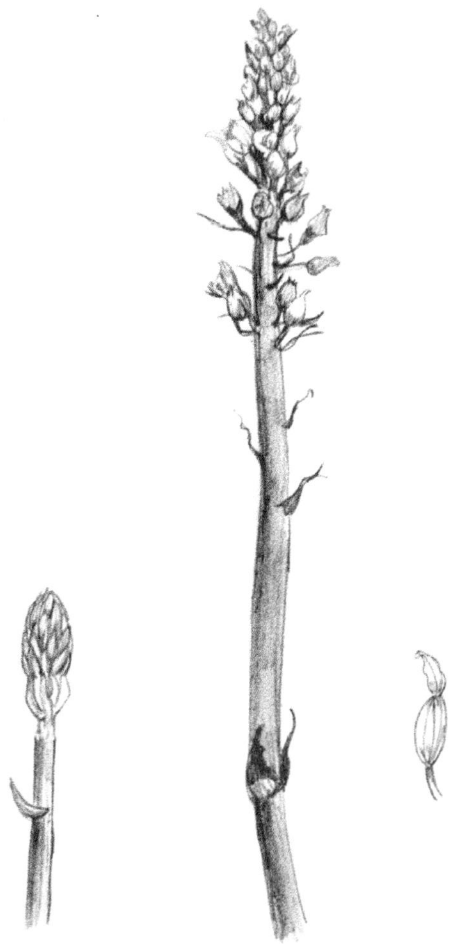

a

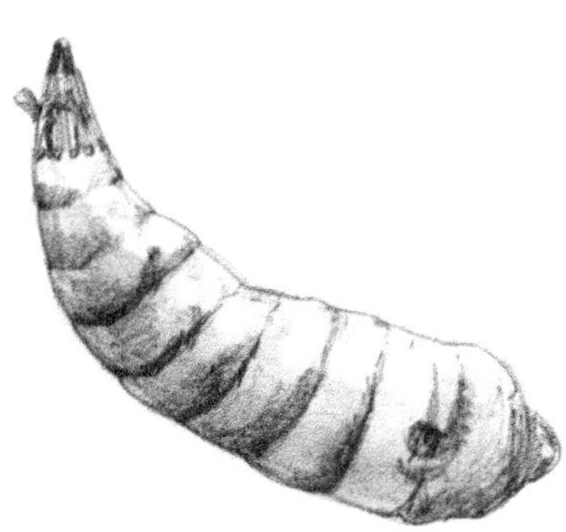

b

Original Reference: *Shen Nong Ben Cao Jing* (*Shen Nong's Materia Medica*, 1st century BCE) 神农本草经

Part Used: Tuber, rhizome

Name:
Pharmaceutical: Gastrodiae Elatae, Rhizoma
Botanical: Gastrodia Elata
Common: Gastrodia Tuber
Wade-Giles: *T'ien-Ma*
Translation: Heavenly Hemp

Energy/Taste: Neutral, sweet

Channel-Organ: Liver

Actions:
1. Eliminate Endogenous Wind and stop spasm and seizure
2. Pacify the Liver and subdue the raised *Yang*
3. Invigorate the Channels and stop pain

Form and Preparation: Powder, decoction, or pill

Dosage:
Horses and Cattle: 20–45 g
Llamas, Alpacas, Goats, Sheep, and Pigs: 5–10 g
Dogs: 1–3 g
Cats and Rabbits: 0.5–1 g
Birds: 0.1–1.5 g

Cautions and Contraindications: None known

Side Effects: May cause allergic skin reactions

Clinical Application
1. Spasm and convulsion due to Internal Stirring of Liver Wind
   Combine with: Uncaria *Gou Teng* And Buthus *Quan Xie*
2. Seizure, headache, and dizziness due to Liver *Yang* Rising
   Combine with: Uncaria *Gou Teng*, Scutellaria *Huang Qin*, and Achyranthes *Niu Xi*
   Classical herbal formula: *Tian Ma Gou Teng Yin*
3. Pain or numbness of limbs due to Wind Damp obstruction
   Combine with: Olibanum *Ru Xiang*, Buthus *Quan Xie*, Gentiana *Qin Jiao* and Notopterygium *Qiang Huo*

History and Comments:
1. Gastrodia *Tian Ma* has been used as an herbal medicine in China for two thousand years. One winter long ago, Shen Long traveled to a mountain to collect medicinal herbs. While searching for plants, he tripped and fell. As he stood back up, he glimpsed

an unusual plant growing among the grasses. Shen Long thought the plant looked like an arrow; it had a dark red stalk and no green leaves. He dug up the plant and ate its huge, dark yellow root bulb. He discovered that this herb could cure many diseases, so he named the herb "Magical Arrow" or "Red Arrow" due to the plant's appearance. Later, that herb was called *Tian Ma* (Heavenly Hemp) to reflect its strong, almost magical calming effects.

2. Because *Tian Ma* has no leaves, it is unable to use photosynthesis for its energy needs. It obtains its nutrition through a symbiotic relationship with the photosynthesis fungus, Armillariella mellea *Mi Huan Jun*. The highest-quality *Tian Ma* is collected during winter.
3. Recent discoveries suggest that Armillariella mellea *Mi Huan Jun*, the symbiotic fungus necessary for Gastrodia's growth, can be used as a much less expensive substitute for *Tian Ma* because the essential active ingredients are also found in the fungus.

Pharmaceutical Ingredients:[1–4]
1. Gastrodin,gastrodioside(p-hydroxybezol),4-hydroxybenzyl alcohol, daucosterol, vanillyl alcohol, vanillin, β-sitosterol
2. Succinic acid, citric acid, palmitic acid, p-hydroxybezaldehyde, alkaloids

Uncaria *Gou Teng* 钩藤

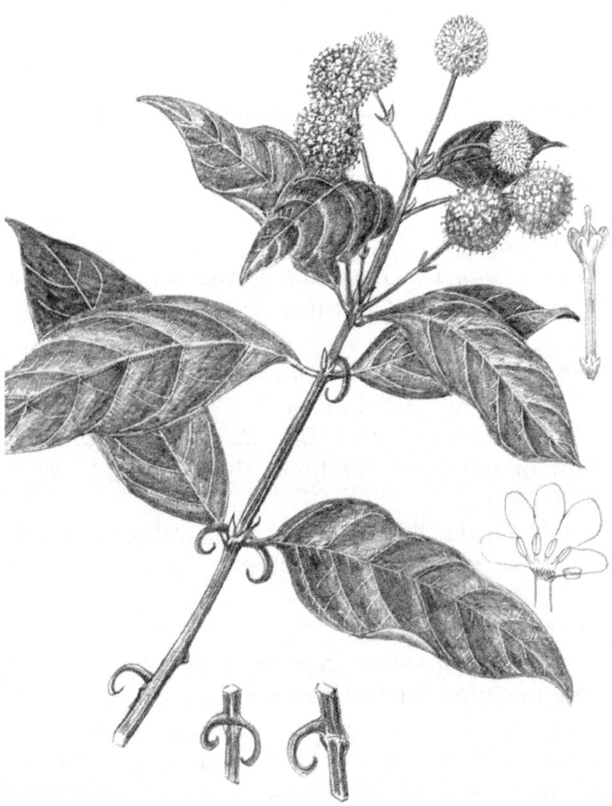

Original Reference: *Ming Yi Bie Lu* (*Miscellaneous Records of Famous Physicians*) by *Tao Hong-Jing*, North and South Kingdoms (5th century) 名医别录

Part Used: Stem with hooks

Name:
Pharmaceutical: Uncariae, Ramulus Cum Uncis
Botanical: Uncaria Rhynchophylia
Common: Uncaria Stem
Wade-Giles: *Kou-T'eng*
Translation: Hook Vine

Energy/Taste: Cool, sweet

Channel-Organ: Liver, Pericardium

Actions:
1. Eliminate Endogenous Wind and stop spasm and seizure
2. Clear Heat and pacify the Liver

Form and Preparation: Powder, decoction, or pill

Dosage:
Horses and Cattle: 30–60 g
Llamas, Alpacas, Goats, Sheep, and Pigs: 5–15 g
Dogs: 2–8 g
Cats and Rabbits: 0.5–1 g
Birds: 0.2–2.5 g

Cautions and Contraindications: None known

Side Effects: May cause bradycardia, dizziness, and allergic skin reactions in patients with hypertension

Clinical Application
1. Seizure or spasm due to Stirring Up of Liver Wind
   Combine with: Chrysanthemum *Ju Hua*, Haliotis *Shi Jue Ming* and Buthus *Quan Xie*
2. Dizziness and headache due to Liver *Yang* Rising
   Combine with: Scutellaria *Huang Qin*, Prunella *Xia Ku Cao*, Haliotis *Shi Jue Ming*, and Chrysanthemum *Ju Hua*

History and Comments:
1. In the Chinese literary masterpiece, *A Dream of Red Mansions* (*Hong-Lou-Meng*), there is a scene in which the character Ms. Xia was so angry that she yelled at her mother-in-law, Mrs. Xue, at the dinner table. This upset Mrs. Xue, and she later felt great pain in her right side. Mrs. Xue's intelligent and well-educated daughter Xue Bao Cai cooked ounces

of *Gou Teng* into a concentrated herbal tea and immediately served it to her mother. Soon after, Mrs. Xue felt calmer and even took a short nap. Her Liver *Qi* and temper were soothed.
2. *Gou Teng* was recognized as a "pediatric herb" because of its light property. It is widely used for treating seizures.
3. *Gou Teng* is used to treat hypertension because it is "Soothing to Liver *Qi*." *Gou Teng* lowers blood pressure. After administering a decoction of *Gou Teng* for 2–7 days, the patients' blood pressure started to decrease. The optimal effects were achieved at day 10 of treatment. As the blood pressure decreased, the associated clinical signs such as headache, dizziness, vertigo, shortness of breath, or insomnia gradually disappeared. This herb is good for early stages of hypertension.

Pharmaceutical Ingredients:[1–4]
1. Indole alkaloids (rhynchophylline, iso-rhynchophylline)
2. Corynoxeine, iso-corynoxeine, corynoneine, isocorynoneine, corynantheine, dihydrocorynatheine, isocorynantheine, hirsutine, hirsuteine
3. Flavonoids (hyperin, trifolin)

Margarita *Zhen Zhu Mu* 珍珠母

Original Reference: *Ben Cao Tu Jing* (*Illustrated Classic of Materia Medica*) by *Su Song* and *Su Zi-rong* in 1061 本草图经

Part Used: Ignited or charred shell

Name:
Pharmaceutical: Margaritifera, Concha
Zoological: Pterla Margaritiferia; P. Martenseii; Hyriopsis Cumingii; Cristaria Plicata
Common: Margarita Shell
Wade-Giles: *Chen-Chu-Mu*
Translation: Treasured Pearl Mother

Energy/Taste: Cold, salty

Channel-Organ: Liver, Heart

Actions:
1. Pacify the Liver and subdue the Rising *Yang*
2. Calm the *Shen* and brighten the eyes

Form and Preparation: Powder, decoction, or pill

Dosage:
Horses and Cattle: 30–60 g
Llamas, Alpacas, Goats, Sheep, and Pigs: 10–30 g
Dogs: 2–8 g
Cats and Rabbits: 0.5–1 g
Birds: 0.1–1.5 g

Cautions and Contraindications: Caution during pregnancy

Side Effects: Overdosage may cause diarrhea.

Margarita *Zhen Zhu* 珍珠

Original Reference: *Ri Hua-Zi Ben Cao* (*Materia Medica of Ri Hua-Zi*) by Ri Hua-Zi in 713 日华子本草

Part Used: Pearl

Name:
Pharmaceutical: Pteria Martensii
Zoological: Pterla Margaritiferia; Hyriopsis Cumingii; Cristaria Plicata
Common: Pearl
Wade-Giles: *Chen-Chu*
Translation: Treasured Pearl

Energy/Taste: Cold, salty

Channel-Organ: Liver, Heart

Actions:
1. Pacify the Liver and subdue the rising *Yang*
2. Calm the *Shen* and brighten the eyes
3. Promote healing and generate flesh

Form and Preparation: Powder, decoction, or pill

Dosage:
Horses and Cattle: 20–60 g
Llamas, Alpacas, Goats, Sheep, and Pigs: 5–15 g
Dogs: 2–6 g
Cats and Rabbits: 0.5–1 g
Birds: 0.1–1.5 g

Cautions and Contraindications: Caution during pregnancy

Side Effects: Overdosage may cause diarrhea.

Hematite *Dai Zhe Shi* 代赭石

Original Reference: *Shen Nong Ben Cao Jing* (*Shen Nong's Materia Medica*, 1st century BCE) 神农本草经

Part Used: Rock

Name:
Pharmaceutical: Haematitum
Mineral Name: Hematite

Common: Iron Ore
Wade-Giles: *Tai-Che-Shih*
Translation: Red Stone From Dai County

Energy/Taste: Cold, bitter

Channel-Organ: Liver, Heart

Actions:
1. Pacify the Liver and subdue the Rising *Yang*
2. Conduct Rebellious *Qi* downward and stop vomiting
3. Cool Blood and stop bleeding

Form and Preparation: Powder, decoction, pill, or topical application

Dosage:
Horses and Cattle: 30–120 g
Llamas, Alpacas, Goats, Sheep, and Pigs: 10–30 g
Dogs: 2–8 g
Cats and Rabbits: 0.5–1 g
Birds: 0.1–1.5 g

Cautions and Contraindications:
1. Caution during pregnancy
2. Caution in patients with Spleen *Qi* Deficiency
3. May counteract Aconite *Fu Zi*

Side Effects: Prolonged use can lead to toxic effects.

Apocynum *Luo Bu Ma* 罗布麻

Original Reference: *Jiu Huang Ben Cao* (*Materia Medica for Relief of Famine*) by *Zhu Su* in 1404 救荒本草

Part Used: Leaf or root

Name:
Pharmaceutical: Apocynum Folium et Radix
Botanical: Apocynum venetum L.
Common: Dogbane
Wade-Giles: *Luo-Pu-Mu*
Translation: Wild-Spread Hemp

Energy/Taste: Cool, sweet, bitter, slightly toxic

Channel-Organ: Liver

Actions:
1. Calm and pacify the Liver *Yang*
2. Clear Heat and benefit urination

Form and Preparation: Powder, decoction, or pill

Dosage:
Horses and Cattle: 30–45 g
Llamas, Alpacas, Goats, Sheep, and Pigs: 3–15 g
Dogs: 1–5 g

Cautions and Contraindications: Avoid long-term use or overdose.

Side Effects: Overdose or long-term use may cause nausea, vomiting, diarrhea, and palpitations.

Celosia *Qing Xiang Zi* 青葙子

Original Reference: *Shen Nong Ben Cao Jing* (*Shen Nong's Materia Medica*, 1st century BCE) 神农本草经

Part Used: Seed

Name:
Pharmaceutical: Celosiae Argenteae, Semen
Botanical: Celosia argentea, C. cristata
Common: Celosia argentea
Wade-Giles: *Ch'ing-Hsiang-Tzu*
Translation: Green Cabinet Seed

Energy/Taste: Cool, bitter

Channel-Organ: Liver

Actions:
1. Clear Liver Heat and brighten eyes
2. Reduce corneal opacity, clear Wind-Heat in the skin

Form and Preparation: Powder, decoction, or pill

Dosage:
Horses and Cattle: 30–60 g
Llamas, Alpacas, Goats, Sheep, and Pigs: 5–15 g
Dogs: 2–4 g
Cats and Rabbits: 0.5–1 g
Birds: 0.1–1.5 g

Cautions and Contraindications:
1. Caution in patients with Liver or Kidney Deficiency
2. Contraindicated in patients with glaucoma

Side Effects: Because it may induce pupil dilatation and affect eye pressure, Celosia *Qing Xiang Zi* should not be given to patients with glaucoma.

Buddleia *Mi Meng Hua* 密蒙花

Original Reference: *Kai Bao Ben Cao* (*Materia Medica of the Kai Bao Era*) by *Ma Zhi* in 973 开宝本草

Part Used: Flower and flower bud

Name:
Pharmaceutical: Buddleiae Officinalis Immaturus, Flos
Botanical: Buddleia officinalis
Common: Buddleia flower
Wade-Giles: *Mi-Meng-Hua*
Translation: Thick Mongolian Flower

Energy/Taste: Cool, sweet

Channel-Organ: Liver

Actions:
1. Clear Liver Heat
2. Brighten eyes and reduce corneal opacity

Form and Preparation: Powder, decoction, or pill

Dosage:
Horses and Cattle: 30–60 g
Llamas, Alpacas, Goats, Sheep, and Pigs: 5–15 g
Dogs: 2–5 g
Cats and Rabbits: 0.5–1 g
Birds: 0.1–1.5 g

Cautions and Contraindications: None known

Side Effects: None known

Equisetum *Mu Zei* 木贼

Original Reference: *Jia You Ben Cao* (*Materia Medica of the Jia You Era*) by *Zhang Yu-xi* and *Su Song* in 1061 嘉佑本草

Part Used: Whole plant above the ground

Name:
Pharmaceutical: Equiseti hiemalis Herba
Botanical: Equisetum hiemale L.
Common: Equisetum
Wade-Giles: *Mu-Tsei*
Translation: Wood Thief

Energy/Taste: Neutral, sweet, bitter

Channel-Organ: Liver and Lung

Actions:
1. Clear Liver, stop bleeding
2. Disperse Wind-Heat and brighten the eyes

Form and Preparation: Powder, decoction, or pill

Dosage:
Horses and Cattle: 20–60 g
Llamas, Alpacas, Goats, Sheep, and Pigs: 5–15 g
Dogs: 2–8 g
Cats and Rabbits: 0.5–1 g
Birds: 0.1–1.5 g

Cautions and Contraindications: None known

Side Effects: None known

Eriocaulon *Gu Jing Cao* 谷精草

Original Reference: *Kai Bao Ben Cao* (*Materia Medica of the Kai Bao Era*) by *Ma Zhi* in 973 开宝本草

Part Used: Flower

Name:
Pharmaceutical: Eriocauli, Flos
Botanical: Eriocaulon buergerianum Koern
Common: Eriocaulon
Wade-Giles: *Ku-Ching-Ts'ao*
Translation: Grain Essence Grass

Energy/Taste: Neutral, sweet, pungent

Channel-Organ: Liver and Lung

Actions:
1. Clear Liver and disperse Wind-Heat
2. Brighten the eyes and eliminate visual opacity

Form and Preparation: Powder, decoction, or pill

Dosage:
Horses and Cattle: 30–60 g
Llamas, Alpacas, Goats, Sheep, and Pigs: 5–15 g
Dogs: 2–8 g
Cats and Rabbits: 0.5–2 g
Birds: 0.3–3 g

Cautions and Contraindications: Caution in patients with Liver *Yin* and Blood Deficiency

Side Effects: None known

Vespertilio *Ye Ming Sha* 夜明沙

Original Reference: *Ri Hua-Zi Ben Cao* (*Materia Medica of Ri Hua-Zi*) by Ri Hua-Zi in 713 日华子本草

Part Used: Feces

Name:
Pharmaceutical: Vespertilionis Faeces

Zoological: Vespertilio superans Thomas
Common: Bat feces
Wade-Giles: *Yeh-Ming-Sha*
Translation: Night Brightness Sand

Energy/Taste: Cold, pungent

Channel-Organ: Liver

Actions:
1. Clear Liver and brighten the eyes
2. Disperse Blood Stasis and reduce accumulations

Form and Preparation: Powder, decoction, or pill

Dosage:
Horses and Cattle: 30–45 g
Llamas, Alpacas, Goats, Sheep, and Pigs: 5–15 g
Dogs: 2–8 g
Cats and Rabbits: 0.5–1 g
Birds: 0.1–1.5 g

Cautions and Contraindications: Caution during pregnancy

Side Effects: May cause nausea and vomiting

Pheretima *Di Long* 地龙

Original Reference: *Shen Nong Ben Cao Jing* (*Shen Nong's Materia Medica*, 1st century BCE) 神农本草经

Part Used: Dried body

Name:
Pharmaceutical: Pheretima
Zoological: Pheretima aspergillum, P. vulgaris Chen, or P. guillelmi
Common: Earthworm
Wade-Giles: *Ti-Lung*
Translation: Earth Dragon

Energy/Taste: Cold, salty

Channel-Organ: Liver, Spleen, Bladder

Actions:
1. Clear Heat and subdue Endogenous Wind
2. Stop asthma and promote urination
3. Activate the Channels

Form and Preparation: Powder, decoction, or pill

Dosage:
Horses and Cattle: 30–60 g
Llamas, Alpacas, Goats, Sheep, and Pigs: 5–15 g
Dogs: 1–3 g
Cats and Rabbits: 0.5–1 g
Birds: 0.1–1 g

Cautions and Contraindications:
1. Caution during pregnancy
2. Caution in patients with Spleen Deficiency

Side Effects: Overdosage may cause dizziness, headache, hypertension followed by hypotension, abdominal pain, gastrointestinal hemorrhage, palpitations, and dyspnea.

Bombyx *Jiang Can* 僵蚕

Original Reference: *Shen Nong Ben Cao Jing* (*Shen Nong's Materia Medica*, 1st century BCE) 神农本草经

Part Used: Dried dead stiffened silkworm body

Name:
Pharmaceutical: Bombyx Batryticatus
Zoological: Bombyx Mori
Common: Mummified Silkworm
Wade-Giles: *Chiang-Ts'an*
Translation: Stiff Silkworm
Alternative: *Bai Jiang Can*

Energy/Taste: Neutral, salty, pungent

Channel-Organ: Liver, Lung

Actions:
1. Extinguish Endogenous Wind and stop spasm
2. Expel Wind and stop pain
3. Dispel toxin and disperse nodules

Form and Preparation: Powder, decoction, or pill

Dosage:
Horses and Cattle: 30–60 g
Llamas, Alpacas, Goats, Sheep, and Pigs: 5–15 g
Dogs: 2–8 g
Cats and Rabbits: 0.5–1 g
Birds: 0.1–1.5 g

Cautions and Contraindications: May antagonize Platycodon *Jie Geng*, Poria *Fu Ling*, Dioscorea *Bei Xie*, and Mantidis *Sang Piao Xiao*

Side Effects: May cause allergic skin reactions, dry throat and mouth, nausea, anorexia, and lethargy

Vitex *Man Jing Zi* 蔓荆子

Original Reference: *Shen Nong Ben Cao Jing* (*Shen Nong's Materia Medica*, 1st century BCE) 神农本草经

Part Used: Fruit

Name:
Pharmaceutical: Viticis, Fructus
Botanical: Vitex trifolia; V. rotundifolia
Common: Vitex seed
Wade-Giles: *Man-Ching-Tzu*

Energy/Taste: Cool, bitter, spicy

Channel-Organ: Bladder, Liver, Stomach

Actions:
1. Soothe the Liver and clear Wind-Heat from the surface
2. Benefit the eyes and act as a transporter to the head
3. Drain Damp and expel Wind to stop pain

Form and Preparation: Powder, decoction, or pill

Dosage:
Horses and Cattle: 15–45 g
Llamas, Alpacas, Goats, Sheep, and Pigs: 5–10 g
Dogs: 2–3 g
Cats and Rabbits: 0.5–1 g
Birds: 0.3–2.5 g

Cautions and Contraindications:
1. Caution in patients with *Yin* or Blood Deficiency
2. May antagonize Aconite *Wu Tou* and Gypsum *Shi Gao*

Side Effects: None known

Buthus *Quan Xie* 全蝎

Original Reference: *Kai Bao Ben Cao* (*Materia Medica of the Kai Bao Era*) by *Ma Zhi* in 973 开宝本草

Part Used: Dried body

Name:
Pharmaceutical: Buthus Martensi
Zoological: Buthus Martensi
Common: Scorpion
Wade-Giles: *Ch'ueh-Hsieh*
Translation: Whole Scorpion

Energy/Taste: Neutral, pungent, toxic

Channel-Organ: Liver

Actions:
1. Extinguish Endogenous Wind and stop spasm
2. Remove a harmful substance and dissipate nodules
3. Activate the Channels to relieve pain

Form and Preparation: Powder, decoction, or pill

Dosage:
Horses and Cattle: 15–30 g
Llamas, Alpacas, Goats, Sheep, and Pigs: 3–9 g
Dogs: 1–3 g
Cats and Rabbits: 0.2–0.5 g
Birds: 0.1–1 g

Cautions and Contraindications:
1. Caution in patients with seizures due to Blood Deficiency
2. Contraindicated during pregnancy, but safe for use in infants
3. **It is toxic**, so do not overdose.

Side Effects: Overdoses can cause respiratory paralysis.

Scolopendra *Wu Gong* 蜈蚣

Original Reference: *Shen Nong Ben Cao Jing* (*Shen Nong's Materia Medica*, 1st century BCE) 神农本草经

Part Used: Dried body with legs removed

Name:
Pharmaceutical: Scolopendra Subspinipes
Zoological: Scolopendra Subspinipes
Common: Centipede
Wade-Giles: *Wu-Kung*
Translation: Centipede

Energy/Taste: Warm, salty, pungent, toxic

Channel-Organ: Liver

Actions:
1. Subdue Endogenous Wind and stop spasm
2. Dispel Toxin and dissipate Nodules
3. Activate the Channels and relieve pain

Form and Preparation: Powder, decoction, or pill

Dosage:
Horses and Cattle: 5–10 g
Llamas, Alpacas, Goats, Sheep, and Pigs: 1–1.5 g
Dogs: 0.5–1 g

Cautions and Contraindications:
1. Contraindicated during pregnancy
2. Avoid overdose.

Side Effects: Overdose may cause nausea, vomiting, abdominal pain, diarrhea, dyspnea, hypotension, allergic skin reactions, or even shock.

Antelopis *Ling Yang Jiao* 羚羊角

This substance is prohibited as is from an endangered species. The following information is just for educational purposes.

Original Reference: *Shen Nong Ben Cao Jing* (*Shen Nong*'s *Materia Medica*, 1st century BCE) 神农本草经

Part Used: Horn

Name:
Pharmaceutical: Antelopis, Cornu
Zoological: Saigatatarica
Common: Antelope Horn
Wade-Giles: *Ling-Yang-Chiao*
Translation: Antelope Horn

Energy/Taste: Cold, salty

Channel-Organ: Liver, Heart

Actions:
1. Pacify the Liver and extinguish Endogenous Wind
2. Clear Heat and brighten eyes
3. Release toxins and anchor *Yang*

Form and Preparation: Powder, decoction, or pill

Dosage: This substance is prohibited as it is from an endangered species.
Horses and Cattle: 6–9 g
Llamas, Alpacas, Goats, Sheep, and Pigs: 1–3 g

Cautions and Contraindications: None known

Side Effects: None known

Note: Although used for thousands of years to control seizures, Antelopis *Ling Yang Jiao* is now prohibited because this antelope is an endangered species. To substitute goat horn *Shan Yang Jiao* for Antelopis *Ling Yang Jiao* in classical herbal formulas, use five times the amount of goat horn for every unit of antelope horn.

SUMMARY OF HERBS THAT PACIFY THE LIVER AND EXTINGUISH ENDOGENOUS WIND

Table 13.1 summarizes and compares the herbs that pacify the Liver and extinguish Endogenous Wind.

REFERENCES

1. Chen JK, Chen TT. Chinese Medical Herbology and Pharmacology. City of Industry, CA: Art of Medicine Press, 2004.
2. Brinker FJ. The Toxicology of Botanical Medicines. Sandy, OR: Eclectic Medical Publications, 2000.
3. Duke JA. Handbook of Medicinal Herbs. New York: Chemical and Rubber Company Press, 2001.
4. Huang KC. The Pharmacology of Chinese Herbs, 2nd Edition. New York: Chemical and Rubber Company Press, 1999.

14 Herbs to Stabilize and Bind (Astringents) 收敛药

Huisheng Xie, Vanessa Preast, Min Su Kim

The sour and astringent (gathering) nature of the astringent herbs allows them to stabilize, constrict, and bind substances; thus, they are used to consolidate *Jing* (Essence) and to stop sweating, chronic diarrhea, fecal or urinary incontinence, bleeding, asthma, and coughing. These herbs may be warm or cold, and they affect the Lung, Spleen, Large Intestine, and Kidney Channels. Combining astringent herbs with tonifying herbs permits simultaneous treatment of both the symptoms and underlying causes of disease. However, astringent herbs are contraindicated when 1) pathogenic factors are lodged in the Exterior or 2) excessive Dampness or Heat has accumulated in the Interior.

Schisandra *Wu Wei Zi* 五味子

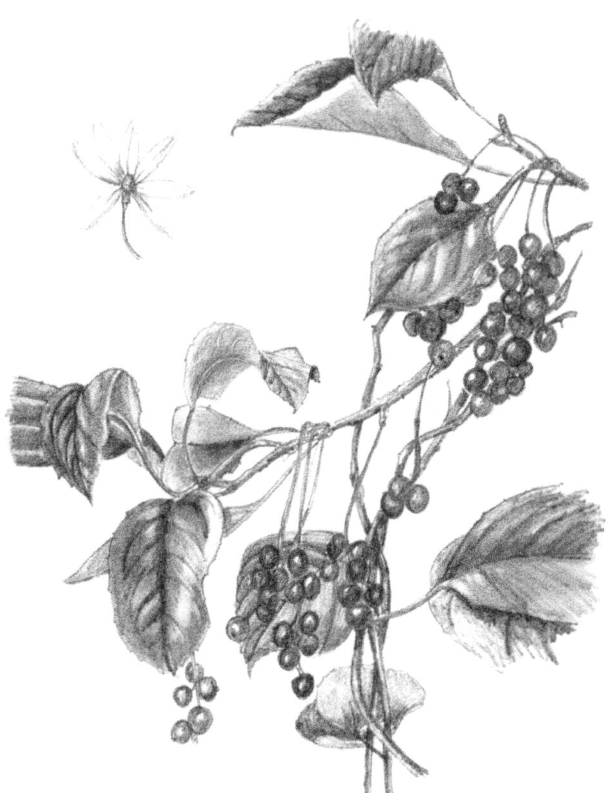

Original Reference: *Shen Nong Ben Cao Jing* (*Shen Nong's Materia Medica*, 1st century BCE) 神农本草经

Part Used: Fruit

Name:
Pharmaceutical: Schizandrae Chinensis, Fructus
Botanical: Schisandra chinensis
Common: Schisandra seed
Wade-Giles: *Wu-Wei-Tzu*
Translation: Five-Taste Seed

Energy/Taste: Warm, sour, pungent, bitter, salty, sweet

Channel-Organ: Lung, Heart, Kidney

Actions:
1. Astringe the Lung, nourish the Kidney
2. Generate Body Fluids, stop excessive sweating
3. Restrain essence, stop diarrhea
4. Calm *Shen*, stop coughing

Form and Preparation: Powder, decoction, or pill

Dosage:
Horses and Cattle: 15–30 g
Llamas, Alpacas, Goats, Sheep, and Pigs: 3–8 g
Dogs: 2–3 g
Cats and Rabbits: 0.5–1 g
Birds: 0.2–1.5 g

Cautions and Contraindications:
1. Contraindicated for acute cough or skin rashes
2. Caution in patients suffering from excessive Internal Heat with unrelieved Exterior Pattern

Side Effects: May occasionally cause vomiting

Clinical Application:
1. Chronic cough and asthma due to rebellion of Lung *Qi* caused by Deficiency of the Lung and Kidney

Combine with: Ginseng *Ren Shen*, Cornus *Shan Zhu Yu*, Prepared Rehmannia *Shu Di Huang*, Ophiopogon *Mai Men Dong*, and Dioscorea *Shan Yao*
Classical herbal formula: *Ren Shen Ge Jie San*

2. Deficiency of *Qi* and Body Fluids (i.e., after profuse fluid loss in febrile disease)
   Clinical signs: Night sweats, spontaneous sweating, thirst, palpitation, dyspnea, deficient and forceless pulse, cough
   Combine with: Ginseng *Ren Shen* and Ophiopogon *Mai Men Dong*
   Classical herbal formula: *Sheng Mai Yin*
3. Diabetes (wasting and thirsting disorder) due to Kidney *Yin* Deficiency
   Clinical signs: Thirst, excessive fluid intake, dyspnea, lassitude, deficient and forceless pulse
   Combine with: Astragalus *Huang Qi*, Rehmannia *Shu Di*, Ophiopogon *Mai Men Dong*, and Trichosanthes *Tian Hua Fen*
   Classical herbal formula: *Xiao Ke Fang*
4. Urinary leakage due to Kidney *Qi* Deficiency
   Combine with: Draconis *Long Gu* and Mantidis *Sang Piao Xiao*
5. Chronic diarrhea due to Spleen and Kidney Deficiency; chronic dysenteric disorders and daybreak diarrhea due to Kidney *Yang* Deficiency
   Combine with: Myristica *Rou Dou Kou*, Evodia *Wu Zhu Yu*, and Psoralea *Bu Gu Zhi*
   Classical herbal formula: *Si Shen Wan*
6. Deficient *Yin* and Blood of the Heart and Kidney
   Clinical signs: Palpitation, irritability, restlessness, anxiety, dream-filled sleep
   Combine with: Rehmannia *Sheng Di Huang*, Ophiopogon *Mai Men Dong*, and Ziziphus *Suan Zao Ren*
   Classical herbal formula: *Tian Wan Bu Xin Dan*

History and Comments:

1. Schisandra *Wu Wei Zi* is known as the "Five-Taste Fruit" because its components have different tastes and different medicinal properties. The whole fruit is salty and is good at storing fluids. The sour peel is a Lung *Qi* astringent, which treats deficient and chronic cough. The pungent and bitter kernel has recently been used for allergic skin disorders. The sweet pulp tonifies Kidney and Lung *Qi*.
2. Good quality Schisandra *Wu Wei Zi* is large, thick, fleshy, oily, shiny, and purplish-red.
3. Although classified as an astringent, Schisandra *Wu Wei Zi* is primarily used as a *Yin* tonic.
4. *Wu Wei Zi* is effective for neurasthenia when combined with Pseudostellaria *Tai Zi Shen*.
5. *Wu Wei Zi* has recently been used to treat allergic skin disorders and to improve liver function in patients with hepatitis. It can decrease the liver enzyme GPT.

Pharmaceutical Ingredients:[1–4]

1. Lignan compounds (schizandrin, deoxyschizandrin, kadsuranin, schisanhenol, schisanhenol acetate, gomisin, angeloygomisin, tiggoylgomisin, benzoylgomisin, rubschisandrin, epigomisin, schisantherin, andeloygomisin, tigloylgomisin, binankadsurin, angeloylbinankadsurin, isobutyroylibinankadsurin, benzoylbinankadsurin, rubschisantherin, r-schizandrin, schizandrol, pseudo-r-schizandrin, gomisin A-J, N-Q wuweizi A,B
2. Palmitic acid, stearic acid, anthocyanin

Chebula *He Zi* 诃子

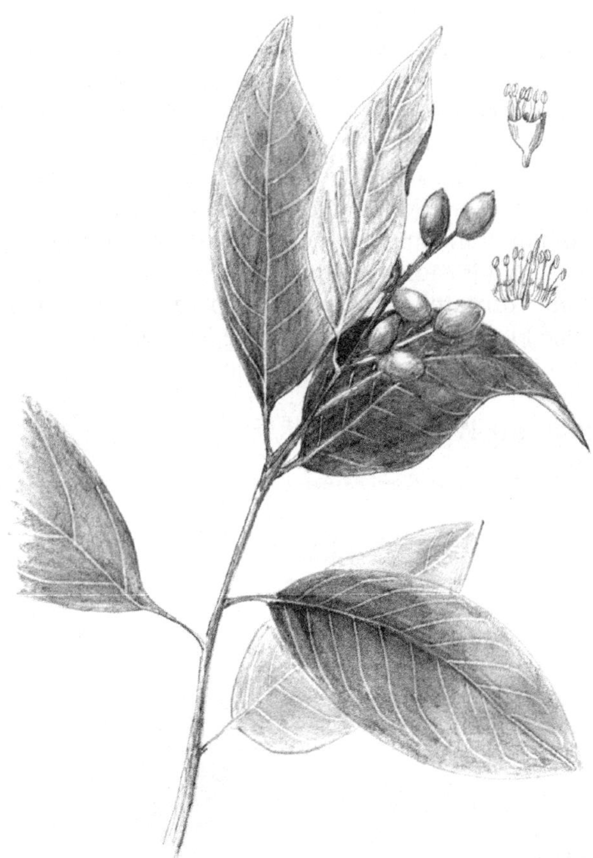

Original Reference: *Yao Xing Lun* (*Discussion of Medicinal Properties*) by *Chen Zhou* in 19th century 药性论

Part Used: Ripe fruit

Name:
Pharmaceutical: Terminaliae Chebulae, Fructus
Botanical: Terminalia chebula Retz
Common: Terminalia fruit
Wade-Giles: *He-Tzu*

Energy/Taste: Neutral, sour, astringent, bitter

Channel-Organ: Lung, Stomach, Large Intestine

Actions:
1. Astringe the intestines and stop diarrhea
2. Astringe the Lung to stop coughing
3. Benefit throat

Form and Preparation: Powder, decoction, or pill

Dosage:
Horses and Cattle: 30–60 g
Llamas, Alpacas, Goats, Sheep, and Pigs: 3–10 g
Dogs: 2–3 g
Cats and Rabbits: 0.5–1 g
Birds: 0.2–1.5 g

Cautions and Contraindications:
1. Caution in patients with Exterior Pattern or accumulation of Internal Damp Heat
2. Caution in patients with Spleen *Qi* Deficiency

Side Effects: May inhibit digestive function.

Clinical Application:
1. Chronic diarrhea, or chronic dysentery
   Combine with: Coptis *Huang Lian*, Saussurea *Mu Xiang* and Mume *Wu Mei*
   Classical herbal formula: *Wu Mei San*
2. Cough and asthma due to Deficiency of Lung or chronic cough with chronic hoarse voice
   Combine with: Platycodon *Jie Geng*, Schisandra *Wu Wei Zi*, Glehnia *Sha Shen*, Lily *Bai He*

History and Comments:
1. Good quality Chebula *He Zi* is yellowish brown, shiny, solid, and hard.
2. *He Zi* is the most commonly prescribed herb in Ayurvedic and Tibetan medicine. Similar to the use of Licorice *Gan Cao* in Chinese medicine, these systems use *He Zi* as a tonic and harmonizing agent in formulas.
3. *He Zi* is often combined with Mume *Wu Mei*.
4. Raw *He Zi* is useful for chronic cough and loss of voice. Roasted *He Zi* is good for chronic diarrhea and dysenteric disorders.

Pharmaceutical Ingredients:[1–4]
1. Triterpene, gallyl glucose, gallic acid
2. Tannin (chebulagic acid, chebulinic acid, corilagin, chebulic acid, terchebulin, punicalagin, terflavin A, terchebin, ellagic acid, gallic acid, glucogallin, chebulin)
3. Triterpenoids (Terminoic acid, arjugenin, arjunoic acid, chebupentol)
4. Shikimic acid, dehydroshikimic acid, arabinose, fructose, glucose, sucrose, rhamnose, amino acids, quinic acid, ethyl gallate, daucosterol, β-sitosterol, triacontanoic acid palmitic acid
5. Sennoside A, tannase, polyphenol oxidase, peroxydase, oxidase, ascorbic acid oxidase, Se, Mg, Fe, Cu, vitamin C

Mume *Wu Mei* 乌梅

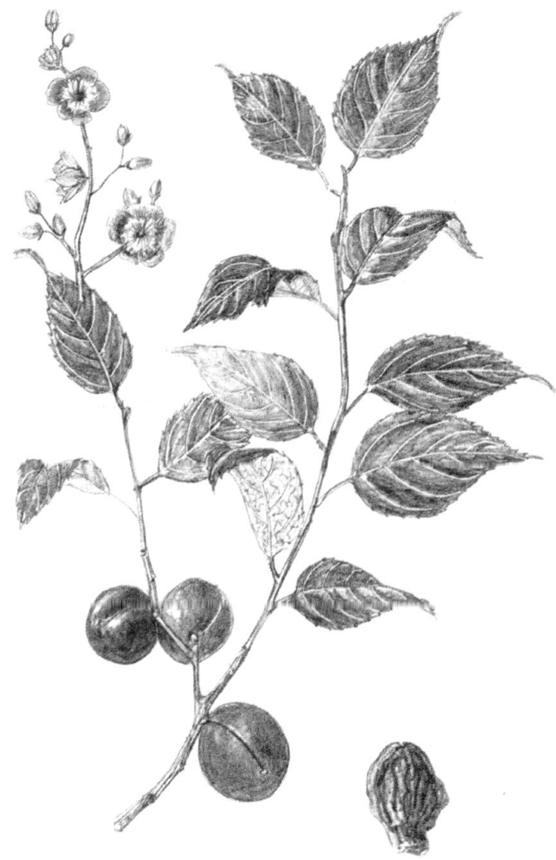

Original Reference: *Shen Nong Ben Cao Jing* (*Shen Nong's Materia Medica*, 1st century BCE) 神农本草经

Part Used: Immature fruit (smoked to black color)

Name:
Pharmaceutical: Pruni Mume, Fructus
Botanical: Prunus Mume
Common: Black Plum
Wade-Giles: *Wu-Mei*
Translation: Dark Plum

Energy/Taste: Neutral, sour

Channel-Organ: Liver, Spleen, Lung, large intestine

Actions:
1. Astringe the Lung to stop cough
2. Restrain the intestines to stop diarrhea
3. Generate Body Fluids to relieve thirst
4. Expel roundworms, alleviate pain
5. Topically as a plaster to treat corns and warts

Form and Preparation: Powder, decoction, or pill

Dosage:
Horses and Cattle: 15–30 g
Llamas, Alpacas, Goats, Sheep, and Pigs: 3–10 g
Dogs: 2–5 g
Cats and Rabbits: 0.5–1 g
Birds: 0.2–1.5 g

Cautions and Contraindications: Caution in patients with unresolved Exterior Pattern or accumulation of Interior Excess Heat

Side Effects: None known

Clinical Application:
1. Chronic cough due to Lung Deficiency
   Combine with: Papaver *Ying Su Ke*, Asinum Gelatinum *E Jiao*, Armenica *Xing Ren*, and Pinellia *Ban Xia*
2. Chronic diarrhea or dysentery
   Combine with: Myristica *Kou Dou Kou*, Chebula *He Zi*, Papaver *Ying Su Ke*, and Schisandra *Wu Wei Zi*
3. Acute dysentery or diarrhea due to Damp-Heat in pediatric animals
   Combine with: Coptis *Huang Lian*, Saussurea *Mu Xiang*
   Classical herbal formula: *Wu Mei San*
4. Diabetes due to *Qi-Yin* Deficiency
   Combine with: Trichosanthes *Tian Hua Fen*, Ophiopogon *Mai Men Dong*, Ginseng *Ren Shen*, and Patrinia *Bai Jiang Cao*, and Pueraria *Ge Gen*

History and Comments:
1. Good quality *Wu Mei* is whole, large, soft, moist, and sour. It should be black on the outside, have thick flesh, and contain small seeds. In Japan, this commonly used herb is called umeboshi and is a prized health tonic for protection against or treatment of indigestion, intestinal parasites, and many other diseases.
2. *Wu Mei* is often combined with Chebula *He Zi*.
3. *Wu Mei* has antibiotic effects and benefits the biliary system.

Pharmaceutical Ingredients:[1–4]
1. Citric acid, oleanolic acid, malic acid, succinic acid, carbohydrates, triterpenoids, sitosterol
2. Picric acid, amygdalin

Cornus *Shan Zhu Yu* 山茱萸

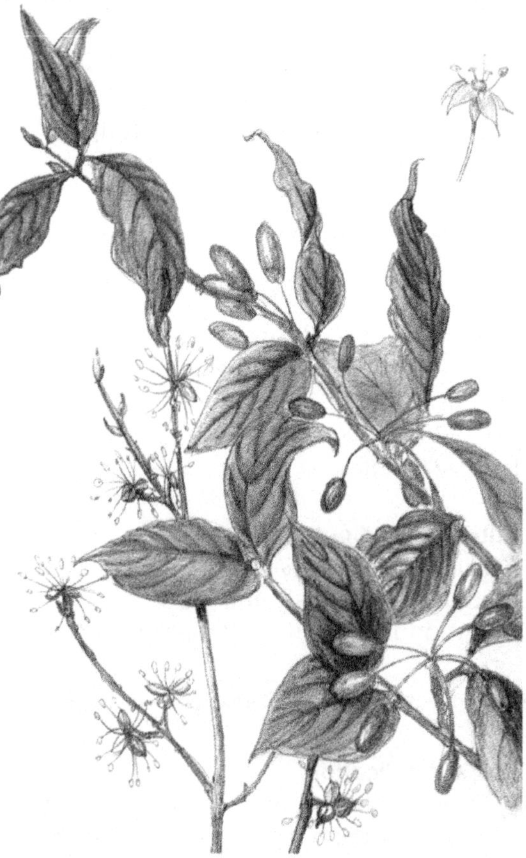

Original Reference: *Shen Nong Ben Cao Jing* (*Shen Nong's Materia Medica*, 1st century BCE) 神农本草经

Part Used: fruit

Name:
Pharmaceutical: Fructus cornus
Botanical: Corni Officinalis, Fructus
Common: Dogwood fruit
Wade-Giles: *Shan-Chu-Yu*
Translation: Mountain Dogwood

Energy/Taste: Slightly warm, sour

Channel-Organ: Liver and Kidney

Actions:
1. Tonify Liver and Kidney
2. Astringe *Jing* and bind substances

Form and Preparation: Powder, decoction, or pill

Dosage:
Horses and Cattle: 30–60 g
Llamas, Alpacas, Goats, Sheep, and Pigs: 5–15 g
Dogs: 3–6 g
Cats and Rabbits: 1–3 g
Birds: 0.3–5 g

Cautions and Contraindications: Due to its warmth, the herb is contraindicated for dysuria due to Excess Heat or Damp-Heat Pattern.

Side Effects: None known

Clinical Application:
1. Liver and Kidney *Yin* Deficiency
   Clinical signs: Dizziness, blurred vision, soreness and weakness of the lower back and rear limbs, urinary leakage, infertility, abnormal sweating, palpitations, shortness of breath
   Combine with: Rehmannia *Shu Di Huang*, Cuscuta *Tu Si Zi*, Lycium *Gou Qi Zi*, Eucommia *Du Zhong*, and Schisandra *Wu Wei Zi*
   Classical herbal formula: *Zuo Gui Wan*
2. Impotence, night sweating, frequent urination or incontinence
   Combine with: Ginseng *Ren Shen*, Ostrea *Mu Li*, Draconis *Long Gu*
3. Uterine bleeding due to False Heat from *Yin* Deficiency
   Combine with: Paeonia *Bai Shao* and Asinum Gelatin *E Jiao*

History and Comments:
1. Good quality Cornus *Shan Zhu Yu* is fat, thick, soft, seedless, and purplish red.
2. Cornus *Shan Zhu Yu* can increase estrogen to balance the patient's endocrine condition. It can also improve absorption of calcium and increase the ratio of HDL/LDL.

Pharmaceutical Ingredients:[1–4]
1. Cornin, verbenalin, saponin, tannin
2. Ursolic acid, gallic acid, morroniside, sweroside, loganin, tellmagrandin, malic acid, tartraric acid, oleanolic acid, strychnine, vitamin A
3. Isoterchebin, gemin D, cornusin A, B, Al, Ma

Euryale *Qian Shi* 芡实

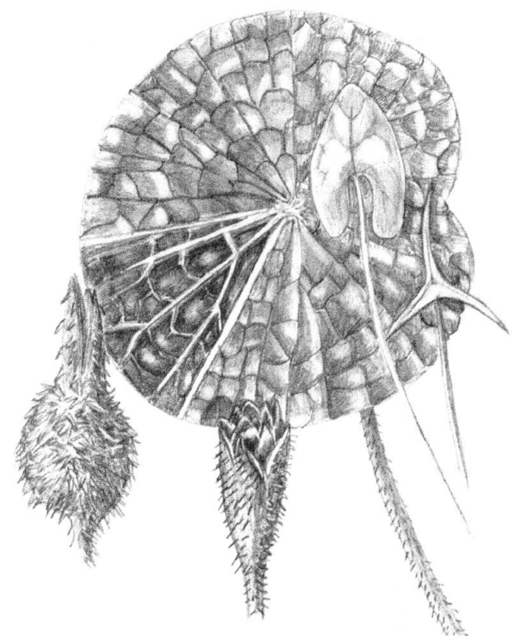

Original Reference: *Shen Nong Ben Cao Jing* (*Shen Nong*'s *Materia Medica*, 1st century BCE) 神农本草经

Part Used: Seed

Name:
Pharmaceutical: Euryales Ferocis, Semen
Botanical: Euryale ferox Salisb.
Common: Euryale seed
Wade-Giles: *Ch'ien-Shih*
Translation: Euryale Solid

Energy/Taste: Neutral, sweet, astringent

Channel-Organ: Spleen, Kidney

Actions:
1. Tonify the Spleen to remove dampness
2. Tonify the Kidney to control *Jing*
3. Stabilize the exterior-surface

Form and Preparation: Powder, decoction, or pill

Dosage:
Horses and Cattle: 30–60 g
Llamas, Alpacas, Goats, Sheep, and Pigs: 3–10 g

Dogs: 1–3 g
Cats and Rabbits: 0.5–1 g
Birds: 0.2–1.5 g

Cautions and Contraindications: None known

Side Effects: None known

Clinical Application:
1. Chronic diarrhea due to Spleen *Qi* Deficiency
   Combine with: Atractylodes *Bai Zhu* and Dioscorea *Shan Yao*, or Codonopsis *Dang Shen*, Poria *Fu Ling*
2. Urinary frequency or leakage
   Combine with: Astragalus *Sha Yuan Zi* and Rosa *Jin Ying Zi*
3. Excessive vaginal discharge due to Damp Heat or Kidney *Qi* Deficiency
   Combine with: Phellodendon *Huang Bai*, Plantago *Che Qian Zi*, Dioscorea *Shan Yao*

History and Comments: Good quality Euryale *Qian Shi* is full, round, and powdery.

Pharmaceutical Ingredients:[1–4]
1. Starch, protein, lipid, carbohydrates, fiber
2. Thiamine, riboflavine, nicotinic acid, carotene, tryptophane, cysteine, cystine, amylose, amylopectin

Mantidis *Sang Piao Xiao* 桑螵蛸

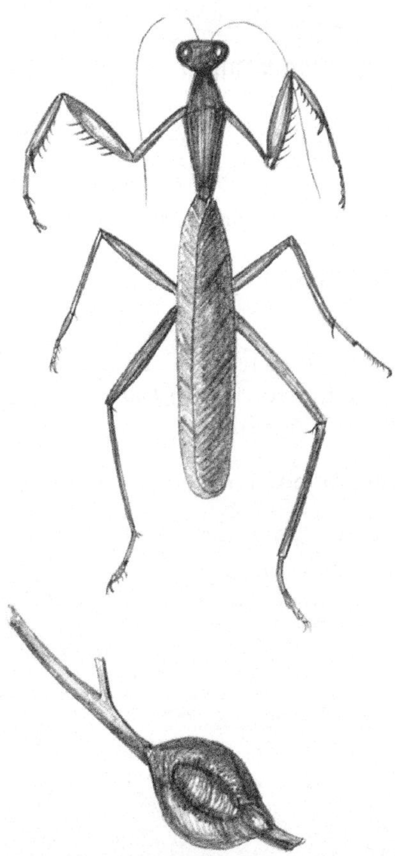

Original Reference: *Shen Nong Ben Cao Jing* (*Shen Nong's Materia Medica*, 1st century BCE) 神农本草经

Part Used: Egg case

Name:
Pharmaceutical: Mantidis, Ootheca
Zoological: Paratenodera Sinensis, P. augustipennis Saussure, Statilia maculata
Common: Mantis egg case
Wade-Giles: *Sang-P'iao-Hsiao*
Translation: Mulberry Egg Case

Energy/Taste: Neutral, sweet, salty

Channel-Organ: Liver, Kidney

Actions:
1. Tonify Kidney and astringe *Jing*
2. Strengthen *Yang* and decrease urination

Form and Preparation: Powder, decoction, or pill

Dosage:
Horses and Cattle: 15–30 g
Llamas, Alpacas, Goats, Sheep, and Pigs: 3–15 g
Dogs: 2–3 g
Cats and Rabbits: 0.5–1 g
Birds: 0.2–1 g

Cautions and Contraindications:
1. Caution in patients with Bladder Damp-Heat
2. May counteract Inula *Xuan Fu Hua*

Side Effects: None known

Clinical Application:
1. Urinary leakage or incontinence due to Kidney *Qi* or *Jing* Deficiency, especially in young patients
   Combine with: Draconis *Long Gu*, Ostrea *Mu Li*, Cornus *Shan Zhu Yu*, Astragalus *Sha Yuan Ji Li*
2. Infertility due to Kidney *Yang* Deficiency
   Combine with: Euryale *Qian Shi*, Cynomorium *Suo Yang* and Cuscuta *Tu Si Zi*

History and Comments:
1. Good quality Mantidis *Sang Piao Xiao* is dry, lightweight, intact, yellow, and without bark.
2. Mantidis *Sang Piao Xiao* may be used as a long-term, mild tonic for pediatric and geriatric patients.

Pharmaceutical Ingredients:[1–4] Ca, Fe, amino acid, protein

Sepia *Hai Piao Xiao* 海螵蛸

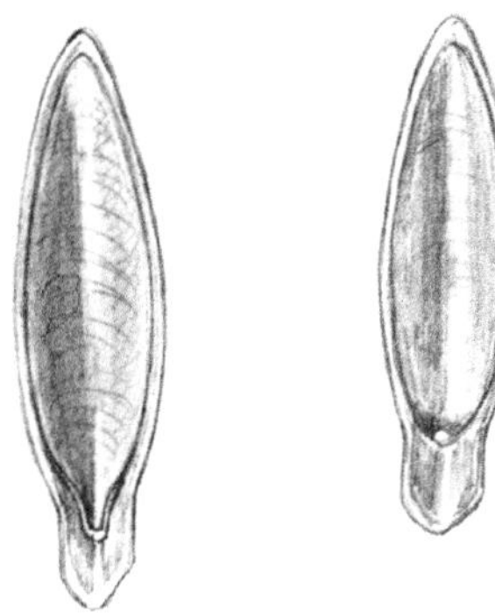

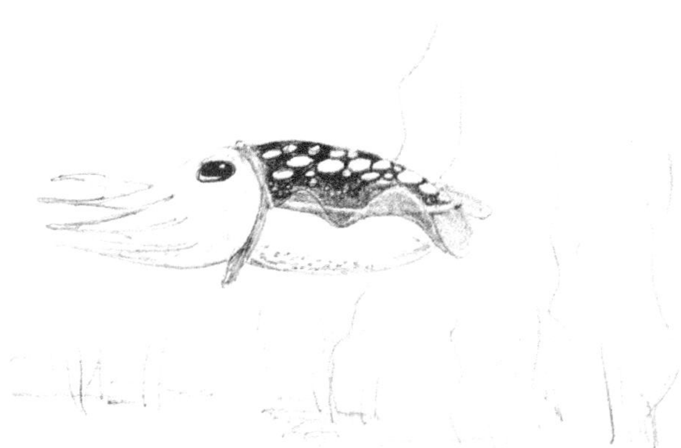

Original Reference: *Shen Nong Ben Cao Jing* (*Shen Nong's Materia Medica*, 1st century BCE) 神农本草经

Part Used: Bone or internal shell

Name:
Pharmaceutical: Sepiae seu Sepiellae, Os
Zoological: Sepia esculenta, Sepiella maindroni
Common: Cuttlefish bone, cuttlebone
Wade-Giles: *Hai-P'iao-Hsiao*
Translation: Ocean Cuttlefish Bone
Alternative: *Wu Zei Gu* 乌贼骨 cuttle-bone

Energy/Taste: Slightly warm, salty, astringent

Channel-Organ: Liver, Kidney

Actions:
1. Stop bleeding, control *Jing*
2. Restrain gastric acidity, stop pain
3. Dry Damp and promote healing of ulcers

Form and Preparation: Powder, decoction, or pill

Dosage:
Horses and Cattle: 30–60 g
Llamas, Alpacas, Goats, Sheep, and Pigs: 3–15 g
Dogs: 2–5 g
Cats and Rabbits: 0.5–1 g
Birds: 0.2–1.5 g

Cautions and Contraindications: Because it is slightly warm and might injure *Yin* and generate Heat, Sepia *Hai Piao Xiao* is not recommended for patients with *Yin* Deficiency or Interior Heat.

Side Effects: Long-term use can lead to constipation.

Clinical Application:
1. Hemorrhage from Stomach, Lung, uterus, or trauma
   Combine with: Rubia *Qian Cao Gen*, Asinum Gelatinum *E Jiao*, Astragalus *Huang Qi*, Melaphis *Wu Bei Zi*, and Trachycarpus *Zong Lu Tan*; can be used alone for bleeding from external injuries
2. Urinary leakage due to Kidney Deficiency
   Combine with: Cornus *Shan Zhu Yu*, Dioscorea *Shan Yao*, Cuscuta *Tu Si Zi*, Ostrea *Mu Li*, and Astragalus *Sha Yuan Ji Li*
3. Stomach pain and acid regurgitation
   Combine with: Fritillaria *Zhe Bei Mu*, Fritillaria *Chuan Bei Mu*
4. Chronic nonhealing ulcerations
   Combine with: Gypsum *Shi Gao*, Draconis *Duan Long Gu*, Borneol *Bing Pian* topically for chronic nonhealing ulcerations

History and Comments: Good quality Sepia *Hai Piao Xiao* is dry, white, large, and intact.

Pharmaceutical Ingredients:[1–4] Ca, NaCl, calcium phosphate, magnesium chloride, chitin

Ephedra *Ma Huang Gen* 麻黄根

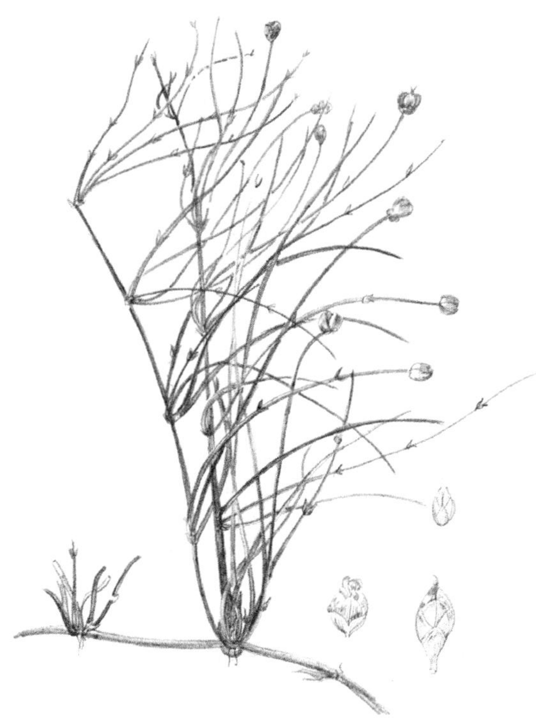

Original Reference: *Ming Yi Bie Lu* (Miscellaneous Records of Famous Physicians) by *Tao Hong-Jing*, North and South Kingdoms (5th century) 名医别录

Part Used: Root

Name:
Pharmaceutical: Ephedrae, Radix
Botanical: Ephedra sinica staph., E. equisetina Bge, E intermedia Shrenk et Meg.
Common: Ephedra root
Wade-Giles: *Ma-Huang*
Translation: Hemp Yellow Root

Energy/Taste: Neutral, sweet

Channel-Organ: Lung

Actions: Astringe surface to stop sweating

Form and Preparation: Powder, decoction, or pill

Dosage:
Horses and Cattle: 15–30 g
Llamas, Alpacas, Goats, Sheep, and Pigs: 3–10 g

Cautions and Contraindications: Contraindicated in patients with Exterior Pattern

Side Effects: None known

Clinical Application: Spontaneous sweating or night sweating
Combine with: Astragalus *Huang Qi*, Angelica *Dang Gui*, Schisandra *Wu Wei Zi*, Biota *Bai Zi Ren*

History and Comments:
1. The root of Ephedra *Ma Huang* stops the sweating caused by Deficiency while the aboveground part of the plant induces sweating that is blocked by excess.
2. The root, *Ma Huang Gen*, contains almost no alkaloids, but the aboveground part, *Ma Huang*, contains alkaloids, including ephedrine.

Pharmaceutical Ingredients:[1–4]
1. Maokonine, ephedradines A, B, C, D, ephedrannin
2. Tyrosine betaine, mahuannins A, B, C, D

Myristica *Rou Dou Kou* 肉豆蔻

Original Reference: *Yao Xing Lun* (*Discussion of Medicinal Properties*) by Chen Zhou in 19th century 药性论

Part Used: Fruit

Name:
Pharmaceutical: Myristicae Fragrantis, Semen
Botanical: Myristica fragrans Houtt
Common: Nutmeg
Wade-Giles: *Jou-Tou-K'ou*
Translation: Fleshy Cardamom

Energy/Taste: Warm, pungent

Channel-Organ: Spleen, Stomach, Large Intestine

Actions:
1. Astringe the intestines to stop diarrhea
2. Warm the Spleen, promote *Qi* to stop pain

Form and Preparation: Powder, decoction, or pill

Dosage:
Horses and Cattle: 15–30 g
Llamas, Alpacas, Goats, Sheep, and Pigs: 3–10 g
Dogs: 2–5 g
Cats and Rabbits: 0.5–1 g
Birds: 0.2–1.5 g

Cautions and Contraindications:
1. Caution in patients with Damp-Heat dysentery or diarrhea
2. Caution in patients during pregnancy

Side Effects: Overdose may cause dizziness and hypersomnia

Ginkgo *Bai Guo* 白果

Original Reference: *Ri Yong Ben Cao* (*Household Materia Medica*) by *Wu Rui* in 1350 日用本草

Part Used: Seed

Name:
Pharmaceutical: Ginkgo Bilobae, Semen
Botanical: Ginkgo biloba L.
Common name: Ginkgo nut
Wade-Giles: *Pai-Kuo*
Translation: Silver Almond

Energy/Taste: Neutral, sweet, bitter, astringent, slightly toxic

Channel-Organ: Lung, Kidney

Actions:
1. Strengthen the Lung and soothe asthma
2. Expel Phlegm and stop wheezing
3. Eliminate Damp and stop discharge

Form and Preparation: Powder, decoction, or pill

Dosage:
Horses and Cattle: 15–45 g
Camel: 30–60 g

Llamas, Alpacas, Goats, Sheep, and Pigs: 3–10 g
Dogs: 2–5 g
Cats and Rabbits: 0.5–1 g
Birds: 0.2–1.5 g

Cautions and Contraindications: Caution in patients with excessive Phlegm or Damp

Side Effects:
1. Overdosage may cause poisoning. The poisoning symptoms include headache, fever, tremors, irritability, and dyspnea.
2. The antidote for the poisoning is a decoction of 30 grams of Glycyrrhiza *Gan Cao* in people.

Papaveris *Ying Su Ke* 罂粟壳
Original Reference: *Ben Cao Gang Mu* (*Materia Medica Compendium*) by *Li Shi-Zhen* in 1590 本草纲目

Part Used: Seed husk

Name:
Pharmaceutical: Papaveris Somniferi, Pericarpium
Botanical: Papaver somniferum L.
Common: Poppy husk
Wade-Giles: *Ying-Su-K'e*
Translation: Poppy Husk

Energy/Taste: Neutral, sour, astringent, toxic

Channel-Organ: Lung, Large Intestine, Kidney

Actions:
1. Astringes the Lung and astringes the intestines
2. Stop pain, stabilize the Lower *Jiao*

Form and Preparation: Powder, decoction, or pill

Dosage:
Horses and Cattle: 30–60 g
Llamas, Alpacas, Goats, Sheep, and Pigs: 3–15 g
Dogs: 2–5 g
Cats and Rabbits: 0.5–1 g
Birds: 0.2–1.5 g

Cautions and Contraindications: Contraindicated in patients with early stages of coughing or dysentery (acute)

Side Effects: Overdose may cause dizziness, nausea, vomiting, constipation, difficulty urinating, and biliary colic.

Halloysite *Chi Shi Zhi* 赤石脂
Original Reference: *Shen Nong Ben Cao Jing* (*Shen Nong's Materia Medica*, 1st century BCE) 神农本草经

Part Used: Mineral resin

Name:
Pharmaceutical: Halloysitum Rubrum
Common: Halloysite
Wade-Giles: *Ch'ih-Shih-Chih*
Translation: Red Stone Resin

Energy/Taste: Warm, sweet, sour, astringent

Channel-Organ: Spleen, Stomach, Large Intestine

Actions:
1. Astringe intestines to stop diarrhea
2. Contain blood to stop bleeding
3. Promote healing of wounds

Form and Preparation: Powder, decoction, or pill

Dosage:
Horses and Cattle: 15–45 g
Llamas, Alpacas, Goats, Sheep, and Pigs: 3–15 g
Dogs: 2–6 g
Cats and Rabbits: 0.5–1 g
Birds: 0.2–1.5 g

Cautions and Contraindications:
1. Caution during pregnancy
2. Caution in patients with hot diarrhea, early stages of dysentery, or accumulation of Damp Heat
3. May antagonize Rheum *Da Huang* and counteract Genkwa *Yuan Hua* and Scutellaria *Huang Qin*

Side Effects: None known

Melaphis *Wu Bei Zi* 五倍子
Original Reference: *Ben Cao Shi Yi* (*Supplement to Materia Medica*) by *Chen Cang-Qi* in 8th century 本草拾遗

Part Used: The insect, which induces gall production by laying its eggs in the branches of the trees (Rhus chinensis Mill or Rhus potaninii Maxim)

Name:
Pharmaceutical: Galla chinensis
Botanical: Melaphis chinensis (Bell) Baker
Common: Gallnut of Chinese sumac
Wade-Giles: *Wu-Pei-Tzu*
Translation: Five Multiple Seed

Energy/Taste: Cold, sour, astringent

Channel-Organ: Lung, Large Intestine, Kidney

Actions:
1. Astringe intestines to stop diarrhea

2. Stop coughing, stop hemorrhage
3. Kill parasites

Form and Preparation: Powder, decoction, or pill

Dosage:
Horses and Cattle: 10–35 g
Llamas, Alpacas, Goats, Sheep, and Pigs: 3–10 g
Dogs: 1–2 g
Cats and Rabbits: 0.5–1 g
Birds: 0.2–0.6 g

Cautions and Contraindications: Caution in patients with diarrhea due to Damp-Heat or coughing due to Lung Heat

Side Effects: None known

Punica *Shi Liu Pi* 石榴皮

Original Reference: *Ming Yi Bie Lu* (*Miscellaneous Records of Famous Physicians*) by *Tao Hong-Jing*, North and South Kingdoms (5th century) 名医别录

Part Used: Husk

Name:
Pharmaceutical: Granati Pericarpium
Botanical: Punica granatum L.
Common: Pomegranate husk
Wade-Giles: *Shih-Liu-P'i*
Translation: Pomegranate Peel

Energy/Taste: Warm, sour, astringent

Channel-Organ: Large Intestine

Actions:
1. Astringe intestines to stop diarrhea
2. Contain Blood to stop bleeding
3. Kill parasites

Form and Preparation: Powder, decoction, or pill

Dosage:
Horses and Cattle: 15–30 g
Camel: 25–45 g
Llamas, Alpacas, Goats, Sheep, and Pigs: 3–15 g
Dogs: 2–5 g
Cats and Rabbits: 0.5–1 g
Birds: 1–2 g

Cautions and Contraindications: Caution in patients with Excess Heat and Food Stagnation

Side Effects: None known

Nelumbo *Lian Zi* 莲子

Original Reference: *Shen Nong Ben Cao Jing* (*Shen Nong's Materia Medica*, 1st century BCE) 神农本草经

Part Used: Seed

Name:
Pharmaceutical: Nelumbinis Nuciferae, Semen
Botanical: Nelumbo nucifera
Common: Lotus seed
Wade-Giles: *Lien-Tzu*
Translation: Lotus Seed

Energy/Taste: Neutral, sweet, astringent

Channel-Organ: Heart, Spleen, Kidney

Actions:
1. Tonify the Spleen to stop diarrhea
2. Reinforce the Kidney to control *Jing*
3. Nourish the Heart Blood and calm *Shen*
4. Clear Heart Fire

Form and Preparation: Powder, decoction, or pill

Dosage:
Horses and Cattle: 60–90 g
Llamas, Alpacas, Goats, Sheep, and Pigs: 10–50 g
Dogs: 2–10 g
Cats and Rabbits: 0.5–2 g
Birds: 0.2–2 g

Cautions and Contraindications: Caution in patients with constipation or abdominal distention

Side Effects: None known

Rubus *Fu Pen Zi* 覆盆子

Original Reference: *Ming Yi Bie Lu* (*Miscellaneous Records of Famous Physicians*) by *Tao Hong-Jing*, North and South Kingdoms (5th century) 名医别录

Part Used: Fruit

Name:
Pharmaceutical: Rubi Chingii, Fructus
Botanical: Rubus Chingii Hu
Common: Raspberry
Wade-Giles: *Fu-P'en-Tzu*
Translation: Overturned Bowl Fruit

Energy/Taste: Slightly warm, sweet, astringent

Channel-Organ: Kidney, Liver

Actions:
1. Augment and stabilize the Kidney
2. Astringe *Jing* and restrain urine
3. Assist the *Yang* and improve vision

Form and Preparation: Powder, decoction, or pill

Dosage:
Horses and Cattle: 15–45 g
Llamas, Alpacas, Goats, Sheep, and Pigs: 3–15 g
Dogs: 2–5 g
Cats and Rabbits: 0.5–1 g
Birds: 0.2–1.5 g

Cautions and Contraindications:
1. Caution in patients with *Yin* Deficiency with Heat
2. Contraindicated in patients with urinary difficulty

Side Effects: None known

Ailanthus *Chun Pi* 椿皮

Original Reference: *Tang Ben Cao* (*Tang Materia Medica*) by *Su Jing* et al., Tang Dynasty 唐本草

Part Used: Bark of root, or stem of tree

Name:
Pharmaceutical: Ailanthi Altissimae, Cortex
Botanical: Ailanthus altissima (Mill.) Swingle
Common: Ailanthus bark
Wade-Giles: *Ch'un-Pi*
Translation: Ailanthus bark

Energy/Taste: Cold, bitter, astringent

Channel-Organ: Liver, Stomach, Large Intestine

Actions:
1. Clear Heat, dry up Damp
2. Astringe the intestines, stop bleeding
3. Kill worms/parasites

Form and Preparation: Powder, decoction, or pill

Dosage:
Horses and Cattle: 15–60 g
Llamas, Alpacas, Goats, Sheep, and Pigs: 3–15 g

Cautions and Contraindications: Caution in patients with Spleen *Qi* or *Yang* Deficiency

Side Effects: None known

Rosa *Jin Ying Zi* 金樱子

Original Reference: *Lei Gong Pao Zhi Lun* (*Lei's Method of Preparing Drugs*) by *Lei Xiao*, 5th century 雷公炮炙论

Part Used: Fruit

Name:
Pharmaceutical: Rosae Laevigatae, Fructus
Botanical: Rosa laevigata Michx.
Common: Rose hip
Wade-Giles: *Chin-Ying-Tzu*
Translation: Golden Cherry Fruit

Energy/Taste: Neutral, sour, astringent

Channel-Organ: Kidney, Bladder, Large Intestine

Actions:
1. Control *Jing*, stabilize the Kidney
2. Astringe the intestines to stop diarrhea
3. Decrease urination

Form and Preparation: Powder, decoction, or pill

Dosage:
Horses and Cattle: 20–45 g
Llamas, Alpacas, Goats, Sheep, and Pigs: 3–15 g
Dogs: 2–5 g
Cats and Rabbits: 0.5–1 g
Birds: 0.2–1.5 g

Cautions and Contraindications: Caution in patients with Excess Heat or Fire

Side Effects: Overdose or long-term use may cause abdominal pain and constipation.

Triticum *Fu Xiao Ma* 浮小麦

Original Reference: *Ben Cao Gang Mu* (*Materia Medica Compendium*) by *Li Shi-Zhen* in 1590 本草纲目

Part Used: Immature wheat grain

Name:
Pharmaceutical: Tritici Aestivi Levis, Fructus
Botanical: Triticum aestivum L.
Common: Light wheat grain
Wade-Giles: *Fu-Hsiao-Mai*
Translation: Floating Little Wheat

Energy/Taste: Cool, sweet, salty

Channel-Organ: Heart

Actions:
1. Stop sweating

Table 14.1. Herbs to stabilize and bind: A quick overview and comparison.

Herbs	Special Actions	Common Characteristics
Herbs to astringe the Lung and Intestines		
Wu Wei Zi	Nourish the Kidney, restrain essence Generate Body Fluid, stop excessive sweating, calm *Shen*	Action: Astringe the Lung to stop cough or asthma, astringe the Intestines to stop diarrhea Indications: Cough, asthma, diarrhea, or dysentery
He Zi	Benefit throat	
Wu Mei	Generate body fluid to relieve thirst Expel roundworms, alleviate pain	
Rou Dou Kou	Warm the Spleen, promote *Qi* to stop pain	
Bai Guo	Expel Phlegm and stop wheezing, eliminate Damp and stop discharge	
Ying Su Ke	Stop pain, stabilize the Lower *Jiao*	
Chi Shi Zhi	Contain Blood to stop bleeding, promote healing	
Wu Bei Zi	Stop hemorrhage, kill parasites	
Shi Liu Pi	Contain Blood to stop bleeding, kill parasites	
Herbs to astringe *Jing* to stop urinary leakage		
Shan Zhu Yu	Tonify Liver *Yin*	Action: Strengthen Kidney, astringe *Jing*, stop urinary leakage Indications: Urinary incontinence, Impotence, premature ejaculation
Qian Shi	Tonify the Spleen to remove Dampness	
Sang Piao Xiao	Tonify Kidney and Strengthen *Yang*	
Hai Piao Xiao	Stop bleeding, restrain gastric acidity, dry Damp and promote healing of ulcers	
Lian Zi	Tonify the Spleen, nourish the Heart Blood, clear Heart Fire and calm *Shen*	
Fu Pen Zi	Strengthen Kidney *Yang*, improve vision	
Chun Pi	Astringe the intestines, stop bleeding, clear Damp-Heat, kill worms/parasites	
Jin Ying Zi	Astringe the intestines to stop diarrhea	
Herbs to stop sweating		
Ma Huang Gen	Astringe the surface to stop sweating	Action: Stop sweating Indication: Excessive sweating
Fu Xiao Ma	Calm *Shen*, tonify *Qi* and clear Heat	

2. Nourish the Heart and calm *Shen*
3. Tonify *Qi* and clear Heat

Form and Preparation: Powder, decoction, or pill

Dosage:
Horses and Cattle: 60–90 g
Llamas, Alpacas, Goats, Sheep, and Pigs: 8–30 g
Dogs: 5–8 g
Cats and Rabbits: 0.5–3 g
Birds: 0.2–5 g

Cautions and Contraindications: None known

Side Effects: None known

SUMMARY OF HERBS THAT STABILIZE AND BIND

Table 14.1 summarizes and compares the herbs that stabilize and bind (astringents).

REFERENCES

1. Chen JK, Chen TT. Chinese Medical Herbology and Pharmacology. City of Industry, CA: Art of Medicine Press, 2004.
2. Brinker FJ. The Toxicology of Botanical Medicines. Sandy, OR: Eclectic Medical Publications, 2000.
3. Duke JA. Handbook of Medicinal Herbs. New York: Chemical and Rubber Company Press, 2001.
4. Huang KC. The Pharmacology of Chinese Herbs, 2nd Edition. New York: Chemical and Rubber Company Press, 1999.

15 Herbs to Open Orifices (Senses) 开窍药

Huisheng Xie, Vanessa Preast, Min Su Kim

The herbs in this chapter treat *Bi Zheng* (Closed Syndrome or Unconsciousness Syndrome) by opening the orifices and senses (Table 15.1). The orifices are called *Qiao* in Traditional Chinese Veterinary Medicine (TCVM). *Qiao* organs include the nose, ears, brain, eyes, and skin. When *Qiao* organs are open, the body has normal senses and perception. When *Qiao* organs are closed, *Bi Zheng* results and the animal loses consciousness. In general, the herbs to open the orifices are strongly aromatic, which has a remarkable ability to stimulate sense organs, restore consciousness, stimulate the central nervous system and revive patients in a coma. Some herbs have a tranquilizing effect, which can treat irritability and stop spasms. These herbs treat the clinical signs of a disease rather than the underlying root cause of the illness. Because cooking or boiling can destroy their effectiveness, most of these herbs are administered in powder or pill form.

These herbs are used only as an immediate therapy for emergency conditions and for a short period of time. Additionally, some of these herbs are contraindicated during pregnancy. Because of the potency and penetration of these herbs, *Yuan* (Source) *Qi* consumption may occur with overdoses or long-term administration.

As listed in Table 15.1, *Bi Zheng* can be divided into Heat or Cold Closed Syndromes. A Heat Closed Syndrome is treated with the appropriate herbs to open the orifices in combination with herbs to clear Heat and resolve toxins. Similarly, for a Cold Closed Syndrome, herbs that dispel Cold and promote *Qi* are combined with herbs that open the orifices (see Table 15.1). Herbs that open the orifices should be avoided when treating *Tuo Zheng* Collapsing or Flaccid Syndrome, a Deficiency Pattern characterized by cold sweating, cold limbs, and a feeble pulse. *Tuo Zheng* may be seen with shock, hemorrhage, loss of Body Fluids, or coma. To treat *Tuo Zheng*, substances that tonify the *Qi* and resuscitate the *Yang* are required.

Bovis Calculus *Niu Huang* 牛黄

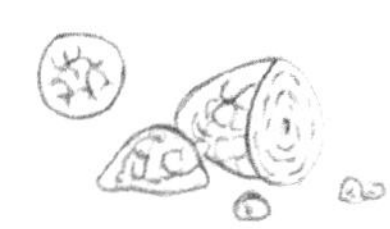

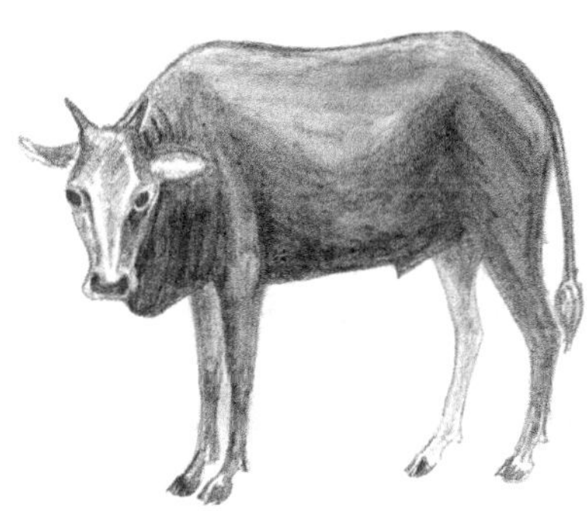

Original Reference: *Shen Nong Ben Cao Jing* (*Shen Nong's Materia Medica*, 1st century BCE) 神农本草经

Part Used: Gallbladder stone of an ox (natural or artificial)

Name:
Pharmaceutical: Bovis, Calculus
Zoological: Bos Taurus domesticus
Common: Ox gallbladder stone
Wade-Giles: *Niu-Huang*
Translation: Ox Yellow

Energy/Taste: Cool, bitter

Channel-Organ: Liver, Heart

Table 15.1. *Bi Zheng* (Closed Syndrome): Differentiation and examples of herbs.

Type	Pathology	Clinical Signs	Examples of Herbs
Heat Closed Syndrome	Corresponds to warm febrile disease entering the *Ying* level (toxemia, meningitis), or Heat collapsing into the Pericardium; may also include heatstroke, strokes, and severe liver disease	Heavy breathing, or dyspnea High fever or hot body Red skin Tongue: yellow tongue coat Pulse: forceful or rapid forceful	Bovis Calculus *Niu Huang*
Cold Closed Syndrome	Seen in poisonings and certain cerebrovascular accidents	Loss of consciousness Cold body Skin/complexion: purple or blue Tongue: pale wet Pulse: slow	Acorus *Shi Chang Pu*

Actions:
1. Open the orifices
2. Clear Heat
3. Detoxify (resolve toxins)
4. Extinguish endogenous Wind to stop spasms
5. Transform Phlegm

Form and Preparation: Powder or pill

Dosage:
Horses and Cattle: 3–12g
Llamas, Alpacas, Goats, and Pigs: 0.5–2g
Dogs: 0.3–1g
Cats and Rabbits: 0.1–0.5g
Birds: 0.1–1g

Cautions and Contraindications:
1. Caution during pregnancy
2. Caution with Spleen *Qi* Deficiency or Stomach *Yin* Deficiency and use only for Excess-Heat Patterns

Side Effects: Overdose or long-term use may cause thrombocytopenia, gastrointestinal hemorrhage, cystitis, asthma, allergic skin reactions, and anaphylaxis.

Clinical Applications:
1. Coma or unconsciousness with convulsions due to high fever
   Combine with: Coptis *Huang Lian*, Rhinoceros *Xi Jiao*, and Moschus *She Xiang*
2. Sore throat or ulcers and boils due to accumulation of Heat Toxins
   Combine with: Indigo *Qing Dai* and Lonicera *Jin Yin Hua*
3. *Shen* disturbances and irritability due to Heat crushing the Pericardium as in warm febrile diseases
   Combine with: Coptis *Huang Lian*, Cinnabaris *Zhu Sha*, Gardenia *Zhi Zi*

Pharmaceutical Ingredients:[1–4]
1. Bile acids, bilirubin
2. Cholic acid, deoxycholic acid
3. Taurine, cholesterol, ergosterol, lecithine

Acorus *Shi Chang Pu* 石菖蒲

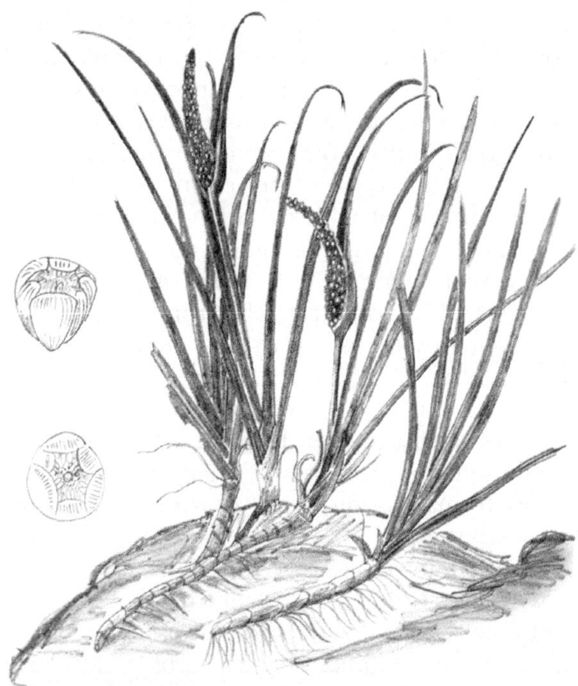

Original Reference: *Shen Nong Ben Cao Jing* (*Shen Nong*'s *Materia Medica*, 1st century BCE) 神农本草经

Part Used: Root and Rhizome

Name:
Pharmaceutical: Acori Graminei, Rhizoma
Botanical: Acorus gramineus

Common: Sweet flag
Wade-Giles: *Shih-Ch'ang-P'u*
Translation: Stone Acorus

Energy/Taste: Warm, pungent, aromatic

Channel-Organ: Heart, Spleen, Stomach

Actions:
1. Open the orifices
2. Pacify *Shen*
3. Remove Damp
4. Harmonize the Stomach

Form and Preparation: Powder, decoction, or pill

Dosage:
Horses and Cattle: 20–45 g
Camels: 30–60 g
Llamas, Alpacas, Goats, and Pigs: 5–15 g
Dogs: 3–5 g
Cats and Rabbits: 1–1.5 g
Birds: 0.1–1.5 g

Cautions and Contraindications:
1. Caution in *Yin* Deficiency with Heat
2. May antagonize the effects of Ephedra *Ma Huang*

Side Effects: None known

Clinical Applications:
1. Mental disorders or coma due to turbid Phlegm blocking the Pericardium or accumulation of Damp-Heat
   Combine with: Bambusa *Zhu Li*, and Curcuma *Yu Jin*
2. Dampness in the Middle Burner (*Zhong Jiao*)
   Clinical signs: Bloat, distension and pain in the chest and abdomen
   Combine with: Citrus *Chen Pi* and Magnolia *Huo Po*
3. Insomnia or heart palpitations due to Heart *Qi* deficiency
   Combine with: Poria *Fu Ling* and Polygala *Yuan Zhi*
   Classical herbal formula: *An Shen Ding Zhi Wan*

Comments:
1. Acorus *Shi Chang Pu* is used widely in Ayurveda as a consciousness-raising herb for meditation.
2. Acorus *Shi Chang Pu* increases the appetite and improves digestion.
3. The ethanol extract of *Acorus gramineus* Soland (EEAGS) has an anticonvulsant effect in mice and rats.

Pharmaceutical Ingredients:[1–4]
1. Essential oils (β-asarone, α-asarone)
2. Caryophyllene
3. α-humulene
4. Seikishone
5. Asarylaldehyde
6. Glucose
7. Amino acids

Borneol *Bing Pian* 冰片

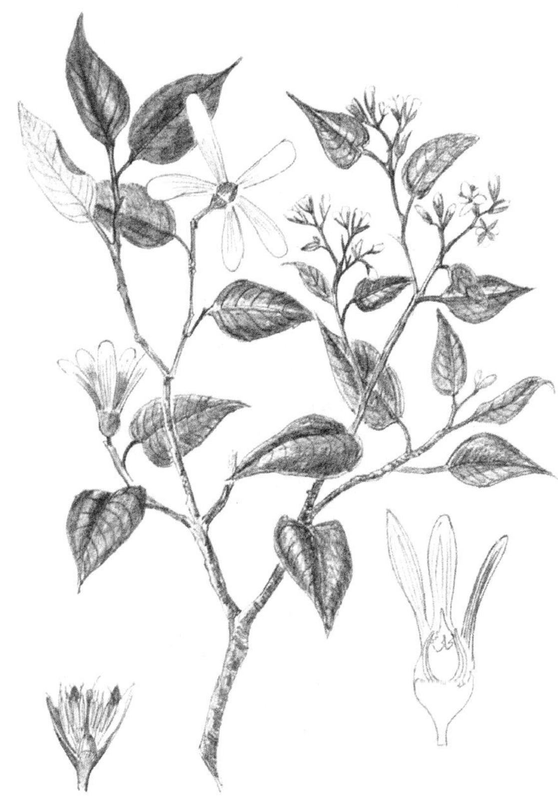

Original Reference: *Tang Ben Cao* (*Tang Materia Medica* by *Su Jing* et al., Tang Dynasty) 唐本草

Part Used: Crystal

Name:
Pharmaceutical: Borneolum
Botanical: Dryobalanops aromatica
Common: Borneol
Wade-Giles: *Ping-P'ien*
Translation: Ice Slice
Alternative: *Mei Pian* or *Long Nao*

Energy/Taste: Slightly cold, pungent, bitter

Channel-Organ: Heart, Spleen, Lung

Actions:
1. Open the orifices

2. Wake up *Shen*
3. Clear Heat and relieve pain
4. Dissipate nodules
5. Alleviate itching (antiinflammatory)

Form and Preparation: Powder for topical use or pill for oral use. *Bing Pian* is the crystal obtained from the plant Dryobalanops aromatica. Natural *Bing Pian* is formed by tapping the tree trunk of *Dryobalanops aromatica* and steaming and distilling the sap to form a hard crystalline substance. Synthetic Borneol *Bing Pian* is chemically created from Turpentine Oil *Song Jie You* and Camphor *Zhang Lao*.

Dosage:
Horses and Cattle: 3–6 g
Llamas, Alpacas, Goats, and Pigs: 0.5–1.5 g
Dogs: 0.5–0.75 g
Cats and Rabbits: 0.03–0.05 g
Birds: 0.01–0.1 g

Cautions and Contraindications:
1. Caution during pregnancy
2. Caution for *Qi* or Blood Deficiency

Side Effects: Overdose may cause nausea and headache.

Clinical Applications:
1. Coma or unconsciousness due to high fever
   Combine with: Moschus *She Xiang*
   Classical herbal formula: *An Gong Niu Huang Wan*
2. Red, swollen and painful eyes, photophobia or excessive tearing
   Use alone: Externally as eye drops
3. Ulceration in the mouth or sore throat
   Combine with: Mirabilitum *Mang Xiao* and Borax *Peng Sha*
   Classical herbal formula: *Bing Beng San*

History and Comments:
1. Borneol *Bing Pian* is a common component of patented formulas for the treatment of gingivitis or stomatitis, and nervousness.
2. Because of the volatile nature of Borneol *Bing Pian*, it is usually not included in a decoction, but is taken separately in the form of a pill or used topically.
3. Its topical use can Clear Heat and stop pain and itching. It has antibacterial and antiinflammatory effects.

Pharmaceutical Ingredients:[1–4]
1. Borneol, isoborneol, α-borneol
2. Sesquiterpenoids humulene, β-elemene, caryophyllene)
3. Triterpenoids (oleanolic acid, asiatic acid, erythrodid)
4. Cineole, camphor, humulene, l-camphor

Styrax *Su He Xiang* 苏合香

Original Reference: *Ming Yi Bie Lu* (*Miscellaneous Records of Famous Physicians* by *Tao Hong-Jing*, North and South Kingdoms, 5th century) 名医别录

Part Used: Resin

Name:
Pharmaceutical: Styrax, liquidus
Botanical: Liquidambar orientalis Mill
Common: Styrax
Wade-Giles: *Su-He-Hsiang*
Translation: Revive and join fragrance

Energy/Taste: Warm, pungent, sweet, aromatic

Channel-Organ: Heart, Spleen

Actions:
1. Open the orifices and clear the mind
2. Penetrate through turbidity
3. Stop pain
4. Open areas of constraint

Form and Preparation: Powder or pill

Dosage:
Horses and Cattle: 5–24 g
Llamas, Alpacas, Goats, and Pigs: 1–5 g
Dogs: 0.5–2 g
Cats and Rabbits: 0.1–0.5 g
Birds: 0.05–0.1 g

Cautions and Contraindications:
1. Caution during pregnancy
2. Caution in patients experiencing sudden collapse with profuse sweating

Side Effects: None known

Moschus *She Xiang* 麝香

Original Reference: *Shen Nong Ben Cao Jing* (*Shen Nong's Materia Medica*, 1st century BCE)

Part Used: Secretion. It comes from a gland found near the navel of the male musk deer. This substance is rare and expensive. Today, the synthesized substitute is used for similar effect.

Name:
Pharmaceutical: Moschus, secretio
Zoological: Moschus moschiferus, M. sifanicus, M. berezovskii
Common: Musk gland secretion
Wade-Giles: *She-Hsiang*
Translation: Musk Fragrance

Table 15.2. Herbs to open orifices: An overview and comparison.

Herb	Special Actions	Common Characteristics
Bovis Calculus *Niu Huang*	Clear Heat, detoxify (resolve toxins) Extinguish endogenous Wind to stop spasm	Taste: Strong aromatic odor Action: Stimulate sense organs, restore consciousness, stimulate the central nervous system and promote revival from coma Indication: Unconsciousness or coma
Acorus *Shi Chang Pu*	Remove Damp and harmonize stomach	
Borneol *Bing Pian*	Clear Heat and relieve pain Dissipate nodules and alleviate itching	
Styrax *Su He Xiang*	Penetrate through turbidity, stop pain Open up areas of constraint	
Moschus *She Xiang*	Invigorate Blood and stop pain Disperse nodules and expel the placenta	

Energy/Taste: Warm, pungent, aromatic

Channel-Organ: Heart, Spleen, Liver

Actions:
1. Open the orifices and clear the mind intensely
2. Invigorate Blood and stop pain
3. Disperse nodules and remove swelling
4. Expel a placenta and stillborn fetus

Form and Preparation: Never decocted; used only in pills or as a powder

Dosage:
Horses and Cattle: 0.5–1.5 g
Llamas, Alpacas, Goats, and Pigs: 0.1–0.2 g
Dogs: 0.05–0.1 g

Cautions and Contraindications:
1. Contraindicated during pregnancy
2. Caution in patients with hypertension

Side Effects:
1. May cause renal failure when administered orally
2. May cause a skin allergy when applied topically

Comments:
1. *She Xiang* is a rare and expensive substance, which comes from the preputial sac of the male musk deer.
2. A synthetic form of *She Xiang* is currently available and may have similar effects.

SUMMARY OF HERBS THAT OPEN THE ORIFICES

Table 15.2 summarizes and compares the herbs that open the orifices.

REFERENCES

1. Chen JK, Chen TT. Chinese Medical Herbology and Pharmacology. City of Industry, CA: Art of Medicine Press, 2004.
2. Brinker FJ. The Toxicology of Botanical Medicines. Sandy, OR: Eclectic Medical Publications, 2000.
3. Duke JA. Handbook of Medicinal Herbs. New York: Chemical and Rubber Company Press, 2001.
4. Huang KC. The Pharmacology of Chinese Herbs, 2nd Edition. New York: Chemical and Rubber Company Press, 1999.

16 Herbs to Expel Parasites
驱虫药

Huisheng Xie, Min Su Kim, Cheryl Chrisman

Because there is a variety of parasites, different methods are available to expel them. In general, conventional pharmaceutical drugs that kill parasites are more effective and expedient, but the herbs discussed in this chapter can also be useful to expel intestinal parasites, including roundworms, hookworms, tapeworms, and pinworms. These herbs often have a bitter taste and most enter the Spleen, Stomach, and Large Intestine Channels; some, however, also enter the Lung Channels.

Herbs to expel parasites are often combined with other herbs, and the ones selected will vary with the underlying disease Pattern. For Cold Patterns, either Zanthoxylum *Chuan Jiao* or Dry Ginger Zingiberis *Gan Jiang* is added to formulas. For Heat Patterns, either Coptis *Huang Lian* or Phellodendron *Huang Bai* is added. For Food Stagnation, herbs such as Crataegus *Shan Zha* and Massa Fermentata *Shen Qu* are added.

When using herbs to expel parasites, the following should be considered: 1) oily foods should be avoided and the herbs should be administered on an empty stomach; 2) some antiparasitic herbs including Melia *Ku Lian Pi* are toxic, and overdosing can cause side effects; 3) some herbs, such as Omphalia *Lei Wan*, should be used with caution during pregnancy or for patients with weak constitutions; and 4) herbs to strengthen the Spleen and Stomach should be used for patients with Spleen *Qi* Deficiency prior to or while taking herbs that expel parasites.

Dryopteris *Guan Zhong* 贯众

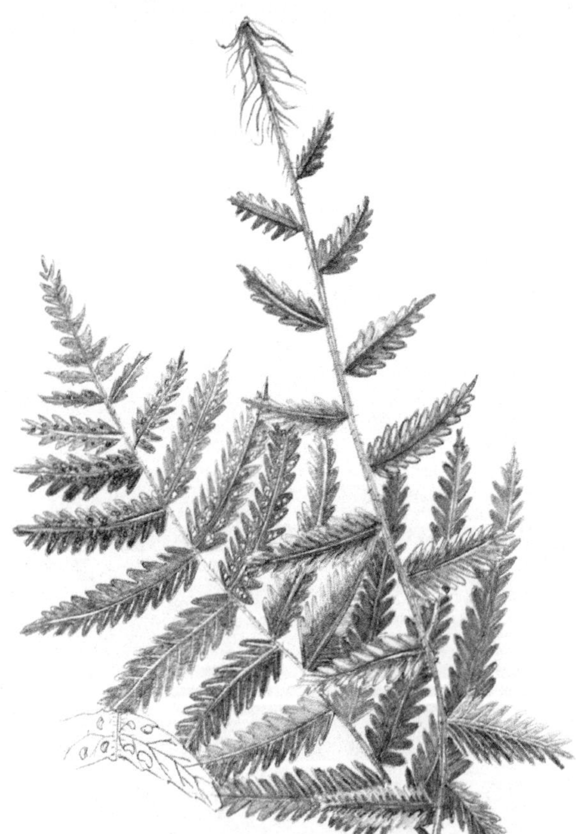

a

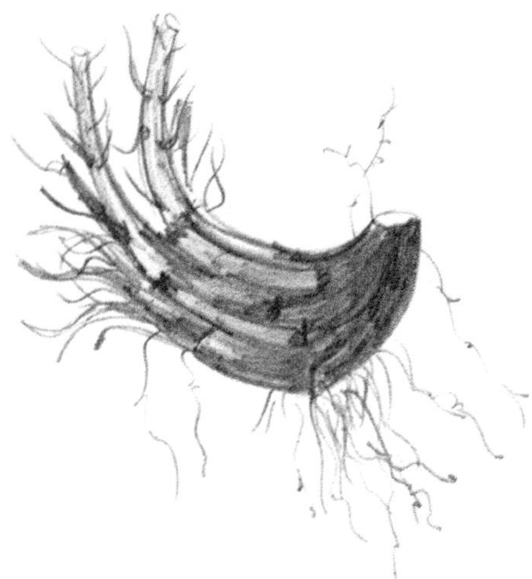

b

Original Reference: *Shen Nong Ben Cao Jing* (*Shen Nong's Materia Medica*, 1st century BCE) 神农本草经

Part Used: Rhizome

Name:
Pharmaceutical: Dryopteris, Rhizoma
Botanical: Dryopteris crassirhizoma Nakai, Lunathyrium-acrosticholides, Woodwardia unigemmata
Common: Dryopteris root
Translation: Link the Multitude

Energy/Taste: Slightly cold, bitter, slightly toxic

Channel-Organ: Stomach, Spleen, Liver

Actions:
1. Kill parasites
2. Clear Heat and resolve toxins
3. Cool Blood and stop bleeding

Form and Preparation: Powder or decoction

Dosage:
Horses and Cattle: 30–90 g
Llamas, Alpacas, Goats, and Pigs: 3–10 g
Dogs: 2–5 g
Cats and Rabbits: 0.5–1 g
Birds: 0.1–1.5 g

Cautions and Contraindications: Caution in patients with a weak constitution or gastric or duodenal ulcers

Side Effects: May cause vomiting, diarrhea, and visual disturbances

Clinical Applications:
1. Various types of gastrointestinal parasites
   Combine with: Omphalia *Lei Wan* and Areca *Bing Lang*, and Quisqualis *Shi Jun Zi* for tapeworms and roundworms
   Combine with: Torreya *Fei Zi* and Areca *Bing Lang* for hookworm
   Combine with: Melia *Ku Lian Pi* and Carpesium *He Shi* for pinworms
2. Wind-Heat invasion, epidemic influenza, and acute inflammation of the parotid glands
   Combine with: Lonicera *Jin Yin Hua*, Forsythia *Lian Qiao*, Isatis *Da Qing Ye* and Isatis *Ban Lan Gen*
3. Bleeding due to Blood Heat
   Clinical signs: Vomiting with blood, epistaxis, bloody diarrhea, or functional uterine bleeding
   Combine with: Biota *Ce Bai Ye*, Agrimony *Xian He Cao* and Eclipta *Han Lian Cao*, and Trachycarpus *Zong Lu Tan*

History and Comments:
1. Good quality Dryopteris *Guan Zhong* is large and firm with a brownish green cross-section. It is extensively used in farm animals in China for general health and deworming programs.
2. When charred, Dryopteris *Guan Zhong* has been shown to be effective to arrest uterine bleeding.
3. Dryopteris *Guan Zhong* has been prescribed for influenza prevention during influenza epidemics in both animals and humans.

Pharmaceutical Ingredients:[1–4]
1. Filmarone, dryocrassin, filic acid, flavaspidic acids
2. Fibaspidins, aspidinol, filicinic acid, ferene, diploptene, diplopterol

Areca *Bing Lang* 槟榔

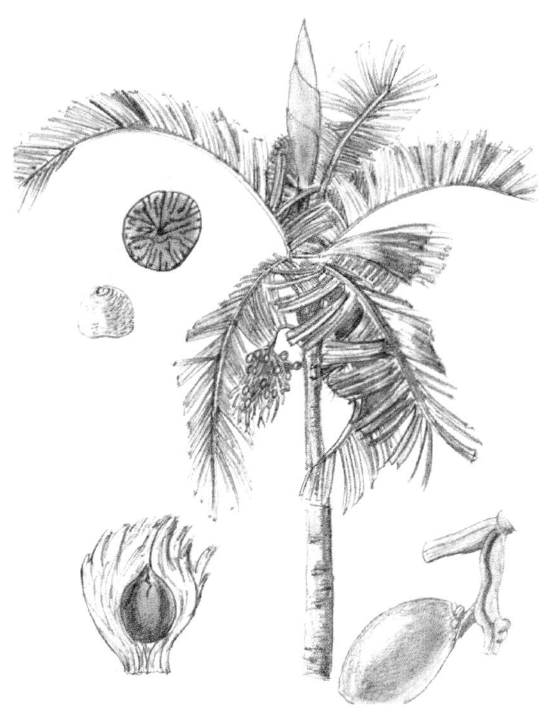

Original Reference: *Ming Yi Bie Lu* (*Miscellaneous Records of Famous Physicians*) by *Tao Hong-Jing*, North and South Kingdoms (5th century) 名医别录

Part Used: Seed

Name:
Pharmaceutical: Arecae Catechu, Semen
Botanical: Areca catechu L.
Common: Betel nut; Areca seed
Alternative: *Da Fu Zi* (*Da Fu Pi* is its peel)

Energy/Taste: Warm, pungent, bitter

Channel-Organ: Stomach, Large Intestine

Actions:
1. Kill parasites, especially tapeworms
2. Move *Qi* and resolve Food Stagnation
3. Promote diuresis

Form and Preparation: Powder or decoction

Dosage:
Horses: 5–15 g
Cattle: 12–60 g
Llamas, Alpacas, Goats, and Pigs: 3–10 g
Dogs: 1–3 g
Cats and Rabbits: 0.5–1 g
Birds: 0.3–3 g

Cautions and Contraindications: Caution in patients with Spleen *Qi* Deficiency

Side Effects: May cause diarrhea

Clinical Applications:
1. Intestinal parasites, especially tapeworms
   Combine with: Curcubita *Nan Gua Zi*
2. Food retention with abdominal distention and constipation or tenesmus associated with dysentery
   Combine with: Saussurea *Mu Xiang*, Rheum *Da Huang*, and Aurantium *Zhi Ke*
   Classical herbal formula: *Mu Xiang Bing Lang Wan*
3. Edema and pain in the paws, hooves, and feet
   Combine with: Poria *Fu Ling*, Phytolacca *Shang Lu*, Akebia *Mu Tong*, Alisma *Ze Xie*
4. Swollen and painful limbs
   Combine with: Chaenomeles *Mu Gua*, Perilla *Zi Su Ye* and Evodia *Wu Zhu Yu*

Pharmaceutical Ingredients:[1–4]
1. Alkaloids (areca red, arecoline, arecaine, guvacoline, guracine, guvacoline, aecolidine, homoarecoline)
2. Lauric acid, myristic acid, palmitic acid, stearic acid, oleic acid
3. Catechol, tannin, fats, areca red, proline, tyrosine, arginine

Quisqualis *Shi Jun Zi* 使君子

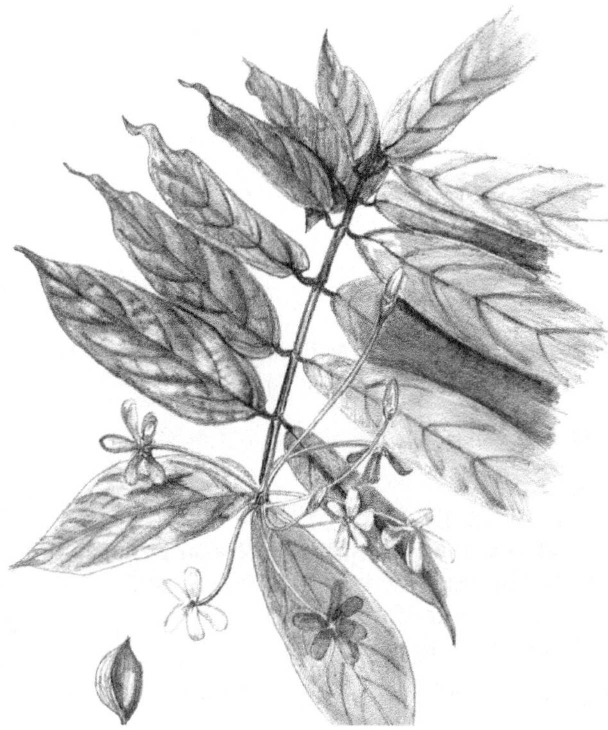

Original Reference: *Kai Bao Ben Cao* (*Materia Medica of the Kai Bao Era*) by *Ma Zhi* in 973 CE 开宝本草

Part Used: Seed and fruit

Name:
Pharmaceutical: Quisqualis Indicae, Fructus
Botanical: Quisqualis indica L.
Common: Quisqualis fruit
Translation: Envoy Seeds

Energy/Taste: Warm, sweet

Channel-Organ: Spleen, Stomach

Actions:
1. Kill parasites, especially roundworms
2. Resolve food accumulation due to intestinal parasites

Form and Preparation: Powder; do *not* prepare as a hot tea

Dosage:
Horses and Cattle: 30–90g
Llamas, Alpacas, Goats, and Pigs: 5–20g
Dogs: 5–10g
Cats and Rabbits: 1–2g
Birds: 0.2–2g

Cautions and Contraindications: Avoid overdosing

Side Effects:
1. Overdosing may induce hiccups, dizziness, lack of energy, nausea, even vomiting, and diarrhea.
2. Administering as a hot tea may induce hiccups or diarrhea.
3. Adverse clinical side effects will subside once administration is stopped.
4. If a toxic reaction occurs, a decoction of cloves (*Ding Xiang*) can be used as an antidote.

Clinical Applications:
1. Roundworms (ascariasis)
   Combine with: Areca *Bing Lang* and Melia *Ku Lian Pi*
2. Pinworms
   Combine with: Stemona *Bai Bu*
3. Nutritional problems in young animals
   Combine with: Codonopsis *Dang Shen*, Atractylodes *Bai Zhu*

History and Comments:
1. A good quality fruit peel is large, dark purple, and shiny, and the seeds should be full, round, and pale yellow.
2. Fruits, leaves, and roots can be used for expelling roundworms and for improving digestion. The fruits and seeds are best at expelling roundworms, but the roots can be used to stop coughing or hiccups and possess antiinflammatory and antibiotic effects. The roots are also used in otitis and prolapsed rectum.
3. Dry-frying until aromatic can reduce the toxicity of Quisqualis *Shi Jun Zi*.
4. A water extract of Quisqualis *Shi Jun Zi* can be used to inhibit some skin fungi.

Pharmaceutical Ingredients:[1–4] Quisqualic acid, potassium quisqualate, cyaniding monoglycoside, trigonelline

Allium *Da Suan* 大蒜

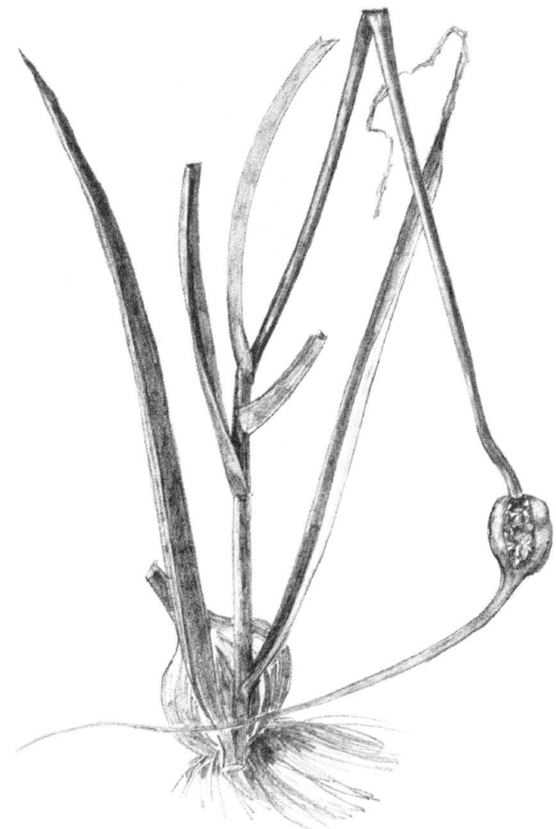

Original Reference: *Ming Yi Bie Lu* (Miscellaneous Records of Famous Physicians) by *Tao Hong-Jing*, North and South Kingdoms (5th century) 名医别录

Part Used: Bulb

Name:
Pharmaceutical: Allii Sativi, Bulbus
Botanical: Allium sativum L.
Common: Garlic bulb
Translation: Large Garlic

Energy/Taste: Warm, pungent

Channel-Organ: Spleen, Stomach, Large Intestine, Lung

Actions:
1. Kill parasites, resolve swelling
2. Relieve toxicity from food poisoning
3. Used to prevent influenza

Form and Preparation: Powder, decoction, or raw; may be used as indirect moxibustion; sliced or properly squeezed garlic may be used for topical administration

Dosage:
Horses and Cattle: 60–120 g
Llamas, Alpacas, Goats, and Pigs: 5–30 g
Dogs: 2–3 g
Cats and Rabbits: 0.5–1 g
Birds: 0.1–1 g

Cautions and Contraindications:
1. Caution in patients with *Yin* Deficiency with Heat
2. Can be a skin irritant so should not be applied topically as a long-term treatment
3. Caution when administering internally to patients with problems of the mouth, tongue, and throat
4. Topical application around the perianal area or enema administration contraindicated during pregnancy

Side Effects: May irritate the skin and eyes

Clinical Applications:
1. Hookworms and roundworms
   Combine with: Areca *Bing Lang*, Carpesium *He Shi*, Melia *Ku Lian Pi*
2. Toxic swellings
   Combine with: Sesame oil and apply topically
3. Food poisoning especially associated with seafood
   Administer alone: Orally

History and Comments:
1. Allium *Da Suan* (garlic) has a purple skin and has a relatively strong effect against toxicity and parasites.
2. For pinworms, it may be applied topically to the perianal area and combined with sesame oil to prevent irritation.
3. Allium *Da Suan* (garlic) can be used as an enema for dysenteric diarrhea.
4. Allium *Da Suan* (garlic) is often used for the prevention of influenza.
5. Allium *Da Suan* (garlic) has antiparasitic, antimicrobial and antifungal effects.

Pharmaceutical Ingredients:[1–4] Alliin, allicin, alliinase, diallyl disulfide, allistatin, glucominol, diallyl thiosulfonate

Melia *Ku Lian Pi* 苦楝皮

Original Reference: *Ming Yi Bie Lu* (*Miscellaneous Records of Famous Physicians*) by *Tao Hong-Jing*, North and South Kingdoms (5th century) 名医别录

Part Used: Bark of the stem or root

Name:
Pharmaceutical: Meliae Radicis, Cortex
Botanical: Melia axedarach L.; M. toosendan Sieb et Zucc.
Common: Chinaberry bark
Translation: Bitter Tree Bark

Energy/Taste: Cold, bitter, toxic

Channel-Organ: Stomach, Spleen, Liver

Actions:
1. Kill parasites (stronger than Quisqualis *Shi Jun Zi*)
2. Treat fungal infection (topical use)

Form and Preparation: Powder or decoction

Dosage:
Horses and Cattle: 50–150 g
Llamas, Alpacas, Goats, and Pigs: 10–50 g
Dogs: 2–5 g
Cats and Rabbits: 0.5–2 g
Birds: 0.1–1.5 g

Cautions and Contraindications:
1. Should not be taken over a prolonged period. **It is toxic.**
2. Caution in patients with weak constitutions or hepatic disorders

Side Effects:
1. May cause dizziness, sleepiness, nausea, and abdominal pain within 1–6 hours after administration
2. May cause internal bleeding, especially of the Lung, Spleen, and Stomach

History and Comments:
1. The half-life of Melia *Ku Lian Pi* is long. It takes over 1 week to be eliminated from the body. Therefore, it should not be prescribed for long-term use.
2. Dead roundworms are often found in the feces 4–9 hours after administration of Melia *Ku Lian Pi*. Administering Melia *Ku Lian Pi* for 3 days can often eliminate roundworms completely.

Curcubita *Nan Gua Zi* 南瓜子

Original Reference: *Zhong Yao Xue* (*Chinese Materia Medica*) by *Gao Xue-ming* in 2002 中药学

Part Used: Seed

Name:
Pharmaceutical: Curcurbitae Moschatae, Semen
Botanical: Curcubita moschata Duch.
Common: Pumpkin seeds
Translation: Southern Melon Seeds

Energy/Taste: Neutral, sweet

Channel-Organ: Stomach, Large Intestine

Actions:
1. Expel parasites and alleviate pain
2. Benefit postpartum fluid metabolism

Form and Preparation: Powder, raw, or decoction

Dosage:
Horses and Cattle: 60–120 g
Llamas, Alpacas, Goats, and Pigs: 5–30 g
Dogs: 2–5 g
Cats and Rabbits: 0.5–2 g
Birds: 0.1–1.5 g

Cautions and Contraindications: None known

Side Effects: None known

Omphalia *Lei Wan* 雷丸

Original Reference: *Shen Nong Ben Cao Jing* (*Shen Nong's Materia Medica*, 1st century BCE) 神农本草经

Part Used: Fungus of omphalia

Name:
Pharmaceutical: Omphaliae, Sclerotium
Botanical: Polyporus mylittae Cooket Mass.; Omphalia lapidescens
Common: Fruiting Body of Omphalia
Translation: Thunder Pill

Energy/Taste: Cold, bitter, slightly toxic

Channel-Organ: Stomach, Large Intestine

Actions: Kill parasites

Form and Preparation: Powder or decoction

Dosage:
Horses and Cattle: 30–60 g
Camels: 45–90 g
Llamas, Alpacas, Goats, and Pigs: 3–20 g
Dogs: 2–5 g
Cats and Rabbits: 0.5–2 g
Birds: 0.1–1.5 g

Cautions and Contraindications:
1. Caution during pregnancy
2. May antagonize Pueraria *Ge Gen* and Polygonum *Bian Ku*

Side Effects: May damage Spleen and Stomach

Carpesium *He Shi* 鹤虱

Original Reference: *Tang Ben Cao* (*Tang Materia Medica*) by *Su Jing* et al., *Tang* Dynasty (618–907 CE) 唐本草

Part Used: Fruit

Name:
Pharmaceutical: Carpesii seu Daucusi, Fructus
Botanical: Carpesium abrotanoides L.; Daucus carota L.
Common: Carpesium fruit
Translation: Crane's Louse

Energy/Taste: Neutral, bitter, pungent, slightly toxic

Channel-Organ: Stomach, Spleen, Liver

Actions:
1. Kill parasites
2. Alleviate pain

Form and Preparation: Powder or decoction

Dosage:
Horses and Cattle: 15–30 g
Llamas, Alpacas, Goats, and Pigs: 3–6 g
Dogs: 2–3 g
Cats and Rabbits: 0.5–1 g
Birds: 0.2–2 g

Cautions and Contraindications: Caution in weak or geriatric patients

Side Effects: May cause nausea, dizziness, and abdominal pain

Torreya *Fei Zi* 榧子

Original Reference: *Ming Yi Bie Lu* (*Miscellaneous Records of Famous Physicians*) by *Tao Hong-Jing*, North and South Kingdoms (5th century) 名医别录

Part Used: Seed

Name:
Pharmaceutical: Torreyae Semen
Botanical: Torreya grandis fort
Common: Torreya seeds

Energy/Taste: Neutral, sweet, astringent

Channel-Organ: Lung, Stomach, Large Intestine

Actions:
1. Kill parasites
2. Moisten the Lung and stop cough

Table 16.1. Herbs to expel parasites: A quick overview and comparison.

Herbs	Special Actions	Common Characteristics
Guan Zhong	Clear Heat and resolve toxins Cool Blood and stop bleeding	Taste: Bitter Action: Expel GI worms
Bing Lang	Kill GI parasites, especially tapeworms Move *Qi* and resolve food stagnation	Indication: GI worms Cautions:
Shi Jun Zi	Kill parasites, especially roundworms Resolve accumulation due to intestinal parasites	1) Take on an empty stomach to increase their activity 2) Avoid oily food
Da Suan	Relieve toxicity for treating food poisons Used to prevent influenza	3) Immediately use herbs to strengthen the Spleen and Stomach after using these "parasite-expelling" herbs
Ku Lian Pi	Kill parasites stronger than Quisqualis *Si Jun Zi* Treat fungal infection (topical use), **toxic**	
Nan Gua Zi	Alleviate pain, benefit postpartum fluid metabolism	
Lei Wan	Slightly **toxic**	
He Shi	Alleviates pain, slightly **toxic**	
Fei Zi	Moisten the Lung and stop cough	

Form and Preparation: Powder or decoction

Dosage:
Horses and Cattle: 60–90 g
Llamas, Alpacas, Goats, and Pigs: 10–30 g
Dogs: 2–8 g
Cats and Rabbits: 0.5–1 g
Birds: 0.1–1.5 g

Cautions and Contraindications: None known

Side Effects: None known

SUMMARY OF HERBS TO EXPEL PARASITES

Table 16.1 summarizes and compares the herbs that expel parasites.

REFERENCES

1. Chen JK, Chen TT. Chinese Medical Herbology and Pharmacology. City of Industry, CA: Art of Medicine Press, 2004.
2. Brinker FJ. The Toxicology of Botanical Medicines. Sandy, OR: Eclectic Medical Publications, 2000.
3. Duke JA. Handbook of Medicinal Herbs. New York: Chemical and Rubber Company Press, 2001.
4. Huang KC. The Pharmacology of Chinese Herbs, 2nd Edition. New York: Chemical and Rubber Company Press, 1999.

17 Herbs for Topical Application 外用药

Huisheng Xie, Min Su Kim, Cheryl Chrisman

Topical herbal applications are some of the oldest therapies in Traditional Chinese Veterinary Medicine (TCVM). Some herbs can be absorbed locally and systemically through the skin, rectum, nasal and oral mucosas, and the Lungs to treat local or generalized diseases. Topical herbal applications not only provide relief of the clinical signs, but can treat the underlying etiology as well. Some of the topical herbs can also be administered orally (internally), but they must be used with caution; patients receiving them must be closely monitored.

The vehicles (carriers) for external application of herbs include water, vegetable oil, wax, tincture, vinegar, and polymers such as hydroxpropyl methylcellulose (HPMC).

Camphor *Zhang Nao* 樟脑

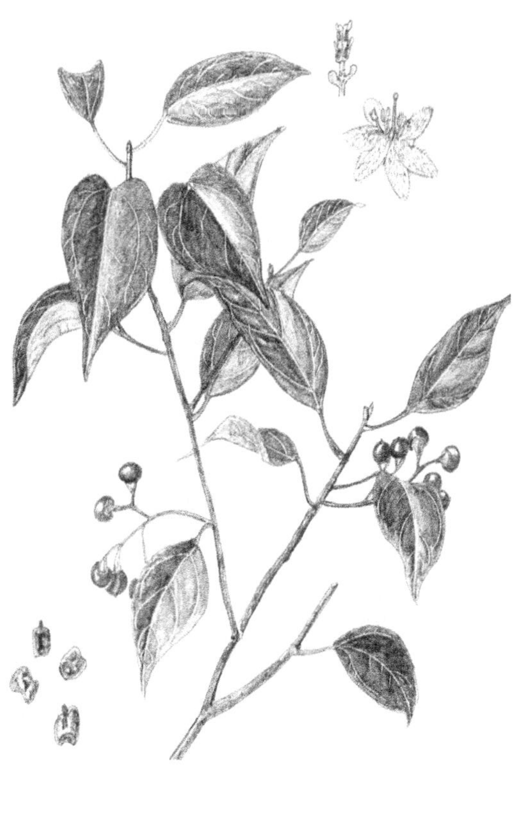

Original Reference: *Ben Cao Gang Mu* (*Materia Medica Compendium*) by *Li Shi-Zhen* in 1590 本草纲目

Part Used: Extracts of the volatile oil derived from twigs, roots, or leaves of Cinnamomum Camphora using steam-distilling techniques

Name:
Pharmaceutical: Camphora ($C_{10}H_{16}O$)
Botanical: Cinnamomum camphora (L.)
Common: Camphor
Wade-Giles: *Chang-Nao*
Translation: Camphor

Energy/Taste: Hot, pungent, toxic

Channel-Organ: Heart

Actions:
1. Remove Wind-Damp and alleviate pain (topically)
2. Kill external parasites and relieve pruritis (topically)
3. Open the orifices and expel turbidity (orally)
4. Invigorate Blood and alleviate pain (orally)

Form and Preparation: Powder or alcohol tincture

Dosage:
Horses and Cattle: 9–15 g
Llamas, Alpacas, Goats, and Pigs: 0.5–3 g
Dogs, cats, rabbits, and birds: only topical use

Cautions and Contraindications:
1. Contraindicated during pregnancy
2. Caution when administering orally

Side Effects:
1. May cause dizziness and hyperactivity
2. Overdose may cause extreme excitement, seizures, and death.

Clinical Applications:
1. Scabies and pruritis
   Combine with: Alum *Bai Fan* (topically)

2. Sudden loss of consciousness or abdominal pain
   Combine with: Borneol *Bing Pian* (orally)
3. Toothaches or other pain and swelling due to trauma or injury
   Use alone: topically

History and Comments:
1. Camphor *Zhang Nao* can stimulate the central nervous system and increase respirations and blood pressure.

Pharmaceutical Ingredients:[1–2] d-camphora

Alum *Bai Fan* 白矾 (or *Ming Fan*) (明矾)

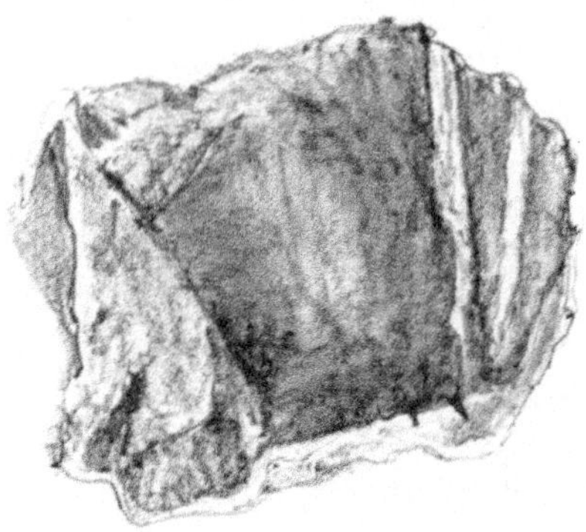

Original Reference: *Shen Nong Ben Cao Jing* (*Shen Nong's Materia Medica*, 1st century BCE) 神农本草经

Part Used: Mineral

Name:
Pharmaceutical: Alum
Mineral: Potassium aluminum sulfate
Common: Alum
Ward-Giles: *Pai-Fan*
Translation: White Alum

Energy/Taste: Cold, sour, astringent

Channel-Organ: Large Intestine, Liver, Lung, Spleen

Actions:
1. Relieve toxicity, kill external parasites, and dry Damp to relieve pruritis (topically)
2. Stop bleeding and alleviate diarrhea (orally)
3. Clear Heat and expel Phlegm (orally)

Form and Preparation: Powder or decoction; fine powder for topical use; powder or decoction for oral administration use

Dosage:
Horses and Cattle: 15–30 g
Llamas, Alpacas, Goats, and Pigs: 3–9 g
Dogs: 0.5–2 g
Cats and Rabbits: 0.2–0.5 g
Birds: 0.1–1 g

Cautions and Contraindications:
1. Caution when administering orally
2. Caution when the gastrointestinal (GI) system is weak
3. Do not use if the patient has GI Damp-Heat.
4. May antagonize Ostrea *Li Mu* and counteract Ephedra *Ma Huang*

Side Effects: May irritate the mouth, throat, and GI tract and cause vomiting, diarrhea, and shock

Clinical Applications:
1. Chronic vaginal discharge with pruritis and eczema
   Combine with: Cnidium *She Chuang Zi* (as an external wash)
2. Pain, redness, and swelling of middle ear
   Combine with: Borneol *Bing Pian* (topically in the ear)
3. Skin Damp-Heat
   Combine with: Stemona *Bai Bu* as a topical external wash
4. Nosebleeds or bleeding due to trauma
   Combine with: Acacia *Er Cha* (topically in the nose or on the wound)
5. Chronic, recalcitrant diarrhea in geriatric patients
   Combine with: Chebula *He Zi* as a powder (orally)

History and Comments:
1. Alum *Bai Fan* (aluminum potassium sulfate) becomes anhydrous Alum *Ku Fan* after being burnt and dehydrated.
2. Alum *Bai Fan* is used as a topical external wash for scabies, ringworm, or skin infections.
3. Alum *Bai Fan* has a strong astringent effect.

Pharmaceutical Ingredients:[1–2] $KAl_2(SO_4)_2(OH)_6$[2]

Calamina *Lu Gan Shi* 炉甘石

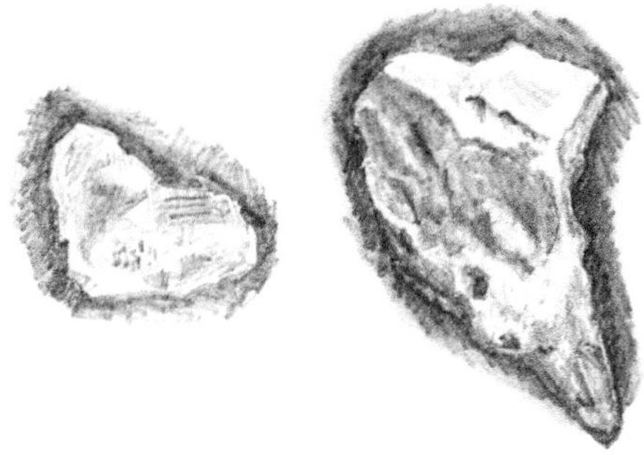

Original Reference: *Ben Cao Gang Mu* (*Materia Medica* Compendium) by *Li Shi-Zhen* in 1590 本草纲目

Part Used: Mineral

Name:
Pharmaceutical: Smithsonitum
Common: Calamine
Wade-Giles: *Lu-Kan-Shih*
Translation: Stove sweet Stone

Energy/Taste: Neutral, sweet

Channel-Organ: Liver, Stomach

Actions:
1. Brighten eyes, remove corneal opacity
2. Dry Damp and promote tissue regeneration

Form and Preparation: Powder

Dosage: For topical use only

Cautions and Contraindications: Do not administer orally (internally).

Side Effects:
1. Contains lead, which can cause lead toxicity
2. Contraindicated as an oral medication

Clinical Applications:
1. Any eye problems
   Combine with: Borax *Peng Sha* as a powder (topically in eyes)
2. Chronic skin ulcerations and moist dermatitis (Damp Heat)
   Combine with: Draconis *Duan Long Gu*, Gypsum *Duan Shi Gao* and Borneol *Bing Pian* (topically)

Pharmaceutical Ingredients:[1–4] Zinc carbonate, calcium oxide, magnesium oxide, ferric oxide, manganese oxide, lead

Borax *Peng Sha* 硼砂

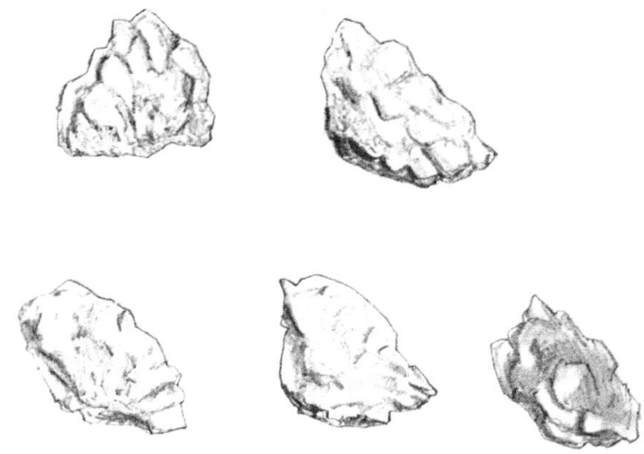

Original Reference: *Ri Hua-Zi Ben Cao* (*Materia Medica of Ri Hua-Zi*) by *Ri Hua-Zi* in 713 日华子本草

Part Used: Mineral

Name:
Pharmaceutical: Borax
Mineral: Borax
Common: Borax
Wade-Giles: *P'eng-Sha*

Energy/Taste: Cool, salty, sweet

Channel-Organ: Lung, Stomach

Actions:
1. Relieve toxicity and prevent putrefaction
2. Clear Heat and dissolve Phlegm
3. Dry Damp

Form and Preparation: Powder for topical use; powder or decoction for oral use

Dosage:
Horses and Cattle: 15–30 g
Llamas, Alpacas, Goats, and Pigs: 2–5 g
Dogs: 0.2–1 g
Cats and Rabbits: 0.1–0.3 g
Birds: 0.01–0.5 g

Cautions and Contraindications: Caution when administering orally (internally)

Side Effects: Renal dysfunction can occur with long-term oral use.

Clinical Applications:
1. Swelling and ulcerations of mouth, tongue, and throat

Combine with: Borneol *Bing Pian* and Alum *Ming Fan* (topically swab the mouth and throat)
2. Phlegm Heat–induced cough with difficult expectoration
Combine with: Trichosanthes *Gua Lou* and Fritillaria *Zhe Bei Mu* (orally)

History and Comments:
1. Borax *Peng Sha* can be used topically for mouth and throat sores.
2. Borax *Peng Sha* is administered orally for Heated Phlegm.

Pharmaceutical Ingredients:[1–4]Sodium tetraborate

Pseudolarix *Tu Jing Pi* 土荆皮

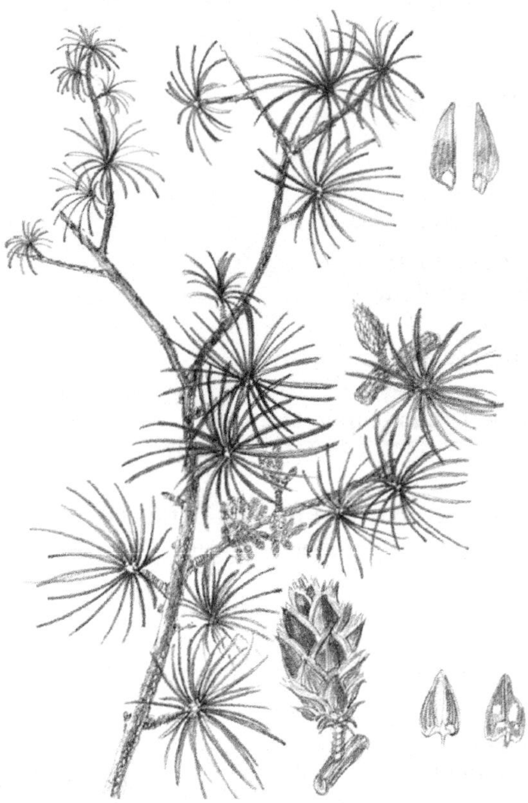

Original Reference: *Ben Cao Gang Mu Shi Yi* (*Omissions for the Materia Medica Compendium*) by *Zhao Xue-min* et al., in 1765 本草纲目拾遗

Part Used: Bark of the root

Name:
Pharmaceutical: Psedolaricis Cortex
Botanical: Pseudolarix kaempferi Gord
Common: Gold larch bark
Wade-Giles: *T'u-Ching-P'i*
Translation: Vulgar Thornwood Bark

Energy/Taste: Warm, pungent, toxic

Channel-Organ: Lung, Spleen

Actions: Kill external parasites and alleviate pruritis

Form and Preparation: Powder mixed with vinegar or alcohol tincture

Dosage: Topical use only

Cautions and Contraindications: Contraindicated for internal use

Side Effects: Internal use may irritate the gastrointestinal tract and cause diarrhea and hemorrhage.

Clinical Applications:
1. Various fungal infections
Single use: with 10–50% alcohol extract (tincture) (topically), or powder mixed with vinegar (topically)
2. Skin Damp Heat, eczema, or other causes of itching
Single use, or combine with: Rheum *Da Huang*, Sophora *Ku Shen* and Phellodendron *Huang Bai* (topically)

Pharmaceutical Ingredients:[1–4] Starch, fat

Cnidium *She Chuang Zi* 蛇床子

Original Reference: *Shen Nong Ben Cao Jing* (*Shen Nong's Materia Medica*, 1st century BCE) 神农本草经

Part Used: Seed

Name:
Pharmaceutical: Cnidii Monnieri, Fructus
Botanical: Cnidium monnieri (L.)
Common: Cnidium seeds
Wade-Giles: *She-Ch'uang-Tzu*
Translation: Snake's Bed Seeds

Energy/Taste: Warm, bitter, pungent, slightly toxic

Channel-Organ: Kidney

Actions:
1. Kill external parasites and alleviate pruritis (topically)
2. Warm Kidney and Tonify *Yang* (orally)
3. Disperse Cold and Wind-Damp (orally)

Form and Preparation: Powder for topical use; powder or decoction administered orally (internally)

Dosage:
Horses and Cattle: 30–90 g
Llamas, Alpacas, Goats, and Pigs: 5–30 g
Dogs: 0.5–2 g
Cats and Rabbits: 0.2–0.5 g
Birds: 0.1–1 g

Cautions and Contraindications:
1. Caution in the presence of Damp-Heat in Lower Burner (*Xia Jiao*) or *Yin* Deficiency with Heat signs
2. May antagonize Moutan *Mu Dan Pi* and Croton *Ba Dou*

Side Effects: Long-term use may cause a skin rash, pruritus, lethargy, abdominal pain, and diarrhea.

Acacia *Er Cha* 儿茶

Original Reference: *Ben Cao Gang Mu* (*Materia Medica Compendium*) by *Li Shi-Zhen* in 1590 本草纲目

Part Used: A paste made from a dried concentrated decoction of black cutch (Acacia) or brown (white) cutch (Uncaria)

Name:
Pharmaceutical: Acacia seu Uncariae, Pasta
Botanical: Acacia catechu (L.) Willd or Uncaria gambier Roxb.
Common: Catechu
Wade-Giles: *Erh-Ch'a*
Translation: Child's Tea

Energy/Taste: Neutral, bitter, astringent

Channel-Organ: Lung

Actions:
1. Drain Damp, absorb seepage, stop bleeding
2. Clear the Lung, transform Phlegm, generate Body Fluids, and alleviate diarrhea

Form and Preparation: Powder for topical use; powder or decoction for oral (internal) use

Dosage:
Horses and Cattle: 15–30 g
Llamas, Alpacas, Goats, and Pigs: 3–9 g
Dogs: 1–3 g
Cats and Rabbits: 0.5–1 g
Birds: 0.1–2 g

Cautions and Contraindications: None

Side Effects: None known

Bufonis *Chan Su* 蟾酥

Original Reference: *Yao Xing Lun* (*Discussion of Medicinal Properties*) by *Chen Zhou* in the 19th century 药性论

Part Used: Dried skin secretions of the toad (toad venom)

Name:
Pharmaceutical: Bufonis, Secretio
Zoological: Bufo bufo gargarizans Cantor or B. Melanostictus Schneider
Common: Poison toad skin secretion
Wade-Giles: *Ch'an-Su*
Translation: Toad

Energy/Taste: Warm, sweet, pungent, toxic

Channel-Organ: Kidney, Stomach

Actions:
1. Relieve toxicity, reduce swelling, and alleviate pain
2. Expel Summer Heat and Damp
3. Open the orifices

Form and Preparation: Powder for topical use; powder or decoction for oral (internal) use

Dosage:
Horses and Cattle: 0.1–0.2 g
Llamas, Alpacas, Goats, and Pigs: 0.03–0.06 g
Dogs: 0.01–0.03 g
Cats, rabbits, and birds: only topical use

Cautions and Contraindications:
1. Contraindicated during pregnancy
2. Caution when administering orally
3. Avoid contact with the eyes.

Side Effects: Oral overdose may cause dyspnea, muscle spasms, arrhythmia and even death. The antidote is Lithospermum *Zi Cao*.

Realgar *Xiong Huang* 雄黄

Original Reference: *Shen Nong Ben Cao Jing* (*Shen Nong's Materia Medica*, 1st century BCE) 神农本草经

Part Used: Mineral

Name:
Pharmaceutical: Realgar
Common: Arsenic disulfide
Wade-Giles: *Hsiung-Huang*
Translation: Male Yellow

Energy/Taste: Warm, pungent, bitter, toxic

Table 17.1. Herbs for topical application: A quick overview and comparison.

Herbs	Special Actions	Common Characteristics
Camphora *Zhang Nao*	Topical use Remove Wind-Damp and stop pain, kill parasites and stop itching, take internally to open orifices and expel turbidity, invigorate Blood and stop pain	Usage: topical application Carrier for external use: Water, vegetable oil, wax, tincture, vinegar, and polymers such as hydroxpropyl methylcellulose (HPMC) Indication: Etiological resolution and symptomatic relief Cautioned for internal use: *Zhang Nao* *Bai Fan* *Peng Sha* *She Chuang Zi* *Chan Su* *Xiong Huang* Contraindicated for internal use: *Lu Gan Shi* *Tu Jing Pi*
Alum *Bai Fan*	Relieve toxicity, kill parasites, dry up dampness to stop itching (topically) Stop bleeding and alleviate diarrhea, clear heat and expel Phlegm (taken orally)	
Calamina *Lu Gan Shi*	Brighten eyes, remove corneal opacity, dry up Damp and generate flesh	
Borax *Peng Sha*	Relieve toxicity and prevent putrefaction Clear Heat and dissolve Phlegm, dry up Damp	
Psuedolarix *Tu Jing Pi*	Kill parasites and stop itching	
Cnidium *She Chuang Zi*	Kill parasites and stop itching Warm Kidney and tonify *Yang*	
Acacia *Er Cha*	Drain Damp, absorb seepage, stop bleeding Clear the Lung, transform Phlegm, generate fluids, stop diarrhea	
Bufonis *Chan Su*	Relieve toxicity, reduce swelling, alleviate pain Expel Summer Heat, open the orifices	
Realgar *Xiong Huang*	Relieve toxicity and kill parasites Dry up Damp and transform Phlegm	

Channel-Organ: Heart, Liver, Stomach

Actions:

1. Relieve toxicity and kill external parasites (topically)
2. Dry Damp and transform Phlegm (orally)

Form and Preparation: Powder for topical use; powder or decoction for oral (internal) use

Dosage:

Horses and Cattle: 10–30 g
Camels: 15–35 g
Llamas, Alpacas, Goats, and Pigs: 0.3–1 g
Dogs, cats, rabbits, and birds: only topical use

Cautions and Contraindications:

1. Contraindicated during pregnancy or when patient has *Yin*/Blood Deficiency
2. Use with caution orally (internal use); use for a short time (no more than 3 days) and at lowest dose

Side Effects: Large or repeated doses are toxic.

SUMMARY OF HERBS FOR TOPICAL APPLICATION

Table 17.1 summarizes and compares the herbs for topical application.

REFERENCES

1. Chen JK, Chen TT. Chinese Medical Herbology and Pharmacology. City of Industry, CA: Art of Medicine Press, 2004.
2. Brinker FJ. The Toxicology of Botanical Medicines. Sandy, OR: Eclectic Medical Publications, 2000.
3. Duke JA. Handbook of Medicinal Herbs. New York: Chemical and Rubber Company Press, 2001.
4. Huang KC. The Pharmacology of Chinese Herbs, 2nd Edition. New York: Chemical and Rubber Company Press, 1999.

Part 2 Chinese Veterinary Herbal Formulation
中兽医方剂

18 Herbal Formulas to Tonify Deficiency 补益剂

Dalu Song, Huisheng Xie, Justin Shmalberg

The formulas in this chapter are used to treat Deficiency Patterns. *Huang Di Nei Jing* states that "no disease occurs if *Yin* and *Yang* maintain a relative balance" and "disease occurs when there is loss of the balance between *Yin* and *Yang*." According to the Eight Principles theory, any disease may be categorized as either Excess or Deficiency when the *Yin* and *Yang* equilibrium is broken.

The Deficiency Pattern is often seen in older patients with chronic illnesses. The typical clinical signs of a Deficiency Pattern include general weakness, fatigue, lethargy, weak pulse, and a pale or red tongue. The Deficiency Patterns are divided into *Qi* Deficiency, Blood Deficiency, *Yin* Deficiency, and *Yang* Deficiency. Tongue and Pulse diagnosis are considered along with the patient's clinical signs in diagnosing the specific Deficiency Pattern (Table 18.1). Treatment involves restoring the *Yin* and *Yang* equilibrium by treating the Deficiency with tonification. Each of the four Deficiency Patterns are treated with a tonifying Chinese herbal formula, each formula having a corresponding characteristic energy, taste, and activity (Table 18.1).

A *Qi* tonic focuses on an Upper Burner and Middle Burner Deficiency (Lung, Heart, and Spleen) because the Spleen generates *Qi* and the Lung distributes *Qi*. For example, *Si Jun Zi Tang* tonifies Spleen *Qi*, Lung *Qi*, and Heart *Qi*. A Blood tonic, on the other hand, primarily focuses on the Lower and Middle Burners (Kidney and Liver) because these influence Blood. The Liver stores the Blood, which enriches the *Jing* stored by the Kidney. Conversely, the *Jing* may also transform into Blood. For example, *Si Wu Tang* acts as a basic Blood tonic by tonifying Kidney *Jing* and Liver Blood. For the remaining forms of herbal tonification, *Yang* tonics are in essence a warm tonification (such as *Jin Gui Shen Qi Wan*), and *Yin* tonics are a cool tonification (such as *Liu Wei Di Huang Wan*).

The tonifying formulas can enhance the physiological activities of internal organs (*Qi* tonics), moisten and nourish the body (Blood and *Yin* tonics), increase disease resistance and immune response, and improve the healing process.

A tonic formula is generally composed of multiple herbs that interact together to produce a certain desired effect while avoiding adverse effects. Using a tonic formula increases the essential substances of the body, but using only tonifying herbs in that formula may generate Stagnation. To prevent Stagnation, herbs that move *Qi* and/or Blood are typically added to the tonic formula. For example, the basic Blood Tonic formula, *Si Wu Tang*, contains the herb Ligusticum *Chuan Xiong* to move *Qi* and Blood to prevent Stagnation. Furthermore, because a Deficiency Pattern is often combined with an Excess Pattern caused by pathogenic factors, a tonic herbal formula may include one or more herbs that resolve pathogenic factors, such as Damp, Heat, Cold, Dryness, Summer Heat, or Wind. For example, in the basic *Qi* tonic formula, *Si Jun Zi Tang*, the herb Poria (*Fu Ling*) is used to drain the pathogenic factor Dampness.

FORMULAS TO TONIFY *QI*

Qi tonic herbal formulas treat *Qi* Deficiency Patterns by enhancing the physiological functions of the *Zang-Fu* organs. There are four *Qi* Deficiency Patterns, including Spleen *Qi* Deficiency, Lung *Qi* Deficiency, Kidney *Qi* Deficiency, and Heart *Qi* Deficiency. One can use the patient's clinical signs to differentiate the Deficiency Pattern and then choose the appropriate herbal formula (Table 18.2). The most common *Qi* Deficiency Patterns are found in the Spleen and Lung because these two "*Zang*" organs are primarily responsible for forming *Qi* from food and air (universe) and transporting *Qi* within the body. Because *Qi* is partly responsible for the generation and movement of Blood, the *Qi* herbal formulas can also be used for Blood Deficiency Patterns.

Qi tonic herbs generally have a sweet taste and neutral or warm temperature. Excessive or long-term

Table 18.1. Tonic and indications.

Deficiency Pattern	Clinical Signs	Tonic Categories	Tonic Characteristics
Qi Deficiency	Weakness, fatigue, or shortness of breath Depression, anorexia Chronic diarrhea, urinary incontinence Tongue: pale/wet Pulse: weak	*Qi* Tonic	Energy: Warm/neutral Taste: Sweet Activity: Tonify the Upper/Middle Burner
Blood Deficiency	Dry and cracked paws/hooves Epidermal scaling Poor stamina Tongue: pale/dry Pulse: thin/weak	Blood Tonic	Energy: Neutral Taste: Sweet Activity: Tonify the Lower/Middle Burner
Yin Deficiency	Cool-seeking, hot, panting, thirsty Epidermal scaling Hyperactivity Tongue: red/dry Pulse: thin/fast	*Yin* Tonic	Energy: Cool Taste: Sweet/bitter Activity: Moisten Body Fluids/clear Heat
Yang Deficiency	*Qi* Deficiency with Cold signs (warm-seeking, cold ear/nose/back/extremity) Tongue: pale purple/swollen/wet Pulse: deep/slow/weak	*Yang* Tonic	Energy: Warm/hot Taste: Sweet Activity: Tonify Yang/warm the interior

Table 18.2. *Qi* Tonic herbal formulas.

Deficiency Patterns	Clinical Signs	Herbal Formulas
Spleen *Qi* Deficiency	Poor appetite, loose stool, muscle atrophy, abdominal distention, fatigue, lassitude, edema, prolapsed rectum	*Shen Ling Bai Zhu San*
Lung *Qi* Deficiency	Cough/asthma, dyspnea, shortness of breath, weak voice, exercise intolerance, recurrent respiratory infections, spontaneous sweating	*Bu Fei San*
Kidney *Qi* Deficiency	Urinary incontinence, infertility, back pain or weakness, intervertebral disc disease	*Jin Suo Gu Jing Wan*
Heart *Qi* Deficiency	Sweating, palpitation, arrhythmia listlessness, anxiety	*Yang Xin San* (Heart *Qi* Tonic)

use of *Qi* tonics can lead to Stagnation or a sense of fullness in the chest and diaphragm. Therefore, a *Qi* tonic formula often contains a small amount of herbs that move *Qi*, such as Citrus (*Chen Pi*). Eleven herbal tonic formulas are discussed in further detail below: *Si Jun Zi Tang, Yi Gong San, Liu Jun Zi Tang, Xiang Sha Liu Jun Zi Tang, Bu Zhong Yi Qi Tang, Shen Ling Bai Zhu San, Sheng Mai Yin, Bu Fei San, Yang Xin Tang*, and *Wei Qi Bu*, and *Wan Dai Fang*.

Si Jun Zi Tang (Four Gentlemen) 四君子汤

Si means four. *Jun Zi* means gentleman. *Tang* means decoction, the form of herbal administration. *Si Jun Zi* is literally translated as Four Gentlemen.

Table 18.3. Ingredients and actions of *Si Jun Zi Tang*.

%	English Names	Chinese *Pin-Yin*	Actions
27.3%	Ginseng root	*Ren Shen*	Tonify *Qi*
27.3%	Atractylodes rhizome	*Bai Zhu*	Strengthen Spleen, tonify *Qi*
27.3%	Poria	*Fu Ling*	Drain Damp, strengthen Spleen
18.1%	Prepared Glycyrrhiza root	*Zhi Gan Cao*	Harmonize and tonify *Qi*

Source: *Tai Ping Hui Min He Ji Ju Fang* (*Imperial Grace Formulary of the Tai Ping Era*), written by *Chen Shi-Wen* et al. and published by the *Song* Dynasty government in 1078 CE

Ingredients: The original formula is composed of 9 g *Ren Shen* (Ginseng), 9 g *Bai Zhu* (Atractylodes), 9 g *Fu Ling* (Poria), and 6 g *Gan Cao* (Glycyrrhiza) (Table 18.3).[1]

Preparation:

1. Powder or capsule method: Herbs are ground into a fine powder. Powder can be encapsulated.
2. Decoction or teapill method: Raw herbs are mixed together and decocted. Herbal water extract (decoction) can be concentrated as granules or teapills.

Actions: Tonify *Qi*, strengthen Spleen and Lung

Indications: General *Qi* Deficiency, Spleen *Qi* Deficiency, Lung *Qi* Deficiency, general weakness, fatigue, weight loss, anorexia, loose stool, pale tongue, weak pulse

Dosage and Usage:
Horses and Cattle: 15–60 g, twice daily
Camels: 30–75 g, twice daily
Llamas, Alpacas, Pigs, Goats, and Sheep: 5–15 g, twice daily
Dogs: 0.5–5 g (or 0.1 g per kg body weight), twice daily
Cats and Rabbits: 0.2–0.5 g (or 0.1 g per kg body weight), twice daily
Birds: 0.1–0.2 g per kg body weight, twice daily
Use 3–8 weeks until primary clinical signs resolve.

Analysis of Formula: *Si Jun Zi Tang* is the basic *Qi* Tonic formula, especially for treating Spleen *Qi* Deficiency. Ginseng, a sweet and warm herb, is the King herb because it can tonify *Qi* and strengthen the Spleen. Atractylodes, which is bitter and warm, serves as the Minister herb to reduce pathogenic Dampness and strengthen the Spleen. Poria, a sweet and neutral herb, is the Adjuvant Herb, which excretes Dampness and strengthens the Spleen. Combining Atractylodes and Poria further enhances the formula's ability to invigorate and tonify the Spleen, dispel Dampness, and promote the Spleen's transportation and transformation functions. Poria also disperses Heat to balance the warm nature of Ginseng and Atractylodes. Glycyrrhiza root, which is sweet and warm, is the Messenger Herb; it harmonizes the actions of the other herbs in the formula while invigorating the Spleen. All the herbs can gently tonify the *Qi* and invigorate the Spleen, resulting in Spleen *Qi* harmony and proper function.

Cautions and Contraindications: Do not use in patients with high blood pressure or *Yin* Deficiency.

Dr. Xie's Comments: I have used this herbal formula in treating general weakness (exercise intolerance or fatigue, pale and wet tongue, and weak pulse) in geriatric patients, especially horses and dogs, with great success.

Clinical and Pharmacological Studies: Much research has been done on this herbal formula. Clinical and animal studies showed that *Si Jun Zi Tang* had no influence on the pH or amount of gastric secretions. It did promote villus growth of gastric enterocytes, and it increased the activity of pepsin, the content of enzyme precursor particles in chief cells, and the level of serum D-xylose.[2] Poorly adaptive young animals readily develop Stomach and Spleen *Qi* Deficiency Pattern if the environment changes or if they are fed or managed poorly. *Zou* reported that 26 of 30 (86%) young dogs with Spleen and Stomach *Qi* Deficiency treated with *Si Jun Zi Tang* recovered.[3] Another clinical study reported a recovery rate of 92.3% when *Si Jun Zi Tang* was used to treat functional dyspepsia and malabsorption, abdominal distension, loose stool, and debilitation.[4] This study also showed that *Si Jun Zi Tang* improved serum interferon activity and immune function. Taken together, these results indicate that the Spleen controls digestion and a vigorous Spleen is able to resist pathogenic invasion. These results suggest conducting further research into *Si Jun Zi Tang*'s ability to strengthen resistance to cancer and to treat immune disease and weakness. *Ren* et al. researched the effect of *Si Jun Zi Tang* on gastric emptying in rats with weak Spleen and Stomach *Qi*; they found that when the Spleen *Qi* was weak, *Si Jun Zi Tang* increased the rate of gastric emptying.[5] They also found that *Si Jun Zi Tang* regulates the electrical activity of the Stomach and duodenum via its regulation of motilin (MOT), cholecystokinin (CCK), and somatostatin (SS) in the hypothalamus and in the plasma. Overall this herbal formula improves Spleen and Stomach weakness and treats dyspepsia caused by various factors.

Regulation of Gastrointestinal Tract Function *Si Jun Zi Tang* does not affect small intestinal activity in normal rats, but it does inhibit hyperactivity and reduce hypoactivity that has been artificially induced by various substances. For example, *Si Jun Zi Tang* inhibited hyperactivity caused by neostigmine and Apoplon (Reserpine).[6] *Si Jun Zi Tang* in other situations inhibited hyperactivity and diarrhea caused by Senna Leaf (*Fan Xie Ye*), widely recognized to increase small intestinal motility and cause diarrhea.[7] In experimental models of Spleen *Qi* Deficiency induced by vinegar, *Si Jun Zi Tang* promoted gastrointestinal motility.[8] Both hypermotile and hypomotile gastrointestinal disorders adversely affect digestion and absorption. Rapid gastrointestinal motility prevents food from remaining in the stomach and intestines for a sufficient amount of time; slow gastrointestinal motility inhibits transportation and the mixing of chyme with digestive secretions. *Si Jun Zi Tang* can be used to treat gastrointestinal motility disorders induced by various diseases due to its ability to stimulate or decrease motility depending on the condition.

Digestion and Absorption Research Using a model of Spleen *Qi* Deficiency, *Si Jun Zi Tang* increased the concentration of MOT in plasma and the small intestine, strengthened gastrointestinal motility, decreased the concentration of PGE2 in the large intestine, and prevented hypermotility of the large intestine.[8,9] These effects promote the digestion and absorption of food in the Intestines. In Spleen *Qi* Deficiency, *Si Jun Zi Tang* increases gastric mucosal cell concentrations of carbonic anhydrase (CA), succinate dehydrogenase (SDH), and Na^+–K^+ adenosine triphosphate enzyme.[10] *Si Jun Zi Tang* also strengthens the barrier function of the intestinal mucosa and promotes enteric epithelial growth to support mucosal integrity.[11] These findings indicate that *Si Jun Zi Tang* can revive digestion and absorption by regulating the concentration and activity of various hormones and enzymes.

Immunopharmacology Research The effect of *Si Jun Zi Tang* was conducted on a T-Lymphocyte study of a Spleen *Qi* Deficiency model.[12] The study showed that the function of T-Lymphocytes in the Spleen *Qi* Deficient group was significantly lower than in the control group, and the group treated with *Si Jun Zi Tang* was significantly higher than the Spleen Deficient group. Another study also revealed that *Si Jun Zi Tang* affected weak Spleen *Qi* by strengthening T-Lymphocyte activity and enhancing the level of IgM.[13] This demonstrates that *Si Jun Zi Tang* can invigorate the Spleen, tonify *Qi*, improve the body's vitality, and enhance immune function via T-Lymphocyte activities.

Si Jun Zi Tang also improved T-Lymphocyte and Natural Killer (NK) cell activity, and increased the neutrophil cytophagic index in patients with weak Spleen *Qi*.[14] Therefore, *Si Jun Zi Tang* improves immune function, especially the cellular immune function of patients with weak Spleen *Qi*.

Si Jun Zi Tang was also studied on red blood cell (RBC) immune function, specifically Red Blood Cell C3b Receptor Rosette (RBC-C3bRR) and Circulating Immune Complex (CIC) Rosette in rats.[15] The research showed that the RBC-3bRR in rats given *Si Jun Zi Tang* was higher than those given normal saline. These results established that *Si Jun Zi Tang* increased RBC immune function, specifically the adherence function of RBC. The above stated research highlights the ability of *Si Jun Zi Tang* to enhance the activity of T-Lymphocytes and RBCs and thus improve the immune function to prevent and treat disease.

Cancer Research *Si Jun Zi Tang* supports *Qi*, regulates digestive function, revives and promotes proper immune function, and causes cancer cell apoptosis.[16] *Si Jun Zi Tang* also slowed Bladder tumor growth in BTTT739 tumor-bearing mice.[17] In additional research, *Si Jun Zi Tang* maintained or increased the concentration of serum selenium (Se) and decreased the concentration of Serum Lipid Peroxidate (LPO).[18] Researchers in this study hypothesized that *Si Jun Zi Tang's* antioxidant feature was the most important factor in its ability to support healthy energy and prolong the survival time of tumor-bearing mice.

Si Jun Zi Tang and mitomycin C (MMC) were used for the treatment of carcinoma of the Bladder. Researchers found that this combination synergistically restrained the growth of mouse Bladder tumors, and *Si Jun Zi Tang* decreased toxic side effects of the mitomycin C.[19] *Si Jun Zi Tang* is an important treatment for patients with late-stage malignant neoplastic disease. It controls tumor growth and improves the quality of life.

It is important to study current and new Chinese formulas that might further prevent as well as treat refractory or malignant disease. *Si Jun Zi Tang* can assist in the treatment of malignant neoplasia and other challenging diseases. Further experimental research may reveal that *Si Jun Zi Tang* has additional actions and benefits.

Yi Gong San (Extraordinary Action) 异功散

Yi Gong San was based on *Si Jun Zi Tang* (Four Gentlemen), adding Citrus *Chen Pi* with an extraordinary action to promote the flow of *Qi*. *Yi* refers to extraordinary, or special. *Gong* means action, or function. *San* is powder, the form of herbal administration.

Source: *Xiao Er Yao Zheng Zhi Jue* (*Craft of Medicinal Treatment for Childhood Disease Patterns*), written by *Qian Yi* and published in 1119

Ingredients: *Si Jun Zi Tang* (9 g *Ren Shen*, 9 g *Bai Zhu*, 9 g *Fu Ling*, and 6 g *Zhi Gan Cao*), adding 6 g *Chen Pi* (Citrus)

Preparation:

1. Powder or capsule method: Herbs are ground into a fine powder. Powder can be encapsulated.
2. Decoction or teapill method: Raw herbs are mixed together and decocted. Herbal water extract (decoction) can be concentrated as granules or teapills.

Actions: Tonify *Qi*, strengthen the Spleen, promote the flow of *Qi*

Indications: Spleen *Qi* Deficiency with Stomach *Qi* Stagnation; Spleen *Qi* Deficiency (general weakness, fatigue, weight loss, anorexia, loose stool, pale tongue, weak pulse) leading to Stomach *Qi* Stagnation (discomfort in the Stomach, sensitivity on palpation of the chest and abdomen, sometimes nausea and vomiting)

Dosage and Usage:

Horses and Cattle: 15–60 g, twice daily
Camels: 30–75 g, twice daily
Llamas, Alpacas, Pigs, Goats, and Sheep: 5–15 g, twice daily
Dogs: 0.5–5 g (or 0.1 g per kg body weight), twice daily
Cats and Rabbits: 0.2–0.5 g (or 0.1 g per kg body weight), twice daily
Birds: 0.1–0.2 g per kg body weight, twice daily

Use 3–8 weeks until primary clinical signs resolve.

Analysis of Formula: *Si Jun Zi Tang* is the basic *Qi* herbal formula that tonifies Spleen *Qi*. *Chen Pi* (Citrus) promotes the flow of *Qi* and harmonizes the Stomach to stop vomiting. Thus, *Yi Gong San* can be used for Spleen *Qi* Deficiency with mild Stomach *Qi* Stagnation.

Cautions and Contraindications: Do not use in patients with *Yin* Deficiency.

Dr. Xie's Comments: *Yi Gong San* can be very useful for patients with *Qi* Deficiency with mild Stomach *Qi* Stagnation (general weakness, occasional vomiting, and abdominal fullness or bloat).

Liu Jun Zi Tang (Six Gentlemen) 六君子汤

Liu Jun Zi Tang is based on *Si Jun Zi Tang* (Four Gentlemen) and adding two ingredients (Two Gentlemen). *Liu* is six. *Jun Zi* refers to gentlemen. *Tang* is decoction, the form of herbal administration.

Source: *Tai Ping Hui Min He Ji Ju Fang (Imperial Grace Formula of the Tai Ping Era)*, written *by Chen Shi Wen* et al. and published in 1078

Ingredients: *Liu Jun Zi Tang* (Six Gentlemen) is composed of *Si Jun Zi Tang* (9 g *Ren Shen*, 9 g *Bai Zhu*, 9 g *Fu Ling*, and 6 g *Zhi Gan Cao*), adding 6 g *Ban Xia* (Pinellia) and 6 g *Chen Pi* (Citrus).

Preparation:

1. Powder or capsule method: Herbs are ground into a fine powder. Powder can be encapsulated.
2. Decoction or teapill method: Raw herbs are mixed together and decocted. Herbal water extract (decoction) can be concentrated as granules or teapills.

Actions: Strengthen Spleen *Qi*, transform Phlegm, stop vomiting

Indications: Spleen *Qi* Deficiency with Phlegm; Spleen *Qi* Deficiency (general weakness, fatigue, weight loss, anorexia, loose stool, pale tongue, weak pulse) leading to accumulation of Dampness, which transforms into Phlegm (coughing of copious sputum, nausea and vomiting)

Dosage and Usage:

Horses and Cattle: 15–60 g, twice daily
Camels: 30–75 g, twice daily
Llamas, Alpacas, Pigs, Goats, and Sheep: 5–15 g, twice daily
Dogs: 0.5–5 g (or 0.1 g per kg body weight), twice daily
Cats and Rabbits: 0.2–0.5 g (or 0.1 g per kg body weight), twice daily
Birds: 0.1–0.2 g per kg body weight, twice daily

Use 1–4 weeks until primary clinical signs resolve.

Analysis of Formula: *Liu Jun Zi Tang* combines *Si Jun Zi Tang* (tonifying Spleen *Qi*) with principle ingredients of *Er Chen Tang* (Chapter 19). *Chen Pi* promotes the flow of *Qi* and harmonizes the Stomach to stop vomiting. *Ban Xia* transforms Phlegm and dries up Dampness. Thus, *Liu Jun Zi Tang* can tonify Spleen *Qi*, transform Phlegm, and stop vomiting, and it is often used for the treatment of Spleen *Qi* Deficiency with Stagnation of Phlegm.

Cautions and Contraindications: Do not use in patients with *Yin* Deficiency.

Dr. Xie's Comments: *Liu Jun Zi Tang* is effective for the treatment of combined *Qi* Deficiency and accumulation of Phlegm (general weakness, excessive salivation, wet cough, and vomiting).

Xiang Sha Liu Jun Zi Tang (Eight Gentlemen) 香砂六君子汤

Xiang Sha Liu Jun Zi Tang was named on the basis of *Liu Jun Zi Tang* (Six Gentlemen) and adding two ingredients (Two Gentlemen): *Mu Xiang* (Saussurea) and *Sha Ren* (Amomum).

Source: *Ping Hui Min He Ji Ju Fang (Imperial Grace Formulary of the Tai Ping Era)*, written by *Chen Shi-Wen* et al. and published by the *Song* Dynasty government in 1078 CE

Ingredients: *Xiang Sha Liu Jun Zi Tang*: 3 g *Mu Xiang* (Saussurea) and 3 g *Sha Ren* (Amomum), in addition to *Liu Jun Zi Tang* (9 g *Ren Shen*, 9 g *Bai Zhu*, 9 g *Fu Ling*, 6 g *Zhi Gan Cao*, 6 g *Ban Xia*, and 6 g *Chen Pi*)

Preparation:

1. Powder or capsule method: Herbs are ground into a fine powder. Powder can be encapsulated.
2. Decoction or teapill method: Raw herbs are mixed together and decocted. Herbal water extract (decoction) can be concentrated as granules or teapills.

Actions: Strengthen Spleen *Qi*, harmonize the Stomach, promote *Qi* flow, relieve pain

Indications: Spleen and Stomach *Qi* Deficiency with Damp-Cold stagnating in the Middle Burner, no appetite, no thirst, abdominal distention or pain, sometimes nausea and vomiting, pale purple and wet tongue, weak or soft wiry pulse

Dosage and Usage:

Horses and Cattle: 15–45 g, twice daily
Camels: 30–60 g, twice daily
Llamas, Alpacas, Pigs, Goats, and Sheep: 7–10 g, twice daily
Dogs: 0.5–5 g (or 0.1 g per kg body weight), twice daily
Cats and Rabbits: 0.2–0.5 g (or 0.1 g per kg body weight), twice daily
Birds: 0.1–0.2 g per kg body weight, twice daily

Use 2–8 weeks until primary clinical signs resolve.

Analysis of Formula: As stated above, *Si Jun Zi Tang* tonifies Spleen *Qi*. *Chen Pi* and *Ban Xia* transform Phlegm and dry up Dampness. *Mu Xiang* and *Sha Ren* promote the flow of *Qi* to relieve pain and harmonize the Stomach to stop vomiting.

Cautions and Contraindications: Do not use in patients with *Yin* Deficiency.

Dr. Xie's Comments: I have used this herbal formula for Spleen *Qi* Deficiency cases presenting with poor appetite and have had great success. I also favor employing this herbal medicine for the long-term maintenance of chronic inflammatory bowel disease (IBD) cases after the initial complaints are eliminated. It can also be used in cancer patients for the treatment and prevention of the side effects of chemotherapy or radiotherapy.

Bu Zhong Yi Qi Tang (Tonifying the Middle and Reinforcing *Qi*) 补中益气汤

This formula was named after its functions. *Bu* means tonifying. *Zhong* is middle (referring to the Middle Burner). *Yi* means reinforcing, or benefitting. *Tang* is decoction, the form of herbal administration. Literally, *Bu Zhong Yi Qi* can be translated as Tonifying the Middle and reinforcing *Qi*.

Source: *Nei Wai Shang Bian Huo Lun* (*Clarifying Doubts about Injury from Internal and External Causes*), written by *Li Ao* and published in 1247

Ingredients: The original formula is composed of 18g *Huang Qi* (Astragalus), 9g *Gan Cao* (Glycyrrhiza), 6g *Ren Shen* (Ginseng), 3g *Dang Gui* (Angelica), 5g *Chen Pi* (Citrus), 6g *Sheng Ma* (Cimicifuga), 6g *Chai Hu* (Bupleurum), and 9g *Bai Zhu* (Atractylodes). Its ingredients, by percentage and action, are listed in Table 18.4.

Preparation:

1. Powder or capsule method: Herbs are ground into a fine powder. Powder can be encapsulated.
2. Decoction or teapill method: Raw herbs are mixed together and decocted. Herbal water extract (decoction) can be concentrated as granules or teapills.

Actions: Replenish *Qi* of the Middle Burner, raise Spleen *Yang* to treat the prolapsed organs

Indications: Prolapse due to deficient *Qi*, which is marked by poor appetite, lassitude, loose stool, and thirst with preference for heated liquids. The formula is also used for prolapse of the rectum, prolapse of the uterus, prolonged diarrhea, protracted dysentery, pale and large tongue with thin white coating, deep and weak pulse.

Table 18.4. Ingredients and actions of *Bu Zhong Yi Qi Tang*.

%	English Names	Chinese *Pin-Yin*	Actions
29	Astragalus	*Huang Qi*	Tonify *Qi* to invigorate *Yang*, benefit the Lung to strengthen the body, promote diuresis and relieve edema
14.5	Glycyrrhiza	*Gan Cao*	Harmonize the effects of other herbs
9.7	Ginseng	*Ren Shen*	Replenish the source (*Yuan*) *Qi*, tonify the Spleen and Lung
4.8	Angelica	*Dang Gui*	Nourish Blood and activate Blood circulation
8	Citrus	*Chen Pi*	Regulate Spleen *Qi*, dry up Dampness, transform Phlegm
9.7	Cimicifuga	*Sheng Ma*	Clear Heat and toxins and lift up Spleen *Qi*
9.7	Bupleurum	*Chai Hu*	Disperse the stagnant Liver *Qi* and raise *Yang Qi*
14.6	Atractylodes	*Bai Zhu*	Strengthen the Spleen, dry up Dampness, tonify *Qi*

Dosage and Usage:

Horses and Cattle: 15–60g, twice daily
Camels: 30–75g twice daily
Llamas, Alpacas, Pigs, Goats, and Sheep: 5–15g, twice daily
Dogs: 0.5–5g (or 0.1g per kg body weight), twice daily
Cats and Rabbits: 0.2–0.5g (or 0.1g per kg body weight), twice daily
Birds: 0.1–0.2g per kg body weight, twice daily
Use 1–4 weeks as needed.

Analysis of Formula: Spleen and Stomach *Qi* Deficiency could cause the failure of *Yang* to ascend or the prolapse of Middle-Burner *Qi*. The treatment should be based on supplementing *Qi* and lifting *Yang*. *Huang Qi* (Astragalus) is used in a larger dosage as the King herb, and it reinforces *Qi* of the Middle-Burner and lifts *Yang* to strengthen the *Wei Qi*. *Ren Shen* (Ginseng), *Bai Zhu* (Atractylodes), and *Gan Cao* (Glycyrrhiza) are used as Minister herbs to replenish *Qi* and strengthen the Spleen, and they are combined with *Huang Qi* (Astragalus) to get a better effect. *Dang Gui* (Angelica) helps *Ren Shen* and *Huang Qi* to invigorate *Qi* and nourish Blood. *Chen Pi* (Citrus) regulates *Qi* and the Stomach and also prevents Stagnation, which may be generated from other tonic herbs. Both *Dang Gui* and *Chen Pi* serve as Adjuvant herbs. *Sheng Ma* (Cimicifuga) and *Chai Hu* (Bupleurum), as the transporter herbs, bear the function of lifting collapsed Middle-Burner *Qi*.

Cautions and Contraindications: This formula is contraindicated for cases with fever due to *Yin* Deficiency.

Dr. Xie's Comments: I have used *Bu Zhong Yi Qi Tang* for fecal incontinence due to Spleen *Qi* Deficiency in dogs, along with an adjunct stimulation of acupuncture. It can also be used for chronic diarrhea in elder patients. Long-term use of this herbal formula may cause Interior Heat and *Yin* Deficiency.

Clinical and Pharmacological Studies: Several case studies showed that *Bu Zhong Yi Qi Tang* is effective for the treatment of chronic diarrhea due to Spleen *Qi* Deficiency in horses[20], cattle[21,22] and dogs[23]. This herbal formula was also proven to have a dual regulating effect on smooth muscles, including those of the intestines and uterus by reducing the movement of hyperactive smooth muscles and increasing the movement of hypoactive smooth muscles.[24] This formula increases the peripheral plasma concentration of T-Lymphocytes, WBC and RBC, and has anti-neoplastic effects.[24] *Bu Zhong Yi Qi Tang* was also successfully used for the treatment of penile paralysis in the bull and paralysis of the urinary bladder[25] and prolapse of the rectum, uterus, and vagina in cows.[26] *Hu* summarized that *Bu Zhong Yi Qi Tang* had a positive influence on improving protein metabolism, preventing anemia, enhancing physical strength, and enhancing phagocytic function of reticuloendothelial, nonspecific immunity, and cellular immunity.[27]

Shen Ling Bai Zhu San (Ginseng, Poria, and Atractylodes) 参苓白术散

This formula was named after its two King herbs and one of its Minister herbs. The two King herbs are *Ren Shen* (Ginseng) and *Bai Zhu* (Atractylodes), the Minister herb is *Fu Ling* (Poria). Therefore, the formula *Shen Ling Bai Zhu San* is literally translated as Ginseng, Poria, and Atractylodes.

Source: *Tai Ping Hui Min He Ji Ju Fang* (*Imperial Grace Formulary of the Tai Ping Era*), written by *Chen Shiwen* et al. and published in 1078

Ingredients: The original formula is composed of 500 g *Lian Zi* (Nelumbo), 500 g *Yi Yi Ren* (Coix), 500 g *Sha Ren* (Amomum), 500 g *Jie Geng* (Platycodon), 750 g *Bai Bian Dou* (Dolichos), 1000 g *Fu Ling* (Poria), 1000 g *Ren Shen* (Ginseng), 1000 g *Gan Cao* (Glycyrrhiza), 1000 g *Bai Zhu* (Atractylodes), and 1000 g *Shan Yao* (Dioscorea). Its ingredient percentages and actions are listed in Table 18.5.

Preparation:

1. Powder or capsule method: Herbs are ground into a fine powder. Powder can be encapsulated.
2. Decoction or teapill method: Raw herbs are mixed together and decocted. Herbal water extract (decoction) can be concentrated as granules or teapills.

Table 18.5. Ingredients and actions of *Shen Ling Bai Zhu San.*

%	English Names	Chinese *Pin-Yin*	Actions
6.45	Nelumbo	*Lian Zi*	Invigorate *Qi*, strengthen the Spleen, stop diarrhea
6.45	Coix	*Yi Yi Ren*	Strengthen the Spleen, promote diuresis, excrete Dampness and calm the mind
6.45	Amomum	*Sha Ren*	Promote Stomach *Qi* flow to improve appetite, facilitate digestion and stop vomiting
6.45	Platycodon	*Jie Geng*	Open the Lung to relieve cough, dissolve Phlegm, guide other herbs to the upper part of the body
9.6	Dolichos	*Bai Bian Dou*	Strengthen the Spleen, eliminate Dampness
12.9	Poria	*Fu Ling*	Strengthen the Spleen, induce diuresis, excrete Dampness
12.9	Ginseng	*Ren Shen*	Replenish the Source (*Yuan Qi*), tonify the Spleen and Lung
12.9	Glycyrrhiza	*Gan Cao*	Harmonize the effects of other herbs
13.0	Atractylodes	*Bai Zhu*	Strengthen the Spleen, dry up Dampness, tonify *Qi* and promote diuresis
12.9	Dioscorea	*Shan Yao*	Tonify the Spleen and Lung

Actions: Replenish *Qi*, tonify the Spleen, remove Dampness, stop diarrhea

Indications: Dampness due to *Qi* Deficiency of the Spleen and Stomach, which is characterized by loose stool or diarrhea, generalized weakness, poor appetite, vomiting or abdominal distention, pale tongue with white and greasy coating, feeble or weak pulse

Dosage and Usage:

Horses and Cattle: 15–60 g, twice daily
Camels: 30–75 g, twice daily
Llamas, Alpacas, Pigs, Goats, and Sheep: 5–15 g, twice daily
Dogs: 0.5–5 g (or 0.1 g per kg body weight), twice daily
Cats and Rabbits: 0.2–0.5 g (or 0.1 g per kg body weight), twice daily
Birds: 0.1–0.2 g per kg body weight, twice daily

Use 3–6 weeks until primary clinical signs resolve.

Analysis of Formula: Dampness results from a disorder in transportation and transformation of the Spleen functions. Spleen *Qi*, in this instance, is weak or deficient and fails to transform water and fluids leading to generation of Dampness in the Interior. It should be treated by means of replenishing *Qi*, strengthening the Spleen and eliminating Dampness to stop diarrhea. *Ren Shen* (Ginseng) and *Bai Zhu* (Atractylodes) act together as the King herbs to tonify *Qi*, strengthen the Spleen, and eliminate Dampness. *Shao Yao* (Dioscorea) and *Lian Zi* (Nelumbo) help *Ren Shen* replenish *Qi* and strengthen the Spleen, while *Bai Bian Dou* (Dolichoris), *Yi Yi Ren* (Coix) and *Fu Ling* (Poria) help *Bai Zhu* reinforce the Spleen and promote diuresis. These four ingredients are used together as Minister herbs. *Sha Ren* (Amomum) can regulate the Stomach and invigorate the Spleen, and *Jie Geng* (Platycodon) disperses the Lung *Qi*, promotes diuresis, and leads other herbs upward to the Lung and upper portion of the body. *Gan Cao* (Glycyrrhiza) supplements *Qi*, reinforces the Spleen, and mediates the properties of other herbs. These three ingredients serve as Messenger herbs.

Cautions and Contraindications: This formula is contraindicated for cases with fever due to *Yin* Deficiency.

Dr. Xie's Comments: I commonly use *Shen Ling Bai Zhu San* for chronic diarrhea due to Spleen *Qi* Deficiency in horses, dogs, and cats.

Clinical and Pharmacological Studies: *Lu* reported that 22 of 25 bovine cases of chronic diarrhea were cured after administration of *Shen Ling Bai Zhu San*.[28] The effective rate of 97.5% (1120 patients) was found when *Shen Ling Bai Zhu San* was used for the treatment of chronic dyspepsia in piglets.[29]

Another study reported that 34 of 36 foal cases of diarrhea were cured by *Shen Ling Bai Zhu San* and two were improved.[30]

An additional study showed that 111 of 138 weanling piglets with refractory diarrhea had completely recovered after using *Shen Ling Bai Zhu San* medication.[31]

Sheng Mai Yin (Generating the Pulse)
生脉散

Sheng means generating. *Mai* means pulse. *Sheng Mai* literally means Generating the Pulse. This formula was named because of its main function of tonifying *Qi* to activate the pulse.

Source: *Jing Yue Quan Shu* (*Collected Treatises of Zhang Jingyue*), written by *Zhang Jiebing* and published in 1624

Ingredients: The formula is composed of 9 g *Ren Shen* (Gingseng), 9 g *Mai Men Dong* (Ophiopogon), and 6 g *Wu Wei Zi* (Schisandra). Its ingredients and actions are listed in Table 18.6.

Table 18.6. Ingredients and actions of *Sheng Mai Yin*.

%	English Names	Chinese *Pin-Yin*	Actions
37.5	Ginseng	*Ren Shen*	Replenish the Source (*Yuan*) *Qi*, tonify the Spleen and Lung, promote the production of Body Fluid, calm the mind
37.5	Ophiopogon	*Mai Men Dong*	Nourish *Yin*, clear false Heat and promote production of Body Fluid to relieve thirst
25	Schisandra	*Wu Wei Zi*	Restrain dissipation of Lung *Qi*, promote production of Body Fluids, preserve the *Jing* and restrain excessive sweating

Preparation:
1. Powder or capsule method: Herbs are ground into a fine powder. Powder can be encapsulated.
2. Decoction or teapill method: Raw herbs are mixed together and decocted. Herbal water extract (decoction) can be concentrated as granules or teapills.

Actions: Tonify *Qi* and promote the production of body fluids, astringe *Yin* and stop cough

Indications: Both *Qi* and *Yin* Deficiency, which are characterized by lethargy, shortness of breath, physical and mental fatigue, and thirst, or prolonged cough with little, but sticky sputum, red and dry tongue, feeble, rapid pulse

Dosage and Usage:
Horses and Cattle: 15–30 g, twice daily
Camels: 30–60 g, twice daily
Llamas, Alpacas, Pigs, Goats, and Sheep: 7–15 g, twice daily
Dogs: 0.5–5 g (or 0.1 g per kg body weight), twice daily
Cats and Rabbits: 0.2–0.5 g (or 0.1 g per kg body weight), twice daily
Birds: 0.1 g per kg body weight, twice daily
Use 2–4 weeks until primary clinical signs resolve.

Analysis of Formula: *Qi* and *Yin* Deficiency results from impairment of *Yin* by Excess Heat and Summer-Heat, or impairment of *Qi* and *Yin* due to chronic overwork, poor nutrition, or chronic illness including prolonged cough. This Pattern should be treated by means of tonifying *Qi* and nourishing *Yin*, promoting production of Body Fluids, and relieving cough. *Ren Shen* (Gingseng) acts as the King herb to tonify *Qi* and promote the production of Body Fluids. *Mai Men Dong*

(Ophiopogon) is used as the Minister herb to nourish *Yin* and clear Heat for moistening the Lung. *Wu Wei Zi* (Schisandra) not only astringes *Yin*, but also astringes the Lung to relieve cough, acting as an Adjuvant herb. Respectively, by tonifying, moistening, and astringing, the three ingredients are used to achieve the results of tonifying *Qi* and nourishing *Yin*, moistening the Lung to stop the cough, and promoting the production of Body Fluids to stop thirst.

Cautions and Contraindications: This formula is contraindicated for cases with Excess Heat or for those with both a cough and profuse sputum.

Dr. Xie's Comments: I have used *Sheng Mai Yin* successfully for the treatment of heart failure, behavioral problems, and chest discomfort due to Heart *Qi* and *Yin* Deficiency.

Clinical and Pharmacological Studies: *Sheng Mai Yin* was successfully used for treatment of collapse due to heatstroke or sunstroke in farm cattle.[32] *Fan* summarized the following effects of *Sheng Mai Yin*: prevention of acute cardiac insufficiency, improvement of circulation of myocardium and coronary vessels, and an anti-inflammatory effect and immuno-stimulating function.[33]

Bu Fei San (Tonifying the Lung) 补肺散

Bu means tonifying, and *Fei* is the Lung. *Bu Fei* literally means Tonifying the Lung. Consequently, this formula was named because of its main function of tonifying the functions of the Lung.

Source: *Chinese Veterinary Herbal Handbook*, written by *Huisheng Xie* and published by the Chi Institute of Chinese Medicine, 2004

Ingredients: *Bu Fei San* is modified from *Bu Fei Tang* from *Yong Lei Qian Fang* (*Everlasting Categorization of Seal Formulas*). The original *Bu Fei Tang* consists of 24 g *Huang Qi* (Astragalus), 9 g *Ren Shen* (Ginseng), 24 g *Shu Di Huang* (Rehmannia), 6 g *Wu Wei Zi* (Schisandra), 9 g *Zi Wan* (Aster), and 12 g *Sang Bai Pi* (Morus). The ingredients and actions of *Bu Fei San* are listed in Table 18.7.

Table 18.7. Ingredients and actions of *Bu Fei San*.

%	English Names	Chinese *Pin-Yin*	Actions
38	Astragalus	*Huang Qi*	Tonify Lung *Qi*
8	Codonopsis	*Dang Shen*	Tonify *Qi*
8	Ginkgo	*Bai Guo*	Astringently consolidate Lung, stop asthma/cough
8	Pheretima	*Di Long*	Activate the Channel, stop asthma
8	Platycodon	*Jie Geng*	Open the Lung, transform Phlegm
8	Schisandra	*Wu Wei Zi*	Astringently consolidate the Lung
8	Perilla	*Zi Su Ye*	Clear Wind-Heat, stop cough
8	Aster	*Zi Wan*	Moisten Lung, stop cough/asthma
6	Glycyrrhiza	*Gan Cao*	Harmonize

Preparation:

1. Powder or capsule method: Herbs are ground into a fine powder. Powder can be encapsulated.
2. Decoction or teapill method: Raw herbs are mixed together and decocted. Herbal water extract (decoction) can be concentrated as granules or teapills.

Actions: Tonify Lung *Qi*, stop cough and asthma

Indications: Chronic cough or asthma due to Lung *Qi* Deficiency. Shortness of breath, chronic cough or asthma, fatigue, exercise intolerance, deep and weak pulse, pale and wet tongue

Dosage and Usage:

Horses and Cattle: 15–60 g, twice daily
Camels: 30–75 g, twice daily
Llamas, Alpacas, Pigs, Goats, and Sheep: 5–15 g, twice daily
Dogs: 0.5–5 g (or 0.1 g per kg body weight), twice daily
Cats and Rabbits: 0.2 0.5 g (or 0.1 g per kg body weight), twice daily
Birds: 0.1–0.2 g per kg body weight, twice daily
Use 3–8 weeks until primary clinical signs resolve.

Analysis of Formula: Lung *Qi* Deficiency is often caused by chronic overwork, poor nutrition, or chronic illness. When the Lung is too deficient to descend and inhale the cosmic *Qi* (*Qing Qi*), it causes rebellious Lung *Qi*, leading to asthma or cough. The King herbs in this formula are *Huang Qi* (Astragalus) and *Dang Shen* (Codonopsis), which work synergistically to tonify *Qi* for the treatment of the root problem, *Qi* Deficiency. *Bai Guo* (Ginkgo) and *Wu Wei Zi* (Schisandra) work as the Minister herbs to consolidate astringently the Lung *Qi* to stop asthma or cough. *Zi Su Ye* (Perilla), *Zi Wan* (Aster), and *Di Long* (Pheretima) are used as the Adjuvant herbs to treat the secondary symptoms (cough and asthma). *Jie Geng* (Platycodon), which opens the Lung as a transporter, and *Gan Cao* (Glycyrrhiza) a harmonizer, are the Messenger herbs.

Cautions and Contraindications: This formula is contraindicated for cough or asthma due to Lung *Yin* Deficiency.

Dr. Xie's Comments: I have used this herbal formula for COPD, heaves, chronic asthma, and cough due to Lung *Qi* Deficiency in horses, dogs, and cats.

Yang Xin Tang (Heart *Qi* Tonic) 养心汤

Yang means tonifying or nourishing. *Xin* is Heart. *Yang Xin* literally means Tonifying the Heart, or Heart *Qi* tonic. Therefore, the name of this formula comes from its main action to tonify the Heart *Qi*.

Source: *Chinese Veterinary Herbal Handbook*, by *Huisheng Xie* and published by the Chi Institute of Chinese Medicine, 2004

Ingredients: The ingredients and actions of *Yang Xin Tang* are listed in Table 18.8.

Preparation:

1. Powder or capsule method: Herbs are ground into a fine powder. Powder can be encapsulated.
2. Decoction or teapill method: Raw herbs are mixed together and decocted. Herbal water extract (decoction) can be concentrated as granules or teapills.

Actions: Tonify Heart *Qi* and invigorate Blood

Indications: Congestive Heart failure, or cardiomyopathy due to Heart *Qi* Deficiency, chronic fatigue, lethargy, listlessness, palpitations, shortness of breath, spontaneous sweating, weak or (irregularly or regularly) intermittent pulse, pale tongue with white coating

Dosage and Usage:

Horses and Cattle: 15–60 g, twice daily
Camels: 30–75 g, twice daily
Llamas, Alpacas, Pigs, Goats, and Sheep: 5–15 g, twice daily
Dogs: 0.5–5 g (or 0.1 g per kg body weight), twice daily
Cats and Rabbits: 0.2–0.5 g (or 0.1 g per kg body weight), twice daily
Birds: 0.1–0.2 g per kg body weight, twice daily
Use 3–8 weeks until primary clinical signs resolve.

Table 18.8. Ingredients and actions of *Yang Xin Tang*.

%	English Name	Chinese *Pin-Yin*	Action
12	Codonopsis	*Dang Shen*	Tonify *Qi*
16	Astragalus	*Huang Qi*	Tonify *Qi*
8	Glycyrrhiza	*Gan Cao*	Tonify *Qi*
10	Poria	*Fu Ling*	Drain Damp, strengthen Spleen
8	Ligusticum	*Chuan Xiong*	Move Blood
8	Angelica	*Dang Gui*	Nourish Blood
8	Biota	*Bai Zi Ren*	Tonify Heart
10	Polygala	*Yuan Zhi*	Tonify Heart
10	Schisandra	*Wu Wei Zi*	Astringently consolidate
10	Cinnamomum	*Rou Gui*	Warm *Yang*

Analysis of Formula: The King herbs in this formula are *Huang Qi* (Astragalus) and *Dang Shen* (Codonopsis), which work synergistically to tonify *Qi* for the treatment of the root problem *Qi* Deficiency. *Bai Zi Ren* (Biota), *Yuan Zhi* (Polygala), and *Wu Wei Zi* (Schisandra) are the Minister herbs to tonify the Heart. *Qi* Deficiency may lead to Blood Deficiency with Stagnation or *Yang* Deficiency with Dampness. Therefore, the Adjuvant herbs include *Chuan Xiong* (Ligusticum) and *Dang Gui* (Angelica), which tonify and move Blood to resolve Stagnation, and *Rou Gui* (Cinnamomum) and *Fu Ling* (Poria), which warm the Heart *Yang* and eliminate Dampness to tonify *Qi*. *Gan Cao* (Glycyrrhiza) is the Messenger herb to harmonize other herbs in the formula.

Cautions and Contraindications: This formula is not used in patients with *Yin* Deficiency

Dr. Xie's Comments: I have used *Yang Xin Tang* for heart failure due to Heart *Qi* Deficiency with great success. The patients can be medicated indefinitely if required. There are no known contraindications with conventional western heart medications, and the formula may exert a synergistic effect when used in combination.

Wei Qi Bu (*Wei Qi* Booster) 卫气补

Wei Qi refers to Defense *Qi*, which is associated with immune functions. *Bu* means tonifying, or boosting.

Source: *Chinese Veterinary Herbal Handbook* by *Huisheng Xie* and published by the Chi Institute of Chinese Medicine, 2004

Ingredients: The ingredients and actions of *Wei Qi Bu* are listed in Table 18.9.

Table 18.9. Ingredients and actions of *Wei Qi Bu*.

%	English Name	Chinese *Pin-Yin*	Action
21	Astragalus	*Huang Qi*	Tonify *Qi* in the whole body and *Wei Qi*
18	Angelica	*Dang Gui*	Tonify and move Blood to resolve Stagnation
21	Codonopsis	*Dang Shen*	Tonify *Qi* and boost *Wei Qi*
5	Lindera	*Wu Yao*	Move *Qi* and clear stagnation
5	Citrus	*Chen Pi*	Move *Qi* to resolve stagnation
10	Lobelia	*Ban Bian Lian*	Clear Heat, inhibit cell mutation
10	Oldenlandia	*Bai Hua She She Cao*	Clear Heat, inhibit cell mutation
10	Scrophularia	*Xuan Shen*	Cool Blood and nourish *Yin*, resolve Stagnation

Preparation:
1. Powder or capsule method: Herbs are ground into a fine powder. Powder can be encapsulated.
2. Decoction or teapill method: Raw herbs are mixed together and decocted. Herbal water extract (decoction) can be concentrated as granules or teapills.

Actions: Tonify *Qi* and Blood, enhancement therapy *Wei Qi,* inhibit mutation

Indications: General weakness, fatigue, apathy, poor appetite, weight loss in senior animals, chronic viral infections, FIV and FeLV in cats, immune boost and general support for postchemo or radiation therapy, anemia, hypothyroidism, chronic arthritis or renal failure in aged dogs, prevention of frequent recurrence of upper respiratory infections

Dosage and Usage:
Horses and Cattle: 15–60 g, twice daily
Camels: 30–75 g, twice daily
Llamas, Alpacas, Pigs, Goats, and Sheep: 5–15 g, twice daily
Dogs: 0.5–5 g (or 0.1–0.2 g per kg body weight), twice daily
Cats and Rabbits: 0.2–0.5 g (or 0.1 g per kg body weight), twice daily
Birds: 0.1 g per kg body weight, twice daily
Use up to 56 weeks as needed

Analysis of Formula: In TCVM, the host defense system is Defense *Qi* or *Wei Qi*. As long as *Wei Qi* is strong enough to keep pathogenic factors (including viruses and bacteria) from invading the body, the animal is healthy. In other words, the TCVM emphasis is on the immune system defense, not on the bacteria and viruses as may be true in the conventional approach. These pathogens are in the environment and even within the animal's body, but they are unable to cause any pathology as long as *Wei Qi* is strong enough to overcome them. However, as soon as *Wei Qi* weakens (or is insufficient), the pathogenic factors (e.g., bacteria and viruses) easily invade the body and cause disease. Failure of the host defense system is a *Wei Qi* Deficiency. *Huang Qi* (Astragalus) and *Dang Shen* (Codonopsis) are the King herbs, which work synergistically to tonify *Wei Qi*. *Wei Qi* Deficiency with invasion of the exogenous pathogens easily leads to *Qi*-Blood Stagnation. Therefore, the Minister herbs include *Dang Gui* (Angelica) and *Xuan Shen* (Scrophularia), which tonify Blood and *Yin* and move Blood to resolve Stagnation, and *Wu Yao* (Lindera) and *Chen Pi* (Citrus), which Move *Qi* to resolve Stagnation. The exogenous pathogens may cause Heat and cell mutation, thereby promoting neoplasia. Therefore, *Ban Bian Lian* (Lobelia) and *Bai Hua She She Cao* (Oldenlandia) work synergistically as the Adjuvant herbs to clear Heat, remove toxins, and inhibit cell mutation.

Cautions and Contraindications: This is one of the safest herbal formulas in veterinary practice. It can be used for a long time period. No side effects have been noticed.

Dr. Xie's Comments: I have used this herbal formula for general immune Deficiency and have combined it with Phlegm or Blood Stasis formulas including *Nei Xiao Luo Li San* for the treatment of neoplasia. With respect to the latter, survival length greater than the median may suggest a strong role in an integrative approach to the oncology patient.

Wan Dai Fang (Ending Vaginal Discharge) 完带方

Wan means ending. *Dai* refers to vaginal discharge. *Fang* means a formulation.

Source: *Fu Qing Zhu Nü Ke* (*Women's Diseases According to Fu Qing-Zhu*), written by *Fu Shan* and published in 1827

Ingredients: The formula is composed of the following ingredients: 30 g *Bai Zhu* (Atractylodes), 30 g *Shan Yao* (Dioscorea), 6 g *Ren Shen* (Ginseng), 15 g *Bai Shao* (Paeonia), 9 g *Cang Zhu* (Atractylodes), 2 g *Chen Pi* (Citrus), 9 g *Che Qian Zi* (Plantago), 2 g *Chai Hu* (Bupleurum), 2 g *Jing Jie* (Schizonepeta), and 3 g *Gan Cao* (Glycyrrhiza) (Table 18.10).

Preparation:
1. Powder or capsule method: Herbs are ground into a fine powder. Powder can be encapsulated.
2. Decoction or teapill method: Raw herbs are mixed together and decocted. Herbal water extract (decoction) can be concentrated as granules or teapills.

Table 18.10. Ingredients and actions of *Wan Dai Fang*.

%	English Name	Chinese *Pin-Yin*	Action
27.8	Atractylodes	*Bai Zhu*	Dry Damp and tonify the Spleen
27.8	Dioscorea	*Shan Yao*	Tonify *Qi* and *Jing*
5.6	Ginseng	*Ren Shen*	Tonify primary *Qi*
13.8	Paeonia	*Bai Shao*	Nourish Liver *Yin* and Blood
8.3	Atractylodes	*Cang Zhu*	Dry Damp and strengthen the Spleen
1.9	Citrus	*Chen Pi*	Move *Qi* and relieve pain
8.2	Plantago	*Che Qian Zi*	Clear Damp-Heat and benefit urination
1.9	Bupleurum	*Chai Hu*	Soothe Liver *Qi*
1.9	Schizonepeta	*Jing Jie*	Clear Wind-cold and move *Qi*
2.8	Glycyrrhiza	*Gan Cao*	Harmonize the formula

Actions: Strengthen the Spleen and tonify *Qi*, soothe the Liver *Qi*, eliminate Damp to end vaginal discharge

Indications: Vaginal or genital discharge due to Spleen *Qi* Deficiency, genital discharge without odor, weak pulse, pale and wet tongue

Dosage and Usage:
Horses and Cattle: 15–60 g, twice daily
Llamas, Alpacas, Pigs, Goats, and Sheep: 5–15 g, twice daily
Dogs: 0.5–5 g (or 0.1 g per kg body weight), twice daily
Use 4–6 weeks until primary clinical signs resolve.

Analysis of Formula: Genital or vaginal discharge is associated with three factors: 1) Spleen *Qi* Deficiency, 2) dysfunction of *Dai Mai* (Girdle Channel), and 3) Liver *Qi* Stagnation. Spleen *Qi* Deficiency fails to transform water and fluids, leading to generation of Dampness in the Interior, which becomes the source of genital discharge.

Physiologically, the *Dai Mai* wraps the lower trunk like a belt, securing all the Channels that traverse the area. Pathogenically, when the *Dai Mai* is Stagnant or dysfunctional in female animals, it fails to secure and hold the Channels, leading to genital or vaginal discharge from the lowest part of the trunk. The Liver controls the free flow of *Qi* in the entire body. When Liver *Qi* is Stagnant, it overwhelms the Spleen and further weakens the transformation process of water and fluids, which leads to an increase in production of Dampness. Even though the genital or vaginal discharge is associated with the above three factors, the core cause is Dampness, which comes from Spleen *Qi* Deficiency. Therefore, the main treatment principle is to tonify Spleen *Qi* and dry up Damp. In the formula, *Bai Zhu* (Atractylodes) and *Shan Yao* (Dioscorea) work synergistically as the King herbs to tonify Spleen *Qi* and dry up Damp. The Minister herbs are *Ren Shen* (Ginseng) and *Cang Zhu* (Atractylodes) to tonify the Source (*Yuan*) *Qi*, strengthen the Spleen, and dry Damp. *Bai Shao* (Paeonia) soothes Liver *Qi* and nourishes *Yin* and Blood, *Chen Pi* (Citrus) moves *Qi* to relieve pain, *Che Qian Zi* (Plantago) clears Damp-Heat and promotes urination, *Chai Hu* (Bupleurum) soothes the Liver, and *Jing Jie* (Schizonepeta) moves *Qi* and clears Wind-Cold. These herbs are Adjuvant herbs to soothe Liver *Qi* and also secure the *Dai Mai*. *Gan Cao* (Glycyrrhiza) is the great harmonizer, which helps all the herbs work together toward a common goal.

Cautions and Contraindications: It is designed for genital or vaginal discharge due to Spleen *Qi* Deficiency. It should be contraindicated with vaginal discharge due to Damp-Heat (dark yellow, bloody, thick, sticky, and foul-smelling discharge from the uterus).

Dr. Xie's Comments: The formula is helpful both with cleansing the uterus and vaginal tract prior to breeding/conception and with inflammation in the uterus and vagina.

FORMULAS TO TONIFY BLOOD

The formulas in this section are used for the treatment of Blood Deficiency. The main signs of Blood Deficiency Pattern include dry haircoat with dandruff, cracked paws or hooves, dizziness, dry and pale tongue, and thin pulse. The most common King ingredients are *Shu Di Huang* (Rehmannia), *Dang Gui* (Angelica), and *Bai Shao* (Paeonia). Because *Qi* generates Blood and causes it to circulate, Blood tonic herbal formulas often include *Qi* tonic herbs such as *Ren Shen* (Ginseng) and *Huang Qi* (Astragalus). Often, Blood Deficiency may lead to Blood Stasis or Stagnation. Therefore, tonic herbal formulas may also contain herbals to move Blood, such as *Chuan Xiong* (Ligusticum) and *Hong Hua* (Carthamus).

Herbs to tonify Blood are rich and tend to generate Dampness and Stagnation, which block the flow of Spleen and Stomach *Qi*. Thus, herbs to move Stomach *Qi* and strengthen the Spleen (Citrus *Chen Pi* or Saussurea *Mu Xiang*) are often added to prevent this problem. Four Blood tonic formulas to be discussed in detail below are *Si Wu Tang, Dang Gui Bu Xue Tang, Gui Qi Yi Mu Tang, Gui Pi Tang.*

Si Wu Tang (Four Substances) 四物汤

Si is four. *Wu* refers to substance. Thus, *Si Wu* literally means Four Substances, or Four Ingredients. This formula consists of four herbal ingredients as the name implies.

Source: *Tai Ping Hui Min He Ji Ju Fang* (*Imperial Grace Formula of the Tai Ping Era*), written by *Chen Shiwen* et al. and published in 1078

Ingredients: The original formula is composed of 12 g *Shu Di Huang* (Rehmannia), 9 g *Dang Gui* (Angelica), 9 g *Bai Shao* (Paeonia), and 6 g *Chuan Xiong* (Ligusticum) (Table 18.11).

Preparation:
1. Powder or capsule method: Herbs are ground into a fine powder. Powder can be encapsulated.
2. Decoction or teapill method: Raw herbs are mixed together and decocted. Herbal water extract (decoction) can be concentrated as granules or teapills.

Actions: Nourish and regulate Blood

Indications: Blood Deficiency, palpitations, anemia, general weakness, pale tongue, thready pulse

Table 18.11. Ingredients and actions of *Si Wu Tang*.

%	English Name	Chinese *Pin-Yin*	Action
34	Rehmannia	*Shu Di Huang*	Enrich and tonify Blood and nourish *Yin*
24	Angelica	*Dang Gui*	Nourish Blood and activate Blood circulation
24	Paeonia	*Bai Shao*	Nourish Blood and soothe the Liver
18	Ligusticum	*Chuan Xiong*	Move *Qi* and Blood, alleviate pain

Dosage and Usage:

Horses and Cattle: 15–60 g, twice daily
Camels: 30–75 g, twice daily
Llamas, Alpacas, Pigs, Goats, and Sheep: 5–15 g, twice daily
Dogs: 0.5–5 g (or 0.1 g per kg body weight), twice daily
Cats and Rabbits: 0.2–0.5 g (or 0.1 g per kg body weight), twice daily
Birds: 0.1–0.2 g per kg body weight, twice daily

Use 4–12 weeks until primary clinical signs resolve.

Analysis of Formula: Blood Deficiency often results from an insufficiency of Blood and/or obstructed Blood circulation. It should be treated by nourishing and regulating Blood. In this formula, *Shu Di Huang* (Rehmannia) nourishes *Yin* and Blood as the King herb. *Dang Gui* (Angelica) and *Bai Shao* (Paeonia) act as Minister herbs with effects of nourishing Blood and the Liver, which stores the Blood. *Chuan Xiong* (Ligusticum) works as an Adjuvant herb to promote circulation of both *Qi* and Blood. In summary, *Shu Di Huang* and *Bai Shao* are designed to nourish Blood, while *Dang Gui* and *Chuan Xiong* are included for nourishing and regulating Blood. The compatibility of this formula aims to nourish Blood without inducing Stasis, and to promote Blood circulation without impairing it.

Cautions and Contraindications: This formula cannot be used for abdominal pain due to Blood Stagnation or *Qi* Deficiency with Dampness.

Dr. Xie's Comments: I have used *Si Wu Tang* for general anemia due to Blood Deficiency, and have combined it with *Gui Pi Tang* for the treatment of autoimmune hemolytic anemia and immune-mediated thrombocytopenia. Clinical results for the latter appear consistent with the reported laboratory and animal model investigations described below.

Clinical and Pharmacological Study:

Effects on Blood and the Hematopoietic System of a Blood Deficient model in irradiated mice suggests some of the effects of the formula. The treatment group was immediately administered 0.2 ml of *Si Wu Tang* (1 g/ml) orally following radiation. The control group and model group were drenched with the same dose of normal saline. Samples of 20 µl blood each were collected from the vena caudalis of the mice on the 1st, 3rd, 5th, and 7th days before and after radiation. The blood was analyzed by a Sysmex-800 globulimeter. The number of WBC and platelets in the *Si Wu Tang* group were significantly higher than the control group ($P < 0.05$). Meanwhile, the hemopoietic progenitor cells of the marrow were cultivated. Progenitor cell colony formation of CFU-GM and CFU-meg declined with radiation; however, after treatment with *Si Wu Tang* the number of cell colonies was significantly increased compared to the control groups.[34]

In another study using a Blood Deficient mouse model, a positive effect was demonstrated on NFS-60 cell propagation after treatment with *Si Wu Tang*, and the propagation of NFS-60 cells was strongest when given *Si Wu Tang* at 4 mg/ml. This may be the molecular basis by which *Si Wu Tang* increases peripheral WBCs of Blood Deficient mice and promotes the colonial propagation of CF-GM and CFU-meg of hematopoietic cells. The WBCs, RBCs, and Hgb were lower in the control groups on the 7th and 14th days, but with several different doses of *Si Wu Tang* (5, 10, and 20 g/kg/day) the number of WBCs, RBCs and Hgb increased. *Si Wu Tang* can also promote the marrow cells by converting them from the C0/1 stage to S stage of cell growth, promoting the synthesis of marrow cell DNA, repressing the apoptosis of marrow cells, and reducing the compensation of myeloid elements. Thus, the low level of hemopoiesis of the Blood Deficient model can be reversed and the hematogenesis improved after the *Si Wu Tang* treatment.[35]

In another laboratory investigation, *Si Wu Tang* promoted the regeneration of peripheral blood and the marrow production of colony-forming unit-erythroid (CFU-E or precursors of erythrocytes), burst-forming unit-erythroid (BFU-E), and colony-forming unit-granulocyte macrophage (CFU-GM) of Blood Deficient mice treated by cyclophosphamide.[36] After cyclophosphamide treatment the number of ancestral progenitor cells decreased in the bone marrow. Treatment with *Si Wu Tang* promoted the regeneration of hematopoietic ancestral cells. *Si Wu Tang* also increased the thymic functions and strengthened the immune function of the Blood Deficient mice. This research suggests that the mechanism of action of *Si Wu Tang* to treat Blood Deficiency in mice is due to the promotion of the number of hematopoietic ancestral cells in the bone marrow and enhancement of the immune function.

In another study, aqueous and alcohol extracts of *Si Wu Tang* were respectively either lavaged or injected subcutaneously into mice to determine the effect on serum lipids.[37,38] The results displayed that both herbal extracts increased HDL-C and decreased LDL-C, serum cholesterol and triglycerides of the mice. This experiment implies that the Blood-promoting and Stagnation-dissolving functions of *Si Wu Tang* may result in decreased lipemia and blood viscosity. *Si Wu Tang* may also decrease the absorption of cholesterol in the intestinal tract, speed up the metabolic rate and transform types of cholesterol, thereby diminishing the risk of coronary heart disease (CHD) and atherosclerosis. Compared with the control group, mice treated with *Si Wu Tang* had significantly improved left ventricular systolic pressure (LVSP) peak value and myofibril contraction velocity. The mean arterial pressure (MAP), isovolumetric contraction (IC) pressure, and heart rate were minimally changed in the SWT group. These results showed that *Si Wu Tang* can enhance the cardiac contractility and strengthen the circulatory function of the heart.[39]

Effects on Immune Function *Si Wu Tang* at the concentration of 0.01–1.00µg/ml significantly promoted the propagation of splenic cells in mice and enhanced the function of T-Lymphocytes leading to immune activation.[40] The activated lymphocytes enhanced cellular immune activities. *Si Wu Tang* also promoted LPS to activate IL-1 produced by macrophages.[41] IL-1 is an important factor in immunity against infections and tumors and can also stimulate hematogenesis, particularly increasing the number of neutrophils. *Shuping Bai* discovered that *Si Wu Tang* can remarkably increase the phagocytosis of macrophages in mice, increase the weight of the thymus and pancreas, and elevate antibody titers. All of these findings indicated that *Si Wu Tang* had an effect on humoral and cell immunity.[42]

RBCs have important functions not only in oxygenation, but also in identifying and storing antigens, removing immune complexes, and reinforcing the dependent reactions of T cells. *Ting Zhang*[43] and *Ruquan Chen*[44], respectively, experimented with mice exposed to ionization and Blood-Deficient rabbits. They found that the damaged receptors of RBC-C3b were repaired, their regeneration capability improved, and the ability to remove immune complexes had been enhanced significantly by *Si Wu Tang*.

The Antiradiation Effects of *Si Wu Tang* Intragastric administration of *Si Wu Tang* (20mg/kg) for 7 days increased peripheral RBCs, WBCs, platelets, and HCT in mice receiving whole body radiation.[45] Another experiment used 60Co to radiate mice. The result was a reduction of CD34+ in the bone marrow; decreased numbers of CFU-GM, BFU-E, colony-forming unit-megakaryocyte (CFU-Meg, or precursors of megakaryocytes) and CFU-Mix; decreased peripheral Blood cells; apoptosis of marrow cells; and chaos of the cycle of cell growth.[46] This study showed that *Si Wu Tang* promoted the number of CFU-GM, CFU-E, BFU-E, CFU-Mix. Similarly, Paeonia from the herb *Bai Shao* promoted marrow stromal cells to excrete hematogenic factors such as granulocyte colony-stimulating factor (G-CSF), granulocyte-macrophage colony-stimulating factor (GM-CSF), and platelet-derived growth factor–α (PDGF-α).[47]

Other Si Wu Tang Effects *Si Wu Tang* is shown to be protective against and a treatment for lidocaine toxicity.[48] The toxicity to the heart caused by lidocaine suppresses myocardial contractility. *Si Wu Tang* inhibited arrhythmias and increased the heart's tolerance to anoxia and hypoxia. The protection against lidocaine toxicity by *Si Wu Tang* is clinically relevant, and *Si Wu Tang* can be used as an antidote to lidocaine toxicity in some instances.

A study on the effect of *Si Wu Tang* and each single herb component on the metabolism of free radicals indicated that *Si Wu Tang* significantly increased the content of RBC superoxide dismutase (SOD) in mice in contrast with both the control group and each single herb tested individually.[49] *Si Wu Tang* also significantly decreased the content of leukopoietin (LPO) in plasma. These results suggest that *Si Wu Tang* has antioxidant functions and each component herb of *Si Wu Tang* has a synergistic effect, so the combined whole is more effective than its parts, which is consistent with ancient theories regarding herbal administration.

Li experimented with the effect of *Si Wu Tang* on uterine smooth muscles.[50] The results of this study indicated that *Si Wu Tang* can repress a spastic uterus and stimulate an inhibited uterus, and thus promote self-regulation. The type of regulatory effect on the uterus was dictated by its dysfunctional state, again consistent with ancient teachings. Ferulaic acid found in *Dang Gui* and *Chuan Xiong* from *Si Wu Tang* is the main compound believed to have an effect on the uterus.[51] Other reports suggested that *Si Wu Tang* can be used for the treatment of leiomyoma of the uterus and dysfunctional uterine bleeding.[52] A clinical trial indicated that 24 out of 26 bovine cases of anemia from postsurgical uterine torsion were cured after using modified *Si Wu Tang*.[53] Additionally, positive outcomes were found using *Si Wu Tang* for the treatment of hematochezia in cattle.[54]

Dang Gui Bu Xue Tang (Angelica to Tonify Blood) 当归补血汤

Dang Gui is the King herb Angelica. *Bu Xue* literally means Tonify Blood. *Bu* is tonify. *Xue* means Blood. *Tang* is decoction, the form of herbal administration.

Source: *Nei Wai Shang Bian Huo Lun* (*Clarifying Doubts about Injury from Internal and External Causes*), written by *Li Ao* and published in 1247

Table 18.12. Ingredients and actions of *Dang Gui Bu Xue Tang.*

%	English Name	Chinese *Pin-Yin*	Action
83	Astragalus	*Huang Qi*	Replenish *Qi* to invigorate *Yang*, benefit the Lung to strengthen the body
17	Angelica	*Dang Gui*	Nourish Blood and activate Blood circulation

Ingredients: The original formula is composed of 30 g *Huang Qi* (Astragalus) and 6 g *Dang Gui* (Angelica). The ingredient percentages and actions are listed in Table 18.12.

Preparation:
1. Powder or capsule method: Herbs are ground into a fine powder. Powder can be encapsulated.
2. Decoction or teapill method: Raw herbs are mixed together and decocted. Herbal water extract (decoction) can be concentrated as granules or teapills.

Actions: Tonify *Qi* to promote generation of Blood

Indications: Blood Deficiency with *Yang* floating marked by fever, polydipsia, large but weak pulse when pressed, or acute Blood loss after parturition or trauma

Dosage and Usage:
Horses and Cattle: 15–60 g, twice daily
Camels: 30–75 g, twice daily
Llamas, Alpacas, Pigs, Goats, and Sheep: 5–15 g, twice daily
Dogs: 0.5–5 g (or 0.1 g per kg body weight), twice daily
Cats and Rabbits: 0.2–0.5 g (or 0.1 g per kg body weight), twice daily
Birds: 0.1–0.2 g per kg body weight, twice daily
Use 3–8 weeks until primary clinical signs resolve.

Analysis of Formula: *Qi* and Blood have a close relationship. *Qi* is the generator of Blood while Blood is the carrier of *Qi*, a vehicle to bring *Qi* to the whole body. When acute loss of Blood leads to Blood Deficiency, deficient Blood fails to carry *Qi*, leading to *Qi* Deficiency with *Yang* floating. *Yang* floating causes fever and polydipsia; this should be treated by replenishing *Qi* and promoting production of Blood. Used as the King herb, *Huang Qi* (Astragalus) in larger doses is capable of tonifying the Spleen and Lung *Qi*, which leads to production of Blood and consolidating superficial resistance to astringe the floating *Yang*. *Dang Gui* (Angelica) acts as the Minister herb with the effect of nourishing Blood. The two herbs work synergistically to promote generation of *Qi* and Blood and astringently consolidate the floating *Yang*. When they are taken by patients that are febrile due to Blood Deficiency, the abundance of Blood may enrich and hold *Yang*. When they are taken by patients with Blood and *Qi* Deficiency, the abundance of *Qi* ensures regeneration of Blood.

Cautions and Contraindications: This formula is contraindicated for patients of *Yin* Deficiency with hectic fever.

Dr. Xie's Comments: I have successfully used this herbal formula for the treatment of anemia due to blood loss as a result of surgery or parturition. Combined with *Gui Pi Tang*, this herbal formula can be used for the treatment of immune-mediated thrombocytopenia.

Clinical and Pharmacological Studies: *Dang Gui Bu Xue Tang* is successfully used for the treatment of anemia due to prolonged labor and postpartum complications as well as chronic nonhealing lesions or ulcerations.[55]

Gui Qi Yi Mu Tang (Angelica, Astragalus, and Leonurus) 归芪益母汤

Gui Qi refers to *Dang Gui* (Angelica). *Qi* refers to *Huang Qi* (Astragalus). They are the two main ingredients of this formula. *Yi Mu* refers to *Yi Mu Cao* (Leonurus).

Source: *Niu Jing Bei Yao Yi Fang* (*Ready-for-Use Classical Prescriptions in Cattle*) was published in 1815. The authors are unknown.

Ingredients: This formula is *Dang Gui Bu Xue Tang* with added *Yi Mu Cao* (Leonurus). The original formula is composed of 30 g *Dang Gui* (Angelica), 120 g *Huang Qi* (Astragalus), and 60 g *Yi Mu Cao* (Leonurus) (Table 18.13).

Preparation:
1. Powder or capsule method: Herbs are ground into a fine powder. Powder can be encapsulated.
2. Decoction or teapill method: Raw herbs are mixed together and decocted. Herbal water extract (decoction) can be concentrated as granules or teapills.

Table 18.13. Ingredients and actions of *Gui Qi Yi Mu Tang.*

%	English Name	Chinese *Pin-Yin*	Action
14.5	Angelica	*Dang Gui*	Nourish Blood and activate Blood circulation
56.5	Astragalus	*Huang Qi*	Tonify *Qi* and warm the Middle Burner, strengthen superficial resistance of the body, lift the sunken *Yang*
29	Leonurus	*Yi Mu Cao*	Activate Blood circulation to relieve Blood stasis in the uterus

Actions: Replenish *Qi* and promote production of Blood, activate Blood circulation to relieve Stasis

Indications: Deficiency of *Qi* and Blood, postpartum anemia, postpartum Blood Stasis, exercise intolerance, general weakness, pale tongue, weak and thin pulse

Dosage and Usage:
Horses and Cattle: 15–60g, twice daily
Camels: 30–75g, twice daily
Llamas, Alpacas, Pigs, Goats, and Sheep: 5–15g, twice daily
Dogs: 0.5–5g (or 0.1g per kg body weight), twice daily
Cats and Rabbits: 0.2–0.5g (or 0.1g per kg body weight), twice daily
Birds: 0.1–0.2g per kg body weight, twice daily
Use 3–8 weeks until primary clinical signs resolve.

Analysis of Formula: Used as the King herb, *Huang Qi* (Astragalus) in larger dosages is capable of tonifying Spleen and Lung *Qi* to enrich the source of Blood. *Dang Gui* (Angelica) acts as the Minister herb with the effect of nourishing Blood. Therefore, these two ingredients used together both tonify *Qi* and promote the generation of Blood. *Yi Mu Cao* (Leonurus) is the Adjuvant herb to promote circulation of Blood and to relieve Stasis, especially Blood Stasis in the uterus. The compatibility of this formula aims to nourish Blood without inducing Stasis—that is, to promote Blood circulation without impairing it.

Cautions and Contraindications: This formula is contraindicated for patients displaying *Yin* Deficiency with hectic fever.

Dr. Xie's Comments: This herbal formula can be used for the treatment of postpartum complications (general weakness, anemia, uterine discharge, and pain) in mares and dairy cows.

Clinical and Pharmacological Studies: *Chuan* reported that all 23 dairy cows of postpartum paresis and/or paralysis were improved after taking *Gui Qi Yi Mu Tang*.[56]

Gui Pi Tang (Restoring the Spleen) 归脾汤

Gui means returning, or restoring. *Pi* is the Spleen. *Tang* is the decoction, the original form of herbal medication. *Gui Pi* literally means Returning the Spleen.

Source: *Ji Sheng Fang* (*Formulas to Aid the Living*), written by *Yan Yonghe* and published in 1253

Ingredients: The original formula is composed of 9g *Bai Zhu* (Atractylodes), 9g *Fu Shen* (Poria), 12g *Huang Qi* (Astragalus), 12g *Long Yan Rou* (Longan), 12g *Suan Zao Ren* (Ziziphus), 6g *Ren Shen* (Ginseng), 6g *Mu Xiang* (Saussurea), 3g *Gan Cao* (Glycyrrhiza), 9g *Dang Gui* (Angelica), and 6g *Yuan Zhi* (Polygala) (Table 18.14).

Preparation:
1. Powder or capsule method: Herbs are ground into a fine powder. Powder can be encapsulated.
2. Decoction or teapill method: Raw herbs are mixed together and decocted. Herbal water extract (decoction) can be concentrated as granules or teapills.

Actions: Replenish *Qi* and Nourish Blood, tonify the Spleen and Heart

Indications: Deficiency Pattern of both *Qi* and Blood within the Spleen and Heart; the Pattern characterized by the failure of the Spleen to control Blood, marked by palpitation, poor appetite and weakness, pale tongue with thin white coating, thready and weak pulse

Dosage and Usage:
Horses and Cattle: 15–60g, twice daily
Camels: 30–75g, twice daily
Llamas, Alpacas, Pigs, Goats, and Sheep: 5–15g, twice daily

Table 18.14. Ingredients and actions of *Gui Pi Tang*.

%	English Name	Chinese *Pin-Yin*	Action
11	Atractylodes	*Bai Zhu*	Tonify the Spleen *Qi*, dry Dampness, promote diuresis
11	Poria	*Fu Shen*	Eliminate Dampness to strengthen the Spleen, calm the Mind
14	Astragalus	*Huang Qi*	Replenish *Qi*, benefit the Lung to strengthen the body, promote diuresis to relieve edema
14	Longan	*Long Yan Rou*	Nourish Blood and tonify the Heart
14	Ziziphus	*Suan Zao Ren*	Nourish the Heart to calm the Mind, arrest sweating
7	Ginseng	*Ren Shen*	Replenish *Yuan Qi*, tonify the Spleen and Lung, promote the production of Body Fluids, calm the Mind
7	Saussurea	*Mu Xiang*	Disperse stagnant *Qi* to relieve abdominal pain
4	Glycyrrhiza	*Gan Cao*	Harmonize the effect of other herbs
11	Angelica	*Dang Gui*	Nourish Blood and activate Blood circulation
7	Polygala	*Yuan Zhi*	Keep Heart-*Yang* and Kidney-*Yin* in balance, calm the mind

Dogs: 0.5–5 g (or 0.1 g per kg body weight), twice daily
Cats and Rabbits: 0.2–0.5 g (or 0.1 g per kg body weight), twice daily
Birds: 0.1–0.2 g per kg body weight, twice daily

Use 3–10 weeks until primary clinical signs resolve.

Analysis of Formula: The Heart stores the Mind (Spirit) and governs Blood; the Spleen controls the emotional sense of *Si* (thinking, worrying, or sympathizing) and holds Blood. Chronic overthinking or preoccupation, overwork, or other chronic illness may injure the Spleen leading to Spleen *Qi* Deficiency. The Spleen is the source of production of Blood. In this case, Deficient Spleen fails to generate Blood that is governed by the Heart, consequently leading to Spleen *Qi* Deficiency and Heart Blood Deficiency. The key to treating this condition is to tonify Spleen *Qi*. Therefore, the King herbs in this herbal formula are *Huang Qi* (Astragalus) and *Dang Shen* (Codonopsis) to tonify Spleen *Qi*. The Minister herbs include *Bai Zhu* (Atractylodes) and *Fu Shen* (Poria) to eliminate Dampness to tonify Spleen *Qi*; *Dang Gui* (Angelica) and *Long Yan Rou* (Longan) are included to nourish Blood and calm the Mind. *Suan Zao Ren* (Ziziphus), *Yuan Zhi* (Polygala), and *Mu Xiang* (Saussurea) act as the Adjuvant herbs, which tonify the Heart Blood, calm the Mind, and move *Qi* to resolve Stagnation. *Gan Cao* (Glycyrrhiza) is used as the Messenger herb to supplement *Qi* and harmonize the properties and functions of other herbs.

Cautions and Contraindications: Do not use in patients with Excess Heat.

Dr. Xie's Comments: I have used *Gui Pi Tang* for treatment of chronic gastrointestinal hemorrhage, anemia, thrombocytopenia, immune-mediated thrombocytopenia, and autoimmune hemolytic anemia with great success. This herbal formula is often used for the treatment of behavioral problems due to Heart Blood Deficiency and Spleen *Qi* Deficiency.

Clinical and Pharmacological Studies: *Gui Pi Tang* Modification was used for the treatment of chronic immune thrombocytopenic purpura in 10 patients. After the herbal administration, platelet count was increased in 7 of 10 patients ($P < 0.05$). Platelet-associated IgG was decreased in 8 of 10 patients ($P < 0.05$). This study indicated that *Gui Pi Tang* appeared to promote the suppression of autoantibodies in patients with chronic immune thrombocytopenic purpura. No side effects were observed in any patient.[57]

FORMULAS TO TONIFY BOTH *QI* AND BLOOD

The herbal formulas in this section are used for the treatment of both *Qi* and Blood Deficiency Pattern. Both the *Qi* and Blood are closely related. *Qi* is the General of Blood and Blood is the mother of *Qi*. Deficient *Qi* often fails to move and generate Blood, and thus leads to Blood Deficiency. On the other hand, Deficient Blood fails to carry *Qi*, causing *Qi* Deficiency. Common signs of both *Qi* and Blood Deficiency are fatigue, anorexia, shortness of breath, dizziness, palpitation, restlessness, depression, pale tongue, and thin and weak pulse. When this occurs, a proper treatment is to tonify both *Qi* and Blood. The common herbal formulas to tonify *Qi* and Blood are *Ba Zhen Tang* and *Zhi Gan Cao Tang*.

Ba Zhen Tang (Eight Treasures) 八珍汤

Ba means eight. *Zhen* means treasure. *Ba Zhen* refers to eight precious ingredients, which are highly valued for their effect of tonifying both *Qi* and Blood.

Source: *Zheng Ti Lei Yao* (*Catalogue Essentials for Correcting the Body*), written by *Bi Lizhai* and published in 1529

Ingredients: The original formula is composed of 9 g *Dang Gui* (Angelica), 6 g *Chuan Xiong* (Ligusticum), 9 g *Bai Shao* (Paeonia), 12 g *Shu Di Huang* (Prepared Rehmannia), 6 g *Ren Shen* (Gingseng), 9 g *Bai Zhu* (Atractylodes), 6 g *Fu Ling* (Poria), and 3 g *Gan Cao* (Glycyrrhiza) (Table 18.15).

Preparation:

1. Powder or capsule method: Herbs are ground into a fine powder. Powder can be encapsulated.

Table 18.15. Ingredients and actions of *Ba Zhen Tang*.

%	English Name	Chinese *Pin-Yin*	Action
15	Angelica	*Dang Gui*	Nourish Blood and activate Blood circulation
10	Ligusticum	*Chuan Xiong*	Move *Qi* and Blood to alleviate pain
15	Paeonia	*Bai Shao*	Nourish Blood and nourish *Yin*
20	Prepared Rehmannia	*Shu Di Huang*	Tonify Blood and nourish *Yin*
10	Ginseng	*Ren Shen*	Replenish *Yuan Qi*, tonify the Spleen and Lung, promote production of Body Fluids, calm the Mind
15	Atractylodes	*Bai Zhu*	Tonify the Spleen, tonify *Qi* and dry Dampness
10	Poria	*Fu Ling*	Strengthen the Spleen, drain Dampness, promote urination
5	Glycyrrhiza	*Gan Cao*	Harmonize effects of other herbs

2. Decoction or teapill method: Raw herbs are mixed together and decocted. Herbal water extract (decoction) can be concentrated as granules or teapills.

Actions: Tonify *Qi* and nourish Blood

Indications: Deficiency of both *Qi* and Blood, marked by lethargy, shortness of breath, dry skin, poor appetite, pale tongue, thready and weak pulse

Dosage and Usage:
Horses and Cattle: 15–60g, twice daily
Camels: 30–75g, twice daily
Llamas, Alpacas, Pigs, Goats, and Sheep: 5–15g, twice daily
Dogs: 0.5–5g (or 0.1g per kg body weight), twice daily
Cats and Rabbits: 0.2–0.5g (or 0.1g per kg body weight), twice daily
Birds: 0.1–0.2g per kg body weight, twice daily
Use 4–12 weeks until primary clinical signs resolve.

Analysis of Formula: *Qi*-Blood Deficiency is mostly caused by a prolonged duration of chronic illness. It should be treated by means of nourishing *Qi* and Blood. As a result, in this formula *Ren Shen* (Ginseng) and *Shu Di Huang* (Rehmannia) work as the King herbs to respectively tonify *Qi* and Blood. *Bai Zhu* (Atractylodes), *Fu Ling* (Poria), *Dang Gui* (Angelica), and *Bai Shao* (Paeonia) act as Minister herbs to help the effect of the King herbs to reinforce *Qi* and Blood. *Chuan Xiong* (Ligusticum), with the action of promoting the circulation of *Qi* and Blood, is used as the Adjuvant herb. *Gan Cao* (Glycyrrhiza or Licorice) serves as the Messenger herb to regulate the Middle Burner and to mediate the properties of other herbs. *Ba Zhen Tang* is actually the combination of two classical herbal formulas, *Si Jun Zi Tang* (a basic *Qi* tonic) and *Si Wu Tang* (a basic Blood tonic), and thus achieves the result of nourishing both *Qi* and Blood.

Cautions and Contraindications: This formula is contraindicated for patients of *Yin* Deficiency with hectic fever.

Dr. Xie's Comments: I have commonly used *Ba Zhen Tang* in clinical practice for the treatment of chronic illness due to both *Qi* and Blood Deficiency.

Shi Quan Da Bu Tang (Ten Large Tonifications) 十全大补汤

Shi means ten, *Quan* refers to everything or all, *Da* means big or great, *Bu* refers to tonification. This formula is *Ba Zhen Tang* (Eight Treasures) with the addition of two more herbs: *Huang Qi* (Astragalus) and *Rou Gui* (Cinnamomum).

Source: *Tai Ping Hui Min He Ji Ju Fang (Imperial Grace Formulary of the Tai Ping Era)*, written by *Chen Shiwen* et al. and published in 1078

Ingredients: The original formula is composed of 9g *Dang Gui*, 6g *Chuan Xiong*, 9g *Bai Shao Yao*, 12g *Shu Di Huang*, 6g *Ren Shen*, 9g *Bai Zhu*, 6g *Fu Ling*, 3g *Zhi Gan Cao*, 9g *Huang Qi*, and 6g *Rou Gui*.

Preparation:
1. Powder or capsule method: Herbs are ground into a fine powder. Powder can be encapsulated.
2. Decoction or teapill method: Raw herbs are mixed together and decocted. Herbal water extract (decoction) can be concentrated as granules or teapills.

Actions: Tonify *Qi* and Blood, warm *Qi*, tonify *Yang*

Indications: Deficiency of *Qi*, Blood, and *Yang* leading to general weakness, poor appetite, exercise intolerance, cold cutaneous temperature in the lumbar region and extremities, pale and swollen tongue, deep and weak pulse

Dosage and Usage:
Horses and Cattle: 15–60g, twice daily
Camels: 30–75g, twice daily
Llamas, Alpacas, Pigs, Goats, and Sheep: 5–15g, twice daily
Dogs: 0.5–5g (or 0.1g per kg body weight), twice daily
Cats and Rabbits: 0.2–0.5g (or 0.1g per kg body weight), twice daily
Birds: 0.1–0.2g per kg body weight, twice daily
Use 4–12 weeks until primary clinical signs resolve.

Analysis of Formula: *Shi Quan Da Bu Tang* is composed of *Si Jun Zi Tang* (containing *Ren Shen*, *Bai Zhu*, *Fu Ling*, and *Zhi Gan Cao*) and *Si Wu Tang* (containing *Dang Gui*, *Chuan Xiong*, *Bai Shao Yao*, and *Shu Di Huang*), *Huang Qi*, and *Rou Gui*. *Si Jun Zi Tang* is a basic *Qi* tonic. *Si Wu Tang* is a basic Blood tonic. *Huang Qi* and *Rou Gui* tonify and warm *Yang Qi*. Therefore, the whole formulation tonifies *Qi*, Blood, and *Yang* and is often used for Deficiency of *Qi*, Blood, and *Yang*.

Cautions and Contraindications: This formula is contraindicated for patients of *Yin* Deficiency with hectic fever.

Dr. Xie's Comments: I have often used *Shi Quan Da Bu Tang* for treatment of general weakness in geriatric patients, especially those with neoplasia.

Clinical and Pharmacological Studies: T-cells identify and destroy antigens such as toxins and tumor cells, and they trigger a host of other immune responses. With age, the body tends to produce fewer of these crucial agents, but *Shi Quan Da Bu Tang* shows the potential to reverse that trend. Studies found that elderly mice given the formula daily were able to generate new T-cells, correct their impaired T-cell activity, and restore the strength of their immune systems.[58]

It is easy to see how geriatric osteoporosis would qualify as a Deficiency disease. Here, too, *Shi Quan Da Bu Tang* is showing promise in the research lab. In Japan, researchers performed ovariectomies on rats to simulate the bone loss associated with menopause. Their bone density had declined to 20% of the control group's. A second test group received *Shi Quan Da Bu Tang*, effectively preventing bone loss secondary to ovariectomy. Electron microscopy confirms that their tibias (herbal treatment group) remained relatively fine and smooth compared to the porous and corroded tibias of the untreated group of rats. Finally, a third group of ovariectomized rats received hormone-replacement therapy (17-beta-estradiol), which similarly protected these rats from the bone loss seen in the untreated group of rats. Clearly, the herbs proved to be as effective as hormone-replacement therapy in preventing bone loss. As with the immune-system studies; human clinical trials are urgently needed.[59]

One group of Japanese researchers investigated what effect the formula would have on the growth of fibrosarcomas in mice. They administered *Shi Quan Da Bu Tang* to a group of mice for 7 days after inoculating them with *QR-32* tumor cells. Compared to the control group, their tumors grew far more slowly and their lives were significantly prolonged.[60] As measured on day 25, the beneficial effects proved to be dose dependent (4–40 mg/day). In separate tests, the researchers found that pretreating a group of mice with *Shi Quan Da Bu Tang* for 7 days before inoculating them with the tumor cells proved equally effective, whereby on day 25 tumor growth was significantly impaired.[61] Another laboratory studied the preventive effects of *Shi Quan Da Bu Tang* on endometrial carcinogenesis in mice. They removed the ovaries from their test animals and introduced controlled carcinogens such as 17-beta-estradiol into their uteri. Two weeks of subsequent treatment with *Shi Quan Da Bu Tang* reduced the measurable levels of certain oncoproteins, which are precursors to tumor formation. In a subsequent experiment, researchers injected a different carcinogen into the left ovaries of 93 mice, and an inert saline solution into the right ovaries. They then tested various dietary additives involving both estrogen and *Shi Quan Da Bu Tang*, and found that the herbal compound actually inhibited the formation of tumors.[62]

Shi Quan Da Bu Tang enhanced its potential to inhibit mouse tumors and resist the debilitating effects of chemotherapy. Subjects treated with the herbal formulation displayed higher white blood cell counts and healthier lymphatic systems than a control group treated with chemotherapy alone.[63,64] *Shi Quan Da Bu Tang* has been tested in a number of settings for its efficacy as a tonifying agent. It was found to readily inhibit laboratory-induced tumors from metastasizing in rat livers.[61,62] Indications were that it accomplished this by activating macrophages and/or T-cells in the infected animals.

These actions as an immune-enhancing agent supported further investigation of the synergy between *Shi Quan Da Bu Tang* and western immune enhancers. Interferon is one candidate for such multidrug applications. One laboratory studied its impact on mouse kidney tumors' ability to metastasize to the lungs. At a dosage of 100,000 IU/mouse, Interferon Alpha significantly inhibited such metastasis, but at the cost of a marked loss in body weight.[65,66] At the experimental dosage of 50 mg/mouse, a similar group of subjects showed a metastatic decline that was barely measurable. However, a combination therapy consisting of suboptimal doses of Interferon Alpha and *Shi Quan Da Bu Tang* together managed an effective synergy, containing most of the tumor cells with no loss of body weight at all. These results were later replicated using Interferon Gamma, with substantially the same results.[66] *Shi Quan Da Bu Tang* enhances phagocytosis, cytokine induction, and the production of antibodies.[67]

Zhi Gan Cao Tang (Prepared Glycyrrhiza) 炙甘草汤

Zhi refers to processing preparation of herbs. *Gan Cao* refers to Glycyrrhiza. *Tang* is decoction.

Source: *Shang Han Za Bing Lun (Discussion of Cold-Induced Disorders and Miscellaneous Diseases)*, written by *Zhang Zhong-Jing* and published in 220

Ingredients: The original formula is composed of 12 g *Zhi Gan Cao* (Glycyrrhiza), 50 g *Sheng Di Huang* (Rehmannia), 6 g *Ren Shen* (Ginseng), 9 g *Sheng Jiang* (Zingiberis), 9 g *Gui Zhi* (Cinnamomum), 6 g *E Jiao* (Asinum), 10 g *Mai Men Dong* (Ophiopogon), 10 g *Huo Ma Ren* (Cannabis), and 10 g *Da Zao* (Jujube) (Table 18.16).

Preparation:

1. Powder or capsule method: Herbs are ground into a fine powder. Powder can be encapsulated.
2. Decoction or teapill method: Raw herbs are mixed together and decocted. Herbal water extract (decoction) can be concentrated as granules or teapills.

Actions: Replenish *Qi* to enrich Blood, nourish to restore pulse

Indications: Palpitation, arrhythmia or heart murmur due to Deficiency of *Qi* and Blood, which is charac-

Table 18.16. Ingredients and actions of *Zhi Gan Cao Tang*.

%	English Name	Chinese *Pin-Yin*	Action
9.8	Glycyrrhiza	*Zhi Gan Cao*	Tonify *Qi* and harmonize the effect of all other herbs
7.4	Zingiberis	*Sheng Jiang*	Disperse pathogenic Wind-Cold, warm *Yang*
4.9	Ginseng	*Ren Shen*	Tonify *Yuan* (Source) *Qi*, tonify the Spleen and Lung, promote production of Body Fluids
41.0	Rehmannia	*Sheng Di Huang*	Nourish *Yin* and Blood, clear Heat
7.4	Cinnamomum	*Gui Zhi*	Warm the Channel and activate *Yang Qi*
4.9	Asinum	*E Jiao*	Nourish Blood to moisten dryness and stop bleeding
8.2	Ophiopogon	*Mai Men Dong*	Nourish *Yin*, clear false Heat from the body
8.2	Cannabis	*Huo Ma Ren*	Moisten dryness and loosen the bowels
8.2	Jujube	*Da Zao*	Tonify *Qi* and moderate the actions of other herbs

terized by intermittent pulse, lassitude, shortness of breath, pale tongue, or prolonged cough

Dosage and Usage:
Horses and Cattle: 15–60g, twice daily
Camels: 30–75g, twice daily
Llamas, Alpacas, Pigs, Goats, and Sheep: 5–15g, twice daily
Dogs: 0.5–5g (or 0.1–0.2g per kg body weight), twice daily
Cats and Rabbits: 0.2–0.5g (or 0.1g per kg body weight), twice daily
Birds: 0.1g per kg body weight, twice daily
Use as needed from 3–10 weeks.

Analysis of Formula: *Zhi Gan Cao* (Glycyrrhiza) and *Sheng Di Huang* (Rehmannia) act as the King herbs to tonify *Qi* and Blood. The Minister herbs include *Ren Shen* (Ginseng) and *Da Zao* (Jujube), which help the King herbs to tonify *Qi*, and *E Jiao* (Asinum), *Mai Men Dong* (Ophiopogon), and *Huo Ma Ren* (Cannabis), which nourish Blood. *Gui Zhi* (Cinnamomun) and *Sheng Jiang* (Zingiberis) function as Adjuvant herbs with the effect of warming the Heart *Yang* and promoting Blood flow. In addition, *Zhi Gan Cao* also mediates the properties of other herbs and is used as the Messenger herb. All herbs in combination tonify *Qi* and enrich the Blood, thereby restoring the normal pulse to relieve palpitation.

Cautions and Contraindications: Do not use in patients with Excess Heat or *Yin* Deficiency.

Dr. Xie's Comments: I have often used *Zhi Gan Cao Tang* for treatment of arrhythmia or heart murmur in the early stage of heart failure due to *Qi* and Blood Deficiency.

Clinical and Pharmacological Studies: *Gao* reported that *Zhi Gan Cao Tang* was successfully used for the treatment of palpitations and arrhythmia in dogs.[68] *Zhi Gan Cao Tang* improved the structure of myocardium to promote and restore cellular function.

Bai Zhu San (Atractylodes Powder) 白术散

Bai Zhu is Atractylodes, the King herb of this formula. *San* here refers to powder.

Source: *Yuan Heng Liao Ma Ji* (*Yuan-Heng's Therapeutic Treatise of Horses*), written by *Yu Benyuan* and *Yu Benheng* and published in 1608

Ingredients: The original formula is composed of 30g *Bai Zhu* (Atractylodes), 30g *Dang Gui* (Angelica), 30g *Shu Di Huang* (Rehmannia), 30g *Dang Shen* (Codonopsis), 60g *E Jiao* (Asinum), 30g *Chen Pi* (Citrus), 20g *Zi Su Ye* (Perilla), 20g *Huang Qin* (Scutellaria), 20g *Sha Ren* (Amomum), 20g *Chuan Xiong* (Ligusticum), 15g *Sheng Jiang* (Zingiberis), 20g *Bai Shao* (Paeonia), and 15g *Gan Cao* (Glycyrrhiza) (Table 18.17).

Preparation:
1. Powder or capsule method: Herbs are ground into a fine powder. Powder can be encapsulated.
2. Decoction or teapill method: Raw herbs are mixed together and decocted. Herbal water extract (decoction) can be concentrated as granules or teapills.

Actions: Tonify Blood and soothe the fetus

Indications: Fetal restlessness due to *Qi* and Blood Deficiency, prevention of abortion

Dosage and Usage:
Horses and Cattle: 15–60g, twice daily
Camels: 30–75g, twice daily
Llamas, Alpacas, Pigs, Goats, and Sheep: 5–15g, twice daily
Dogs: 0.5–5g (or 0.1g per kg body weight), twice daily
Cats and Rabbits: 0.2–0.5g (or 0.1g per kg body weight), twice daily
Birds: 0.1–0.2g per kg body weight, twice daily
Use 4–12 weeks until primary clinical signs resolve.

Analysis of Formula: In TCVM, abortion is often caused by the Spleen *Qi* being too weak to hold the

Table 18.17. Ingredients and actions of *Bai Zhu San*.

%	English Name	Chinese *Pin-Yin*	Action
8.6	Atractylodes	*Bai Zhu*	Tonify the Spleen, dry up Dampness, tonify *Qi*
8.6	Angelica	*Dang Gui*	Nourish Blood and activate Blood circulation
8.6	Rehmannia	*Shu Di Huang*	Nourish Blood and *Yin*
8.6	Codonopsis	*Dang Shen*	Tonify the Middle Burner (*Zhong Jiao*) and replenish *Qi*
17	Asinum	*E Jiao*	Nourish Blood, secure the fetus, stop bleeding
8.6	Citrus	*Chen Pi*	Move *Qi*, dry up Dampness and transform Phlegm
6	Perilla	*Zi Su Ye*	Transform Phlegm, keep the adverse Lung *Qi* downward
6	Scutellaria	*Huang Qin*	Clear Heat from the Lung
6	Amomum	*Sha Ren*	Promote Stomach *Qi* flow and appetite, secure the fetus
6	Ligusticum	*Chuan Xiong*	Promote flow of *Qi* and Blood, alleviate pain
5	Zingiberis	*Sheng Jiang*	Disperse Wind-Cold, dissipate Stomach Cold
6	Paeonia	*Bai Shao*	Nourish Blood, pacify the Liver and relieve pain
5	Glycyrrhiza	*Gan Cao*	Harmonize the effects of other herbs

fetus. The fetal restlessness stems from a lack of nourishment due to Blood Deficiency. These conditions should be treated by tonifying *Qi* and nourishing Blood to secure the fetus. Therefore, *Bai Zhu* (Atractylodes) and *Dang Shen* (Codonopsis) work synergistically as the King herbs to tonify *Qi* and strengthen the Spleen's physiological action of holding the fetus. *Shu Di Huang* (Rehmannia), *Bai Shao* (Paeonia), *Dang Gui* (Angelica), and *E Jiao* (Asinum) together serve as the Minister herbs to tonify Blood and secure the fetus. The Adjuvant herbs include *Sha Ren* (Amomum) and *Zi Su Ye* (Perilla) to calm the fetus, *Chen Pi* (Citrus) and *Chuan Xiong* to move *Qi* and Blood to resolve Stagnation and to relieve pain, and *Huang Qin* (Scutellaria) to clear Heat from the uterus. Both *Sheng Jiang* (Zingiberis) and *Gan Cao* (Glycyrrhiza) harmonize and regulate the effects of other herbs and work as the Messenger herbs. The combination of all ingredients works to tonify *Qi*, nourish Blood, activate *Qi* and Blood, clear Heat from the uterus, and secure the fetus.

Cautions and Contraindications: Do not use in patients with internal excessive Heat.

Dr. Xie's Comments: I have used this herbal formula for treatment of pregnant mares that have a history of early abortion. Many of the mares have carried foals to term following prophylactic administration.

Clinical and Pharmacological Studies: Fetal restlessness due to Deficiency of *Qi* and Blood is successfully treated by *Bai Zhu San*.[69] Another study indicated that *Bai Zhu San* was an effective therapy for abortion caused by Deficiency of *Qi* and Blood or sudden trauma. *Bai Zhu* (Atractylodes) and *Huang Qin* (Scutellaria) in this formula were the key herbs responsible for the reported effects.[70]

Dang Gui Shao Yao San (Angelica and Paeonia) 当归芍药散

Dang Gui refers to Angelica and *Shao Yao* is Paeonia, which are the King herbs in this formula. *San* is powder, an original form of herbal delivery.

Source: *Dang Gui Shao Yao San* from *Jin Gui Yao Lue Fang Lun* (*Synopsis of Prescriptions from the Golden Cabinet*), written by *Zhang Zhong-Jing* in 220

Ingredients: The ingredients and actions of *Dang Gui Shao Yao San* are listed in Table 18.18.

Preparation:
1. Powder or capsule method: Herbs are ground into a fine powder. Powder can be encapsulated.
2. Decoction or teapill method: Raw herbs are mixed together and decocted. Herbal water extract (decoction) can be concentrated as granules or teapills.

Actions: Nourish Liver Blood, soothe Liver *Qi*, strengthen Spleen, resolve Damp

Indications: Edema, pruritus, abdominal pain due to Liver Blood Deficiency

Dosage and Usage:
Horses and Cattle: 15–60 g, twice daily
Camels: 30–75 g, twice daily

Table 18.18. Ingredients and actions of *Dang Gui Shao Yao San*.

%	English Name	Chinese *Pin-Yin*	Action
10.5	Angelica	*Dang Gui*	Nourish Liver Blood
21.1	Paeonia	*Bai Shao*	Nourish Liver Blood and soothe Liver *Qi*
15.8	Atractylodes	*Cang Zhu*	Strengthen the Spleen and dry up Damp
15.8	Lophatherum	*Dan Zhu Ye*	Drain Damp-Heat
15.8	Crataegus	*Sha Zha*	Promote appetite, resolve food stasis
10.5	Cnidium	*She Chuang Zi*	Dry up Damp, kill parasites
10.5	Polyporous	*Zhu Ling*	Drain Damp

Llamas, Alpacas, Pigs, Goats, and Sheep: 5–15 g, twice daily
Dogs: 0.5–5 g (or 0.1 g per kg body weight), twice daily
Cats and Rabbits: 0.2–0.5 g (or 0.1 g per kg body weight), twice daily
Birds: 0.1–0.2 g per kg body weight, twice daily
Use 3–8 weeks until primary clinical signs resolve.

Analysis of Formula: In TCVM, the Liver stores the Blood, which in turn nourishes the fetus. Liver *Qi* Stagnation together with Blood Deficiency causes pruritus and abdominal pain. When the Liver overcontrols the Spleen, the water metabolism is damaged, leading to Damp accumulation and edema. Therefore, *Dang Gui* (Angelica) and *Bai Shao* (Paeonia) work synergistically as the King herbs to soothe Liver *Qi* and to tonify Liver Blood. The Minister herbs are *Zhu Ling* (Polyporous), *Cang Zhu* (Atractylodes), and *Dan Zhu Ye* (Lophatherum). Together they strengthen the Spleen and drain Dampness. *Sha Zha* (Crataegus) and *She Chuang Zi* (Cnidium) are the adjunct and Messenger herb that harmonizes the Stomach to promote appetite, and a transporter to the skin to stop itching, respectively.

Cautions and Contraindications: None known

Dr. Xie's Comments: I have used *Dang Gui Shao Yao San* for treatment of pregnant mares that tend to have skin problems and colic.

Qi Sai Fang (*Qi* Performance) 气赛方

Sai refers to competition, or performance. *Fang* means formulation.

Source: *Chinese Veterinary Herbal Handbook* by *Huisheng Xie* and published by the Chi Institute of Chinese Medicine, 2004

Ingredients: The ingredients and actions of *Qi Sai Fang* are listed in Table 18.19.

Preparation:
1. Powder or capsule method: Herbs are ground into a fine powder. Powder can be encapsulated.
2. Decoction or teapill method: Raw herbs are mixed together and decocted. Herbal water extract (decoction) can be concentrated as granules or teapills.

Actions: Tonify *Qi* and Blood, move Blood, relieve pain

Indications: Poor performance due to *Qi*-Blood Deficiency with *Qi* Stagnation, exercise intolerance, muscle pain, weight loss, pale purple and wet tongue, deep and weak pulse

Table 18.19. Ingredients and actions of *Qi Sai Fang*.

%	English Name	Chinese *Pin-Yin*	Action
13	Paeonia	*Bai Shao*	Tonify Blood and soothe Liver
6	Angelica	*Dang Gui*	Tonify and move Blood, resolve Stagnation, relieve pain
16	Astragalus	*Huang Qi*	Tonify *Qi*
13	Codonopsis	*Dang Shen*	Tonify *Qi*
16	Apis	*Feng Hua Fen*	Tonify *Qi* and *Yin* tonic
6	Moutan	*Mu Dan Pi*	Cool and move Blood, relieve pain
13	Crataegus	*Shan Zha*	Strengthen Stomach, promote appetite
13	Polygonum	*He Shou Wu*	Tonify Blood
4	Glycyrrhiza	*Gan Cao*	Harmonize

Dosage and Usage:
Horses and Cattle: 15–60 g, twice daily
Camels: 30–75 g, twice daily
Llamas, Alpacas, Pigs, Goats, and Sheep: 5–15 g, twice daily
Dogs: 0.5–5 g (or 0.1 g per kg body weight), twice daily
Cats and Rabbits: 0.2–0.5 g (or 0.1 g per kg body weight), twice daily
Birds: 0.1–0.2 g per kg body weight, twice daily
Use 4–12 weeks until primary clinical signs resolve.

Analysis of Formula: Athletic performance refers to the ability of an athlete to complete a task. In the racing community, performance is often assessed in terms of speed. There are three major factors that can limit an athlete's speed: physiological fatigue, psychogenic stress, and pain. The key to improving performance is to reinforce and tonify *Qi*, thus eliminating physiological fatigue. The King herbs in this formula are *Huang Qi* (Astragalus) and *Dang Shen* (Codonopsis), which work synergistically to tonify *Qi* for the treatment of the root problem of poor performance. *Qi* Deficiency tends to lead to Blood Deficiency. Therefore, the Minister herbs include *Bai Shao* (Paeonia), *Dang Gui* (Angelica), and *He Shou Wu* (Polygonum), which synergistically work to tonify Blood and the Liver (the storage of Blood), and *Feng Hua Fen* (Apis) to tonify *Qi*. The athletic psychogenic stress and pain are caused by *Qi*-Blood Stagnation. Therefore, *Mu Dan Pi* (Moutan) and *Shan Zha* (Crataegus) work as the Adjuvant herbs to move Stagnation in order to relieve pain. *Gan Cao* (Glycyrrhiza), a harmonizer, is the Messenger herb.

Cautions and Contraindications: This formula is not used in patients with *Yin* Deficiency.

Dr. Xie's Comments: I have used this herbal formula for general poor performance, muscle atrophy, or loss of body weight in horses. The formula may also be used in small animal patients for *Qi* tonification and peripheral neuropathy.

FORMULAS TO TONIFY *YIN*

The herbal formulas in this section are used for the treatment of *Yin* Deficiency Pattern. Common signs of *Yin* Deficiency are cool-seeking behavior, panting, hot ears/nose, restlessness or hyperactivity, irritability, low fever, red and dry tongue, thin and fast pulse. The King ingredients of these formulas include *Sheng Di Huang* (Rehmannia), *Mai Men Dong* (Ophiopogon), *Bai He* (Lily), and *Shan Zhu Yu* (Cornus). *Yin* Deficiency often leads to generation of false Heat or Fire in the Interior. Therefore, the herbal formulas to tonify *Yin* are often added with the herbs to clear Heat such as *Zhi Mu* (Anemarrhena) and *Huang Bai* (Phellodendron).

Liu Wei Di Huang Wan (Rehmannia 6)
六味地黄丸

Liu Wei refers to six ingredients of this formula. *Di Huang* refers to *Shu Di Huang*, or Rehmannia, which is the King herb in this formula.

Source: *Xiao Er Yao Zheng Zhi Jue* (*Craft of Medicinal Treatment for Childhood Disease Patterns*), written by *Qian Yi* and published in 1119

Ingredients: The original formula is composed of 24g *Shu Di Huang* (Rehmannia), 12g Shan *Zhu Yu* (Cornus), 12g *Shan Yao* (Dioscorea), 9g *Ze Xie* (Alisma), 9g *Mu Dan Pi* (Moutan), and 9g *Fu Ling* (Poria) (Table 18.20).

Preparation:
1. Powder or capsule method: Herbs are ground into a fine powder. Powder can be encapsulated.
2. Decoction or teapill method: Raw herbs are mixed together and decocted. Herbal water extract (decoction) can be concentrated as granules or teapills.

Table 18.20. Ingredients and actions of *Liu Wei Di Huang Wan*.

%	English Name	Chinese *Pin-Yin*	Action
32	Rehmannia	*Shu Di Huang*	Tonify Kidney *Jing*, nourish *Yin* and Blood
16	Cornus	*Shan Zhu Yu*	Tonify the Liver and Kidney *Yin*, tonify Blood
16	Dioscorea	*Shan Yao*	Tonify Spleen *Qi*
12	Alisma	*Ze Xie*	Eliminate water retention and purge false Fire
12	Moutan	*Mu Dan Pi*	Dissipate the Blood Stagnation
12	Poria	*Fu Ling*	Strengthen the Spleen, induce diuresis, excrete Dampness

Actions: Nourish *Yin* and tonify Kidney

Indications: Deficiency of Kidney *Yin*, which is characterized by soreness and weakness of the back and stifles, premature ejaculation, diabetes, osteomyelitis, low-grade fever, *lin* syndrome, red and dry tongue with little coating, thready and rapid pulse

Dosage and Usage:
Horses and Cattle: 15–60g, twice daily
Camels: 30–75g, twice daily
Llamas, Alpacas, Pigs, Goats, and Sheep: 5–15g, twice daily
Dogs: 0.5–5g (or 0.1g per kg body weight), twice daily
Cats and Rabbits: 0.2–0.5g (or 0.1g per kg body weight), twice daily
Birds: 0.1–0.2g per kg body weight, twice daily
Use 4–16 weeks until primary clinical signs resolve.

Analysis of Formula: *Liu Wei Di Huang Wan* is one of the most important basic herbal tonics for Kidney *Yin* Deficiency Pattern. *Shu Di Huang* (Rehmannia) in a larger dosage is the King herb to tonify Kidney Essence (*Jing*) and *Yin*. *Shan Zhu Yu* (Cornus) and *Shan Yao* (Dioscorea) act as the Minister herbs. *Shan Zhu Yu* nourishes the Liver and Kidney *Yin* and retains Kidney Essence, and *Shan Yao* reinforces the Spleen and Kidney and consolidates Kidney Essence. *Ze Xie* (Alisma), *Mu Dan Pi* (Moutan), and *Fu Ling* (Poria) play the roles of being the Adjuvant herbs. *Ze Xie* can promote diuresis to eliminate Dampness and prevent *Shu Di Huang* from generating Dampness. *Mu Dan Pi* possesses the functions of clearing Heat from the Liver and inhibiting the warm property of *Shan Zhu Yu*. *Fu Ling* eliminates Dampness from the Spleen and helps *Shan Yao* promote transportation and transformation of the Spleen. The combination of all ingredients results in "three tonic effects and three sedative effects" to ensure the tonification of Kidney and Liver *Yin* without any Stagnation. Thus, this herbal formula is safe to be used long term.

Cautions and Contraindications: This formula is used with caution with Spleen *Qi* or *Yang* Deficiency.

Dr. Xie's Comments: I have often used *Liu Wei Di Huang Wan* for maintenance in *Yin* Deficiency Patterns of chronic renal failure, skin diseases, and hyperadrenocorticism.

Clinical and Pharmacological Studies: Zi reported that 12 cases of constipation due to *Yin* Deficiency in dairy cows were cured by *Liu Wei Di Huang Wan*.[71] Another clinical study indicated that a positive outcome was seen in treatment of diabetes insipidus in horses using *Liu Wei Di Huang Wan*.[72]

Zhi Bai Di Huang Wan (Anemarrhena, Phellodendron, and Rehmannia) 知柏地黄丸

Zhi refers to *Zhi Mu* or Anemarrhena. *Bai* is *Huang Bai* or Phellodendron. *Di Huang* refers to all ingredients of *Liu Wei Di Huang Wan*. *Wan* is teapill. Thus, *Zhi Bai Di Huang Wan* is *Liu Wei Di Huang Wan*, adding *Zhi Mu* and *Huang Bai*.

Source: *Yi Fang Kao* (*Investigations of Medical Formulas*), written by *Wu Kun* and published in 1584

Ingredients: The original formula is composed of *Liu Wei Di Huang Wan* (24 g *Shu Di Huang*, 12 g *Shan Zhu Yu*, 12 g *Shan Yao*, 9 g *Ze Xie*, 9 g *Mu Dan Pi*, and 9 g *Fu Ling*), adding 12 g *Zhi Mu* and 12 g *Huang Bai*.

Preparation:

1. Powder or capsule method: Herbs are ground into a fine powder. Powder can be encapsulated.
2. Decoction or teapill method: Raw herbs are mixed together and decocted. Herbal water extract (decoction) can be concentrated as granules or teapills.

Actions: Tonify *Yin* and clear False Heat

Indications: False Heat with *Yin* Deficiency characterized by heat intolerance, panting, cool-seeking behavior, low-grade fever, red skin, red and dry tongue, and fast pulse. It is applicable to the treatment of chronic renal failure, chronic dermatological issues, hypertension, diabetes, hyperthyroidism, and other chronic diseases, which pertain to Kidney *Yin* Deficiency with Heat. *Liu Wei Di Huang* is the basic Kidney *Yin* tonic. *Zhi Mu* (Anemarrhena) and *Huang Bai* (Phellodendron) synergistically work together to enhance the actions of tonifying *Yin* and clearing Heat.

Dosage and Usage:

Horses and Cattle: 15–60 g, twice daily
Camels: 30–75 g, twice daily
Llamas, Alpacas, Pigs, Goats, and Sheep: 5–15 g, twice daily
Dogs: 0.5–5 g (or 0.1 g per kg body weight), twice daily
Cats and Rabbits: 0.2–0.5 g (or 0.1 g per kg body weight), twice daily
Birds: 0.1–0.2 g per kg body weight, twice daily

Use 4–12 weeks until primary clinical signs resolve.

Analysis of Formula: *Liu Wei Di Huang* is the basic *Yin* Tonic. *Zhi Mu* (Anemarrhena) clears Heat. *Huang Bai* (Phellodendron) clears Damp-Heat. *Zhi Mu* and *Huang Bai* synergistically tonify *Yin* and clear false Heat due to *Yin* Deficiency. *Zhi Bai Di Huang Wan* is designed for false Heat (or false Fire) due to *Yin* Deficiency.

Cautions and Contraindications: This formula is cautioned with Spleen *Qi* or *Yang* Deficiency.

Dr. Xie's Comments: I have often used *Zhi Bai Di Huang Wan* for the treatment of chronic skin lesions and endocrine disorders presenting with false Heat due to *Yin* Deficiency. It is often used for balancing the excessive Heat in the Fire constitution animals.

Qi Ju Di Huang Wan (Lycium, Chrysanthemum and Rehmannia) 杞菊地黄丸

Qi refers to *Gou Qi Zi* or Lycium. *Ju* is *Ju Hua* or Chrysanthemum. *Di Huang* refers to all ingredients of *Liu Wei Di Huang Wan*. *Wan* is teapill. Thus, *Qi Ju Di Huang Wan* is *Liu Wei Di Huang Wan*, adding *Gou Qi Zi* and *Ju Hua*.

Source: *Yi Zong Jin Jian* (*Golden Mirror of the Medical Tradition*), written by *Wu Qian* et al. and published in 1742

Ingredients: The original formula is composed of *Liu Wei Di Huang Wan* (24 g *Shu Di Huang*, 12 g *Shan Zhu Yu*, 12 g *Shan Yao*, 9 g *Ze Xie*, 9 g *Mu Dan Pi*, and 9 g *Fu Ling*), adding 9 g *Gou Qi Zi* (Lycium) and 6 g *Ju Hua* (Chrysanthemum).

Preparation:

1. Powder or capsule method: Herbs are ground into a fine powder. Powder can be encapsulated.
2. Decoction or teapill method: Raw herbs are mixed together and decocted. Herbal water extract (decoction) can be concentrated as granules or teapills.

Actions: Nourish Liver and Kidney *Yin*, brighten eyes

Indications: Eye problems due to Liver Heat with *Yin* Deficiency, which are characterized by photophobia, dry, painful and red eyes, wiry pulse and red tongue. This herbal formula can be used for the treatment of Keratoconjunctivitis Sicca (KCS), chronic conjunctivitis, hypertension.

Dosage and Usage:

Horses and Cattle: 15–60 g, twice daily
Camels: 30–75 g, twice daily
Llamas, Alpacas, Pigs, Goats, and Sheep: 5–15 g, twice daily
Dogs: 0.5–5 g (or 0.1 g per kg body weight), twice daily
Cats and Rabbits: 0.2–0.5 g (or 0.1 g per kg body weight), twice daily
Birds: 0.1–0.2 g per kg body weight, twice daily

Use 4–10 weeks until primary clinical signs resolve.

Analysis of Formula: *Liu Wei Di Huang* is the basic *Yin* Tonic. *Gou Qi Zi* (Lycium) nourishes Liver *Yin* and Blood and brightens the eyes. *Ju Hua* (Chrysanthemum) clears Liver Heat and brightens eyes. *Qi Ju Di Huang Wan* is designed for any chronic eye problems due to Liver Heat with *Yin* Deficiency.

Cautions and Contraindications: This formula is used with caution in patients with Spleen *Qi* or *Yang* Deficiency.

Dr. Xie's Comments: I have often used *Qi Ju Di Huang Wan* for the treatment of chronic uveitis and Keratoconjunctivitis Sicca (KCS) with Liver Heat and *Yin* Deficiency.

Mai Wei Di Huang Wan (Rehmannia 8) 麦味地黄丸

Mai refers to *Mai Men Dong* or Ophiopogon. *Wei* is *Wu Wei Zi* or Schisandra. *Di Huang* refers to all ingredients of *Liu Wei Di Huang Wan*. *Wan* is teapill. Thus, *Mai Wei Di Huang Wan* is *Liu Wei Di Huang Wan* with the addition of *Mai Men Dong* and *Wu Wei Zi*. This herbal formula is also called *Ba Wei Di Huang*. *Ba* means eight and *Wei* refers to ingredients.

Source: *Ti Ren Hui Bian* (*Compilation of Material of Benevolence for the Body*), written by *Peng Yong-Guang* and published in 1549

Ingredients: The original formula is composed of *Liu Wei Di Huang Wan* (24 g *Shu Di Huang*, 12 g *Shan Zhu Yu*, 12 g *Shan Yao*, 9 g *Ze Xie*, 9 g *Mu Dan Pi*, and 9 g *Fu Ling*), adding 9 g *Mai Men Dong* (Ophiopogon) and 9 g *Wu Wei Zi* (Schisandra).

Preparation:
1. Powder or capsule method: Herbs are ground into a fine powder. Powder can be encapsulated.
2. Decoction or teapill method: Raw herbs are mixed together and decocted. Herbal water extract (decoction) can be concentrated as granules or teapills.

Actions: Nourish and tonify Kidney and Lung *Yin*

Indications: Chronic dry cough or dyspnea due to Lung *Yin* Deficiency

Dosage and Usage:
Horses and Cattle: 15–60 g, twice daily
Camels: 30–75 g, twice daily
Llamas, Alpacas, Pigs, Goats, and Sheep: 5–15 g, twice daily
Dogs: 0.5–5 g (or 0.1 g per kg body weight), twice daily
Cats and Rabbits: 0.2–0.5 g (or 0.1 g per kg body weight), twice daily
Birds: 0.1–0.2 g per kg body weight, twice daily
Use 3–10 weeks until primary clinical signs resolve.

Analysis of Formula: *Liu Wei Di Huang Wan* is the basic *Yin* Tonic. *Mai Men Dong* (Ophiopogon) nourishes Lung *Yin* and moistens the dryness. *Wu Wei Zi* (Schisandra) clears Heat and nourishes *Yin*. *Mai Wei Di Huang Wan* is designed for chronic dry cough, dyspnea or asthma due to Lung *Yin* Deficiency.

Cautions and Contraindications: This formula is used with caution in patients with Spleen *Qi* or *Yang* Deficiency.

Dr. Xie's Comments: I have often used *Mai Wei Di Huang Wan* for the treatment of dry cough with Lung *Yin* Deficiency.

Du Qi Wan (Capital *Qi*) 都气丸

Du refers to capital. *Du Qi* refers to the Capital *Qi* (or Source *Qi*), which originates from the Kidney to grasp the Lung *Qi* to maintain its normal inhaling and exhaling functions. *Wan* refers to pill, the form of herbal administration. This formula is *Liu Wei Di Huang Wan* with the addition of *Wu Wei Zi* (Schisandra) for improving inhalation by tonifying the Kidney *Qi*.

Source: *Zheng Yin Mai Zhi* (Pattern, Cause, Pulse, and Treatment), written by *Qin Jing-Ming* and published in 1702

Ingredients: The original formula is composed of *Liu Wei Di Huang Wan* (24 g Shu Di Huang, 12 g *Shan Zhu Yu*, 12 g *Shan Yao*, 9 g *Ze Xie*, 9 g *Mu Dan Pi*, and 9 g *Fu Ling*) adding 9 g *Wu Wei Zi* (Schisandra).

Preparation:
1. Powder or capsule method: Herbs are ground into a fine powder. Powder can be encapsulated.
2. Decoction or teapill method: Raw herbs are mixed together and decocted. Herbal water extract (decoction) can be concentrated as granules or teapills.

Actions: Nourish Kidney *Yin* to grasp *Qi*

Indications: Kidney *Yin* Deficiency when the Kidney is so deficient it fails to grasp the Lung *Qi* leading to chronic wheezing or asthma, cough, and dyspnea. Thus, *Wu Wei Zi* (Schisandra) is added to astringently consolidate both the Lung and Kidney to strengthen respiration and relieve wheezing or asthma.

Dosage and Usage:
Horses and Cattle: 15–60 g, twice daily
Camels: 30–75 g, twice daily
Llamas, Alpacas, Pigs, Goats, and Sheep: 5–15 g, twice daily
Dogs: 0.5–5 g (or 0.1 g per kg body weight), twice daily
Cats and Rabbits: 0.2–0.5 g (or 0.1 g per kg body weight), twice daily
Birds: 0.1–0.2 g per kg body weight, twice daily
Use 3–10 weeks until primary clinical signs resolve.

Analysis of Formula: *Du Qi Wan* is composed of *Liu Wei Di Huang Wan* and *Wu Wei Zi* (Schisandra). *Liu Wei Di Huang Wan* is used for nourishing and reinforcing *Yin*. *Wu Wei Zi* astringently consolidates both the Lung and Kidney to ensure normal respiration and relieve dyspnea, wheezing, or asthma.

Cautions and Contraindications: This formula is used with caution in patients with Spleen *Qi* or *Yang* Deficiency.

Dr. Xie's Comments: I have often used *Du Qi Wan* for the treatment of chronic asthma, dyspnea, and heaves with Lung/Kidney *Yin* Deficiency.

Zuo Gui Wan (Restoring the Left) 左归丸

Zuo means left. *Gui* refers to return, or restore. *Wan* is teapill. The Kidney is divided into Kidney *Yin* and Kidney *Yang*. According to the TCVM pulse theory, Kidney *Yin* is associated with the left side of the pulse and the Kidney *Yang* is related to the right side of the pulse. Thus, *Zuo Gui Wan* basically refers to Restoring Kidney *Yin*.

Source: *Jing Yue Quan Shu* (*Collected Treatises of Zhang Jing-yue*), written by *Zhang Jiebing* and published in 1624

Ingredients: The original formula (Table 18.21) is composed of 240g *Shu Di Huang* (Rehmannia), 120g *Shan Yao* (Dioscorea), 120g *Gou Qi Zi* (Lycium), 120g *Shan Zhu Yu* (Cornus), 90g *Chuan Niu Xi* (Cyathula), 120g *Tu Si Zi* (Cuscuta), 120g *Lu Jiao Jiao* (Cervus), and 120g *Gui Ban Jiao* (Testudinus).

Table 18.21. Ingredients and actions of *Zuo Gui Wan*.

%	English Name	Chinese *Pin-Yin*	Action
22.9	Rehmannia (Prepared)	*Shu Di Huang*	Enrich Blood and nourish *Yin*, tonify *Jing*
11.4	Dioscorea (baked)	*Shan Yao*	Tonify Spleen *Qi* and secure Kidney *Jing*
11.4	Lycium	*Gou Qi Zi*	Nourish Liver *Yin* and Blood
11.4	Cornus	*Shan Zhu Yu*	Tonify Liver and Kidney *Yin*
8.7	Cyathula	*Chuan Niu Xi*	Strengthen the bones and joints, relieve pain
11.4	Cuscuta	*Tu Si Zi*	Tonify Liver and Kidney *Yin*, strengthen Kidney *Yang*
11.4	Cervus	*Lu Jiao Jiao*	Nourish the Kidney and Blood
11.4	Testudinis	*Gui Ban Jiao*	Tonify the Kidney *Jing* to strengthen the bones, nourish Blood to nurture the Heart

Preparation:
1. Powder or capsule method: Herbs are ground into a fine powder. Powder can be encapsulated.
2. Decoction or teapill method: Raw herbs are mixed together and decocted. Herbal water extract (decoction) can be concentrated as granules or teapills.

Actions: Nourish *Yin* and reinforce the Kidney, replenish the Essence to benefit the Marrow

Indications: *Yin* Deficiency with soreness or weakness at the back and knees, premature ejaculation, dry and red tongue with little coating

Dosage and Usage:
Horses and Cattle: 15–60g, twice daily
Camels: 30–75g, twice daily
Llamas, Alpacas, Pigs, Goats, and Sheep: 5–15g, twice daily
Dogs: 0.5–5g (or 0.1g per kg body weight), twice daily
Cats and Rabbits: 0.2–0.5g (or 0.1g per kg body weight), twice daily
Birds: 0.1–0.2g per kg body weight, twice daily
Use 3–12 weeks until primary clinical signs resolve.

Analysis of Formula: Kidney *Yin* Deficiency, along with consumption of *Jing* (Essence) and marrow, should be treated by nourishing Kidney *Yin* to replenish Essence and supplement marrow. In this formula, *Shu Di Huang* (Rehmannia) is the King herb, which replenishes Kidney Essence. Acting as the Minister herbs, *Shan Zhu Yu* (Cornus) and *Gou Qi Zi* (Lycium) tonify the Liver and Kidney *Yin*, preserve the Essence, and improve eyesight. *Lu Jiao Jiao* (Cervus) and *Gui Ban Jiao* (Testudinus) are the key herbs for replenishing Essence and marrow. Additionally, *Lu Jiao Jiao* can also tonify the Kidney *Yang*, which, used in conjunction with herbs for nourishing *Yin*, enhances such an effect: This is known as "treating *Yin* within *Yang*." *Shan Yao* (Dioscorea) strengthens the Spleen and consolidates Kidney Essence. *Tu Si Zi* (Cuscuta) tonifies the Kidney and Liver *Yin* and improves eyesight, and *Chuan Niu Xi* (Cyathula) tonifies the Liver and Kidney and strengthens the back and knees. The five ingredients above assume the role of Adjuvant herbs. All ingredients together greatly reinforce genuine *Yin* and Kidney Essence without any purgative effect.

Cautions and Contraindications: This formula should not be used with Spleen Deficiency, *Qi* Stagnation, and Damp-Heat because the ingredients are likely to generate Dampness.

Dr. Xie's Comments: I have often used *Zuo Gui Wan* for *Yin* Deficiency Pattern with some degree of *Yang* Deficiency (panting, cool-seeking, warm ears and body, but pale purple tongue and deep and weak pulse) in geriatric conditions, including chronic renal failure, endocrine disorders, and *Wei* syndrome.

Clinical and Pharmacological Studies: *Zuo Gui Wan* was reported to be used for the treatment of more than 50 diseases according to the published academic journals of Chinese and Western medicine in the last 10 years. In spite of the complexity and diversity of the clinical disorders that *Zuo Gui Wan* is applicable to, they are all closely related to the diminution or disturbance of neuro-endocrine-immunological network function. The main complaints are Deficiency (*Xu*) of the body and depletion of the Essence. Experimental research initially showed that *Zuo Gui Wan* might integrate and adjust actions of these systems.[73]

Da Bu Yin Wan (Greatly Replenishing *Yin*) 大补阴丸

Da means great or big. *Bu* refers to tonify or replenish. *Wan* is pill, the form of original herbal administration. Thus, *Da Bu Yin Wan* was named after its function of greatly replenishing the *Yin*.

Source: *Dan Xi Xin Fa* (*Teachings of Dan-Xi*), written by *Zhu Dan-Xi* and published in 1481

Ingredients: The original formula (Table 18.22) is composed of 180g *Shu Di Huang* (Rehmannia Prepared), 180g *Gui Ban Jiao* (Testudinus Prepared), 120g *Huang Bai* (Phellodendron parched), and 120g *Zhi Mu* (Anemarrhena parched).

Preparation:
1. Originally and traditionally, all above ingredients are ground into fine powder and mixed with porcine spinal cord and honey to make paste and pill.
2. Powder or capsule method: Herbs are ground into a fine powder. Powder can be encapsulated.
3. Decoction or teapill method: Raw herbs are mixed together and decocted. Herbal water extract (decoction) can be concentrated as granules or teapills.

Table 18.22. Ingredients and actions of *Da Bu Yin Wan*.

%	English Name	Chinese *Pin-Yin*	Action
30	Rehmannia Prepared	*Shu Di Huang*	Nourish Blood and *Yin*
30	Testudinis Prepared	*Gui Ban Jiao*	Nourish *Yin* to suppress excess Liver *Yang*, reinforce the Kidney to strengthen the bones
20	Phellodendron Parched	*Huang Bai*	Nourish *Yin* and clear Kidney false fire
20	Anemarrhena Parched	*Zhi Mu*	Moisten dryness through nourishing *Yin*

Actions: Nourish *Yin* and clear Fire

Indications: Severe false Fire due to *Yin* Deficiency accompanied by what is described in humans as a steaming sensation in bones, hectic fever, cough, hemoptysis, feverish and sore knees and feet, red tongue with little coating, rapid and forceful pulse

Dosage and Usage:
Horses and Cattle: 15–60g, twice daily
Camels: 30–75g, twice daily
Llamas, Alpacas, Pigs, Goats, and Sheep: 5–15g, twice daily
Dogs: 0.5–5g (or 0.1g per kg body weight), twice daily
Cats and Rabbits: 0.2–0.5g (or 0.1g per kg body weight), twice daily
Birds: 0.1–0.2g per kg body weight, twice daily
Use 3–12 weeks until primary clinical signs resolve.

Analysis of Formula: This formula nourishes *Yin* and clears Heat. It is used when Liver and Kidney *Yin* Deficiency cause upward flaring of false Heat. *Shu Di Huang* (Rehmannia) and *Gui Ban Jiao* (Testudinus) are the King herbs; both nourish *Yin* to suppress flaring up of false Heat (floating *Yang*). *Huang Bai* (Phellodendron) and *Zhi Mu* (Anemarrhena) are cold in nature and bitter in flavor, and are used as Minister herbs to purge the Heat and preserve *Yin*. Porcine spinal cord and honey are sweet and moist in nature and are employed as Adjuvant herbs, which can help the King herb to replenish Essence and inhibit the bitter and dry nature of *Huang Bai*.

Cautions and Contraindications: This formula should not be used too frequently or for a prolonged period of time due to its likelihood of promoting Damp.

Dr. Xie's Comments: I have often used *Da Bu Yin Wan* for severe *Yin* Deficiency Patterns with false Fire (Heat) (red and dry tongue, a fast and strong pulse, panting, cool-seeking behavior, warm ears and body) and in geriatric conditions including hyperthyroidism, hyperadrenocorticism, and *Wei* syndrome. *Da Bu Yin Wan* can be used when *Zhi Bai Di Huang Wan* is not strong enough to treat false Heat due to *Yin* Deficiency. Both herbal formulas may be used interchangeably in the clinical setting.

Clinical and Pharmacological Studies: A lab animal study indicated *Da Bu Yin Wan* could regulate the proliferation of T- and B-Lymphocytes in autoimmunodeficient mice induced by Campylobacter jejuni.[74]

Bai He Gu Jin Tang (Lily Strengthening the Lung) 百合固金汤

Bai He is Lily bulb, the King herb of this formula. *Gu* means consolidate or strengthen. *Jin* is the Metal (of the Five Elements) which refers to the Lung. *Tang* is decoction, the form of herbal administration. *Bai He Gu Jin* is translated as Lily Strengthening the Lung.

Source: *Yi Fang Ji Jie* (*Collected Analysis of Medical Formula*), written by *Wang Ang* and published in 1682

Ingredients: The original formula (Table 18.23) is composed of 12 g *Bai He* (Lily), 9 g *Sheng Di Huang* (Rehmannia), 9 g *Shu Di Huang* (Rehmannia), 9 g *Dang Gui* (Angelica), 6 g *Bai Shao* (Paeonia), 3 g *Gan Cao* (Glycyrrhiza), 6 g *Jie Geng* (Platycodon), 3 g *Xuan Shen* (Scrophularia), 6 g *Chuan Bei Mu* (Fritillaria), and 10 g *Mai Men Dong* (Ophiopogon).

Preparation:

1. Powder or capsule method: Herbs are ground into a fine powder. Powder can be encapsulated.
2. Decoction or teapill method: Raw herbs are mixed together and decocted. Herbal water extract (decoction) can be concentrated as granules or teapills.

Table 18.23. Ingredients and actions of *Bai He Gu Jin Tang*.

%	English name	Chinese *Pin-Yin*	Action
16.7	Lily	*Bai He*	Nourish *Yin* to moisten the Lung
12.5	Rehmannia Fresh	*Sheng Di Huang*	Clear Heat, cool Blood and nourish *Yin*
12.5	Rehmannia Prepared	*Shu Di Huang*	Nourish Blood and *Yin*
12.5	Angelica	*Dang Gui*	Nourish Blood and activate Blood circulation
8.3	Paeonia	*Bai Shao*	Nourish Blood, soothe the Liver and relieve pain
4.2	Glycyrrhiza	*Gan Cao*	Harmonize the effect of other herbs
8.3	Platycodon	*Jie Geng*	Open the Lung *Qi* to relieve cough, dissolve Phlegm and transporter to the Upper Burner
4.2	Scrophularia	*Xuan Shen*	Nourish *Yin* to clear Kidney false Fire
8.3	Fritillaria	*Chuan Bei Mu*	Nourish the Lung, transform Phlegm to stop cough
12.5	Ophiopogon	*Mai Men Dong*	Nourish *Yin*, clear Heat and promote production of Body Fluids to relieve thirst

Actions: Tonify the Lung and Kidney *Yin*, transform Phlegm and stop cough

Indications: Lung and Kidney *Yin* Deficiency with cough, dyspnea, hemoptysis, pharyngitis, laryngitis, fever, red and dry tongue with little coating, thready and rapid pulse

Dosage and Usage:

Horses and Cattle: 15–60 g, twice daily
Camels: 30–75 g, twice daily
Llamas, Alpacas, Pigs, Goats, and Sheep: 5–15 g, twice daily
Dogs: 0.5–5 g (or 0.1 g per kg body weight), twice daily
Cats and Rabbits: 0.2–0.5 g (or 0.1 g per kg body weight), twice daily
Birds: 0.1–0.2 g per kg body weight, twice daily

Use 3–10 weeks until primary clinical signs resolve.

Analysis of Formula: *Bai He Gu Jin Tang* is originally designed to be used for Lung and Kidney *Yin* Deficiency. Kidney and Lung *Yin* Deficiency causes Fire flaring up, which impairs the Lung collaterals, resulting in a failure of the Lung *Qi* to disperse and descend, and thus leads to dry cough and dyspnea. The key treatment for such conditions is to tonify the Lung and Kidney *Yin* to stop cough and transform Phlegm. The following three are the King herbs of the formula: *Bai He* (Lily) nourishes the Lung *Yin* and promotes the production of body fluid to relieve cough, and *Sheng Di Huang* (Rehmannia Fresh) and *Shu Di Huang* (Rehmannia, Prepared) nourish Kidney *Yin* and clear the Heat from the Blood. Both *Mai Men Dong* (Ophiopogon) and *Xuan Shen* (Scrophularia) act as Minister herbs. *Mai Men Dong* assists *Bai He* in nourishing the Lung *Yin* and clearing the Heat. *Xuan Shen* assists *Sheng Di Huang* and *Shu Di Huang* in nourishing Kidney *Yin* and cooling Blood. Functioning as Adjuvant herbs, *Dang Gui* (Angelica) and *Bai Shao* (Paeonia) nourish the Blood. *Chuan Bei Mu* (Fritillaria) moistens the Lung and transforms Phlegm, and *Jie Geng* (Platycodon) improves the condition of the throat and guides other herbs upward. *Gan Cao* (Glycyrrhiza) purges Fire, harmonizes the properties of other herbs, and serves as a Messenger herb.

Cautions and Contraindications: This formula is contraindicated if there are signs of Phlegm-Damp with wet cough and a greasy tongue with white coating.

Dr. Xie's Comments: I have used *Bai He Gu Jin Tang* for chronic dry cough due to Lung and Kidney *Yin* Deficiency in horses, dogs, and cats, resulting in significant clinical improvement.

Clinical and Pharmacological Studies: *Chen* reported positive outcomes using *Bai He Gu Jin Tang* for the treatment of chronic cough and chronic bronchitis in domestic animals.[75]

Fan also showed that *Bai He Gu Jin Tang* can enhance the immune system to relieve cough and resolve Phlegm, and to clear Heat.[76]

Ge Jie San (Gecko Powder) 蛤蚧散

Ge Jie (Gecko) is the King herb of this formula. *San* means powder, the original form of this herbal formula.

Source: *Yuan Heng Liao Ma Ji* (*Yuan-Heng's Therapeutic Treatise of Horses*), written by *Yu Benyuan* and *Yu Benheng* in 1608

Ingredients: The ingredients and actions of *Ge Jie San* are listed in Table 18.24.

Preparation:

1. Historically, all the above herbs are ground into fine powder and mixed with 120 g of honey to make a paste.
2. Powder or capsule

Actions: Nourish *Yin* and moisten the Lung, stop cough and asthma

Indications: Chronic cough or asthma due to Lung *Yin* Deficiency with Kidney *Qi* Deficiency, dyspnea or heaves, chronic cough or asthma, exercise intolerance, edema in the limbs, deep and weak pulse, red and dry tongue

Table 18.24. Ingredients and actions of Ge *Jie San*.

%	English	Chinese *Pin-Yin*	Action
8	Gecko	*Ge Jie*	Tonify Lung and Kidney, stop cough and asthma
7	Ophiopogon	*Mai Men Dong*	Nourish Lung *Yin*
7	Asparagus	*Tian Men Dong*	Nourish Heart *Yin*
7	Lily	*Bai He*	Moisten the Lung
7	Trichosanthes	*Gua Lou*	Promote Body Fluid and transform Phlegm
5	Eriobotrya	*Pi Pa Ye*	Open the Upper Burner and benefit Lung
7	Aristolochia	*Ma Dou Ling*	Stop asthma and cough
7	Perilla	*Zi Su Ye*	Clear Wind-Heat, stop cough
5	Fritillaria	*Chuan Bei Mu*	Eliminate Phlegm and nourish Lung *Yin*
5	Anemarrhena	*Zhi Mu*	Clear Heat, promote Body Fluid and *Yin*
5	Trichosanthes	*Tian Hua Fen*	Promote Body Fluid, clear Heat
5	Gardenia	*Zhi Zi*	Clear Heat
5	Stephania	*Bai Yao Zi*	Cool Blood, clear Heat
5	Gentiana	*Qin Jiao*	Clear Wind-Damp and nourish *Yin*
5	Cimcifuga	*Sheng Ma*	Clear Wind-Heat
5	Myrrh	*Mo Yao*	Activate Blood to stop pain
5	Stephania	*Han Fang Ji*	Eliminate Damp and Phlegm

Dosage and Usage:

Horses and Cattle: 15–60 g, twice daily
Camels: 30–75 g, twice daily
Llamas, Alpacas, Pigs, Goats, and Sheep: 5–15 g, twice daily
Dogs: 0.5–5 g (or 0.1 g per kg body weight), twice daily
Cats and Rabbits: 0.2–0.5 g (or 0.1 g per kg body weight), twice daily
Birds: 0.1–0.2 g per kg body weight, twice daily

Use 3–8 weeks until primary clinical signs resolve.

Analysis of Formula: This herbal formula is designed for chronic asthma and cough due to Lung *Yin* Deficiency with Kidney *Qi* Deficiency. *Ge Jie* (Gecko) is the King herb to tonify Kidney and Lung to stop heaves and cough. The Minister ingredients include *Mai Men Dong* (Ophiopogon), *Tian Men Dong* (Asparagus), *Bai He* (Lily), and *Gua Lou* (Trichosanthes), which nourish *Yin*, clear Heat, and Moisten the Lung to stop cough; *Pi Pa Ye* (Eriobotrya), *Ma Dou Ling* (Aristolochia), *Zi Su Ye* (Perilla), and *Chuan Bei Mu* (Fritillaria), which transform Phlegm to stop cough and descend *Qi*; and *Zhi Mu* (Anemarrhena) and *Tian Hua Fen* (Trichosanthes), which clear Heat from the Lung. The Adjuvant herbs include *Zhi Zi* (Gardenia) and *Bai Yao Zi* (Stephania) to cool Blood and remove toxins, *Qin Jiao* (Gentiana) and *Sheng Ma* (Cimcifuga) to clear false Heat, *Mo Yao* (Myrrh) to move Blood to stop pain, and *Han Fang Ji* (Stephania) to move fluids to eliminate Phlegm. *Feng Mi* (Honey) works as a Messenger herb to moisten the Lung and harmonize all herbal ingredients.

Cautions and Contraindications: This formula is contraindicated for cough due to Lung Excess Heat.

Dr. Xie's Comments: *Ge Jie San* was a very important classical formula for chronic heaves and lower airway diseases due to Lung *Yin* and Kidney *Qi* Deficiency in horses. However, some of the ingredients carry concerns, given either their reported toxicity or scarcity. For example, *Han Fang Ji* (Stephania) is believed to contain aristolochic acid, which is associated with renal toxicity and possibly urinary neoplasia. In addition, *Ge Jie* (Gecko) is an animal product and is very limited in availability. In order to avoid these problems and concerns, a new modern formula called *Hu Xi Cang* (see Formula #35) has been created.

Yi Guan Jian (One for All) 一贯煎

Yi is the number "1." *Guan* refers to all. *Jian* is decoction, an herbal form of administration. Basically *Yi Guan Jian* is named for its use in treating all the disorders

Table 18.25. Ingredients and actions of *Yi Guan Jian*.

%	English Name	Chinese *Pin-Yin*	Action
15.3	Glehnia	*Bei Sha Shen*	Nourish Lung and Stomach *Yin*
15.5	Ophiopogon	*Mai Men Dong*	Nourish *Yin*, clear Heat and promote production of Body Fluids
15.3	Angelica	*Dang Gui*	Nourish Blood and activate Blood circulation
30.5	Rehmannia	*Sheng Di Huang*	Nourish *Yin*, clear Heat, cool and nourish Blood
15.4	Lycium	*Gou Qi Zi*	Nourish Liver and Kidney, improve eyesight and moisten Lung
8.4	Melia	*Chuan Lian Zi*	Promote the flow of Liver *Qi* to relieve pain

(regurgitation, pain in the chest, hypochondria, and dry throat) resultant from Liver *Yin* Deficiency. Thus, *Yi Guan Jian* refers to one decoction for the treatment of all Liver *Yin* Deficiency conditions.

Source: *Xu Ming Yi Lei An* (*Continuation of Famous Physician's Cases Organized by Categories*), written by *Wei Zhi-Xiu* and published in 1770

Ingredients: The original formula (Table 18.25) is composed of 9 g *Bei Sha Shen* (Glehnia), 9 g *Mai Men Dong* (Ophiopogon), 9 g *Dang Gui* (Angelica), 18 g *Sheng Di Huang* (Rehmannia), 9 g *Gou Qi Zi* (Lycium), and 5 g *Chuan Lian Zi* (Melia).

Preparation:

1. Powder or capsule method: Herbs are ground into a fine powder. Powder can be encapsulated.
2. Decoction or teapill method: Raw herbs are mixed together and decocted. Herbal water extract (decoction) can be concentrated as granules or teapills.

Actions: Nourish *Yin* and soothe Liver *Qi*

Indications: Liver *Qi* Stagnation due to *Yin* Deficiency, accompanied by chest discomfort, epigastric and hypochondriac pain, acid reflux, dry throat and mouth, red and dry tongue, thready and wiry pulse

Dosage and Usage:

Horses and Cattle: 15–60 g, twice daily
Camels: 30–75 g, twice daily
Llamas, Alpacas, Pigs, Goats, and Sheep: 5–15 g, twice daily
Dogs: 0.5–5 g (or 0.1 g per kg body weight), twice daily
Cats and Rabbits: 0.2–0.5 g (or 0.1 g per kg body weight), twice daily
Birds: 0.1–0.2 g per kg body weight, twice daily

Use 3–10 weeks until primary clinical signs resolve.

Analysis of Formula: This herbal formula is designed for Liver and Kidney *Yin* Deficiency, Liver *Qi* Stagnation, and invasion of the Stomach by Stagnant Liver *Qi*. It acts by nourishing *Yin* and dispersing Liver *Qi* Stagnation. *Sheng Di Huang* (Rehmannia) is used as the King herb to nourish Y*in* and Blood so as to invigorate the Liver and Kidney. *Bei Sha Shen* (Glehnia), *Mai Men Dong* (Ophiopogon), *Dang Gui* (Angelica), and *Gou Qi Zi* (Lycium) act as the Minister herbs to reinforce the effects of the King herb. *Chuan Lian Zi* (Melia), which serves as the Adjuvant herb, is aimed at dispersing Liver *Qi* Stagnation and purging Heat, promoting the flow of *Qi* and relieving pain.

Cautions and Contraindications: This formula is contraindicated if there are signs of Spleen *Qi* Deficiency and a greasy tongue with white coating.

Dr. Xie's Comments: I typically employ *Yi Guan Jian* for the treatment of chronic hepatitis due to Liver *Yin* Deficiency.

Clinical and Pharmacological Studies: Positive results were reported when *Yi Guan Jian* was used to treat pregnancy toxemia in mules and hepatic jaundice in cows.[77] *Yi Guan Jian* also has a significant hepatoprotectant effect.[78]

Hu Qian Wan (Hidden Tiger) 虎潜丸

Hu is tiger. *Qian* refers to hidden. *Wan* is the pill, the form of the herbal administration. In Chinese culture, the hidden tiger lying on the ground becomes even stronger and more powerful as it receives the *Yin* from both heaven and earth. *Hu Qian* is named for its *Yin*-tonifying actions which enhance bone and tendon strength.

Source: *Dan Xi Xin Fa* (*Teachings of Zhu Dan-Xi*), written by *Zhu Zhen-Heng* and published in 1481

Ingredients: The original formula (Table 18.26) is composed of 150 g *Huang Bai* (Phellodendron), 120 g *Gui Ban Jiao* (Testudinus Prepared), 60 g *Zhi Mu* (Anemarrhena baked), 60 g *Shu Di Huang* (Rehmannia Prepared), 60 g *Chen Pi* (Citrus), 60 g *Bai Shao* (Paeonia), 45 g *Suo Yang* (Cynomorium), 50 g *Chuan Niu Xi* (Cyathula), and 15 g *Gan Jiang* (Zingiberis).

Preparation:

1. Powder or capsule method: Herbs are ground into a fine powder. Powder can be encapsulated.

Table 18.26. Ingredients and actions of *Hu Qian Wan.*

%	English Name	Chinese *Pin-Yin*	Action
25	Phellodendron	*Huang Bai*	Clear fire from the Kidney and resolve Damp-Heat
20	Testudinis (Prepared)	*Gui Ban Jiao*	Nourish *Yin* to soothe Liver *Yang*, tonify the Kidney, strengthen the bones, nourish Blood
5	Anemarrhena (baked)	*Zhi Mu*	Clear Lung and Stomach Heat, moisten dryness through nourishing *Yin*
10	Rehmannia (Prepared)	*Shu Di Huang*	Nourish Blood and *Yin*
10	Citrus	*Chen Pi*	Regulate Spleen *Qi*, dry up Dampness
10	Paeonia	*Bai Shao*	Nourish Blood, pacify the Liver and relieve pain
7.5	Cynomorium	*Suo Yang*	Warm *Yang* and replenish Essence
10	Cyathula	*Chuan Niu Xi**	Strengthen the Kidney and benefit the knees
2.5	Zingiberis	*Gan Jiang*	Disperse Spleen and Stomach Cold for the treatment of abdominal pain

*Tiger bone *Hu Gu* (Os tigris) was originally used in this formulation. *Chuan Niu Xi* (Cyathula) is substituted because the tiger is endangered and can no longer be used.

2. Decoction or teapill method: Raw herbs are mixed together and decocted. Herbal water extract (decoction) can be concentrated as granules or teapills.

Actions: Nourish *Yin* and purge Fire, strengthen tendons and bones

Indications: Soreness and weakness of the lumbar spine and stifles, tendonopathies, osteopenia, muscle atrophy of the limbs, altered ambulation or ataxia, red tongue with little coating, thready and weak pulse

Dosage and Usage:
Horses and Cattle: 15–60 g, twice daily
Camels: 30–75 g, twice daily
Llamas, Alpacas, Pigs, Goats, and Sheep: 5–15 g, twice daily
Dogs: 0.5–5 g (or 0.1 g per kg body weight), twice daily
Cats and Rabbits: 0.2–0.5 g (or 0.1 g per kg body weight), twice daily
Birds: 0.1–0.2 g per kg body weight, twice daily
Use 4–12 weeks until primary clinical signs resolve.

Analysis of Formula: This formula is indicated for Liver and Kidney *Yin* Deficiency, causing interior False Heat and lack of nourishment in tendons and bones. It acts by nourishing *Yin*, purging Fire, and strengthening tendons and bones. *Gui Ban* (Testudinus) nourishes Kidney *Yin* and Essence, and *Huang Bai* (Phellodendron) with its bitter and cold nature, clears the Heat and purges Fire to preserve *Yin*. *Gui Ban* and *Huang Bai* are the King herbs and have the effects of nourishing *Yin* and purging Fire. *Shu Di Huang* (Rehmannia) and *Bai Shao* (Paeonia) nourish *Yin* and Blood, *Zhi Mu* (Anemarrhena) nourishes *Yin* and clears the Heat; these three herbs function as the Minister herbs. Cyathula (*Chuan Niu Xi*) tonifies the Kidney and strengthens the tendons and bones, and *Suo Yang* (Cynomorium) warms *Yang* and replenishes Essence; *Gan Jiang* (Zingiberis) and *Chen Pi* (Citrus), by warming the Middle Burner and regulating the Stomach, can protect the stomach from the bitter and cold nature of *Huang Bai* and *Zhi Mu* and prevent *Yin* tonics from creating Dampness and causing Stagnation. The last four herbs play the role of Adjuvant herbs.

Cautions and Contraindications: This formula is contraindicated in paresis of the hind limbs due to Dampness or invasion by exogenous pathogenic factors.

Dr. Xie's Comments: I have used *Hu Qian Wan* for the treatment of hind limb paresis (*Wei* Syndrome) due to *Yin* Deficiency. This formula may also be appropriate for clinical Patterns resulting from degenerative myelopathy.

Clinical and Pharmacological Studies: Experimental research has proved that *Hu Qian Wan* enhances bone density of patients with Kidney Deficiency and regulates cortisol and sexual hormones, which helps to lend credence to the historically acknowledged relationship between Kidney Deficiency and bone density.[79]

Zheng Ye Tang (Regenerating Body Fluids) 增液汤

This formula was named after its function of regenerating Body Fluids. *Zheng* means regenerate or enrich. *Ye* refers to Body Fluids. *Tang* is decoction.

Source: *Wen Bing Tiao Bian* (*Systematic Difference of Warm Diseases*), written by *Wu Ju-tong* and published in 1798

Ingredients: The original formula (Table 18.27) is composed of 100 g *Xuan Shen* (Scrophularia), 80 g *Sheng Di Huang* (Rehmannia), and 80 g *Mai Men Dong* (Ophiopogon).

Preparation:
1. Powder or capsule method: Herbs are ground into a fine powder. Powder can be encapsulated.
2. Decoction or teapill method: Raw herbs are mixed together and decocted. Herbal water extract (decoction) can be concentrated as granules or teapills.

Table 18.27. Ingredients and actions of *Zheng Ye Tang*.

%	English Name	Chinese *Pin-Yin*	Action
40	Scrophularia	*Xuan Shen*	Nourish *Yin* to subdue Kidney Fire
30	Rehmannia	*Sheng Di Huang*	Clear the Heat, cool the Blood and nourish *Yin*
30	Ophiopogon	*Mai Men Dong*	Nourish *Yin*, clear the Heat and promote production of Body Fluids to relieve thirst

Actions: Promote production of Body Fluids, specifically to exert a laxative effect

Indications: Heat with dry stool or constipation resulting from fluid Deficiency of the Intestines in aged animals or arising from *Yin* Deficiency

Dosage and Usage:
Horses and Cattle: 15–60g, twice daily
Camels: 30–75g, twice daily
Llamas, Alpacas, Pigs, Goats, and Sheep: 5–15g, twice daily
Dogs: 0.5–5g (or 0.1g per kg body weight), twice daily
Cats and Rabbits: 0.2–0.5g (or 0.1g per kg body weight), twice daily
Birds: 0.1–0.2g per kg body weight, twice daily
Use 4–12 weeks until primary clinical signs resolve.

Analysis of Formula: This formula treats the impairment of fluids caused by Heat, by promoting production of Body Fluids. Used as the King herb, *Xuan Shen* (Scrophularia) nourishes *Yin* to produce Body Fluids and clears Heat to moisten dryness. *Sheng Di Huang* (Rehmannia) and *Mai Men Dong* (Ophiopogon) function as Minister and Adjuvant herbs to improve the effects of the King herb. All ingredients together can restore *Yin* and Body Fluids.

Cautions and Contraindications: Use with caution if there is fever and abdominal pain.

Dr. Xie's Comments: I have used *Zheng Ye Tang* for feline megacolon and in cases presenting with chronic dehydration due to global prolonged *Yin* Deficiency.

Clinical and Pharmacological Studies: *Zheng Ye Tang* was effectively used for the treatment of large animal chronic pharyngitis.[80] *Zheng Ye Tang* also has significant antibiotic and antitoxic effects, which may be the pharmacological basis of possible additional functions.[81]

Wu Shen San (Five *Shen* Powder) 五参散

Wu is the number five. *Shen* stands for the name of five ingredients ending with *shen*, which are *Ren Shen* (Ginseng), *Ku Shen* (Sophora), *Xuan Shen* (Scrophularia), *Zi Shen* (Polygonum), and *Bei Sha Shen* (Glehnia).

Table 18.28. Ingredients and actions of *Wu Shen San*.

%	English Name	Chinese *Pin-Yin*	Action
12.5	Ginseng	*Ren Shen*	Replenish the *Yuan* (Source) *Qi*, promote the production of Body Fluids, calm the Mind
12.5	Sophora	*Ku Shen*	Clear Heat, expel Dampness and kill intestinal parasite
12.5	Scrophularia	*Xuan Shen*	Nourish *Yin* to subdue Kidney Fire
12.5	Polygonum	*Zi Shen*	Clear Heat and toxin, cool Blood to resolve nodules
12.5	Glehnia	*Bei Sha Shen*	Nourish Lung and Stomach *Yin*
12.5	Gentiana	*Qin Jiao*	Dispel Wind and Dampness and clear internal Heat
12.5	Polygonum	*He Shou Wu*	Tonify Blood and Kidney *Jing*, clear toxins
12.5	Gleditsia	*Zao Jiao Ci*	Eliminate Phlegm, benefit the bowel movements

Source: *Yuan Heng Liao Ma Ji* (*Yuan-Heng's Therapeutic Treatise of Horses*), written by *Yu Benyuan* and *Yu Benheng* and published in 1608

Ingredients: The original formula (Table 18.28) is composed of 30g *Ren Shen* (Ginseng), 30g *Ku Shen* (Sophora), 30g *Xuan Shen* (Scrophularia), 30g *Zi Shen* (Polygonum) (or *Quan Shen*), 30g *Bei Sha Shen* (Glehnia), 30g *Qin Jiao* (Gentiana), 30g *He Shou Wu* (Polygonum), 30g *Zao Jiao Ci* (Gleditsia), and 100cc *Feng Mi* (Honey).

Preparation:
1. Historically, all herbs above are ground into fine powder and added to 100g of honey to make paste.
2. Powder or capsule method: Herbs are ground into a fine powder. Powder can be encapsulated.
3. Decoction or teapill method: Raw herbs are mixed together and decocted. Herbal water extract (decoction) can be concentrated as granules or teapills.

Actions: Tonify *Qi* and nourish Blood, activate Blood circulation and disperse Wind, moisten the skin

Indications: Chronic skin dryness and pruritus due to the invasion of Wind-Heat with underlying *Yin* and Blood Deficiency; clinical signs of pruritus, alopecia, pale or red tongue

Dosage and Usage:
Horses and Cattle: 15–60 g, twice daily
Camels: 30–75 g, twice daily
Llamas, Alpacas, Pigs, Goats, and Sheep: 5–15 g, twice daily
Dogs: 0.5–5 g (or 0.1 g per kg body weight), twice daily
Cats and Rabbits: 0.2–0.5 g (or 0.1 g per kg body weight), twice daily
Birds: 0.1–0.2 g per kg body weight, twice daily
Use 3–10 weeks until primary clinical signs resolve.

Analysis of Formula: This herbal formula is used for the treatment of pruritus due to Lung *Qi* Stagnation, disharmony of *Yin* and *Wei Qi* along with Blood Stagnation due to external invasion of Wind-Heat. It acts by tonifying *Qi* and nourishing Blood, activating Blood circulation and dispersing Wind, clearing pores, and moistening the skin. *Ren Shen* (Ginseng), *Ku Shen* (Sophora), *Xuan Shen* (Scrophularia), *Zi Shen* (Polygonum), and *Bai Sha Shen* (Glehnia) are the King herbs and function by invigorating *Qi*, promoting Blood circulation and clearing Heat. *He Shou Wu* (Polygonum) helps the King herbs to nourish Blood, and *Qin Jiao* (Gentiana) dispels Wind and Dampness and clears Heat; both act as Minister herbs. *Zao Jiao Ci* (Gleditsia) clears orifices and *Feng Mi* (Honey) moistens the skin; both are Adjuvant and Messenger herbs.

Cautions and Contraindications: This formula is used with caution in patients with Spleen *Qi* Deficiency.

Dr. Xie's Comments: I have used *Wu Shen San* to treat chronic pruritus and alopecia due to general Blood and/or *Yin* Deficiency with Heat.

Clinical and Pharmacological Studies: Good clinical results were found when *Wu Shen San* was used to treat equine cases of urticaria.[82]

Chen reported that *Wu Shen San* was successfully used to treat pruritus and alopecia in domestic animals.[83]

Hu Xi Cang (Breathe Easier) 呼吸畅

Hu is exhale and *Xi* means inhale. *Hu Xi* together refers to breathe. *Cang* means ease, or easier.

Source: *Chinese Veterinary Herbal Handbook* by *Huisheng Xie* and published by the Chi Institute of Chinese Medicine, 2004

Ingredients: The ingredients and actions of *Hu Xi Cang* are listed in Table 18.29.

Preparation:
1. Powder or capsule method: Herbs are ground into a fine powder. Powder can be encapsulated.
2. Decoction or teapill method: Raw herbs are mixed together and decocted. Herbal water extract (decoction) can be concentrated as granules or teapills.

Table 18.29. Ingredients and actions of *Hu Xi Cang*.

%	English Name	Chinese *Pin-Yin*	Action
10	Platycodon	*Jie Geng*	Open the Lung and transform Phlegm to stop cough
10	Lily	*Bai He*	Moisten the Lung and tonify Lung *Yin*
10	Peucedanum	*Qian Hu*	Transform Phlegm, stop asthma
10	Cinnamomum	*Rou Gui*	Warm Kidney and dispel Cold
10	Perilla	*Zi Su Zi*	Descend *Qi* to stop asthma, transform Phlegm to stop cough
10	Armeniaca	*Xing Ren*	Stop cough and asthma
10	Codonopsis	*Dang Shen*	Tonify *Qi*
10	Schisandra	*Wu Wei Zi*	Consolidate and nourish Lung *Yin*
10	Ophiopogon	*Mai Men Dong*	Nourish Lung *Yin*
10	Fritillaria	*Zhe Bei Mu*	Transform Phlegm and clear Lung Heat

Actions: Nourish Lung *Yin*, tonify Lung and Kidney *Qi*, stop asthma and cough

Indications: Dyspnea, asthma, cough due to Kidney and Lung Deficiency, deep and weak pulse, pale and swollen tongue

Dosage and Usage:
Horses and Cattle: 15–60 g, twice daily
Camels: 30–75 g, twice daily
Llamas, Alpacas, Pigs, Goats, and Sheep: 5–15 g, twice daily
Dogs: 0.5–5 g (or 0.1 g per kg body weight), twice daily
Cats and Rabbits: 0.2–0.5 g (or 0.1 g per kg body weight), twice daily
Birds: 0.1–0.2 g per kg body weight, twice daily
Use 3–10 weeks until primary clinical signs resolve.

Analysis of Formula: Chronic obstructive pulmonary disease (COPD), also known as "heaves" or recurrent airway obstruction (RAO), is a big problem in horses. COPD is believed to be induced by chronic exposure to dust, mold, and fungal elements. In TCVM, COPD is caused by invasion of Wind-Toxin with an underlying Lung *Yin* Deficiency and Kidney and Lung *Qi* Deficiency. Normal breathing requires cooperation of both the Lung and Kidney. The Lung dominates respiration from its location in the Upper Burner; it has the highest position of the Five *Zang* Organs. The Kidney has the lowest position of the Five Organs, and it functions by grasping *Qi* from the Upper Burner and bringing it to the Lower Burner. The key to treating this type of COPD is tonification of both the Lung and Kidney. Thus, *Bai He* (Lily) and *Mai Men Dong* (Ophiopogon) are used as the King herbs to nourish Lung *Yin*, moisten dryness in the Lung, and clear Heat. *Wu Wei Zi* (Schisandra), *Dang Shen* (Codonopsis), and *Rou Gui* (Cinnamomum) are Minister herbs to tonify the Lung and Kidney. *Wu Wei Zi* consolidates the Kidney and Lung and nourishes Lung *Yin*. *Dang Shen* nourishes *Qi*, and *Rou Gui* warms the Kidney and brings the Source *Qi* and Fire to the Lower Burner and Kidney. *Xing Ren* (Armeniaca), *Qian Hu* (Peucedanum), *Zi Su Ye* (Perilla), and *Zhe Bei Mu* (Fritillaria) work synergistically as the Adjuvant herbs to stop the symptomatic dyspnea, cough, or heaves. *Jie Geng* (Platycodon), the Messenger herb, opens the Lung *Qi* and brings the effect of all other herbs to the Lung and Upper Burner.

Cautions and Contraindications: Use with caution during pregnancy.

Dr. Xie's Comments: I have used *Hu Xi Cang* for the treatment of recurrent airway obstruction (RAO) and summer pasture–associated obstructive pulmonary disease (SPAOPD) in horses with clinical success.

Xiao Ke Fang (Polyuria-Polydipsia Formula) 消渴方

Xiao means wasting and polyuria (PU) and *Ke* refers to thirsting polydipsia (PD). *Xiao Ke* together refers to PU/PD syndrome or diabetes. *Fang* means an herbal formula or recipe.

Source: *Chinese Veterinary Herbal Handbook* by *Huisheng Xie* and published by the Chi Institute of Chinese Medicine, 2004

Ingredients: The ingredients and actions of *Xiao Ke Fang* are listed in Table 18.30.

Preparation:

1. Powder or capsule method: Herbs are ground into a fine powder. Powder can be encapsulated.
2. Decoction or teapill method: Raw herbs are mixed together and decocted. Herbal water extract (decoction) can be concentrated as granules or teapills.

Actions: Nourish *Yin* and resolve thirst, reinforce Kidney Essence, nourish Liver Blood

Indications: *Xiao Ke* (Diabetes) syndrome, polyuria, glucosuria due to Kidney *Yin* Deficiency, which is characterized by polydipsia, polyuria, panting, cool-seeking behavior, thready and fast pulse, red and dry tongue

Table 18.30. Ingredients and actions of *Xiao Ke Fang*.

%	English Name	Chinese *Pin-Yin*	Action
7	Trichosanthes	*Tian Hua Fen*	Promote Body Fluids, clear Heat
7	Ophiopogon	*Mai Men Dong*	Nourish *Yin*
7	Schisandra	*Wu Wei Zi*	Nourish *Yin*, astringently consolidate *Yin*
7	Angelica	*Dang Gui*	Nourish Blood
7	Ligusticum	*Chuan Xiong*	Activate Blood and resolve stagnation
7	Rehmannia Fresh	*Sheng Di Huang*	Cool Blood, clear Heat and nourish *Yin*
7	Rehmannia Prepared	*Shu Di Huang*	Nourish *Yin* and reinforce *Jing*
7	Paeonia	*Bai Shao*	Nourish Blood and soothe Liver *Qi*
5	Platycodon	*Jie Geng*	Open the Lung and transform Phlegm
5	Astragalus	*Huang Qi*	Tonify *Qi*
5	Codonopsis	*Dang Shen*	Tonify *Qi*
5	Pueraria	*Ge Gen*	Promote Body Fluids, clear Wind-Heat
5	Coptis	*Huang Lian*	Clear Heat, detoxify
5	Lycium	*Gou Qi Zi*	Nourish *Yin*
5	Chrysanthemum	*Ju Hua*	Clear Heat and Fire
5	Juncus	*Deng Xin Cao*	Clear Heat
4	Glycyrrhiza	*Gan Cao*	Harmonize

Dosage and Usage:

Horses and Cattle: 15–60 g, twice daily
Camels: 30–75 g, twice daily
Llamas, Alpacas, Pigs, Goats, and Sheep: 5–15 g, twice daily
Dogs: 0.5–5 g (or 0.1 g per kg body weight), twice daily
Cats and Rabbits: 0.2–0.5 g (or 0.1 g per kg body weight), twice daily
Birds: 0.1–0.2 g per kg body weight, twice daily

Use 4–16 weeks until primary clinical signs resolve.

Analysis of Formula: *Yin* Deficiency with Heat and Dryness is the main pathological mechanism of diabetes. In this formula, *Shu Di Huang* (Rehmannia) and *Sheng Di Huang* (Rehmannia) are the King herbs, which tonify *Yin* and replenish the Kidney Essence. Acting as the Minister herbs, *Mai Men Dong* (Ophiopogon), *Bai Shao* (Paeonia), *Dang Gui* (Angelica), *Ge Gen* (Pueraria), *Wu Wei Zi* (Schisandra), and *Gou Qi Zi* (Lycium) tonify Kidney *Yin*, moisten dryness and promote body fluids, and clear Heat. *Bai Shao* and *Dang Gui* tonify Liver Blood. Additional herbs function as the Adjuvant herbs; *Huang Qi* (Astragalus) and *Dang Shen* (Codonopsis) tonify *Qi*. *Huang Lian* (Coptis), *Deng Xin Cao* (Juncus), *Ju Hua* (Chrysanthemum), and *Jie Geng* (Platycodon) clear Heat. *Gan Cao* (Glycyrrhiza) harmonizes all other herbs and serves as the Messenger herb.

Cautions and Contraindications: Use with caution for *Qi* Deficiency.

Dr. Xie's Comments: I have used *Xiao Ke Fang* for the treatment of diabetes due to Kidney *Yin* Deficiency in dogs and cats.

FORMULAS TO TONIFY *YANG*

The herbal formulas in this section are used for the treatment of *Yang* Deficiency. Common signs of *Yang* Deficiency Pattern are cold back and extremities; warm-seeking behavior; soreness and weakness of the back and rear limbs; urinary incontinence; female infertility; premature ejaculation; pale, wet and swollen tongue; and deep and weak pulse. *Yang* Deficiency Patterns include Heart *Yang* Deficiency, Spleen *Yang* Deficiency, and Kidney *Yang* Deficiency. Because the Kidney controls the fire of "Ming-men" (the gate of life), which is the base of the whole body's *Yang* (or global *Yang*), the Kidney *Yang* is often called the true *Yang*, or Source *Yang*. All of these formulas focus on tonifying the Kidney *Yang* because various *Yang* Deficiency Patterns originate from or at least are associated with the Kidney. The herbs to tonify *Yang* are often hot and tend to cause dryness. To counter this adverse effect, *Yang* tonic formulas often include *Yin* tonic herbs such as *Shu Di Huang* (Rehmannia) and *Shan Zhu Yu* (Cornus). Kidney *Yang* Deficiency fails to control water metabolism, leading to edema or ascites. For this reason, *Fu Ling* (Poria) and *Ze Xie* (Alisma) are often used to drain Dampness in the herbal formulas to tonify *Yang*.

Bao Yuan Tang (Protecting Source *Yang*) 保元汤

Bao means protecting, or preserving. *Yuan* refers to *Yuan* (Source) *Qi* (*Yang*). *Tang* is the decoction, the form of herbal administration.

Source: *Jing Yue Quan Shu* (*Collected Treatises of Zhang Jing-Yue*), written by *Zhang Jie-Bing* and published in 1624

Ingredients: The original formula (Table 18.31) is composed of 6 g *Huang Qi* (Astragalus), 6 g *Ren Shen* (Ginseng), 1.5 g *Rou Gui* (Cinnamomum), and 3 g *Gan Cao* (Glycyrrhiza).

Table 18.31. Ingredients and actions of *Bao Yuan Tang*.

%	English Name	Chinese *Pin-Yin*	Action
36	Astragalus	*Huang Qi*	Tonify *Qi*
36	Ginseng	*Ren Shen*	Tonify *Yuan Qi* and resuscitate *Yang*
10	Cinnamomum	*Rou Gui*	Tonify *Yang*
18	Glycyrrhiza	*Gan Cao*	Harmonize

Preparation:
1. Powder or capsule method: Herbs are ground into a fine powder. Powder can be encapsulated.
2. Decoction or teapill method: Raw herbs are mixed together and decocted. Herbal water extract (decoction) can be concentrated as granules or teapills.

Actions: Tonify Heart *Qi* and *Yang*

Indications: *Qi* and *Yang* Deficiency with symptoms such as congestive heart failure, cardiomyopathy, chronic fatigue, cold ears and nose, shortness of breath, spontaneous sweating, collapse, syncope, weak or irregular pulse, pale or purple tongue

Dosage and Usage:
Horses and Cattle: 15–30 g, twice daily
Camels: 30–60 g, twice daily
Llamas, Alpacas, Pigs, Goats, and Sheep: 5–10 g, twice daily
Dogs: 0.5–5 g (or 0.1 g per kg body weight), twice daily
Cats and Rabbits: 0.2–0.5 g (or 0.1 g per kg body weight), twice daily
Birds: 0.1 g per kg body weight, twice daily
Use as needed from 4–12 weeks.

Analysis of Formula: *Yang Qi* collapse leads to fainting or syncope. The treatment strategy is to resuscitate the *Yang Qi* and to allow normal physiologic functions. Thus, the King herb in this formula is *Ren Shen* (Ginseng), which tonifies *Yuan Qi* and revives *Yang*. Used as the Minister herbs, *Huang Qi* (Astragalus) and *Rou Gui* (Cinnamomum) tonify *Qi* and warm *Yang*. *Gan Cao*, the Adjuvant and Messenger herb, tonifies *Qi* and harmonizes the effects of the other herbs.

Cautions and Contraindications: Do not use in patients with *Yin* Deficiency.

Dr. Xie's Comments: I have successfully used *Bao Yuan Tang* for congestive heart failure and syncope due to Heart *Yang* Deficiency.

Shen Qi Wan (Kidney *Qi* Pill) 肾气丸

Shen here refers to the Kidney. *Wan* is pill. This formula was named after its function of tonifying Kidney *Qi*. Since it originates from *Jin Gui Yao Lue Fang Lun* (or *Jin Gui* for short), this herbal formula is also called *Jin Gui Shen Qi Wan*. *Jin Gui* means golden cabinet or bookcase and here refers to the text *Jin Gui Yao Lue Fang Lun*.

Source: *Jin Gui Yao Lue Fang Lun* (*Synopsis of Prescription from the Golden Cabinet*), written by *Zhang Zhong-Jing* and published in 220

Ingredients: The original formula (Table 18.32) is composed of 240 g *Sheng Di Huang* (Rehmannia), 120 g *Shan*

Table 18.32. Ingredients and actions of *Shen Qi Wan.*

%	English Name	Chinese *Pin-Yin*	Action
25.9	Rehmannia Fresh	*Sheng Di Huang*	Clear heat, cool Blood and nourish *Yin*
15.6	Dioscorea	*Shan Yao*	Strengthen the Spleen and tonify *Jing*
15.6	Cornus	*Shan Zhu Yu*	Tonify Liver and Kidney *Yin*, nourish the *Jing* and Blood
11.7	Alisma	*Ze Xie*	Eliminate water retention and clear False Fire
11.7	Poria	*Fu Ling*	Strengthen the Spleen, promote diuresis, excrete Dampness
11.7	Moutan	*Mu Dan Pi*	Cool Blood, resolve Blood Stagnation, clear Heat
3.9	Cinnamomum	*Gui Zhi*	Warm the channels to dispel Cold, tonify *Yang*
3.9	Aconite	*Fu Zi*	Warm the Kidney, tonify *Yang*, relieve pain and dispel Cold

Yao (Dioscorea), 120g *Shan Zhu Yu* (Cornus), 90g *Ze Xie* (Alisma), 90g *Fu Ling* (Poria), 90g *Mu Dan Pi* (Moutan), 30g *Gui Zhi* (Cinnamomum), and 30g *Fu Zi* (Aconite).

Preparation:

1. Powder or capsule method: Herbs are ground into a fine powder. Powder can be encapsulated.
2. Decoction or teapill method: Raw herbs are mixed together and decocted. Herbal water extract (decoction) can be concentrated as granules or teapills.

Actions: Warm and tonify Kidney *Yang*

Indications: Kidney *Yang* Deficiency with hind limb paresis or pain, cold sensations in hind limbs and Kidney (lumbar) regions, dysuria or polyuria, pale and swollen tongue, deep and feeble pulse, as well as Phlegm-retention, edema, and diabetes

Dosage and Usage:

Horses and Cattle: 15–30g, twice daily
Camels: 30–60g, twice daily
Llamas, Alpacas, Pigs, Goats, and Sheep: 5–10g, twice daily
Dogs: 0.5–5g (or 0.1g per kg body weight), twice daily
Cats and Rabbits: 0.2–0.5g (or 0.1g per kg body weight), twice daily
Birds: 0.05g per kg body weight, twice daily

Use 3–8 weeks until primary clinical signs resolve.

Analysis of Formula: Kidney *Yang* Deficiency leads to internal coldness and Stagnation, which blocks *Qi* flow and urination. The key treatment strategy is to warm and tonify Kidney *Yang*. *Fu Zi* (Aconite) and *Gui Zhi* (Cinnamomum) are the King herbs with the effects of warming and tonifying Kidney *Yang*. *Yang* tonics are hot and tend to consume *Yin*. Thus, *Sheng Di Huang* (Rehmannia), *Shan Yao* (Dioscorea), and *Shan Zhu Yu* (Cornus) are Minister herbs to nourish Kidney *Yin* and harmonize the hot energy of *Fu Zi* and *Gui Zhi*. The combination of the King and Minister herbs warms and tonifies Kidney *Yang* while avoiding unnecessary damage to the Kidney *Yin*. Used as Adjuvant herbs, *Ze Xie* (Alisma), *Fu Ling* (Poria) and *Mu Dan Pi* (Moutan) can promote diuresis and Blood circulation and prevent the tonic herbs from generating Dampness. The combined application of all ingredients, which are warm but not drying and tonifying without Damp-generating, activates Kidney *Yang* and *Qi*.

Cautions and Contraindications: This formula is contraindicated for *Yin* Deficiency with dry throat and mouth, red tongue with little coating.

Dr. Xie's Comments: I have used *Shen Qi Wan* for the treatment of renal failure, infertility, hypothyroidism, and other chronic illnesses due to Kidney *Yang* Deficiency.

Clinical and Pharmacological Studies: *Fan* pointed out that *Jin Gui Shen Qi Wan* was effective for the treatment of impotence of the horse.[84]

Chen et al. reported that the effects of *Jin Gui Shen Qi Wan* included an enhanced immune recovery in rats, an increase in the action of SOD in large rats, an increased ACTH level in plasma in rats with Kidney Deficiency, and a promotion of hematopoiesis in bone marrow.[85]

You Gui Wan (Restoring the Right) 右归丸

You means right. *Gui* refers to returning, or restoring. *Wan* is teapill. The Kidney is divided into Kidney *Yin* and Kidney *Yang*. According to the TCVM pulse theory, Kidney *Yin* is associated with the left side of pulse and the Kidney *Yang* is related to the right side of the pulse. Thus, *You Gui Wan* basically refers to Restoring Kidney *Yang*.

Source: *Jing Yue Quan Shu* (*Collected Treatises of Zhang Jing Yue*), written by *Zhang Jing Yue* and published in 1624

Ingredients: The original formula (Table 18.33) is composed of 240g *Shu Di Huang* (Rehmannia), 120g *Shan Yao* (Dioscorea), 90g *Shan Zhu Yu* (Cornus), 120g *Gou Qi Zi* (Lycium), 120g *Tu Si Zi* (Cuscuta), 120g *Lu Jiao Jiao* (Cervus), 120g *Du Zhong* (Eucommia), 90g *Dang Gui* (Angelica), 60g *Rou Gui* (Cinnamomum), and 60g *Fu Zi* (prepared Aconite).

Table 18.33. Ingredients and actions of *You Gui Wan*.

%	English Name	Chinese *Pin-Yin*	Action
21.1	Rehmannia	*Shu Di Huang*	Nourish *Yin* and Blood
10.5	Dioscorea	*Shan Yao*	Tonify Spleen and Lung
7.9	Cornus	*Shan Zhu Yu*	Tonify Liver and Kidney *Yin*, nourish *Jing*
10.5	Lycium	*Gou Qi Zi*	Nourish Liver and Kidney *Yin*, improve eyesight
10.5	Cuscuta	*Tu Si Zi*	Tonify Liver and Kidney *Yin*, Strengthen Kidney *Yang*
10.5	Cervus	*Lu Jiao Jiao*	Nourish Kidney and Blood
10.5	Angelica	*Dang Gui*	Tonify Liver and Kidney *Yang*, strengthen tendons and bones
7.9	Eucommia	*Du Zhong*	Nourish Blood and activate Blood circulation
5.3	Cinnamomum	*Rou Gui*	Warm and tonify the Kidney and Spleen *Yang*, disperse Internal Cold
5.3	Prepared Aconite	*Fu Zi*	Warm and tonify *Yang*, relieve pain and dispel Cold

Preparation:

1. Powder or capsule method: Herbs are ground into a fine powder. Powder can be encapsulated.
2. Decoction or teapill method: Raw herbs are mixed together and decocted. Herbal water extract (decoction) can be concentrated as granules or teapills.

Actions: Warm and nourish Kidney *Yang*, replenish *Jing* and marrow

Indications: Kidney *Yang* Deficiency and a decline in Fire of the *Ming Men* (gate of life), as well as physical and mental fatigue from chronic illness in geriatric patients; main clinical signs of warm-seeking behavior, cold back and limbs, soreness and paresis of the back and rear limbs, or infertility due to *Yang* Deficiency, pale tongue with white coating, deep and slow pulse

Dosage and Usage:

Horses and Cattle: 15–30g, twice daily
Camels: 30–60g, twice daily
Llamas, Alpacas, Pigs, Goats, and Sheep: 5–10g, twice daily
Dogs: 0.5–5g (or 0.1g per kg body weight), twice daily
Cats and Rabbits: 0.2–0.5g (or 0.1g per kg body weight), twice daily
Birds: 0.05g per kg body weight, twice daily

Use 3–8 weeks until primary clinical signs resolve.

Analysis of Formula: *You Gui Wan* is used for Kidney *Yang* Deficiency and decline of Fire in the *Ming Men*. The key treatment strategy is to warm and tonify Kidney *Yang* and replenish Kidney Essence. *Fu Zi* (Prepared Aconite), *Rou Gui* (Cinnamomum), and *Lu Jiao Jiao* (Cervus) are the King herbs that warm and tonify Kidney *Yang*. *Shu Di Huang* (Rehmannia), *Shan Zhu Yu* (Cornus), *Gou Qi Zi* (Lycium), and *Shan Yao* (Dioscorea) act as Minister herbs, which nourish Kidney *Yin*, strengthen the Liver and Spleen, and replenish Kidney Essence. Used as Adjuvant herbs, *Tu Si Zi* (Cuscuta) and *Du Zhong* (Eucommia) tonify Kidney *Yang* and strengthen the back and rear limbs, while *Dang Gui* (Angelica) nourishes and regulates Blood. The herbs of this formula combined together have a tonic action without any purgative effect, and they activate Kidney *Yang* while nourishing Kidney *Yin*. *You Gui Wan* also replenishes Kidney *Jing* (Essence).

Cautions and Contraindications: This formula can generate Dampness and therefore should not be used in patients with edema, watery diarrhea, and ascites due to *Yang* Deficiency.

Dr. Xie's Comments: I have used *You Gui Wan* for renal failure, infertility, and hyperadrenocorticism due to Kidney *Yang* Deficiency in horses, dogs, and cats.

Clinical and Pharmacological Studies: Studies indicate that *You Gui Wan* increased the plasma concentration of testosterone in experimental rats with Kidney *Yang* Deficiency.[86]

Ba Ji San (Morinda Powder) 巴戟散

Ba Ji Tian is Morinda, the King herb of this formula. *San* refers to powder, the original form of herbal administration.

Source: *Yuan Heng Liao Ma Ji* (*Yuan-Heng's Therapeutic Treatise of Horses*), written by *Yu Benyuan* and *Yu Benheng* and published in 1608

Ingredients: The original formula (Table 18.34) is composed of 45g *Ba Ji Tian* (Morinda), 45g *Rou Cong Rong* (Cistanche), 45g *Bu Gu Zhi* (Psoralea), 45g *Hu Lu Ba* (Trigonella), 30g *Xiao Hui Xiang* (Foeniculum), 30g *Rou Dou Kou* (Myristica), 30g *Chen Pi* (Citrus), 30g *Qing Pi* (Citrus), 20g *Rou Gui* (Cinnamomum), 20g *Mu Tong* (Akebia), 20g *Chuan Lian Zi* (Melia), and 15g *Bing Lang* (Areca).

Table 18.34. Ingredients and actions of *Ba Ji San.*

%	English Name	Chinese *Pin-Yin*	Action
12	Morinda	*Ba Ji Tian*	Tonify Kidney *Yang* and strengthen the back
12	Cistanche	*Rou Cong Rong*	Tonify Kidney *Yang*, moisten the bowels
12	Psoralea	*Bu Gu Zhi*	Replenish Kidney *Qi* and strengthen tendons and bones
12	Trigonella	*Hu Lu Ba*	Replenish Kidney *Qi* and strengthen tendons and bones
8	Foeniculum	*Xiao Hui Xiang*	Dispel cold, relieve pain, regulate *Qi* flow
8	Myristica	*Rou Dou Kou*	Warm the Spleen and Stomach
8	Citrus	*Chen Pi*	Regulate Spleen *Qi*, dry up Dampness
8	Citrus	*Qing Pi*	Soothe Liver *Qi* to resolve Stagnation
5.4	Cinnamomum	*Rou Gui*	Warm Kidney and Spleen *Yang*, disperse internal Cold
5.3	Akebia	*Mu Tong*	Remove Dampness and Heat
5.3	Melia	*Chuan Lian Zi*	Promote *Qi* flow to relieve pain
4	Areca	*Bing Lang*	Promote Stomach *Qi* flow

Preparation:
1. Powder or capsule method: Herbs are ground into a fine powder. Powder can be encapsulated.
2. Decoction or teapill method: Raw herbs are mixed together and decocted. Herbal water extract (decoction) can be concentrated as granules or teapills.

Actions: Warm and tonify Kidney *Yang*

Indications: Lumbar pain and/or hind limb paresis due to Kidney *Yang* Deficiency

Dosage and Usage:
Horses and Cattle: 15–30 g, twice daily
Camels: 30–60 g, twice daily
Llamas, Alpacas, Pigs, Goats, and Sheep: 5–10 g, twice daily
Dogs: 0.5–5 g (or 0.1 g per kg body weight), twice daily
Cats and Rabbits: 0.2–0.5 g (or 0.1 g per kg body weight), twice daily
Birds: 0.05 g per kg body weight, twice daily
Use 4–12 weeks until primary clinical signs resolve.

Analysis of Formula: The key to treating Kidney *Yang* Deficiency is to warm and tonify Kidney *Yang*. *Ba Ji Tian* (Morinda) is the King herb, which warms and tonifies Kidney *Yang*. *Rou Cong Rong* (Cistanche), *Bu Gu Zhi* (Psoralea), *Hu Lu Ba* (Trigonella), *Xiao Hui Xiang* (Foeniculum), and *Rou Gui* (Cinnamomum) are the Minister herbs, which enhance *Ba Ji Tian's* ability to warm and tonify Kidney *Yang* as well as strengthen tendons and bones, relieve Cold, and ameloriate pain. *Chen Pi* (Citrus), *Qing Pi* (Citrus), *Bing Lang* (Areca), and *Chuan Lian Zi* (Melia) are Adjuvant herbs, which warm the Spleen and Stomach and activate *Qi* to relieve symptomatic stiffness and pain. *Mu Tong* (Akebia) is a Messenger herb that activates the meridians and works to drain Damp. The combination of these herbs produces the following results: warming and tonifying Kidney *Yang*, activating the meridians and relieving pain, dispelling Cold and draining Damp.

Cautions and Contraindications: This formula is contraindicated for patients with *Yin* Deficiency with fever.

Dr. Xie's Comments: *Ba Ji Tian* is especially good for the treatment of *Bi* syndrome of the back due to Kidney *Yang* Deficiency.

Clinical and Pharmacological Studies: *Li* reported that 63 out of 67 sows with postpartum paralysis of the hind limbs recovered after administration of *Ba Ji San* and acupuncture with vitamin B12 at *Shen-Shu*.[87]

Jie Gu San (Reuniting Fracture) 接骨散

Jie means continuing. *Gu* is bone. *San* means powder. *Jie Gu* together means reuniting fracture.

Source: *Jie Gu San* from *Zhong Shou Yi Xue* (*Traditional Chinese Veterinary Medicine*), written by *Yu Chuan* and published in 1979[88]

Ingredients: The ingredients and actions of *Jie Gu San* are listed in Table 18.35.

Preparation:
1. Powder or capsule method: Herbs are ground into a fine powder. Powder can be encapsulated.
2. Decoction or teapill method: Raw herbs are mixed together and decocted. Herbal water extract (decoction) can be concentrated as granules or teapills.

Actions: Tonify Kidney; tonify *Yang*, *Qi*, and Blood; promote bone healing

Indications: Prevention and treatment of fracture, degenerative joint disease (DJD), OCD, and osteopenia accompanied by Kidney *Qi*, *Yang* or *Jing* Deficiency with deep and weak pulse and pale tongue

Dosage and Usage:
Horses and Cattle: 15–30 g, twice daily
Camels: 30–60 g, twice daily

Table 18.35. Ingredients and actions of *Jie Gu San*.

%	English Name	Chinese *Pin-Yin*	Action
7.7	Dipsacus	*Xu Duan*	Tonify Kidney, promote bone healing process
7.7	Psoralea	*Bu Gu Zhi*	Tonify Kidney *Yang*
5.1	Cyathula	*Chuan Niu Xi*	Tonify Kidney *Yang*, strengthen rear limbs, direct *Qi* and Blood downward
7.7	Drynaria	*Gu Sui Bu*	Promote bone healing process, tonify Kidney *Yang*
2.6	Cervus	*Lu Jiao Jiao*	Tonify Kidney *Yang* and *Qi*
7.7	Atractylodes	*Bai Zhu*	Tonify *Qi*
7.7	Codonopsis	*Dang Shen*	Tonify *Qi*
7.7	Astragalus	*Huang Qi*	Tonify *Qi*
7.7	Angelica	*Dang Gui*	Move and nourish Blood
7.7	Rehmannia	*Shu Di Huang*	Nourish Blood
10.3	Draconis	*Long Gu*	Pacify the Mind, dissipate swelling
10.2	Ostrea	*Mu Li*	Pacify the Liver *Yang*, soften the hardness
5.1	Morus	*Sang Zhi*	Move *Qi* and smooth limb movement
5.1	Pyrite	*Zi Ran Tong*	Move Blood and strengthen bones

Llamas, Alpacas, Pigs, Goats, and Sheep: 5–10g, twice daily
Dogs: 0.5–5g (or 0.1g per kg body weight), twice daily
Cats and Rabbits: 0.2–0.5g (or 0.1g per kg body weight), twice daily
Birds: 0.05g per kg body weight, twice daily

Use 4–16 weeks until primary clinical signs resolve.

Analysis of Formula: The Kidney controls the bones and cartilage. Any bony changes and pathology are related to the Kidney. Fracture is often directly caused by traumatic injuries, leading to local *Qi*-Blood Stagnation and pain. However, when Kidney *Qi/Yang* is deficient, the bones and joints lack nourishment, leading to failure of healing of injured bones (malunion) or ongoing articular damage. Thus, the key treatment strategy for fracture and bony changes is to tonify Kidney *Qi* and *Yang* and move *Qi* and Blood to resolve Stagnation. *Xu Duan* (Dipsacus), *Bu Gu Zhi* (Psoralea), and *Gu Sui Bu* (Drynaria) are the King herbs, which tonify Kidney *Yang*, strengthen bones, and promote bone healing. Used as the Minister herbs, *Chuan Niu Xi* (Cyathula), *Lu Jiao Jiao* (Cervus), *Bai Zhu* (Atractylodes), *Dang Shen* (Condonopsis), and *Huang Qi* (Astragalus) tonify *Qi* and *Yang* to enhance the King herbs' ability to tonify Kidney. *Dang Gui* (Angelica), *Shu Di Huang* (Rehmannia), *Long Gu* (Draconis), and *Mu Li* (Ostrea) are the Adjuvant herbs. *Dang Gui* and *Shu Di Huang* work synergistically to move and nourish Blood. *Long Gu* and *Mu Li* pacify the Mind, soften the hardness and dissipate swelling. Functioning as the Messenger herbs, *Sang Zhi* (Morus) moves *Qi* and serves as the transporter to the limbs and *Zi Ran Tong* (Pyrite) moves Blood and is the transporter to the bones.

Cautions and Contraindications: Use with caution for *Yin* Deficiency.

Dr. Xie's Comments: *Jie Gu San* can be used for the treatment and prevention of fractures and OCD lesions, or postsurgical therapy to promote bone healing.

FORMULAS TO TONIFY *YIN, YANG, AND JING*

The herbal formulas in this section are used in treating Patterns of both *Yin* Deficiency and *Yang* Deficiency. Common signs of both *Yin* and *Yang* Deficiency Patterns are dizziness, soreness and weakness of the back and rear limbs, premature ejaculation, coldness at the back and extremities, afternoon fever, panting, heat and/or cold intolerance. The King ingredients of these formulas are *Shu Di Huang* (Rehmannia) and *Shan Zhu Yu* (Cornus) to tonify *Yin*, and *Fu Zi* (Aconite) and *Rou Gui* (Cinnamomum) to tonify *Yang*.

Di Huang Yin Zi (Rehmannia Decoction)
地黄饮子

Di Huang refers to Rehmannia, one of the King herbs in this formula. *Yin Zi* means decoction.

Source: *Zheng He Sheng Ji Zong Lu (Comprehensive Recording of Sage-like Benefit from the Zheng He Era)*, written by *Shen Fu* et al. and published in 1117

Ingredients: The ingredients and actions of *Di Huang Yin Zi* are listed in Table 18.36.

Preparation:
1. Powder or capsule method: Herbs are ground into a fine powder. Powder can be encapsulated.
2. Decoction or teapill method: Raw herbs are mixed together and decocted. Herbal water extract (decoction) can be concentrated as granules or teapills.

Actions: Tonify Kidney *Yin*, tonify Kidney *Yang*

Indications: Both Kidney *Yin* and Kidney *Yang* Deficiency. Severe hind limb weakness, paresis or paralysis due to intervertebral disc disease (IVDD), coldness at the back and extremities with hot ears and head, thirsty but too weak to drink or swallow water, weak voice or unable to vocalize, weak and thin pulse, red or pale tongue

Table 18.36. Ingredients and actions of *Di Huang Yin Zi.*

%	English Name	Chinese *Pin-Yin*	Action
8	Rehmannia Prepared	*Shu Di Huang*	Nourish Blood, tonify Kidney *Jing* and *Yin*
8	Cornus	*Shan Zhu Yu*	Tonify *Yin*
8	Cistanche	*Rou Cong Rong*	Tonify Kidney *Yin* and *Yang*, replenish *Jing*
8	Morinda	*Ba Ji Tian*	Tonify Kidney *Yang*
8	Aconite	*Fu Zi*	Tonify and warm *Yang*, relieve pain and dispel Cold
8	Cinnamomum	*Rou Gui*	Tonify *Yang*, warm the Spleen, disperse internal Cold
8	Dendrobium	*Shi Hu*	Nourish *Yin*, clear false Heat, generate fluids
8	Ophiopogon	*Mai Men Dong*	Nourish *Yin*
8	Acorus	*Shi Chang Pu*	Open orifices, excrete Phlegm, calm the Mind
8	Polygala	*Yuan Zhi*	Keep Heart-*Yang* and Kidney-*Yin* in balance, calm the Mind
8	Poria	*Fu Ling*	Strengthen the Spleen, promote diuresis, excrete Dampness
8	Schisandra	*Wu Wei Zi*	Astringently consolidate
2	Zingiberis	*Sheng Jiang*	Harmonize the Stomach
2	Jujube	*Da Zao*	Strengthen the Spleen and Stomach

Dosage and Usage:

Horses and Cattle: 15–30g, twice daily

Camels: 30–60g, twice daily

Llamas, Alpacas, Pigs, Goats, and Sheep: 5–10g, twice daily

Dogs: 0.5–5g (or 0.1g per kg body weight), twice daily

Cats and Rabbits: 0.2–0.5g (or 0.1g per kg body weight), twice daily

Birds: 0.05g per kg body weight, twice daily

Use 4–16 weeks until primary clinical signs resolve.

Analysis of Formula: *Di Huang Yin Zi* is designed for both Kidney *Yin* and Kidney *Yang* Deficiency leading to rear weakness and false Heat in the Upper Burner. *Shu Di Huang* (Rehmannia) and *Shan Zhu Yu* (Cornus), which tonify Kidney *Yin* and strengthen Kidney Water to control the Fire in the Heart, are the King herbs. *Rou Cong Rong* (Cistanche) and *Ba Ji Tian* (Morinda) are ministers and tonify Kidney *Yang* while strengthening the back. *Fu Zi* (Aconite) and *Rou Gui* (Cinnamomum) warm and tonify Kidney *Yang* and restore the Ming-men Fire (Source *Yang*). *Shi Hu* (Dendrobium), *Mai Men Dong* (Ophiopogon), and *Wu Wei Zi* (Schisandra) nourish *Yin* and enrich Body Fluids to clear false Heat, which simultaneously counters the drying and hot actions of *Fu Zi* and *Rou Gui*. *Shi Chang Pu* (Acorus), *Yuan Zhi* (Polygala), and *Fu Ling* (Poria) harmonize the relationship between the Fire (Heart) and the Water (Kidney). *Sheng Jiang* (Zingiberis) and *Da Zao* (Jujube) are the Messenger herbs to harmonize all other herbs.

Cautions and Contraindications: Use with caution for accumulation of Damp in the Interior.

Dr. Xie's Comments: It is commonly used for the treatment of *Qi-Yin* Deficiency paresis and paralysis due to intervertebral disc disease (IVDD) or degenerative myelopathy.

Yin Yang Huo San (Epimedium Powder) 淫羊藿散

Yin Yang Huo is Epimedium, the King herb of this formulation. *San* refers to powder, the original form of the medication.

Source: *Chinese Veterinary Herbal Handbook* by *Huisheng Xie* and published by the Chi Institute of Chinese Medicine, 2004

Ingredients: The ingredients and actions of *Yin Yang Huo San* are listed in Table 18.37.

Table 18.37. Ingredients and actions of *Yin Yang Huo San.*

%	English Name	Chinese *Pin-Yin*	Action
7	Epimedium	*Yin Yang Huo*	Tonify Kidney *Yang/Jing*, promote productive functions
7	Cuscuta	*Tu Si Zi*	Tonify Kidney *Yang*, *Jing*, and *Yin*
5	Paeonia	*Bai Shao*	Nourish Liver *Yin* and Blood
8	Polygonum	*He Shou Wu*	Nourish Blood and *Jing*, benefit hair
6	Actinolite	*Yang Qi Shi*	Tonify Kidney *Yang*
7	Cynomorium	*Suo Yang*	Tonify Kidney *Yang*
7	Psoralea	*Bu Gu Zhi*	Tonify Kidney *Yang* and strengthen the bones
5	Dipsacus	*Xu Duan*	Tonify Kidney *Yang* and promote healing of fracture
8	Lycium	*Gou Qi Zi*	Nourish Liver *Yin*, benefit the eyes
5	Codonopsis	*Dang Shen*	Tonify *Qi*
7	Astragalus	*Huang Qi*	Tonify *Qi*
8	Rehmannia Prepared	*Shu Di Huang*	Nourish Kidney *Yin* and *Jing*
7	Angelica	*Dang Gui*	Nourish Blood
5	Ophiopogon	*Mai Men Dong*	Moisten and nourish *Yin*
5	Scrophularia	*Xuan Shen*	Cool Blood and clear Heat
3	Citrus	*Chen Pi*	Move *Qi* and relieve pain

Preparation:

1. Powder or capsule method: Herbs are ground into a fine powder. Powder can be encapsulated.
2. Decoction or teapill method: Raw herbs are mixed together and decocted. Herbal water extract (decoction) can be concentrated as granules or teapills.

Actions: Tonify Kidney *Yang*, nourish *Yin/Jing*

Indications: Male and female infertility due to Kidney *Jing* or *Yang* Deficiency, weak and deep pulse and pale and swollen tongue

Dosage and Usage:

Horses and Cattle: 15–30g, twice daily
Camels: 30–60g, twice daily
Llamas, Alpacas, Pigs, Goats, and Sheep: 5–10g, twice daily
Dogs: 0.5–5g (or 0.1g per kg body weight), twice daily
Cats and Rabbits: 0.2–0.5g (or 0.1g per kg body weight), twice daily
Birds: 0.05g per kg body weight, twice daily

Use 4–16 weeks until primary clinical signs resolve.

Analysis of Formula: Kidney *Jing* Deficiency leads to poor growth or development, premature aging, and infertility. Kidney *Jing* can be divided into the *Yang* portion (Ming-men fire or Life Gate Fire, Kidney *Yang*) and *Yin* portion (source *Yin* or Kidney *Yin*). Therefore, *Yin Yang Huo* (Epimedium) and *Shu Di Huang* (Rehmannia) are used as the King herbs to tonify Kidney *Jing* and *Yang* and to promote reproductive functions. Used as the Minister herbs, *Tu Si Zi* (Cuscuta), *He Shou Wu* (Polygonum), *Yang Qi Shi* (Actinolite), *Suo Yang* (Cynomorium), *Bu Gu Zhi* (Psoralea), and *Xu Duan* (Dipsacus) function to enhance the King herbs' ability to tonify Kidney *Jing*, Kidney *Yin*, and Kidney *Yang*. Serving as the Adjuvant herbs, *Bai Shao* (Paeonia) and *Gou Qi Zi* (Lycium) nourish Liver *Yin* and Blood and benefit the eyes; *Huang Qi* (Astragalus) and *Dang Shen* (Codonopsis) tonify Spleen *Qi* to generate the postnatal *Jing* to supplement the prenatal *Jing* (Kidney *Jing*); *Mai Men Dong* (Ophiopogon) and *Xuan Shen* (Scrophularia) cool Blood, clear Heat, and nourish *Yin* to balance the Heat from Kidney *Yang* and *Jing* tonics; *Dang Gui* (Angelica) moves Blood and *Chen Pi* (Citrus) moves *Qi*, which ensures that Stagnation is not generated as a result of the tonification.

Cautions and Contraindications: Use with caution for accumulation of Damp in the Interior.

Dr. Xie's Comments: I have often used *Yin Yang Huo* for the treatment of infertility, premature aging, and maintenance of general Kidney *Yin* and *Yang* Deficiency.

REFERENCES

1. Zhang X. The clinical application of *Si Jun Zi Tang*. Practical Journal of Integration of Chinese Medicine and Western Medicine 1997;6:555.
2. Peng C, Lei ZQ. The empirical study of *Si Jun Zi Tang* on digestion, activity and absorption. Pharmacology and Clinics of Chinese Materia Medica 1995;5:6–8.
3. Zou YK. The treatment of spleen *Qi* deficiency in puppies. Journal of Traditional Chinese Veterinary Medicine 1995;5:6–8.
4. Wang WB, Xie XF. Analysis of 26 examples of treatment of functional dyspepsia with *Si Jun Zi Tang*. Journal of Chinese Medicine 2003;11:1961.
5. Ren P, Huang X, Zhang L. The effect of *Si Jun Zi Tang* to emptying rate of experimental spleen deficient rat. Chinese Journal of Integrated Traditional and Western Medicine 2000;20:596–598.
6. Huang SM, Liang M, Sun ET. The effect of *Si Jun Zi Tang* to driving function of rat stomach and intestine. Journal of Chinese Herbs 1989;9:60.
7. Zhang M, Ye FQ, Chen WW. The effect of *Si Jun Zi Tang* abstraction to diarrhea caused by Senna Leaf. Pharmacology and Clinical use of Chinese Herbs 2002;5:12–13.
8. Ren P, Huang X, Xie LJ. The effect of *Si Jun Zi Tang* to the content of motilin and PGE2 in rat model of spleen deficiency. Pharmacology and Clinics of Chinese Materia Medica 1994;6:7–8.
9. Wei YM, Zong RQ, Yang XP. Content changes of rat model of spleen deficiency and adjusting function of *Si Jun Zi Tang*. Chinese Veterinary Newsletter 2001;3:281–283.
10. Yi CQ, Ye BK, Jin JS. The effect of *Si Jun Zi Tang* to gastric mucosa cell enzymohistochemistry and plasma gut hormone of spleen deficient rat. Beijing University of Chinese Medicine Journal 1997;6:31–34.
11. Peng C, Xie ZQ. The mechanism research of *Si Jun Zi Tang* resisting experimental damage of stomach and intestine cell in Spleen Deficient animals. Pharmacology and Clinics of Chinese Materia Medica 1996;1:1–4.
12. Xu CM, Wang ZY, Xia T. The research of *Si Jun Zi Tang* to regulate the t-lymphocyte proliferating function in spleen deficient rat. Shang Hai Medicine 1996;7:23–24.
13. Li JB, Chen S, Li LX. The effect of *Si Jun Zi Tang* on lymphocyte function of spleen *qi* deficient rat model. Chengdu University of Chinese Medicine Journal 2001;3:31–32.
14. Xu DS, Shen ZY, Wang WJ. The observation of *You Gui Yin*, *Si Jun Zi Tang* and *Tao Hong Si Wu Tang* to regulate immune function of patients with renal deficiency, spleen deficiency, blood stagnation. Integration of Chinese Medicine and Western Medicine Magazine 1999;12:712–714.
15. Ji ZB, Fu YY, Hu XM. The effect of *Si Jun Zi Tang* to RBC immune function of tumor-bearing mice. Heilongjiang College of Commerce Journal (Natural Science Edition) 2000;16:1–4.
16. Guo WJ, Yu EX, Zheng SG. The research of invigorating spleen herbs to induce the apoptosis of human HCC SMM7721. Digestive Magazine of World Chinese People 2000;1:52–53.
17. Li CG, Li ML, Shu XH. Research on *Si Jun Zi Tang* resisting tumor of mice bladder cancer. Journal of Chinese Herbs 2004;2:316–317.
18. Li CG, Shu XH, Li ML. Effect of *Si Jun Zi Tang* to antioxidant ability of bladder cancer mice. Journal of Chinese Herbs 2003;21:1902–1903.
19. Li CG, Li ML, Shu XH. The function of *Si Jun Zi Tang* to diminish toxins and enhance effect in chemotherapy of bladder cancer mice. Combination of Chinese Medicine and Western Medicine Journal 2005;4:354–357.

20. Liu JY. Seven methods for chronic diarrhea in horses. Chinese Journal of Traditional Veterinary Science 1989;3:39–41. (In Chinese)
21. Shi YX. Clinical application of *Bu-zhong-yi-qi-tang* in veterinary medicine. Chinese Journal of Veterinary Medicine 1985;6:41–42. (In Chinese)
22. Xue SB, et al. Experiment to treat syndrome of diarrhea due to deficiency of the spleen in large domestic animals with added *Bu Zhong Yi Qi Tang*. Shandong Journal of Livestock and Veterinary Medicine 1998;2:40–41.
23. Liu ZJ. Canine chronic diarrhea was treated with *Bu Zhong Yi Qi Tang*. Chinese Journal of Veterinary Medicine 2003;1:33.
24. Yan ZT, Luo YJ, Zhong WX. A review of *Bu Zhong Yi Qi Tang* on veterinary medicine. Chinese Journal of Veterinary Medicine 1995;7:52–54. (In Chinese)
25. Li ZX. Application to prevent and treat diseases in cows with *Bu Zhong Yi Qi Tang*. Chinese Journal of Dairy Cows 1994;5:36–37.
26. Yu JX. Prolapse of uterus in dairy cattle was treated with *Bu Zhong Yi Qi Tang*. Advisory of Breeding Technique 2003;7:32.
27. Hu YL. Traditional Chinese Veterinary Medicine. Beijing: Chinese Agriculture Press, 2006:445–446.
28. Lu TY. Specific effect for chronic diarrhea in calf was treated by modified *Shen Ling Bai Zhu San*. Livestock of Present Era 1996;3:30.
29. Hui ZR. Chronic dyspeptic diarrhea in piglets was treated with *Shen Ling Bai Zhu San*. Gansu Livestock—Veterinary 2002;1:23.
30. Shang EM. Diarrhea in foal was treated with added *Shen Ling Bai Zhu San*. Chinese Veterinary Science and Technique 2001;5:42.
31. Sun N. Refractory Diarrhea in weanling piglets was treated with *Shen Ling Bai Zhu San*. Journal of Traditional Chinese Veterinary Medicine 2003;6:34.
32. Qian Y. *Sheng Mai Yin* possessed a magical effect to treat the collapse due to sunstroke in farm cattle. Journal of TCVM and Medica 1996;4:38–39.
33. Fan K, et al. Differential Application and Analysis of TCVM Prescription. Beijing: Chemical Industry Press, 2006: 146–147.
34. Cho CH, Mei QB, Shang P, Lee SS, So HL, Guo X, Li Y. Study of the gastrointestinal protective effects of polysaccharides from Angelica sinensis in rats. Planta Medica 2000;66: 348–351.
35. Yuan JR, Lu YW, Rong R. The research analyzed by computer on compatible mechanism of *Si Wu Tang* to nourish blood. Chinese Journal of Experimental Traditional Medical Formula 2000;1:36–39.
36. Duan MR. New application of *Tao Hong Si Wu Tang*. Gansu Journal of Chinese Medicine 2005;7:8–9.
37. Tan Wei, Song CS, Tan HL, Liu LL, Ma ZC, Wang YG, Gao Y. The effect of *Si Wu Tang* on hematogenesis of blood deficient mice caused by depletion method. Chinese Journal of Chinese Materia Medica 2005;12:926–929.
38. Ma ZC, Gao Y, Liu YX, Tan HL, Lu XQ, Zhang L. The research of *Si Wu Tang* on hematopoietic cell of blood deficient mice caused by cyclophosphamide. Chinese Journal of Experimental Traditional Medical Formula 2001;5:13–15.
39. Deng CL. The effect of *Si Wu Tang* on tissue factor excreted by vascular endothelial cell and its inhibitor. Journal of Nanhua University (Medical Edition) 2001;2:120–121.
40. Huang SL, Peng T, Gong CM, Guan XW. The effect of *Si Wu Tang* on HDL-C and LDL-C of normal animal. Journal of Liberation Army Medical High Training School 1999; 1:37–38.
41. Jin W, Yan JJ. The pharmacological research proceeding of *Si Wu Tang*. Guangdong Pharmaceutical Journal 2004;1:64–67.
42. Bai SP, Guan XW, Gong CM, Guan M. The effect of *Si Wu Tang* on microcirculation of mice earflap and mesenterium. Chinese Journal of Microcirculation 1997;4:37–38.
43. Zhang T, Tan YY, Pan YS. The effect of *Si Wu Tang* on propagation of RBC and spinal cord stem cell. Journal of Beijing University of Traditional Chinese Medicine 2000;1:36–38.
44. Chen RQ, Liang Y, Ou M. Research on immune function of blood deficient RBC, transformation of deformable lymphocyte and metabolism of free radical. Integrated Traditional Chinese and Western Medicine in Practice of Critical Care Medicine 1999;4:151–153.
45. Bai SP. The effect of *Si Wu Tang* on mice immune function. Journal of Cellular and Molecular Immunology 1998;3:22.
46. Lu XQ, Ma ZC, Gao Y. The pharmacological research proceeding of *Si Wu Tang*. Chinese Journal of Experimental Traditional Medical Formula 2001;4:56–59.
47. Hsu HY, Ho YH, Lin CC. Protection of mouse bone marrow by *Si Wu Tang* against whole body irradiation. Journal of Ethnopharmacology 1996;52:113–117.
48. Wang HL, Song YJ, Zhao GD, Feng X, Gong CM. Research of *Si Wu Tang* on toxicity of lidocaine. Pharmacology and Clinics of Chinese Materia Medica 1997;3:7–8.
49. *Yang* Y, Rong R, Lu YW, Yuan JY. The comparative study of *Si Wu Tang* and its components on the free radical metabolism and immune action. Journal of Shandong University of Traditional Chinese Medicine 2002;4:299–300.
50. Li AY. The effect of *Si Wu Tang* on uterus of smooth muscle. Yunnan Journal of Traditional Chinese Medicine and Materia Medica 2003;3:36–37.
51. Liu GY. The clinical observation of *Si Wu Tang* formula change on 45 cases of hysteromyoma. Guiding Journal of Traditional Chinese Medicine and Pharmacology 2005;2:33–34.
52. Er Tu BY, Wang AJ. Clinical observation of *Tao Hong Si Wu Tang* formula change on 45 cases of woman dysfunction uterine bleeding. Journal of Chinese Physician 2005;4:56.
53. Liu CY. Syndrome of blood deficiency after uterus torsion in the cattle was treated by modified *Si Wu Tang*. Journal of TCVM 1997;4:42.
54. Wang XW. Diagnosis and treatment of hematochezia in cattle. Journal of TCVM 2003;2:15.
55. Fan K. Differential Application and Analysis of TCVM Prescription. Beijing: Chemical Industry Press, 2006:149–150.
56. Chuan WJ. Added *Gui Qi Yi Mu Tang* was used to treat milk cow postpartum paralysis. Journal of TCVM and Medica 2004;2:45–46.
57. Yamaguchi K, et al. Effects of kami-kihi-to (*jia-wei-gui-pi-tang*) on autoantibodies in patients with chronic immune thrombocytopenic purpura. American Journal of Chinese Medicine 1993;21(3–4):251–255.
58. Iijma K, et al. *Juzen-taiho-to* (*Shi Quan Da Bu Tang*), a Japanese herbal medicine, modulates type 1 and type 2 T cell responses in old BALB/c mice. American Journal of Chinese Medicine 1999;27(2):191–203.
59. Hidaka S, et al. Preventive effects of TCM on experimental osteoporosis induced by ovariectomy in rats. Calcified Tissue International 1997;61(3):239–246.
60. Ohnishi Y et al. Dept. of Pathogenic biochemistry, Research Institute for Waken-Yaku, Toyama: Inhibitory effect of a TCM herbal formula on progressive growth of weakly malignant clone cells derived from murine fibrosarcoma. Japan Journal of Cancer Research 1996;87(10):1039–1044.
61. Ohnishi Y, et al. Oral administration of a TCM *Shi Quan Da Bu Tang* inhibits Liver metastasis of colon 26-L-5 carcinoma cells. Japan Journal of Cancer Research 1998;89(2):206–213.
62. Niwa K, et al. Preventive effects of *Shi Quan Da Bu Tang* on N-methyl-N-nitrosourea and estradiol-17 beta induced endo-

metrial carcinogenesis in mice. Carcinogenesis 2001;22 (4):587–591.
63. Qi C, et al. Effects of *Shi Quan Da Bu Tang* on detoxifying from chemotherapy: clinical and laboratory studies. Journal of Zhe Jiang TCM College 2000;24(4):16–18.
64. Wang YR. Effect of *Shi Quan Da Bu Tang* on immune function after chemotherapy and radiotherapy in tumor patients. Journal of Hubei TCM 1997;19(5):21–22.
65. Niu HH. Review of TCM on tumor metastasis. Journal of TCM 2002;48(2):150–152.
66. Muraishi Y, et al. The effect of interferon-alpha A/D in combination with the Japanese herbs and TCM *Shi Quan Da Bu Tang* on lung metastasis of murine renal carcinoma. Anticancer Research 2000;20(5A):2931 2937.
67. Saiki I, et al. A Kampo medicine *Shi Quan Da Bu Tang*—prevention of malignant progression and metastasis of tumor cells and the mechanism of action. Biological Pharmaceutical Bulletin 2000;23(6):677–688.
68. Gao PE. Clinical case was treated by *Zhi Gan Cao Tang*. Journal of TCVM 1997;4:23.
69. Zhao WH. Clinical characterization of equine conditions. Chinese Domestic Animal and Poultry Studies Enterprise, 1 2008:53.
70. Liu HR. Research progress to prevent reproductive diseases in female animals with TCM herbs. Henan Journal of Animal Husbandry and Veterinary Medicine 2001;(22)3:8–10.
71. Zi ZF. *Liu Wei Di Huang Wan* for the treatment of constipation due to deficiency of *Yin* in the dairy cows. Feeding and Breeding of Livestock and Poultry 2000;1:30.
72. Chen ZJ, et al. Effect of herbal treatment for diabetes insipidus in horses. Journal of TCVM 2004;3:42–43.
73. Li HW. Progresses in modern clinical applications and experimental researches of *Zuo Gui Wan*. Chinese Journal of Experimental Traditional Medicinal Formulae 2004;10(1):58.
74. Zhao Y, et al. Serum-pharmacological study of *Da Bu Yin Wan* (Pill) on proliferation of T and B lymphocytes in autoimmune mice induced by campylobacter Jejuni (CJ) Journal of Wannan Medicine College 2006;01(25):8–10.
75. Chen XD. *Bai He Gu Jin Tang* was used to treat cough due to Interior Deficiency for domestic animals. Journal of TCVM 2005;6:26–27.
76. Fan K. Application and Analysis of Differentiation on TCVM Prescriptions. Beijing: Chemical Industry Press, 2006:91–92.
77. Chen XD. Clinical application of *Yi Guan Jian*. Journal of TCVM 2004;2:42–43.
78. Wang K, et al. Research summary on *Yi Guan Jian* to protect the liver. Chinese and Western Medicine 2007;4(114):89–91.
79. Li HC. *Hu Qian Wan* to influence bone density in patients with kidney deficiency. Chinese Journal of Integrated Traditional and Western Medicine 1997;27(9):669–670.
80. Wen JM, et al. Modified *Zheng Ye Tang* for the treatment of chronic pharyngitis in large animals. Journal of TCVM Medica 2003;22(6):35.
81. Fan K. Differential Application and Analysis of Differentiation on Prescription of TCVM. Beijing: Chemical Industry Press, 2006:154.
82. Yun GZ. Bian Shen Huang (urticaria) was treated with integrated Chinese traditional and Western veterinary medicine. Journal of TCVM and Medica 2007;1:62.
83. Chen WX. Two cases for clinical treatment—verification on domestic animals dermatonosis. Journal of TCVM 2005;4 (125):30.
84. Fan K. Differential Application and Analysis of TCVM Prescriptions. Beijing: Chemical Industry Press, 2006;155.
85. Chen M, et al. Discussion of obtaining *Yang* from *Yin* using *Shen Qi Wan*. Journal of Henan University of Chinese Medicine 2007;3:12–14.
86. Liu TC, et al. Experimental research for the influence of *You Gui Wan* on hypothalamus-pituitary-adrenocortical axis (HPA axis) of large rats. Medicine and Medica of TCM 2007;4(27):56–57.
87. Li CQ. *Ba Ji San* and aquapuncture at Shen-shu were used to treat paralysis in sows. Journal of TCVM and Medica 2005; (24):511–512.
88. Yu C. Zhong Shou Yi Xue (Traditional Chinese Veterinary Medicine). Beijing, China Agricultural Press, 1979:552–555.

19 Herbal Formulas to Release the Exterior 解表剂

Dalu Song, Justin Shmalberg, Huisheng Xie

The herbal formulas in this chapter are designed to treat Exterior Patterns. An Exterior Pattern is characterized by nasal congestion and discharge, fever and chills, lethargy and depression, and a superficial pulse. It is often caused by exogenous pathogenic Wind-Cold or Wind-Heat. Treatment requires the use of a sweating method to release the pathogens from the Exterior. All herbal formulas in this chapter have some degree of ability to open the skin pores to induce sweating and release the Exterior. In Traditional Chinese Veterinary Medicine (TCVM), the skin pores include the sweat glands. When they are open, the body sweats. These open skin pores can also allow for invasion by pathogens, especially Wind, into the body. Therefore, the patient should avoid exposure to Wind after taking an herbal formula to release the Exterior.

Ma Huang Tang (Ephedra Decoction) 麻黄汤

This formula was named after its King herb, so it is called *Ma Huang Tang*, which is literally translated as Ephedra Decoction.

Source: *Shang Han Lun* (*The Treatise of Cold-Induced Disorders*), written by *Zhang Zhong-Jing* and published during the East *Han* Dynasty at the beginning of 3 CE

Ingredients: The original formula is composed of 9g *Ma Huang* (Ephedra), 6g *Gui Zhi* (Cinnamomum), 9g *Xing Ren* (Armeniaca), and 3g *Gan Cao* (Glycyrrhiza). The ratio of ingredients and their actions are listed in Table 19.1.

Preparation:

1. Powder or capsule method: Herbs are ground into a fine powder. The powder can be encapsulated.
2. Decoction or teapill method: Raw herbs are mixed together and decocted. An herbal water extract (decoction) can be concentrated as granules or teapills.

Actions: Promote sweating to dispel Exterior pathogenic factors, disperse the Lung *Qi* to relieve asthma

Indications: This formula is recommended for an Excess Exterior Pattern due to exogenous Wind-Cold. Exogenous Wind-Cold is characterized by a marked aversion to Cold, a slight fever, generalized pain and stiffness, a short-stride gait, an arched back, dyspnea or tachypnea without panting, no sweating, a thin, white coating of the tongue, and a superficial pulse. It often occurs in young patients with a strong constitution.

Dosage and Usage:
Horses and Cattle: 15–45g twice daily
Use 2–3 days until primary clinical signs resolve.

Analysis of Formula: Invasion of Wind-Cold at the Exterior leads to obstruction of *Wei Qi* (Defensive *Qi*), Stagnation of skin pores, and failure of Lung *Qi* to disperse. This condition should be treated by inducing sweating to expel the pathogenic factor Wind-Cold from the Exterior and by dispersing Lung *Qi* to relieve asthma. *Ma Huang* (Ephedra), the King herb in this formula, provides both of these actions. *Gui Zhi* (Cinnamomum), as the Minister herb, disperses pathogenic Cold by warming the Channels. *Xing Ren* (Armeniaca) relieves stagnant Lung *Qi* and serves as an Adjuvant herb to enhance the King herb's effect to relieve cough and asthma. *Gan Cao* (Glycyrrhiza) is the Messenger herb, capable of mediating the properties of the other herbs in this formula. *Gan Cao* (Glycyrrhiza) tonifies *Qi* and enriches the Middle Burner (*Zhong Jiao*) to prevent *Ma Huang* (Ephedra) and *Gui Zhi* (Cinnamomum) from inducing excessive sweating and impairing the *Zheng Qi*.

Cautions and Contraindications: The formula is a very potent diaphoretic and produces intense sweating, which may damage Body Fluids and Blood. It is only

Table 19.1. Ingredients and actions of *Ma Huang Tang*.

%	English Name	Chinese *Pin-Yin*	Actions
33.3	Ephedra	*Ma Huang*	Dispel Exterior pathogenic factors, induce sweating
22.3	Cinnamomun	*Gui Zhi*	Dispel Exterior pathogenic factors, warm the Channels to relieve pain
33.3	Armeniaca	*Xing Ren*	Relieve cough and asthma
11.1	Glycyrrhiza	*Gan Cao*	Harmonize and moderate the properties of other herbs

used for an Excess Exterior Pattern, when no sweating is apparent. It should be used for a short time only and no more than 5 days. It is contraindicated for patients that are already sweating, are weak, and have Blood Deficiency or Interior Heat.

Dr. Xie's Comments: *Ma Huang Tang* is a very important classical formula to treat excessive Wind-Cold Patterns in horses and domestic animals, but it is not commonly used in dogs and cats.

Clinical and Pharmacological Studies: *Ma Huang Tang* has been successfully used to treat upper respiratory diseases and asthma in domestic animals and horses.[1,2] In his TCVM book, Dr. Hu states that *Ma Huang Tang* has antipyretic effects and promotes secretion, relieves cough, resolves Phlegm and promotes bronchodilation.[3]

Gui Zhi Tang (Cinnamomum Decoction) 桂枝汤

Gui Zhi Tang (Cinnamomum Decoction) is named after the King herb: *Gui Zhi* (Cinnamomum). *Tang* means decoction for the form of administration. Thus, *Gui Zhi Tang* literally translates to Cinnamomum Decoction.

Source: *Shang Han Lun* (*The Treatise of Cold-Induced Disorders*), written by *Zhang Zhong-Jing* and published during the East *Han* Dynasty in early 3 CE

Ingredients: The original formula (Table 19.2) is composed of 9 g *Gui Zhi* (Cinnamomum), 9 g *Bai Shao Yao* (Paeonia), 6 g *Gan Cao* (Glycyrrhiza), 9 g *Sheng Jiang* (Zingiberis), and 6 g *Da Zao* (Jujube).

Preparation:

1. Powder or capsule method: Herbs are ground into a fine powder. The powder can be encapsulated.
2. Decoction or teapill method: Raw herbs are mixed together and decocted. An herbal water extract (decoction) can be concentrated as granules or teapills.

Table 19.2. Ingredients and actions of *Gui Zhi Tang*.

%	English Name	Chinese *Pin-Yin*	Action
23	Cinnamomum	*Gui Zhi*	Dispel Exterior pathogenic factors, warm the Channels to relieve pain
23	Paeonia	*Bai Shao Yao*	Nourish *Yin* and Blood
16	Glycyrrhiza	*Gan Cao*	Moderate the properties of other herbs, harmonize
23	Zingiberis	*Sheng Jiang*	Dispel Cold, regulate the Stomach
15	Jujube	*Da Zao*	Replenish *Yin*, reinforce the Spleen

Actions: Expel pathogenic factors from the muscles and skin, regulate *Ying Qi* to relieve the Exterior

Indications: This formula is indicated for an Exterior Deficiency Pattern due to exogenous Wind-Cold. The clinical signs include a marked aversion to Wind, sweating, mild fever, nasal congestion or discharge, a thin white coating of the tongue, and a superficial and slow pulse. An Exterior Deficiency Pattern often occurs in geriatric or weak patients.

Dosage and Usage:

Horses and Cattle: 15–60 g, twice daily
Camels: 30–75 g, twice daily
Llamas, Alpacas, Pigs, Goats, and Sheep: 5–15 g, twice daily
Dogs: 0.5–5 g (or 0.1 g per kg body weight), twice daily
Cats and Rabbits: 0.2–0.5 g (or 0.1 g per kg body weight), twice daily
Birds: 0.1–0.2 g per kg body weight, twice daily

Use for 1–2 weeks until the primary clinical signs resolve.

Analysis of Formula: When *Zheng Qi* is weak, pathogenic Wind-Cold invades. For this condition, the key to successful treatment is to expel the pathogenic factor Wind-Cold from the muscles and skin and to regulate *Ying Qi* and *Wei Qi* to restore *Zheng Qi*. *Gui Zhi* (Cinnamomum) is the King herb and can expel pathogenic Wind-Cold from the muscles and skin and warm the Channels to enhance *Yang*. *Bai Shao Yao* (Paeonia), the Minister herb, will nourish *Yin* to promote the production of Body Fluids and astringe *Ying Qi* to suppress sweating. Together, the combination of these first two ingredients in the same proportions remove Wind-Cold, consolidate *Yin*, and harmonize *Ying Qi* and *Wei Qi*. *Sheng Jiang* (Zingiberis) in combination with *Gui Zhi* (Cinnamomum) has the double action of dispelling Cold and regulating the Stomach. *Da Zao* (Jujube) with *Bai Shao Yao* (Paeonia) replenishes *Yin* and reinforces the Spleen. Therefore,

Da Zao (Jujube) and *Bai Shao Yao* (Paeonia) together serve as Adjuvant herbs, enhancing the effect of the King and Minister herbs to regulate *Ying Qi*, *Wei Qi*, *Yin*, and *Yang*. By reinforcing the Spleen and Stomach, these two herbs also support the generation and transportation of *Ying Qi* and *Wei Qi*. *Gan Cao* (Glycyrrhiza) is an Adjuvant herb, which replenishes *Qi* and regulates the Stomach. When combined with *Gui Zhi* (Cinnamomum), it expels pathogenic factors from the body's surface. With *Bai Shao Yao* (Paeonia), it transforms *Yin* to regulate *Ying Qi*. *Gan Cao* (Glycyrrhiza) is also a Messenger herb and mediates and harmonizes the other herbs.

Cautions and Contraindications: *Gui Zhi Tang* (Cinnamomum Decoction) should not be used in animals affected by an Excess Exterior Pattern due to exogenous Wind-Cold or Wind-Heat. An Excess Exterior Pattern is often present in young or strong patients with fever, strong pulse, and no sweat.

Dr. Xie's Comments: I have effectively used *Gui Zhi Tang* for respiratory disease in weak and/or pregnant cattle and horses with an acute onset of runny nose, aching body, thin and white tongue coating, and weak pulses.

Clinical and Pharmacological Studies: Good results have been obtained when *Gui Zhi Tang* was used to treat upper respiratory infections, influenza caused by Wind-Cold invading the Lung, abdominal pain from external pathogens, Wind-Cold invasion of the limbs, and low-grade fever after parturition.[4] *Gui Zhi Tang* has been shown to induce sweating and clear Heat.[5]

Jing Fang Bai Du San (Schizonepeta and Ledebouriella for Detoxification) 荆防败毒散

This formula was named after its King herb and function: *Jing* refers to *Jing Jie* (Schizonepeta), and *Fang* refers to *Fang Feng* (Ledebouriella). *Bai* means anti, and *Du* means toxin. *Bai Du* refers to the function of the formula to detoxify (remove toxins). San means powder. Thus, *Jing Fang Bai Du San* means Schizonepeta and Ledebouriella for Detoxification Powder.

Source: *She Sheng Zhong Miao Fang* (*Marvelous Formula for the Health of the Multitudes*), written by *Zhang Shi-Che* and published in 1550

Ingredients: The original formula (Table 19.3) is composed of 9 g of each of the following ingredients: *Jing Jie* (Schizonepeta), *Fang Feng* (Ledebouriella), *Chai Hu* (Bupleurum), *Qian Hu* (Peucedanum), *Chuan Xiong* (Ligusticum), *Zhi Ke* (Aurantium), *Qiang Huo* (Notopterygium), *Du Huo* (Angelica), *Fu Ling* (Poria), *Jie Geng* (Platycodon), and 5 g of *Gan Cao* (Glycyrrhiza).

Table 19.3. Ingredients and actions of *Jing Fang Bai Du San*.

%	English Name	Chinese *Pin-Yin*	Action
9.7	Schizonepeta	*Jing Jie*	Disperse Exterior Wind-Cold or Wind-Heat
9.7	Ledebouriella	*Fang Feng*	Expel Wind, eliminate Damp, relieve pain
9.7	Bupleurum	*Chai Hu*	Mediate *Shao Yang* Channel, disperse Liver *Qi* Stagnation, raise Spleen *Yang*
9.7	Peucedanum	*Qian Hu*	Clear Lung Heat, disperse Lung *Qi*, alleviate cough, transform Phlegm
9.7	Ligusticum	*Chuan Xiong*	Move *Qi* and Blood, disperse Wind, alleviate pain
9.7	Aurantium	*Zhi Ke*	Move *Qi*
9.7	Notopterygium	*Qiang Huo*	Disperse Cold, expel Wind and Damp, relieve pain
9.7	Angelica	*Du Huo*	Expel Wind and Damp, relieve pain
9.7	Poria	*Fu Ling*	Strengthen the Spleen, promote diuresis, eliminate Damp
9.7	Platycodon	*Jie Geng*	Open the Lung *Qi*, relieve cough, dissolve Phlegm
3	Glycyrrhiza	*Gan Cao*	Harmonize

Preparation:

1. Powder or capsule method: Herbs are ground into a fine powder. The powder can be encapsulated.
2. Decoction or teapill method: Raw herbs are mixed together and decocted. An herbal water extract (decoction) can be concentrated as granules or teapills.

Actions: Dissipate Wind-Cold and eliminate Damp

Indications: This formula is indicated for invasion by Wind, Cold and Damp, marked by inflammatory swelling such as urticaria, allergic dermatitis, bronchitis, eczema, ulcerations of the skin and upper respiratory tract, a red tongue, and a fast and strong pulse.

Dosage and Usage:

Horses and Cattle: 15–60 g, twice daily
Camels: 30–75 g, twice daily
Llamas, Alpacas, Pigs, Goats, and Sheep: 5–15 g, twice daily
Dogs: 0.5–5 g (or 0.1 g per kg body weight), twice daily
Cats and Rabbits: 0.2–0.5 g (or 0.1 g per kg body weight), twice daily
Birds: 0.1–0.2 g per kg body weight, twice daily

Use for 1–4 weeks until the primary clinical signs have resolved.

Analysis of Formula: Invasion by pathogenic Wind, Cold, and Damp leads to failure of the Lung to disperse and descend. The formula is designed to relieve the Exterior and dispel Cold and Damp. *Jing Jie* (Schizonepeta), *Fang Feng* (Ledebouriella), *Qiang Huo* (Notopterygium), and *Du Huo* (Angelica) act as King herbs, dispersing pathogenic Wind, Cold, and Damp. *Chuan Xiong* (Ligusticum) eliminates pathogenic factors, removes obstruction in Channels, and relieves pain. *Chai Hu* (Bupleurum) eliminates pathogenic factors from muscles and skin. Together they are the Minister herbs. *Jie Geng* (Platycodon), *Zhi Ke* (Aurantium), *Qian Hu* (Peucedanum), and *Fu Ling* (Poria) are Adjuvant herbs and they disperse the Lung *Qi*, resolve Phlegm, and relieve cough. *Gan Cao* (Glycyrrhiza) serves as the Messenger herb, mediating the properties of other herbs.

Cautions and Contraindications: None known

Dr. Xie's Comments: This formula is mild, and therefore it can be used for pregnant, weak, or geriatric patients, but a higher dosage is needed when treating severe cases.

Clinical and Pharmacological Studies: Good outcomes have been achieved when *Jing Fang Bai Du San* was used to treat influenza in horses.[6] Positive results have been achieved when the modified *Jing Fang Bai Du San* was used to treat food poisoning due to rotten rice straw fed to cows.[7] *Jing Fang Bai Du San* has also been found to inhibit influenza virus in vitro.[8]

Sang Ju Yin (Morus and Chrysanthemum) 桑菊饮

This formula was named after its two King herbs. *Sang* refers to *Sang Ye* (Morus), *Ju* refers to *Ju Hua* (Chrysanthemum), and *Yin* means decoction. *Sang Ju Yin* therefore means Morus and Chrysanthemum Decoction.

Source: *Wen Bing Tiao Bian* (*Detailed Analysis of Seasonal Febrile Diseases*), written by *Wu Jutong* and published in 1798

Ingredients: The original formula (Table 19.4) is composed of 7.5 g *Sang Ye* (Morus), 3 g *Ju Hua* (Chrysanthemum), 6 g *Xing Ren* (Armeniaca), 5 g *Lian Qiao* (Forsythia), 2.5 g *Bo He* (Mentha), 6 g *Jie Geng* (Platycodon), 2.5 g *Gan Cao* (Glycyrrhiza), and 6 g *Lu Gen* (Phragmites).

Table 19.4. Ingredients and actions of *Sang Ju Yin*.

%	English Name	Chinese *Pin-Yin*	Action
20	Morus	*Sang Ye*	Dispel Wind and Heat, clear Liver Heat, improve vision
8	Chrysanthemum	*Ju Hua*	Expel Wind, improve vision, clear Heat and toxins
15	Armeniaca	*Xing Ren*	Disperse the Lung *Qi* to relieve cough and dyspnea
13	Forsythia	*Lian Qiao*	Clear Heat and toxins, subdue swelling
7	Mentha	*Bo He*	Disperse Wind and Heat
15	Platycodon	*Jie Geng*	Open the Lung *Qi*, relieve cough, clear Phlegm
7	Glycyrrhiza	*Gan Cao*	Harmonize
15	Phragmites	*Lu Gen*	Clear Heat, promote Body Fluids and prevent vomiting

Preparation:

1. Powder or capsule method: Herbs are ground into a fine powder. The powder can be encapsulated.
2. Decoction or teapill method: Raw herbs are mixed together and decocted. An herbal water extract (decoction) can be concentrated as granules or teapills.

Actions: Expel Wind-Heat, disperse the Lung to relieve cough

Indications: This formula is indicated for mild Exterior Heat or Wind-Heat Patterns, which are seen at the early stage of invasion of exogenous pathogenic Wind-Heat. Clinical signs include a cough, mild fever, slight thirst, red tongue tip and margins, and a superficial, rapid pulse. *Sang Ju Yin* (Morus and Chrysanthemum) is used for upper respiratory infections, influenza, acute bronchitis, and acute tonsillitis.

Dosage and Usage:

Horses and Cattle: 15–60 g, twice daily
Camels: 30–75 g, twice daily
Llamas, Alpacas, Pigs, Goats, and Sheep: 5–15 g, twice daily
Dogs: 0.5–5 g (or 0.1 g per kg body weight), twice daily
Cats and Rabbits: 0.2–0.5 g (or 0.1 g per kg body weight), twice daily
Birds: 0.1–0.2 g per kg body weight, twice daily
Use 1–4 weeks until primary clinical signs resolve.

Analysis of Formula: Exogenous Wind-Heat invades the Lung and leads to Lung *Qi* Stagnation. The main effect is to eliminate Wind and Heat and to disperse the Lung *Qi* and relieve cough. *Sang Ye* (Morus) and *Ju Hua* (Chrysanthemum), the King herbs, expel Wind to relieve the Exterior Pattern and disperse Lung *Qi* to relieve cough. *Xing Ren* (Armeniaca) and *Jie Geng* (Platycodon) function as Minister herbs and enhance the effect of the King herbs. *Lian Qiao* (Forsythia), *Bo*

He (Mentha), and *Lu Gen* (Phragmites) serve as Adjuvant herbs to eliminate Heat and toxins, dispel Wind-Heat to clear Heat, and promote the production of Body Fluids respectively. *Gan Cao* (Glycyrrhiza), the Messenger herb, clears Lung Heat, relieves cough, and mediates the other herbs' properties.

Caution and Contraindications: None known

Dr. Xie's Comments: I have successfully used *Sang Ju Yin* for upper airway infections in weak and/or pregnant cattle and horses. The dosage should be doubled when treating severe cases.

Clinical and Pharmacological Studies: Good clinical results have been achieved when *Sang Ju Yin* was used to treat influenza in cows.[9] *Sang Ju Yin* has also been useful to treat influenza, acute bronchitis, and pharyngitis caused by Wind-Heat.[10]

Yin Qiao San (Lonicera and Forsythia) 银翘散

This formula was named after the two King herbs. *Yin* refers to *Jing Yin Hua* (Lonicera), *Qiao* refers to *Lian Qiao* (Forsythia), and *San* means powder. Thus, *Yin Qiao San* is translated as Lonicera and Forsythia Powder.

Source: *Wen Bing Tiao Bian* (*Detailed Analysis of Seasonal Febrile Diseases*), written by *Wu Jutong* and published in 1798

Ingredients: The original formula (Table 19.5) is composed of 30g *Jin Yin Hua* (Lonicera), 30g *Lian Qiao* (Forsythia), 18g *Jie Geng* (Platycodon), 18g *Bo He* (Mentha), 18g *Niu Bang Zi* (Arctium), 12g *Dan Zhu Ye* (Lophatherum), 12g *Jing Jie Sui* (Schizonepeta), 15g *Dan Dou Chi* (Soja), and 15g *Gan Cao* (Glycyrrhiza).

Table 19.5. Ingredients and actions of *Yin Qiao San*.

%	English Name	Chinese *Pin-Yin*	Action
17.9	Lonicera	*Jin Yin Hua*	Clear Heat and toxins
17.9	Forsythia	*Lian Qiao*	Clear Heat and toxins, subdue swelling
10.7	Platycodon	*Jie Geng*	Open the Lung *Qi*, relieve cough, dissolve Phlegm
10.7	Mentha	*Bo He*	Disperse Wind and Heat
10.7	Arctium	*Niu Bang Zi*	Disperse Wind-Heat in the Lung channel, relieve sore throat
7.1	Lophatherum	*Dan Zhu Ye*	Clear Heat, relieve restlessness, promote diuresis
7.1	Schizonepeta	*Jing Jie Sui*	Open the surface to relieve the Exterior pathogen
8.95	Soja	*Dan Dou Chi*	Relieve the Exterior
8.95	Glycyrrhiza	*Sheng Gan Cao*	Harmonize

Preparation:

1. Powder or capsule method: Herbs are ground into a fine powder. The powder can be encapsulated.
2. Decoction or teapill method: Raw herbs are mixed together and decocted. Most ingredients contain volatile oils, which could be lost with extended decoction. Thus, the formula should be boiled for a short time (about 10 to 15 minutes). A special procedure is used to collect the volatile oils during decoction, and then the collected volatile oils are added at the end of the process. The herbal water extract (decoction) can be concentrated as granules or teapills.

Actions: Relieve exogenous pathogenic factors, clear Heat, eliminate toxins

Indications: Used to treat the early stage of an Exterior Pattern due to Wind-Heat invasion

Dosage and Usage:

Horses and Cattle: 15–60g, twice daily
Camels: 30–75g, twice daily
Llamas, Alpacas, Pigs, Goats, and Sheep: 5–15g, twice daily
Dogs: 0.5–5g (or 0.1g per kg body weight), twice daily
Cats and Rabbits: 0.2–0.5g (or 0.1g per kg body weight), twice daily
Birds: 0.1–0.2g per kg body weight, twice daily
Use 1–4 weeks until primary clinical signs resolve.

Analysis of Formula: Wind-Heat invasion leads to Stagnation of defensive *Qi* and failure of the Lung's purifying and descending functions. The key treatment is to relieve the Exterior by expelling Wind and clearing Heat and toxins. *Jin Yin Hua* (Lonicera) and *Lian Qiao* (Forsythia) act as the King herbs to clear Heat, eliminate toxins, and expel Exterior pathogenic factors. *Bo He* (Mentha), *Niu Bang Zi* (Arctium), and *Dan Dou Chi* (Soja) act together as Minister herbs, enhancing the expulsion of pathogenic factors without impairment of the Body Fluids. *Dan Zhu Ye* (Lophatherum) and *Lu Gen* (Phragmites) clear Heat and promote the production of Body Fluids, and *Jie Geng* (Platycodon) disperses the Lung to relieve cough. These last three ingredients are the Adjuvant herbs. *Sheng Gan Cao* (Glycyrrhiza) acts as a Messenger herb to clear Heat and toxins, mediate properties of other herbs, and—when combined with *Jie Geng* (Platycodon)—soothe the throat.

Cautions and Contraindications: This formula is not indicated for Exterior Patterns due to Wind-Cold.

Dr. Xie's Comments: I have effectively used *Yin Qiao San* for the treatment and prevention of upper airway infections and influenza in horses, dogs, and cats.

Clinical and Pharmacological Studies: *Yin Qiao San* has been successfully used for the treatment of pneumonia in cows.[11] *Yin Qiao San* has also been found to be effective for contagious pleuropneumonia of cattle.[12] Studies have shown that *Yin Qiao San* has strong antipyretic, antiinflammatory, and antiallergenic effects.[13]

Xiao Qing Long Tang (Small Blue Dragon) 小青龙汤

Xiao means small, *Qing* means blue, *Long* means dragon, and *Tang* refers to decoction for the original form of the herbal formula administration. *Xiao Qing Long* is literally translated as Small Blue Dragon. In Chinese folklore, *Xiao Qing Long* was responsible for generating rain. This herbal formula will produce sweating and resolve retained fluids just as the dragon (*Xiao Qing Long*) generates rain.

Source: *Shang Han Lun* (*The Treatise of Cold Induced Disorders*), written by *Zhang Zhong-Jing* and published during the East *Han* Dynasty at the beginning of 3 CE

Ingredients: The original formula (Table 19.6) is composed of 9g *Ma Huang* (Ephedra), 9g *Bai Shao Yao* (Paeonia), 6g *Xi Xin* (Asarum), 6g *Gan Jiang* (Zingiberis), 6g *Zhi Gan Cao* (Glycyrrhiza), 9g *Gui Zhi* (Cinnamomum), 6g *Ban Xia* (Pinellia), and 6g *Wu Wei Zi* (Schisandra).

Preparation:
1. Powder or capsule method: Herbs are ground into a fine powder. The powder can be encapsulated.
2. Decoction or teapill method: Raw herbs are mixed together and decocted. The herbal water extract (decoction) can be concentrated as granules or teapills.

Table 19.6. Ingredients and actions of *Xiao Qing Long Tang*.

%	English Name	Chinese *Pin-Yin*	Action
15	Ephedra	*Ma Huang*	Dispel Exterior pathogenic factors, promote sweating
15	Paeonia	*Bai Shao Yao*	Nourish *Yin* and Blood
10	Asarum	*Xi Xin*	Disperse Wind-Cold, transform Phlegm
10	Zingiberis	*Gan Jiang*	Disperse Wind-Cold
10	Glycyrrhiza	*Zhi Gan Cao*	Moderate the properties of other herbs, harmonize
15	Cinnamomum	*Gui Zhi*	Dispel Wind-Cold, warm the Channels to relieve pain
15	Pinellia	*Ban Xia*	Dry Damp, transform Phlegm
10	Schisandra	*Wu Wei Zi*	Conserve Lung *Qi*, promote production of Body Fluids

Actions: Relieve the pathogenic factors Wind-Cold from the Exterior, warm the Lung to resolve retained fluids

Indications: Cough and dyspnea in the Exterior caused by Wind-Cold invasion with excessive fluid retention in the Interior, accompanied by aversion to Cold, thin sputum, swollen extremities, a wet and pale tongue, and a superficial pulse

Dosage and Usage:
Horses and Cattle: 15–30g, twice daily
Camels: 30–45g, twice daily
Llamas, Alpacas, Pigs, Goats, and Sheep: 5–10g, twice daily
Dogs: 0.5–5g (or 0.1g per kg body weight), twice daily
Cats and Rabbits: 0.2–0.5g (or 0.1g per kg body weight), twice daily
Use for 3–5 days until the primary clinical signs have resolved.

Analysis of Formula: This formula is used for a Wind-Cold invasion of the Exterior, accumulation of fluid in the Lungs, and failure of the Lung *Qi* to descend. The main effect is to relieve the Exterior signs and dissipate Cold, as well as warm the Lung and resolve fluid retention. The King herbs *Ma Huang* (Ephedra) and *Gui Zhi* (Cinnamomum) induce sweating to relieve the Exterior and disperse Lung *Qi* to relieve asthma. *Xi Xin* (Asarum) and *Gan Jiang* (Zingiberis), the Minister herbs, warm the Lung and remove Cold and help the *Yang* remove retained fluids. Serving as the two Adjuvant herbs, *Bai Shao Yao* (Paeonia) nourishes Blood and astringes *Yin*, while *Wu Wei Zi* (Schisandra) astringes the Lung to relieve asthma. *Bai Shao Yao* (Paeonia) and *Wu Wei Zi* (Schisandra) also prevent pungent, warm, and dry ingredients such as *Ma Huang* (Ephedra), *Xi Xin* (Asarum), and *Gan Jiang* (Zingiberis) from impairing Body Fluids and consuming *Qi*. Thus, they eliminate the pathogenic factors without impairing *Zheng Qi*. *Ban Xia* (Pinellia) acts as the third Adjuvant herb, drying Damp and resolving Phlegm. *Zhi Gan Cao* (Glycyrrhiza) acts as the Messenger herb, replenishing *Qi* and mediating the properties and actions of the other herbs.

Cautions and Contraindications: This formula is warm and dry and should not be used in patients that have cough or asthma with yellow sputum and Interior Heat.

Dr. Xie's Comments: The formula is potent and should be used for a short time only (no more than 5 days). It is contraindicated for patients that are weak or have Interior Heat.

Clinical and Pharmacological Studies: Animal studies have shown that *Xiao Qing Long Tang* is diaphoretic and relieves cough.[14] It is used for the treatment of pneumonia and pleural effusion accompanied by aversion to Cold, fever without perspiration, cough, asthma, profuse thin Phlegm, a white and wet tongue coating, and a superficial pulse. *Xiao Qing Long Tang* can also relieve bronchial spasms in cats.[15]

Fang Feng Tong Sheng San (Ledebouriella Passing the God) 防风通圣散

Fang Feng is Ledebouriella, one of the King herbs. *Tong* means pass, *Sheng* refers to God, and *San* means powder for the form of herbal administration. *Fang Feng Tong Sheng* can be translated literally as Ledebouriella Passing the God.

Source: *Xuan Ming Lun Fang* (*Formula from Discussion Illuminating*), written by *Liu Yuan-Su*, and published in 1172 CE

Ingredients: The original formula (Table 19.7) is composed of 3 g *Fang Feng* (Ledebouriella), 3 g *Jing Jie* (Schizonepeta), 3 g *Lian Qiao* (Forsythia), 3 g *Ma Huang* (Ephedra), 3 g *Bo He* (Mentha) , 3 g *Chuan Xiong* (Ligusticum), 3 g *Dang Gui* (Angelica), 3 g *Bai Shao Yao* (Paeonia), 3 g *Bai Zhu* (Atractylodes), 3 g *Zhi Zi* (Gardenia), 3 g *Da Huang* (Rheum), 3 g *Mang Xiao* (Mirabilitum), 6 g *Shi Gao* (Gypsum), 6 g *Huang Qin* (Scutellaria), 6 g *Jie Geng* (Platycodon), 6 g *Gan Cao* (Glycyrrhiza), and 12 g *Hua Shi* (Talcum).

Preparation:

1. Powder or capsule method: Herbs are ground into a fine powder. The powder can be encapsulated.
2. Decoction or teapill method: Raw herbs are mixed together and decocted. The herbal water extract (decoction) can be concentrated as granules or teapills.

Actions: Relieve Exterior Wind-Heat and purge Interior Heat

Indications: Excess Patterns of both the Interior and Exterior due to Wind invasion and internal accumulation of Heat, manifested as aversion to Cold, high fever, constipation, dark yellow urine, papules, pustules, eczema and pruritus, red and dry tongue, and fast pulse

Dosage and Usage:

Horses and Cattle: 15–60 g, twice daily
Camels: 30–75 g, twice daily
Llamas, Alpacas, Pigs, Goats, and Sheep: 5–15 g, twice daily
Dogs: 0.5–5 g (or 0.1 g per kg body weight), twice daily
Cats and Rabbits: 0.2–0.5 g (or 0.1 g per kg body weight), twice daily
Birds: 0.1–0.2 g per kg body weight, twice daily
Use 1–4 weeks until primary clinical signs resolve.

Analysis of Formula: This formula is used for Interior and Exterior Excess Patterns due to Wind invasion and internal accumulation of Heat. The treatment strategy is to expel Wind and clear Internal Heat. *Fang Feng* (Ledebouriella), *Jing Jie* (Schizonepeta), *Ma Huang* (Ephedra), and *Bo He* (Mentha) relieve the Exterior by expelling Wind and inducing sweating. *Da Huang* (Rheum) and *Mang Xiao* (Mirabilitum) clear Heat and relax the bowels and combine with *Zhi Zi* (Gardenia) and *Hua Shi* (Talcum) to drain Internal Heat. These eight herbs together serve as the King herbs. As the Minister herbs, *Jie Gen* (Platycodon), *Shi Gao* (Gypsum), *Huang Qin* (Scutellaria), and *Lian Qiao* (Forsythia) relieve Lung and Stomach Heat. The three Adjuvant herbs

Table 19.7. Ingredients and actions of *Fang Feng Tong Sheng San*.

%	English Name	Chinese *Pin-Yin*	Action
4.1	Ledebouriella	*Fang Feng*	Expel Wind, eliminate Damp, relieve pain
4.1	Schizonepeta	*Jing Jie*	Disperse Wind-Cold
4.1	Forsythia	*Lian Qiao*	Clear Heat and toxin, subdue inflammatory swelling
4.1	Ephedra	*Ma Huang*	Promote sweating, relieve asthma
4.1	Mentha	*Bo He*	Clear Wind-Heat, relieve sore throat, eliminate Heat and toxin
4.1	Ligusticum	*Chuan Xiong*	Move *Qi* and Blood, relieve pain
4.1	Angelica	*Dang Gui*	Nourish Blood, move Blood
4.1	Paeonia	*Bai Shao Yao*	Nourish Blood, restrain *Yin*, pacify the Liver
4.1	Atractylodes	*Bai Zhu*	Strengthen the Spleen, dry Damp, tonify *Qi*
4.1	Gardenia	*Zhi Zi*	Clear Heat and Fire away from Three Burners (*San Jiao*)
4.1	Rheum	*Da Huang*	Purge the Large Intestine, clear Heat
4.1	Mirabilitum	*Mang Xiao*	Purge Fire, loosen the bowels
8.2	Gypsum	*Shi Gao*	Clear Heat or Fire in the Lung and Heat in the muscles
8.2	Scutellaria	*Huang Qin*	Clear Heat in the Lung
8.2	Platycodon	*Jie Geng*	Transform Phlegm, guide other herbs to the upper part of the body
8.2	Glycyrrhiza	*Gan Cao*	Harmonize
18	Talcum	*Hua Shi*	Drain Damp-Heat

Dang Gui (Angelica), *Chuan Xiong* (Ligusticum), and *Bai Shao Yao* (Paeonia) mediate Blood and expel Wind. The fourth Adjuvant herb *Bai Zhu* (Atractylodes) strengthens the Spleen and eliminates Damp. *Gan Cao* (Glycyrrhiza) harmonizes the effect of other herbs, making it the Messenger herb. Therefore, all herbs mutually cooperate to create the effects of the formula, which are to have diaphoretic and purgative effects without hurting the Interior and to relieve superficial symptoms by dispelling Wind and purging Interior Heat.

Cautions and Contraindications: This formula is contraindicated in patients with constitutional *Qi* and *Yin* Deficiency, in geriatric patients, and during pregnancy.

Dr. Xie's Comments: *Fang Feng Tong Sheng San* is often used for the treatment of upper airway infections, influenza, and dermatitis due to both Exterior and Interior Excess Heat.

Clinical and Pharmacological Studies: A modified *Fang Feng Tong Sheng San* was successfully used for the treatment of 20 cases of upper respiratory infection and influenza, 8 cases of orchitis, 5 cases of urticaria, 4 cases of neck pain, and 8 cases of generalized pain and swelling.[16]

Xin Yi San (Magnolia Powder) 辛夷散

This formula was named after the King herb *Xin Yi* (Magnolia). *San* means powder. *Xin Yi San* literally translates to Magnolia Powder.

Source: *Zhong Shou Yi Zhi Liao Xue* (*Therapeutics of Traditional Chinese Veterinary Medicine*), written by the China Academy of Agricultural Sciences and published by China Agricultural Press in 1972

Ingredients: The original formula (Table 19.8) is composed of 45 g *Xin Yi* (Magnolia), 30 g *Zhi Mu* (Anemarrhena), 30 g *Huang Bai* (Phellodendron), 21 g *Bei Sha Shen* (Glehnia), 15 g *Yu Jin* (Curcuma), 9 g *Mu Xiang* (Saussurea), and 9 g *Ming Fan* (Alum).

Preparation:
1. Powder or capsule method: Herbs are ground into a fine powder. The powder can be encapsulated.
2. Decoction or teapill method: Raw herbs are mixed together and decocted. The herbal water extract (decoction) can be concentrated as granules or teapills.

Actions: Nourish *Yin* to expel Fire and dissolve Phlegm, clear congested nasal passages

Table 19.8. Ingredients and actions of *Xin Yi San*.

%	English Name	Chinese *Pin-Yin*	Action
28	Magnolia	*Xin Yi*	Clear Wind-Cold, open congested nose
18.5	Anemarrhena	*Zhi Mu*	Clear Lung and Stomach Heat, moisten dryness
18.5	Phellodendron	*Huang Bai*	Clear Kidney False Fire and Damp-Heat
13	Glehnia	*Bei Sha Shen*	Clear Heat, nourish *Yin*, relieve dry cough
12	Curcuma	*Yu Jin*	Clear Blood Heat, dissipate Blood stasis, alleviate pain
5	Saussurea	*Mu Xiang*	Disperse *Qi* Stagnation in the Stomach and intestines to relieve pain
5	Alum	*Ming Fan*	Astringe the Lung to relieve asthma, clear Heat to dissolve Phlegm

Indications: Nasal congestion or sinusitis, characterized by unilateral continual production of a malodorous and purulent nasal discharge

Dosage and Usage:
Horses and Cattle: 15–60 g, twice daily
Camels: 30–75 g, twice daily
Llamas, Alpacas, Pigs, Goats, and Sheep: 5–15 g, twice daily
Dogs: 0.5–5 g (or 0.1 g per kg body weight), twice daily
Cats and Rabbits: 0.2–0.5 g (or 0.1 g per kg body weight), twice daily
Birds: 0.1–0.2 g per kg body weight, twice daily
Use 4–8 weeks until primary clinical signs resolve

Analysis of Formula: *Xin Yi* (Magnolia) is the King herb, dissipating Wind-Cold and clearing congested nasal passages. *Zhi Mu* (Anemarrhena) and *Huang Bai* (Phellodendrom) serve as Minister herbs for clearing Kidney False Fire and Damp Heat. *Bei Sha Shen* (Glehnia) clears Heat and nourishes *Yin*. *Yu Jin* (Curcuma) cools Blood to clear Heat and resolve *Qi* Stagnation. *Mu Xiang* (Saussurea) moves *Qi* to resolve Stagnation. *Ming Fan* (Alum) dissolves Phlegm. These four herbs act as Adjuvant and Messenger herbs. Together, all ingredients nourish *Yin* to clear Heat and dissolve Phlegm, clear congested nasal passages, and resolve the nasal discharge.

Cautions and Contraindications:
This formula should be used only with Excess Fire.

Dr. Xie's Comments: I have successfully used *Xin Yi San* for chronic nasal congestion, sinusitis, and nasal discharge in cats, dogs, and horses.

Clinic and Pharmacological Studies: In a clinical trial *Xin Yi San* was successfully used to treat empyema of the frontal sinus in horses and mules. Eighteen cases were treated with an average dose of 5 g of formula for an average of 9.5 days. For complete resolution of clinical signs, the mild cases required 3–5 g of the formula as the treatment dose, and severe cases needed 8–10 g of the formula as the treatment dose.[17] *Xin Yi San* was also found to relieve bronchial spasms.[18]

REFERENCES

1. Shen ZJ. *Ma Huang Tang* modification for the treatment of common cold of domestic animals. Journal of Traditional Chinese Veterinary Medicine and Medica 2003;22(2):33.
2. Ma YB. *Ma Huang Tang* for the treatment of asthma in horses. Journal of China Veterinary Science and Technology 2002;36 (6):43.
3. Hu YL. Traditional Chinese Veterinary Medicine. Beijing: China Agricultural Press, 2006:386.
4. Veterinary Hospital of Kelan County Shanxi Province. Application of *Gui Zhi Tang* in veterinary clinics. In: Compiled Treatises on All TCVM Experiences in China. Beijing: Science Press, 1977:393–395.
5. Li F. Literature Review on Studies of Herbal Prescriptions. Nanjing: Jiangsu Science and Technology Press 1981:541–542.
6. Su DC, et al. Application of *Jing Fang Bai Du San* for the treatment of influenza in horses. Qinghai Livestock 2004;(2):47.
7. Yan XZ. Modified *Jing Fang Bai Du San* for the treatment of food poisoning due to rotten rice straw in cows. Guizhou Livestock and Veterinary Medicine 2001;25(1):31.
8. Hu YL. Traditional Chinese Veterinary Medicine. Beijing: China Agriculture Press, 2006:387.
9. Zhang YK. *Sang Ju Yin* modification for the treatment of influenza in cows. Journal of Traditional Chinese Veterinary Medicine and Medica 1997;(4):33.
10. Fan K, et al. Differentiation of Syndromes and Analysis of Prescriptions of TCVM. Beijing: Chemical Industry Press, 2006:75.
11. Wang XM. *Yin Qiao San* modification for the treatment of pneumonia in cows. Advisory of Breed 2004;(5):12–13.
12. Zhao JH. *Yin Qiao San* for the treatment of contagious pleuropneumonia of cattle. Traditional Chinese Veterinary Medicine and Medica 1996(4):26–27.
13. Hu YL. Traditional Chinese Veterinary Medicine. Beijing: China Agriculture Press, 2006:389.
14. Li F. Literature Review on Studies of Herbal Prescriptions. Nanjing: Jiangsu Science and Technology Press, 1981:71–73.
15. Guangzhou TCM College. Science of Prescriptions. Shanghai: Shanghai Science and Technology Press, 1979:18–19.
16. Wang Y. Application of *Fang Feng Tong Sheng San* in clinic. Journal of Traditional Chinese Veterinary Medicine and Medica 1991;(3):19.
17. Wu YL. The modified *Xin Yi San* for the treatment of empyema of frontal sinus in equine and mule. Journal of Traditional Chinese Veterinary Medicine and Medica 1995;14(1):33.
18. Hu YL. Traditional Chinese Veterinary Medicine. Beijing: Agriculture Press, 2006:416.

20 Herbal Formulas to Transform Phlegm and to Relieve Cough and Asthma 祛痰止咳平喘剂

Dalu Song, Justin Shmalberg, Huisheng Xie

There are close relationships between Phlegm, cough, and asthma. Accumulation of Phlegm in the Lung often leads to coughing. Chronic coughing often causes Lung *Qi* to rebel upward, leading to asthma. Therefore, the herbal formulas to transform Phlegm may also stop coughing and asthma. Phlegm can be divided into five types based on different causes and sources: Damp-Phlegm, Heat-Phlegm, Dry-Phlegm, Cold-Phlegm, and Wind-Phlegm.

Damp-Phlegm is the primary source of Phlegm, which is associated with disruption of the transformation and transportation functions of the Spleen. The deficient Spleen fails to transform water and fluids and leads to an accumulation of Damp, which then transforms into Phlegm. For this reason, herbs that strengthen the Spleen and dry Damp are often included in these herbal formulas. The typical herbal formula in this category is *Er Chen Tang*.

Heat or Fire boils and scorches Body Fluids and transforms them into Heat-Phlegm. Clinical signs associated with Heat-Phlegm include a thick yellow Phlegm, a red tongue with a yellow coating, and a slippery and fast pulse. *Qing Qi Hua Tan Wan* was formulated for this condition.

Dryness consumes and dries Body Fluids and transforms the thickened fluids into Dry-Phlegm. The clinical signs associated with Dry-Phlegm include a dry or bloody type of Phlegm, a dry cough, chest pain, dry nose, dry tongue, and choppy pulse. *Qing Zao Jiu Fei Tang* is effective for this condition.

Cold can injure the Upper Burner (*Shang Jiao*) and/or Middle Burner (*Zhong Jiao*). Cold also will cause fluids to congeal, leading to Cold-Phlegm, which is treated with *San Zi Yang Qin Tang*.

Damp-Phlegm, Heat-Phlegm, Dry-Phlegm, and Cold-Phlegm are forms of Substantial Phlegm. Wind-Phlegm is classified as Non-substantial Phlegm that disturbs the flow of *Qi* and causes tremors, seizures, or internal Wind. The herbal formulas to resolve Wind-Phlegm, *Di Tan Tang* and *Ding Xian Wan*, are discussed in Chapter 31, "Herbal Formulas to Expel Wind."

Substantial Phlegm can eventually accumulate in the body, leading to nodules, lumps, and masses. The formulas to treat this form of Substantial Phlegm include *Hai Zao Yu Hu Tang* and *Nei Xiao Luo Li San*.

Er Chen Tang (Two Aged Herbs) 二陈汤

The name of this formula comes from two herbs, the King herb *Ban Xia* (Pinellia), and the Minister herb *Ju Pi* (Citrus). *Er* means two, *Chen* means aged or old-fashioned. Like an aged fine wine, the older (longer they are processed or stored) these two herbs are, the more effective they become with fewer side effects. *Tang* means decoction. *Er Chen Tang* can literally be translated as Two Aged Herbs Decoction.

Source: *Tai Ping Hui Min He Ji Ju Fang* (*Imperial Grace Formulary of the Tai Ping Era*), written by *Chen Shi-Wen* et al. and published in 1078 CE

Ingredients: The original formula (Table 20.1) is composed of 15 g *Ban Xia* (Pinellia), 15 g *Ju Pi* or *Chen Pi* (Citrus), 9 g *Fu Ling* (Poria), and 5 g *Gan Cao* (Glycyrrhiza).

Preparation:

1. Powder or capsule method: Herbs are ground into a fine powder. The powder can be encapsulated.
2. Decoction or teapill method: Raw herbs are mixed together and decocted. The herbal water extract (decoction) can be concentrated as granules or teapills.

Actions: Dry Damp to resolve Phlegm, regulate *Qi*, normalize the Spleen and Stomach

Indications: Damp-Phlegm with productive cough and profuse white sputum with associated white, wet tongue coating and slippery pulse

Table 20.1. Ingredients and actions of *Er Chen Tang*.

%	English Name	Chinese *Pin-Yin*	Action
34	Pinellia	*Ban Xia*	Dry Damp, transform Phlegm
34	Citrus	*Ju Pi* or *Chen Pi*	Regulate Spleen *Qi*, dry Damp, transform Phlegm
20	Poria	*Fu Ling*	Strengthen the Spleen, drain Damp, calm the mind
12	Glycyrrhiza	*Gan Cao*	Harmonize

Dosage and Usage:

Horses and Cattle: 15–60 g, twice daily

Camels: 30–75 g, twice daily

Llamas, Alpacas, Pigs, Goats, and Sheep: 5–15 g, twice daily

Dogs: 0.5–5 g (or 0.1 g per kg body weight), twice daily

Cats and Rabbits: 0.2–0.5 g (or 0.1 g per kg body weight), twice daily

Birds: 0.1–0.2 g per kg body weight, twice daily

Use 2–6 weeks until primary clinical signs resolve.

Analysis of Formula: A dysfunction of the Spleen in transportation and transformation leads to the accumulation of Damp, which transforms into Phlegm. The key treatment is to reduce Damp, resolve Phlegm, and regulate the Middle Burner (*Zhong Jiao*) and the circulation of *Qi*. *Ban Xia* (Pinellia), the King herb, resolves cough by drying Damp and transforming Phlegm. It also suppresses rebellious *Qi* and regulates the Stomach to relieve vomiting. *Chen Pi* (Citrus), used as a Minister herb, promotes the effects of *Ban Xia* (Pinellia), as well as increases the flow of *Qi* to eliminate Phlegm. *Fu Ling* (Poria) is the Adjuvant herb, which strengthens the Spleen and drains Damp to stop "the source of Phlegm production." Additionally, *Fu Ling* treats both the superficial clinical signs and the root cause of the disease, when combined with the King and Minister herbs. *Gan Cao* (Glycyrrhiza) serves as a Messenger herb to regulate the Spleen and mediate the properties of the other herbs.

Cautions and Contraindications: This formula is contraindicated in cases showing Dryness of the Lung due to *Yin* Deficiency.

Dr. Xie's Comments: I have successfully used *Er Chen Tang* for the treatment of wet cough in horses, dogs, and cattle. With modifications, it can be used as the basic herbal formula for treating any other Phlegm conditions.

Clinical and Pharmacological Studies: Chen reported on 456 cases of domestic animals with cough that were treated with *Er Chen Tang*. Among those cases there were 178 horses, 143 cows, 97 sheep, and 38 pigs.[1] After the herbal treatment, 398 cases were cured and 58 cases improved. Dr. Hu found that *Er Chen Tang* reduces hypersalivation and gastric acidity.[2]

Wen Dan Tang (Warming the Gallbladder) 温胆汤

Wen means warming, *Dan* refers to Gallbladder, and *Tang* means decoction. Thus, *Wen Dan Tang* literally translates to Warming the Gallbladder Decoction.

Source: *San Yin Ji Yi Bing Zheng Fang Lun* (*Treatise on the Three Categories of Pathogenic Factors of Diseases*), written by *Chen Yan* and published in 1174 CE

Ingredients: The original formula (Table 20.2) is composed of 6 g *Ban Xia* (Pinellia), 6 g *Zhu Ru* (Bambusa), 6 g *Zhi Shi* (Aurantium), 9 g *Ju Pi* or *Chen Pi* (Citrus), 3 g *Gan Cao* (Glycyrrhiza), and 5 g *Fu Ling* (Poria).

Preparation:

1. Powder or capsule method: Herbs are ground into a fine powder. The powder can be encapsulated.
2. Decoction or teapill method: Raw herbs are mixed together and decocted. The herbal water extract (decoction) can be concentrated as granules or teapills.

Actions: Regulate the flow of *Qi* to remove Phlegm, clear Gallbladder Heat, regulate the Stomach

Indications: Stagnation of Gallbladder *Qi* with Phlegm or disharmony between the Gallbladder and Stomach with clinical signs of timidity; being easily frightened; anxiety; vomiting; seizures; greasy, white tongue coating; wiry or slippery pulse

Dosage and Usage:

Horses and Cattle: 15–60 g, twice daily

Camels: 30–75 g, twice daily

Table 20.2. Ingredients and actions of *Wen Dan Tang*.

%	English Name	Chinese *Pin-Yin*	Action
17	Pinellia	*Ban Xia*	Dry Damp, transform Phlegm
17	Bambusa	*Zhu Ru*	Clear Lung Phlegm-Heat, clear Stomach Heat
17	Aurantium	*Zhi Shi*	Break up *Qi* Stagnation in the intestines
26	Citrus	*Ju Pi* or *Chen Pi*	Regulate Spleen *Qi*, dry Damp, transform Phlegm
9	Glycyrrhiza	*Gan Cao*	Harmonize
14	Poria	*Fu Ling*	Strengthen the Spleen, drain Damp

Llamas, Alpacas, Pigs, Goats, and Sheep: 5–15 g, twice daily
Dogs: 0.5–5 g (or 0.1 g per kg body weight), twice daily
Cats and Rabbits: 0.2–0.5 g (or 0.1 g per kg body weight), twice daily
Birds: 0.1–0.2 g per kg body weight, twice daily
Use 1–4 weeks until primary clinical signs resolve.

Analysis of Formula: Physiologically, the Gallbladder is responsible for making decisions or judgments. A lack of Gallbladder *Qi* gradually leads to timidity and further *Qi* Stagnation. *Qi* Stagnation causes generation of Phlegm, which disturbs *Shen* and leads to anxiety, being easily frightened, insomnia, other behavioral changes, dizziness, or seizures. When Gallbladder *Qi* Stagnation is present, the Gallbladder fails to descend and excrete bile into the gastrointestinal tracts, leading to disharmony between the Gallbladder and Stomach and vomiting. The resulting disharmony is treated by moving *Qi*, transforming Phlegm, clearing the Gallbladder, and regulating the Stomach. *Ban Xia* (Pinellia), the King herb, eliminates Damp and transforms Phlegm, descends *Qi*, and regulates the Stomach. *Zhu Ru* (Bambusa), the Minister herb, clears Gallbladder Heat and regulates the Stomach to stop vomiting. *Zhi Shi* (Aurantium), and *Chen Pi* (Citrus) regulate the flow of *Qi* to reduce Phlegm. *Fu Ling* (Poria) strengthens the Spleen and induces diuresis to eliminate Damp and prevent the generation of Phlegm. These last three ingredients are the Adjuvant herbs. *Gan Cao* (Glycyrrhiza) is the Messenger herb to invigorate the Spleen and mediate the properties of the other herbs.

Cautions and Contraindications: This formula should not be used in patients with *Yin* and/or Blood Deficiency.

Dr. Xie's Comments: I have successfully used *Wen Dan Tang* for behavior problems (especially irrational fear), due to lack of Gallbladder *Qi* in horses and dogs. *Wen Dan Tang* is also useful in treating canine distemper associated with Phlegm-Heat in the Interior and disharmony between the Gallbladder and Stomach.

Clinical and Pharmacological Studies: This formula has been useful in treating epilepsy, acute and chronic gastritis, enteritis, and chronic bronchitis associated with Phlegm-Heat in the Interior and disharmony between the Gallbladder and the Stomach.[3]

Zhi Sou San (Stopping Cough) 止嗽散

Zhi means stop, *Sou* refers to cough, and *San* means powder. Thus, *Zhi Sou San* means Stop Cough Powder.

Source: *Yi Xue Xin Wu* (*Medical Revelations*), written by *Chen Guo Peng*, published in 1732 CE

Table 20.3. Ingredients and actions for *Zhi Sou San*.

%	English Name	Chinese *Pin-Yin*	Action
18	Stemona	*Bai Bu*	Descend Lung *Qi* to relieve cough
18	Aster	*Zi Wan*	Moisten the Lung, stop cough
15.1	Cynanchum	*Bai Qian*	Clear Wind-Heat, dispel Phlegm, stop cough
12.3	Platycodon	*Jie Geng*	Open the Lung, transform Phlegm, stop cough
12.3	Citrus	*Chen Pi*	Regulate Spleen *Qi*, dry Damp, transform Phlegm
18	Schizonepeta	*Jing Jie*	Relieve the Exterior
6.3	Glycyrrhiza	*Gan Cao*	Harmonize

Ingredients: The original formula (Table 20.3) is composed of 60 g *Bai Bu* (Stemona), 60 g *Zi Wan* (Aster), 50 g *Bai Qian* (Cynanchum), 40 g *Jie Geng* (Platycodon), 40 g *Chen Pi* (Citrus), 60 g *Jing Jie* (Schizonepeta), and 20 g *Gan Cao* (Glycyrrhiza).

Preparation:

1. Powder or capsule method: Herbs are ground into a fine powder. The powder can be encapsulated.
2. Decoction or teapill method: Raw herbs are mixed together and decocted. The herbal water extract (decoction) can be concentrated as granules or teapills.

Actions: Open the Lung, expel pathogenic factors from the Exterior, relieve cough, transform Phlegm

Indications: This formula is indicated for exogenous Wind invasion of the Lung, with cough, white Phlegm, thin white tongue coating, superficial pulse.

Dosage and Usage:
Horses and Cattle: 15–60 g, twice daily
Camels: 30–75 g, twice daily
Llamas, Alpacas, Pigs, Goats, and Sheep: 5–15 g, twice daily
Dogs: 0.5–5 g (or 0.1 g per kg body weight), twice daily
Cats and Rabbits: 0.2–0.5 g (or 0.1 g per kg body weight), twice daily
Birds: 0.1–0.2 g per kg body weight, twice daily
Use 4–8 weeks until primary clinical signs resolve.

Analysis of Formula: This formula acts by expelling Wind and dispersing the Lung *Qi*, as well as relieving cough and resolving Phlegm. *Zi Wan* (Aster) and *Bai Bu* (Stemona), the King herbs, relieve cough and dissolve Phlegm. *Jie Geng* (Platycodon) and *Bai Qian* (Cynanchum), the Minister herbs, open the Lung to descend Lung *Qi*, relieve coughing, and resolve sputum. *Jing Jie* (Schizonepeta), which expels residual pathogenic factors from the Exterior, and *Chen Pi* (Citrus), which regulates the flow of *Qi* and dissolves Phlegm, act together as Adjuvant herbs. Used as a Messenger herb, *Gan Cao* (Glycyrrhiza) mediates the properties of the other herbs and, with *Jie Geng* (Platycodon), relieves a sore throat.

Cautions and Contraindications: Avoid using this formula alone in animals with Lung *Yin* Deficiency and in those with excessive Lung Heat with cough, dyspnea, and thick yellow Phlegm.

Dr. Xie's Comments: I have successfully used *Zhi Sou San* for chronic coughs. This herbal formula is designed to treat coughing and dyspnea. As soon as these clinical signs are resolved, patients with *Yin* Deficiency should be treated with *Bai He Gu Jing Tang*; patients with Lung Heat should be treated with *Qing Fei San*.

Clinical and Pharmacological Studies: In one clinical study *Zhi Sou San* was used to treat 58 patients with upper respiratory infections, tracheal inflammation, acute bronchitis, and acute pneumonia. After the herbal treatment, 52 patients had completely recovered, and the remaining 6 cases had significantly improved.[4] *Zhi Sou San* has been shown to relax the smooth muscles of the bronchi and increase bronchial mucus secretions.[5]

Ma Xing Shi Gan Tang (Ephedra, Armeniaca, Gypsum, and Glycyrrhiza) 麻杏石甘汤

The names of the ingredients are abbreviated in this formula. *Ma Huang* (Ephedra) is abbreviated to *Ma*, *Xing Ren* (Armeniaca) to *Xing*, *Shi Gao* (Gypsum) to *Shi*, *Gan Cao* (Glycyrrhiza) to *Gan*, and *Tang* means decoction. Thus, *Ma Xing Shi Gan Tang* means Ephedra, Armeniaca, Gypsum and Glycyrrhiza Decoction.

Source: *Shang Han Lun* (*The Treatise of Cold-induced Disorders*), written by *Zhang Zhong-Jing* and published during the East *Han* Dynasty at the beginning of 3 CE

Ingredients: The original formula (Table 20.4) is composed of 9g *Ma Huang* (Ephedra), 9g *Xing Ren* (Armeniaca), 18g *Shi Gao* (Gypsum), and 6g *Gan Cao* (Glycyrrhiza).

Preparation:

1. Powder or capsule method: Herbs are ground into a fine powder. The powder can be encapsulated.
2. Decoction or teapill method: Raw herbs are mixed together and decocted. The herbal water extract (decoction) can be concentrated as granules or teapills.

Table 20.4. Ingredients and Actions of *Ma Xing Shi Gan Tang.*

%	English Name	Chinese *Pin-Yin*	Action
21	Ephedra	*Ma Huang*	Induce sweating, relieve the Exterior, stop asthma
21	Armeniaca	*Xing Ren*	Disperse Lung *Qi* to relieve cough and dyspnea
16	Gypsum	*Shi Gao*	Clear Heat in the Lung, Stomach, or muscles
42	Glycyrrhiza	*Gan Cao*	Harmonize

Actions: Clear Lung Heat, alleviate cough and dyspnea

Indications: This formula is used to resolve exogenous pathogenic factors such as Heat in the Lung leading to cough and asthma with fever, thirst, flaring nares, abnormal sweating Patterns, a thin white or yellow tongue coating, and a rapid, superficial pulse.

Dosage and Usage:

Horses and Cattle: 15–60g, twice daily
Camels: 30–75g, twice daily
Llamas, Alpacas, Pigs, Goats, and Sheep: 5–15g, twice daily
Dogs: 0.5–5g (or 0.1g per kg body weight), twice daily
Cats and Rabbits: 0.2–0.5g (or 0.1g per kg body weight), twice daily
Birds: 0.1–0.2g per kg body weight, twice daily
Use 3–7 days until primary clinical signs resolve.

Analysis of Formula: Excess Heat, transformed from exogenous Wind, accumulates in the Lung and causes failure of the Lung's purifying and descending functions. The main effects of the formula are to disperse Heat and relieve cough and asthma. *Ma Huang* (Ephedra) and *Shi Gao* (Gypsum) are the King herbs, supporting each other to clear Lung Heat. *Xing Ren* (Armeniaca), the Minister herb, causes the Lung *Qi* to descend, and it also enhances the King herbs' functions of relieving cough and asthma. *Gan Cao* (Glycyrrhiza) acts as the Adjuvant and Messenger herb to replenish *Qi*, regulate the Middle-Burner (*Zhong Jiao*), and mediate the other herbs' properties.

Cautions and Contraindications: Avoid in cases of cough and asthma due to Wind-Cold or to Excessive Phlegm-Heat.

Dr. Xie's Comments: Even though *Ma Xing Shi Gan Tang* is a very important classical formula to treat an Excess Lung Heat Pattern in horses and domestic animals, it is not commonly used in dogs and cats.

Clinical and Pharmacological Studies: Good clinical outcomes were achieved when *Ma Xing Shi Gang Tang* was used to treat asthma due to Lung Heat in sheep and goats.[6] *Ma Xing Shi Gan Tang* has also been used successfully to treat asthma due to Lung Heat with Lung *Qi* Deficiency.[7] The antiasthmatic effect of *Ma Xing Shi Gan Tang* is due to relaxation of bronchial smooth muscles from a release of histamine caused by degranulation of mast cells.[8]

Su Zi Jiang Qi Tang (Perilla for Descending *Qi*) 苏子降气汤

The formula was named after its King herb *Su Zi* (Perilla) and its main function. *Jiang* means descending, which refers to the ability of this formula to descend *Qi*, and *Tang* means decoction—thus, the name Perilla for Descending *Qi* Decoction.

Source: *Tai Ping Hui Min He Ji Ju Fang (Imperial Grace Formula of the Tai Ping Era)*, written by *Chen Shiwen* et al. and published by the *Song* Dynasty government in 1078 CE

Ingredients: The original formula (Table 20.5) is composed of 75 g *Su Zi* (Perilla), 75 g *Ban Xia* (Pinellia), 15 g *Dang Gui* (Angelica), 60 g *Gan Cao* (Glycyrrhiza), 30 g *Qian Hu* (Peucedanum), 30 g *Hou Po* (Magnolia), and 30 g *Rou Gui* (Cinnamomum).

Preparation:

1. Powder or capsule method: Herbs are ground into a fine powder. The powder can be encapsulated.
2. Decoction or teapill method: Raw herbs are mixed together and decocted. The herbal water extract (decoction) can be concentrated as granules or teapills.

Table 20.5. Ingredients and actions of *Su Zi Jiang Qi Tang*.

%	English Name	Chinese *Pin-Yin*	Action
24	Perilla	*Su Zi*	Descend Lung *Qi*, disperse Phlegm
24	Pinellia	*Ban Xia*	Dry Damp, transform Phlegm, descend Stomach *Qi*
5	Angelica	*Dang Gui*	Nourish and move Blood
20	Glycyrrhiza	*Gan Cao*	Harmonize
9	Peucedanum	*Qian Hu*	Clear Lung Heat, transform Phlegm, alleviate cough
9	Magnolia	*Hou Po*	Move *Qi*, resolve Stomach *Qi* Stagnation
9	Cinnamomum	*Rou Gui*	Warm the Spleen and Stomach, disperse Internal Cold

Actions: Direct the rebellious *Qi* downward, relieve asthma, expel Phlegm, stop cough

Indications: This formula is indicated for cough and asthma with Excess in the Upper Burner (*Shang Jiao*) and Deficiency in the Lower Burner (*Xia Jiao*). The Upper Burner (*Shang Jiao*) mainly refers to the Lung, and the Lower Burner (*Xia Jiao*) refers to the Kidney. The main signs of this condition are copious amounts of white Phlegm and dyspnea (Excess in the Upper Burner) with rear weakness and Coldness (Deficiency in the Lower Burner); a white, wet, or greasy tongue coating; and a slippery or superficial pulse.

Dosage and Usage:

Horses and Cattle: 15–60 g, twice daily
Camels: 30–75 g, twice daily
Llamas, Alpacas, Pigs, Goats, and Sheep: 5–15 g, twice daily
Dogs: 0.5–5 g (or 0.1 g per kg body weight), twice daily
Cats and Rabbits: 0.2–0.5 g (or 0.1 g per kg body weight), twice daily
Birds: 0.1–0.2 g per kg body weight, twice daily
Use 4–12 weeks until primary clinical signs resolve.

Analysis of Formula: Excessive accumulation of Phlegm and saliva and dysfunction of ascension and descension of the Lung are associated with the Deficiency of Kidney *Yang*. A Deficient Kidney fails to grasp and receive *Qi* from the Lung, leading to Stagnation of Lung *Qi*, generation of Phlegm, and dyspnea. The treatment of this Pattern focuses on descending the abnormally rising *Qi* and eliminating Phlegm to relieve asthma and cough. *Su Zi* (Perilla), as the King herb, descends *Qi* and eliminates Phlegm to relieve cough, dyspnea, and asthma. The following are used as Minister herbs: *Ban Xia* (Pinellia) dries Damp, eliminates Phlegm, and descends *Qi*; *Hou Po* (Magnolia) sends *Qi* down and eliminates Phlegm to stop asthma; and *Qian Hu* (Peucedanum) disperses Lung *Qi* and eliminates Phlegm to relieve cough. The King and Minister herbs focus on the Excess Pattern in the Upper Burner *(Shang Jiao)* Lung. *Rou Gui* (Cinnamomum) warms the Kidney *Yang* to benefit the reception of *Qi* and relieve asthma. *Dang Gui* (Angelica) nourishes Blood, moistens dryness, and also helps *Rou Gui* (Cinnamomum) treat the Deficiency Pattern in the Lower Burner (*Xia Jiao*) and Kidney. These two herbs are the Adjuvant herbs. *Gan Cao* (Glycyrrhiza) mediates the properties of other herbs and is the Messenger herb.

Cautions and Contraindications: Most of the ingredients are warm and dry in nature, so this formula is contraindicated for cough and asthma due to Lung and Kidney *Yin* Deficiency or Lung Heat.

Dr. Xie's Comments: I have successfully used *Su Zi Jiang Qi Tang* for chronic dyspnea, cough, or asthma in cats, dogs, and horses. It works especially well for older patients. It can also be used for chronic Stomach *Qi* Rebellion (nausea or vomiting).

Clinical and Pharmacological Studies: *Su Zi Jiang Qi Tang* has been successfully used to control respiratory system disease in chickens.[9] The formula's effectiveness to alleviate cough and asthma is connected to its ability to reduce bronchial secretions, relax bronchial spasms, relieve cough, mediate digestive fluid secretion, and moderate immune response.[10–11]

Qing Qi Hua Tan Wan (Clearing Heat and Transforming Phlegm) 清气化痰丸

This formula is named after its function: *Qing Qi* means clearing (Lung) Heat, *Hua Tan* means transforming Phlegm, and *Wan* means pill. Thus, *Qing Qi Hua Tan* translates as Clearing Heat and Transforming Phlegm.

Source: *Yi Fang Kao* (*Investigation of Medicine Formula*), written by *Wu Kun* and published in 1584 CE

Ingredients: The original formula (Table 20.6) is composed of 30 g *Gua Lou Ren* (Trichosanthes), 30 g *Chen Pi* (Citrus), 30 g *Huang Qin* (Scutellaria), 30 g *Xing Ren* (Armeniaca), 30 g *Zhi Shi* (Aurantium), 30 g *Fu Ling* (Poria), 45 g *Dan Nan Xing* (Arisaema), and 45 g *Ban Xia* (Pinellia).

Table 20.6. Ingredients and actions of *Qing Qi Hua Tan Wan*.

%	English Name	Chinese *Pin-Yin*	Action
11.1	Trichosanthes	*Gua Lou Ren*	Clear Heat, disperse Phlegm, moisten Lung to relieve cough
11.1	Citrus	*Chen Pi*	Regulate Spleen *Qi*, dry Damp, transform Phlegm
11.1	Scutellaria	*Huang Qin*	Clear Lung Heat or Fire
11.1	Armeniaca	*Xing Ren*	Disperse Lung *Qi*, relieve cough and dyspnea
11.1	Aurantium	*Zhi Shi*	Break up *Qi* Stagnation, dissipate masses in the abdomen
11.1	Poria	*Fu Ling*	Strengthen the Spleen, promote diuresis, drain Damp
16.7	Arisaema	*Dan Nan Xing*	Clear Heat, remove Phlegm
16.7	Pinellia	*Ban Xia*	Dry Damp, transform Phlegm

Preparation:
1. Powder or capsule method: Herbs are ground into a fine powder. The powder can be encapsulated.
2. Decoction or teapill method: Raw herbs are mixed together and decocted. The herbal water extract (decoction) can be concentrated as granules or teapills.

Actions: Clear Heat and resolve Phlegm, regulate the flow of *Qi* and stop cough

Indications: This formula is indicated for cough due to Phlegm-Heat characterized by difficult expectoration of thick yellowish sputum, dyspnea, nausea, a red tongue with a greasy yellow coating, and a slippery and rapid pulse. It is used for diseases such as pneumonia, acute bronchitis, and acute exacerbation of chronic bronchitis, with thick yellow Phlegm related to a Phlegm Heat Pattern.

Dosage and Usage:
Horses and Cattle: 15–60 g, twice daily
Camels: 30–75 g, twice daily
Llamas, Alpacas, Pigs, Goats, and Sheep: 5–15 g, twice daily
Dogs: 0.5–5 g (or 0.1 g per kg body weight), twice daily
Cats and Rabbits: 0.2–0.5 g (or 0.1 g per kg body weight), twice daily
Birds: 0.1–0.2 g per kg body weight, twice daily
Use 2–6 weeks until primary clinical signs resolve.

Analysis of Formula: Lung Heat scorches and converts Body Fluids into Phlegm, further obstructing the flow of *Qi* and leading to cough, dypsnea, or asthma. This Pattern is treated by clearing Heat to remove Phlegm, regulating the flow of *Qi* and arresting the cough. *Dan Nan Xing* (Arisaema), as the King herb, clears the Heat and removes Phlegm. *Huang Qin* (Scutellaria), clears Lung Fire, and *Gua Lou Ren* (Trichosanthes) clears Lung Heat and removes Phlegm. They are used as Minister herbs and promote the effects of the King herb. *Zhi Shi* (Aurantium) and *Chen Pi* (Citrus) regulate the *Qi* flow to relieve congestion and remove Phlegm, while *Fu Ling* (Poria) reinforces the Spleen and induces diuresis so that Phlegm is never generated. *Xing Ren* (Armeniaca) redirects the adverse flow of *Qi* downward to relieve cough, while *Ban Xia* (Pinellia) eliminates Damp and removes Phlegm. These five ingredients play the role of Adjuvant herbs.

Cautions and Contraindications: Cold in nature, this formula should be used with caution in debilitated animals with diarrhea due to Spleen *Qi* or *Yang* Deficiency.

Dr. Xie's Comments: I have successfully used *Qing Qi Hua Tan Wan* to treat lower airway infections due to Lung Heat in horses and dogs.

Clinical and Pharmacological Studies: Researchers at Guangzhou TCM college have reported good results when *Qing Qi Hua Tan Wan* was used to treat pneumonia and chronic bronchitis with Excessive Heat and thick, yellow Phlegm.[12]

Qing Zao Jiu Fei Tang (Eliminating Dryness to Let the Lung Survive) 消燥救肺汤

This formula is named after its function. *Qing* translates to clearing or eliminating and *Zao* means dryness; *Qing Zao* means eliminating dryness. *Jiu* means to allow someone to survive or to resuscitate; *Jiu Fei* means resuscitating the Lung or letting the Lung survive. The Lung likes moisture, so the Dry pathogen is the worst enemy of the Lung. Dryness can damage and kill the Lung. Thus, eliminating the Dryness makes the Lung survive. *Tang* means decoction. Thus, *Qing Zao Jiu Fei Tang* means Eliminating Dryness to Let the Lung Survive.

Source: *Yi Men Fa Lu* (*Precepts for Physicians*), written by *Yu Chang* and published in 1658 CE

Ingredients: The original formula (Table 20.7) is composed of 9g *Sang Ye* (Morus), 15g *Shi Gao* (Gypsum), 3g *Gan Cao* (Glycyrrhiza), 2g *Ren Shen* (Ginseng), 3g *Huo Ma Ren* (Cannabis), 3g *E Jiao* (Asinum), 4g *Mai Men Dong* (Ophiopogon), 2g *Xing Ren* (Armeniaca), and 6g *Pi Pa Ye* (Eriobotrya).

Table 20.7. Ingredients and Actions of *Qing Zao Jiu Fei Tang.*

%	English Name	Chinese *Pin-Yin*	Actions
19.1	Morus	*Sang Ye*	Dispel Wind-Heat, clear Liver Heat
31.9	Gypsum	*Shi Gao*	Clear Lung Heat
6.4	Glycyrrhiza	*Gan Cao*	Harmonize
4.3	Ginseng	*Ren Shen*	Tonify *Yuan Qi*, promote the production of Body Fluids
6.4	Cannabis	*Huo Ma Ren*	Moisten the Lung, nourish *Yin*
6.4	Asinum	*E Jiao*	Nourish Blood and *Yin*, moisten dryness, stop bleeding
8.5	Ophiopogon	*Mai Men Dong*	Nourish *Yin*, clear Heat, promote production of Body Fluids
4.3	Armeniaca	*Xing Ren*	Disperse the Lung to relieve cough and dyspnea
12.7	Eriobotrya	*Pi Pa Ye*	Clear Lung Heat, transform Phlegm

Preparation:

1. Powder or capsule method: Herbs are ground into a fine powder. The powder can be encapsulated.
2. Decoction or teapill method: Raw herbs are mixed together and decocted. The herbal water extract (decoction) can be concentrated as granules or teapills.

Actions: Eliminate Dryness and moisten the Lung to stop cough

Indications: Impairment of the Lung by Dry-Heat with fever; dry cough, mouth and throat; red tongue with little coating; fast pulse

Dosage and Usage:

Horses and Cattle: 15–60g, twice daily
Camels: 30–75g, twice daily
Llamas, Alpacas, Pigs, Goats, and Sheep: 5–15g, twice daily
Dogs: 0.5–5g (or 0.1g per kg body weight), twice daily
Cats and Rabbits: 0.2–0.5g (or 0.1g per kg body weight), twice daily
Birds: 0.1–0.2g per kg body weight, twice daily
Use 4–8 weeks until primary clinical signs resolve.

Analysis of Formula: Invasion of Heat-Dry in the Lung and consumption of both *Yin*, Body Fluids, and *Qi* should be treated by eliminating Heat-Dry and moistening the Lung. *Sang Ye* (Morus) disperses the Lung *Qi* to relieve cough; *Shi Gao* (Gypsum) clears Lung Heat; *Sang Ye* (Morus) *and Shi Gao* (Gypsum) act together as King herbs. *E Jiao* (Asinum), *Mai Men Dong* (Ophiopogon), and *Huo Ma Ren* (Cannabis), as Minister herbs, moisten the Lung and nourish *Yin*. *Ren Shen* (Ginseng) tonifies *Qi* and promotes the production of Body Fluids. *Xing Ren* (Armeniaca) and *Pi Pa Ye* (Eriobotrya) disperse Lung *Qi* and moisten Dryness in the Lung. These three herbs are the Adjuvant herbs. *Gan Cao* (Glycyrrhiza) acts as a Messenger herb and harmonizes the effects of the other herbs.

Cautions and Contraindications: *Qing Zao Jiu Fei Tang* is the main formula used to treat impairment of the Lung by Dryness and Heat. Therefore, it must be used with caution or modified when it is used to treat Lung *Qi* Deficiency or a wet cough.

Dr. Xie's Comments: *Qing Zao Jiu Fei Tang* is especially effective for dry cough due to Lung *Yin* Deficiency in the fall or other dry seasons and when environmental conditions are dry.

Clinical and Pharmacological Studies: *Qing Zao Jiu Fei Tang* has been successfully used to treat acute bronchitis in animals, with fever, dry cough without Phlegm, dry mouth and throat, and a red tongue with little coating.[13]

San Zi Yang Qin Tang (Three Seeds to Nourish Elders) 三子养亲汤

San means "three," *Zi* is translated as seed or son, *Yang* means to nourish or tonify and *Qin* means parents or elders. *Yang Qin* translates to nourish one's parents, or elders and *Tang* is Decoction. *San Zi Yang Qin* means Three Seeds to Nourish Elders.

Source: *Han Shi Yi Tong* (Comprehensive Medicine According to Master *Han*), written by *Han Mao* and published in 1522 CE

Ingredients: The original formula (Table 20.8) is composed of 9 g *Zi Su Zi* (Perilla), 9 g *Bai Jie Zi* (Sinapsis) and 9 g *Lai Fu Zi* (Raphanus).

Preparation:
1. Powder or capsule method: Herbs are ground into a fine powder. The powder can be encapsulated.
2. Decoction or teapill method: Raw herbs are mixed together and decocted. The herbal water extract (decoction) can be concentrated as granules or teapills.

Actions: Warm the Lung to transform Phlegm and descend *Qi* to promote the appetite

Indications: Accumulation of Phlegm, Rebellious *Qi*, Food Stagnation with wet cough, dyspnea, hypersalivation, poor appetite, greasy white tongue coating, slippery pulse

Dosage and Usage:
Horses and Cattle: 15–60 g, twice daily
Camels: 30–75 g, twice daily
Llamas, Alpacas, Pigs, Goats, and Sheep: 5–15 g, twice daily
Dogs: 0.5–5 g (or 0.1 g per kg body weight), twice daily
Cats and Rabbits: 0.2–0.5 g (or 0.1 g per kg body weight), twice daily
Birds: 0.1–0.2 g per kg body weight, twice daily
Use 4–16 weeks until primary clinical signs resolve.

Table 20.8. Ingredients and actions of *San Zi Yang Qin Tang*.

%	English Name	Chinese *Pin-Yin*	Actions
33.4	Sinapsis	*Bai Jie Zi*	Warm the Lung to transform Phlegm, move *Qi* to resolve Stagnation
33.3	Perilla	*Zi Su Zi*	Descend *Qi* to transform Phlegm, relieve cough and asthma
33.3	Raphanus	*Lai Fu Zi*	Promote appetite, descend *Qi*, transform Phlegm

Analysis of Formula: Geriatric patients tend to have Cold in the Interior with *Qi* Deficiency in the Middle Burner (*Zhong Jiao*). Spleen *Qi* Deficiency leads to generation of Phlegm. Cold blocks *Qi* flow and allows Phlegm to gather and accumulate in the Lung. As a result, the Lung *Qi* rebels, leading to a wet cough, dyspnea, or wheezing. Spleen *Qi* Deficiency also causes loss of appetite and poor digestion. This condition is treated by warming the Lung to transform Phlegm and descending *Qi* to promote digestion. Thus, *Bai Jie Zi* (Sinapsis) works as the King herb to warm the Lung to dispel Cold, transform Phlegm to stop cough, and move *Qi* to resolve Stagnation. Serving as a Minister herb, *Zi Su Zi* (Perilla) descends Lung *Qi* to stop wheezing and transforms Phlegm to stop coughing. *Lai Fu Zi* (Raphanus) promotes digestion and descends *Qi* to stop Rebellious *Qi*, and it works as both an Adjuvant and Messenger herb.

Cautions and Contraindications: This formula is warm and should be used with caution in patients with *Yin* Deficiency.

Dr. Xie's Comments: *San Zi Yang Qin Tang* is effective for the symptomatic treatment of wet cough and wheezing in geriatric patients, but as soon as these clinical signs resolve, the herbal formula is combined with other herbal formulas to treat the underlying Deficiency. Patients with Lung *Qi* Deficiency should be treated with *Bu Fei San*; those with Lung *Yin* Deficiency need to be treated with *Bai He Gu Jing Tang*.

Hai Zao Yu Hu Tang (Sargassum Jade Pot) 海澡玉壶汤

Hai Zao is Sargassum, the King herb. *Yu Hu* means jade pot. The formula is of great value, like a jade pot. *Tang* means decoction, which was the original form of administration. Thus, *Hai Zao Yu Hu* means Sargassum Jade Pot.

Source: *Wai Ke Zheng Zong* (*True Lineage of External Medicine*), written by *Chen Shigong* and published in 1617 CE

Ingredients: The original formula (Table 20.9) is composed of 30 g *Hai Zao* (Sargassum), 30 g *Zhe Bei Mu* (Fritillaria), 30 g *Chen Pi* (Citrus), 30 g *Kun Bu* (Laminaria), 30 g *Qin Pi* (Citrus), 30 g *Chuan Xiong* (Ligusticum), 30 g *Dang Gui* (Angelica), 30 g *Lian Qiao* (Forsythia), 30 g *Ban Xia* (Pinellia), 30 g *Gan Cao* (Glycyrrhiza), 30 g *Du Huo* (Angelica),and 15 g *Hai Dai* (Zostera).

Table 20.9. Ingredients and actions of *Hai Zao Yu Hu Tang*.

%	English Name	Chinese *Pin-Yin*	Actions
8.6	Sargassum	*Hai Zao*	Resolve Heat-Phlegm, soften hard nodules
8.6	Fritillaria	*Zhe Bei Mu*	Transform Phlegm, relieve cough
8.6	Citrus	*Chen Pi*	Move *Qi*, dry Damp and transform Phlegm
8.6	Laminaria	*Kun Bu*	Resolve Heat-Phlegm, soften hard nodules
8.6	Citrus	*Qing Pi*	Soothe Liver *Qi* to resolve stagnation
8.6	Ligusticum	*Chuan Xiong*	Move Blood and *Qi*, disperse Wind, alleviate pain
8.6	Angelica	*Dang Gui*	Nourish and move Blood
8.6	Forsythia	*Lian Qiao*	Clear Heat and toxins, subdue swelling
8.6	Pinellia	*Ban Xia*	Dry Damp, transform Phlegm
8.6	Glycyrrhiza	*Gan Cao*	Harmonize
8.6	Angelica	*Du Huo*	Expel Wind-Damp, relieve pain
5.4	Zostera	*Hai Dai*	Resolve Heat-Phlegm, soften hard nodules

Preparation:

1. Powder or capsule method: Herbs are ground into a fine powder. The powder can be encapsulated.
2. Decoction or teapill method: Raw herbs are mixed together and decocted. The herbal water extract (decoction) can be concentrated as granules or teapills.

Actions: Resolve Phlegm and soften hardness, move *Qi* and Blood, dissipate masses

Indications: Goiter, hyperthyroidism or thyroid nodules

Dosage and Usage:

Horses and Cattle: 15–60 g, twice daily
Camels: 30–75 g, twice daily
Llamas, Alpacas, Pigs, Goats, and Sheep: 5–15 g, twice daily
Dogs: 0.5–5 g (or 0.1 g per kg body weight), twice daily
Cats and Rabbits: 0.2–0.5 g (or 0.1 g per kg body weight), twice daily
Birds: 0.1–0.2 g per kg body weight, twice daily

Use for 4–16 weeks until the primary clinical signs resolve.

Analysis of Formula: Stagnation of *Qi*, Stasis of Blood, and accumulation of Phlegm can be treated by moving *Qi* and Blood and transforming Phlegm to eliminate nodules. The King herbs, *Hai Zao* (Sargassum), *Kun Bu* (Laminaria) and *Hai Dai* (Zostera) resolve Heat-Phlegm and soften hard nodules. The Minister herbs *Lian Qiao* (Forsythia), *Ban Xia* (Pinellia), and *Zhe Bei Mu* (Fritillaria) enhance the resolution of Heat-Phlegm and soften hard nodules. *Chen Pi* (Citrus) and *Qing Pi* (Citrus) relieve *Qi* Stagnation. *Chuan Xiong* (Ligusticum) and *Dang Gui* (Angelica) move Blood to resolve Stagnation. *Du Huo* (Angelica) expels Wind-Damp and resolves Stagnation. These five herbs are Adjuvant herbs. *Gan Cao* (Glycyrrhiza) acts as the Messenger herb, harmonizing the effects of other herbs.

Cautions and Contraindications: Do not use in patients with *Qi* or Blood Deficiency

Dr. Xie's Comments: I have successfully used *Hai Zao Yu Hu Tang* for hyperthyroidism in cats.

Clinical and Pharmacological Studies: *Hai Zao Yu Hu Tang* has been successfully used to treat autoimmune thyroiditis, thyroid adenoma, and carcinoma.[14] A controlled study was conducted on the effects of *Hai Zao Yu Hu Tang* in 14 cats with feline hyperthyroidism.[15] *Hai Zao Yu Hu Tang* was compared to methimazole and the herbal formula produced statistically significant ($P < 0.05$) greater improvement in every parameter measured except the circulating serum T4 levels.[15]

Xiao Ying San (Eliminating Goiter) 消瘿散

This formula was named after its function. *Xiao* means "eliminating," *Ying* refers to goiter, and San is powder, the form of administration. Thus, *Xiao Ying San* translates literally to Eliminating Goiter Powder.

Source: *Zheng Zhi Zhun Sheng* (Standards of Patterns and Treatments), written by *Wang Ken-Tang* and published in 1602 CE

Ingredients: The original formula (Table 20.10) is composed of 30 g *Hai Zao* (Sargassum), 30 g *Hai Dai* (Zostera), 30 g *Kun Bu* (Laminaria), 30 g *Hai Ma* (Hippocampus), 30 g *Hai Ge Ke* (Cyclina), 30 g *Shi Yan* (Spirifera), and 30 g *Hai Piao Xiao* (Sepia).

Preparation:

1. Powder or capsule method: Herbs are ground into a fine powder. The powder can be encapsulated.
2. Decoction or teapill method: Raw herbs are mixed together and decocted. The herbal water extract (decoction) can be concentrated as granules or teapills.

Actions: Resolve Phlegm, soften hard nodules, tonify Kidney Jing

Indications: Goiter, hypothyroidism, hyperthyroidism

Table 20.10. Ingredients and actions of *Xiao Ying San.*

%	English Name	Chinese *Pin-Yin*	Action
14.3	Sargassum	*Hai Zao*	Resolve Heat-Phlegm, soften hard nodules
14.3	Zostera	*Hai Dai*	Resolve Heat-Phlegm, soften hard nodules
14.3	Laminaria	*Kun Bu*	Resolve Heat-Phlegm, soften hard nodules
14.3	Hippocampus*	*Hai Ma*	Warm the Kidney and tonify *Yang Qi*, eliminate Blood Stasis
14.3	Cyclina	*Hai Ge Ke*	Resolve Heat-Phlegm, soften hard nodules
14.3	Spirifera	*Shi Yan*	Clear Heat, soften the hardness
14.2	Sepia	*Hai Piao Xiao*	Consolidate astringently

**Hai Ma* (Hippocampus) in the original formula should be substituted with *Rou Cong Rong* (Cistanche) and *Tu Si Zi* (Cuscuta) because *Hai Ma* (Hippocampus or Seahorse) is endangered and no longer used.

Dosage and Usage:

Horses and Cattle: 15–60 g, twice daily
Camels: 30–75 g, twice daily
Llamas, Alpacas, Pigs, Goats, and Sheep: 5–15 g, twice daily
Dogs: 0.5–5 g (or 0.1 g per kg body weight), twice daily
Cats and Rabbits: 0.2–0.5 g (or 0.1 g per kg body weight), twice daily
Birds: 0.1–0.2 g per kg body weight, twice daily

Use for 4–16 weeks until primary clinical signs resolve.

Analysis of Formula: *Qi* and Blood Stagnation and the accumulation of Phlegm are treated by resolving Phlegm and moving *Qi* and Blood. *Hai Zao* (Sargassum), *Kun Bu* (Laminaria), *Hai Dai* (Zostera), and *Hai Ge Ke* (Cyclina) act as the King herbs, resolving Heat-Phlegm and softening the hardness. *Shi Yan* (Spirifera), as the Minister herb, resolves Damp-Heat and acts as a diuretic, which can enhance the softening of hard nodules. *Hai Ma* (Hippocampus) warms the Kidney and reinforces *Yang Qi*. *Hai Piao Xiao* (Sepia) acts as an astringent to consolidate Kidney *Jing* (Essence). These two herbs act together as Adjuvant and Messenger herbs, and they restore the Kidney Deficiency.

Cautions and Contraindications: Do not use in patients with hypertension or *Yin* Deficiency

Dr. Xie's Comments: *Xiao Ying San* can be used for both hyperthyroidism and hypothyroidism, especially in patients with renal failure. But *Hai Ma* (Hippocampus) in the original formula should be substituted with *Rou Cong Rong* (Cistanche) and *Tu Si Zi* (Cuscuta) because *Hai Ma* (Hippocampus) is a Seahorse, which is endangered and no longer used.

Clinical and Pharmacological Studies: This formula is similar to *Hai Zao Yu Hu Tang*, but it has been adapted for patients with renal insufficiency.[16]

Nei Xiao Luo Li San (Eliminating Internal Lumps) 内消瘰疬散

Nei means internal. *Xiao* means eliminating. *Luo Li* translates as lumps, nodules and tumor masses. San is powder, the original form of administration. Thus, *Nei Xiao Luo Li San* means Eliminating Internal Lumps Powder.

Source: *Nei Xiao Luo Li San* from *Yi Xue Fa Ming* (*Medical Innovations*), by *Li Ao* in 1115–1234 CE

Ingredients: The original formula (Table 20.11) is composed of 240 g *Xia Ku Cao* (Prunella), 150 g *Xuan Shen* (Scrophularia), 150 g *Shi Yan* (Spirifera), 30 g *Hai Zao* (Sargassum), 30 g *Zhe Bei Mu* (Fritillaria), 30 g *Bo He*

Table 20.11. Ingredients and Actions of *Nei Xiao Luo Li San.*

%	English Name	Chinese *Pin-Yin*	Action
25	Prunella	*Xia Ku Cao*	Clear Liver Fire, resolve masses
15.8	Scrophularia	*Xuan Shen*	Nourish *Yin* to subdue the false Kidney-Fire
15.8	Spirifera	*Shi Yan*	Soften and resolve hard masses
3.1	Sargassum	*Hai Zao*	Resolve Phlegm, soften and resolve hard masses
3.1	Fritillaria	*Zhe Bei Mu*	Transform Phlegm, clear Heat, dispel *Qi* and Blood Stagnation
3.1	Mentha	*Bo He*	Dispel Wind and Heat
3.1	Trichosanthes	*Tian Hua Fen*	Remove Heat, promote Body Fluids, relieve swelling
3.1	Cyclina	*Hai Ge Ke*	Remove Phlegm, soften hard masses
3.1	Ampelopsis	*Bai Lian*	Clear Heat, cool Blood
3.1	Forsythia	*Lian Qiao*	Clear Heat, detoxify, subdue swelling
3.1	Rheum	*Da Huang*	Purge Heat, promote defecation
3.1	Glycyrrhiza	*Gan Cao*	Clear Heat, remove toxins, harmonize
3.1	Rehmannia	*Sheng Di Huang*	Clear Heat, cool Blood, nourish *Yin*
3.1	Platycodon	*Jie Geng*	Transform Phlegm
3.1	Aurantium	*Zhi Ke*	Move *Qi* to relieve pain
3.1	Angelica	*Dang Gui*	Nourish Blood, activate blood circulation
3.1	Niter	*Xiao Shi*	Soften hard masses

(Mentha), 30g *Tian Hua Fen* (Trichosanthes), 30g *Hai Ge Ke* (Cyclina), 30g *Bai Lian* (Ampelopsis), 30g *Lian Qiao* (Forsythia), 30g *Da Huang* (Rheum), 30g *Gan Cao* (Glycyrrhiza), 30g *Sheng Di Huang* (Rehmannia), 30g *Jie Geng* (Platycodon), 30g *Zhi Ke* (Aurantium), 30g *Dang Gui* (Angelica), and 30g *Xiao Shi* (Niter).

Preparation:

1. Powder or capsule method: Herbs are ground into a fine powder. The powder can be encapsulated.
2. Decoction or teapill method: Raw herbs are mixed together and decocted. The herbal water extract (decoction) can be concentrated as granules or teapills.

Actions: Resolve Phlegm, soften hard nodules, eliminate goiter

Indications: Nodules, lumps, tumor masses associated with a purple tongue, slippery pulse

Dosage and Usage:

Horses and Cattle: 15–60g, twice daily
Camels: 30–75g, twice daily
Llamas, Alpacas, Pigs, Goats, and Sheep: 10–15g, twice daily
Dogs: 0.5–5g (or about 0.1g per kg body weight), twice daily
Cats and Rabbits: 0.2–0.5g (or about 0.1g per kg body weight), twice daily
Birds: 0.1 per kg body weight, twice daily

Use for 4–16 weeks until primary clinical signs have resolved.

Analysis of Formula: Lumps and nodules are often caused by Stagnation of *Qi* and Stasis of Blood leading to accumulated Phlegm. This is treated by resolving Phlegm and activating the circulation of *Qi* and Blood to eliminate the nodules. Ingredients *Hai Zao* (Sargassum), *Shi Yan* (Spirifera), *Hai Ge Ke* (Cyclina), and *Xiao Shi* (Niter) act as King herbs to resolve Phlegm and soften hardness to alleviate nodules. Serving as the Minister herbs, *Xia Ku Cao* (Prunella), *Xuan Shen* (Scrophularia), *Zhe Bei Mu* (Fritillaria), *Tian Hua Fen* (Trichosanthes), *Bai Lian* (Ampelosis), *Lian Qiao* (Forsythia), and *Shen Di Huang* (Rehmannia), will transform Phlegm, clear Heat, and soften hard nodules. *Jie Geng* (Platycodon) and *Zhi Ke* (Aurantium) move *Qi* and resolve Stagnation. *Dang Gui* (Angelica) and *Da Huang* (Rheum) move Blood to resolve Stasis, and *Bo He* (Mentha) expels Wind and disperses Stagnation. These five herbs serve as Adjuvant herbs. *Gan Cao* (Glycyrrhiza) acts as the Messenger and guiding herb, which enhances the effect of softening hard nodules to eliminate masses and harmonizes other herbs.

Cautions and Contraindications: This formula should be used with caution in patients with *Qi* Deficiency.

Dr. Xie's Comments: *Nei Xiao Luo Li San* is a very important classical formula to treat the generalized lumps and masses in dogs, cats, and horses.

REFERENCES

1. Chen XD. *Er Chen Tang* for the treatment of cough in domestic animals. Journal of Traditional Chinese Veterinary Medicine and Medica 2000;19(1):36–37.
2. Hu YL. Traditional Chinese Veterinary Medicine. Beijing: China Agriculture Press, 2006:413.
3. Li F. Literature Review on Studies of Herbal Prescriptions. Nanjing: Jiangsu Science and Technology Press, 1981: 605–611.
4. Niu YN. *Zhi Sou San* for the treatment of chronic cough in domestic animals. Journal of Traditional Chinese Veterinary Medicine 2005;(5):20–22.
5. Hu YL. Traditional Chinese Veterinary Medicine. Beijing: China Agriculture Press, 2006:414.
6. Wang QS. *Ma Xing Shi Gan Tang* for the treatment of asthma due to Lung Heat in sheep and goats. Journal of Traditional Chinese Veterinary Medicine 2005;(3):42–43.
7. E ZH. *Ma Xing Shi Gan Tang* was used to treat Patterns of lung heat with lung *Qi* deficiency. Journal of Traditional Chinese Veterinary Medicine and Medica 2001;20(3):24.
8. Hu YL. Traditional Chinese Veterinary Medicine. Beijing: China Agriculture Press, 2006:390.
9. Hou K. *Su Zi Jiang Qi Tang* has a better effect to control respiration system disease in chickens. An Hui Agriculture 2004;(11):35.
10. Li F. Literature Review on Studies of Herbal Prescriptions. Nanjing: Jian Su Science and Technology Press, 1981.
11. Hu YL. Traditional Chinese Veterinary Medicine. Beijing: China Agriculture Press, 2006:414–415.
12. Guangzhou TCM College. TCM Science of Prescriptions. Shanghai: Shanghai Science and Technology Press, 1979:186–187.
13. Hu YL. Traditional Chinese Veterinary Medicine. Beijing: China Agriculture Press, 2006:415.
14. Li F. Literature Review on Studies of Chinese Herbal Prescriptions. Nanjing: Jiangsu Science and Technology Press, 1981:71–73.
15. Wilcox DL, Liu HR, Ma Y, Xie H, Tangjitjaroen W. Comparison of the Chinese herbal formula *Hai Zao Yu Hu Tang* and methimazole for the treatment of feline hyperthyroidism. American Journal of Traditional Chinese Veterinary Medicine 2009;4(1):27–38.
16. Guangzhou TCM College, Science of Chinese Herbal Formulas. Shanghai: Shanghai Science and Technology Press, 1979: 18–19.

21 Herbal Formulas to Clear Heat 清热方

Xiujun Wang, Michael Bartholomew, Huisheng Xie

Herbal formulas to clear Heat are used to clear Damp-Heat, Summer-Heat, Heat Toxin, and Interior Heat Patterns. Interior Heat conditions include Heat in the *Zang-Fu* organs, Heat in the *Qi* Level, *Ying* (Nutrient) Level, and *Xue* (Blood) Level. Differentiation of these Heat Patterns is discussed in Chapter 4. *Wei, Qi, Ying and Xue*, the Four Levels (or Four Stages), are a Pattern Identification system established by Ye Tianshi and described in his book, *Wai Gan Wen Re Pian* (*Treatise on Exogenous Epidemic Fevers*), published in 1746. This system is recommended when the initial clinical signs of disease include acute febrile conditions (Excess Heat). *Wei, Qi, Ying, and Xue* represent Four Levels of a disease's pathological development (Table 21.1). The most superficial is the *Wei* Level (Exterior), the next level is the *Qi* Level (Internal organs), deeper still is the *Ying* level (Nutrient Stage), and the deepest level is the *Xue* Level (Blood Stage). *Ying* and *Xue* Patterns usually refer to deep and severe conditions, and together they are called the *Ying-Xue* level. Cool herbal formulas to release the Exterior (Chapter 19) are used to treat Heat in the *Wei* Level.

Among the Eight Methods (*Ba-Fa*) of TCVM therapeutics, herbal formulas to clear Heat utilize a clearing method (*Qing-Fa*). The term "clear" refers to the elimination and purification of Heat Pathogens out of the body. Because of their Heat-clearing nature, these formulas are cold and can easily injure Spleen and Stomach *Yang Qi*. Therefore, the formulas often include ingredients that protect the functions of the Stomach and Spleen and are often used for only a short time.

Bai Hu Tang (White Tiger) 白虎汤

Bai means white, *Hu* means tiger, and *Tang* means decoction. Therefore, *Bai Hu Tang* is translated as White Tiger Decoction. In Chinese, *Bai Hu* is another name of *Shi Gao* (Gypsum) with its white color and potent action like a tiger.

Source: *Shang Han Za Bing Lun* (*Treatise on Cold-Induced Disorders and Miscellaneous Diseases*), written by *Zhang Zhong-Jing* in 220 CE

Ingredients: The original formula for *Bai Hu Tang* is composed of 250 g *Shi Gao* (Gypsum), 45 g *Zhi Mu* (Anemarrhena), 25 g *Gan Cao* (Glycyrrhiza), and 45 g *Jing Mi* (Oryza) (Table 21.2).

Preparation:

1. Powder or capsule method: Herbs are ground into a fine powder. The powder can be encapsulated.
2. Decoction or teapill method: Raw herbs are mixed together and decocted. The herbal water extract

Table 21.1. The Four Levels (Four Stages) of an illness.

Stage	Level or Stage	Location	Herbal Formula
1	*Wei* (Defense)	Body Surface, Body Fluids, muscles, joints	*Yin Qiao San*
2	*Qi*	Lung, Stomach, Large Intestine	*Bai Hu Tang*
3	*Ying* (Nutrient)	*Shen*, Heart, Pericardium	*Qing Ying Tang*
4	*Xue* (Blood)	Blood Heat and hemorrhage	*Xi Jiao Di Huang Tang*

Table 21.2. Ingredients and actions of *Bai Hu Tang*.

%	English Name	Chinese *Pin-Yin*	Actions
68.5	Gypsum	*Shi Gao*	Clear Stomach Heat
12.3	Anemarrhena	*Zhi Mu*	Clear Stomach Heat and Lung Fire, produce Body Fluids
6.9	Glycyrrhiza	*Gan Cao*	Harmonize other herbs
12.3	Oryza	*Jing Mi*	Nourish Stomach *Yin*

(decoction) can be concentrated as granules or teapills.

Actions: Clear Heat and produce Body Fluids

Indications: Excess Heat in *Qi* Stage/Level with a high fever, easy/profuse sweating, excessive thirst, dry mouth and red tongue, and big and strong pulse

Dosage and Usage:
Horses and Cattle: 15–60 g, twice daily
Camels: 30–75 g, twice daily
Llamas, Alpacas, Goats, Sheep, and Pigs: 5–15 g, twice daily
Dogs: 0.5–5 g (or 0.1 g per kg body weight), twice daily
Cats and Rabbits: 0.2–0.5 g (or 0.1 g per kg body weight), twice daily
Birds: 0.1–0.2 g per kg body weight, twice daily
Use for 1–2 weeks until the primary clinical signs have resolved.

Analysis of Formula: *Bai Hu Tang* is the most common formula for the treatment of Excess Heat of the *Yang Ming* Channels (Large Intestine and Stomach) and Heat at the *Qi* Stage/Level. In this formula, *Shi Gao* (Gypsum), a pungent, sweet, and very cold herb, is the King herb, which can clear Heat in the *Yang Ming* or *Qi* Level. *Zhi Mu* (Anemarrhena), which is bitter, cold, and moistening, serves as the Minister herb, which clears Heat and moistens Dryness. *Gan Cao* (Glycyrrhiza) and *Jing Mi* (Oryza), the Adjuvant and Messenger herbs, tonify the Stomach and nourish *Yin*. They also moderate the coldness of *Shi Gao* (Gypsum) and *Zhi Mu* (Anemarrhena), which can damage the Spleen and Stomach *Qi*. All of the herbs together clear Heat and the produce Body Fluids.

Cautions and Contraindications: *Bai Hu Tang* is contraindicated in patients with *Yin* Deficiency or Spleen *Qi* Deficiency.

Dr. Xie's Comments: *Bai Hu Tang* is often used for the so called "Four Excessive Signs," which include excessively high fever, excessive thirst, excessive sweating in horses or panting in dogs, and an excessive pulse. The Pattern differentiation of Heat in the *Qi* Level (Stage) is made on the basis of these four excessive signs.

Clinical and Pharmacological Studies: *Bai Hu Tang* has been effectively used to treat high fever of unknown origin in pigs.[1] *Bai Hu Tang* has also been used for the treatment of 48 cases in human patients with high fever caused by the exogenous pathogens Heat or Damp Heat. Forty-four patients (91.6%) clinically recovered with *Bai Hu Tang* medication.[2]

Qing Ying Tang (Clearing *Ying* Heat) 清营汤

Qing means to clear or remove, *Ying* refers to Heat in the *Ying* Stage (Nutrient Level) and *Tang* is decoction, the original form of this formula. Together, *Qing Ying Tang* is a formula to clear *Ying* Heat (Heat in *Ying* Level of the body).

Source: *Wen Bing Tiao Bian* (*Systematic Difference of Warm Diseases*), written by *Wu Ju-Tong* and published in 1798

Ingredients: The original formula of *Qing Ying Tang* (Table 21.3) was composed of 10 g *Xi Jiao* (Rhinoceros), 60 g *Sheng Di Huang* (Rehmannia), 45 g *Xuan Shen* (Scrophularia), 15 g *Zhu Ye* (Bambusa), 45 g *Jin Yin Hua* (Lonicera), 30 g *Lian Qiao* (Forsythia), 25 g *Huang Lian* (Coptis), 30 g *Dan Shen* (Salvia), and 45 g *Mai Men Dong* (Ophiopogon). Today, *Xi Jiao* (Rhinoceros) horn is substituted with *Shui Niu Jiao* (Bubali) Water buffalo horn because of the endangered status of the rhinoceros.

Preparation:
1. Powder or capsule method: Herbs are ground into a fine powder. The powder can be encapsulated.
2. Decoction or teapill method: Raw herbs are mixed together and decocted. The herbal water extract (decoction) can be concentrated as granules or teapills.

Actions: Cool Blood and detoxify, clear Heat and nourish *Yin*

Indications: Pathologic Heat just entering the *Ying* Stage with a high fever, increased thirst, faint macular

Table 21.3. Ingredients and actions of *Qing Ying Tang*.

%	English Name	Chinese *Pin-Yin*	Actions
3.3	Rhinoceros*	*Xi Jiao*	Cool Blood, remove toxins
19.7	Rehmannia	*Sheng Di Huang*	Nourish *Yin*, eliminate Heat, cool Blood
14.8	Scrophularia	*Xuan Shen*	Clear Heat and nourish *Yin*
4.9	Bambusa	*Zhu Ye*	Clear Heat, promote diuresis
14.8	Lonicera	*Jin Yin Hua*	Clear Heat and remove toxins
9.8	Forsythia	*Lian Qiao*	Clear Heat and remove toxins
8.2	Coptis	*Huang Lian*	Clear Heat, expel Damp
9.8	Salvia	*Dan Shen*	Cool Blood
14.7	Ophiopogon	*Mai Men Dong*	Nourish *Yin* and clear Heat

*The original formulation used *Xi Jiao* (Rhinoceros horn). Its use is now prohibited because the rhinoceros is endangered. Today, water buffalo horn, or *Shui Niu Jiao* (Bubali), is used instead.

eruptions, restlessness or coma, red tongue, dry mouth, slippery and fast pulse

Dosage and Usage:
Horses and Cattle: 15–60 g, twice daily
Camels: 30–75 g, twice daily
Llamas, Alpacas, Goats, Sheep, and Pigs: 5–15 g, twice daily
Dogs: 0.5–5 g (or 0.1 g per kg body weight), twice daily
Cats and Rabbits: 0.2–0.5 g (or 0.1 g per kg body weight), twice daily
Birds: 0.1–0.2 g per kg body weight, twice daily
Use for 1–4 weeks until the primary clinical signs have resolved.

Analysis of Formula: This formula is effective to treat Heat in the *Ying* Level or Heat moving from the *Qi* Level into the *Ying* Level. *Xi Jiao* (Rhinoceros), as the King herb, can cool and relieve toxic Heat from the *Ying* Level, as can its modern-day substitute, *Shui Niu Jiao* (Bubali). Excessive Heat can damage *Yin*; *Sheng Di Huang* (Rehmannia), *Xuan Shen* (Scrophularia), *Mai Men Dong* (Ophiopogon), as the Minister herbs, can protect *Yin* and eliminate Heat by nourishing *Yin*. *Huang Lian* (Coptis), *Jin Yin Hua* (Lonicera), *Lian Qiao* (Forsythia), and *Zhu Ye* (Bambusa) are the Adjuvant herbs used to clear and relieve *Qi* Level Heat. This can prevent further invasion by pathogenic Heat. *Dan Shen* (Salvia), the Messenger herb, cools Blood, promotes Blood flow, eliminates Stasis to activate Blood circulation, and can guide other herbs to the Heart Channel to clear Heat in the Heart and Pericardium. All of the herbs together function to cool the *Ying* Level, clear Heat, remove toxins, and nourish *Yin*.

Cautions and Contraindications: This formula should be used with caution in cases with Spleen *Qi* Deficiency.

Dr. Xie's Comments: *Qing Ying Tang* is used to treat Heat in the *Ying* Level/Stage. In veterinary practice, it is often used in treating encephalitis, meningitis, and other neurological disorders with Heat as well as behavior changes occurring after an infectious disease, including parvovirus and distemper.

Clinical and Pharmacological Studies: In one clinical study, *Li* used *Qing Ying Tang* to treat 20 bovine cases of postpartum fever, noting a positive clinical response within 2 doses.[3] *Qing Ying Tang* has also been successfully used to treat a True-Heat with False-Cold Pattern in cattle, in which Cold signs (cold limbs and extremities), were seen in Excess Heat patients (high fever, slippery and forceful pulse).[4]

Xi Jiao Di Huang Tang (Horn and Rehmannia) 犀角地黄汤

Xi Jiao refers to rhinoceros horn, *Di Huang* refers to *Sheng Di Huang* (Rehmannia), and Tang means decoction. Thus, *Xi Jiao Di Huang Tang* is translated as Rhinoceros Horn and Rehmannia Decoction. Historically, *Xi Jiao* (Rhinoceros) was used in this formulation, but now the rhinoceros is endangered, so its use is prohibited and water buffalo horn or *Shui Niu Jiao* (Bubali) is used instead.

Source: *Qian Jin Yao Fang* (*Thousand Ducat Formulas*), written by *Sun Si-Miao* and published in 652 CE

Ingredients: The original formula of *Xi Jiao Di Huang Tang* is composed of 10 g *Xi Jiao* (Rhinoceros), 150 g *Sheng Di Huang* (Rehmannia), 60 g *Bai Shao Yao* (Paeonia), and 45 g *Mu Dan Pi* (Moutan). *Xi Jiao* (Rhinoceros) is substituted with a higher dose of water buffalo horn (3–4 times as much as *Xi Jiao*) or *Shui Niu Jiao* (Bubali) (Table 21.4).

Preparation:
1. Powder or capsule method: Herbs are ground into a fine powder. The powder can be encapsulated.
2. Decoction or teapill method: Raw herbs are mixed together and decocted. The herbal water extract (decoction) can be concentrated as granules or teapills.

Actions: Clear Heat and remove toxins, cool Blood, activate Blood to eliminate Stasis

Indications: Excess Blood Heat or Heat in the Blood Level

Dosage and Usage:
Horses and Cattle: 15–60 g, twice daily
Camels: 30–75 g, twice daily
Llamas, Alpacas, Goats, Sheep, and Pigs: 5–15 g, twice daily

Table 21.4. Ingredients and actions of *Xi Jiao Di Huang Tang*.

%	English Name	Chinese *Pin-Yin*	Actions
12	Bubali*	*Shui Niu Jiao*	Cool Blood, remove toxins
50	Rehmannia	*Sheng Di Huang*	Nourish *Yin*, eliminate Heat, cool Blood to stop bleeding
22	Paeonia	*Bai Shao Yao*	Astringe *Yin*, relieve pain
16	Moutan	*Mu Dan Pi*	Cool Blood, promote Blood flow

*The original formulation used *Xi Jiao* (Rhinoceros horn). Its use is now prohibited because the rhinoceros is endangered. Today, water buffalo horn, or *Shui Niu Jiao* (Bubali), is used instead.

Dogs: 0.5–5 g (or 0.1 g per kg body weight), twice daily
Cats and Rabbits: 0.2–0.5 g (or 0.1 g per kg body weight), twice daily
Birds: 0.1–0.2 g per kg body weight, twice daily
Use for 2–6 weeks until the primary clinical signs have resolved.

Analysis of Formula: The formula is used to treat diseases with pathogenic warm factors or Heat in the Blood Level. Aggressive toxic Heat can damage Blood and *Ying* and Heat can disturb the Heart spirit *(Shen)*. *Shui Niu Jiao* (Bubali) is used as the King herb to cool the *Ying* Level, clear Heat, and detoxify. *Sheng Di Huang* (Rehmannia), the Minster herb, is also used to eliminate Heat by nourishing *Yin* and cooling the Blood to stop bleeding. *Bai Shao Yao* (Paeonia) is used to nourish Yin, and *Mu Dan Pi* (Moutan) is used to cool Blood and promote Blood circulation. Both *Bai Shao Yao* and *Mu Dan Pi* are the Adjuvant and Messenger herbs. All four herbs of the formula together clear Heat, nourish *Yin*, cool Blood, and activate Blood circulation to eliminate Stasis.

Cautions and Contraindications: This formula should be used cautiously in patients with Spleen *Qi* Deficiency.

Dr. Xie's Comments: Since *Xi Jiao Di Huang Tang* is used to treat Heat in the Blood Level or Stage, it is often used to treat hemorrhage or other disorders of hemostasis, such as disseminated intravascular coagulation (DIC), that occur secondarily to infectious or other disease processes in veterinary practice.

Clinical and Pharmacological Studies: The formula not only treats Excess Heat in the Blood Level, but has other functions as well. In one clinical study Fang used *Xi Jiao Di Huang Tang* to treat patients with diabetic peripheral neuropathy, which is due to Dry-Heat burning Body Fluids and *Qi* Deficiency. The patients had redness of the skin, lassitude, dry mouth, constipation, yellow and greasy coating of the tongue, and slippery and fast pulse, which improved in 10 days after 1 dose per day of *Xi Jiao Di Huang Tang*.[5] Another application of *Xi Jiao Di Huang Tang* has been to treat snake bites.[6]

Huang Lian Jie Du Tang (Coptis for Detoxification) 黄连解毒汤

Huang Lian refers to Coptis, the King herb of this formula. *Jie* means anti, and *Du* is toxins; so *Jie Du* means detoxification. Thus, *Huang Lian Jie Du* translates literally to Coptis for Detoxification.

Source: *Wai Tai Mi Yao (Arcane Essentials from the Imperial Library)*, written by *Wang Tao* in 752 CE

Ingredients: The original formula of *Huang Lian Jie Du Tang* is composed of 30 g *Huang Lian* (Coptis), 60 g *Huang Qin* (Scutellaria), 60 g *Huang Bai* (Phellodendron), and 45 g *Zhi Zi* (Gardenia) (Table 21.5).

Table 21.5. Ingredients and actions of *Huang Lian Jie Du Tang*.

%	English Name	Chinese *Pin-Yin*	Actions
15.5	Coptis	*Huang Lian*	Purge Heart Fire and Middle Burner Fire
31	Scutellaria	*Huang Qin*	Purge the Upper Burner Fire
31	Phellodendron	*Huang Bai*	Purge Lower Burner Fire
22.5	Gardenia	*Zhi Zi*	Purge Triple Burner Fire

Preparation:
1. Powder or capsule method: Herbs are ground into a fine powder. The powder can be encapsulated.
2. Decoction or teapill method: Raw herbs are mixed together and decocted. The herbal water extract (decoction) can be concentrated as granules or teapills.

Actions: Purge Fire to remove toxins

Indications: Heat in the Triple Burner (the *San Jiao* or Triple Heater) with excessive Heat or Heat Toxins all over the body with clinical signs of swollen lymph nodes, edema, high fever, restlessness, red tongue, and full pulse

Dosage and Usage:
Horses and Cattle: 15–60 g, twice daily
Camels: 30–75 g, twice daily
Llamas, Alpacas, Goats, Sheep, and Pigs: 5–15 g, twice daily
Dogs: 0.5–5 g (or 0.1 g per kg body weight), twice daily
Cats and Rabbits: 0.2–0.5 g (or 0.1 g per kg body weight), twice daily
Birds: 0.1–0.2 g per kg body weight, twice daily
Use for 1–2 weeks until the primary clinical signs have resolved.

Analysis of Formula: This formula is used to treat diseases with Excess Toxic Heat by purging Fire to remove toxins. *Huang Lian* (Coptis), the King herb, purges Excess Fire in the Heart and Middle Burner (*Zhong Jiao*). *Huang Qin* (Scutellaria) purges Fire from the Upper Burner *(Shang Jiao)*, *Huang Bai* (Phellodendron) purges Fire from the Lower Burner (*Xia Jiao*), and *Zhi Zi* (Gardenia) purges Triple Burner *(San Jiao)* Fire as it drains through the Bladder Channels to the bladder. These three herbs are all Minister herbs. The four herbs together expel pathogens and toxic Heat.

Cautions and Contraindications: Use only to treat Excess Heat (*Shi Re*) or virulent Fire. *Huang Lian Jie Du Tang* is contraindicated for patients with False Heat or *Yin* Deficiency Heat (*Xu Re*).

Dr. Xie's Comments: Since *Huang Lian Jie Du Tang* is used to treat Heat or Damp Heat in the entire body, in veterinary practice, it is often used to treat bacterial infections of the urinary tract, Lungs, and skin.

Clinical and Pharmacological Studies: Enterotoxemia is an acute and fatal infectious disease of sheep and goats. *Huang Lian Jie Du Tang* has been used successfully to treat enterotoxemia in both sheep and goats.[7] *Huang Lian Jie Du Tang* has been shown to enhance the humoral immunity of tumor-bearing mice by strengthening the action of the natural killer cells (NK) cells and stimulating T-cells to excrete Interleukin-4 (IL-4).[8]

Pu Ji Xiao Du Yin (Universal Detoxification) 普济消毒饮

Pu Ji means universal or global, *Xiao* means clearing or eliminating, *Du* means toxin, and *Yin* refers to decoction, the form of herbal administration. *Pu Ji Xiao Du* can therefore be literally translated as Universal Detoxification.

Source: *Dong Yuan Shi Xiao Fang* (*Effective Formulas of Li Dong-Yuan*), written by *Li Dong-Yuan* and published during the *Jin-Yuan* Dynasty (1115–1368 CE)

Ingredients: The original formula of *Pu Ji Xiao Du Yin* is composed of 15 g *Huang Qin* (Scutellaria), 15 g *Huang Lian* (Coptis), 6 g *Chen Pi* (Citrus), 6 g *Gan Cao* (Glycyrrhiza), 6 g *Xuan Shen* (Scrophularia), 6 g *Chai Hu* (Bupleurum), 6 g *Jie Geng* (Platycodon), 3 g *Lian Qiao* (Forsythia), 3 g *Ban Lan Gen* (Isatis), 3 g *Ma Bo* (Lasiosphaera), 3 g *Niu Bang Zi* (Arctium), 3 g *Bo He* (Mentha), 2 g *Jiang Can* (Bombyx), and 2 g *Sheng Ma* (Cimicifuga) (Table 21.6).

Preparation:

1. Powder or capsule method: Herbs are ground into a fine powder. The powder can be encapsulated.
2. Decoction or teapill method: Raw herbs are mixed together and decocted. The herbal water extract (decoction) can be concentrated as granules or teapills.

Actions: Clear Heat, remove toxins, expel Wind

Indications: Excess Heat in the Upper Burner (*Shang Jiao*), Lung Heat with clinical signs of redness, swelling and sensitivity of the head and face, dyspnea or asthma, fever, thirst, a red tongue, and a fast and forceful pulse

Table 21.6. Ingredients and actions of *Pu Ji Xiao Du Yin.*

%	English Name	Chinese *Pin-Yin*	Actions
19	Scutellaria	*Huang Qin*	Purge Upper Burner Fire
19	Coptis	*Huang Lian*	Purge Heart Fire and Middle Burner Fire
7.6	Citrus	*Chen Pi*	Invigorate Spleen and regulate *Qi*, dry Damp to eliminate Phlegm
7.6	Glycyrrhiza	*Gan Cao*	Harmonize and tonify *Qi*
7.6	Scrophularia	*Xuan Shen*	Nourish *Yin* to lessen Fire and detoxify
7.6	Bupleurum	*Chai Hu*	Expel Wind and relieve Heat, soothe the Liver *Qi*
7.6	Platycodon	*Jie Geng*	Open the Lung, relieve sore throat
3.8	Forsythia	*Lian Qiao*	Clear Heat, remove toxins, and remove Stasis
3.8	Isatis	*Ban Lan Gen*	Clear Heat, remove toxins, and cool Blood
3.8	Lasiosphaera	*Ma Bo*	Clear Heat, stop bleeding and remove toxins
3.8	Arctium	*Niu Bang Zi*	Dispel Wind and Heat
3.8	Mentha	*Bo He*	Expel Wind and dissipate Heat
2.5	Bombyx	*Jiang Can*	Dispel Wind and relieve convulsions, dissipate Phlegm and remove Stasis
2.5	Cimicifuga	*Sheng Ma*	Clear Heat and remove toxins, ascend *Yang-Qi*

Dosage and Usage:

Horses and Cattle: 15–60 g, twice daily
Camels: 30–75 g, twice daily
Llamas, Alpacas, Goats, Sheep, and Pigs: 5–15 g, twice daily
Dogs: 0.5–5 g (or 0.1 g per kg body weight), twice daily
Cats and Rabbits: 0.2–0.5 g (or 0.1 g per kg body weight), twice daily
Birds: 0.1–0.2 g per kg body weight, twice daily

Use for 3–6 weeks until the primary clinical signs have resolved.

Analysis of Formula: The formula is used to treat acute contagious diseases characterized by swelling and redness of the face and head, caused by Wind-Heat or Heat Toxin attacking the head and face. *Huang Lian* (Coptis) and *Huang Qin* (Scutellaria), the King herbs, clear Heat, purge pathogenic Fire, and expel Upper Burner *(Shang Jiao)* toxic Heat. *Niu Bang Zi* (Arctium), *Lian Qiao* (Forsythia), *Bo He* (Mentha), and *Jiang Can* (Bombyx), the Minister herbs, disperse Wind-Heat of the head and face. *Xuan Shen* (Scrophularia), *Ma Bo* (Lasiosphaera), and *Ban Lan Gen* (Isatis) enhance the King herbs' functions of clearing Heat and removing toxins. *Gan Cao* (Glycyrrhiza) and *Jie Geng* (Platycodon) relieve soreness of the throat and *Chen Pi* (Citrus) regulates *Qi* to disperse Stagnation. These six herbs function as Adjuvant herbs. *Sheng Ma* (Cimicifuga) and *Chai Hu* (Bupleurum) dispel Wind-Heat and guide the other herbs to the head as the Messenger herbs. All of the herbs work together to clear Heat, remove toxins, and dispel Wind-Heat.

Cautions and Contraindications: Since *Pu Ji Xiao Du Yin* is normally used to treat Excess Heat in the Upper Burner (*Shang Jiao*), it must be used with caution in patients with False Heat due to *Yin* Deficiency.

Dr. Xie's Comments: In veterinary practice, *Pu Ji Xiao Du Yin* is often used to treat equine adenitis (strangles), otitis, cellulitis, and lymphangitis due to Excess Damp-Heat.

Clinical and Pharmacological Studies: *Pu Ji Xiao Du Yin* has been used to treat 74 human cases of epidemic parotitis (mumps). After taking the herbal medication, 72 cases (97.3%) had clinically recovered.[9] Similar results were found in another clinical trial, in which *Pu Ji Xiao Du Yin* was used to treat 56 human cases of epidemic parotitis (mumps).[10]

Qing Wen Bai Du Yin (Clearing Epidemics to Defeat Toxins) 清瘟败毒饮

Qing means clearing and expelling, *Wen* means epidemics or infectious diseases, *Bai* means to defeat or overcome, *Du* means toxins and *Yin* is decoction. Thus, *Qing Wen Bai Du* is translated as Clearing Epidemics to Defeat Toxins.

Source: *Yi Zhen Yi De* (*Achievement Regarding Epidemic Rashes*), written by *Yu Shi-Yu* and published in 1794 CE

Ingredients: *Qing Wen Bai Du Yin* is composed of 120g *Shi Gao* (Gypsum), 30g *Zhi Mu* (Anemarrhena), 6g *Xi Jiao* (Rhinoceros), 30g *Sheng Di Huang* (Rehmannia), 20g *Mu Dan Pi* (Moutan), 25g *Xu Shen* (Scrophularia), 25g *Chi Shao Yao* (Paeonia), 20g *Huang Lian* (Coptis), 30g *Zhi Zi* (Gardenia), 25g *Huang Qin* (Scutellaria), 30g *Lian Qiao* (Forsythia), 25g *Jie Geng* (Platycodon), 25g *Dan Zhu Ye* (Lophatherum), and 15g *Gan Cao* (Glycyrrhiza) (Table 21.7).

Preparation:
1. Powder or capsule method: Herbs are ground into a fine powder. The powder can be encapsulated.
2. Decoction or teapill method: Raw herbs are mixed together and decocted. The herbal water extract (decoction) can be concentrated as granules or teapills.

Actions: Clear Heat of the *Qi* Level, cool Blood, purge Fire, remove toxins

Table 21.7. Ingredients and actions of *Qing Wen Bai Du Yin*.

%	English Name	Chinese *Pin-Yin*	Actions
28.2	Gypsum	*Shi Gao*	Clear Heat, purge Fire
7	Anemarrhena	*Zhi Mu*	Clear Heat, nourish *Yin*
1.4	Rhinoceros*	*Xi Jiao*	Cool Blood, calm mind
7.	Rehmannia	*Sheng Di Huang*	Cool Blood, nourish *Yin*
4.7	Moutan	*Mu Dan Pi*	Cool Blood, disperse Stasis
5.9	Scrophularia	*Xuan Shen*	Clear heat, nourish *Yin*
5.9	Paeonia	*Chi Shao Yao*	Remove Heat to cool Blood
4.7	Coptis	*Huang Lian*	Purge Heart Fire and Middle Burner Fire
7	Gardenia	*Zhi Zi*	Purge Triple Burner Fire
5.9	Scutellaria	*Huang Qin*	Purge Upper Burner Fire
7	Forsythia	*Lian Qiao*	Clear Heat and remove toxins
5.9	Platycodon	*Jie Geng*	Open the Lung, eliminate Phlegm
5.9	Lophatherum	*Dan Zhu Ye*	Promote urination to drain Heat
3.5	Glycyrrhiza	*Gan Cao*	Harmonize and tonify *Qi*

*The original formulation used *Xi Jiao* (Rhinoceros horn) Its use is now prohibited because the rhinoceros is endangered. Today, water buffalo horn, or *Shui Niu Jiao* (Bubali), is used instead.

Indications: Excessive toxic Heat, Heat in both *Qi* and Blood Levels with signs of a high fever, restlessness or manic behavior, increased thirst, macules, dark red tongue, and fast pulse

Dosage and Usage:
Horses and Cattle: 15–60g, twice daily
Camels: 30–75g, twice daily
Llamas, Alpacas, Goats, Sheep, and Pigs: 5–15g, twice daily
Dogs: 0.5–5g (or 0.1g per kg body weight), twice daily
Cats and Rabbits: 0.2–0.5g (or 0.1g per kg body weight), twice daily
Birds: 0.1–0.2g per kg body weight, twice daily

Use for 2–4 weeks until the primary clinical signs have resolved.

Analysis of Formula: This was a common formula to treat epidemic diseases in ancient times. It is still commonly used to treat toxic Excess Heat in both the *Qi* and Blood Levels. The formula is based on three other classical formulations including *Bai Hu Tang*, *Huang Lian Jie Du Tang*, and *Qing Ying Tang*. In the formula, *Shi Gao* (Gypsum) and *Zhi Mu* (Anemarrhena) are the King herbs and clear the Heat in the *Qi* Level. *Shui Niu Jiao* (Bubali), which is substituted for Rhinoceros; *Sheng Di Huang* (Rehmannia); *Mu Dan Pi* (Moutan); *Xuan Shen* (Scrophularia); and *Chi Shao Yao* (Paeonia) clear Heat of the *Ying* Level and cool Blood to remove pathogenic Heat. *Huang Lian* (Coptis), *Zhi Zi* (Gardenia), *Huang Qin* (Scutellaria), and *Lian Qiao* (Forsythia) purge Excess Fire or Heat of the Triple Burner (*San Jiao*). These nine herbs are all Minister herbs. *Dan Zhu Ye* (Lophatherum) promotes urination to drain Heart Fire, which can lead Heat downward. Conversely, *Jie Geng* (Platycodon) can carry the action of other herbs upward. Together, these two herbs act as Adjuvant herbs. The Messenger herb is *Gan Cao* (Glycyrrhiza), which clears Heat, removes toxins, and coordinates the other herbs' actions. Working synergistically these herbs make up a potent formula for clearing Heat from *Qi* and Blood Levels and removing toxic Heat.

Cautions and Contraindications: Only use *Qing Wen Bai Du Yin* to treat Excess Fire or Excess Heat (*Shi Re*). This formula is contraindicated in patients with False Heat (*Xu Re*).

Dr. Xie's Comments: *Qing Wen Bai Du Yin* has similar actions to *Huang Lian Jie Du Tang* to clear Heat and remove toxins. *Qing Wen Bai Du Yin* uses a high dose of *Shi Gao* (Gypsum) to clear Heat and is combined with *Shui Niu Jiao* (Bubali) and *Sheng Di Huang* (Rehmannia) to cool Blood. These actions make this formula useful for treating meningitis, septicemia, distemper, and parvovirus due to Heat in both the *Qi* and Blood Levels. *Huang Lian Jie Du Tang* is a fundamental formula to clear Heat-Toxin from the *Qi* Level, and *Qing Wen Bai Du Yin* is used more commonly when the Heat-Toxin has reached the Blood Level from the *Qi* Level.

Clinical and Pharmacological Studies: Research has confirmed that *Qing Wen Bai Du Yin* has strong antibiotic, antiviral, and antipyretic effects. Streptococcosis often causes significant toxic Excess Heat and in these cases, *Qing Wen Bai Du Yin* can produce a good therapeutic effect with fewer side effects and less bacterial drug resistance than antibiotics.[11] Hemorrhagic fever with renal syndrome (HFRS, caused by hantaviruses) is a warm disease according to TCVM theory. Its progression, like others, can also be divided into the four stages: *Wei*, *Qi*, *Ying* (Nutrient), and *Xue* (Blood). The virus invades and stays in the Interior to produce Heat, thereby damaging the blood vessels and leading to hemorrhage. Bao successfully treated 40 cases of HFRS with this formula.[12]

Wu Wei Xiao Du Yin (Five Herbs to Eliminate Toxins) 五味消毒饮

Wu means five, *Wei* refers to ingredient or herb, *Xiao* means eliminate and *Du* means toxins. *Yin* has the same meaning as *Tang*, decoction. Together, they mean Five Herbs to Eliminate Toxins.

Source: *Yi Zong Jin Jian* (*Golden Mirror of Medicine*), written by *Wu Qian* and published in 1742 CE

Table 21.8. Ingredients and actions of *Wu Wei Xiao Du Yin*.

%	English Name	Chinese *Pin-Yin*	Actions
22.2	Lonicera	*Jin Yin Hua*	Clear Heat and remove toxins
22.2	Chrysanthemum	*Ju Hua*	Clear Heat and remove toxins
22.2	Taraxacum	*Pu Gong Ying*	Clear Heat and remove toxins
22.2	Viola	*Zi Hua Di Ding*	Cool Blood, dissipate swelling
11.2	Begonia	*Zi Bei Tian Kui*	Cool Blood, remove toxins

Ingredients: *Wu Wei Xiao Du Yin* consists of 60 g *Jin Yin Hua* (Lonicera), 60 g *Ju Hua* (Chrysanthemum), 60 g *Pu Gong Ying* (Taraxacum), 60 g *Zi Hua Di Ding* (Viola), and 30 g *Zi Bei Tian Kui* (Begonia) (Table 21.8).

Preparation:

1. Powder or capsule method: Herbs are ground into a fine powder. The powder can be encapsulated.
2. Decoction or teapill method: Raw herbs are mixed together and decocted. The herbal water extract (decoction) can be concentrated as granules or teapills.

Actions: Clear Heat and remove toxins, eliminate ulcers, dissipate swelling

Indications: Excessive Heat Toxin in the Exterior and Interior or all types of ulcerations and boils marked with erythema, swelling, Heat, and pain. The main clinical signs are typical of septicemia and may include localized redness, swelling, Heat and pain of the skin or joints, fever, a red tongue, and a fast and forceful pulse.

Dosage and Usage:

Horses and Cattle: 15–60 g, twice daily
Camels: 30–75 g, twice daily
Llamas, Alpacas, Goats, Sheep, and Pigs: 5–15 g, twice daily
Dogs: 0.5–5 g (or 0.1 g per kg body weight), twice daily
Cats and Rabbits: 0.2–0.5 g (or 0.1 g per kg body weight), twice daily
Birds: 0.1–0.2 g per kg body weight, twice daily

Use for 2–6 weeks until the primary clinical signs have resolved.

Analysis of Formula: Excessive Heat or Fire and Damp-Heat are generated from environmental conditions, seasonal changes, or foods. They damage blood vessels and cause Stagnation, which accumulates in the Interior and in turn generates more Heat. As this cycle continues, the Excess Fire/Heat Toxin deepens and gradually forms very hard and deep-seated lesions and wounds, which cause swelling and pain. *Zheng Qi* pushes out toxins, leading to ulceration and boils. The goal of treatment is to clear Heat and detoxify. *Jin Yin Hua* (Lonicera), the King herb, is used to clear Heat, detoxify and dissipate swelling. *Zi Hua Di Ding* (Viola), *Zi Bei Tian Kui* (Begonia), *Pu Gong Ying* (Taraxacum), and *Ju Hua* (Chrysanthemum) clear Heat, detoxify, and disperse ulcers, swelling and toxins as the Adjuvant herbs. All of the herbs together clear Heat, remove toxins, and disperse ulcers and swelling.

Cautions and Contraindications: Caution in Spleen *Qi* Deficiency

Dr. Xie's Comments: *Wu Wei Xiao Du Yin* has strong actions to clear Heat and remove toxins on the surface. It is also used for fever of unknown origin, mastitis, feline infectious peritonitis (FIP), feline leukemia virus (FeLV), and folliculitis/furunculosis.

Clinical and Pharmacological Studies: Nephrotic syndrome is a group of clinical signs including albuminuria, hematuria, hypoproteinemia, edema, hyperlipemia, abdominal distension, blushing, a yellow and greasy tongue coating, and a slippery, fast pulse. *Wu Wei Xiao Du Yin* has been successfully used to treat this Heat Toxin Pattern. In previous studies, the formula was decocted with water, and 1 dose was taken daily by humans with nephropathy from a Heat Toxin Pattern with edema. After 10 doses, their edema decreased; and after 5 months, the urine and serum lipids and albumin all normalized.[13,14]

Xiao Huang San (Clearing Yellow Swelling) 消黄散

Xiao means removing, *Huang* means yellow and here refers to a swelling that is painful, hot, and yellow. San means powder. Thus, *Xiao Huang San* is translated as Clearing Yellow Swelling Powder.

Source: *Yuan Heng Liao Ma Ji* (*Yuan-Heng's Therapeutic Treatise of Horses*), written by *Yu Benyun* and *Yu Benheng* during the *Ming* Dynasty and published in 1608 and distributed all over the world

Ingredients: The formula of *Xiao Huang San* is composed of 25 g *Huang Yao Zi* (Dioscorea), 25 g *Bai Yao Zi* (Stephania), 25 g *Zhi Mu* (Anemarrhena), 20 g *Zhi Zi* (Gardenia), 20 g *Huang Qin* (Scutellaria), 30 g *Da Huang* (Rheum), 20 g *Zhe Bei Mu* (Fritillaria), 25 g *Lian Qiao* (Forsythia), 20 g *Yu Jin* (Curcuma), 90 g *Mang Xiao* (Mirabilite), 30 g *Huang Lian* (Coptis), 15 g *Gan Cao* (Glycyrrhiza), 20 g *Fang Feng* (Ledebouriella), 20 g *Chan Tui* (Cicada), and 20 g *Huang Qi* (Astragalus) (Table 21.9).

Table 21.9. Ingredients and actions of *Xiao Huang San*.

%	English Name	Chinese *Pin-Yin*	Actions
6.25	Dioscorea	*Huang Yao Zi*	Clear Heat and remove toxins
6.25	Stephania	*Bai Yao Zi*	Clear Heat and remove toxins
6.25	Anemarrhena	*Zhi Mu*	Cool Blood, clear Heat
5	Gardenia	*Zhi Zi*	Clear Heat, purge Fire
5	Scutellaria	*Huang Qin*	Clear Heat and remove toxins
7.5	Rheum	*Da Huang*	Cool Blood, detoxify
5	Fritillaria	*Zhe Bei Mu*	Relieve cough and reduce sputum
6.25	Forsythia	*Lian Qiao*	Clear Heat and remove toxins
5	Curcuma	*Yu Jin*	Cool Blood
22.5	Mirabilite	*Mang Xiao*	Clear Heat, purge Fire
7.5	Coptis	*Huang Lian*	Clear Heat and remove toxins
3.75	Glycyrrhiza	*Gan Cao*	Harmonize and tonify *Qi*
5	Ledebouriella	*Fang Feng*	Eliminate Wind
3.75	Cicada	*Chan Tui*	Clear Heat, expel Wind
5	Astragalus	*Huang Qi*	Nourish *Qi*

Preparation:

1. Powder or capsule method: Herbs are ground into a fine powder. The powder can be encapsulated.
2. Decoction or teapill method: Raw herbs are mixed together and decocted. The herbal water extract (decoction) can be concentrated as granules or teapills.

Actions: Clear Heat, purge Fire, cool Blood to remove toxins.

Indications: Excess Heat in the Triple Burner (*San Jiao*) or Heat Toxin in the whole body with hot painful swellings, red tongue with yellow coating, fast and forceful pulse

Dosage and Usage:

Horses and Cattle: 15–60 g, twice daily
Camels: 30–75 g, twice daily
Llamas, Alpacas, Goats, Sheep, and Pigs: 5–15 g, twice daily
Dogs: 0.5–5 g (or 0.1 g per kg body weight), twice daily
Cats and Rabbits: 0.2–0.5 g (or 0.1 g per kg body weight), twice daily
Birds: 0.1–0.2 g per kg body weight, twice daily

Use for 2–6 weeks until the primary clinical signs have resolved.

Analysis of Formula: *Xiao Huang San* is used to treat surface swelling due to Heat Toxins or Excess Heat in animals. In the formula, *Huang Yao Zi* (Dioscorea), *Bai Yao Zi* (Stephania) and *Huang Qin* (Scutellaria) are the King herbs that clear Heat and detoxify. *Da Huang* (Rheum) and *Mang Xiao* (Mirabilite) clear toxic Heat of the Stomach and Large Intestine, and *Lian Qiao* (Forsythia) has the function of clearing Heat and removing toxins. These three are the Minister herbs. *Yu Jin* (Curcuma) cools Blood and *Zhe Bei Mu* (Fritillaria) clears Heat and transforms Phlegm. *Zhi Mu* (Anemarrhena) nourishes *Yin* to lessen Fire, and *Huang Qi* (Astragalus) tonifies *Qi* to disperse ulceration and promote tissue regeneration. These four herbs are all Adjuvant herbs. *Fang Feng* (Ledebouriella), and *Chan Tui* (Cicada) expel Wind and guide other herbs to the skin and surface. Together with *Gan Cao* (Glycyrrhiza), which harmonizes all of the other herbs, these three herbs are the Messenger herbs. All of the herbs together clear Heat, cool Blood, remove toxins, and expel Wind.

Cautions and Contraindications: Use only to treat excessive Heat and Heat Toxins. This formula is contraindicated in patients with False Heat or Spleen *Qi* Deficiency.

Dr. Xie's Comments: *Xiao Huang San* is the fundamental veterinary formula to treat the swelling, redness, heat, and pain associated with various types of dermatitis.

Clinical and Pharmacological Studies: Mastitis, called *Nai Huang* in TCVM, is often caused by Heat Toxin. *Xiao Huang San* has been used to treat 89 bovine mastitis cases. After 5–10 daily oral treatments with this herbal medicine, 86 of the cases (96.6%) had clinically recovered.[15]

Xian Fang Huo Ming Yin (Immortal Formula for Saving Life) 仙方活命饮

Xian means immortal, Fang refers to a formula or recipe, *Huo* means surviving or saving. and *Ming* means life. *Huo Ming* implies that the formula is so good that it can save one's life from the edge of death. *Yin* means decoction. *Xian Fang Huo Ming* can be translated as Immortal Formula for Saving Life.

Source: *Jiao Zhu Fu Ren Liang Fang* (*Revised Fine Formulas for Women*), written by *Bi Li-Zhi* and published in the 16th century

Ingredients: *Xian Fang Huo Ming Yin* consists of 90 g *Jin Yin Hua* (Lonicera), 25 g *Dang Gui* (Angelica), 25 g *Chen Pi* (Citrus), 20 g *Fang Feng* (Ledebouriella), 20 g *Bai Zhi* (Angelica), 15 g *Gan Cao* (Glycyrrhiza), 20 g *Zhe Bei Mu* (Fritillaria), 20 g *Tian Hua Fen* (Trichosanthes), 15 g *Ru Xiang* (Olibanum), 15 g *Mo Yao* (Myrrh), 15 g *Zao Jiao Ci* (Gleditsia), and 30 g *Chuan Shan Jia* (Manitis) (Table 21.10).

Table 21.10. Ingredients and actions of *Xian Fang Huo Ming Yin*.

%	English Name	Chinese *Pin-Yin*	Actions
29	Lonicera	*Jin Yin Hua*	Clear Heat and remove toxins
8	Angelica	*Dang Gui*	Tonify Blood
8.1	Citrus	*Chen Pi*	Move *Qi*, transform Damp
6.5	Ledebouriella	*Fang Feng*	Disperse Wind
6.5	Angelica	*Bai Zhi*	Disperse Wind, relieve pain
4.8	Glycyrrhiza	*Gan Cao*	Tonify *Qi* and harmonize
6.5	Fritillaria	*Zhe Bei Mu*	Transform Phlegm to relieve cough
6.5	Trichosanthes	*Tian Hua Fen*	Transform Phlegm and produce Body Fluids
4.8	Olibanum	*Ru Xiang*	Move Blood to relieve pain
4.8	Myrrh	*Mo Yao*	Move Blood to remove Stasis
4.8	Gleditsia	*Zao Jiao Ci*	Promote the discharge of pus, reduce swelling
9.7	Manitis*	*Chuan Shan Jia*	Move Blood to remove Stagnation

**Chuan Shan Jia* (Manitis) is endangered. Today, *Zao Jiao Ci* (Gleditsia) is used as a substitute.

Preparation:
1. Powder or capsule method: Herbs are ground into a fine powder. The powder can be encapsulated.
2. Decoction or teapill method: Raw herbs are mixed together and decocted. The herbal water extract (decoction) can be concentrated as granules or teapills.

Actions: Clear Heat, remove toxins, move Blood to reduce swelling and promote the drainage of pus

Indications: *Yang* Pattern of sores, boils, and carbuncles with erythematous, swollen, hot, and painful skin lesions and fever; red tongue; and fast and forceful pulse

Dosage and Usage:
Horses and Cattle: 15–60 g, twice daily
Camels: 30–75 g, twice daily
Llamas, Alpacas, Goats, Sheep, and Pigs: 5–15 g, twice daily
Dogs: 0.5–5 g (or 0.1 g per kg body weight), twice daily
Cats and Rabbits: 0.2–0.5 g (or 0.1 g per kg body weight), twice daily
Birds: 0.1–0.2 g per kg body weight, twice daily

Use for 2–4 weeks until the primary clinical signs have resolved.

Analysis of Formula: The *Yang* Pattern of sores, boils, and carbuncles, is usually caused by the collection of toxic Heat (Heat Toxin) or Phlegm-Fire and local Stagnation of *Qi*-Blood. The therapeutic principle is to clear Heat and detoxify, regulate *Qi*, promote Blood flow, reduce swelling, and relieve pain. *Jin Yin Hua* (Lonicera) acts as the King herb to clear Heat and detoxify. Serving as the Minister herbs, *Fang Feng* (Ledebouriella) and *Bai Zhi* (Angelica) eliminate Damp, expel Wind, and promote the drainage of pus. *Dang Gui* (Angelica), *Ru Xiang* (Olibanum), and *Mo Yao* (Myrrh), move Blood and eliminate Stasis to relieve pain. *Tian Hua Fen* (Trichosanthes) and *Zhe Bei Mu* (Fritillaria) transform Phlegm, remove Stasis, and reduce swelling. *Chen Pi* (Citrus) moves *Qi* to resolve Stagnation. The three herbs together are the Adjuvant herbs. The Messenger Herbs are *Chuan Shan Jia* (Manitis), *Zao Jiao Ci* (Gleditsia), and *Gan Cao* (Glycyrrhiza). *Chuan Shan Jia* (Manitis) and *Zao Jiao Ci* (Gleditsia) penetrate the Channels and open the surface to promote the drainage of pus. *Gan Cao* (Glycyrrhiza) harmonizes other herbs and also clears Heat and detoxifies.

Cautions and Contraindications: *Xian Fang Huo Ming Yin* is used to treat the early stage of sores and boils associated with *Yang* Excess or the accumulation of Heat-toxin in the skin. Therefore, it is contraindicated with *Yin* Pattern of boils and sores, which present as chronic nonhealing wounds without redness and Heat. The side effects are few and generally limited to nausea and vomiting. Thus, use *Xian Fang Huo Ming Yin* with caution in patients with Spleen *Qi* Deficiency, or modify the formula by adding herbs such as *Huang Qi* (Astragalus) to tonify Spleen *Qi*.

Dr. Xie's Comments: *Xian Fang Huo Ming Yin* is often used for the treatment of carbuncles, boils, and open wounds in horses and dogs.

Clinical and Pharmacological Studies: In one study, *Xian Fang Huo Min Yin* was used to treat 76 human cases of ulcerated carbuncles. After 7–12 doses of the oral herbal medication administered once daily, 61 patients recovered and all skin lesions were completely healed.[16]

Wei Jing Tang (Phragmites Decoction) 苇茎汤

Wei Jing is another name for *Lu Gen* or Phragmites, which is the King herb of this formula. *Tang* means decoction, the form of herbal administration. Thus, *Wei Jing Tang* translates to Phragmites Decoction.

Source: *Wai Tai Mi Yao* (*Arcane Essentials from the Imperial Library*), written by *Wang Tao* and published in 752 CE

Ingredients: *Wei Jing Tang* is composed of 150g *Lu Gen* (Phragmites), 120g *Dong Gua Ren* (Benincasa), 150g *Yi Yi Ren* (Coix) seed, and 45g *Tao Ren* (Persica) (Table 21.11).

Table 21.11. Ingredients and actions of *Wei Jing Tang*.

%	English Name	Chinese *Pin-Yin*	Actions
32.3	Phragmites	*Wei Jing or Lu Gen*	Clear Lung Heat, promote purulent drainage
25.8	Benincasa	*Dong Gua Ren*	Clear Heat, disperse Phlegm
32.2	Coix	*Yi Yi Ren*	Tonify the Spleen, eliminate Damp
9.7	Persica	*Tao Ren*	Remove Blood Stasis

Preparation:
1. Powder or capsule method: Herbs are ground into a fine powder. The powder can be encapsulated.
2. Decoction or teapill method: Raw herbs are mixed together and decocted. The herbal water extract (decoction) can be concentrated as granules or teapills.

Actions: Clear the Lung, transform Phlegm, resolve Stagnation, promote purulent drainage

Indications: Pulmonary abscess or purulent pneumonia due to Excess Heat with fever, cough, yellow and malodorous Phlegm, dry mouth, red tongue with yellow and greasy coat, slippery and fast pulse

Dosage and Usage:
Horses and Cattle: 15–60g, twice daily
Camels: 30–75g, twice daily
Llamas, Alpacas, Goats, Sheep, and Pigs: 5–15g, twice daily
Dogs: 0.5–5g (or 0.1g per kg body weight), twice daily
Cats and Rabbits: 0.2–0.5g (or 0.1g per kg body weight), twice daily
Birds: 0.1–0.2g per kg body weight, twice daily
Use for 2–4 weeks until the primary clinical signs have resolved.

Analysis of Formula: Pulmonary abscess or purulent pneumonia is usually caused by Excess Heat Toxins or Phlegm Heat accumulated in the Lung. The therapeutic principle is to clear Heat, transform Phlegm and remove the purulent discharge. *Wei Jing* (Phragmites), the King herb, is the principle herb to treat pneumonia. Its function is to clear the Lung and to disperse Heat. The Minister herb is *Dong Gua Ren* (Benincasa), which removes Blood Stasis and expels the purulent discharge. *Tao Ren* (Persica) promotes Blood flow and disperse Stasis, and *Yi Yi Ren* (Coix) promotes diuresis and drains purulence. The two herbs together are the Adjuvant and Messenger Herbs. This formula acts to transform Phlegm, clear Lung Heat, and remove purulent discharges.

Cautions and Contraindications: This formula is contraindicated during pregnancy because of strong blood-moving actions of *Tao Ren* (Persica).

Dr. Xie's Comments: *Wei Jing Tang* is often used for the treatment of pneumonia and lower airway diseases due to Lung Excess Heat in horses and dogs.

Clinical and Pharmacological Studies: *Wei Jing Tang* has been applied extensively to lobar pneumonia, mycoplasmal pneumonia, right middle Lung lobe syndrome, chronic bronchitis, nasosinusitis, and chronic colitis in human clinics. These diseases are mainly caused by the accumulation of toxic Heat with Phlegm. In one study, 30 cases were treated with *Wei Jing Tang* at 1 dose once a day, while severe cases were given 2 doses daily, and 26 cases made a full recovery and 4 cases improved.[17,18]

Long Dan Xie Gan Tang (Gentiana for Purging the Liver) 龙胆泻肝汤

Long Dan refers to *Long Dan Cao* (Gentiana), *Xie* means purging or clearing the Fire, *Gan* means the Liver and *Tang* means decoction, the form of herbal administration. Thus, *Long Dan Xie Gan* translates to Gentiana for Purging the Liver (Fire).

Source: *Yi Fang Ji Jie* (*Analytic Collection of Medical Formulas*), written by *Wang Ang* and published in 1682

Ingredients: The original formula of *Long Dan Xie Gan Tang* is composed of 45 g *Long Dan Cao* (Gentiana), 30 g *Huang Qin* (Scutellaria), 30 g *Zhi Zi* (Gardenia), 30 g *Ze Xie* (Alisma), 30 g *Mu Tong* (Akebia), 20 g *Che Qian Zi* (Plantago), 25 g *Dang Gui* (Angelica), 30 g *Chai Hu* (Bupleurum), 15 g *Gan Cao* (Glycyrrhiza), and 45 g *Sheng Di Huang* (Rehmannia) (Table 21.12).

Table 21.12. Ingredients and actions of *Long Dan Xie Gan Tang*.

%	English Name	Chinese *Pin-Yin*	Actions
15	Gentiana	*Long Dan Cao*	Clear Heat, eliminate Damp
10	Scutellaria	*Huang Qin*	Clear Heat, eliminate Damp
10	Gardenia	*Zhi Zi*	Clear Heat in the Liver and Triple Burner
10	Alisma	*Ze Xie*	Drain Damp
10	Akebia	*Mu Tong*	Drain Damp-Heat, alleviate water retention
6.8	Plantago	*Che Qian Zi*	Promote diuresis to drain Damp-Heat
8.7	Angelica	*Dang Gui*	Move Blood
10	Bupleurum	*Chai Hu*	Soothe Liver *Qi* to resolve Stagnation
5	Glycyrrhiza	*Gan Cao*	Tonify *Qi*, harmonize
15	Rehmannia	*Sheng Di Huang*	Cool Blood, nourish *Yin*

Preparation:

1. Powder or capsule method: Herbs are ground into a fine powder. The powder can be encapsulated.
2. Decoction or teapill method: Raw herbs are mixed together and decocted. The herbal water extract (decoction) can be concentrated as granules or teapills.

Actions: Purge Heat and Fire in the Liver and Gallbladder, clear Damp Heat in the Triple Burner (*San Jiao*)

Indications:

1. Excessive Liver Fire or Heat flaring up characterized by aggression, irritability, conjunctivitis, red and swollen eyelids, pain in the anterior abdomen, inflamed and swollen ears, red tongue with yellow coating, wiry pulse
2. Liver Damp-Heat flowing down characterized by excessive genital discharge; moist dermatitis in the lower abdomen, inguinal, perianal, and/or genital areas; swollen scrotum; interdigital dermatitis; red tongue with a yellow, greasy coating; wiry or slippery pulse

Dosage and Usage:

Horses and Cattle: 15–60 g, twice daily
Camels: 30–75 g, twice daily
Llamas, Alpacas, Goats, Sheep, and Pigs: 5–15 g, twice daily
Dogs: 0.5–5 g (or 0.1 g per kg body weight), twice daily
Cats and Rabbits: 0.2–0.5 g (or 0.1 g per kg body weight), twice daily
Birds: 0.1–0.2 g per kg body weight, twice daily

Use for 2–6 weeks until the primary clinical signs have resolved.

Analysis of Formula: *Long Dan Xie Gan Tang* was formulated to treat excessive Liver Fire/Heat or Liver Damp-Heat. In the formula, *Long Dan Cao* (Gentiana) is the King herb, purging Excess Heat/Fire from the Liver and eliminating Damp Heat of the Lower Burner (*Xia Jiao*). *Zhi Zi* (Gardenia) and *Huang Qin* (Scutellaria) have the function of purging pathogenic Fire and clearing Heat, which assists *Long Dan Cao* (Gentiana) to clear Excess Fire of the Liver and Gallbladder. *Ze Xie* (Alisma), *Mu Tong* (Akebia) and *Che Qian Zi* (Plantago) are diuretics that drain Damp Heat and enhance the ability of *Long Dan Cao's* (Gentiana's) to clear Liver Heat. These five herbs are the Minister herbs. *Dang Gui* (Angelica) promotes Blood flow, *Sheng Di Huang* (Rehmannia) nourishes Blood, and *Chai Hu* (Bupleurum) soothes

Liver *Qi* and disperses Stagnation. These three herbs are the Adjuvant herbs. *Gan Cao* (Glycyrrhiza), as the Messenger Herb, coordinates the herbal actions of the formula. All of the herbs together purge Excess Liver Fire, drain Damp, and nourish Blood.

Cautions and Contraindications: This formula is used to treat Excess Fire and Damp-Heat of the Liver and Gallbladder. It is a very cold herbal formula and may harm the Spleen. Therefore, it is contraindicated in patients with Spleen *Qi* Deficiency unless it is modified by herbs to tonify the Spleen *Qi*, such as *Dang Shen* (Codonopsis) and *Bai Zhu* (Atractylodes).

Dr. Xie's Comments: *Long Dan Xie Gan Tang* is often used for the treatment of hepatitis, moist dermatitis, or otitis due to Liver Excess Heat in veterinary practice.

Clinical and Pharmacological Studies:
Long Dan Xie Gan Tang has been used to treat tinnitus, flank pain, impotence, and vaginal pruritis caused by Excess Fire of the Liver-Gallbladder and Damp-Heat of the Liver. In a study of scrotal dermatitis, treatment involved washing the scrotum with a decoction of the formula twice a day and after 4 doses the pruritis had lessened.[19] After 3 more doses, the swelling and pruritis were gone. Since in this study the tongue continued to show a thin, light, yellow coating, treatment was continued orally at 6g daily for 10 days and then complete resolution occurred.[19] Additionally, this formula has been used for the treatment of glaucoma, otitis, and keratitis with satisfactory results.[20]

Qing Fei San (Clearing the Lung) 清肺散

Qing means to clear, *Fei* refers to the Lung and *San* means powder. Thus, *Qing Fei* means Clearing the Lung.

Source: *Yuan Heng Liao Ma Ji* (*Yuan-Heng's Therapeutic Treatise of Horses*), written by *Yu Benyun* and *Yu Benheng* during the *Ming* Dynasty, published in 1608 and distributed throughout the world

Ingredients: The original formula of *Qing Fei San* is composed of 90g *Ban Lan Gen* (Isatis), 50g *Ting Li Zi* (Lepidium), 25g *Gan Cao* (Glycyrrhiza), 50g *Zhe Bei Mu* (Fritillaria), and 30g *Jie Geng* (Platycodon) (Table 21.13).

Preparation:
1. Historically, all herbs were mixed and ground into a powder and then mixed with 120g of honey to form a paste.
2. Powder or capsule method: Herbs are ground into a fine powder. The powder can be encapsulated.
3. Decoction or teapill method: Raw herbs are mixed together and decocted. The herbal water extract (decoction) can be concentrated as granules or teapills.

Table 21.13. Ingredients and actions of *Qing Fei San*.

%	English Name	Chinese *Pin-Yin*	Actions
36.8	Isatis	*Ban Lan Gen*	Clear Heat and detoxify
20.4	Lepidium	*Ting Li Zi*	Clear Lung Heat
10.2	Glycyrrhiza	*Gan Cao*	Clear Heat and detoxify
20.4	Fritillaria	*Zhe Bei Mu*	Transform Phlegm to relieve cough
12.2	Platycodon	*Jie Geng*	Open the Lung, transform Phlegm

Actions: Clear the Lung to stop asthma or dyspnea, transform Phlegm to stop cough

Indications: This formula is used to treat excessive Lung Heat Pattern characterized by a sore throat with swelling and dysphagia, shortness of breath, cough, dyspnea or asthma, a dry mouth, a red tongue, and a forceful pulse.

Dosage and Usage:
Horses and Cattle: 15–60g, twice daily
Camels: 30–75g, twice daily
Llamas, Alpacas, Goats, Sheep, and Pigs: 5–15g, twice daily
Dogs: 0.5–5g (or 0.1g per kg body weight), twice daily
Cats and Rabbits: 0.2–0.5g (or 0.1g per kg body weight), twice daily
Birds: 0.1–0.2g per kg body weight, twice daily

Use for 2–6 weeks until the primary clinical signs have resolved.

Analysis of Formula: Heat Toxins invade the body and accumulate in the Lung. Heat boils Body Fluids and transforms them into Phlegm. The combination of Heat and Phlegm obstruct the Lung and airways, leading to a sore throat, cough, dyspnea, or asthma. The treatment principle for this condition is to clear Lung Heat and transform Phlegm to stop coughing, asthma, or dyspnea. *Ban Lan Gen* (Isatis) and *Zhe Bei Mu* (Fritillaria) are the King herbs, which clear Lung Heat and relieve asthma and cough. *Ting Li Zi* (Lepidium) and *Jie Geng* (Platycodon) are the Minister herbs that open the Lung, clear Lung Heat, and transform Phlegm to stop dyspnea and cough. *Gan Cao* (Glycyrrhiza), the Messenger herb, clears Heat, removes toxins, and harmonizes the other herbs. Honey moistens the Lung to stop coughing, clear Heat, and detoxify. All of the herbs together clear the Lung Heat and transform Phlegm to stop the cough and asthma.

Cautions and Contraindications: Side effects are rare. It should be used with caution in patients with Spleen *Qi* Deficiency because it is a cold herbal formula.

Dr. Xie's Comments: *Qing Fei San* is often used for bronchitis, disease of the lower airways, and pneumonia due to Excess Lung Heat.

Clinical and Pharmacological Studies: Excess Lung Heat, if failed to be treated properly, can shift to the Large Intestine, leading to constipation. Lin treated 50 horses with constipation due to Lung Heat. After the herbal medication was administered once daily for 7–14 days, all the horses recovered.[21] Cough is a common symptom of Lung disorders. Qin used *Qing Fei San* to treat 270 cases of cough in humans and 97.8% showed a positive response to treatment.[22]

Yu Nü Jian (Jade Lady) 玉女煎

Yu means jade, *Nü* means lady and *Jian* means decoction, the form of herbal administration. Thus, *Yu Nü* is translated as Jade Lady. *Yu Nü* refers to *Shi Gao* (Gypsum), the King ingredient of the formula, which, like jade, is cold and *Yin* in nature.

Source: *Jing Yue Quan Shu* (*Collected Treatises of Zhang Jing-Yue*), written by *Zhang Jiebing* and published in 1624

Ingredients: *Yu Nü Jian* is composed of 10g *Shi Gao* (Gypsum), 15g *Shu Di Huang* (Rehmannia), 6g *Mai Men Dong* (Ophiopogon),5g5g *Zhi Mu* (Anemarrhena), and 5g *Niu Xi* (Achyranthis) (Table 21.14).

Preparation:

1. Powder or capsule method: Herbs are ground into a fine powder. The powder can be encapsulated.
2. Decoction or teapill method: Raw herbs are mixed together and decocted. The herbal water extract (decoction) can be concentrated as granules or teapills.

Actions: Clear Stomach Heat and nourish Kidney *Yin*

Indications: Stomach Heat with *Yin* Deficiency characterized by toothache or loose teeth, bleeding gums, stomatitis, gingivitis, halitosis, signs of head pain, irritability or restlessness, red and dry tongue with a yellow coating thin and fast pulse

Table 21.14. Ingredients and actions of *Yu Nü Jian*.

%	English Name	Chinese *Pin-Yin*	Actions
24.4	Gypsum	*Shi Gao*	Clear Heat, purge Fire
36.6	Rehmannia	*Shu Di Huang*	Tonify Blood
14.6	Ophiopogon	*Mai Men Dong*	Nourish Lung *Yin*, produce Body Fluids
12.2	Anemarrhena	*Zhi Mu*	Clear Heat, nourish *Yin*
12.2	Achyranthis	*Niu Xi*	Tonify the Kidney and Liver, descend *Qi*-Blood to the Lower Burner and stifles

Dosage and Usage:

Horses and Cattle: 15–60g, twice daily
Camels: 30–75g, twice daily
Llamas, Alpacas, Goats, Sheep, and Pigs: 5–15g, twice daily
Dogs: 0.5–5g (or 0.1g per kg body weight), twice daily
Cats and Rabbits: 0.2–0.5g (or 0.1g per kg body weight), twice daily
Birds: 0.1–0.2g per kg body weight, twice daily

Use for 3–8 weeks until the primary clinical signs have resolved.

Analysis of Formula: *Yu Nü Jian* was formulated to treat Excess Stomach Heat (*Yang-Ming*) with Kidney *Yin* Deficiency (*Shao Yin*). Excess Heat in the Stomach flares up along the Stomach Channel to the gums and cheek, leading to bleeding gums, gingivitis, or stomatitis. Persistent Stomach Heat injures Kidney *Yin*. The Kidney controls the bones and teeth. Thus, Stomach Heat with Kidney *Yin* Deficiency may cause toothache and loose teeth. The principle of treatment is to clear Stomach Heat and nourish Kidney *Yin*. *Shi Gao* (Gypsum), the King herb, clears the Excess Fire and Heat from the *Yang-Ming* (Stomach) with its pungent, sweet, and very cold nature. *Shu Di Huang* (Rehmannia), as the Minister herb, nourishes Kidney *Yin* with its sweet and mildly warm nature. The King and Minister herbs together clear Heat and strengthen the Kidney (Water Element) to help treat both Excess Fire and *Yin* Deficiency. *Zhi Mu* (Anemarrhena) has a bitter, cold, and moisturizing nature that assists *Shi Gao* (Gypsum) in clearing Stomach Heat. This herb also assists *Shu Di Huang* (Rehmannia) in nourishing Kidney *Yin*. *Mai Men Dong* (Ophiopogon) supports *Shu Di Huang* (Rehmannia) in nourishing Kidney *Yin* and moistening Stomach Dryness. *Zhi Mu* (Anemarrhena) and *Mai Men Dong* (Ophiopogon) are Adjuvant herbs. *Niu Xi* (Achyranthis) is the Messenger herb that ensures downward flow of Blood, thereby reinforcing the Liver and Kidney.

Cautions and Contraindications: *Yu Nü Jian* is contraindicated for patients with Spleen *Qi* Deficiency or chronic diarrhea.

Dr. Xie's Comments: *Yu Nü Jian* is most often used for the treatment of stomatitis and gingivitis due to Stomach Heat.

Clinical and Pharmacological Studies: Most cases of chronic atrophic gastritis occur in geriatric patients. The longer the course of disease, the more opportunity there is to develop Stomach *Yin* Deficiency (False Heat in the Stomach) with stomach pain, dry stool, a red and dry tongue, and a thin and fast pulse. *Rui* used 1 dose/day of *Yu Nü Jian* to treat 63 human patients with chronic atrophic gastritis. A positive response to treatment was seen in 2–5 months, with the fastest response occurring in 50 days and the longest taking 6 months. Type 2 diabetes is a common endocrine disease.[23] Since 2003 Chen has used *Yu Nü Jian* to treat 42 cases of diabetes and has had favorable results after 8 weeks of treatment with 1 dose of the formula decocted twice in 500 ml of water and taken twice a day.[24]

Yu Jin San (Curcuma Powder) 郁金散

Yu Jin refers to Curcuma, the King ingredient of the formula. *San* is powder, the original form of herbal administration. Thus, *Yu Jin San* translates literally into Curcuma Powder.

Source: *Yuan Heng Liao Ma Ji* (*Yuan-Heng's Therapeutic Treatise of Horses*), written by *Yu Benyun* and *Yu Benheng* during the *Ming* Dynasty, published in 1608 and spread throughout the world

Ingredient: The formula of *Yu Jin San* is composed of 45 g *Yu Jin* (Curcuma), 30 g *He Zi* (Chebula), 30 g *Huang Qin* (Scutellaria), 45 g *Da Huang* (Rheum), 20 g *Huang Lian* (Coptis), 20 g *Zhi Zi* (Gardenia), 30 g *Bai Shao Yao* (Paeonia), and 30 g *Huang Bai* (Phellodendron) (Table 21.15).

Preparation:

1. Powder or capsule method: Herbs are ground into a fine powder. The powder can be encapsulated.
2. Decoction or teapill method: Raw herbs are mixed together and decocted. The herbal water extract (decoction) can be concentrated as granules or teapills.

Table 21.15. Ingredients and actions of *Yu Jin San*.

%	English Name	Chinese *Pin-Yin*	Actions
17.4	Curcuma	*Yu Jin*	Cool Blood, disperse Stasis
11.5	Chebula	*He Zi*	Astringently consolidate intestines to stop diarrhea
11.5	Scutellaria	*Huang Qin*	Clear Heat, eliminate Damp
17.3	Rheum	*Da Huang*	Clear Heat, move Blood to disperse Stasis
7.8	Coptis	*Huang Lian*	Clear Heat, eliminate Damp
11.5	Gardenia	*Zhi Zi*	Clear Liver Heat
11.5	Paeonia	*Bai Shao Yao*	Nourish *Yin*, tonify Blood
11.5	Phellodendron	*Huang Bai*	Clear Heat, eliminate Damp

Actions: Clear Damp-Heat and remove toxins, astringently consolidate the intestines to stop diarrhea

Indications: Heat Toxin, Damp-Heat in the intestines or Damp-Heat in the Spleen characterized by diarrhea, watery stool with mucous and blood, abdominal pain, thirst, red tongue with a yellow coating, and strong and fast pulse

Dosage and Usage:
Horses and Cattle: 15–60 g, twice daily
Camels: 30–75 g, twice daily
Llamas, Alpacas, Goats, Sheep, and Pigs: 5–15 g, twice daily
Dogs: 0.5–5 g (or 0.1 g per kg body weight), twice daily
Cats and Rabbits: 0.2–0.5 g (or 0.1 g per kg body weight), twice daily
Birds: 0.1–0.2 g per kg body weight, twice daily

Use for 1–4 weeks until the primary clinical signs have resolved.

Analysis of Formula: *Yu Jin San* (Curcuma Powder) is mainly used to treat enteritis, colitis, or inflammatory bowel disease due to excessive Damp Heat or Heat Toxins. *Yu Jin* (Curcuma), the King herb of the formula, cools Blood to clear Heat, and moves *Qi* and Blood to eliminate Stagnation and Stasis. *Huang Lian* (Coptis), Huang Qin (Scutellaria), *Huang Bai* (Phellodendron), and *Zhi Zi* (Gardenia), are the Minister herbs that clear the Stagnant Fire of the Triple Burner (*San Jiao*) and eliminate Damp-Heat. *Bai Shao Yao* (Paeonia) and *He Zi* (Chebula) stop diarrhea by retaining *Yin* and astringing the intestines, and *Da Huang* (Rheum) clears Heat in the Blood and removes toxins, and they are the Adjuvant herbs. All of the herbs combined clear Heat, detoxify, and have antidiarrheal and astringent properties.

Cautions and Contraindications: Since *Yu Jin San* (Curcuma Powder) is very cold and good at clearing excessive Damp-Heat or Heat Toxin in the intestines, it can harm the Spleen if it is overdosed or used long term. Use with caution for a short duration or with herbs to supplement the Spleen in patients with underlying Spleen *Qi* Deficiency.

Dr. Xie's Comments: *Yu Jin San* is a classical veterinary formula that treats any bloody, mucoid diarrhea due to Damp-Heat in the gastrointestinal tract.

Clinical and Pharmacological Studies: Canine parvovirus is an infectious disease that often infects puppies and is characterized by vomiting, bloody diarrhea, dehydration, anemia, and fever. *Yu Jin San* was used to successfully treat canine parvovirus in an 8-month-old puppy. One dose of the formula was decocted three times and administered orally 3 times a day. The dog recovered after 2 days.[25] *Chang Huang* syndrome (Intestinal Heat Toxin) is a common internal disease in cattle, with clinical signs of diarrhea, fishy smelling stool, and abdominal pain. *Yu Jin San* was used to treat 98 cases of *Chang Huang* syndrome (62 buffalo, 24 beef cattle, and 12 dairy cows) and 1 dose of a decoction of the formula was drenched once a day for 2–3 days. A positive effect was achieved in 98.1% of cases.[26]

Bai Tou Weng San (Pulsatilla Powder) 白头翁散

Bai Tou Weng refers to Pulsatilla, the King ingredient of the formula, and *San,* which is powder, the original form of herbal administration. Thus, *Bai Tou Weng San* translates literally to Pulsatilla Powder.

Source: *Shang Han Za Bing Lun* (*Treatise on Cold-Induced Disorders and Miscellaneous Diseases*), written by *Zhang Zhong-Jing* and published in 220 CE

Ingredients: *Bai Tou Weng San* consists of 90 g *Bai Tou Weng* (Pulsatilla), 45 g *Huang Bai* (Phellodendron), 45 g *Huang Lian* (Coptis), and 45 g *Qin Pi* (Fraxinus) (Table 21.16).

Preparation:
1. Powder or capsule method: Herbs are ground into a fine powder. The powder can be encapsulated.
2. Decoction or teapill method: Raw herbs are mixed together and decocted. The herbal water extract (decoction) can be concentrated as granules or teapills.

Actions: Clear Heat, eliminate Dampness, remove toxins, cool Blood to stop diarrhea

Indications: Bloody dysentery or Damp Heat in the Large Intestine characterized by rectal tenesmus; urgency to defecate; bloody, purulent stool with a fishy smell; fever; colic; thirst; red tongue with a yellow coating, and fast pulse

Table 21.16. Ingredients and actions of *Bai Tou Weng San.*

%	English Name	Chinese *Pin-Yin*	Actions
40	Pulsatilla	*Bai Tou Weng*	Clear Heat, cool Blood to stop diarrhea
20	Phellodendron	*Huang Bai*	Clear Heat, eliminate Damp
20	Coptis	*Huang Lian*	Clear Heat, eliminate Damp
20	Fraxinus	*Qin Pi*	Clear Heat, eliminate Damp

Dosage and Usage:
Horses and Cattle: 15–60 g, twice daily
Camels: 30–75 g, twice daily
Llamas, Alpacas, Goats, Sheep, and Pigs: 5–15 g, twice daily
Dogs: 0.5–5 g (or 0.1 g per kg body weight), twice daily
Cats and Rabbits: 0.2–0.5 g (or 0.1 g per kg body weight), twice daily
Birds: 0.1–0.2 g per kg body weight, twice daily

Use for 1–4 weeks until the primary clinical signs have resolved.

Analysis of Formula: *Bai Tou Weng San* (Pulsatilla Powder) is mainly composed of highly bitter and cold herbs that effectively treat an acute onset of enteritis or inflammatory bowel disease caused by accumulation of Damp Heat in the Large Intestine. *Bai Tou Weng* (Pulsatilla), as the King herb, cools Blood, clears Heat and removes toxins in the Large Intestine. Working as the Minister herbs, *Huang Lian* (Coptis) clears Damp-Heat and removes toxins of the large intestine and *Huang Bai* (Phellodendron) clears Damp Heat in the Lower Burner (*Xia Jiao*). As an Adjuvant herb, *Qin Pi* (Fraxinus) clears Damp-Heat in the Liver and cools Blood. All of the herbs together clear Heat, remove toxins, and cool Blood to stop diarrhea.

Cautions and Contraindications: *Bai Tou Weng San* (Pulsatilla Powder) was formulated to treat bloody dysentery, acute onset of colitis, or inflammatory bowel disease. Since it consists of herbs that are bitter and cold in nature, it can easily harm Spleen *Qi* and *Yang*, and it should not be used long-term; caution should be used against overdosing. *Bai Tou Weng San* (Pulsatilla Powder) is contraindicated in Spleen *Qi* or *Yang* Deficiency.

Dr. Xie's Comments: *Bai Tou Weng Tang* and *Yu Jin San* both clear Damp-Heat in the gastrointestinal tract and are used for Bloody diarrhea. *Bai Tou Weng Tang* uses *Bai Tou Weng* (Pulsatilla) as the King herb to cool Blood and clear Damp Heat, and is good for treating dysentery and relieving tenesmus. It is used more for acute onset colitis. *Yu Jin San* uses *Yu Jin* (Curcuma) as its King herb to cool Blood and resolve Stagnation; it is good at astringently consolidating the intestines to stop diarrhea and is often used for subacute or chronic bloody diarrhea.

Clinical and Pharmacological Studies: Diarrhea is a common gastrointestinal tract disease in calves. *Bai Tou Weng San* prepared as a powder was used to treat 25 calves with chronic bacillary diarrhea at a dose of 70 g/patient, twice a day, for 2 days; 88% of patients showed a positive response.[27] Additionally, dysentery of young pigs is caused by the invasion of the pathogen Damp-Heat. Clinical signs include bloody, purulent, and fishy smelling diarrhea. In one study, *Bai Tou Weng San*, prepared as a powder, was administered at 4–6g every day to 30 cases, and 27 cases responded well to treatment.[28]

Zhi Li San (Red Back Door) 止痢散

Zhi means stopping, *Li* means dysentery or bloody diarrhea, and *San* means powder, the form of herbal administration. Thus, *Zhi Li San* can literally be translated to Stop Dysentery Powder. It is a very potent formula to treat bloody diarrhea due to Damp Heat in the gastrointestinal tract. Therefore, it is also called Red Back Door because the back door refers to the anus, the door of defecation, as compared with the front door, or penis or vulva, the door for urination.

Source: *Chinese Veterinary Herbal Handbook* compiled by Dr. Huisheng Xie and published by the Chi Institute of Chinese Medicine 2004

Ingredients: The ingredients and actions of *Zhi Li San* are listed in Table 21.17.

Preparation:

1. Capsule method: Herbs are ground into a fine powder and encapsulated.
2. Teapill method: Raw herbs are mixed together and decocted.
3. It can be administered as a suppository if oral medication causes vomiting.

Table 21.17. Ingredients and actions of *Zhi Li San*.

%	English Name	Chinese *Pin-Yin*	Action
7.4	Phellodendron	*Huang Bai*	Clear Heat toxin, detoxify
5.0	Coptis	*Huang Lian*	Clear Damp Heat, detoxify
7.4	Scutellaria	*Huang Qin*	Clear Damp Heat, detoxify
7.4	Gardenia	*Zhi Zi*	Clear Damp Heat, detoxify
14.6	Sanguisorba	*Di Yu*	Cool Blood, stop bleeding
7.3	Pinellia	*Ban Xia*	Transform Phlegm, stop vomiting
4.9	Atractylodes	*Cang Zhu*	Dry Damp, strengthen Spleen
3.9	Angelica	*Dang Gui*	Nourish Blood
7.3	Paeonia	*Bai Shao Yao*	Nourish Blood
7.4	Astragulus	*Huang Qi*	Tonify *Qi*
7.4	Dioscorea	*Shan Yao*	Tonify *Qi*
3.9	Saussurea	*Mu Xiang*	Move *Qi*, resolve pain
4.9	Aurantium	*Zhi Ke*	Move *Qi*, resolve pain
7.3	Bambusa	*Zhu Ru*	Transform Phlegm, stop vomiting
3.9	Glycyrrhiza	*Gan Cao*	Harmonize

Actions: Clear Damp-Heat, move *Qi* to relieve pain, tonify Spleen *Qi* to stop diarrhea

Indications: The major use for *Zhi Li San* (Red Back Door) is the treatment of canine parvovirus or Damp-Heat in the GI tract with Spleen *Qi* Deficiency with diarrhea containing blood and mucous, vomiting, anorexia, Damp-Heat in the large intestines, red tongue, and a fast or weak pulse.

Dosage and Usage:

Horses and Cattle: 15–60g, twice daily
Camels: 30–75g, twice daily
Llamas, Alpacas, Goats, Sheep, and Pigs: 5–15g, twice daily
Dogs: 0.5–5g (or 0.1g per kg body weight), twice daily
Cats and Rabbits: 0.2–0.5g (or 0.1g per kg body weight), twice daily
Birds: 0.1–0.2g per kg body weight, twice daily

Use for 1–2 weeks until the primary clinical signs have resolved.

Analysis of Formula: *Zhi Li Tang* is effective for canine parvovirus or other causes of Damp-Heat in GI tract. *Huang Lian* (Coptis) and *Huang Bai* (Phellodendron), the King herbs, clear Damp-Heat and remove toxins from the intestinal tract. Working as Minister herbs, *Huang Qin* (Scutellaria), *Zhi Zi* (Gardenia), and *Di Yu* (Sanguisorba) clear Damp-Heat and cool Blood to remove toxins. Toxic Damp-Heat often causes diarrhea and vomiting. Thus, *Ban Xia* (Pinellia), *Cang Zhu* (Atractylodes), and *Zhu Ru* (Bambusa) are added to strengthen the Spleen, to dry Damp to stop diarrhea, and to transform Phlegm to stop vomiting. Toxic Damp-Heat also leads to Stagnation and colic. Therefore, *Mu Xiang* (Saussurea) and *Zhi Ke* (Aurantium) are used to move *Qi* to resolve Stagnation and pain. *Qi* and Blood are also consumed during the course of disease. *Huang Qi* (Astragulus), *Shan Yao* (Dioscorea), *Dang Gui* (Angelica), and *Bai Shao Yao* (Paeonia) tonify *Qi* and Blood. These nine ingredients together are the Adjuvant herbs. *Gan Cao* (Glycyrrhiza) harmonizes the other herbs and works as the Messenger herb.

Cautions and Contraindications: *Zhi Li San* (Red Back Door) should be used cautiously in patients with *Yin* Deficiency.

Dr. Xie's Comments: *Zhi Li Tang* (Red Back Door) is effective for parvovirus infections and can be used as a suppository if the patient is vomiting.

Yin Chen Hao Tang (Artemisia Decoction) 茵陈蒿汤

Yin Chen Hao means Artemisia, the King ingredient of the formula, and *tang* means decoction, the original

Table 21.18. Ingredients and actions of *Yin Chen Hao Tang*.

%	English Name	Chinese *Pin-Yin*	Actions
70	Artemisia	*Yin Chen Hao*	Clear Damp-Heat
17	Gardenia	*Zhi Zi*	Clear Liver Heat
13	Rheum	*Dai Huang*	Purge Fire, cool Blood

form of herbal administration. Thus, *Yin Chen Hao Tang* translates literally to Artemisia Decoction.

Source: *Shang Han Za Bing Lun* (*Treatise on Cold-Induced Disorders and Miscellaneous Diseases*), written by *Zhang Zhong-Jing* in 220 CE

Ingredients: *Yin Chen Hao Tang* is composed of 250g *Yin Chen Hao* (Artemisia), 60g *Zhi Zi* (Gardenia), and 45g *Da Huang* (Rheum) (Table 21.18).

Preparation:
1. Powder or capsule method: Herbs are ground into a fine powder. The powder can be encapsulated.
2. Decoction or teapill method: Raw herbs are mixed together and decocted. The herbal water extract (decoction) can be concentrated as granules or teapills.

Actions: Clear Heat, eliminate Damp, resolve jaundice

Indications: Jaundice with Damp-Heat (*Yang* jaundice) characterized by bright yellow eyelids and lips, scant and dark yellow urine, dry stool, yellow and greasy coating of the tongue, and a slippery pulse

Dosage and Usage:
Horses and Cattle: 15–60g, twice daily
Camels: 30–75g, twice daily
Llamas, Alpacas, Goats, Sheep, and Pigs: 5–15g, twice daily
Dogs: 0.5–5g (or 0.1g per kg body weight), twice daily
Cats and Rabbits: 0.2–0.5g (or 0.1g per kg body weight), twice daily
Birds: 0.1–0.2g per kg body weight, twice daily
Use for 1–2 weeks until the primary clinical signs have resolved.

Analysis of Formula: *Yang* jaundice is caused by the accumulation of Damp-Heat in the Liver and Gallbladder. Damp-Heat evaporates Body Fluids and steams the body, causing the Liver to fail to maintain the normal flow of *Qi* and bile. Consequently, bile escapes and flows through the entire body, which turns a bright yellow color. In the formula, *Yin Chen Hao* (Artemisia), as the King herb, clears Damp-Heat from the Liver and eliminates the jaundice. *Zhi Zi* (Gardenia) clears Damp-Heat from the Triple Burner (*San Jiao*) and *Da Huang* (Rheum) cools Blood to disperse Heat accumulation. These two herbs are the Minister and Adjuvant herbs. All of the herbs together clear Heat, eliminate Damp, and resolve jaundice.

Cautions and Contraindications: Since this formula was designed for the treatment of *Yang* Jaundice (Excess Damp-Heat in the Liver), it is contraindicated or must be modified in patients with *Yin* Jaundice due to Cold-Damp.

Dr. Xie's Comments: *Yin Chen Hao Tang* is effective to treat hepatitis due to Liver Damp-Heat in horses and dogs.

Clinical and Pharmacological Studies: In a clinical study, *He* compared *Yin Chen Hao Tang* with the conventional western medical (WM) treatment of cholestatic jaundice. *Yin Chen Hao Tang* (treatment group, 57 cases) significantly resolved jaundice and reduced liver enzymes better than the WM treatment (control group, 53 cases).[29] *Yin Chen Hao Tang* has also been successfully used for the treatment of 18 cases of biliary atresia.[30]

Dao Chi San (Guiding Out Heat) 导赤散

Dao means draining, conducting, or guiding out; *Chi* means red (referring to Heat in the Heart and/or Small Intestine); and *San* means powder, the original form of herbal administration. Thus, *Dao Chi San* is translated as Guiding the Heat Out Powder. The color red (Chi) corresponds to the Fire element (Heat, Heart, and Small Intestine). *Dao Chi* refers to the fact that the formula drains and conducts Heat out of the Heart or/and Small Intestine through the Bladder (or urination).

Source: *Xiao Er Yao Zheng Zhi Jue* (*Craft of Medicinal Treatment for Childhood Disease Patterns*), written by *Qian Yi* in 1119 CE

Ingredients: The ingredients of *Dao Chi San* are 6g *Dan Zhu Ye* (Lophatherum), 6g *Gan Cao* (Glycyrrhiza), 9g *Mu Tong* (Akebia), and 15g Sheng Di Huang (Rehmannia) (Table 21.19).

Preparation:
1. Powder or capsule method: Herbs are ground into a fine powder. The powder can be encapsulated.
2. Decoction or teapill method: Raw herbs are mixed together and decocted. The herbal water extract (decoction) can be concentrated as granules or teapills.

Actions: Clear Heat from Heart and Small Intestine and benefit urination

Table 21.19. Ingredients and actions of *Dao Chi San.*

%	English Name	Chinese *Pin-Yin*	Actions
16.7	Lophatherum	*Dan Zhu Ye*	Clear Heat, drain Damp, benefit urination
16.7	Glycyrrhiza	*Gan Cao*	Harmonize
25	Akebia	*Mu Tong*	Clear Heart Fire, drain Small Intestine Heat
41.6	Rehmannia	*Sheng Di Huang*	Cool Blood, nourish *Yin*, clear Heat

Indications: Heat of the Heart and Small Intestine characterized by dysuria, restlessness, anxiety, ulceration or sores of the oral cavity, gingivitis, increased thirst, red tongue, and deep pulse

Dosage and Usage:
Horses and Cattle: 15–60g, twice daily
Camels: 30–75g, twice daily
Llamas, Alpacas, Goats, Sheep, and Pigs: 5–15g, twice daily
Dogs: 0.5–5g (or 0.1g per kg body weight), twice daily
Cats and Rabbits: 0.2–0.5g (or 0.1g per kg body weight), twice daily
Birds: 0.1–0.2g per kg body weight, twice daily
Use for 2–4 weeks until the primary clinical signs have resolved.

Analysis of Formula: The Heart and Small Intestine belong to the same element (Fire). They share a *Yin* (Wife) and *Yang* (Husband) relationship. The Small Intestine Channel is also related to the Bladder Channel because both belong to *Tai-Yang*. Heat in the Heart flares up and leads to restlessness, stomatitis, and gingivitis. Heat migrates down from the Heart to the Small Intestine via the Husband-Wife relationship and then goes to the Bladder through the *Tai-Yang* connection; dysuria, hematuria, and/or cystitis results. *Mu Tong* (Akebia) and *Sheng Di Huang* (Rehmannia), as the King herbs, drain and conduct Heat out of the Heart and Small Intestine through urination, thereby cooling Blood and nourishing *Yin*. Working as the Minister herb, *Dan Zhu Ye* (Lophatherum) promotes urination and drains Heat out of the Heart. *Gan Cao* (Glycyrrhiza) regulates the Stomach and harmonizes all other herbs, and serves as the Adjuvant and Messenger herb.

Cautions and Contraindications: *Dao Chi San* should be used with caution in patients with Spleen *Qi* Deficiency.

Dr. Xie's Comments: I have often used *Dao Chi San* for the treatment of cystitis, hematuria, stomatitis, and gingivitis due to excessive Heat or Fire in the Heart or Small Intestine in dogs cats, and horses.

Xi Xin San (Cleansing the Heart) 洗心散

Xi means cleansing, *Xin* means the Heart and *San* means powder, the form of herbal administration. Thus, *Xi Xin San* translates literally to Cleansing the Heart Powder.

Source: *Yuan Heng Liao Ma Ji* (*Yuan-Heng's Therapeutic Treatise of Horses*), written by *Yu Benyun* and *Yu Benheng* and published in 1608

Ingredients: *Xi Xin San* is composed of 30g *Tian Hua Fen* (Trichosanthes), 30g *Huang Qin* (Scutellaria), 20 *Huang Lian* (Coptis), 30g *Lian Qiao* (Forsythia), 25g *Fu Shen* (Poria), 20g *Huang Bai* (Phellodendron), 30g *Jie Geng* (Platycodon), 30g *Zhi Zi* (Gardenia), 20g *Niu Bang Zi* (Arctium), 15g *Mu Tong* (Akebia), and 15g *Bai Zhi* (Angelica) (Table 21.20).

Preparation:
1. Powder or capsule method: Herbs are ground into a fine powder. The powder can be encapsulated.
2. Decoction or teapill method: Raw herbs are mixed together and decocted. The herbal water extract (decoction) can be concentrated as granules or teapills.

Actions: Clear Fire, remove toxins and eliminate Stasis to subdue swelling

Indications: Excessive Heat in the Heart characterized by boils or ulcers of the tongue, restlessness, irritability, red tongue, and fast and forceful pulse

Table 21.20. Ingredients and actions of *Xi Xin San.*

%	English Name	Chinese *Pin-Yin*	Actions
11	Trichosanthes	*Tian Hua Fen*	Produce Body Fluids to stop thirst
11	Scutellaria	*Huang Qin*	Clear Heat, eliminate Damp
8	Coptis	*Huang Lian*	Clear Heat, eliminate Damp
11	Forsythia	*Lian Qiao*	Clear Heat and remove toxins
9	Poria	*Fu Shen*	Calm Heart and *Shen* (spirit)
8	Phellodendron	*Huang Bai*	Clear Heat, eliminate Damp
11	Platycodon	*Jie Geng*	Open the Lung and guide other herbs to the Upper Burner
11	Gardenia	*Zhi Zi*	Clear Heat of the Triple Burner
8	Arctium	*Niu Bang Zi*	Subdue swelling and remove toxins
6	Akebia	*Mu Tong*	Drain Fire out of the Heart, benefit urination
6	Angelica	*Bai Zhi*	Move *Qi* to relieve pain

Dosage and Usage:

Horses and Cattle: 15–60 g, twice daily
Camels: 30–75 g, twice daily
Llamas, Alpacas, Goats, Sheep, and Pigs: 5–15 g, twice daily
Dogs: 0.5–5 g (or 0.1 g per kg body weight), twice daily
Cats and Rabbits: 0.2–0.5 g (or 0.1 g per kg body weight), twice daily
Birds: 0.1–0.2 g per kg body weight, twice daily

Use for 2–6 weeks until the primary clinical signs have resolved.

Analysis of Formula: The formula is used to treat stomatitis or gingivitis due to excessive Heart Heat and Fire. The treatment strategy is to clear Fire to remove toxins. *Huang Qin* (Scutellaria), *Huang Lian* (Coptis), *Huang Bai* (Phellodendron), and *Zhi Zi* (Gardenia) are the King herbs, and they clear Fire from the Triple Burner (*San Jiao*) and purge the Heat from the Heart. The Minister herbs are *Lian Qiao* (Forsythia), *Mu Tong* (Akebia), and *Tian Hua Fen* (Trichosanthes), which assist the King herbs in purging Fire to remove toxins and draining Heat out of the Heart. *Niu Bang Zi* (Arctium) subdues swelling and detoxifies. *Bai Zhi* (Angelica) relieves pain and promotes tissue regeneration. *Fu Shen* (Poria) calms the Heart and Shen. These three herbs are the Adjuvant herbs. *Jie Geng* (Platycodon) is the Messenger herb, which guides other herbs upward to the Upper Burner (*Shang Jiao*), where the Heart is located. All of the herbs together have the function of purging Fire to remove toxins and clearing Heart Heat to subdue swelling.

Cautions and Contraindications: *Xi Xin San* is used only for stomatitis or gingivitis due to excessive Heart Heat and Fire, and it is contraindicated in patients with False Heat due to Heart *Yin* Deficiency.

Dr. Xie's Comments: *Xi Xin San* is a fundamental veterinary herbal formula to clear Excess Fire and Heat out of the Heart. It is often used for the treatment of *Shen* Disturbances, stomatitis, and gingivitis due to excessive Heat or Fire in the Heart.

Clinical and Pharmacological Studies: *Du Huang* is local swelling, which originates from the umbilicus and then spreads to the whole abdomen if not treated. In a clinical study, Li used *Xi Xin San* to treat 32 cases of *Du Huang* in horses, and all clinically recovered. The herbs were ground into a powder and administered once daily with warm water 2–4 times. Acupuncture was also used in these cases to augment the herbal treatment.[31]

Qing Hao Bie Jia Tang (Artemisia and Amyda) 青蒿鳖甲汤

The formula is named for two ingredients: *Qing Hao* or Artemisia and *Bie Jia* or Amyda. *Tang* means decoction, the original formulation of the herb. Thus, *Qing Hao Bie Jia Tang* translates as Artemisia and Amyda Decoction.

Source: *Wen Bing Tiao Bian* (*Systematic Difference of Warm Diseases*), written by *Wu Ju-Tong* and published in 1798 CE

Ingredients: *Qing Hao Bie Jia Tang* is composed of 45 g *Qing Hao* (Artemisia), 90 g *Bie Jia* (Amyda), 60 g *Sheng Di Huang* (Rehmannia), 145 g *Zhi Mu* (Anemarrhena), and 60 g *Mu Dan Pi* (Moutan) (Table 21.21).

Preparation:

1. Powder or capsule method: Herbs are ground into a fine powder. The powder can be encapsulated.
2. Decoction or teapill method: Raw herbs are mixed together and decocted. The herbal water extract (decoction) can be concentrated as granules or teapills.

Actions: Nourish *Yin* to vent Heat

Indications: Residual Heat in a chronic febrile disease with *Yin* Deficiency characterized by a low-grade lingering fever, night fever and morning chills, dry mouth, red tongue with less coating, and thin and fast pulse

Dosage and Usage:

Horses and Cattle: 15–60 g, twice daily
Camels: 30–75 g, twice daily
Llamas, Alpacas, Goats, Sheep, and Pigs: 5–15 g, twice daily
Dogs: 0.5–5 g (or 0.1 g per kg body weight), twice daily
Cats and Rabbits: 0.2–0.5 g (or 0.1 g per kg body weight), twice daily

Table 21.21. Ingredients and actions of *Qing Hao Bie Jia Tang*.

%	English Name	Chinese *Pin-Yin*	Actions
11	Artemisia	*Qing Hao*	Clear False Heat and eliminate Summer-Heat
23	Amyda	*Bie Jia*	Nourish *Yin* to suppress *Yang*
15	Rehmannia	*Sheng Di Huang*	Nourish *Yin*, cool Blood, clear Heat
36	Common anemarrhena rhizome	*Zhi Mu*	Clear Heat, nourish *Yin*, moisten the Lung
15	Moutan	*Mu Dan Pi*	Clear Heat, cool Blood

Birds: 0.1–0.2 g per kg body weight, twice daily

Use for 2–6 weeks until the primary clinical signs have resolved.

Analysis of Formula: *Qing Hao Bie Jia Tang* is a common formula used to treat residual Heat with *Yin* Deficiency in the late stage of a febrile disease. The principle is to nourish *Yin* and vent Heat. *Qing Hao* (Artemisia) penetrates and nourishes *Yin* to clear hidden residual Heat, while *Bie Jia* (Amyda) goes straight to the *Yin* to nourish it and reduce fever. These two herbs are the King herbs. *Sheng Di Huang* (Rehmannia) and *Zhi Mu* (Anemarrhena) assist the King herbs to nourish *Yin* and clear Heat. *Mu Dan Pi* (Moutan) assists *Qing Hao* (Artemisia) to relieve and eliminate the hidden residual Heat in the deeper body. These three herbs together are the Minister herbs and Adjuvant herbs.

Cautions and Contraindications: Because *Qing Hao Bie Jia Tang* is designed for residual Heat in the deeper levels of the body associated with the late stage of febrile diseases, it is contraindicated for Heat in the *Qi* Level (early stage) of febrile or warm diseases.

Dr. Xie's Comments: *Qing Hao Bie Jia Tang* is effective for treating the residual Heat with *Yin* Deficiency, which is often the Pattern of the late stages of febrile or warm disease in horses, pigs, and cattle.

Clinical and Pharmacological Studies: *Qing Hao Bie Jia Tang* has been used for the treatment of Heat with *Yin* Deficiency in different diseases with favorable outcomes. The formula was used to treat a person with fever of unknown origin and the body temperature became normal after 1 dose per day for 3 days.[32] *Qing Hao Bie Jia Tang* has also been successfully used to treat night sweats in humans with residual Heat from febrile illness, and in these patients the sweating decreased after 3 doses and they recovered after 5 doses.[33]

Xiang Ru San (Mosla Powder) 香薷散

Xiang Ru means Mosla, the King ingredient of the formula, and *San* means powder, the form of herbal administration. *Xiang Ru San* therefore translates literally to Mosla Powder.

Source: *Yuan Heng Liao Ma Ji* (*Yuan-Heng's Therapeutic Treatise of Horses*), written by *Yu Benyun* and *Yu Benheng* and published in 1608

Ingredients: *Xiang Ru San* is composed of 60 g *Xiang Ru* (Mosla), 30 g *Huang Qin* (Scutellaria), 25 g *Huang Lian* (Coptis), 20 g *Gan Cao* (Glycyrrhiza), 30 g *Chai Hu* (Bupleurum), 30 g *Dang Gui* (Angelica), 45 g *Lian Qiao* (Forsythia), 60 g *Tian Hua Fen* (Trichosanthes), and 30 g *Zhi Zi* (Gardenia) (Table 21.22).

Table 21.22. Ingredients and actions of *Xiang Ru San.*

%	English Name	Chinese *Pin-Yin*	Actions
18	Mosla	*Xiang Ru*	Remove Summer-Heat to relieve the Exterior
9	Scutellaria	*Huang Qin*	Clear Heat, eliminate Damp
8	Coptis	*Huang Lian*	Clear Heat, eliminate Damp
6	Glycyrrhiza	*Gan Cao*	Tonify *Qi*, harmonize
9	Bupleurum	*Chai Hu*	Soothe Liver *Qi* to resolve Stagnation
9	Angelica	*Dang Gui*	Move Blood, nourish Blood
14	Forsythia	*Lian Qiao*	Clear Heat and detoxify
18	Trichosanthes	*Tian Hua Fen*	Clear Lung Heat, expel Phlegm
9	Gardenia	*Zhi Zi*	Clear Heat in the Triple Burner

Preparation:

1. Powder or capsule method: Herbs are ground into a fine powder. The powder can be encapsulated.
2. Decoction or teapill method: Raw herbs are mixed together and decocted. The herbal water extract (decoction) can be concentrated as granules or teapills.

Actions: Clear Heat and remove Summer-Heat, nourish Blood, promote production of Body Fluids

Indications: Summer Heat characterized by high fever, heat intolerance, anhydrosis, tachypnea, heaves or dyspnea, depression, lethargy and weakness, dry feces, dry mouth and red tongue, and strong and fast pulse

Dosage and Usage:

Horses and Cattle: 15–60 g, twice daily

Camels: 30–75 g, twice daily

Llamas, Alpacas, Goats, Sheep, and Pigs: 5–15 g, twice daily

Dogs: 0.5–5 g (or 0.1 g per kg body weight), twice daily

Cats and Rabbits: 0.2–0.5 g (or 0.1 g per kg body weight), twice daily

Birds: 0.1–0.2 g per kg body weight, twice daily

Use for 2–8 weeks until the primary clinical signs have resolved.

Analysis of Formula: Summer-Heat is mainly caused by scorching Body Fluids in hot weather or by high humidity in the summer (Damp Heat). The treatment strategy is to clear Summer-Heat, nourish Blood, and promote the production of Body Fluids. *Xiang Ru* (Mosla), as the King herb, relieves the Exterior, eliminates Summer-Heat, disperses Damp, and clears Heat. *Chai Hu* (Bupleurum), *Huang Lian* (Coptis), *Huang Qin* (Scutellaria), *Zhi Zi* (Gardenia), and *Lian Qiao* (Forsythia) are the Minister herbs that clear Heat out of the entire body and all the Channels. *Dang Gui* (Angelica) and *Tian Hua Fen* (Trichosanthes) are the Adjuvant herbs, which nourish Blood and promote the production of Body Fluids. *Gan Cao* (Glycyrrhiza), as the Messenger herb, removes toxins and harmonizes all the other herbs. Together, these ingredients eliminate Summer-Heat by cooling and nourishing Blood to promote the production of Body Fluids.

Cautions and Contraindications: Use with caution in patients with Spleen *Qi* Deficiency.

Dr. Xie's Comments: *Xiang Ru San* can be used for the treatment of heatstroke or sunstroke. It can also be modified and used to treat anhydrosis in horses.

Clinical and Pharmacological Studies: Ma used *Xiang Ru San* to treat Heatstroke in German Shepherd Dogs. The formula was decocted and administered as a liquid, 1 dose daily for 4 days. In addition, one session of hemoacupuncture was performed on *Er-jian* (the tip of the ear). Patients recovered within 4 days.[34] Postparturient swine are easily affected by Summer Heat. Xu treated heatstroke and sunstroke in a postpartum pig with a decoction of the formula.[35] The patient responded well after 3 days of 1 dose daily.

Jue Ming San (Haliotis Powder) 决明散

Jue Ming refers to Haliotis, the King ingredient of the formula and *San* means powder, the form of herbal administration. Thus, *Jue Ming San* translates literally as Haliotis Powder.

Source: *Yuan Heng Liao Ma Ji* (*Yuan-Heng's Therapeutic Treatise of Horses*), written by *Yu Benyun* and *Yu Benheng* and published in 1608

Ingredients: *Jue Ming San* is composed of 45 g *Shi Jue Ming* (Haliotis), 45 g *Jue Ming* Zi (Cassia), 30 g *Zhi Zi* (Gardenia), 30 g *Da Huang* (Rheum), 30 g *Bai Yao Zi* (Stephania), 30 g *Huang Yao Zi* (Dioscorea), 30 g *Huang Qi* (Astragalus), 20 g *Huang Qin* (Scutellaria), 20 g *Mo Yao* (Myrrh), 20 g *Huang Lian* (Coptis), and 20 g *Yu Jin* (Curcuma) (Table 21.23).

Preparation:

1. Historically, all the ingredients are mixed and ground into a fine powder and then mixed with honey to form a paste.
2. Capsule method: Herbs are ground into a fine powder and encapsulated.
3. Teapill method: Raw herbs are mixed together and decocted. The herbal water extract (decoction) can be concentrated as granules or teapills.

Actions: Clear Liver Heat to brighten the eyes and resolve Stagnation to eliminate opacity

Indications: Eye problems due to the accumulation of Heat in the Liver associated with conjunctivitis; swollen, painful eyes; diffuse or focal cloudiness of the cornea; red tongue with a yellow coating; and wiry or strong pulse

Table 21.23. Ingredients and actions of *Jue Ming San.*

%	English Name	Chinese *Pin-Yin*	Actions
14.1	Haliotis	*Shi Jue Ming*	Calm the Liver and suppress *Yang*
14.1	Cassia	*Jue Ming Zi*	Clear Liver Heat to improve eyesight
9.4	Gardenia	*Zhi Zi*	Clear Liver Heat
9.4	Rheum	*Da Huang*	Purge Fire, cool Blood
9.4	Stephania	*Bai Yao Zi*	Clear Heat and remove toxins
9.4	Dioscorea	*Huang Yao Zi*	Remove Heat to cool Blood
9.4	Astragalus	*Huang Qi*	Tonify *Qi*
6.3	Scutellaria	*Huang Qin*	Clear Heat, eliminate Damp
6.3	Myrrh	*Mo Yao*	Promote Blood flow, remove Blood Stasis
6.3	Coptis	*Huang Lian*	Clear Heat, eliminate Damp
6.3	Curcuma	*Yu Jin*	Cool Blood, clear Heat

Dosage and Usage:

Horses and Cattle: 15–60 g, twice daily
Camels: 30–75 g, twice daily
Llamas, Alpacas, Goats, Sheep, and Pigs: 5–15 g, twice daily
Dogs: 0.5–5 g (or 0.1 g per kg body weight), twice daily
Cats and Rabbits: 0.2–0.5 g (or 0.1 g per kg body weight), twice daily
Birds: 0.1–0.2 g per kg body weight, twice daily

Use for 4–8 weeks until the primary clinical signs have resolved.

Analysis of Formula: *Jue Ming San* is mainly used to improve acuity of vision and remove nebula or opacity from the cornea. In the formula, *Shi Jue Ming* (Haliotis) and *Jue Ming Zi* (Cassia) are the King herbs, used to clear Liver Heat, disperse swelling, relieve pain, and diminish corneal opacity or nebula. *Huang Lian* (Coptis), *Huang Qin* (Scutellaria), and *Zhi Zi* (Gardenia) clear Heat and purge pathogenic Fire; *Huang Yao Zi* (Dioscorea) and *Bai Yao Zi* (Stephania), cool Blood to remove pathogenic Heat. These five herbs are the Minister herbs that serve to strengthen the effects of clearing Liver Heat and detoxification. *Da Huang* (Rheum), *Yu Jin* (Curcuma), and *Mo Yao* (Myrrh) eliminate Stasis to subdue swelling and relieve pain, and Huang *Qi* (Astragalus) tonifies Spleen *Qi*. These four herbs are the Adjuvant herbs. When honey is used in the formulation, it serves as the Messenger herb. All the herbs together clear Liver Heat to brighten the eyes and resolve Stagnation to clear opacity.

Cautions and Contraindications: *Jue Ming San* (Haliotis Powder) is contraindicated in patients with Spleen *Qi* Deficiency.

Dr. Xie's Comments: *Jue Ming San* is effective for treating uveitis and other eye conditions due to Liver Heat in horses and dogs.

Clinical and Pharmacological Studies: Immune-mediated transplant rejection is the main reason for surgical failure in corneal transplants. In one clinical study, 24 patients with corneal transplantation immune rejection were treated with a modified *Jue Ming San*: oral administration twice a day, for 7 days. After 2 weeks, all patients had relief from bulbar conjunctival congestion and swelling and decreased cloudiness of the cornea. Three cases had complete regression of the rejection reaction and sight was significantly improved.[36]

REFERENCES

1. Wang QS, Yuan SQ, Ge SH, Zhao QL. The application of *Bai Hu Tang* in the veterinary clinic. Journal of Traditional Chinese Veterinary Medicine 2005;(3):54.
2. Pu YX. The observation of curative effect of *Bai Hu Tang* to treat 48 cases with fever caused by exogenous pathogens. Yunnan Journal of Traditional Chinese Medicine and Materia Medica 2005;26(2):33.
3. Li PY. Treatment of postpartum fever of cattle with *Qing Ying Tang*. Journal of Traditional Chinese Veterinary Medicine 1997;(1):29.
4. Zhang SY, *Yang* ZM. Treatment of true heat with pseudo-cold using *Qing Ying Tang*. Yunnan Journal of Animal Science and Veterinary Medicine 2000;9(3):43.
5. Fang DJ, Jiang Q. New application of *Xi Jiao Di Huang Tang*. Shanxi Journal of Traditional Chinese Medicine 2005;25(6): 584–585.
6. Zeng Zhongyi, Zhang Lifen, Feng Jianlai, Qu Jinglai. Treatment effects of *Xi Jiao Di Huang Tang* on TT,PT,APTT in plasma of snakebite patients. Journal of Snake 2005;17(2):76–78.
7. Tang SG. Treatment on enterotoxaemia with *Huang Lian Jie Du Tang*. Journal of Traditional Chinese Veterinary Medicine 2007;26(2):45–46.
8. Zhou G, Zhang Y, Kong DY. Experimental study of effect on immunifaction in of *Huang Lian Jie Du Tang* in tumor-bearing mice, Chinese Journal of Experimental Traditional Medical Formulae 2007;(13)3:56–57.
9. Zhou XS. The treatment on 74 cases of epidemic parotitis with *Pu Ji Xiao Du Yin*. Guangming Journal of Chinese Medicine 2006;(6):51–52.
10. Wang HY, Wei XL. The treatment on 56 cases of epidemic parotitis with *Pu Ji Xiao Du Yin*. Liaoning Journal of Traditional Chinese Medicine 2006;33(3):339.
11. Li RY. The treatment of streptococcosis with *Qing Wen Bai Du Yin*. Journal of Traditional Chinese Veterinary Medicine 2003;22(6):23–24.
12. Bao HJ. The treatment of 40 cases of hemorrhagic fever with renal syndrome with *Qing Wen Bai DuYin*. Clinical Journal of Traditional Chinese Medicine 2004;16(4):329.
13. Liu J, Li Q. The experience of *Wu Wei Xiao Du Yin* to treat kidney diseases. Shandong Journal of Chinese Medicine 2007; 26(2):275–276.
14. Hu L, Chang Z. The clinical application examples of *Wu Wei Xiao Du Yin* in treatment of kidney internal diseases. Beijing Journal of Traditional Chinese Medicine 2007;26(5): 305–306.
15. Wang YK. *Xiao Huang San* for the treatment of mastitis in cows. Journal of Traditional Chinese Veterinary Medicine 2004;23(4):19.
16. Cai YS. *Xian Fang Huo Min Yin* for the treatment of 76 cases of ulcerated carbuncles. Journal of Traditional Chinese Medicine 2000;41(6):362.
17. Wang GM. New application of *Wei Jing Tang* in clinic. Li Shi Zhen Medicine and Materia Medica Research 2006;17(4): 646–647.
18. Wang LL, Xu J. Treatment of 50 cases of pulmonary diseases with *Qian Jin Wei Jing Tang*. Journal of Practical Traditional Chinese Internal Medicine 2007;21(2):58.
19. Li BG. The clinical application of *Long Dan Xie Gan Tang*. Forum on Traditional Chinese Medicine 2006;21(2):31–32.
20. Zhang X. Clinical application of *Long Dan Xie Gan Tang*— China Tropical Medicine 2003;3(5):656–657.
21. Lin MX. The treatment of constipation caused by excessive lung heat in horses. Journal of Traditional Chinese Veterinary Medicine 1998;17(3):46.
22. Qin CH, Li F. The observation of curative effect on infantile cough with *Qing Fei San*. Practical Pharmacy and Clinical Remedies 2006;9(5):299–300.
23. Rui QG. The curative effect of *Yu Nü Jian* on 63 cases of chronic atrophic gastritis. Chinese Journal of Prime Medicine Pharmacy 2004;11(9):1140.
24. Chen Y. Treatment of 42 cases of type 2-diabetes due to stomach heat and *Yin* deficiency using *Yu Nü Jian*. Henan Traditional Chinese Medicine 2006;26(12):35–36.
25. Deng GD, Zhu YF. Treatment of canine parvovirus with *Yu Jin San*. Journal of Traditional Chinese Veterinary Medicine 2003;22(3):43.
26. *Yang* Y, Pi JC. Treatment of chordapsus in cattle with *Yu Jin San*. Journal of Traditional Chinese Veterinary Medicine 2004;23(1):27–28.
27. Wei JX, Zhao CP, Zhang JW. Treatment of chronic bacillary diarrhea in calves with *Bai Tou Weng San*. Journal of Yellow Cattle Science 2004;(3):4.
28. Wang W, *Yang* QX, Ye GH. Treatment of white dysentery in piglets with *Bai Tou Weng San*. Jilin Journal of Animal Husbandry and Veterinary Medicine 2003;(2):9.
29. He RL. Therapeutic effect of *Yin Chen Hao Tang* on infant hepatitis syndrome. Integrated Traditional Chinese and Western Medicine in Practice of Critical Care Medicine 1998;5(1):10–11.
30. Kobayashi H, Horikoshi K, Yamataka A, et a1. Beneficial effect of a traditional herbal medicine in postoperative biliary atresia patients. Pediatric Surgery International 2001;17(5):386–389.
31. Li SL. Treatment of equine *Du Huang* with *Xi Xin San*. Journal of Traditional Chinese Veterinary Medicine 1998;17(2):13.
32. Liang XS. *Qing Hao Bie Jia Tang* for the treatment of heat with *Yin* deficiency. Journal of Practical Traditional Chinese Medicine 2005;21(5):295.
33. Liu XY. Comprehension of *Qing Hao Bie Jia Tang* for the treatment of night sweats. Journal of Practical Traditional Chinese Medicine 2005;21(12):759.
34. Ma ZW. Treatment of heatstroke in German shepherd dogs with *Xiang Ru San*. Journal of Traditional Chinese Veterinary Medicine 2003;22(4):35.
35. Xu SD. Treatment of swine heatstroke after delivery with *Xiang Ru San*. Chinese Journal of Traditional Veterinary Medicine 1998;(2):37.
36. Ma DL, Pan ZQ, Jie Y. The role of the traditional Chinese medicine in the modified *Jue Ming San* preventing and treating corneal transplantation immune rejection. Journal of Traditional Chinese Ophthalmology 2003;16(3):139–140.

22 Herbal Formulas to Warm the Interior 温里剂

Xiujun Wang, Hanru Liu, Michael Bartholomew, Justin Shmalberg

Formulas to warm the Interior and formulas to expel Cold are mainly composed of herbs that are energetically warming and therefore good at expelling Cold. The main functions of these formulas are warming the Interior, dispelling Cold, and reviving *Yang*. They are used to treat Interior Cold Patterns.

Based on the location of herb action and the character of clinical application, formulas which warm the Interior can be divided into formulas that warm the Interior and dispel Cold, formulas that warm and activate meridians, and formulas that revive *Yang* for resuscitation.

FORMULAS TO WARM THE MIDDLE BURNER TO DISPEL COLD

The formulas in this section treat Cold in the Middle Burner, which is often caused by Spleen *Yang* Deficiency. The main symptoms include abdominal pain; nausea or vomiting; anorexia; abdominal fullness or distention; exercise intolerance; cold extremities; a pale purple tongue with white, greasy coating; and a deep, slow, and weak pulse.

Li Zhong Tang (Regulating the Middle) 理中汤

Li is regulating. *Zhong* refers to the Middle. *Tang* is decoction. Thus, *Li Zhong Tang* translates literally to Regulating the Middle Decoction.

Source: *Shang Han Za Bing Lun* (*Treatise on Cold-Induced Disorders and Miscellaneous Diseases*), written by *Zhang Zhongjing* in 220 CE

Ingredients: The formula is composed of 60 g *Dang Shen* (Codonopsis), 60 g *Gan Jiang* (Zingiberis), 60 g *Gan Cao* (Glycyrrhiza), and 60 g *Bai Zhu* (Atractylodes) (Table 22.1).

Table 22.1. Ingredients and actions of *Li Zhong Tang*.

%	English Name	Chinese *Pin-Yin*	Actions
25	Codonopsis*	*Dang Shen*	Strengthen the Middle Burner and tonify *Qi*, promote the transporting and transforming function of the Spleen
25	Zingiberis	*Gan Jiang*	Warm the Interior to dispel Cold
25	Glycyrrhiza	*Gan Cao*	Harmonize the other herbs and tonify *Qi*
25	Atractylodes	*Bai Zhu*	Tonify the Spleen and dry up Damp

*Originally *Ren Shen* (Ginseng) was used in the formula. In modern practice, *Dang Shen* (Codonopsis) is often substituted.

Preparation

1. Powder or capsule method: Herbs are ground into a fine powder. Powder can be encapsulated.
2. Decoction or teapill method: Herbs are mixed together and decocted. Herbal water extract (decoction) can be concentrated as granules or teapills.

Actions: Warm the Middle Burner (*Zhong Jiao*) to dispel Cold, tonify *Qi*, and strengthen the Spleen

Indications: False Cold (Deficiency Cold) of the Spleen and Stomach, characterized by pain in the abdomen; preference for pressure and warmth; vomiting; loose stool; cold limbs and ears; a pale, wet tongue with thick, white coating; and deep, slow, and weak pulse

Dosage and Usage

Horses and Cattle: 15–30 g, twice daily
Camels: 30–45 g, twice daily

Llamas, Alpacas, Goats, Sheep, and Pigs: 5–10 g, twice daily
Dogs: 0.5–5 g (or 0.05 g per kg body weight), twice daily
Cats and Rabbits: 0.1–0.5 g (or 0.05 g per kg body weight), twice daily
Birds: 0.05 g per kg body weight, twice daily
Use 1–3 weeks until primary clinical signs resolve.

Analysis of Formula: This formula is the basic formula to warm the Interior. *Gan Jiang* (Zingiberis), as the King Herb, warms the *Yang* of the Middle Burner (*Zhong Jiao*) and dispels Cold of the Spleen and Stomach. *Dang Shen* (Codonopsis), as the Minister herb, strengthens the Middle Burner, tonifies *Qi*, and promotes the transportation and transformation functions of the Spleen and Stomach. The Adjuvant herb is *Bai Zhu* (Atractylodes), which works to strengthen the Spleen and dry up Damp. *Gan Cao* (Glycyrrhiza) not only assists *Bai Zhu* (Atractylodes) and *Dang Shen* (Codonopsis) to tonify *Qi* and strengthen the Spleen, but also coordinates the actions of the other herbs in the formula. All of the herbs together warm the Interior, disperse Cold, tonify *Qi*, and strengthen the Spleen.

Cautions and Contraindications: Do not use in patients with retention of Damp-Heat in Middle Burner and *Yin* Deficiency generating False Heat.

Dr. Xie's Comments: *Li Zhong Tang* is the important and fundamental formula to treat Spleen *Yang* Deficiency with accumulation of Cold in the Interior. It can be modified to treat any Spleen *Yang* Deficiency Pattern.

Clinical and Pharmacological Studies: *Li Zhong Tang* was successfully used to treat 10 cases of diarrhea in piglets, 1 case of cold cough in sheep, and 1 case of "daybreak" diarrhea in a mule. Daybreak diarrhea refers to episodes that occur early in the morning before the sun rises. Diarrhea during the daybreak time period is often caused by Spleen *Yang* Deficiency.[1] Pharmacological studies show that *Li Zhong Tang* can degrade the concentration of free hydrochloric acid in gastric juices, which relieves pain associated with erosion of the mucosa, reduces the activation of pepsin, and promotes cell regeneration and reparation of mucosa.[2]

Fu Zi Li Zhong Tang (Aconite for Regulating the Middle) 附子理中汤

Fu Zi is Aconite, the King ingredient of the formula. *Li Zhong* refers to regulating the Middle. *Tang* is decoction, the original form of herbal administration. Thus, *Fu Zi Li Zhong* translates directly to Aconite for Regulating the Middle.

Table 22.2. Ingredients and actions of *Fu Zi Li Zhong Tang*.

%	English Name	Chinese *Pin-Yin*	Actions
20	Codonopsis	*Dang Shen*	Strengthen the Middle Burner and tonify *Qi*, promote the transporting and transforming function of the Spleen and Stomach
20	Zingiberis	*Gan Jiang*	Warm the *Yang* of the Middle Burner to dispel Coldness of the Spleen and Stomach
20	Glycyrrhiza	*Gan Cao*	Harmonize the other herbs and tonify *Qi*
20	Atractylodes	*Bai Zhu*	Strengthen the Spleen and dry up Dampness
20	Aconite	*Fu Zi*	Warm the Interior to dispel Cold, tonify Kidney *Yang*

Source: *Tai Ping Hui Min He Ji Ju Fang* (*Imperial Grace Formulary of the Tai Ping Era*), written by *Chen Shi-Wen* et al. and published by the Song Dynasty government 1078 CE.

Ingredients: The formula is composed of 60 g *Dang Shen* (Codonopsis), 60 g *Gan Jiang* (Zingiberis), 60 g *Gan Cao* (Glycyrrhiza), 60 g *Bai Zhu* (Atractylodes), and 60 g *Fu Zi* (Aconite) (Table 22.2).

Preparation

1. Powder or capsule method: Herbs are ground into a fine powder. Powder can be encapsulated.
2. Decoction or teapill method: Herbs are mixed together and decocted. Herbal water extract (decoction) can be concentrated as granules or teapills.

Actions: Warm *Yang* to dispel Cold, tonify *Qi* to invigorate the Spleen

Indications: Severe Deficiency-Cold of the Spleen and Stomach or Spleen *Yang* Deficiency with the Interior Cold characterized by abdominal pain; diarrhea with undigested food; nausea and vomiting; chills; a pale, swollen, and purple tongue; and deep, weak, slow pulse

Dosage and Usage:
Horses and Cattle: 15–30 g, twice daily
Camels: 30–45 g, twice daily
Llamas, Alpacas, Goats, Sheep, and Pigs: 5–10 g, twice daily
Dogs: 0.5–3 g (or 0.05 g per kg body weight), twice daily
Cats and Rabbits: 0.1–0.3 g (or 0.05 g per kg body weight), twice daily
Birds: 0.05 g per kg body weight, twice daily
Use 1 week until primary clinical signs resolve.

Analysis of Formula: The formula is composed of the basic classical formulation *Li Zhong Tang* plus prepared Aconite. *Fu Zi* (Aconite) is very pungent and hot, potently warming the Interior. *Gan Jiang* (Zingiberis) is moderately beneficial in warming the Interior but is good at penetrating and carrying the warm energy to the entire body. *Fu Zi* (Aconite) and *Gan Jiang* (Zingiberis) mutually promote the warming effect in the formula and work as the King herbs. *Dang Shen* (Codonopsis) is sweet and neutral in its nature and, as the Minister herb, strengthens the Middle Burner, tonifies *Qi*, and promotes the transporting and transforming functions of the Spleen and Stomach. The Adjuvant herb is *Bai Zhu* (Atractylodes), strengthening the Spleen and drying up Damp. Working as the Messenger herb, *Gan Cao* (Glycyrrhiza) not only coordinates the herb actions of the formula, but also counters the side effect of Aconite. All of the herbs together tonify *Yang* and warm the Interior to dispel Cold.

Cautions and Contraindications: Do not use to treat patients with *Yin* Deficiency, False Heat (Deficiency Heat), loss of blood, or during pregnancy.

Dr. Xie's Comments: *Fu Zi Li Zhong Tang* is a potent formula to tonify Spleen and Kidney *Yang* to dispel Internal Cold. It is often used to treat diarrhea due to Spleen and Kidney *Yang* Deficiency, "daybreak" diarrhea, or chronic diarrhea in elderly patients with *Yang* Deficiency.

Clinical and Pharmacological Studies: *Fu Zi Li Zhong Tang* was successfully used to treat diarrhea caused by Spleen *Yang* Deficiency secondary to duodenal ulcer, pancreatitis, or postradiotherapy of nasopharyngeal carcinoma. After the herbal treatment, the diarrhea in 13 out of 17 cases was clinically cured, and another 3 cases improved.[3] Pharmacological studies show that *Fu Zi Li Zhong Tang* has the function of relieving pain; regulating movement of the intestinal tract; and improving physical strength, immune function, and resistance to cold.[4]

Lian Li Tang (Coptis for Regulating the Middle) 连理汤

Lian refers to *Huang Lian* or Coptis. *Li* refers to *Li Zhong Tang* (Regulating the Middle). *Tang* is decoction, the form of herbal administration. Thus, *Lian Li* translates to Coptis for Regulating the Middle.

Source: *Zheng Yin Mai Zhi* (*Pattern, Cause, Pulse and Treatment*), written by *Qin Jing-Ming* and published in 1702 CE

Ingredients: The formula is composed of 60g *Dang Shen* (Codonopsis), 60g *Gan Jiang* (Zingiberis), 60g *Gan Cao* (Glycyrrhiza), 60g *Bai Zhu* (Atractylodes), 60g *Huang Lian* (Coptis), and 60g *Fu Ling* (Poria) (Table 22.3).

Table 22.3. Ingredients and actions of *Lian Li Tang*.

%	English Name	Chinese *Pin-Yin*	Actions
16.7	Codonopsis	*Dang Shen*	Strengthen the Middle Burner and tonify *Qi*, promote the transporting and transforming function of the Spleen and Stomach
16.7	Zingiberis	*Gan Jiang*	Warm the *Yang* of the Middle Burner and disperse Cold of the Spleen and Stomach
16.5	Glycyrrhiza	*Gan Cao*	Harmonize the other herbs and tonify *Qi*
16.7	Atractylodes	*Bai Zhu*	Invigorate the Spleen and dry Damp
16.7	Poria	*Fu Ling*	Strengthen the Spleen and drain Damp
16.7	Coptis	*Huang Lian*	Clear Heat, dry Damp, and purge Fire to remove toxins

Preparation:
1. Powder or capsule method: Herbs are ground into a fine powder. Powder can be encapsulated.
2. Decoction or teapill method: Herbs are mixed together and decocted. Herbal water extract (decoction) can be concentrated as granules or teapills.

Actions: Warm the Interior to dispel Cold and clear Damp-Heat

Indications: Deficiency-Cold of Spleen and Stomach with Damp-Heat; stomachache; dysentery; vomiting; abdominal distension, drooling, licking the lips, coldness of the back and ears; yellow coating of the tongue; and deep, slow, weak pulse

Dosage and Usage:
Horses and Cattle: 15–30g, twice daily
Camels: 30–45g, twice daily
Llamas, Alpacas, Goats, Sheep, and Pigs: 5–10g, twice daily
Dogs: 0.5–5g (or 0.05g per kg body weight), twice daily
Cats and Rabbits: 0.1–0.5g (or 0.05g per kg body weight), twice daily
Birds: 0.05g per kg body weight, twice daily
Use 1–2 weeks until primary clinical signs resolve.

Analysis of Formula: The formula is designed for False Cold due to Spleen *Yang* Deficiency with mild

Damp-Heat. Chronic accumulation of coldness in the Middle Burner attracts and bottles up the fluids, which are stagnant and transform into Damp-Heat. Clinically this appears as dysentery (bloody, mucoid diarrhea), and a tongue with a yellow coating. The treatment principle is to tonify Spleen *Qi*, warm the Middle Burner, and clear Damp-Heat. Therefore, *Gan Jiang* (Zingiberis) and *Huang Lian* (Coptis) work together as the King herbs to warm the Interior and dispel Cold, while simultaneously clearing Damp-Heat out of the Middle Burner. *Dang Shen* (Codonopsis) and *Bai Zhu* (Atractylodes) are the Minister herbs that tonify *Qi*, dry up Damp, and promote the transporting and transforming functions of the Spleen and Stomach. The Adjuvant herb is *Fu Ling* (Poria), acting to strengthen the Spleen and drain Damp. Serving as the Messenger, *Gan Cao* (Glycyrrhiza) coordinates the herb actions of the prescription. All of the herbs together warm the Interior to dispel Cold, tonify Spleen *Qi*, and clear Damp-Heat.

Cautions and Contraindications: Do not use to treat patients with excessive Damp-Heat in the Spleen.

Dr. Xie's Comments: The formula is often used to treat chronic dysentery, chronic bacillary diarrhea, and chronic enteritis in which both Cold and Heat are present. Clinically this presents as a patient with a cold back and ears, yellow and greasy coating of the tongue, and bloody dysentery or watery diarrhea.

Clinical and Pharmacological Studies: *Lian Li Tang* was used to treat 36 cases of chronic ulcerative colitis from 2001 to 2006.[5] The treatment group was treated with 170 ml decoction of the formula orally in the morning, and 170 ml as a retention enema at night. The control group was treated with a standard antibiotic procedure. In the herbal treatment group, 97.22% of patients in the herbal treatment group showed a positive response; 85.29% of patients in the Western medicine treatment group had a positive response. Even more significant was that 88.89% of patients in the herbal treatment group had a nonrecurrence rate of 2 years, and only 14.29% of patients in the Western medicine treatment group did not have a reoccurrence for 2 years.

Xiao Jian Zhong Tang (Mildly Strengthening the Middle) 小健中汤

Xiao means small, or mild. *Jian* means strengthening. *Zhong* refers to *Zhong Jiao*, or Middle Burner. *Tang* is decoction, the form of herbal administration. Thus, *Xiao Jian Zhong* translates to Mildly Strengthening the Middle.

Source: *Shang Han Za Bing Lun* (*Treatise on Cold-Induced Disorders and Miscellaneous Diseases*), written by *Zhang Zhongjing* and published in 220 CE

Table 22.4. Ingredients and actions of *Xiao Jian Zhong Tang*.

%	English Name	Chinese Pin-Yin	Actions
10.8	Cinnamomum	*Gui Zhi*	Warm *Yang Qi* and dispel Cold
7.2	Glycyrrhiza	*Gan Cao*	Harmonize the other herbs and tonify *Qi*
14.5	Jujube	*Da Zao*	Tonify Spleen *Qi*
21.7	Paeonia	*Bai Shao Yao*	Nourish *Ying*-Blood, soothe Liver *Qi*
9.6	Zingiberis	*Sheng Jiang*	Warm the Stomach to dispel Cold
36.2	Maltose	*Yi Tang*	Warm and strengthen the Middle Burner, relax spasm to relieve pain

Ingredients: The formula is composed of 9 g *Gui Zhi* (Cinnamomum), 6 g *Gan Cao* (Glycyrrhiza), 12 g *Da Zao* (Jujube), 18 g *Bai Shao Yao* (Paeonia), 8 g *Sheng Jiang* (Zingiberis), and 30 g *Yi Tang* (Maltose) (Table 22.4).

Preparation:

1. Powder or capsule method: Herbs are ground into a fine powder. Powder can be encapsulated.
2. Decoction or teapill method: Herbs are mixed together and decocted. Herbal water extract (decoction) can be concentrated as granules or teapills.

Actions: Warm and tonify the Middle Burner (*Zhong Jiao*), relax spasm to relieve abdominal pain

Indications: Deficiency-Cold in the Middle Burner, disharmony between the Liver and Spleen, spasmodic pain in the abdomen, preference for pressure and warmth, debilitation, general weakness, timid nature

Dosage and Usage:

Horses and Cattle: 15–30 g, twice daily
Camels: 30–45 g, twice daily
Llamas, Alpacas, Goats, Sheep, and Pigs: 5–10 g, twice daily
Dogs: 0.5–5 g (or 0.05 g per kg body weight), twice daily
Cats and Rabbits: 0.1–0.5 g (or 0.05 g per kg body weight), twice daily
Birds: 0.05 g per kg body weight, twice daily
Use 2–6 weeks until primary clinical signs resolve.

Analysis of Formula: This formula is for Deficiency-Cold (False Cold) in the Middle Burner (*Zhong Jiao*), accompanied by disharmony between the Liver and Spleen. *Yi Tang* (Maltose), as the King herb, warms and strengthens the Middle Burner and alleviates urgency and spasm, thereby relieving abdominal pain. The Minister herbs are *Gui Zhi* (Cinnamomum), which is pungent and warming and serves to warm *Yang Qi* to dispel Cold, and *Bai Shao Yao* (Paeonia), which is sour and sweet and nourishes *Ying*-Blood, alleviates the Liver *Qi* Stagnation, and resolves Stomach pain. *Sheng Jiang* (Zingiberis) warms the Stomach and dispels Cold, and *Da Zao* (Jujube) tonifies Spleen *Qi*. Together they are the Adjuvant herbs. *Gan Cao* (Glycyrrhiza) is the Messenger herb that nourishes *Qi*, harmonizes the Middle Burner (*Zhong Jiao*), and coordinates the herb actions in the formula.

Cautions and Contraindications: The formula is sweet and warm, so it is not suitable for *Yin* Deficiency or Excess Heat.

Dr. Xie's Comments: *Xiao Jian Zhong Tang* is a mild and safe formula to treat Coldness in the Middle Burner due to Spleen *Yang* Deficiency. It can be used in elderly or pregnant patients when *Fu Zi Li Zhong Tang* is too potent to be used.

Clinical and Pharmacological Studies: *Xiao Jian Zhong Tang* was used for the treatment of 58 human cases of chronic gastritis.[6] After herbal treatment, 32 cases were cured, 18 case were significantly improved, and 8 cases failed to respond. Another clinical trial indicated similar results.[7]

Huang Qi Jian Zhong Tang (Astragalus for Strengthening the Middle) 黄芪健中汤

Huang Qi refers to Astragalus, the King ingredient of the formula. *Jian* means strengthening. *Zhong* refers to the Middle Burner (*Zhong Jiao*), or the Spleen and Stomach. *Tang* is decoction, the form of herbal administration. *Huang Qi Jian Zhong* translates to Astragalus for Strengthening the Middle.

Source: *Jin Gui Yao Lue Fang Lun* (*Synopsis of Prescriptions from the Golden Cabinet*), written by *Zhang Zhong-Jing* and published in 220 CE

Ingredients: The formula of *Huang Qi Jian Zhong Tang* (Table 22.5) is composed of 30 g *Yi Tang* (Maltose), 9 g *Gui Zhi* (Cinnamomum), 18 g *Bai Shao Yao* (Paeonia), 9 g *Sheng Jiang* (Zingiberis), 6 g *Da Zao* (Jujube), 5 g *Huang Qi* (Astragalus), and 6 g *Gan Cao* (Glycyrrhiza).

Table 22.5. Ingredients and actions of *Huang Qi Jian Zhong Tang*.

%	English Name	Chinese *Pin-Yin*	Actions
10.8	Cinnamomum	*Gui Zhi*	Warm *Yang Qi* to dispel Cold
7.2	Glycyrrhiza	*Gan Cao*	Harmonize the other herbs and tonify *Qi*
7.2	Jujube	*Da Zao*	Nourish Spleen and *Qi*
21.7	Paeonia	*Bai Shao Yao*	Nourish *Yin* and Blood, soothe Liver *Qi*, relieve nausea and abdominal pain
10.8	Zingiberis	*Sheng Jiang*	Warm the Stomach and dispel Cold
36.1	Maltose	*Yi Tang*	Warm and strengthen the Middle Burner, relax spasm and relieve pain
6.2	Astragalus	*Huang Qi*	Tonify Spleen *Qi*

Preparation:

1. Powder or capsule method: Herbs are ground into a fine powder. Powder can be encapsulated.
2. Decoction or teapill method: Herbs are mixed together and decocted. Herbal water extract (decoction) can be concentrated as granules or teapills.

Actions: Warm the Middle Burner, tonify *Yang Qi*, nourish *Yin* and Blood, harmonize the Interior to alleviate pain

Indications: Deficiency of *Qi*, Blood, *Yin*, and *Yang*. Clinical signs include abdominal pain; warm-seeking behavior; preference for external abdominal pressure, thin body, shortness of breath, palpitations or restlessness, spontaneous perspiration or panting at night, damp feet, pale or red tongue, and weak or thin pulse.

Dosage and Usage:

Horses and Cattle: 15–30 g, twice daily
Camels: 30–45 g, twice daily
Llamas, Alpacas, Goats, Sheep, and Pigs: 5–10 g, twice daily
Dogs: 0.5–5 g (or 0.05 g per kg body weight), twice daily
Cats and Rabbits: 0.1–0.5 g (or 0.05 g per kg body weight), twice daily
Birds: 0.05 g per kg body weight, twice daily
Use 2–6 weeks until primary clinical signs resolve.

Analysis of Formula: The formula is comprised of *Xiao Jian Zhong Tang* with additional *Huang Qi* (Astragalus), serving as the King herb. *Huang Qi* (Astragalus) reinforces the power of tonifying *Yang-Qi* and warming the Middle Burner. *Gui Zhi* (Cinnamomum) and *Yi Tang* (Maltose), as the Minister herbs, warm *Yang-Qi* and strengthen the Middle Burner to dispel Cold and alleviate urgency and spasm to relieve abdominal pain. *Bai Shao Yao* (Paeonia) nourishes *Yin* and Blood. *Sheng Jiang* (Zingiberis) has the properties of warming the Stomach and dispelling Cold, while *Da Zao* (Jujube) tonifies Spleen *Qi*. Together they are the Adjuvant herbs. *Gan Cao* (Glycyrrhiza) is the Messenger herb that nourishes *Qi*, harmonizes the Middle Burner (*Zhong Jiao*), and coordinates the herb actions in the formula.

Cautions and Contraindications: Do not use to treat cases with *Yin* Deficiency or excessive Damp-Heat.

Dr. Xie's Comments: *Huang Qi Jian Zhong Tang* is good at warming the Middle Burner, tonifying *Yang-Qi* Deficiency, and alleviating urgency to stop abdominal pain. It is often used to treat general *Yang-Qi* Deficiency and exhaustion with chronic abdominal pain. In modern practice, it is used for the treatment of chronic gastritis, heart murmur, and congestive heart failure.

Clinical and Pharmacological Studies: Modified *Huang Qi Jian Zhong Tang* was used to treat 170 human cases of intestinal ulceration with a good effect. One dose per day was given orally. Thirty-four cases were cured after 70 continuous doses, 57 cases were cured after 90 continuous doses, and 64 cases were cured after 110 doses. The overall effective rate was 91.2%.[8]

Da Jian Zhong Tang (Potent Strengthening of the Middle) 大健中汤

Da means large, major, or potent. *Jian* means strengthening. *Zhong* refers to the Middle Burner (*Zhong Jiao*), or the Spleen and Stomach. *Tang* is decoction, the form of herbal administration. Thus, *Da Jian Zhong Tang* translates to Potent Decoction to Strengthen the Middle.

Source: *Jin Gui Yao Lue Fang Lun* (*Synopsis of Prescriptions from the Golden Cabinet*), written by *Zhang Zhong-Jing* and published in 220 CE

Ingredients: The formula of *Da Jian Zhong Tang* (Table 22.6) is composed of 6 g *Chuan Jiao* (Zanthoxylum), 12 g *Gan Jiang* (Zingiberis), and 6 g *Ren Shen* (Ginseng).

Preparation:
1. Powder or capsule method: Herbs are ground into a fine powder. Powder can be encapsulated.
2. Decoction or teapill method: Herbs are mixed together and decocted. Herbal water extract (decoction) can be concentrated as granules or teapills.

Actions: Warm the Middle Burner, tonify *Qi*, reverse Rebellious Stomach *Qi*, stop abdominal pain

Table 22.6. Ingredients and actions of *Da Jian Zhong Tang*.

%	English Name	Chinese *Pin-Yin*	Actions
25	Zanthoxylum	*Chuan Jiao*	Warm the Middle Burner to dispel Cold, dry up Damp and stop pain
50	Zingiberis	*Gan Jiang*	Warm the Middle Burner to dispel Cold and relieve pain
25	Ginseng	*Ren Shen*	Tonify Spleen and Lung *Qi*, reinforce Source (*Yuan*) *Qi*

Indications: Acute abdominal pain or vomiting caused by *Yang* Deficiency of the Middle Burner (*Zhong Jiao*). The main clinical signs are abdominal pain; loose stool; vomiting; coldness of the ears and back; a pale purple, wet tongue with a white, greasy coating; and a deep, weak, slow, and deficient pulse.

Dosage and Usage:
Horses and Cattle: 15–30 g, twice daily
Camels: 30–45 g, twice daily
Llamas, Alpacas, Goats, Sheep, and Pigs: 5–10 g, twice daily
Dogs: 0.5–5 g (or 0.05 g per kg body weight), twice daily
Cats and Rabbits: 0.1–0.5 g (or 0.05 g per kg body weight), twice daily
Birds: 0.05 g per kg body weight, twice daily
Use 1–2 weeks until primary clinical signs resolve.

Analysis of Formula: *Da Jian Zhong Tang* consists of purely pungent and hot herbs to warm and tonify Middle Burner *Yang*. Its actions of warming the Middle Burner and dispelling Cold are far stronger than *Xiao Jian Zhong Tang*. *Da Jian Zhong Tang* also has the function of reversing Rebellious Stomach *Qi* to stop vomiting. It is usually used to treat abdominal pain and vomiting caused by *Yang* Deficiency of the Middle Burner accompanied by an abundance of Cold signs. Serving as the King herb, *Gan Jiang* (Zingiberis) warms the Spleen *Yang* to dispel Cold and moves Stomach *Qi* to stop vomiting and abdominal pain. The Minister herb is *Chuan Jiao* (Zanthoxylum), working to enhance the King herb's actions of warming the Interior to dispel Cold. *Ren Shen* (Ginseng) tonifies *Yuan Qi* (Source *Qi*) and the Spleen and works as the Adjuvant herb.

Cautions and Contraindications: Do not use to treat cases with abdominal pain caused from Damp-Heat or cases with False-Heat due to *Yin*-Deficiency.

Dr. Xie's Comments: I often use *Da Jian Zhong Tang* to treat *Yang* Deficiency of the Middle Burner and abundance of Coldness. Patients with this condition typically have cold ears, nose, and lower abdomen and will exhibit heat-seeking behavior; nausea or vomiting; vomiting immediately after eating or drinking cold foods or water; abdominal pain; colic that is worse with exposure to cold; a pale purple tongue; and a weak, slow pulse.

Clinical and Pharmacological Studies: Xu used the modified *Da Jian Zhong Tang* to treat chronic pancreatitis in humans. The result indicated that 1 dose of herbal medication alleviated abdominal pain; after 3 doses patients took food without vomiting, and after 10 doses, the patients fully recovered clinically.[9] In another study, neurotransmitter levels were measured to quantify *Da Jian Zhong Tang*'s effect on pain.

Patients with Spleen *Yang* Deficiency were treated with the formula and serum neurotransmitters were measured. Plasma levels of 5-hydroxytryptamine (5-HT, or serotonin), 5-hydroxytryptophan (5-HTP), and 5-Hydroxyindoleacetic acid (5-HIAA) were all decreased after administration of the formula, suggesting that *Da Jian Zhong Tang* provides pain relief.[10]

Wu Zhu Yu Tang (Evodia Decoction) 吴茱萸汤

Wu Zhu Yu refers to Evodia, the King ingredient of the formula. *Tang* is decoction, the form of herbal administration. Thus, *Wu Zhu Yu Tang* translates literally to Evodia Decoction.

Source: *Shang Han Za Bing Lun* (*Treatise on Cold-Induced Disorders and Miscellaneous Diseases*), written by *Zhang Zhongjing* and published in 220 CE

Ingredients: *Wu Zhu Yu Tang* (Table 22.7) is composed of 30 g *Wu Zhu Yu* (Evodia), 30 g *Dang Shen* (Codonopsis), 30 g *Sheng Jiang* (Zingiberis), and 20 g *Da Zao* (Jujube).

Preparation:

1. Powder or capsule method: Herbs are ground into a fine powder. Powder can be encapsulated.
2. Decoction or teapill method: Herbs are mixed together and decocted. Herbal water extract (decoction) can be concentrated as granules or teapills.

Actions: Warm the Middle Burner, tonify Spleen *Qi*, descend Stomach *Qi* to stop vomiting

Indications: Vomiting due to Spleen *Qi* Deficiency and Stomach Coldness. The main clinical signs are vomiting after eating; sour or dry vomiting; abdominal pain; chills; diarrhea; restlessness; a pale, wet tongue with a white, greasy coating; and a deep, weak pulse.

Dosage and Usage:

Horses and Cattle: 15–30 g, twice daily
Camels: 30–45 g, twice daily
Llamas, Alpacas, Goats, Sheep, and Pigs: 5–10 g, twice daily
Dogs: 0.5–5 g (or 0.05 g per kg body weight), twice daily
Cats and Rabbits: 0.1–0.5 g (or 0.05 g per kg body weight), twice daily
Birds: 0.05 g per kg body weight, twice daily

Use 1–3 weeks until primary clinical signs resolve.

Table 22.7. Ingredients and actions *Wu Zhu Yu Tang*.

%	English Name	Chinese *Pin-Yin*	Actions
27.3	Evodia	*Wu Zhu Yu*	Dispel Cold, move Stomach *Qi* to stop vomiting and pain
27.3	Codonopsis	*Dang Shen*	Tonify Spleen *Qi*
27.3	Zingiberis	*Sheng Jiang*	Warm the Stomach to dispel Cold
18.1	Jujube	*Da Zao*	Nourish Spleen *Qi*

Analysis of Formula: The formula is designed for vomiting due to Spleen *Qi* Deficiency with Cold in the Stomach. *Wu Zhu Yu* (Evodia) is the King herb, which is pungent and hot. It enters the Liver, Spleen, Stomach, and Kidney and consequently warms the Middle Burner while also descending *Qi* to stop vomiting and abdominal pain. A large dose of *Sheng Jiang* (Zingiberis), as Minister herb, warms the Middle Burner to stop vomiting, harmonizes the Stomach, and reverses the Rebellious *Qi*. It assists *Wu Zhu Yu* (Evodia) to dispel Cold and stop vomiting and pain. *Dang Shen* (Codonopsis) tonifies *Qi*, strengthens the Spleen, and is the Adjuvant herb. The sweet flavor of *Da Zao* (Jujube) has the effect of relaxing and regulating the Middle Burner (*Zhong Jiao*). This assists *Dang Shen* (Codonopsis) to tonify Spleen *Qi* and *Sheng Jiang* (Zingiberis) to regulate the Spleen and Stomach. *Da Zao* (Jujube) also restricts the pungent natures of *Wu Zhu Yu* (Evodia) *Sheng Jiang* (Zingiberis), so it is the Messenger herb in the formula.

Cautions and Contraindications: Do not use to treat cases with Excess Heat or False Heat in the Stomach.

Dr. Xie's Comments: *Wu Zhu Yu Tang* is often used for chronic nausea or vomiting due to Spleen *Qi* Deficiency in dogs and cats.

Clinical and Pharmacological Studies: *Zhi Shi* (Aurantium) and *Cang Zhu* (Atractylodes) were added to *Wu Zhu Yu Tang* to treat gastroesophageal reflux disease of geriatric men. In 28 cases, 21 cases had a significantly positive effect, 5 cases showed improvement and 2 cases showed no change after the herbal medication. 93% of patients in this study had a positive response.[11]

FORMULAS TO WARM THE MERIDIANS TO DISPEL COLD

The formulas in this section are used to treat Cold accumulated in the Channels and Meridians, which often occurs in patients with *Yang* or Blood Deficiency. Exogenous Cold invades the body, congeals in the Channels and Meridians, obstructs the flow of *Qi* leading to Stagnation of *Qi* and Blood, and results in pain. The primary actions of these formulas are to warm the Channels to dispel Cold and to resolve Stagnation to relieve pain.

Huang Qi Gui Zhi Wu Wu Tang (Astragalus and Cinnamomum Five) 黄芪桂枝五物汤

Huang Qi refers to Astragalus, the King ingredient of the formula. *Gui Zhi* is Cinnamomum. The first *Wu* means five. The second *Wu* refers to ingredient. *Wu Wu* refers to a total of five ingredients of the formula. *Tang* is decoction, the form of herbal administration.

Source: *Shang Han Za Bing Lun* (*Treatise on Cold-Induced Disorders and Miscellaneous Diseases*), written by *Zhang Zhongjing* and published in 220 CE

Ingredients: *Huang Qi Gui Zhi Wu Wu Tang* (Table 22.8) is composed of 9 g *Huang Qi* (Astragalus), 9 g *Gui Zhi* (Cinnamomum), 9 g *Bai Shao Yao* (Paeonia), 18 g *Sheng Jiang* (Zingiberis), and 4 g *Da Zao* (Jujube).

Preparation:

1. Powder or capsule method: Herbs are ground into a fine powder. Powder can be encapsulated.
2. Decoction or teapill method: Herbs are mixed together and decocted. Herbal water extract (decoction) can be concentrated as granules or teapills.

Actions: Tonify *Qi* and warm the Channels/Meridians, harmonize *Ying-Wei* and relieve joint pain

Indications: *Yang-Qi* Deficiency with joint pain due to Stagnation of Blood. The main clinical signs are pain in the joints; stiffness or numbness in the limbs; cold extremities; a pale, purple tongue; and a weak, tight pulse.

Dosage and Usage:

Horses and Cattle: 15–30 g, twice daily
Camels: 30–45 g, twice daily
Llamas, Alpacas, Goats, Sheep, and Pigs: 5–10 g, twice daily
Dogs: 0.5–5 g (or 0.05 g per kg body weight), twice daily
Cats and Rabbits: 0.1–0.5 g (or 0.05 g per kg body weight), twice daily
Birds: 0.05 g per kg body weight, twice daily
Use 1–3 weeks until primary clinical signs resolve.

Table 22.8. Ingredients and actions of *Huang Qi Gui Zhi Wu Wu Tang*.

%	English Name	Chinese *Pin-Yin*	Actions
18	Astragalus	*Huang Qi*	Tonify Spleen *Qi*
18	Cinnamomum	*Gui Zhi*	Warm *Yang-Qi* to dispel Cold
18	Paeonia	*Bai Shao Yao*	Nourish Blood and harmonize *Ying-Wei*
36	Zingiberis	*Sheng Jiang*	Warm the Stomach to dispel Cold
10	Jujube	*Da Zao*	Nourish Spleen *Qi*

Analysis of Formula: *Yang-Qi* Deficiency leads to a failure of the body's ability to defend itself against Exogenous Pathogens. Pathogenic Wind and Cold invade the body and then migrate to joints. They obstruct the flow of *Qi* and Blood, leading to pain or numbness in the joints. Serving as the King herb, *Huang Qi* (Astragalus) is sweet and warm in the formula. It tonifies *Qi* and reinforces the *Wei Qi* (Defensive *Qi*) at the surface. *Gui Zhi* (Cinnamomum) dispels Wind-Cold and warms the Channels/Meridians, relaxing muscle spasm and relieving pain. *Gui Zhi* (Cinnamomum) also warms the Exterior and supports *Huang Qi* (Astragalus) to stimulate *Wei Qi*; while *Huang Qi* (Astragalus) tonifies the Exterior *Yang-Qi* to enhance *Gui Zhi's* (Cinnamomum's) ability to dispel Cold. *Bai Shao Yao* (Paeonia) nourishes Blood and harmonizes *Ying-Wei* to resolve Stagnation and relieve joint pain. Together with *Gui Zhi* (Cinnamomum), *Bai Shao Yao* (Paeonia) regulates *Ying-Wei* and harmonizes both the Interior and Exterior. These two herbs are Minister herbs. *Sheng Jiang* (Zingiberis) is pungent and warm, which dispels Wind-Cold to assist *Gui Zhi* (Cinnamomum). *Da Zao* (Jujube) is sweet and warm, which nourishes Blood and tonifies *Qi* to support *Huang Qi* (Astragalus) and *Bai Shao Yao* (Paeonia). *Sheng Jiang* (Zingiberis) and *Bai Shao Yao* (Paeonia) together are the Adjuvant and Messenger herbs.

Cautions and Contraindications: Do not use to treat patients with *Yin* Deficiency *Bi* syndrome.

Dr. Xie's Comments: *Huang Qi Gui Zhi Wu Wu Tang* is a famous formula used to treat *Yang-Qi* Deficiency and joint pain due to Stagnation of Blood. In the modern practice, this formula is used for the treatment of peripheral neuritis, lingering effects of cerebral paralysis, arthritis, hip or pelvic pain, myocarditis, bedsores, and acute circumscribed edema.

Clinical and Pharmacological Studies: *Huang Qi Gui Zhi Wu Wu Tang* was used in treating 58 cases of rheumatoid arthritis. In the herbal treatment group, *Huang Qi Gui Zhi Wu Wu Tang* was given orally 3 times/day. After 1 month of herbal treatment, 29 cases were clinically cured, 16 cases showed a significantly positive effect, 9 cases showed some positive effect, and 4 cases showed no effect. In the control group, glucosidorum tripterygll totorum was taken orally, 20 g, 3 times/day. After 1 month of treatment, 11 cases were clinically cured, 7 cases had an obvious positive effect, 6 cases had some positive effect, and 6 cases had no effect.[12]

Yang He Tang (*Yang* Harmonizing) 阳和汤

He means peace or harmonizing. *Tang* is decoction, the form of herbal administration. *Yang He* refers to the fact that this formula is able to warm and harmonize

Table 22.9. Ingredients and actions of *Yang He Tang*.

%	English Name	Chinese *Pin-Yin*	Actions
54.5	Rehmannia	*Shu Di Huang*	Nourish Blood, tonify Kidney *Yin* and *Jing*
5.5	Cinnamomum	*Rou Gui*	Warm and tonify *Yang* to dispel Cold
3.6	Ephedra	*Ma Huang*	Relieve the Exterior, induce diuresis to alleviate edema
16.4	Cervus	*Lu Jiao Jiao*	Tonify *Yang*, strengthen bones and muscles
10.9	Sinapsis	*Bai Jie Zi*	Warm the Lung, activate the Channels to resolve Stagnation
3.6	Zingiberis	*Gan Jiang*	Warm and activate *Yang* to dispel Cold
5.5	Glycyrrhiza	*Gan Cao*	Clear Heat and detoxify, harmonize other herb actions

(comfort) the areas of the body where Cold has accumulated and caused *Yin*-type swellings. This is as the sunlight (*Yang*) warms the earth and dispels Cold (*Yin*) to keep harmony.

Source: *Wai Ke Zheng Zhi Quan Sheng Ji* (*Complete Collection of Patterns and Treatments in External Medicine*), written by *Wang Wei-De* and published in 1740 CE

Ingredients: *Yang He Tang* (Table 22.9) is composed of 30g *Shu Di Huang* (Rehmannia), 3g *Rou Gui* (Cinnamomum), 2g *Ma Huang* (Ephedra), 9g *Lu Jiao Jiao* (Cervus), 6g *Bai Jie Zi* (Sinapsis), 2g *Gan Jiang* (Zingiberis), and 3g *Gan Cao* (Glycyrrhiza).

Preparation:

1. Powder or capsule method: Herbs are ground into a fine powder. Powder can be encapsulated.
2. Decoction or teapill method: Herbs are mixed together and decocted. Herbal water extract (decoction) can be concentrated as granules or teapills.

Actions: Warm *Yang* and nourish Blood, dispel Cold to resolve Stagnation

Indications: *Yin*-type localized swelling (*Yin Ju*) due to Stagnation of Phlegm and *Yang* Deficiency. *Yin Ju* is characterized by local swelling that is not hot to touch and does not affect the color and texture of the skin. The other signs are no thirst; no pain on palpation; a pale tongue with a white, greasy coating; and a deep, thin pulse. *Yu Ju* can be found in discrete areas of the muscles, tendons/ligaments or sinews, bones, or blood vessels.

Dosage and Usage:
Horses and Cattle: 15–30g, twice daily
Camels: 30–45g, twice daily
Llamas, Alpacas, Goats, Sheep, and Pigs: 5–10g, twice daily
Dogs: 0.5–5g (or 0.05g per kg body weight), twice daily
Cats and Rabbits: 0.1–0.5g (or 0.05g per kg body weight), twice daily
Birds: 0.05g per kg body weight, twice daily
Use 1–4 weeks until primary clinical signs resolve.

Analysis of Formula: *Yu Ju* is caused by a combination of Blood Deficiency and *Yang* Deficiency. Deficient Blood fails to nourish the muscles, tendons, ligaments, bones, joints, and blood vessels. *Yang* Deficiency leads to Cold Stagnation, which congeals and transforms to Phlegm. Cold Phlegm is accumulated in the malnourished muscle, bones, tendons, ligaments, and blood vessels, leading to *Yu Ju*. In the formula, *Shu Di Huang* (Rehmannia) nourishes Blood and tonifies Kidney *Yin* and *Jing*, and serves as the King herb. *Lu Jiao Jiao* (Cervus), which tonifies *Yang* and strengthens bones and muscles, is the Minister herb. *Ma Huang* (Ephedra), *Rou Gui* (Cinnamomum), and *Gan Jiang* (Zingiberis), the Adjuvant herbs, enter the Exterior and warm and activate *Yang* to dispel Cold. *Gan Cao* (Glycyrrhiza), as the Messenger herb, clears Heat and detoxifies, coordinating the herb actions of a prescription.

Cautions and Contraindications: *Yang He Tang* is used for swelling that is not open. Do not use for *Yu Ju* when it is open with draining pus. It is also contraindicated in cases with Heat and/or *Yin* Deficiency.

Dr. Xie's Comments: In modern practice, *Yang He Tang* is often use in treating aseptic suppuration in the deep muscle, chronic osteomyelitis, tubercular joint disease, rheumatoid arthritis, and lymphatic tuberculosis.

Clinical and Pharmacological Studies: Ren conducted a clinical trial on the delayed union of bone fractures. In the herbal group, 100 cases (67 cases were men and 33 cases were women) were treated with *Yang He Tang*. The dose was 50ml of herbal water extract given orally 2 times daily for 50 days. In the control group, 50 cases (31 cases were men and 19 cases were women) were treated with 2 calcium tablets and 1 vitamin A/D tablet, 2 times daily for 50 days. The results showed that 94% of patients in the herbal group had a positive response and 68.9% of patients in the control group had a positive response.[13]

Wu Tou Tang (Aconite Decoction) 乌头汤

Wu Tou refers to Aconite, the King ingredient of the formula. *Tang* is decoction, the form of herbal administration.

Table 22.10. Ingredients and actions of *Wu Tou Tang*.

%	English Name	Chinese *Pin-Yin*	Actions
21.4	Ephedra	*Ma Huang*	Relieve the Exterior, induce diuresis to alleviate edema
21.4	Paeonia	*Bai Shao Yao*	Nourish Blood and harmonize *Ying-Wei*
21.4	Astragalus	*Huang Qi*	Tonify Spleen *Qi*
21.4	Glycyrrhiza	*Gan Cao*	Clear Heat, detoxify and harmonize the other herb actions
14.4	Aconite	*Chuan Wu*	Expel Wind-Damp, warm Channels to relieve pain

Source: *Jin Gui Yao Lue Fang Lun* (*Synopsis of Prescriptions from the Golden Cabinet*), written by *Zhang Zhong-Jing* and published in 220 CE

Ingredients: *Wu Tou Tang* (Table 22.10) is composed of 9 g *Ma Huang* (Ephedra), 9 g *Bai Shao Yao* (Paeonia), 9 g *Huang Qi* (Astragalus), 9 g *Gan Cao* (Glycyrrhiza), and 6 g *Chuan Wu* (Aconite).

Preparation:
1. Powder or capsule method: Herbs are ground into a fine powder. Powder can be encapsulated.
2. Decoction or teapill method: Herbs are mixed together and decocted. Herbal water extract (decoction) can be concentrated as granules or teapills.

Actions: Expel Wind-Damp, activate Channels and dispel Cold

Indications: Severe pain due to invasion of Wind-Cold-Damp. The main signs include intense pain in the joints and back, severe stiffness of limbs, a pale purple tongue, and a wiry pulse.

Dosage and Usage:
Horses and Cattle: 15–30 g, twice daily
Camels: 30–45 g, twice daily
Llamas, Alpacas, Goats, Sheep, and Pigs: 5–10 g, twice daily
Dogs: 0.5–3 g (or 0.05 g per kg body weight), twice daily
Cats and Rabbits: 0.1–0.3 g (or 0.05 g per kg body weight), twice daily
Use 2–5 days until primary clinical signs resolve.

Analysis of Formula: Exogenous Wind-Cold-Damp pathogens invade the body, become chronic, and accumulate in the Exterior, including channels, tendons, ligaments, muscles, and joints; this obstructs flow of *Qi* and blood, leading to pain. Therefore, *Chuan Wu* (Aconite), the King herb, expels Wind-Damp and warms *Yang* to dispel Cold and treat the underlying cause. *Ma Huang* (Ephedra) is the Minister herb and serves to warm and relieve the Exterior. Serving as the Adjuvant herbs, *Bai Shao Yao* (Paeonia) and *Huang Qi* (Astragalus) tonify *Qi* and Blood and counter the harsh nature (the too-hot effect) of *Chuan Wu* (Aconite) and *Ma Huang* (Ephedra). *Gan Cao* (Glycyrrhiza) harmonizes all other herbs and works as the Messenger herb.

Cautions and Contraindications: This formula is very potent and toxic and should be not used long term. It should not be used in pregnant, weak, or elderly patients.

Dr. Xie's Comments*:* *Wu Tou Tang* historically is a famous formula to treat intense pain in joints and muscles due to Wind-Cold-Damp.

Clinical and Pharmacological Studies: A study on *Wu Tou Tang's* function of relieving pain and reducing inflammation was conducted in mice.[14] The result showed that *Wu Tou Tang* (40 g of *Wu Tou Tang* per 1 kg of body weight) significantly increased the pain threshold of a mouse to heat stimulation and decreased the incidence rate of writhing response caused by 0.7 acetic acid. *Wu Tou Tang* also significantly reduced the degree of swelling in mouse ears caused by dimethyl benzene.

FORMULAS TO REVIVE *YANG* FOR RESUSCITATION

The formulas in this section are used in treating *Yang* Deficiency and exhaustion and collapse of Heart *Yang* and/or Kidney *Yang*. Exhaustion and collapse is a severe form of *Yang* Deficiency, which is accompanied by accumulation of Cold (*Yin*) Excess, leading to extremely cold extremities, cold ears and back, severe depression or loss of consciousness, a gray or dark tongue, and a feeble pulse.

Si Ni Tang (Four Frigid Extremities) 四逆汤

Si refers to four, or four limbs and extremities. *Ni* means rebelling. *Si Ni* refers to the fact that the four limbs are so cold that they are frigid and stiff. Normally, four limbs and extremities can extend and move easily. But, Cold makes them frigid and stiff (rebelling). *Tang* is decoction, the form of herbal administration.

Source: *Shang Han Za Bing Lun* (*Treatise on Cold-Induced Disorders and Miscellaneous Diseases*), written by *Zhang Zhongjing* and published in 220 CE

Ingredients: The formula is composed of 45 g *Fu Zi* (Aconite), 45 g *Gan Jiang* (Zingiberis), and 30 g *Gan Cao* (Glycyrrhiza) (Table 22.11).

Table 22.11. Ingredients and actions of *Si Ni Tang.*

%	English Name	Chinese *Pin-Yin*	Actions
37.5	Aconite	*Fu Zi*	Warm *Yang-Qi* to dispel Cold, revive *Yang* for resuscitation
37.5	Zingiberis	*Gan Jiang*	Warm the Middle Burner to dispel Cold
25	Glycyrrhiza	*Gan Cao*	Harmonize the other herb actions

Preparation:

1. Powder or capsule method: Herbs are ground into a fine powder. Powder can be encapsulated.
2. Decoction or teapill method: Herbs are mixed together and decocted. Herbal water extract (decoction) can be concentrated as granules or teapills.

Actions: Warm the Middle Burner to dispel Cold, revive *Yang* for resuscitation

Indications: *Yang* exhaustion or collapse. The main signs are coldness in all four limbs, cold extremities, severe depression or loss of consciousness, a gray or dark tongue, and a feeble pulse.

Dosage

Horses and Cattle: 15–30g, twice daily
Camels: 30–45g, twice daily
Llamas, Alpacas, Goats, Sheep, and Pigs: 5–10g, twice daily
Dogs: 0.5–5g (or 0.05g per kg body weight), twice daily
Cats and Rabbits: 0.1–0.5g (or 0.05g per kg body weight), twice daily
Use for 1 week until primary clinical signs resolve.

Analysis of Formula: Severe Kidney *Yang* Deficiency causes accumulation of Cold (*Yin*), which makes whole-body *Yang* collapse further. The treatment strategy is resuscitating *Yang* and reviving *Qi*. In the formula, *Fu Zi* (Aconite) is pungent and hot and acts as the King herb because it warms *Yang-Qi* to dispel Cold. It is the most potent herb to revive *Yang* for resuscitation. *Gan Jiang* (Zingiberis), as the Minister herb, warms the Middle Burner to dispel Cold. *Gan Cao* (Glycyrrhiza) is the Adjuvant and Messenger herb, which tonifies *Qi* and harmonizes other herb actions.

Cautions and Contraindications: Do not use to treat cases with *Qi* Stagnation in the Interior caused by Blood Deficiency or any Heat conditions. This formula is contraindicated in pregnancy.

Dr. Xie's Comments*:* *Si Ni Tang* historically is a famous formula to treat *Yang* Collapse. In modern practice, it is often used after the initial western emergent medical care.

Clinical and Pharmacological Studies: Recent pharmacological studies show that *Si Ni Tang* increases heart functions and blood circulation and promotes metabolic functions. The demethyl coclaurine in *Fu Zi* (Aconite) has the same function as aleudrin in relation to the affinity of adrenergic receptors; it can reinforce myocardial contractility, increase heart rate, and increase coronary artery blood flow.[15] *Si Ni Tang* also improved the life quality of patients with coronary heart disease and angina cordis. The group with Cold accumulation due to *Yang* Deficiency treated with *Si Ni Tang* had a better outcome than other Pattern groups and had an obvious improvement in several dimensions, including physiological functions, body pain, limitations of degree of body activity, and rate of angina pectoris attacks.[16]

Shen Fu Tang (Ginseng and Aconite) 参附汤

Shen Fu refers to *Ren Shen* (Ginseng) and *Fu Zi* (Aconite), the only two ingredients of the formula. *Tang* is decoction, the form of herbal administration. Thus, *Shen Fu* translates literally to Ginseng and Aconite.

Source: *Shi Yi De Xiao Fang* (*Effective Formulas from Generations of Physicians*), written by *Wei Yi-Lin* and published in 1345 CE

Ingredients: *Shen Fu Tang* is composed of 12g *Ren Shen* (Ginseng), and 9g *Fu Zi* (Aconite) (Table 22.12).

Preparation:

1. Powder or capsule method: Herbs are ground into a fine powder. Powder can be encapsulated.
2. Decoction or teapill method: Herbs are mixed together and decocted. Herbal water extract (decoction) can be concentrated as granules or teapills.

Actions: Revive *Yang* for resuscitation, tonify *Qi*

Indications: Sudden collapse of *Yang-Qi*. The main symptoms include acute chest pain, coldness of four limbs, cold extremities, short and weak breath, gray or black tongue, feeble and almost disappearing pulse.

Table 22.12. Ingredients and actions of *Shen Fu Tang.*

%	English Name	Chinese *Pin-Yin*	Actions
57.1	Ginseng	*Ren Shen*	Tonify *Yuan Qi*, strengthen the Spleen and Lung, calm *Shen* (spirit)
42.9	Aconite	*Fu Zi*	Warm *Yang-Qi* to dispel Cold, revive *Yang* for resuscitation

Dosage and Usage:
Horses and Cattle: 15–30 g, twice daily
Camels: 30–45 g, twice daily
Llamas, Alpacas, Goats, Sheep, and Pigs: 5–10 g, twice daily
Dogs: 0.5–5 g (or 0.05 g per kg body weight), twice daily
Cats and Rabbits: 0.1–0.5 g (or 0.05 g per kg body weight), twice daily
Birds: 0.05 g per kg body weight, twice daily
Use 2–5 days until primary clinical signs resolve.

Analysis of Formula: This formula is designed for *Yang-Qi* collapse. In the formula, *Ren Shen* (Ginseng) is sweet and warm, which potently tonifies *Yuan Qi*. *Fu Zi* (Aconite) is very pungent and hot, which warms and strengthens Kidney *Yang*. The two herbs mutually promote one another to resuscitate *Yang* and revive *Qi*. Both synergize to work as the King and Minister herbs.

Cautions and Contraindications: Do not use to treat Heat Patterns or pregnant patients. Avoid excessive use.

Dr. Xie's Comments*:* *Shen Fu Tang* historically is a famous formula to urgently treat acute collapse of *Yang Qi* (chest pain, spontaneous sweating, weak and faint breath, loss of consciousness, feeble or disappearing pulse). In modern veterinary practice, these severely collapsed patients are often sent to the emergency room for treatment using Western medicines.

Qi Fu Tang (Astragalus and Aconite) 芪附汤

Qi Fu refers to the only two ingredients of the formula: *Huang Qi* (Astragalus) and *Fu Zi* (Aconite). *Tang* is decoction, the form of herbal administration. *Qi Fu* translates directly to Astragalus and Aconite.

Source: *Wei Shi Jia Cang Shu* (*Collected Formulas of the Wei Family*), written by *Wei Xianzhuan* and published during the *Song* Dynasty in 1227 CE

Ingredients: *Qi Fu Tang* is composed of equal proportions of *Fu Zi* (Aconite), and *Huang Qi* (Astragalus) (Table 22.13).

Table 22.13. Ingredients and actions of *Qi Fu Tang*.

%	English Name	Chinese *Pin-Yin*	Actions
50	Aconite	*Fu Zi*	Warm *Yang Qi* to dispel Cold, revive *Yang* for resuscitation
50	Astragalus	*Huang Qi*	Tonify *Qi*, strengthen the Spleen, consolidate the surface

Preparation:
1. Powder or capsule method: Herbs are ground into a fine powder. Powder can be encapsulated.
2. Decoction or teapill method: Herbs are mixed together and decocted. Herbal water extract (decoction) can be concentrated as granules or teapills.

Indications: Deficiency of *Wei-Yang*. The clinical signs include prolonged sweating, fatigue or near exhaustion, pale and wet tongue, and a weak pulse.

Actions: Warm *Yang*, tonify *Wei Qi*, consolidate the surface to stop sweating

Dosage and Usage:
Horses and Cattle: 15–30 g, twice daily
Camels: 30–45 g, twice daily
Llamas, Alpacas, Goats, Sheep, and Pigs: 5–10 g, twice daily
Dogs: 0.5–5 g (or 0.05 g per kg body weight), twice daily
Cats and Rabbits: 0.1–0.5 g (or 0.05 g per kg body weight), twice daily
Birds: 0.05 g per kg body weight, twice daily
Use 2–7 days until primary clinical signs resolve.

Analysis of Formula: This formula is used for urgent treatment of persistent and prolonged sweating due to *Wei Qi* Deficiency. *Wei Qi* controls the skin pores and governs the mechanism that "opens and closes" the sweat glands. When *Wei Qi* is deficient, it fails to control this open-close mechanism, leading to continuous sweating. If sweating is not controlled, *Yang-Qi* will become depleted and collapse. Therefore, treat by tonifying *Wei Qi* to stop sweating. In the formula, *Huang Qi* (Astragalus), the King herb, is sweet and warm. It tonifies Wei Qi and consolidates the surface to stop sweating. *Fu Zi* (Aconite), the Minister herb, is very pungent and hot and warms and strengthens the *Yang* to support Wei Qi. The two herbs together mutually promote one another to assist *Yang* and supplement *Wei Qi* to consolidate the surface.

Cautions and Contradictions: This formula is contraindicated in cases with pregnancy, Heat, and *Yin* Deficiency.

Dr. Xie's Comments*:* *Qi Fu Tang* can be used in chronic spontaneous sweating due to *Wei Qi* Deficiency in horses. It is intended for short-term use only because it is very potent. It may not be useful in small animal patients.

Clinical and Pharmacological Studies: The pharmacological research shows that the active component of *Huang Qi* (Astragalus) has antiviral and immune-regulating functions, lessens myocardial inflammatory infiltration and the degree of cellular necrosis, increases the activity of natural killer cells, decreases replication of cardioviruses, improves the immunologic mechanisms of patient cells, strengthens myocardial contractility, boosts the ejection fraction of the left ventricle, improves heart function, decreases the abnormal electrical activity of myocardial cells, and decreases the occurrence of arrhythmias.[17] Another study indicated that *Qi Fu Tang* stimulated the production of antibodies.[18]

Zhen Wu Tang (True Warrior) 真武汤

Zhen means true. *Wu* refers to warrior. According to Chinese folk culture, the *Zhen Wu* represents the god located in the North to control water and prevent flooding. *Zhen Wu* is needed when edema and ascites occur because control of water metabolism is lost in the body. *Tang* is decoction, the form of herbal administration. Thus, *Zhen Wu Tang* translates to True Warrior (or God to Control the Water) Decoction.

Source: *Shang Han Za Bing Lun* (*Treatise on Cold-Induced Disorders and Miscellaneous Diseases*), written by *Zhang Zhongjing* and published in 220 CE

Ingredients: The formula of *Zhen Wu Tang* (Table 22.14) is composed of 9 g *Fu Zi* (Aconite), 9 g *Fu Ling* (Poria), 9 g *Bai Shao Yao* (Paeonia), 9 g *Sheng Jiang* (Zingiberis), and 6 g *Bai Zhu* (Atractylodes).

Preparation:
1. Powder or capsule method: Herbs are ground into a fine powder. Powder can be encapsulated.
2. Decoction or teapill method: Herbs are mixed together and decocted. Herbal water extract (decoction) can be concentrated as granules or teapills.

Actions: Warm *Yang*, drain Damp to resolve water retention.

Table 22.14. Ingredients and actions of *Zhen Wu Tang*.

%	English Name	Chinese *Pin-Yin*	Actions
21.4	Aconite	*Fu Zi*	Warm *Yang-Qi*, dispel Cold, revive *Yang* for resuscitation
21.4	Poria	*Fu Ling*	Drain Damp, strengthen the Spleen
21.4	Paeonia	*Bai Shao Yao*	Tonify *Yin* and harmonize the Interior
21.4	Zingiberis	*Sheng Jiang*	Warm the Stomach to dispel Cold
14.4	Atractylodes	*Bai Zhu*	Tonify Spleen *Qi*, dry Damp

Indications: Water retention due to *Yang* Deficiency. Clinical signs include chills; aversion to Cold; stranguria or dysuria; palpitation; loss of balance or disorientation; edema and pain of four limbs; ascites; diarrhea; pale and swollen tongue with tooth marks (indentation); a white, greasy coating of the tongue; and a deep, weak pulse.

Dosage and Usage:
Horses and Cattle: 15–30 g, twice daily
Camels: 30–45 g, twice daily
Llamas, Alpacas, Goats, Sheep, and Pigs: 5–10 g, twice daily
Dogs: 0.5–5 g (or 0.05 g per kg body weight), twice daily
Cats and Rabbits: 0.1–0.5 g (or 0.05 g per kg body weight), twice daily
Birds: 0.05 g per kg body weight, twice daily
Use 1–3 weeks until primary clinical signs resolve.

Analysis of Formula: This formula treats *Yang* Deficiency, which causes water retention in the Interior. In the formula, *Fu Zi* (Aconite), the King herb, is strongly pungent and hot, and it warms and tonifies Kidney *Yang* to dispel water and Damp in the Interior. The Minister herbs are *Sheng Jiang* (Zingiberis), which warms and scatters accumulated water, and *Fu Ling* (Poria) and *Bai Zhu* (Atractylodes), which strengthen the Spleen and tonify *Qi* to alleviate water retention. Serving as the Adjuvant herb, *Bai Shao Yao* (Paeonia) retains *Yin*, harmonizes the Interior, and serves to balance the pungent and dry nature of *Fu Zi* (Aconite) and *Sheng Jiang* (Zingiberis). Thus, the formula alleviates water retention without damaging *Yin*.

Dr. Xie's Comments: I have often used *Zhen Wu Tang* for the treatment of ascites in congestive heart failure due to *Yang* Deficiency.

Cautions and Contraindications: Avoid feeding pork, peach, and plum when taking this formula. This formula is contraindicated in cases with projectile vomiting and/or pregnancy.

Clinical and Pharmacological Studies: In a study on canine patients with congestive heart failure (CHF), *Zhen Wu Tang* significantly increased urinary output and strengthened myocardial contractility, improved the heart function, and promoted blood circulation.[19] Wang researched the effects of *Zhen Wu Tang* on free radical metabolism in old mice (3-month-old, male, 25 ± 2 g).[20] The results showed that the formula can significantly raise the superoxide dismutase (SOD) activity of red blood cells. The formula also reduced fatigue, improved oxygen perfusion, reduced harmful oxidative processes, and reduced stress.[20]

Hui Xiang San (Foeniculum Powder) 茴香散

Hui Xiang refers to Foeniculum, the King herb of this formula. *San* is powder, the original form of herbal administration. Thus, *Hui Xiang San* translates directly to Foeniculum Powder.

Source: *Yuan Heng Liao Ma Ji* (*Yuan-Heng's Therapeutic Treatise of Horses*), written by *Yu Benyun* and *Yu Benheng* during the *Ming* Dynasty and published in 1608 CE

Ingredients: *Hui Xiang San* (Table 22.15) is composed of 30g *Xiao Hui Xiang* (Foeniculum), 25g *Ba Ji Tian* (Morinda), 25g *Bu Gu Zhi* (Psoralea), 25g *Hu Lu Ba* (Trigonella), 20g *Rou Gui* (Cinnamomum), 25g *Dang Gui* (Angelica), 20g *Chen Pi* (Citrus), 20g *Qing Pi* (Citrus), 25g *Chuan Lian Zi* (Melia), 5g *Hua Jiao* (Zanthoxylum), 15g *Tong Cao* (Tetrapanax), 20g *Rou Dou Kou* (Myristica), 20g *Gao Ben* (Ligusticum), 15g *Niu Bang Zi* (Arctium), and 10g *Xi Xin* (Asarum).

Preparation:
1. Powder or capsule method: Herbs are ground into a fine powder. Powder can be encapsulated.
2. Decoction or teapill method: Herbs are mixed together and decocted. Herbal water extract (decoction) can be concentrated as granules or teapills.

Actions: Tonify Kidney *Yang*, dispel Cold and Damp, resolve pain

Table 22.15. Ingredients and actions of *Hui Xiang San*.

%	English Name	Chinese *Pin-Yin*	Actions
10	Foeniculum	*Xiao Hui Xiang*	Warm Kidney *Yang*, dispel Cold
8.3	Morinda	*Ba Ji Tian*	Warm *Yang*, tonify Kidney, strengthen back/rear
8.3	Psoralea	*Bu Gu Zhi*	Tonify Kidney *Yang* and benefit bones
8.3	Trigonella	*Hu Lu Ba*	Tonify Kidney *Yang*, strengthen rear, dispel Cold
6.7	Cinnamomum	*Rou Gui*	Warm Kidney *Yang*
8.3	Angelica	*Dang Gui*	Move Blood
6.7	Citrus	*Chen Pi*	Move *Qi*, resolve pain
6.7	Citrus	*Qing Pi*	Move *Qi*, resolve pain
8.3	Melia	*Chuan Lian Zi*	Move *Qi*, resolve pain
1.7	Zanthoxylum	*Hua Jiao*	Eliminate Damp, resolve pain
5	Tetrapanax	*Tong Cao*	Drain Damp
6.7	Myristica	*Rou Dou Kou*	Eliminate Damp
6.7	Ligusticum	*Gao Ben*	Clear Wind-Cold
5	Arctium	*Niu Bang Zi*	Clear Wind-Heat
3.3	Asarum	*Xi Xin*	Clear Wind Cold, relieve pain

Indications: Pain in back or rear limbs due to Kidney *Yang* Deficiency with Stagnation of Cold/Damp. The main signs include stiffness or weakness of back or rear limbs; coldness of back or extremities; a pale purple tongue with a white, greasy coating; and deep, weak pulse.

Dosage and Usage:
Horses and Cattle: 15–30g, twice daily
Camels: 30–45g, twice daily
Llamas, Alpacas, Goats, Sheep, and Pigs: 5–10g, twice daily
Dogs: 0.5–5g (or 0.05g per kg body weight), twice daily
Cats and Rabbits: 0.1–0.5g (or 0.05g per kg body weight), twice daily
Birds: 0.05g per kg body weight, twice daily
Use 2–6 weeks until primary clinical signs resolve.

Analysis of Formula: The formula *Hui Xiang San* is designed for Kidney *Yang* Deficiency leading to coldness and weakness of the back and rear limbs. In the formula, *Xiao Hui Xiang* (Foeniculum), the King herb, tonifies Kidney *Yang*, warms the back to dispel Cold, and resolves Stagnation to relive pain. Serving as the Minister herbs, *Ba Ji Tian* (Morinda), *Bu Gu Zhi* (Psoralea), *Hu Lu Ba* (Trigonella), and *Rou Gui* (Cinnamomum) warm *Yang* and tonify Kidney *Qi* to enhance the King herb to dispel Cold. Cold leads to *Qi*-Blood Stagnation and pain. Therefore, the first group of Adjuvant herbs, *Dang Gui* (Angelica), *Chen Pi* (Citrus), *Qing Pi* (Citrus), *Chuan Lian Zi* (Melia), and *Hua Jiao* (Zanthoxylum) move *Qi* and Blood, resolve Stagnation, and relieve pain. The second group of Adjuvant herbs *Tong Cao* (Tetrapanax), *Rou Dou Kou* (Myristica), *Gao Ben* (Ligusticum), *Niu Bang Zi* (Arctium) and *Xi Xin* (Asarum) eliminate the pathogenic factors including Wind, Damp, and Cold to relieve Stagnation.

Cautions and Contraindications: This formula is contraindicated in patients with Heat signs.

Dr. Xie's Comments: *Xiang Hui San* is an effective formula to treat coldness and pain of back and rear limbs due to Kidney *Yang* Deficiency. It can also be used for coldness in the Liver Channel leading to swelling of the scrotum.

Yi Zhi San (Alpinia Powder) 益智散

Yi Zhi refers to *Yi Zhi Ren*, or Alpinia, the King herb of this formula. *San* is powder, the original form of herbal administration. Thus, *Yi Zhi San* translates literally to Alpinia Powder.

Source: *Yuan Heng Liao Ma Ji* (*Yuan-Heng's Therapeutic Treatise of Horses*), written by *Yu Benyun* and *Yu Benheng* and published in 1608 CE.

Table 22.16. Ingredients and actions of *Yi Zhi San*.

%	English	Chinese *Pin-Yin*	Actions
7.2	Alpinia	*Yi Zhi Ren*	Warm Spleen and Kidney, astringently hold Kidney *Qi*/*Jing*
6	Myristica	*Rou Dou Kou*	Warm and strengthen Spleen, clear Damp
4.9	Cinnamomum	*Rou Gui*	Warm and tonify Kidney *Yang*
3.9	Amomum	*Sha Ren*	Strengthen Spleen and clear Damp
2.4	Asarum	*Xi Xin*	Dispel Cold to resolve pain
6	Amomum	*Cao Guo*	Dry up Damp, clear Cold, transform Phlegm
7.2	Atractylodes	*Bai Zhu*	Strengthen and tonify Spleen
7.2	Paeonia	*Bai Shao Yao*	Nourish Blood, soothe Liver *Qi*
6	Angelica	*Dang Gui*	Nourish Blood
6	Citrus	*Qing Pi*	Move *Qi* and relieve pain
2.4	Saussurea	*Mu Xiang*	Move *Qi* and relieve pain
6	Aurantium	*Zhi Ke*	Move *Qi* and relieve pain
7.2	Magnolia	*Hou Po*	Move *Qi* and relieve pain
3.7	Ligusticum	*Chuan Xiong*	Activate and resolve Stagnation
2.5	Areca	*Bing Lang*	Move *Qi* to stop abdominal pain
4.8	Schisandra	*Wu Wei Zi*	Astringently consolidate *Yin* and *Jing*
3.6	Angelica	*Bai Zhi*	Dispel Wind-Cold to relieve pain
2.4	Zingiberis	*Sheng Jiang*	Harmonize the Stomach to stop vomiting
7	Jujube	*Da Zao*	Tonify Spleen *Qi*, harmonize the Stomach
3.6	Glycyrrhiza	*Gan Cao*	Harmonize all other herbs

Ingredients: *Yi Zhi San* (Table 22.16) is composed of 30g *Yi Zhi Ren* (Alpinia), 25g *Rou Dou Kou* (Myristica), 20g *Rou Gui* (Cinnamomum), 15g *Sha Ren* (Amomum), 10g *Xi Xin* (Asarum), 25g *Cao Guo* (Amomum), 30g *Bai Zhu* (Atractylodes), 30g *Bai Shao Yao* (Paeonia), 25g *Dang Gui* (Angelica), 25g *Qing Pi* (Citrus), 10g *Mu Xiang* (Saussurea), 25g *Zhi Ke* (Aurantium), 30g *Hou Po* (Magnolia), 15g *Chuan Xiong* (Ligusticum), 10g *Bing Lang* (Areca), 20g *Wu Wei Zi* (Schisandra), 15g *Bai Zhi* (Angelica), 10g *Sheng Jiang* (Zingiberis), 28g *Da Zao* (Jujube), and 15g *Gan Cao* (Glycyrrhiza).

Preparation:

1. Powder or capsule method: Herbs are ground into a fine powder. Powder can be encapsulated.
2. Decoction or teapill method: Herbs are mixed together and decocted. Herbal water extract (decoction) can be concentrated as granules or teapills.

Actions: Warm and tonify Spleen and Kidney, clear Damp, move *Qi*, relieve pain

Indications: Developmental orthopedic disease (DOD) due to Spleen *Qi* and Kidney *Yang* Deficiency. The main symptoms include DOD in the young patients, nausea or vomiting, depression, weakness of four limbs, atrophied muscles, a pale tongue, and a weak pulse.

Dosage and Usage:

Horses and Cattle: 15–30g, twice daily
Camels: 30–45g, twice daily
Llamas, Alpacas, Goats, Sheep, and Pigs: 5–10g, twice daily
Dogs: 0.5–5g (or 0.05g per kg body weight), twice daily
Cats and Rabbits: 0.1–0.5g (or 0.05g per kg body weight), twice daily
Birds: 0.05g per kg body weight, twice daily
Use 2–6 weeks until primary clinical signs resolve.

Analysis of Formula: This formula is designed for developmental orthopedic disease (DOD). In TCVM, DOD is related to the Spleen and Kidney. The Kidney is the root of prenatal *Jing* and controls bones. The Spleen is the root of postnatal Jing. Although the prenatal *Jing* is continually depleted by the day-to-day *Qi* requirements of the body, the Spleen *Qi* creates postnatal *Jing* from food and uses it to replenish the prenatal *Jing*. Young animals with DOD usually have insufficient prenatal *Jing*, which fails to nourish and support bones. The patients with osteoporosis often have a weak Spleen *Qi*. The key to treating DOD is to tonify both the Kidney and Spleen. Therefore, *Yi Zhi Ren* (Alpinia), the King herb, warms the Middle Burner and strengthens the Spleen. Serving as the Minister herbs, *Rou Dou Kou* (Myristica), *Rou Gui* (Cinnamomum), *Sha Ren* (Amomum), *Bai Zhi* (Angelica), *Cao Guo* (Amomum), and *Xi Xin* (Asarum) warm the Spleen and Kidney and tonify *Yang*, enhancing *Yi Xhi Ren's* (Alpinia's) effect to warm the Middle Burner to dispel Cold. Coldness leads to Stagnation and pain; thus, *Qing Pi* (Citrus), *Mu Xiang* (Saussurea), *Zhi Ke* (Aurantium), *Hou Po* (Magnolia), *Chuan Xiong* (Ligusticum), and *Bing Lang* (Areca) move *Qi* to resolve Stagnation and descend *Qi* to stop vomiting. *Bai Zhu* (Atractylodes) tonifies Spleen *Qi* and dries Dampness. Blood and *Yin* are the essential substances to build the bones. *Bai Shao Yao* (Paeonia), *Dang Gui* (Angelica), and *Wu Wei Zi* (Schisandra) tonify *Yin* and Blood. These 10 ingredients are the Adjuvant herbs. *Sheng Jiang* (Zingiberis), *Da Zao* (Jujube), and *Gan Cao* (Glycyrrhiza) work together as the Messenger herbs to harmonize the Spleen and Stomach and coordinate all other herbs.

Cautions and Contraindications: This formula is contraindicated in patients with False Heat or Stomach Heat.

Dr. Xie's Comments: *Yi Zhi San* was originally formulated to treat developmental orthopedic disease (DOD)

in foals. It can also be used for dogs and other species. DOD is also called metabolic bone disease and is a new general term for orthopedic abnormalities that occur between birth and 18 months of age.[21] DOD includes osteochondrosis, osteochondritis dissecans, subchondral cystic lesions, physitis (epiphysitis), acquired flexure deformities (contracted tendons), cervical vertebral malformation (wobblers), malformation of the cuboidal bones of the carpus and tarsus (angular limb deformity), and juvenile arthritis.

REFERENCES

1. Zhang YX. The application of *Li Zhong Tang* in veterinary clinics. Traditional Chinese Veterinary Medicine 2007;5: 62–63.
2. Bian HM. The effect of *Li Zhong Tang* to the function of intestinal motility of experimental animals. Journal of Nanjing Traditional Chinese Medical College 1993;l9(4):33.
3. He Wei. Treatment on 17 cases long-diarrhea with *Fu Zi Li Zhong Tang* Journal of Practical Traditional Chinese Medicine 2006;22(5):285.
4. Hu YH. Reproduction of the animal model of diarrhea due to spleen deficiency and the regulative function of *Fu Zi Li Zhong Tang*. Journal of Shanghai Traditional Chinese Medicine 1981;8:45.
5. Fan XJ. Treatment on 36 cases of chronic ulcerative colitis with *Jia Wei Lian Li Tang*. Si Chuan Journal of Traditional Chinese Medicine 2006;5:49.
6. Ma SL. *Xiao Jian Zhong Tang* for the treatment of 58 human cases of chronic gastritis. Journal of Integrated Western and Chinese Medicine 1998;1(11):71.
7. Zhang CG. The research of *Xiao Jian Zhong Tang*. Beijing Journal of Traditional Chinese Medicine 1994;(4):43–45.
8. Chen RR. *Huang Qi Jian Zhong Tang* for the treatment of 170 cases of duodenobulbar ulcer. Shandong Journal of Traditional Chinese Medicine 1991;(10):20.
9. Xu L. The clinical application of *Da Jian Zhong Tang*. Practical Journal of Traditional Chinese Internal Medicine 2006;(1):50.
10. Chen JT. The effect of research of *Da Jian Zhong Tang* on serum neurotransmitter of insufficiency of spleen—*YANG* Mice. Zhejiang Journal of Traditional Chinese Medicine 2007; 42(5):300–301.
11. Li JW. Modified *Wu Zhu Yu Tang* for the treatment of 31 cases of functional dyspepsia. Information on Traditional Chinese Medicine 2007;1:30.
12. Wang FC, Zhang HM. Treatment of rheumatoid arthritis with *Huang Qi Gui Zhi Wu Wu Tang*. Practical Journal of Traditional Chinese Internal Medicine 2004;18(5):434.
13. Ren GL. The observance of *Yang He Tang* treating delayed union of bone fracture. The Journal of Traditional Chinese Orthopedics and Traumatology 1999;11(2):11–13.
14. Mao LM, Hong SL, Yu L, Guang H. The pain relief and anti-inflammatory action of *Wu Tou Tang*. Henan Institute of Medical Science 1994;3(4):325–328.
15. Zhu XJ. *Si Ni Tang* and *Sheng Mai San* for the treatment of 37 cases of chronic arrhythmia. Practical Journal of Traditional Chinese Internal Medicine 2007;(21):9,56.
16. *Yang* XJ. The clinical research of *Si Ni Tang* on the life quality of patients with coronary heart disease and angina. Journal of Henan University of Chinese Medicine 2007;22(132):28–30.
17. *Yang* FZ. Treatment of viral myocarditis with *Astragalus*. Journal of Shanghai Medicine 1995;(2):28–31.
18. Dong C, Li JL, Xu QY. The effect of *Qi Fu Tang* on the immune function of an aging mouse. Chinese Journal of Hospital Pharmacy 2002;22(10):605–607.
19. Wang JN, Long ZJ, Wang QM. A study on *Zhen Wu Tang* on its function of strengthening heart and diureses. Journal of Chinese Traditional Patent Medicine 1997;19(3):27–30.
20. Wang YX, Chen KM, Hao W, Zhang W. The pharmacodynamic study of *Zhen Wu Tang*. Liaoning Journal of Traditional Chinese Medicine 2007;27(12):565–566.
21. Ott, EA. Nutritional factors in developmental orthopedic disease. In: N. Edward Robinson (ed), Current Therapy in Equine Medicine. New York: Harcourt Brace Jovanovich, Inc., 1992:720–724.

23 Herbal Formulas to Eliminate Dampness 祛湿剂

Songhua Hu, Huisheng Xie, Justin Shmalberg

The formulas described in this chapter are mainly composed of diuretic herbs that eliminate Dampness, induce diuresis, relieve stranguria, and drain turbidity and are suitable for the treatment of diseases caused by pathogenic Dampness. According to the Eight Therapeutic Principles, eliminating Dampness is a method for dispersing pathogenic factors.

As a disease-causing factor, Dampness may develop Exteriorly or Interiorly, settle in the Exterior or in the Interior, and it might affect either the thoracic limbs, lumbosacral region or pelvic limbs. In nature, there are three different Damp factors: Cold-Damp, Damp-Heat, and Wind-Damp. Based on their use in clinically different diseases, the formulas are generally subdivided into five categories: 1) to dry Damp and harmonize the Spleen and Stomach, 2) to clear Damp-Heat, 3) to drain Damp and promote urination, 4) to dispel Wind-Damp, and 5) to warm the *Yang* to dispel Cold-Damp.

Most of the herbs used in these formulas are pungent and aromatic in flavor, with a warm nature. They also often stimulate diuresis. These features, which are beneficial for draining Damp, also mean that these formulas tend to consume Body Fluids. Therefore, they are not suitable for Patterns with Deficiency of Body Fluids but should only be used when combined with herbs that nourish *Yin*, if necessary. As Dampness has heavy, turbid, viscous, and greasy characteristics and impedes the movement of *Qi*, the formulas are usually supplemented with *Qi*-regulating herbs so as to disperse Dampness by promoting the movement of *Qi*.

FORMULAS TO DRY DAMP AND HARMONIZE THE SPLEEN AND STOMACH

The formulas in this section are used for the treatment of Damp Turbidity seen in digestive disorders due to retention of Dampness inside the body or damage to the Spleen by Dampness. When Dampness lingers in the Interior, it is stagnant, accumulates, and transforms into turbid Damp or Damp Turbidity (*Shi Zhuo*). The clinical signs of *Shi Zhuo* include abdominal distention, nausea or vomiting, poor appetite, diarrhea, weight loss, depression, a greasy or thick white coating of the tongue, and a slippery pulse. The main ingredients used in these formulas are *Cang Zhu* (Atractylodes), *Huo Xiang* (Pogostemon), *Chen Pi* (Citrus), and *Sha Ren* (Amomum).

Ping Wei San (Harmonizing the Stomach) 平胃散

Ping means harmonizing, *Wei* is the Stomach. and *San* means powder, the original form of herbal administration. Thus, *Ping Wei* translates literally as Harmonizing the Stomach.

Source: *Ping Wei San* was originally recorded in *Tai Ping Hui Min He Ji Ju Fang* (*Imperial Grace Formulary of the Tai Ping Era*), written by *Chen Shi-Wen* et al. and published by the *Song* Dynasty government in 1078 CE. It was also recorded in *Yuan Heng Liao Ma Ji* (*Yuan-Heng's Therapeutic Treatise of Horses*), written by *Yuan Beng-yuan* and *Yuan Beng-heng* and published in 1608 CE.

Ingredients: The original formulation of *Ping Wei San* contains 15 g *Cang Zhu* (Atractylodes), 9 g *Hou Po* (Magnolia), 9 g *Chen Pi* (Citrus), 4 g *Gan Cao* (Glycyrrhiza), 2 g *Sheng Jiang* (Zingiberis), and 2 g *Da Zao* (Jujube) (Table 23.1).

Preparation:

1. Powder or capsule method: Herbs are ground into a fine powder. The powder can be encapsulated.
2. Decoction or teapill method: Raw herbs are mixed together and decocted. The herbal water extract (decoction) can be concentrated as granules or teapills.

Table 23.1. Ingredients and actions of *Ping Wei San.*

%	English Name	*Pin-Yin* Name	Actions
36.6	Atractylodes	*Cang Zhu*	Eliminate Damp
22	Magnolia	*Hou Po*	Promote *Qi* flow
22	Citrus	*Chen Pi*	Dry Damp, move *Qi*
9.8	Glycyrrhiza	*Gan Cao*	Harmonize the properties of other herbs
4.8	Zingiberis	*Sheng Jiang*	Harmonize the Stomach
4.8	Jujube	*Da Zao*	Tonify *Qi*, harmonize the Spleen and Stomach

Actions: Dry Dampness and strengthen the Spleen, promote the flow of *Qi* and regulate the Stomach

Indications: Stagnation of Dampness in the Stomach characterized by anorexia; abdominal distention; vomiting or regurgitation; diarrhea; a thick, white, greasy coating of the tongue; and a slow pulse

Dosage and Usage:
Horses and Cattle: 15–60 g, twice daily
Camels: 30–75 g, twice daily
Llamas, Alpacas, Goats, Sheep, and Pigs: 5–15 g, twice daily
Dogs: 0.5–5 g(or 0.1 g per kg body weight), twice daily
Cats and Rabbits: 0.2–0.5 g (or 0.1 g per kg body weight), twice daily
Birds: 0.1–0.2 g per kg body weight, twice daily
Use for 3–8 weeks until the primary clinical signs have resolved.

Analysis of Formula: *Ping Wei San* is the main formula for treatment of Stagnation of Dampness in the Spleen and Stomach. The Pattern should be treated by drying Dampness and reinforcing the Spleen, promoting the flow of *Qi*, and regulating the Stomach. *Cang Zhu* (Atractylodes), being bitter in flavor and warm in nature, is used as the King herb at a large dose to eliminate Dampness and activate the Spleen. Serving as the Minister herb, *Hou Po* (Magnolia) eliminates Dampness and promotes the circulation of *Qi*, enhancing the effect of the King herb and relieving abdominal fullness. As the Adjuvant herb, *Chen Pi* (Citrus) assists *Hou Po* (Magnolia) to promote the flow of *Qi* to relieve abdominal fullness and helps *Cang Zhu* (Atractylodes) eliminate Dampness and regulate the Middle Burner (*Zhong Jiao*). *Gan Cao* (Glycyrrhiza), *Sheng Jiang* (Zingiberis) and *Da Zao* (Jujube) serve as Messenger herbs to mediate the properties of other herbs in the formula and to regulate the Stomach and reinforce the Spleen.

Cautions and Contraindications: *Ping Wei San* should be used with caution in patients with Stomach *Yin* Deficiency.

Dr. Xie's Comments: *Ping Wei San* is the basic herbal formula to treat any disorders of the Spleen and Stomach. It treats Cold accumulated in the Spleen and Stomach. It can be used for Spleen *Qi* Deficiency if *Si Jun Zi Tang* is used concurrently. For Dampness in the Spleen, *Wu Ling San* is added and for Stomach *Yin* Deficiency, *Yu Nü Jian* is added.

Clinical and Pharmacological Studies: In one study, *Ping Wei San* was used to treat 46 human patients with chronic gastritis. After 30 daily herbal treatments, 8 cases had completely recovered, 18 cases had significantly improved, 16 cases had mild improvement, and 4 cases had no improvement.[1]

Bu Huan Jin Zheng Qi San (Not Trade For Gold) 不换金正气散

Bu means do not, *Huan* means trade, *Jin* refers to gold, and *Zheng Qi* means rectifying the *Qi*. *San* is powder for the form of herbal administration. *Bu Huan Jin Zheng Qi* basically means that this formula is so valuable, because of its ability to rectify *Qi*, that it should not be traded for gold.

Source: *Tai Ping Hui Min He Ji Ju Fang* (*Imperial Grace Formula of the Tai Ping Era*), written by *Chen Shi Wen* et al. and published in 1078 CE

Ingredients: *Bu Huan Jin San Ping Wei San* is formulated by the addition of 10 g *Huo Xiang* (Pogostemon) and 10 g *Ban Xia* (Pinellia) to modified *Ping Wei San, which consists of* 10 g *Cang Zhu* (Atractylodes), 10 g *Hou Po* (Magnolia), 10 g *Chen Pi* (Citrus), 10 g *Gan Cao* (Glycyrrhiza), and 5 g *Sheng Jiang* (Zingiberis).

Preparation:
1. Powder or capsule method: Herbs are ground into a fine powder. The powder can be encapsulated.
2. Decoction or teapill method: Raw herbs are mixed together and decocted. The herbal water extract (decoction) can be concentrated as granules or teapills.

Actions: Eliminate Dampness to relieve the Exterior, harmonize the Middle Burner (*Zhong Jiao*) to stop vomiting

Indications: Weak Spleen and Cold Stomach accompanied by the exogenous invasion of Wind-Damp characterized by abdominal distention and pain, vomiting or diarrhea, and thick white greasy coating of the tongue and a soft pulse

Dosage and Usage:
Horses and Cattle: 15–60 g, twice daily
Camels: 30–75 g, twice daily

Llamas, Alpacas, Goats, Sheep, and Pigs: 5–15 g, twice daily
Dogs: 0.5–5 g (or 0.1 g per kg body weight), twice daily
Cats and Rabbits: 0.2–0.5 g (or 0.1 g per kg body weight), twice daily
Birds: 0.1–0.2 g per kg body weight, twice daily

Use for 2–6 weeks until the primary clinical signs have resolved.

Analysis of Formula: The King herb is *Huo Xiang* (Pogostemon), which eliminates Damp, relieves the Exterior, and strengthens the Spleen to stop diarrhea. *Cang Zhu* (Atractylodes) and *Bian Xia* (Pinellia) are the Minister herbs to dry Dampness and harmonize the Stomach to stop vomiting. Serving as the Adjuvant herbs, *Hou Po* (Magnolia) and *Chen Pi* (Citrus) move *Qi* to relieve pain and descend the Stomach *Qi* to stop vomiting. *Gan Cao* (Glycyrrhiza) and *Sheng Jiang* (Zingiberis) work as the Messenger herbs to harmonize the Middle Burner *(Zhong Jiao)* and coordinate all other herbs.

Cautions and Contraindications: *Bu Huan Jin Zheng Qi San* should be used with caution in patients with Interior Dryness from Stomach *Yin* Deficiency.

Dr. Xie's Comments: *Bu Huan Jin Zheng Qi San* is effective for the treatment of exogenous Wind Cold upsetting the Middle Burner *(Zhong Jiao)* with accumulation of Dampness. Clinically, this could present as an acute onset of vomiting or diarrhea after traveling or seasonal changes; abdominal pain or fullness; and a white, greasy coating of the tongue.

Xiao Shi Ping Wei San (Promoting Digestion to Harmonize the Stomach) 消食平胃散

Xiao here means digestion, and *Shi* here means food. Basically *Xiao Shi* means promoting digestion, *Ping* means harmonizing, *Wei* is the Stomach, and *San* is powder for the form of herbal administration. Thus, *Xiao Shi Ping Wei* can be translated as Promoting Digestion to Harmonize the Stomach.

Source: *Veterinary Pharmacopoeia of the People's Republic of China, Part II,* written by the Chinese Veterinary Pharmacopoeia Committee and published by China Agricultural Press in 2005

Ingredients: *Xiao Shi Ping Wei San* is composed of *Ping Wei San* with the addition of *Bing Lang* (Areca) and *Shan Zha* (Crataegus).

Preparation:

1. Powder or capsule method: Herbs are ground into a fine powder. The powder can be encapsulated.
2. Decoction or teapill method: Raw herbs are mixed together and decocted. The herbal water extract (decoction) can be concentrated as granules or teapills.

Actions: Stimulate the appetite and digestion, move *Qi* to relieve Stagnation

Indications: The formula is indicated for the Spleen that is impaired by Cold and Dampness and for indigestion caused by Food Stagnation. The main signs are abdominal fullness or pain, anorexia, vomiting or diarrhea, a pale purple tongue, and deep or slippery pulse.

Dosage and Usage:
Horses and Cattle: 15–60 g, twice daily
Camels: 30–75 g, twice daily
Llamas, Alpacas, Goats, Sheep, and Pigs: 5–15 g, twice daily
Dogs: 0.5–5 g (or 0.1 g per kg body weight), twice daily
Cats and Rabbits: 0.2–0.5 g (or 0.1 g per kg body weight), twice daily
Birds: 0.1–0.2 g per kg body weight, twice daily

Use for 2–4 weeks until the primary clinical signs have resolved.

Analysis of Formula: *Xiao Shi Ping Wei San* combines the actions of *Ping Wei San* (drying Dampness and strengthening the Spleen) with the King ingredients *Shan Zha* (Crataegus) and *Bing Lang* (Areca). *Shan Zha* (Crataegus) promotes digestion, eliminates Food Stagnation to stop diarrhea, and invigorates Blood to disperse Stagnation. *Bing Lang* (Areca) moves *Qi* to resolve Food Stagnation and kills gastrointestinal parasites to stop pain. Thus, *Xiao Shi Ping Wei San* can promote digestion and eliminate Food Stagnation to stop vomiting, dry Dampness, and strengthen Spleen *Qi* to stop diarrhea. It is often used for the treatment of Food Stagnation with Cold-Damp in the Spleen and Stomach.

Cautions and Contraindications: None known

Dr. Xie's Comments: *Xiao Shi Ping Wei San* is effective for the treatment of Cold-Damp accumulated in the Spleen with Food Stagnation in horses, cattle, pigs, goats, and sheep.

Xiao Ji Ping Wei San (Eliminating Food Stagnation to Harmonize the Stomach) 消积平胃散

Xiao here means eliminating or clearing, and *Ji* here means Stagnation of Food. *Ping* means harmonizing, *Wei* is the Stomach, and *San* is powder for the form of herbal administration. Thus, *Xiao Ji Ping Wei* translates to Eliminating Food Stagnation to Harmonize the Stomach.

Source: *Yuan Heng Liao Ma Ji (Yuan-Heng's Therapeutic Treatise of Horses)*, written by *Yuan Beng-Yuan and Yuan Beng-Heng* and published in 1608 CE

Ingredients: *Xiao Ji Ping Wei San* is composed of *Ping Wei San* [15 g *Cang Zhu* (Atractylodes), 9 g *Hou Po* (Magnolia), 9 g *Chen Pi* (Citrus), 4 g *Gan Cao* (Glycyrrhiza), 2 g *Sheng Jiang* (Zingiberis), and 2 g *Da Zao* (Jujube)], plus 15 g *Shan Zha* (Crataegus), 15 g *Xiang Fu* (Cyperus), and 15 g *Sha Ren* (Amomum).

Preparation:
1. Powder or capsule method: Herbs are ground into a fine powder. The powder can be encapsulated.
2. Decoction or teapill method: Raw herbs are mixed together and decocted. The herbal water extract (decoction) can be concentrated as granules or teapills.

Actions: Move *Qi* to relieve Food Stagnation and strengthen the Spleen to stimulate the appetite

Indications: Inappetence due to Food Stagnation characterized by anorexia, abdominal distention, colic, fatigue, vomiting or diarrhea with foul smell, a purple tongue, and a weak or wiry pulse

Dosage and Usage:
Horses and Cattle: 15–60 g, twice daily
Camels: 30–75 g, twice daily
Llamas, Alpacas, Goats, Sheep, and Pigs: 5–15 g, twice daily
Dogs: 0.5–5 g (or 0.1 g per kg body weight), twice daily
Cats and Rabbits: 0.2–0.5 g (or 0.1 g per kg body weight), twice daily
Birds: 0.1–0.2 g per kg body weight, twice daily
Use for 2–4 weeks until the primary clinical signs have resolved.

Analysis of Formula: *Xiao Ji Ping Wei San* combines *Ping Wei San* (tonifying Spleen *Qi*) with three King ingredients: *Shan Zha* (Crataegus), *Xiang Fu* (Cyperus), and *Sha Ren* (Amomum). *Shan Zha* (Crataegus) eliminates Food Stagnation to stimulate the appetite. *Xiang Fu* (Cyperus) smooths Liver *Qi* to resolve Stagnation and disperses Stasis to relieve pain. *Sha Ren* (Amomum) eliminates Damp and strengthens the Spleen to stimulate the appetite. Thus, *Xiao Ji Ping Wei San* can eliminate Food Stagnation to stop pain, dry Dampness, and strengthen Spleen *Qi* to stimulate the appetite. It is often used for the treatment of anorexia due to Food Stagnation.

Cautions and Contraindications: None known

Dr. Xie's Comments: *Xiao Ji Ping Wei San* is often used to treat anorexia or inappetence in any illness. After the appetite has improved, other herbal formulas should be added to treat the underlying causes.

Cheng Qi Ping Wei San (Purging the Bowel to Harmonize the Stomach) 承气平胃散

Cheng Qi means purging of the Large Intestines or defecation. *Ping* means harmonize, *Wei* means the Stomach, and *San* is powder for the form of herbal administration. Thus, *Cheng Qi Ping Wei* translates to Purging the Bowel to Harmonize the Stomach.

Source: *Niu Yi Jin Jian (Golden Guide for Bovine Veterinarians)*, written anonymously and published during the *Qing* Dynasty between the early 18th century and early 19th century CE

Ingredients: *Cheng Qi Ping Wei San* is composed of *Ping Wei San* in combination with *Shen Qu* (Massa Fermentata), *Cao Guo* (Amomum), *Shan Zha* (Crataegus), *Qing Pi* (Citrus), *Ban Xia* (Pinellia), *Bing Lang* (Areca), *Zhi Ke or Zhi Qiao* (Aurantium), *Zhi Shi* (Aurantium), and *Mai Ya* (Hordeum). The ingredients of *Ping Wei San* are *Cang Zhu* (Atractylodes), *Hou Po* (Magnolia), *Chen Pi* (Citrus), *Gan Cao* (Glycyrrhiza), *Sheng Jiang* (Zingiberis), and *Da Zao* (Jujube)

Preparation:
1. Powder or capsule method: Herbs are ground into a fine powder. The powder can be encapsulated.
2. Decoction or teapill method: Raw herbs are mixed together and decocted. The herbal water extract (decoction) can be concentrated as granules or teapills.

Actions: Purge the Large Intestine to remove Food Stagnation, move *Qi* to stop colic, strengthen Spleen *Qi* to stimulate the appetite, dry Damp to stop vomiting

Indications: Food Stagnation with Cold and Damp in the Spleen and Stomach characterized by poor appetite or anorexia, depression, colic, vomiting or diarrhea, a pale purple tongue, and a wiry or deep pulse

Dosage and Usage:
Horses and Cattle: 15–60 g, twice daily
Camels: 30–75 g, twice daily
Llamas, Alpacas, Goats, Sheep, and Pigs: 5–15 g, twice daily
Dogs: 0.5–5 g (or 0.1 g per kg body weight), twice daily
Cats and Rabbits: 0.2–0.5 g (or 0.1 g per kg body weight), twice daily
Birds: 0.1–0.2 g per kg body weight, twice daily
Use for 2–4 weeks until the primary clinical signs have resolved.

Analysis of Formula: *Cheng Qi Ping Wei San* combines *Ping Wei San* (drying Damp and strengthening the

Spleen) with nine additional ingredients. Serving as the King herbs, *Zhi Shi* (Aurantium), *Shen Qu* (Massa Fermentata), *Shan Zha* (Crataegus), *Zhi Qiao* (Aurantium), and *Mai Ya* (Hordeum) purge the Large Intestine to remove Food Stagnation. *Bing Lang* (Areca), *Cao Guo* (Amomum), *Qing Pi* (Citrus), and *Ban Xia* (Pinellia) are the Minister and Adjuvant herbs to move *Qi* to stop pain and dry Dampness to strengthen the Spleen.

Dr. Xie's Comments: *Cheng Qi Ping Wei San* historically has been effectively used to treat Food Stagnation and constipation in cattle. It can also be used to treat chronic constipation in dogs, impactions in horses and megacolon in cats.

Huo Xiang Zheng Qi San (Pogostemon to Rectify the *Qi*) 藿香正气散

Huo Xiang refers to Pogostemon, the King ingredient of the formula, and *Zheng Qi* means to rectify the *Qi*. *San* is powder for the form of herbal administration. Thus, *Huo Xiang Zheng Qi* translates as Pogostemon to Rectify *Qi*.

Source: *Huo Xiang Zheng Qi San* was originally from *Tai Ping Hui Min He Ji Ju Fang (Imperial Grace Formulary of the Tai Ping Era)*, written by *Chen Shi-Wen* et al. and published by the *Song* Dynasty government in 1078 CE

Ingredients: The formula contains 60g *Huo Xiang* Pogostemon), 45g *Zi Su Ye* (Perilla), 15g *Bai Zhi* (Angelica), 30g *Da Fu Pi* (Areca), 30g *Fu Ling* (Poria), 30g Bai *Zhu* (Atractylodes), 20g *Ban Xia* (Pinellia), 30g *Chen Pi* (Citrus), 30g *Hou Po* (Magnolia), 20g *Jie Geng* (Platycodon), and 15g *Gan Cao* (Glycerrhiza) (Table 23.2).

Table 23.2. Ingredients and actions of *Huo Xiang Zheng Qi San.*

%	English Name	*Pin-Yin* Name	Actions
18.6	Pogostemon	*Huo Xiang*	Dispel Wind and Cold, aromatically disperse Damp, stop vomiting
13.8	Perilla	*Zi Su Ye*	Dispel Exterior Wind/ Cold
4.6	Angelica	*Bai Zhi*	Dispel Exterior Wind/ Cold and eliminate Damp
6.2	Pinellia	*Ban Xia*	Dry Damp, harmonize the Stomach, descend rebelling *Qi* to stop vomiting
9.2	Citrus	*Chen Pi*	Harmonize the Stomach, descend rebelling *Qi* to stop vomiting, dry Damp
9.2	Poria	*Fu Ling*	Drain Damp, promote urination
9.2	Atractylodes	*Bai Zhu*	Strengthen the Spleen to remove Damp to stop diarrhea
9.2	Magnolia	*Hou Po*	Dry Damp, move *Qi* to relieve pain
9.2	Areca	*Da Fu Pi*	Move *Qi* to relieve abdominal distention
6.2	Platycodon	*Jie Geng*	Open the inhibited Lung
4.6	Glycyrrhiza	*Gan Cao*	Harmonize herbs, tonify *Qi*

Preparation:

1. Powder or capsule method: Herbs are ground into a fine powder. The powder can be encapsulated.
2. Decoction or teapill method: Raw herbs are mixed together and decocted. The herbal water extract (decoction) can be concentrated as granules or teapills.

Actions: Relieve the Exterior, disperse Dampness, regulate *Qi* of the Middle Burner *(Zhong Jiao)*

Indications: Invasion of the Exterior by Wind and Cold in combination with impairment of the Interior by Dampness characterized by an acute onset of headache, general aching and stiffness, depression, vomiting, diarrhea, abdominal distention, pale purple tongue with thin white coating, and a superficial pulse

Dosage and Usage:

Horses and Cattle: 15–60g, twice daily
Camels: 30–75g, twice daily
Llamas, Alpacas, Goats, Sheep, and Pigs: 5–15g, twice daily
Dogs: 0.5–5g (or 0.1g per kg body weight), twice daily
Cats and Rabbits: 0.2–0.5g (or 0.1g per kg body weight), twice daily
Birds: 0.1–0.2g per kg body weight, twice daily

Use for 2–6 weeks until the primary clinical signs have resolved.

Analysis of Formula: *Huo Xiang Zheng Qi San* was formulated to treat Wind-Cold Pattern together with Interior impairment by Dampness. *Huo Xiang* (Pogostemon), the King herb, dispels Wind-Cold, aromatically disperses Damp, and stops vomiting by regulating the Middle Burner *(Zhong Jiao)*. *Zi Su Ye* (Perilla) and *Bai Zhi* (Angelica), pungent and aromatic in flavor, act as Minister herbs to support the action of the King herb to dispel Wind-Cold and eliminate Damp. *Ban Xia* (Pinellia) and *Chen Pi* (Citrus) remove Dampness, harmonize the Stomach and descend rebelling *Qi* to stop vomiting. *Fu Ling* (Poria) and Bai *Zhu* (Atractylodes) strengthen the Spleen to remove Dampness, and they harmonize the Middle Burner *(Zhong Jiao)* to stop diarrhea. *Hou Po* (Magnolia) and *Da Fu Pi* (Areca) disperse Dampness and relieve abdominal distention by promoting the movement of *Qi*. *Jie Geng* (Platycodon) opens the inhibited Lung and relieves the Exterior Pattern; it also eliminates Damp. The previous seven herbs are all the Adjuvant herbs. Serving as the Messenger, *Gan Cao* (Glycerrhiza) harmonizes all other herbs. All the herbs work together to dispel Wind and Cold from the Exterior and eliminate Dampness in the Interior, normalizing the circulation of *Qi* and function of the Spleen and Stomach.

Cautions and Contraindications: Avoid overcooking if using the formula as a decoction, because this will reduce the effectiveness of the pungent and aromatic herbs.

Dr. Xie's Comments: *Huo Xiang Zheng Qi San* was originally used to treat patients with vomiting and diarrhea due to the external invasion of Cold-Wind together with Internal Dampness. It is often used for traveler's sickness, car or motion sickness, and any infections with the occurrence of both vomiting and diarrhea.

FORMULAS TO CLEAR DAMP-HEAT

The formulas in this section are used to treat Damp-Heat in the Interior. A Damp-Heat Pattern is often caused by the exogenous invasion of Damp-Heat from the environment. It also develops from Dampness in the Interior, which attracts or transforms into Heat. Damp and Heat attract each other, are married, and become the more potent pathogenic factor Damp-Heat. Damp-Heat is stubborn and clings to the body, making it more difficult to clear. Damp-Heat mainly affects the Spleen or gastrointestinal tract, the Liver and Gallbladder, and the Urinary Bladder. The main ingredients to clear Damp-Heat include *Yin Chen Hao* (Artemisia), *Huang Lian* (Coptis), and *Mu Tong* (Akebia).

Ba Zheng San (Eight Rectifying) 八正散

Ba means eight and refers to the eight ingredients in the formula. *Zheng* means rectification or purification. Thus this formula's name comes from the fact that the eight herbal ingredients eliminate pathogenic factors and make the Lower Burner (*Xia Jiao*) have normal and righteous functions.

Source: *Tai Ping Hui Min He Ji Ju Fang* (*Imperial Grace Formulary of the Tai Ping Era*), written by *Chen Shi-Wen* et al. and published by the *Song* Dynasty government in 1078 CE

Ingredients: *Ba Zheng San* contains 30 g *Mu Tong* (Akebia), 30 g *Qu Mai* (Dianthus), 45 g *Che Qian Zi* (Plantago), 30 g *Bian Xu* (Polygonum), 10 g *Hua Shi* (Talcum), 25 g *Zhi Zi* (Gardenia), 25 g *Da Huang* (Rheum), 25 g *Gan Cao* (Glycyrrhiza), and 10 g *Deng Xin Cao* (Juncus) (Table 23.3).

Table 23.3. Ingredients and actions of *Ba Zheng San*.

%	English Name	*Pin-Yin* Name	Actions
13	Akebia	*Mu Tong*	Drain Damp-Heat and induce diuresis
13	Dianthus	*Qu Mai*	Clear Damp-Heat and induce diuresis
20	Plantago	*Che Qian Zi*	Clear Damp-Heat and induce diuresis
13	Polygonum	*Bian Xu*	Clear Damp-Heat and induce diuresis
4	Talcum	*Hua Shi*	Clear Damp-Heat and induce diuresis
11	Gardenia	*Zhi Zi*	Clear Damp-Heat out of the Triple Burner (*San Jiao*)
11	Rheum	*Da Huang*	Purge Fire and expel the pathogenic Heat out of the Lower Burner (*Xia Jiao*)
4	Juncus	*Deng Xin Cao*	Remove Heat from the Heart
11	Glycyrrhiza	*Gan Cao*	Harmonize the properties of other ingredients, relieve spasms and pain

Preparation:

1. Powder or capsule method: Herbs are ground into a fine powder. The powder can be encapsulated.
2. Decoction or teapill method: Raw herbs are mixed together and decocted. The herbal water extract (decoction) can be concentrated as granules or teapills.

Actions: Clear Damp-Heat, purge Fire, promote diuresis

Indications: Stranguria due to Damp-Heat marked by frequent and urgent urination with pain, hematuria, urinary stuttering and bradyuria, turbid and dark urine, uroschesis, a red tongue with greasy yellow coating, and a slippery and rapid pulse

Dosage and Usage:

Horses and Cattle: 15–60 g, twice daily
Camels: 30–75 g, twice daily
Llamas, Alpacas, Goats, Sheep, and Pigs: 5–15 g, twice daily
Dogs: 0.5–5 g (or 0.1 g per kg body weight), twice daily
Cats and Rabbits: 0.2–0.5 g (or 0.1 g per kg body weight), twice daily
Birds: 0.1–0.2 g per kg body weight, twice daily

Use for 2–10 weeks until the primary clinical signs have resolved.

Analysis of Formula: This formula is designed to treat Heat and Dampness that has drained down to the urinary bladder. The King herb, *Mu Tong* (Akebia) drains Damp-Heat out of the body. *Qu Mai* (Dianthus), *Che Qian Zi* (Plantago), *Bian Xu* (Polygonum), *Hua Shi* (Talcum), and *Deng Xin Cao* (Juncus) serve as Minister herbs capable of clearing Damp-Heat and inducing diuresis. As Adjuvant herbs, *Zhi Zi* (Gardenia) and *Da Huang* (Rheum) purge Fire and expel the pathogenic Heat out of the Lower Burner (*Xia Jiao*). *Gan Cao* (Glycyrrhiza) harmonizes the other ingredients and relieves spasms and pain, acting as the Messenger herb.

Cautions and Contraindications: *Ba Zheng San* consists of diuretics with bitter and cold natures and is suitable for excessive Fire or Damp-Heat in the Bladder. Use with caution in patients who have a weak constitution or are pregnant.

Dr. Xie's Comments: *Ba Zheng San* is the classical formula for treating a Bladder Damp-Heat Pattern. It is used for the treatment of cystitis, urethritis, urinary tract infection or inflammation, urinary crystals, and bladder or kidney stones due to Damp-Heat.

Hua Shi San (Talcum Powder) 滑石散

Hua Shi refers to Talcum, the King ingredient of the formula, and *San* is powder for the form of herbal administration. Thus, *Hua Shi San* translates literally to Talcum Powder.

Source: *Yuan Heng Liao Ma Ji* (*Yuan-Heng's Therapeutic Treatise of Horses*), written by *Yu Benyun* and *Yu Benheng* during the *Ming* Dynasty and published in 1608

Ingredients: *Hua Shi San* contains 60 g *Hua Shi* (Talcum), 30 g *Ze Xie* (Alisma), 30 g *Yin Chen Hao* (Artemisia), 30 g *Zhi Mu* (Anemarrhena), 30 g *Huang Bai* (Phellodendron), 30 g *Zhu Ling* (Polyporus), and 10 g *Deng Xin Cao* (Juncus) (Table 23.4).

Table 23.4. Ingredients and actions of *Hua Shi San*.

%	English Name	*Pin-Yin* Name	Actions
27.4	Talcum	*Hua Shi*	Clear Damp-Heat, induce diuresis, remove urinary calculus
13.6	Alisma	*Ze Xie*	Drain Damp, clear False Heat
13.6	Artemisia	*Yin Chen Hao*	Purge Fire, promote diuresis
13.6	Anemarrhena	*Zhi Mu*	Clear Heat, nourish *Yin*
13.6	Phellodendron	*Huang Bai*	Clear Heat, nourish *Yin*
13.6	Polyporus	*Zhu Ling*	Drain Damp
4.6	Juncus	*Deng Xin Cao*	Drain Heat through urination

Preparation:

1. Powder or capsule method: Herbs are ground into a fine powder. The powder can be encapsulated.
2. Decoction or teapill method: Raw herbs are mixed together and decocted. The herbal water extract (decoction) can be concentrated as granules or teapills.

Actions: Clear Damp-Heat, purge Fire, nourish *Yin* and promote diuresis

Indications: Difficulty urinating due to Bladder Damp-Heat, or Bladder *Qi* Stagnation characterized by frequent and urgent urination with pain, abdominal pain, hematuria, a red or purple tongue, and rapid pulse

Dosage and Usage:

Horses and Cattle: 15–60 g, twice daily
Camels: 30–75 g, twice daily
Llamas, Alpacas, Goats, Sheep, and Pigs: 5–15 g, twice daily
Dogs: 0.5–5 g (or 0.1 g per kg body weight), twice daily
Cats and Rabbits: 0.2–0.5 g (or 0.1 g per kg body weight), twice daily
Birds: 0.1–0.2 g per kg body weight, twice daily

Use for 2–4 weeks until the primary clinical signs have resolved.

Analysis of Formula: *Hua Shi San* was formulated for the accumulation of Damp-Heat in the Lower Burner (*Xia Jiao*) leading to dysfunction of the urinary bladder, urinary dripping, or urination with pain and colic. *Hua Shi* (Talcum) is the King herb due to its cold nature and functions to remove Damp-Heat by promoting diuresis. *Ze Xie* (Alisma), *Yin Chen Hao* (Artemisia), and *Zhu Ling* (Polyporus) serve as the Minister herbs, helping the King herb eliminate Damp-Heat. Serving as the Adjuvant herbs, *Zhi Mu* (Anemarrhena) and *Huang Bai* (Phellodendron) clear Heat and nourish *Yin* to restore the Body Fluids, which may be damaged by excessive Heat or Damp Heat. *Deng Xin Cao* (Juncus), as the Messenger herb, guides the Heat and Dampness to go out with urine. Together, these herbs act to clear pathogenic Damp-Heat and promote diuresis to resolve Stagnation in the Bladder.

Cautions and Contraindications: Use with caution in patients with Spleen *Qi* Deficiency.

Dr. Xie's Comments: Both *Hua Shi San* and *Ba Zheng San* clear Damp-Heat and promote urination, and both are used for Bladder Damp Heat. However, *Hua Shi San* can also nourish *Yin* and clear False Heat, and is often used for chronic urinary tract infections (UTI) or cystitis, or in *Yin* Deficient patients. *Ba Zheng San* has a much stronger effect to clear Damp-Heat and purge excessive Fire and hence is often used for severe UTI and cystitis cases.

Yin Chen Zhu Fu San (Artemisia, Atractylodes and Aconite) 茵陈术附散

Yin Chen refers to *Yin Chen Hao* (Artemisia), the King ingredient of the formula. *Zhu* refers to *Bai Zhu* (Atractylodes), and *Fu* refers to *Fu Zi* or Aconite. *San* is powder, for the form of herbal administration. Thus, *Yin Chen Zhu Fu* translates as Artemisia, Atractylodes and Aconite.

Source: *Yi Xue Xin Wu* (*Medical Revelations*), written by *Cheng Guo-Peng* and published in 1732 CE

Ingredients: *Yin Chen Zhu Fu San* is composed of 3g *Yin Chen Hao* (Artemisia), 6g *Bai Zhu* (Atractylodes), 1.5g *Fu Zi* (Aconite), 1.5g *Gan Jiang* (Zingiberis), 1g *Rou Gui* (Cinnamomum), and 3g *Gan Cao* (Glycyrrhiza) (Table 23.5).

Preparation:

1. Powder or capsule method: Herbs are ground into a fine powder. The powder can be encapsulated.
2. Decoction or teapill method: Raw herbs are mixed together and decocted. The herbal water extract (decoction) can be concentrated as granules or teapills.

Actions: Warm and strengthen the Spleen, eliminate Damp to resolve jaundice

Indications: *Yin* Jaundice due to Cold-Damp or Spleen *Qi* Deficiency characterized by chronic icterus or jaundice; gray-yellow color of mucous membranes of the eyes, mouth, and nose; depression; weakness in all four limbs; loss of appetite; cool ears and nose; cold extremities; a pale tongue with a white and greasy coating; and a deep, thready, weak pulse

Dosage and Usage:

Horses and Cattle: 15–60g, twice daily
Camels: 30–75g, twice daily
Llamas, Alpacas, Goats, Sheep, and Pigs: 5–15g, twice daily
Dogs: 0.5–5g (or 0.1g per kg body weight), twice daily
Cats and Rabbits: 0.2–0.5g (or 0.1g per kg body weight), twice daily
Birds: 0.1–0.2g per kg body weight, twice daily

Use for 1–4 weeks until the primary clinical signs have resolved.

Table 23.5. Ingredients and actions of *Yin Chen Zhu Fu San.*

%	English Name	*Pin-Yin* Name	Actions
18.7	Artemisia	*Yin Chen Hao*	Clear Damp-Heat
37.5	Atractylodes	*Bai Zhu*	Tonify the Spleen, dry Damp
9.4	Aconite	*Fu Zi*	Warm the Interior
9.4	Zingiberis	*Gan Jiang*	Warm the Interior
6.3	Cinnamomum	*Rou Gui*	Warm the Kidney
18.7	Glycyrrhiza	*Gan Cao*	Harmonize the properties of other ingredients

Analysis of Formula: *Yin Chen Zhu Fu San* was formulated for *Yin* Jaundice due to Cold-Damp associated with Spleen *Qi* Deficiency. Therefore, *Yin Chen Hao* (Artemisia), *Bai Zhu* (Atractylodes), and *Fu Zi* (Aconite) are selected as the King herbs to eliminate Damp, warm the *Yang* to dispel Cold, and strengthen the Spleen to stop the source of Damp. Working as the Minister herbs, *Gan Jiang* (Zingiberis) and *Rou Gui* (Cinnamomum) warm the Spleen and Kidney *Yang* to dispel Cold. *Gan Cao* (Glycyrrhiza) tonifies Spleen *Qi* and harmonizes the actions of all other herbs, serving as the Adjuvant and Messenger herb.

Cautions and Contraindications: *Yin Chen Zhu Fu San* is contraindicated in patients with *Yang* Jaundice or Liver Damp-Heat.

Dr. Xie's Comments: Jaundice (or *Huang Dan*) is divided into *Yang* Jaundice and *Yin* Jaundice. *Yang* Jaundice is often caused by excessive Heat or Damp-Heat in the Liver and Gallbladder and should be treated with *Yin Chen Hao Tang*. *Yin* Jaundice is often caused by Cold-Damp, is associated with Spleen *Qi* Deficiency, and should be treated with *Yin Chen Zhu Fu Tang*.

FORMULAS TO DRAIN DAMP AND PROMOTE URINATION

The formulas in this section are used to treat accumulation of water and Dampness in the Interior. Dampness is very sticky and clings to the body. Dampness in the Interior tends to block and clog the water pathways leading to disorders of water metabolism. Consequently edema, diarrhea, and difficult urination or urinary obstruction may occur. Urination is the key vehicle to expel Dampness from the body, hence promoting urination and diuresis to drain and leach Damp out is the main treatment strategy for this condition. The principal herbs found in these formulas are *Fu Ling* (Poria), *Zhu Ling* (Polyporus), *Ze Xie* (Alisma), *Che Qian Zi* (Plantago), *Hua Shi* (Talcum), and *Tong Cao* (Tetrapanax).

Wu Ling San (Five Ingredients with Poria) 五苓散

Wu means five and refers to the five ingredients of the formula. *Ling* refers to *Fu Ling* (Poria), one of the key ingredients of the formula. *San* is powder, for the form

Table 23.6. Ingredients and actions of *Wu Ling San.*

%	English Name	*Pin-Yin* Name	Actions
31.3	Alisma	*Ze Xie*	Drain Damp, promote diuresis
18.7	Poria	*Fu Ling*	Drain Damp, promote diuresis
18.7	Polyporus	*Zhu Ling*	Drain Damp, promote diuresis
18.7	Atractylodes	*Bai Zhu*	Strengthen the Spleen and water metabolism, dry Damp
12.6	Cinnamomum	*Gui Zhi*	Promote urinary bladder to excrete urine

of herbal administration. Thus, *Wu Ling* translates to Five Ingredients with Poria.

Source: *Shang Han Za Bing Lun* (*Discussion of Cold-Induced Disorders and Miscellaneous Diseases*), written by *Zhang Zhong-Jing* and published in 220 CE

Ingredients: *Wu Ling San* is composed of 75 g *Ze Xie* (Alisma), 45 g *Fu Ling* (Poria), 45 g *Zhu Ling* (Polyporus), 45 g *Bai Zhu* (Atractylodes), and 30 g *Gui Zhi* (Cinnamomum) (Table 23.6).

Preparation:

1. Powder or capsule method: Herbs are ground into a fine powder. The powder can be encapsulated.
2. Decoction or teapill method: Raw herbs are mixed together and decocted. The herbal water extract (decoction) can be concentrated as granules or teapills.

Actions: Drain Damp, promote diuresis, activate the flow of *Qi*, strengthen the Spleen

Indications: Water retention due to Bladder *Qi* Stagnation characterized by dysuria, edema, diarrhea, a pale tongue with greasy white coating, and a soft pulse

Dosage and Usage:

Horses and Cattle: 15–60 g, twice daily
Camels: 30–75 g, twice daily
Llamas, Alpacas, Goats, Sheep, and Pigs: 5–15 g, twice daily
Dogs: 0.5–5 g (or 0.1 g per kg body weight), twice daily
Cats and Rabbits: 0.2–0.5 g (or 0.1 g per kg body weight), twice daily
Birds: 0.1–0.2 g per kg body weight, twice daily

Use for 4–12 weeks until the primary clinical signs have resolved.

Analysis of Formula: Pathogenic Cold initially enters the Bladder Meridian to cause pain and fever. The external invasion of Cold gradually affects the urinary bladder and blocks the flow of *Qi*, leading to dysuria, water retention (including edema), or diarrhea. This condition should be treated by draining Damp, promoting diuresis, and moving Bladder *Qi* to benefit urination. As the King herb, *Ze Xie* (Alisma) drains Damp and has a strong diuretic effect. *Fu Ling* (Poria) and *Zhu Ling* (Polyporus) act as the Minister herbs, enhancing the King herb's ability to eliminate Dampness by promoting diuresis. *Bai Zhu* (Atractylodes), as the Adjuvant herb, is used to strengthen the Spleen and restore normal water metabolism in the body. *Gui Zhi* (Cinnamomum), as the Messenger herb, encourages the urinary bladder to excrete urine and expels pathogenic factors to relieve the Exterior. All the herbs together strengthen the Spleen and induce diuresis.

Cautions and Contraindications: Do not use *Wu Ling San* to treat Heat Patterns due to the warm nature of the formula.

Dr. Xie's Comments: *Wu Ling San* is a common formula for eliminating the water retention that results from dysfunction of the transportation and transformation functions of the Spleen. In modern veterinary practice, it can be used as an adjunct herbal formula to treat water retention, ascites, or edema caused by congestive heart failure or liver cirrhosis. In cases without Exterior Cold signs (headache or fever), *Rou Gui* (Cinnamomum bark) usually replaces *Gui Zhi* (Cinnamomum twig) in order to reinforce *Qi* and excrete urine.

Si Ling San (Four Ingredients with Poria) 四苓散

Si means four and refers to the four ingredients in the formula. *Ling* refers to *Fu Ling* (Poria), one of the key ingredients of the formula. *San* is powder for the form of herbal administration. Thus, *Si Ling* means Four Ingredients with Poria.

Source: *Dan Xi Xin Fa* (*Teachings of Zhu Dan-Xi*), written by *Zhu Zhen-Heng* and published in 1481 CE

Ingredients: *Si Ling San* is made by removing *Gui Zhi* (Cinnamomum twig) from *Wu Lin San.* It is composed of 75 g *Ze Xie* (Alisma), 45 g *Fu Ling* (Poria), 45 g *Zhu Ling* (Polyporus), and 45 g *Cang Zhu* (Atractylodes).

Preparation:

1. Powder or capsule method: Herbs are ground into a fine powder. The powder can be encapsulated.
2. Decoction or teapill method: Raw herbs are mixed together and decocted. The herbal water extract (decoction) can be concentrated as granules or teapills.

Actions: Strengthen the Spleen to eliminate Damp

Indications: Diarrhea or edema due to Spleen *Qi* Deficiency. characterized by dysuria, edema, a pale tongue, and a weak pulse

Dosage and Usage:
Horses and Cattle: 15–60 g, twice daily
Camels: 30–75 g, twice daily
Llamas, Alpacas, Goats, Sheep, and Pigs: 5–15 g, twice daily
Dogs: 0.5–5 g (or 0.1 g per kg body weight), twice daily
Cats and Rabbits: 0.2–0.5 g (or 0.1 g per kg body weight), twice daily
Birds: 0.1–0.2 g per kg body weight, twice daily
Use for 2–8 weeks until the primary clinical signs have resolved.

Analysis of Formula: *Si Ling San* contains the same ingredients as *Wu Lin San* except that *Gui Zhi* (Cinnamomum) has been removed. As the King herb, *Ze Xie* (Alisma) drains Damp and promotes diuresis. *Bai Zhu* (Atractylodes), as the Minister herb, strengthens the Spleen and restores water metabolism to eliminate Damp. *Fu Ling* (Poria) and *Zhu Ling* (Polyporus) act as the Adjuvant and Messenger herbs, draining Damp and promoting diuresis. All the herbs together strengthen the Spleen to eliminate Damp.

Cautions and Contraindications: Use with caution in patients with *Yin* Deficiency or Heat.

Dr. Xie's Comments: *Si Ling San* is designed for the adjunct treatment of the disorder of water metabolis including pleural effusion, ascites and edema. In cases due to *Yang* or *Qi* Deficiency, *Shi Pi Yin* is usually combined.

Yin Chen Wu Ling San (Artemisia Plus Five Ingredients) 茵陈五苓散

Yin Chen refers to *Yin Chen Hao* (Artemisia). *Wu Ling* refers to the five ingredients of the formula *Wu Ling San*, one of which is *Fu Ling* (Poria), a key ingredient in this formula. *San* is powder for the form of herbal administration. Thus, *Yin Chen Wu Ling San* translates to Artemisia Plus Five Ingredients.

Source: *Jin Gui Yao Lue Fang Lun* (*Synopsis of Prescriptions from the Golden Cabinet*), written by *Zhang Zhong-Jing* in 220 CE

Ingredients: *Yin Chen Wu Ling San* is formed by adding 4 g *Yin Chen Hao* (Artemisia) to 2 g *Wu Ling San* [*Ze Xie* (Alisma), *Fu Ling* (Poria), *Zhu Ling* (Polyporus), *Cang Zhu (Atractylodes)*, and *Gui Zhi* (Cinnamomum)].

Preparation:
1. Powder or capsule method: Herbs are ground into a fine powder. The powder can be encapsulated.
2. Decoction or teapill method: Raw herbs are mixed together and decocted. The herbal water extract (decoction) can be concentrated as granules or teapills.

Actions: Clear Damp-Heat, drain Damp to resolve jaundice

Indications: Jaundice caused by Damp-Heat in the Liver

Dosage and Usage:
Horses and Cattle: 15–60 g, twice daily
Camels: 30–75 g, twice daily
Llamas, Alpacas, Goats, Sheep, and Pigs: 5–15 g, twice daily
Dogs: 0.5–5 g (or 0.1 g per kg body weight), twice daily
Cats and Rabbits: 0.2–0.5 g (or 0.1 g per kg body weight), twice daily
Birds: 0.1–0.2 g per kg body weight, twice daily
Use for 2–10 weeks until the primary clinical signs have resolved.

Analysis of Formula: Jaundice is often caused by Damp-Heat. Therefore, *Yin Chen Hao* (Artemisia) works as the King herb to clear Damp-Heat and resolve jaundice. Serving as the Adjuvant and Messenger herbs, *Wu Ling San* (*Ze Xie* (Alisma), *Fu Ling* (Poria), *Zhu Ling* (Polyporus), *Cang Zhu* (Atractylodes), and *Gui Zhi* (Cinnamomum) promotes urination and drains Damp to resolve jaundice.

Cautions and Contraindications: *Yin Chen Wu Ling San* should be used with caution in patients with *Yin* Deficiency or Heat.

Dr. Xie's Comments: Both *Yin Chen Wu Ling San* and *Yin Chen Hao Tang* (Chapter 21) are used for Jaundice with Damp-Heat, or *Yang* Jaundice, characterized by bright yellow color of eyelids and lips. However, *Yin Chen Wu Ling San* is more effective to drain Damp, and *Yin Chen Hao Tang* is more effective to clear Heat. Therefore, *Yin Chen Wu Ling San* is often used for the Jaundice due to Damp Heat (Damp predominant) with edema, urinary difficulty, a yellow tongue, and soft or slippery pulse. *Yin Chen Hao Tang* is used for the Jaundice due to Damp Heat (Heat predominant) with fever, acute onset, a red tongue, and a fast pulse.

Wei Ling San (Stomach and Poria) 胃苓散

Wei refers to *Ping Wei San* (Harmonizing the Stomach) and Ling refers to *Wu Ling San* (Five Ingredients with Poria). *Wei Ling San* is named after a combination of these two classical formulas.

Source: *Shi Yi De Xiao Fang* (*Effective Formulas from Generations of Physicians*), written by *Wei Yi-Lin* and published in 1345 CE

Ingredients: *Wei Ling San* is formed by combining 10g *Ping Wei San* (Harmonizing the Stomach) with 10g *Wu Ling San* (Five Ingredients with Poria).

Preparations:
1. Powder or capsule method: Herbs are ground into a fine powder. The powder can be encapsulated.
2. Decoction or teapill method: Raw herbs are mixed together and decocted. The herbal water extract (decoction) can be concentrated as granules or teapills.

Actions: Eliminate Damp and harmonize the Stomach, move *Qi*, promote urination

Indications: Cold-Damp accumulated in the Middle Burner (*Zhong Jiao*) characterized by diarrhea, edema, abdominal pain and fullness, pale tongue with greasy coating, and a slow or soft pulse

Dosage and Usage:
Horses and Cattle: 15–60g, twice daily
Camels: 30–75g, twice daily
Llamas, Alpacas, Goats, Sheep, and Pigs: 5–15g, twice daily
Dogs: 0.5–5g (or 0.1g per kg body weight), twice daily
Cats and Rabbits: 0.2–0.5g (or 0.1g per kg body weight), twice daily
Birds: 0.1–0.2g per kg body weight, twice daily
Use for 4–8 weeks until the primary clinical signs have resolved.

Analysis of Formula: *Wei Ling San* was formulated for Cold-Damp in the Spleen and Stomach with Damp accumulated in the Interior. *Wei Ling San* consists of two classical formulas: *Ping Wei San* and *Wu Ling San*. *Ping Wei San* is effective at strengthening the Spleen, drying Damp, and harmonizing and warming the Stomach to dispel Cold. *Wu Ling San* promotes urination and drains Damp to resolve edema. Thus, this combination of two formulas is used to treat both Cold and Damp accumulated in the Spleen and Stomach.

Cautions and Contraindications: Do not use *Wei Ling San* to treat cases of *Yin* Deficiency.

Dr. Xie's Comments: *Ping Wei San* is used to treat Damp and Stagnation in the Spleen and Stomach with Cold. *Wu Ling San* treats Water retention in the Interior. The combination of these two formulas becomes *Wei Ling San*, which is used to treat Cold-Damp in the Spleen and Stomach.

Zhu Ling San (Polyporus Powder) 猪苓散

Zhu Ling refers to Polyporus. *San* is powder for the form of herbal administration. Thus, *Zhu Ling San* translates directly as Polyporus Powder.

Source: *Yuan Heng Liao Ma Ji* (*Yuan-Heng's Therapeutic Treatise of Horses*), written by *Yu Benyuan* and *Yu Benheng* and published in 1608

Ingredients: The original formula of *Zhu Ling San* contains 60g *Zhu Ling* (Polyporus), 60g *Ze Xie* (Alisma), 30g *Qing Pi* (Citrus), 30g *Chen Pi* (Citrus), 15g *Tian Xian Zi* (Scopolia japonica), and 15g *Qian Niu Zi* (Pharbitis). Since *Tian Xian Zi* (Scopolia japonica) is so toxic, the modern formula uses 15g *Mu Xiang* (Saussurea) as a substitute (Table 23.7).

Preparation:
1. Powder or capsule method: Herbs are ground into a fine powder. The powder can be encapsulated.
2. Decoction or teapill method: Raw herbs are mixed together and decocted. The herbal water extract (decoction) can be concentrated as granules or teapills.

Actions: Expel Damp, move *Qi* to resolve pain, remove water to stop diarrhea

Indications: Diarrhea due to Cold attack on the intestines characterized by diarrhea, thirst, abdominal pain, emaciation, pale or purple tongue, and deep and soft pulse

Dosage and Usage:
Horses and Cattle: 15–60g, twice daily
Camels: 30–75g, twice daily

Table 23.7. Ingredients and actions of *Zhu Ling San*.

%	English Name	*Pin-Yin* Name	Actions
28.6	Polyporus	*Zhu Ling*	Drain Damp, promote diuresis
28.6	Alisma	*Ze Xie*	Drain Damp, promote diuresis
14.3	Citrus	*Qing Pi*	Move *Qi* to relieve pain
14.3	Citrus	*Chen Pi*	Move *Qi*, strengthen the Spleen
7.1	Scopolia japonica*	*Tian Xian Zi*	Move *Qi*, resolve spasms, relieve pain
7.1	Pharbitis	*Qian Niu Zi*	Remove water and Damp to stop diarrhea

**Tian Xian Zi* (Scopolia japonica) is no longer used in the modern formula because of its toxic nature. Today, *Mu Xiang* (Saussurea) is substituted.

Llamas, Alpacas, Goats, Sheep, and Pigs: 5–15 g, twice daily
Dogs: 0.5–5 g (or 0.1 g per kg body weight), twice daily
Cats and Rabbits: 0.2–0.5 g (or 0.1 g per kg body weight), twice daily
Birds: 0.1–0.2 g per kg body weight, twice daily
Use for 2–4 weeks until the primary clinical signs have resolved.

Analysis of Formula: This formula was formulated to treat watery diarrhea in horses due to an attack of the Cold Pathogen. *Zhu Ling* (Polyporus) and *Ze Xie* (Alisma), as the King herbs, are able to drain Damp and eliminate water to stop diarrhea. *Qing Pi* (Citrus), *Chen Pi* (Citrus), *Tian Xian Zi* (Scopolia japonica) or *Mu* Xiang (Saussurea), and *Qian Niu Zi* (Pharbitis) move *Qi* to relieve colic and remove water to stop diarrhea. These four ingredients serve as Minister and Adjuvant herbs. The combined effects of the herbs promote normal flow of *Qi*, expel Damp, stimulate diuresis, and relieve diarrhea.

Cautions and Contraindications: *Zhu Ling San* should not be used in pregnant patients.

Dr. Xie's Comments: *Tian Xian Zi* (Scopolia japonica) in the original formula is very toxic. The modern formula uses *Mu Xiang* (Saussurea) as a substitute.

Zhu Ling Ze Xie Yin (Polyporus and Alisma) 猪苓泽泻饮

Zhu Ling refers to Polyporus. *Ze Xie* refers to Alisma. *Yin* means decoction for the form of herbal administration. Thus, *Zhu Ling Ze Xie* translates literally as Polyporus and Alisma.

Source: *Niu Jing Bei Yao Yi Fang* (*Essential Prescriptions for Cattle Diseases*), written by *Shen Lian Fang* in the *Qing* Dynasty (1644–1840 CE)

Ingredients: *Zhu Ling Ze Xie Yin* is composed of equal portions of *Zhu Ling* (Polyporus), *Ze Xie* (Alisma), *Qing Pi* (Citrus), *Chen Pi* (Citrus), *Mu Tong* (Akebia), and *Hua Shi* (Talcum) and *Che Qian Zi* (Plantago).

Preparation:
1. Powder or capsule method: Herbs are ground into a fine powder. The powder can be encapsulated.
2. Decoction or teapill method: Raw herbs are mixed together and decocted. The herbal water extract (decoction) can be concentrated as granules or teapills.

Actions: Drain Damp to resolve edema, move *Qi* to relieve pain

Indications: Abdominal distention due to water retention in cattle characterized by abdominal fullness and distention, colic, diarrhea, edema, greasy coating of the tongue, and a deep pulse

Dosage and Usage:
Horses and Cattle: 15–60 g, twice daily
Camels: 30–75 g, twice daily
Llamas, Alpacas, Goats, Sheep, and Pigs: 5–15 g, twice daily
Dogs: 0.5–5 g (or 0.1 g per kg body weight), twice daily
Cats and Rabbits: 0.2–0.5 g (or 0.1 g per kg body weight), twice daily
Birds: 0.1–0.2 g per kg body weight, twice daily
Use for 2–4 weeks until the primary clinical signs have resolved.

Analysis of Formula: Working as the King herbs, *Zhu Ling* (Polyporus) and *Ze Xie* (Alisma) drain Damp to relieve edema and promote urination to stop diarrhea. Damp blocks *Qi* flow, leading to Stagnation and pain. Serving as the Minister herbs, *Qing Pi* (Citrus) and *Chen Pi* (Citrus) are used to move *Qi* and resolve Stagnation to relieve pain. Damp lingers in the Middle Burner (*Zhong Jiao*) and transforms into Heat. Thus, *Mu Tong* (Akebia), *Hua Shi* (Talcum), and *Che Qian Zi* (Plantago) are the Adjuvant and Messenger herbs to clear Damp-Heat and promote urination.

Cautions and Contraindications: Do not use *Zhu Ling Ze Xie Yin* to treat patients with *Yin* Deficiency.

Dr. Xie's Comments: *Zhu Ling Ze Xie Yin* is useful to treat edema and ascites due to water retention in animals. Since the primary effect of the formula is to reduce water retention, once the signs have improved, an herbal formula to treat the underlying disease Patterns should be added, such as *Shi Pi Yin* for Spleen and Kidney *Qi* Deficiency and *Zhen Wu Tang* for Kidney and Heart *Yang* Deficiency.

Wu Pi Yin (Five Peels) 五皮饮

Wu means five and *Pi* means peel or skin. *Wu Pi* refers to the fact that the five ingredients of the formula are all derived from the peel or skin of the plant. *Yin* is decoction for the form of herbal administration. Thus, *Wu Pi* means Five Peels.

Source: *Hua Shi Zhong Zang Jing* (*Hua Tuo's Treasury Classic*) the exact author and year of publication are unknown. However, this work is attributed to *Hua Tuo*, who lived during the Eastern *Han* Dynasty and Three Kingdoms era of China and died in 208 CE.

Ingredients: *Wu Pi Yin* contains 50 g *Fu Ling Pi* (Poria), 50 g *Chen Pi* (Citrus), 50 g *Da Fu Pi* (Areca), 50 g *Sheng*

Table 23.8. Ingredients and actions of *Wu Pi Yin*.

%	English Name	*Pin-Yin* Name	Actions
20.0	Poria	*Fu Ling Pi*	Promote diuresis, eliminate edema, strengthen Spleen
20.0	Citrus	*Chen Pi*	Move *Qi* and dry Damp
20.0	Areca	*Da Fu Pi*	Move *Qi* and dry Damp
20.0	Zingiberis	*Sheng Jiang Pi*	Dissipate retained water with a pungent flavor
20.0	Morus	*Sang Bai Pi*	Descend the Lung *Qi*, dredge water passage

Jian Pi (Zingiberis), and 50g *Sang Bai Pi* (Morus) (Table 23.8).

Preparation:

1. Powder or capsule method: Herbs are ground into a fine powder. The powder can be encapsulated.
2. Decoction or teapill method: Raw herbs are mixed together and decocted. The herbal water extract (decoction) can be concentrated as granules or teapills.

Actions: Remove Damp to alleviate edema and move *Qi* to strengthen the Spleen

Indications: Edema due to impairment of the Spleen characterized by edema or fluid retention in the limbs or abdomen, a pale tongue, and a soft or weak pulse

Dosage and Usage:

Horses and Cattle: 15–60g, twice daily
Camels: 30–75g, twice daily
Llamas, Alpacas, Goats, Sheep, and Pigs: 5–15g, twice daily
Dogs: 0.5–5g (or 0.1g per kg body weight), twice daily
Cats and Rabbits: 0.2–0.5g (or 0.1g per kg body weight), twice daily
Birds: 0.1–0.2g per kg body weight, twice daily

Use for 4–8 weeks until the primary clinical signs have resolved.

Analysis of Formula: *Wu Pi Yin* is mainly used to treat edema due to accumulation of water caused by Stagnation of *Qi*. *Fu Ling* (Poria) eliminates water to treat edema with a slightly sweet taste as the King herb. *Da Fu Pi* (Areca) and *Chen Pi* (Citrus) serve as the Minister herbs. *Da Fu Pi* (Areca) eliminates Dampness by promoting the movement of *Qi* in the Spleen and Stomach with its warm nature and pungent taste. *Chen Pi* (Citrus) harmonizes the Stomach by encouraging the normal flow of *Qi* in the Lung and Spleen with its warm nature and pungent, bitter taste. *Sheng Jiang Pi* (Zingiberis) and *Sang Bai Pi* (Morus) are the Adjuvant and Messenger herbs. *Sheng Jiang Pi* (Zingiberis) dissipates water in the Spleen, Stomach, and skin with its pungent flavor., *Sang Bai Pi* (Morus) removes retained water by descending Lung *Qi*. The combined effects of the five herbs are to remove Dampness to alleviate edema and regulate the flow of *Qi* to strengthen the Spleen.

Cautions and Contraindications: Overdosing can damage *Yin* due to the elimination of Damp and retained water. Therefore, use *Wu Pi Yin* with caution in patients with *Yin* Deficiency.

Dr. Xie's Comments: *Wu Pi Yin* is effective for the treatment of any type of subcutaneous edema in the limbs and abdomen. All five ingredients come from the peel, skin, or bark of the plants. Therefore, the herbs go to the surface and effectively treat the retained fluids or water in the Exterior.

Si Miao San (Four Wonders) 四妙散

Si means four and refers to the four ingredients in this formula. Miao means wonder or marvel, and *San* is powder for the form of herbal administration. *Si Miao* translates literally as Four Wonders.

Source: *Cheng Fang Bian Du* (*Convenient Reader of Established Formulas*), written by *Zhang Bing-Cheng* and published in 1904 CE

Ingredients: *Si Miao San* contains 240g *Huang Bai* (Phellodendron), 240g *Yi Yi Ren* (Coix), 120g *Cang Zhu* (Atractylodes), and 120g *Niu Xi* (Achyranthes) (Table 23.9).

Preparation:

1. Powder or capsule method: Herbs are ground into a fine powder. The powder can be encapsulated.
2. Decoction or teapill method: Raw herbs are mixed together and decocted. The herbal water extract (decoction) can be concentrated as granules or teapills.

Table 23.9. Ingredients and actions of *Si Miao San*.

%	English Name	*Pin-Yin* Name	Actions
33.3	Phellodendron	*Huang Bai*	Clear Damp-Heat in the Lower Burner *(Xia Jiao)*
33.3	Coix	*Yi Yi Ren*	Smoothen Channels and joints
16.7	Atractylodes	*Cang Zhu*	Dry Damp, strengthen the Spleen
16.7	Achyranthes	*Niu Xi*	Descend the herb's effect to the Lower Burner (*Xia Jiao*) to eliminate Damp-Heat

Actions: Clear Heat and remove Damp, smooth tendons and strengthen the bones

Indications: Damp-Heat in the Middle (*Zhong Jiao*) and Lower (*Xia Jiao*) Burners or *Wei* Syndrome due to Damp-Heat characterized by an acute onset of paresis and numbness of rear limbs, atrophied muscles, painful and swollen hocks and stifles, a red or yellow tongue, and a fast pulse

Dosage and Usage:
Horses and Cattle: 15–60 g, twice daily
Camels: 30–75 g, twice daily
Llamas, Alpacas, Goats, Sheep, and Pigs: 5–15 g, twice daily
Dogs: 0.5–5 g (or 0.1 g per kg body weight), twice daily
Cats and Rabbits: 0.2–0.5 g (or 0.1 g per kg body weight), twice daily
Birds: 0.1–0.2 g per kg body weight, twice daily
Use for 4–10 weeks until the primary clinical signs have resolved.

Analysis of Formula: This formula is mainly used to treat Damp-Heat in the Middle (*Zhong Jiao*) and Lower (*Xia Jiao*) Burners. As the King herb, *Cang Zhu* (Atractylodes) dries Damp and strengthens the Spleen to eliminate Dampness in the Middle Burner (*Zhong Jiao*). *Huang Bai* (Phellodendron) is the Minister herb, predominantly removing the Damp-Heat in the Lower Burner (*Xia Jiao*). *Yi Yi Ren* (Coix), the Adjuvant herb, smooths the channels and joints and removes Damp. *Niu Xi* (Achyranthes) descends the herbs' effects to the Lower Burner (*Xia Jiao*) to eliminate Damp-Heat, serving as the Messenger herb. The four herbs together clear Heat and remove Damp.

Cautions and Contraindications: Do not use *Si Miao San* in patients with *Yin* Deficiency.

Dr. Xie's Comments: *Si Miao San* is based on the classical formula *Er Miao San* (Two Wonders), which consists of two ingredients, 15 g *Huang Bai* (Phellodendron) and 15 g *Cang Zhu* (Atractylodes). *Er Miao San* was originally formulated by *Zhu Dan-Xi* in his book *Dan Xi Xin Fa* (*Teachings of Zhu Dan-Xi*) published in 1481. Its main actions are to clear Heat and dry Damp, and it is used to treat Damp-Heat in the skin, tendons, and joints of the Lower Burner (*Xia Jiao*). *San Miao San* (Three Wonders) is composed of *Er Miao San* [*Huang Bai* (Phellodendron) and *Cang Zhu* (Atractylodes)] plus *Niu Xi* (Achyranthes), which strengthens the back, rear limbs, bones, and tendons/ligaments, and also enhances the "descending" effect to the rear limbs and feet. Thus, *San Miao San* is often used for *Wei* syndrome due to Damp-Heat. Adding *Yi Yi Ren* (Coix) to *San Miao San* makes *Si Miao San*. *Yi Yi Ren* (Coix) drains Damp and removes retained water; strengthens the Spleen; and softens and smooths joints, tendons, and ligaments to resolve stiffness (*Bi* Syndrome). Thus, *Si Miao San* is often used for Damp-Heat in the lower abdomen or rear limbs or *Wei* Syndrome due to Damp-Heat.

FORMULAS TO DISPEL WIND-DAMP

The formulas in this section are used to treat *Bi* Syndrome due to the external invasion of three combining pathogenic factors: Wind, Cold, and Damp. The main signs of *Bi* Syndrome include stiffness and pain. Herbs such as *Du Huo* (Angelica), *Qiang Huo* (Notopterygium), *Qin Jiao* (Gentiana), and *Sang Ji Sheng* (Loranthus) are often used as the main ingredients in these formulas.

Du Huo Ji Sheng Tang (Angelica and Loranthus) 独活寄生汤

The name of this formula is derived from the two King herbs. *Du Huo* refers to Angelica, while *Ji Sheng* refers to Loranthus. *Tang* is decoction for the form of herbal administration. Thus, *Du Huo Ji Sheng* is translated as Angelica and Loranthus.

Source: *Qian Jin Yao Fang* (*Thousand Ducat Formulas*), written by *Sun Si-Miao* in 652 CE

Ingredients: *Du Huo Ji Sheng Tang* contains 9 g *Du Huo* (Angelica), 6 g *Sang Ji Sheng* (Loranthus), 6 g *Du Zhong* (Eucommia), 6 g *Niu Xi* (Achyranthes), 6 g *Qin Jiao* (Gentiana), 6 g *Rou Gui* (Cinnamomum), 6 g *Ren Shen* (Ginseng), 6 g *Chuan Xiong* (Ligusticum), 6 g *Bai Shao Yao* (Paeonia), 6 g *Shu Di Huang* (Rehmannia), 6 g *Fu Ling* (Poria), 6 g *Gan Cao* (Glycyrrhiza), 6 g *Dang Gui* (Angelica), 6 g *Xi Xin* (Asarum), and 6 g *Fang Feng* (Ledebouriella) (Table 23.10).

Preparation:
1. Powder or capsule method: Herbs are ground into a fine powder. The powder can be encapsulated.
2. Decoction or teapill method: Raw herbs are mixed together and decocted. The herbal water extract (decoction) can be concentrated as granules or teapills.

Actions: Expel Wind-Damp, relieve Stagnation and pain, tonify the Liver and Kidney, tonify *Qi* and Blood

Indications: Chronic *Bi* Syndrome or rheumatic pain of the limbs due to Deficiency of the Liver and Kidney complicated by Wind-Cold-Dampness invasion characterized by stiffness and pain of the limbs and back, rear weakness, warm-seeking behavior, shortness of breath, palpitations, pale tongue with a white coating, and a thin and weak pulse.

Table 23.10. Ingredients and actions of *Du Huo Ji Sheng Tang*.

%	English Name	*Pin-Yin* Name	Actions
9.7	Angelica	*Du Huo*	Expel Wind-Cold-Damp, move *Qi* to relieve pain
6.45	Loranthus	*Sang Ji Sheng*	Strengthen the Liver and Kidney to relieve pain
6.45	Asarum	*Xi Xin*	Dissipate Cold-Damp, warm the Channels
6.45	Cinnamomum	*Rou Gui*	Warm the *Yang* to dispel Cold
6.45	Ledebouriella	*Fang Feng*	Expel Wind-Damp
6.45	Gentiana	*Qin Jiao*	Eliminate Wind-Damp, dredge the Channels
6.45	Eucommia	*Du Zhong*	Tonify the Liver and Kidney, strengthen the back
6.45	Achyranthes	*Niu Xi*	Tonify the Liver and Kidney, strengthen the tendons and bones
6.45	Angelica	*Dang Gui*	Nourish and move Blood
6.45	Ligusticum	*Chuan Xiong*	Move *Qi* and Blood to relieve pain
6.45	Paeonia	*Bai Shao Yao*	Nourish Blood
6.45	Rehmannia	*Shu Di Huang*	Nourish Blood, *Yin*, and *Jing*
6.45	Ginseng	*Ren Shen*	Tonify *Qi*
6.45	Poria	*Fu Ling*	Strengthen the Spleen, drain Damp
6.45	Glycyrrhiza	*Gan Cao*	A messenger

Dosage and Usage:

Horses and Cattle: 15–60 g, twice daily

Camels: 30–75 g, twice daily

Llamas, Alpacas, Goats, Sheep, and Pigs: 5–15 g, twice daily

Dogs: 0.5–5 g (or 0.1 g per kg body weight), twice daily

Cats and Rabbits: 0.2–0.5 g (or 0.1 g per kg body weight), twice daily

Birds: 0.1–0.2 g per kg body weight, twice daily

Use for 4–12 weeks until the primary clinical signs have resolved.

Analysis of Formula: The Liver stores Blood and controls *Jin* (includes tendons and ligaments). The Kidney dominates the back and pelvic limbs and controls bones and joints. Chronic invasion of Wind-Cold-Damp eventually damages the Liver and Kidney, leading to Blood, *Yin*, and *Yang* Deficiency. Geriatric patients with Liver and Kidney Deficiency are more susceptible to attack and invasion by External Wind-Cold-Damp. The three combined pathogenic factors, Wind-Cold-Damp, block *Qi* flow in the Channels, *Jin*, and joints, leading to pain and stiffness. Liver and Kidney Deficiency leads to rear weakness, paraparesis, and pain and weakness of the back. The treatment strategy for this condition is to expel Wind-Damp to resolve Stagnation and pain, warm the Kidney to dispel Cold, and nourish Blood to tonify the Liver. Serving as the King herbs, *Du Huo* (Angelica) expels Wind-Cold-Damp to resolve Stagnation and relieve pain, while *Sang Ji Sheng* (Loranthus) tonifies the Liver and Kidney to strengthen the *Jin* and joints and to alleviate pain. *Xi Xin* (Asarum) and *Rou Gui* (Cinnamomum) dissipate Cold-Damp with their pungent flavor and warm the Channels. *Fang Feng* (Ledebouriella) expels Wind-Damp. *Qin Jiao* (Gentiana) eliminates Wind-Damp and dredges the Channels. *Du Zhong* (Eucommia) and *Niu Xi* (Achyranthes) tonify the Liver and Kidney, strengthen the tendons and bones, and relieve pain. These six herbs are the Minister herbs. *Dang Gui* (Angelica), *Chuan Xiong* (Ligusticum), *Bai Shao Yao* (Paeonia), and *Shu Di Huang* (Rehmannia) nourish Blood. *Ren Shen* (Ginseng) and *Fu Ling* (Poria) tonify *Qi* and strengthen the Spleen. These six herbs are Adjuvant herbs. *Gan Cao* (Glycyrrhiza) serves as a Messenger herb.

Cautions and Contraindications: Do not use *Du Huo Ji Sheng Tang* to treat *Bi* Syndrome due to *Yin* Deficiency or Heat *Bi* Syndrome

Dr. Xie's Comments: *Du Huo Ji Sheng Tang* effectively treats chronic *Bi* syndrome, especially due to generalized *Qi*, Blood, and *Yang* Deficiency in geriatric or pregnant patients.

Qiang Huo Sheng Shi Tang (Notopterygium to Defeat Damp) 羌活胜湿汤

Qiang Huo refers to Notopterygium, one of the King ingredients of the formula. *Sheng* means defeat or overcome, *Shi* means Damp, and *Tang* is decoction for the form of herbal administration. Therefore, *Qiang Huo Sheng Shi* translates as Notopterygium to Defeat Damp.

Source: *Nei Wai Shang Bian Huo Lun* (*Clarifying Doubts about Injury from Internal and External Causes*), written by *Li Ao* and published in 1247 CE

Ingredients: *Qiang Huo Sheng Shi Tang* consists of 6 g *Qiang Huo* (Notopterygium), 6 g *Du Huo* (Angelica), 3 g *Fang Feng* (Ledebouriella), 3 g *Chuan Xiong* (Ligusticum), 3 g *Gao Ben* (Ligusticum), 2 g *Man Jing Zi* (Vitex), and 3 g *Gan Cao* (Glycyrrhiza)(Table 23.11).

Preparation:

1. Powder or capsule method: Herbs are ground into a fine powder. The powder can be encapsulated.
2. Decoction or teapill method: Raw herbs are mixed together and decocted. The herbal water extract (decoction) can be concentrated as granules or teapills.

Table 23.11. Ingredients and actions of *Qiang Huo Sheng Shi Tang*.

%	English Name	*Pin-Yin* Name	Actions
24.5	Notopterygium	*Qiang Huo*	Expel Wind-Damp from the Upper Burner (*Shang Jiao*)
24.5	Angelica	*Du Huo*	Expel Wind-Damp from the Lower Burner (*Xia Jiao*)
12.2	Ledebouriella	*Fang Feng*	Dissipate the superficial Wind-Damp
12.2	Ligusticum	*Gao Ben*	Expel Wind-Cold from the head to relieve pain
6.2	Ligusticum	*Chuan Xiong*	Activate Blood circulation to stop pain
8.2	Vitex	*Man Jing Zi*	Dissipate Wind-Damp from the head to relieve pain
12.2	Glycyrrhiza	*Gan Cao*	Harmonize the herbs

Actions: Expel Wind-Damp, relieve pain

Indications: Wind-Damp in the Exterior of the body characterized by aversion to Cold, mild fever, stiffness of the lumbar region or limbs, difficulty walking, white or greasy coating of the tongue, and a superficial pulse.

Dosage and Usage:
Horses and Cattle: 15–60 g, twice daily
Camels: 30–75 g, twice daily
Llamas, Alpacas, Goats, Sheep, and Pigs: 5–15 g, twice daily
Dogs: 0.5–5 g (or 0.1 g per kg body weight), twice daily
Cats and Rabbits: 0.2–0.5 g (or 0.1 g per kg body weight), twice daily
Birds: 0.1–0.2 g per kg body weight, twice daily
Use for 2–8 weeks until the primary clinical signs have resolved.

Analysis of Formula: *Qiang Huo* (Notopterygium) and *Du Huo* (Angelica) are the King herbs that act to remove Wind-Damp from the thoracic limbs or Upper Burner (*Shang Jiao*) of the body and remove Wind-Damp from the pelvic limbs or Lower Burner (*Xia Jiao*) of the body, respectively. *Fang Feng* (Ledebouriella) and *Gao Ben* (Ligusticum) expel superficial Wind-Damp to relieve pain as the Minister herbs. Acting as the Adjuvant herbs, *Man Jing Zi* (Vitex) expels Wind-Damp from the head to relieve pain, while *Chuan Xiong* (Ligusticum) activates blood circulation to stop pain. *Gan Cao* (Glycyrrhiza) acts as the Messenger herb to harmonize all ingredients of the formula. Working together these herbs expel Wind-Damp and resolve Stagnation to relieve pain.

Cautions and Contraindications: Do not use *Qiang Huo Sheng Shi Tang* in patients with *Yin* or Blood Deficiency. Equine and bovine patients should be kept warm and encouraged to produce a mild sweat after taking the formula.

Dr. Xie's Comments: *Qiang Huo Sheng Shi Tang* is effective for the treatment of the early stage or acute onset of Wind (wandering) *Bi*, Cold (painful) *Bi*, or Damp (fixed) *Bi* syndrome.

FORMULAS TO WARM THE *YANG* TO DISPEL COLD-DAMP

The formulas in this section are used to treat the accumulation of Body Fluids or Cold-Damp due to Kidney *Yang* Deficiency or the Interior Cold that arises from lingering Damp because of Spleen *Yang* Deficiency. The main ingredients of each formula include *Gan Jiang* (Zingiberis), *Gui Zhi* (Cinnamomum), and *Fu Zi* (Aconite). The two most commonly used formulas in veterinary practice are *Zhen Wu Tang* (True Warrior) and *Shi Pi Yin* (Strengthening the Spleen). *Zhen Wu Tang* is discussed in Chapter 22 (Herbal Formulas to Warm the Interior).

Shi Pi Yin (Strengthening the Spleen) 实脾饮

Shi means strengthen, *Pi* means the Spleen, and *Yin* means decoction for the form of original administration. Thus, *Shi Pi* translates literally to Strengthening the Spleen.

Source: *Shi Yi De Xiao Fang* (*Effective Formulas from Generations of Physicians*), written by *Wei Yi-Lin* and published in 1345 CE

Ingredients: *Shi Pi Yin* is composed of 30 g *Hou Po* (Magnolia), 30 g *Bai Zhu* (Atractylodes), 30 g *Mu Gua* (Chaenomeles), 30 g *Mu Xiang* (Saussurea), 30 g Cao Guo (Amomum), 30 g *Da Fu Pi* (Areca), 30 g *Fu Zi* (Aconite), 30 g *Fu Ling* (Poria), 30 g *Gan Jiang* (Zingiberis), and 15 g *Gan Cao* (Glycyrrhiza) (Table 23.12).

Preparation:
1. Powder or capsule method: Herbs are ground into a fine powder. The powder can be encapsulated.
2. Decoction or teapill method: Raw herbs are mixed together and decocted. The herbal water extract (decoction) can be concentrated as granules or teapills.

Actions: Warm the *Yang*, strengthen the Spleen, eliminate Damp and retained Body Fluids, move *Qi* to relieve pain

Table 23.12. Ingredients and actions of *Shi Pi Yin.*

%	English Name	*Pin-Yin Name*	Actions
10.6	Magnolia	*Hou Po*	Move *Qi*, dry Damp, resolve Stagnation, relieve pain
10.6	Atractylodes	*Bai Zhu*	Strengthen the Spleen, tonify *Qi*
10.5	Chaenomeles	*Mu Gua*	Dry Damp, expel Wind-Damp, stop vomiting
10.5	Saussurea	*Mu Xiang*	Move *Qi*, relieve pain
10.5	Amomum	*Cao Guo*	Move, strengthen the Spleen, eliminate Damp
10.5	Areca	*Da Fu Pi*	Move *Qi*, remove retained fluid
10.5	Aconite	*Fu Zi*	Warm *Yang*, dispel Cold
10.5	Poria	*Fu Ling*	Drain Damp, promote urination
10.5	Zingiberis	*Gan Jiang*	Warm *Yang*, dispel Cold
5.3	Glycyrrhiza	*Gan Cao*	Harmonize other herbs

Indications: Edema of the lower abdomen and rear limbs due to Spleen and Kidney *Yang* Deficiency characterized by edema especially in the abdomen and pelvic limbs; coldness in the back and extremities; no thirst, vomiting, or diarrhea; a greasy, white coating of the tongue; and a deep, weak, slow pulse

Dosage and Usage:

Horses and Cattle: 15–60g, twice daily

Camels: 30–75g, twice daily

Llamas, Alpacas, Goats, Sheep, and Pigs: 5–15g, twice daily

Dogs: 0.5–5g (or 0.1g per kg body weight), twice daily

Cats and Rabbits: 0.2–0.5g (or 0.1g per kg body weight), twice daily

Birds: 0.1–0.2g per kg body weight, twice daily

Use for 4–12 weeks until the primary clinical signs have resolved.

Analysis of Formula: Edema can be divided into *Yang* and *Yin*. *Yin* edema, also called *Yin Shui* (*Yin* type of retained fluid) is often caused by Kidney and Spleen *Yang* Deficiency. Deficient *Yang* fails to warm the body and transform water and fluids, leading to accumulation of water and fluids in the Interior. Retained fluid also builds up in the Exterior, leading to subcutaneous edema. This fluid is heavy and tends to gravitate into the Lower Burner (*Xia Jiao*); hence, edema occurs in the lower abdomen and extremities. Therefore, *Fu Zi* (Aconite) and *Gan Jiang* (Zingiberis) are the King herbs to warm the Kidney and Spleen *Yang* to dispel Cold and transform fluids to resolve edema. *Bai Zhu* (Atractylodes) and *Fu Ling* (Poria), the Minister herbs, strengthen the Spleen, tonify *Qi*, promote urination, and eliminate Damp. The Adjuvant herbs are *Hou Po* (Magnolia), *Mu Gua* (Chaenomeles), *Cao Guo* (Amomum), *Mu Xiang* (Saussurea), and *Da Fu Pi* (Areca), which tonify the Spleen, eliminate Damp, and move *Qi* to resolve Stagnation and pain. Serving as the Messenger herb, *Gan Cao* (Glycyrrhiza) tonifies *Qi* and harmonizes all other herbs.

Cautions and Contraindications: Do not use *Shi Pi Yin* to treat *Yang* Edema (or *Yang Shui*). *Yang* type of edema occurs when Exogenous Pathogens invade, and it is characterized by swelling, pain, heat, and redness in the limbs and trunk.

Dr. Xie's Comments: *Shi Pi Yin* and *Zhen Wu Tang* both warm the *Yang* to dispel Cold-Damp and are used to treat *Yin* types of edema, or *Yin Shui*. *Yin Shui* is retained water or fluids often caused by Spleen or/and Kidney *Yang* Deficiency. *Yin* Edema presents with coldness in the back and extremities and no Heat or redness. *Zhen Wu Tang* is more focused on tonifying Kidney *Yang* and *Men-Ming* Fire and is often used to treat edema in chronic heart failure. *Shi Pi Yin* is effective to strengthen Spleen *Qi* to eliminate Damp and is often used to treat subcutaneous edema in limbs and abdomen. Both *Zhen Wu Tang* and *Shi Pi Yin* can be used for the treatment of ascites in liver cirrhosis.

REFERENCE

1. Cao YC. Clinical application of Ping Wei San. Acta of Nanjing College of Traditional Chinese Medicine. 1995, 11(2):29.

24 Herbal Formulas to Regulate Stagnation 理气和解剂

Bruce Ferguson

The formulas in this chapter are used to treat dysfunctions of *Qi* that involve inadequate movement of *Qi* and thus result in *Qi* Stagnation or *Qi* Rebellion. These formulas may also be used to regulate *Qi* dysfunction in specific *Zang-Fu* organs.

Pathological processes affecting the body usually interfere with the normal flow of *Qi* first. Normalizing *Qi* flow disturbances in the Channels and Meridians (*Jing-Luo*) is facilitated by acupuncture, *Tui Na*, *Qigong*, and herbal formulas. Restoring normal *Qi* movement in the *Zang-Fu* organs is a powerful aspect of TCVM herbal formulas.

Primary symptoms of *Qi* Stagnation Patterns are Excess in nature. If there is pure Stagnation, pain and distension are primary. If there are also signs of reverse energy flux, as with *Qi* Rebellion, problems such as nausea and coughing may occur.

The primary *Zang-Fu* organs that show *Qi* Stagnation signs are the Liver and Spleen/Stomach. When there is Liver *Qi* Constraint, there may be hypochondriac and lateral costal distension and pain, abnormal estrus cycles, and pain in the Lower *Jiao*. In the case of Spleen and Stomach *Qi* Stagnation, abdominal distention and bloating, discomfort relieved by flatulence, poor appetite, and irregular bowel movements may result.

Qi Rebellion Patterns are most common in the Lung and Stomach. Lung *Qi* Rebellion has signs such as coughing, wheezing, and dyspnea. Stomach *Qi* Rebellion may include belching, borborygmi, hiccoughs, nausea, licking of lips, and vomiting.

Etiological factors involved in *Qi* Stagnation are both exogenous and endogenous. Exogenous factors include constitution (species)-inappropriate diet, invasion of *Liu Qi* or exogenous pathogens, and various forms of trauma. Endogenous factors such as psychological depression, emotional disharmonies, and forms of emotional frustration that lead to Liver *Qi* Stagnation are common causes of *Zang-Fu* organ *Qi* Stagnation. Various types of chronic deficiencies such as Spleen *Qi* and Lung *Qi* Deficiency may also be part of the genesis of *Qi* Stagnation.

The pathogenesis of *Qi* Stagnation commonly involves the Liver since one of its functions is to assure the smooth flow of *Qi*. Various toxic (e.g., environmental toxins, vaccinations) and psychological (e.g., frustration, long standing anger) insults may injure the Liver. *Qi* Stagnation may also arise from Dampness and Phlegm generation from a poorly functioning Spleen. Trauma that leads to Blood Stagnation in the Middle and Upper *Jiao* may also lead to the forms of *Qi* Stagnation and Rebellion mentioned above.

TCVM treatment principles for *Qi* Stagnation are to activate the *Qi* and resolve *Qi* Stagnation. For *Qi* Rebellion the principles also include descending rebellious *Qi*. If *Qi* Stagnation (Excess) presents concurrently with *Qi* Deficiency, the Deficiency must be tonified along with the *Qi*-activating tactics.[1]

Recent research results build a bridge between the TCVM principles and Western biomedical models. For example, the general notion of *Qi* Stagnation may overlap that of inhibited or reduced peristalsis in tubular organs. Reduced diaphragmatic excursions, increased pulmonary mucosal secretions and thickened gastrointestinal secretions may be seen in *Qi* Stagnation and Rebellion. Reduced depth of breathing and abdominal tension common in emotional Stagnation may also be involved in this Stagnation. It is likely that the expanding science of the brain-viscera connection with respect to neurophysiology and endogenously generated peptides will serve to further elucidate these issues in the future.

Western biomedical viewpoints on the herbal formulas used to treat *Qi* Stagnation may note that the herbs are commonly pungent and aromatic, with essential oils that modify tubular organ motility and secretions. Herbs in these formulas may also be warming, which will lead to increased endogenous metabolic functions. Lastly they are drying, which gives them use in modifying the hypersecretory state of enteric and pulmonary tissues.

In TCVM we should observe the general cautions and contraindications that pungent, aromatic, warming, and drying herbs have. They may consume the Body Fluids and disperse the *Qi*, so they should be discontinued as soon as obvious improvement has plateaued. Patients presenting with Blood, *Yin*, or Body Fluids Deficiency should use these formulas with care and, possibly, the addition of appropriate Blood or *Yin* tonics.

Xiao Chai Hu Tang (Minor Bupleurum) 小柴胡汤

This formula is named for the King ingredient, *Chai Hu* (Bupleurum). *Xiao* means small, or minor. *Tang* is decoction, the form of herbal administration. *Xiao Chai Hu Tang* is distinguished from *Da Chai Hu Tang* (Major Bupleurum).

Source: *Shang Han Za Bing Lun* (*Treatise on Cold-Induced Disorders and Miscellaneous Diseases*), written by *Zhang Zhong-Jing* and published in 220 CE

Ingredients: The original ingredients of *Xiao Chai Hu Tang* were decocted together twice and concentrated in a liquid form. The formula contained 24g *Chai Hu* (Bupleurum), 9g *Huang Qin* (Scutellaria), 24g *Ban Xia* (Pinellia), 9g *Sheng Jiang* (Zingiberis), 9g *Ren Shen* (Ginseng), 9g *Gan Cao* (Glycyrrhiza), and 12g *Da Zao* (Jujube) (Table 24.1).[2]

Preparation:

1. Powder or capsule method: Herbs are ground into a fine powder. Powder can be encapsulated.
2. Decoction or teapill method: Raw herbs are mixed together and decocted. Herbal water extract (decoction) can be concentrated as granules or teapills.

Actions: Harmonize and release *Shao Yang* disorders

Indications: This formula is indicated for Shao *Yang* Disease, or Shao *Yang* level disorder when a pathogen lodges halfway between the Exterior and Interior. The main clinical signs are alternating fever and chills; dry throat; chewing or lip-smacking as if there is a bitter taste in the mouth; irritability; mild resistance to thoracic and chondriac compression; nausea and vomiting; reduced appetite; normal or thin, white tongue coating; and a tight or wiry pulse.[2–4]

Table 24.1. Ingredients and actions of *Xiao Chai Hu Tang.*

%	English Name	Chinese *Pin-Yin*	Actions
25	Bupleurum	*Chai Hu*	Relieve Liver *Qi* Stagnation
9.4	Scutellaria	*Huang Qin*	Clear Heat, dry Damp
25	Pinellia	*Ban Xia*	Resolve Phlegm
9.4	Zingiberis	*Sheng Jiang*	Warm the Middle Jiao
9.4	Ginseng	*Ren Shen*	Tonify *Qi*
9.4	Glycyrrhiza	*Gan Cao*	Harmonize, tonify Middle Jiao
12.4	Jujube	*Da Zao*	Harmonize, tonify Middle Jiao

Dosage and Usage:

Horses and Cattle: 15–60g, twice daily
Camels: 30–75g, twice daily
Llamas, Alpacas, Goats, Sheep, and Pigs: 10–15g, twice daily
Dogs: 0.5–5g (or 0.1g per kg body weight), twice daily
Cats and Rabbits: 0.2–0.5g (or 0.1g per kg body weight), twice daily
Birds: 0.1–0.2g per kg body weight, twice daily

Use 1–3 weeks until primary clinical signs resolve.

Analysis of Formula: The King herb, *Chai Hu* (Bupleurum), is the most important herb available to harmonize *Shao Yang* (half Exterior and half Interior) disorders. It is cooling and ascending, and it relieves Liver *Qi* constraint. Serving as the Minister herb, *Huang Qin* (Scutellaria) drains Heat from the *Shao Yang*. *Ban Zia* (Pinellia) and *Sheng Jiang* (Zingiberis) act together to reduce Phlegm and Stagnation in the Middle Burner and reduce vomiting. *Ren Shen* (Ginseng) and *Da Zao* (Jujube) tonify *Qi* and protect the Spleen and Stomach. These four ingredients are the Adjuvant herbs. *Gan Cao* (Glycyrrhiza) harmonizes all other herbs, working as the Messenger herb.[5,6]

Cautions and Contraindications: This formula is contraindicated in patients with Excess above and Deficiency below, Liver *Yang* Rising, Liver Fire, or oral bleeding due to *Yin* Deficiency.

Dr. Xie's Comments: *Xiao Chai Hu Tang* was originally designed for *Shao Yang* Pattern, or the Half Exterior and Half Interior Pattern (*Ban Piao Ban Ni*). If the pathogenic Wind or Wind Cold is affecting only the Exterior, this Pattern is called a *Tai Yang* Pattern. On the other hand, when the pathogenic factors invade to the Interior and affect internal organs, it is called *Yang Ming* Pattern. *Shao Yang* Pattern occurs in the special stage that marks the transition from the *Tai Yang* (Exterior) to the *Yang Ming* (Interior); hence, it is called the Half Exterior and Half Interior Pattern. In modern veterinary practice, *Xiao Chai Hu* Tang is often used in treating acute viral hepatitis, otitis, and chronic hepatitis.

Clinical and Pharmacological Studies: There are numerous recent scientific publications investigating the biological effects of *Xiao Chai Hu San*. Most of the recent research focuses on hepatoprotective and regenerative functions. For example, Chang et al. found that *Xiao Chai Hu San* could inhibit the production of Hepatitis B virus in a stable HBV-producing cell line as well as have antineoplastic effects.[7] In rats, Chen et al. found that *Xiao Chai Hu San* could prevent liver fibrosis induced by bile duct ligation (BDL) by inhibiting collagen accumulation, suppressing procollagen alpha1 types (I) and (III), and tissue inhibition of metalloproteinases 1 (TIMP-1) mRNA expression. After administration of *Xiao Chai Hu Tang*, hyperbilirubinemia reduced approximately fourfold when compared with the BDL-untreated group. *Xiao Chai Hu San* also significantly reduced the collagen content and fibrogenic score, as well as downregulated elevated procollagen alpha1 types (I) and (III) and TIMP-1 mRNA level. Finally, they concluded that *Xiao Chai Hu San* significantly reduced cholestasis in rats with BDL, markedly reduced the collagen content by 50%, and exerted its antifibrogenic effect by downregulation of the mRNA expression of procollagen alpha1 types (I) and (III) and TIMP-1 in liver tissue.[8]

Da Chai Hu Tang (Major Bupleurum) 大柴胡汤

Da means large, or major. This formula is named for the King ingredient, *Chai Hu* (Bupleurum). It is distinguished from *Xiao Chai Hu Tang* (Minor Bupleurum).

Source: *Shang Han Za Bing Lun* (*Treatise on Cold-Induced Disorders and Miscellaneous Diseases*), written by *Zhang Zhong-Jing* and published in 220 CE

Ingredients: The original ingredients of *Da Chai Hu Tang* were decocted together twice and concentrated in a liquid form. The formula contained 24 g *Chai Hu* (Bupleurum), 9 g *Huang Qin* (Scutellaria), 9 g *Zhi Shi* (Aurantium), 6 g *Da Huang* (Rheum), 9 g *Bai Shao Yao* (Paeonia), 24 g *Ban Xia* (Pinellia), 15 g *Sheng Jiang* (Zingiberis), and 12 g *Da Zao* (Jujube) (Table 24.2).[2]

Table 24.2. Ingredients and actions of *Da Chai Hu Tang*.

%	English Name	Chinese *Pin-Yin*	Actions
22.2	Bupleurum	*Chai Hu*	Relieve Liver *Qi* Stagnation
8.4	Scutellaria	*Huang Qin*	Clear Heat, dry Damp
8.3	Aurantium	*Zhi Shi*	Regulate and descend *Qi*
5.6	Rheum	*Da Huang*	Purge accumulation downward
8.3	Paeonia	*Bai Shao Yao*	Tonify Blood and soothe Liver
22.2	Pinellia	*Ban Xia*	Resolve Phlegm
13.9	Zingiberis	*Sheng Jiang*	Warm the Middle *Jiao*
11.1	Jujube	*Da Zao*	Harmonize, tonify the Middle *Jiao*

Preparation:

1. Powder or capsule method: Herbs are ground into a fine powder. Powder can be encapsulated.
2. Decoction or teapill method: Raw herbs are mixed together and decocted. Herbal water extract (decoction) can be concentrated as granules or teapills.

Actions: Harmonize and release the *Shao Yang* and purge Interior Heat accumulation

Indications: This formula is indicated for a combination of *Shao Yang* and *Yang Ming* Patterns. The main signs are alternating fever and chills; resistance to thoracic compression; chewing or lip-smacking as if there is a bitter taste in the mouth; irritability; nausea; vomiting in species that can and colic in those that cannot; hot, putrid stools or firm and dry constipation; a yellow tongue coating; and a tight and excess pulse.[2–4]

Dosage and Usage:

Horses and Cattle: 15–60 g, twice daily
Camels: 30–75 g, twice daily
Llamas, Alpacas, Goats, Sheep, and Pigs: 10–15 g, twice daily
Dogs: 0.5–5 g (or 0.1 g per kg body weight), twice daily
Cats and Rabbits: 0.2–0.5 g (or 0.1 g per kg body weight), twice daily
Birds: 0.1–0.2 g per kg body weight, twice daily
Use 1–3 weeks until primary clinical signs resolve.

Analysis of Formula: The King herb, *Chai Hu* (Bupleurum), harmonizes the *Shao Yang* and releases Liver *Qi* constraint. The Minister herbs are *Huang Qin* (Scutellaria), which facilitates the clearing of Heat from the Liver and Gallbladder, and *Da Huang* (Rheum) and *Zhi Shi* (Aurantium), which drain the Heat Excess from the Middle Burner through the stool. *Ban Xia* (Pinellia) regulates and descends the Middle Burner *Qi* while stopping vomiting. *Bai Shao Yao* (Paeonia) nourishes Blood and softens the Liver to relieve abdominal pain. These two are the Adjuvant herbs. The Messenger herbs are *Da Zao* (Jujube) and *Sheng Jiang* (Zingiberis). With *Bai Shao Yao* (Paeonia), *Da Zao* (Jujube) protects the *Yin* from further injury from pathogenic Heat and the harsh draining properties of *Da Huang* (Rheum). *Sheng Jiang* (Zingiberis) and *Da Zao* (Jujube) further harmonize the Middle Burner and assist in releasing the *Shao Yang* pathogen.[5,6]

Cautions and Contraindications: This formula is contraindicated in Exterior Patterns when there is no Interior Heat.

Dr. Xie's Comments: *Da Chai Hu Tang* is formed by a combination of *Xiao Chai Hu Tang* and *Xiao Cheng Qi Tang*. *Xiao Chai Hu Tang* is for *Shao Yang* Pattern, and

Xiao Cheng Qi Tang clears *Yang Ming* Pattern. Therefore, *Da Chai Hu Tang* is historically used in treating a combination of *Shao Yang* and *Yang Ming* Patterns. In modern veterinary practice, it is often used in treating gastric ulcers and acute pancreatitis.

Clinical and Pharmacological Studies: There are numerous recent scientific publications investigating the biological effects of *Da Chai Hu Tang*. Most of the recent research focuses on suppressing atherosclerotic lesions and modifying cholesterol-induced pathologies. For example, Iizuka et al. delineated the inhibitory effects of *Da Chai Hu Tang* on the progression of atherosclerotic lesions in Kurosawa and Kusanagi-hypercholesterolemic rabbits. Their results suggest that *Da Chai Hu Tang* has inhibitory effects on the development of atheromatous plaque formation in rabbits. They hypothesize that it is possible that the antioxidative effects of *Da Chai Hu Tang* on LDL led to the beneficial effects observed in this study.[9]

Si Ni San (Four for Rebelling) 四逆散

Si means four, and here it refers to four ingredients. *Ni* means rebelling. When the *Yang Qi* is constrained from reaching the distal extremities, they are cold or frigid and cannot move in their normal way. Thus, they are considered to be rebelling. *San* is powder, the original form of herbal administration.

Source: *Shang Han Za Bing Lun* (*Treatise on Cold-Induced Disorders and Miscellaneous Diseases*), written by *Zhang Zhong-Jing* and published in 220 CE

Ingredients: The original formula was made by grinding the herbs into a fine powder. The formula contains 9–12g *Chai Hu* (Bupleurum), 9–12g *Zhi Shi* (Citrus), 12–24g *Bai Shao Yao* (Paeonia), and 6–9g *Gan Cao* (Glycyrrhiza) (Table 24.3).[2]

Preparation:
1. Powder or capsule method: Herbs are ground into a fine powder. Powder can be encapsulated.
2. Decoction or teapill method: Raw herbs are mixed together and decocted. Herbal water extract (decoction) can be concentrated as granules or teapills.

Table 24.3. Ingredients and actions of *Si Ni San*.

%	English Name	Chinese *Pin-Yin*	Actions
21	Bupleurum	*Chai Hu*	Relieve Liver *Qi* Stagnation
21	Aurantium	*Zhi Shi*	Regulate and descend *Qi*
42	Paeonia	*Bai Shao Yao*	Tonify Blood and soothe Liver
16	Glycyrrhiza	*Gan Cao*	Harmonize and tonify *Qi*

Actions: Dispel pathogens, soothe Liver *Qi* and relieve *Qi* Stagnation, regulate the Spleen

Indications: Cold distal extremities with warm central core, thoracic resistance to compression, a red tongue with yellow coating, and a tight or wiry pulse[2–4]

Dosage and Usage:
Horses and Cattle: 15–60g, twice daily
Camels: 30–75g, twice daily
Llamas, Alpacas, Goats, Sheep, and Pigs: 10–15g, twice daily
Dogs: 0.5–5g (or 0.1g per kg body weight), twice daily
Cats and Rabbits: 0.2–0.5g (or 0.1g per kg body weight), twice daily
Birds: 0.1–0.2g per kg body weight, twice daily
Use 1–4 weeks until primary clinical signs resolve.

Analysis of Formula: The King herb, *Chai Hu* (Bupleurum), soothes Liver *Qi*, relieves Stagnation and disperses *Qi* throughout the body. The Minister herb, *Zhi Shi* (Citrus), drains Stagnation from the Middle Burner. The Adjuvant herb, *Bai Shao Yao* (Paeonia), nourishes the Liver *Yin* and Blood to relieve pain and protect the Liver from too much dispersion injury. Serving as the Messenger herb, *Gan Cao* (Glycyrrhiza) harmonizes and nourishes the Spleen while reducing pain from *Qi* constraint.[5,6]

Cautions and Contraindications: None known

Dr. Xie's Comments: *Si Ni San* is historically and originally used in treating collapse due to Stagnation of *Yang-Qi*. In modern veterinary practice, it is often used for the treatment of disharmony between the Liver and Spleen leading to abdominal pain, pain in the hypochondriac area, slightly cold extremities, a purple tongue, and wiry pulse. The name of the formula (*Si Ni **San***) can be confused with the name of *Si Ni **Tang***, which is composed of totally different ingredients, and is used for *Yang* Deficiency.

Clinical and Pharmacological Studies: There are numerous recent scientific publications investigating the biological effects of *Si Ni San*. Most of the recent research focuses on both dermatological and hepatoprotective benefits. For example, Zhang et al. aimed to evaluate the role of the four major active ingredients contained in the prescription (saikosaponins, paeoniflorin, naringin, and glycyrrhizin) in the inhibitory effect to contact sensitivity in mice. When administered during the induction phase, saikosaponin A and glycyrrhizin showed significant inhibitory effects, and paeoniflorin and naringin did not. These components in *Si Ni San* also inhibited the activation and proliferation of T-lymphocytes and the production of cytokines such as tumor necrosis factor-alpha and interferon-gamma to different extents. Saikosaponin A and paeoniflorin dose-dependently reduced the splenocyte adhesion to type I collagen, and glycyrrhizin only showed a slight tendency. Furthermore, treatment with glycyrrhizin or saikosaponin A, rather than paeoniflorin or naringin, moderately inhibited the matrix metalloproteinase (MMP)-2 activity of the splenocytes from PCl-CS mice, and the combination of all four components showed a strong inhibition against MMP-2. Moreover, the components markedly decreased the serum level of nitric oxide in PCl-sensitized mice. The results indicated that saikosaponin A and glycyrrhizin may be the major contributors in the alleviation effect of *Si Ni San* on contact sensitivity, and paeoniflorin and naringin may exhibit a cooperative effect.[10]

With respect to hepatoprotective effects, Jiang et al. examined the effects of *Si Ni San* on various experimental liver injury models and the formula's mechanisms of action. *Si Ni San* showed significant hepatoprotection against CCl(4)-induced hepatic damage, both in vivo and in vitro. To the liver injury induced by Bacillus Calmette-Guerin (BCG) with lipopolysaccharide (LPS), *Si Ni San* also provided significant alleviation through enhancing nitric oxide (NO) release by macrophages. Against the liver injury induced by a delayed-type hypersensitivity reaction to picryl chloride (PCl-DTH), *Si Ni San* alleviated the reaction remarkably when administered during either the induction or effector phase. A significant reduction of in vitro hepatotoxicity, as measured by the inhibition of serum transaminase elevation, was observed in nonparenchymal cells from liver-injured mice treated with *Si Ni San*. *Si Ni San* facilitated apoptosis in nonparenchymal cells from liver-injured mice, as well as in spleen cells activated by PCl in vivo or by concanavalin A (Con A) in vitro. These results suggest that *Si Ni San* decreases liver injury through multiple mechanisms, including protection of the hepatocyte membrane, enhancement of NO release, and dysfunction of liver-infiltrating cells mainly through causing their apoptosis.[11]

An interesting clinical study in humans by Ninomiya evaluated effects more closely related to the original Frigid Extremities use of *Si Ni San*. Palmoplantar hyperhidrosis is common in patients who are susceptible to strains on the autonomic nervous system, and stress and mental strain have been proven to produce sweating in this population. The effect of *Si Ni San* on 40 patients was evaluated based on changes in palmoplantar sweat volume and skin temperature before and after stress loading. Ninomiya also measured changes in the palmoplantar sweat volume and skin temperature due to stress load in 35 healthy control subjects who did not receive *Si Ni San*. Before treatment, the prestress sweat volume in patients was larger than that in healthy controls; however, after *Si Ni San* treatment, their prestress sweat volume decreased. With stress, the sweat volume increased in both patients and controls, but the net increase in the patients was larger than that in the healthy controls. After *Si Ni San* treatment, the net increase of sweat volume due to stress was smaller than that of pretreatment; however, it did not show a significant difference with that of healthy controls. The palmoplantar skin temperature of the patients before treatment was lower than that of healthy controls. Palmoplantar skin temperature rose with stress loading in healthy controls, but decreased in pretreatment patients. *Si Ni San* treatment reduced the palmoplantar perspiration in palmoplantar hidrosis patients at rest and under stress. Furthermore, it also improved other serious complications, especially coldness of the extremities.[12]

Chai Hu Shu Gan San (Bupleurum to Soothe the Liver) 柴胡疏肝散

This formula is named for the primary ingredient, *Chai Hu* (Bupleurum) and its main intended action (*Shu Gan*) in this formula. *Shu* means soothe or smoothen. *Gan* is the Liver and *San* is powder, the original form of herbal administration.

Source: *Jing Yue Quan Shu* (*Collected Treatises of Zhang Jing-Yue*), written by *Zhang Jie-Bing* and published in 1624 CE

Ingredients: The original formula was made by grinding the herbs into a fine powder. The formula contained 6 g *Chen Pi* (Citrus), 6 g *Chai Hu* (Bupleurum), 4.5 g *Chuan Xiong* (Ligusticum), 4.5 g *Zhi Ke* (Aurantium), 4.5 g *Bai Shao Yao* (Paeonia), 1.5 g *Gan Cao* (Glycyrrhiza), and 4.5 g *Xiang Fu Zi* (Cyperus) (Table 24.4).[2]

Preparation:

1. Powder or capsule method: Herbs are ground into a fine powder. Powder can be encapsulated.
2. Decoction or teapill method: Raw herbs are mixed together and decocted. Herbal water extract (decoction) can be concentrated as granules or teapills.

Table 24.4. Ingredients and actions of *Chai Hu Shu Gan San*.

%	English Name	Chinese *Pin-Yin*	Actions
19	Citrus	*Chen Pi*	Regulate *Qi*
19	Bupleurum	*Chai Hu*	Relieve Liver *Qi* Stagnation
14.3	Ligusticum	*Chuan Xiong*	Invigorate *Qi* and Blood
14.3	Aurantium	*Zhi Ke*	Regulate *Qi*
14.3	Paeonia	*Bai Shao Yao*	Tonify Blood and soothe Liver
14.3	Cyperus	*Xiang Fu Zi*	Regulate Liver *Qi*
4.8	Glycyrrhiza	*Gan Cao*	Harmonize and tonify *Qi*

Actions: Spread the Liver *Qi*, harmonize Blood and alleviate pain

Indications: *Chai Hu Shu Gan San* is indicated for Liver *Qi* Stagnation Patterns. The main signs are irritability, anger, hypochondriac pain or painful resistance to thoracic compression, a red tongue or tongue edges, and a tight to wiry pulse.[2–4]

Dosage and Usage:

Horses and Cattle: 15–60g, twice daily
Camels: 30–75g, twice daily
Llamas, Alpacas, Goats, Sheep, and Pigs: 10–15g, twice daily
Dogs: 0.5–5g (or 0.1g per kg body weight), twice daily
Cats and Rabbits: 0.2–0.5g (or 0.1g per kg body weight), twice daily
Birds: 0.1–0.2g per kg body weight, twice daily
Use 3–6 weeks until primary clinical signs resolve.

Analysis of Formula: The King herbs, *Chen Pi* (Citrus) and *Chai Hu* (Bupleurum), act together to spread the Liver *Qi* and regulate *Qi* in the Middle Burner. This function of Liver *Qi* regulation is furthered by the Ministers, *Xiang Fu Zi* (Cyperus) and *Bai Shao Yao* (Paeonia). *Bai Shao Yao* (Paeonia) also relieves pain, soothes the Liver by nourishing Blood and *Yin* and protects it from potential damage by dispersing herbs. *Chuan Xiong* (Ligusticum) and *Zhi Ke* (Aurantium) reduce Stagnation in the Middle Burner, disperse clumping, and work as the Adjuvant herbs. Serving as the Messenger herb, *Gan Cao* (Glycyrrhiza) harmonizes, protects the Stomach, and mildly relieves pain.[5,6]

Dr. Xie's Comments: *Chai Hu Shu Gan San* is an effective herbal formula to treat behavior problems, and hepatitis due to Liver *Qi* Stagnation in horses, dogs and cats.

Xiao Yao San (Free and Easy Wandering) 逍遥散

Xiao Yao San is named after ancient philosophers/monks who had a rambling lifestyle and mindset. *Xiao Yao* means freely and easily wandering around. Because *Xiao Yao San* allows constrained Liver *Qi* to flow freely, it allows freedom to psychoemotional blockages, as well, and thus the opportunity to ramble.

Source: *Tai Ping Hui Min He Ji Ju Fang* (*Imperial Grace Formulary of the Tai Ping Era*), written by *Chen Shi-Wen* et al. and published by the *Song* Dynasty government in 1078 CE

Ingredients: The original formula was made by grinding the herbs into a fine powder and taking with baked *Sheng Jiang* (Zingiberis) and *Bo He* (Mentha). *Xiao Yao San* contains 30g *Chai Hu* (Bupleurum), 30g *Dang Gui* (Angelica), 30g *Bai Shao Yao* (Paeonia), 30g *Bai Zhu* (Atractylodes), 30g *Fu Ling* (Poria), 15g *Gan Cao* (Glycyrrhiza), 6g *Sheng Jiang* (Zingiberis), and 3g *Bo He* (Mentha) (Table 24.5).[2]

Table 24.5. Ingredients and actions of *Xiao Yao San*.

%	English Name	Chinese *Pin-Yin*	Actions
17.2	Bupleurum	*Chai Hu*	Relieve Liver *Qi* Stagnation
17.2	Angelica	*Dang Gui*	Tonify and move Blood
17.2	Paeonia	*Bai Shao Yao*	Tonify Blood and soothe Liver
17.2	Atractylodes	*Bai Zhu*	Tonify *Qi* and dry Damp
17.2	Poria	*Fu Ling*	Drain Damp
8.6	Glycyrrhiza	*Gan Cao*	Harmonize and tonify *Qi*
3.4	Zingiberis	*Sheng Jiang*	Harmonize Stomach
2	Mentha	*Bo He*	Relieve Liver *Qi* Stagnation and clear Heat

Preparation:

1. Powder or capsule method: Herbs are ground into a fine powder. Powder can be encapsulated.
2. Decoction or teapill method: Raw herbs are mixed together and decocted. Herbal water extract (decoction) can be concentrated as granules or teapills.

Actions: Spread Liver *Qi*, relieve Stagnation, tonify Spleen *Qi* and nourish Blood

Indications: Hypochondriac pain or painful resistance to thoracic compression, chewing or lip-smacking as if there is a bitter taste in the mouth, irritability, fatigue, reduced food intake, gastrointestinal upset, abnormal estrus cycle, pale-red tongue, and a tight or wiry but weak pulse[2–4]

Dosage and Usage:

Horses and Cattle: 15–60g, twice daily
Camels: 30–75g, twice daily
Llamas, Alpacas, Goats, Sheep, and Pigs: 10–15g, twice daily
Dogs: 0.5–5g (or 0.1g per kg body weight), twice daily
Cats and Rabbits: 0.2–0.5g (or 0.1g per kg body weight), twice daily
Birds: 0.1–0.2g per kg body weight, twice daily
Use 3–6 weeks until primary clinical signs resolve.

Analysis of Formula: *Xiao Yao San* is constructed to spread constrained Liver *Qi* as well as nourish Spleen *Qi* and tonify Blood. The King herb, *Chai Hu* (Bupleurum), relieves Liver *Qi* Stagnation. The Minister herbs, *Dang Gui* (Angelica) and *Bai Shao Yao* (Paeonia), cofunction to tonify Blood, with the resultant Blood redistributing to the Liver and helping to soften and soothe the Liver. Two of three Adjuvant herbs, *Bai Zhu* (Atractylodes) and

Fu Ling (Poria), work together to tonify the Spleen. The other Adjuvant herb, *Gan Cao* (Glycyrrhiza), is also a Spleen *Qi* tonic and cofunctions with *Bai Shao Yao* (Paeonia) to reduce painful spasms. There are two Messenger herbs: *Wei Jiang* (Zingiberis) harmonizes the Middle Burner, and *Bo He* (Mentha) enhances *Chai Hu's* (Bupleurum's) actions and also has a cooling function for the constrained and Heated Liver.[5,6]

Cautions and Contraindications: None known

Dr. Xie's Comments: Both *Xiao Yao San* and *Chai Hu Shu Gan San* are commonly used in treating Liver *Qi* Stagnation in horses, dogs, and cats. *Xiao Yao San* is used for excessive Liver *Qi* Stagnation causing Spleen impairment and gastrointestinal disorders (poor appetite, vomiting, loose stool). *Chai Hu Shu Gan San* is good at soothing the Liver and used for pure Liver *Qi* Stagnation.

Clinical and Pharmacological Studies: There are numerous recent scientific publications investigating the biological effects of *Xiao Yao San*. Most of the recent research focuses on psychological and dermatological efficacy. For example, Kobayashi. et al. investigated the role of *Xiao Yao San* in human atopic dermatitis (AD). A substantial portion of AD patients treated with conventional therapy become intractable after several cycles of recurrence. Over the last 20 years they have developed an alternative approach to treating many of these patients by diet and herbal medicine. In their review, to demonstrate the effectiveness of the method of individualized herbal therapy, results are presented for a series of patients who had failed with conventional therapy but were treated afterward in their institution. Based on these data, they contend that there exists a definite subgroup of AD patients in whom conventional therapy fails, but the "Diet and Herbal" approach succeeds in healing. Therefore, this approach should be considered seriously as a second-line treatment for AD patients. They emphasize that herbal therapy for AD is more "art" than technology, for which expertise is an essential prerequisite.[13]

Tong Xie Yao Fang (Important Formula for Painful Diarrhea) 痛泻要方

Tong means painful. *Xie* here means diarrhea. *Yao* means important, or key. *Fang* is the formula. Thus, *Tong Xie Yao Fang* is literally translated as Important Formula for Painful Diarrhea, which is simply a direct statement of fact regarding the usefulness and efficacy of this formula.

Source: *Jing Yue Quan Shu* (*Collected Treatises of Zhang Jing-Yue*), written by *Zhang Jie-Bing* and published in 1624 (CE)

Table 24.6. Ingredients and actions of *Tong Xie Yao Fang*.

%	English Name	Chinese *Pin-Yin*	Actions
37.5	Atractylodes	*Bai Zhu*	Tonify *Qi*, dry Damp
25	Paeonia	*Bai Shao Yao*	Tonify Blood and soothe Liver
18.8	Citrus	*Chen Pi*	Regulate *Qi*
18.7	Ledebouriella	*Fang Feng*	Relieve Intestinal Wind and pain

Ingredients: The original formula was made by grinding the herbs into powder and taking them in either powder or pill form. *Tong Xie Yao Fang* contains 90 g *Bai Zhu* (Atractylodes), 60 g *Bai Shao Yao* (Paeonia), 45 g *Chen Pi* (Citrus), and 45 g *Fang Feng* (Ledebouriella) (Table 24.6).[2]

Preparation:
1. Powder or capsule method: Herbs are ground into a fine powder. Powder can be encapsulated.
2. Decoction or teapill method: Raw herbs are mixed together and decocted. Herbal water extract (decoction) can be concentrated as granules or teapills.

Actions: Disperse Liver *Qi*, relieve abdominal pain, tonify Spleen *Qi*, stop diarrhea

Indications: Recurrent abdominal pain with borborygmi; painful diarrhea; thin, white tongue coating; and a tight to wiry, thin pulse[2–4]

Dosage and Usage:
Horses and Cattle: 15–60 g, twice daily
Camels: 30–75 g, twice daily
Llamas, Alpacas, Goats, Sheep, and Pigs: 10–15 g, twice daily
Dogs: 0.5–5 g (or 0.1 g per kg body weight), twice daily
Cats and Rabbits: 0.2–0.5 g (or 0.1 g per kg body weight), twice daily
Birds: 0.1–0.2 g per kg body weight, twice daily
Use 1–3 weeks until primary clinical signs resolve.

Analysis of Formula: This formula is designed to reduce diarrhea from Spleen deficiency with an overacting Liver. The King herb, *Bai Zhu* (Atractylodes), strengthens the Spleen and dries Dampness. The Minister herb, *Bai Shao Yao* (Paeonia) tonifies Liver Blood and *Yin* to soften and soothe the Liver and relieve pain. The Adjuvant herb, *Chen Pi* (Citrus), harmonizes and regulates *Qi* in the Middle Burner and mildly assists in transforming Dampness. The Messenger herb, *Fang Feng* (Ledebouriella), enters the Liver and Spleen channels and thus focuses the formula on the weak Spleen and overcontrolling Liver.[5,6]

Cautions and Contraindications: None known

Dr. Xie's Comments: *Tong Xie Yao Fang* is an effective herbal formula to treat painful diarrhea due to disharmony between the Liver and Spleen.

Clinical and Pharmacological Studies: There are few recent scientific publications investigating the biological effects of *Tong Xie Yao Fang*. Most of the recent research focuses on the efficacy of *Tong Xie Yao Fang* in reducing the symptoms of Inflammatory Bowel Disease (IBD). For example, Bensoussan et al. attempted to determine whether Chinese herbal medicine (CHM) is of any benefit in the treatment of IBD. They used a randomized, double-blind, placebo-controlled trial conducted during 1996 through 1997. A total of 116 patients who fulfilled the Rome criteria, an established standard for diagnosis of IBD, were enrolled. Patients were randomly allocated to 1 of 3 treatment groups: individualized Chinese herbal formulations (n = 38), a standard Chinese herbal formulation (n = 43), or placebo (n = 35). Patients received 5 capsules 3 times daily for 16 weeks and were evaluated regularly by a traditional Chinese herbalist and by a gastroenterologist. Patients, gastroenterologists, and herbalists were all blinded to the treatment group. Change in total bowel symptom scale scores and global improvement was assessed by patients and gastroenterologists, and change in the degree of interference in life caused by IBD symptoms was assessed by patients. Compared with patients in the placebo group, patients in the active treatment groups (standard and individualized CHM) had significant improvement in bowel symptom scores as rated by patients (P = .03) and by gastroenterologists (P = .001), and significant global improvement as rated by patients (P = .007) and by gastroenterologists (P = .002). Patients reported that treatment significantly reduced the degree of interference with life caused by IBD symptoms (P = .03). Chinese herbal formulations individually tailored to the patient proved no more effective than standard CHM treatment. On follow-up 14 weeks after completion of treatment, only the individualized CHM treatment group maintained improvement.[14]

Bian et al. published a systematic review on the effectiveness of *Tong Xie Yao Fang* for irritable bowel syndrome (IBS). The authors set out to systematically review the effectiveness of the Chinese herbal medicine *Tong Xie Yao Fang* (TXYF) and TXYF with different Chinese herbal additions (TXYF-A) in the management of IBS in order to make evidence-based recommendations. METHODS: The authors searched the literature to identify randomized trials of TXYF or TXYF-A for patients with IBS by using MEDLINE, EMBASE, the Cochrane Controlled Trials Register (CCTR), the Cochrane Complementary Medicine Fields Specialized Register from 1966 to 2004, the CMB Disc database from January 1978 to December 1988, and the Full Text Chinese Journal database from January 1994 to December 2004. Standard forms regarding study design, treatment course, outcome measures, and adverse events were used to abstract data. Studies were assigned a quality score based on published methodology. Relative risk (RR) and 95% confidence interval (CI) were analyzed. RESULTS: Twelve studies (n = 1125) that met the criteria for review were identified. There was heterogeneity in the studies with regard to herbal formula, control medicine, treatment course, and outcome measurement. The quality of all studies was low. The pooled analyses of effectiveness for the near term (immediately after finishing the treatment course), short term (3 months after finishing the treatment course), and long term (6 months or more after finishing the treatment course) showed that the effect of TXYF-A was better than that of conventional medicine in four, two, and six studies, respectively. The RRs were 1.34 (95% CI 1.16–1.54, $P < 0.05$), 1.39 (95% CI 1.17–1.64, $P < 0.05$), and 1.34 (95% CI 1.12–1.61, $P < 0.05$), respectively. Overall, combining all data from the 12 studies, the effectiveness of TXYF-As was higher than that in control groups, with statistical significance and RR of 1.35 (95% CI 1.21–1.50, $P < 0.05$).

CONCLUSIONS: There is evidence to indicate the potential usefulness of TXYF-A for IBS patients. The results were limited by the poor quality and heterogeneity of these studies. Further studies with carefully designed, randomized double-blinded placebo-controlled trials will be needed to confirm the effectiveness of TXYF or TXYF-A for IBS.[15]

Yue Ju Wan (Escaping Stagnation) 越鞠丸

Yue means escape. *Ju* here refers to Stagnation. *Wan* is pill, the form of the medication. This formula relieves Stagnation from a number of possible pathoetiological factors and thus allows the patient to "escape" the problems of Stagnation.

Source: *Dan Xi Xin Fa* (*Teachings of Dan-Xi*), written by *Zhu Dan-Xi* and published in 1481 (CE)

Ingredients: The original formula was made by grinding equal amounts of the herbs and forming into pills with water. *Yue Ju Wan* contains 6–12 g *Cang Zhu* (Atractylodes), 6–12 g *Chuan Xiong* (Ligusticum), 6–12 g *Xiang Fu* (Cyperus), 6–12 g *Zhi Zi* (Gardenia), and 6–12 g *Shen Qu* (Massa Fermentata) (Table 24.7).[2]

Preparation:

1. Powder or capsule method: Herbs are ground into a fine powder. Powder can be encapsulated.
2. Decoction or teapill method: Raw herbs are mixed together and decocted. Herbal water extract (decoction) can be concentrated as granules or teapills.

Table 24.7. Ingredients and actions of *Yue Ju Wan*.

%	English Name	Chinese *Pin-Yin*	Actions
20	Atractylodes	*Cang Zhu*	Dry Damp, Strengthen Spleen
20	Ligusticum	*Chuan Xiong*	Invigorate Blood and *Qi*
20	Cyperus	*Xiang Fu*	Regulate Liver *Qi*
20	Gardenia	*Zhi Zi*	Drain Fire
20	Massa Fermentata	*Shen Qu*	Relieve Food Stagnation

Actions: Promote the movement of *Qi* and Blood, dry Damp, relieve Stagnation

Indications: Distension and resistance to thoracoabdominal compression; hypochondriac pain; eructation; vomiting in species that can, mild colic in those that cannot; possible coughing with sputum; and reduced appetite[2–4]

Dosage and Usage:
Horses and Cattle: 15–60 g, twice daily
Camels: 30–75 g, twice daily
Llamas, Alpacas, Goats, Sheep, and Pigs: 10–15 g, twice daily
Dogs: 0.5–5 g (or 0.1 g per kg body weight), twice daily
Cats and Rabbits: 0.2–0.5 g (or 0.1 g per kg body weight), twice daily
Birds: 0.1–0.2 g per kg body weight, twice daily
Use 2–6 weeks until primary clinical signs resolve.

Analysis of Formula: This formula is designed to treat mild to moderate *Qi* Stagnation in the gastrointestinal system. The King herb, *Xiang Fu* (Cyperus), is a key herb to regulate stagnant Liver *Qi*. The rest of the ingredients are the Minister and Adjuvant herbs, which reinforce this effect or ameliorate the adverse consequences suffered by the gastrointestinal system from *Qi* Stagnation. *Cang Zhu* (Atractylodes) dries damp, transforms Phlegm, and tonifies Spleen *Qi*. *Chuan Xiong* (Ligusticum) invigorates *Qi* and Blood and reduces pain. *Zhi Zi* (Gardenia) clears Heat from the three *Jiaos* and thus reduces Heat from the *Qi* Stagnation. *Shen Qu* (Massa Fermentata) resolves Food Stagnation and harmonizes the Stomach.[5,6]

Cautions and Contraindications: This formula is used for Stagnation due to Excess and should not be used for Stagnation due to Deficiency.

Dr. Xie's Comments: *Yue Ju Wan* is used in treating Six types of Stagnation, which include *Qi*, Blood, Phlegm, Fire, Damp, and food. *Qi* Stagnation is the key pathology to treat because it often causes other types of Stagnation, or all other types of Stagnation lead to *Qi* Stagnation.

Table 24.8. Ingredients and actions of *Ju Pi San*.

%	English Name	Chinese *Pin-Yin*	Actions
40	Citrus	*Chen Pi*	Regulate *Qi*, direct *Qi* downward
60	Zingiberis	*Sheng Jiang*	Harmonize and warm Stomach

Ju Pi San (Tangerine Peel) 橘皮散

Ju Pi refers to Tangerine peel, or Citrus, the King ingredient of the formula. *San* is powder, the form of herbal administration. Thus, *Ju Pi San* translates directly to Tangerine Peel Powder.

Source: *Jin Gui Yao Lue Fang Lun* (*Synopsis of Prescription from the Golden Cabinet*), written by *Zhang Zhongjing* and published in 220 CE

Ingredients: The original formula was made by decocting the herbs twice in boiling water and drinking the mixture of each decoction. *Ju Pi San* contains 12 g *Chen Pi* (Citrus) and of *Sheng Jiang* (Zingiberis) (Table 24.8).[2]

Preparation:
1. Powder or capsule method: Herbs are ground into a fine powder. Powder can be encapsulated.
2. Decoction or teapill method: Raw herbs are mixed together and decocted. Herbal water extract (decoction) can be concentrated as granules or teapills.

Actions: Warm the Stomach, invigorate the Middle Burner *Yang* and stop vomiting

Indications: Nausea and/or vomiting with Cold signs such as abdominal pain, cold extremities, white tongue coating, a tight, slow pulse[2–4]

Dosage and Usage:
Horses and Cattle: 15–60 g, twice daily
Camels: 30–75 g, twice daily
Llamas, Alpacas, Goats, Sheep, and Pigs: 10–15 g, twice daily
Dogs: 0.5–5 g (or 0.1 g per kg body weight), twice daily
Cats and Rabbits: 0.2–0.5 g (or 0.1 g per kg body weight), twice daily
Birds: 0.1–0.2 g per kg body weight, twice daily
Use 1–4 weeks until primary clinical signs resolve.

Analysis of Formula: This formula treats rebellious *Qi* from Cold in the Stomach. The King herb, *Chen Pi* (Citrus), regulates and mildly warms the Middle Burner *Qi* and directs rebellious *Qi* downward. The Minister herb, *Sheng Jiang* (Zingiberis), warms the Middle Burner and invigorates the *Yang*.[5,6]

Cautions and Contraindications: This formula is contraindicated in cases of nausea and vomiting from Heat.

Dr. Xie's Comments: Classical veterinary herbal formula *Ju Pi San* is different from the one above. This *Ju Pi San* was originally from *Yuan Heng Liao Ma Ji (Yuanheng's Therapeutic Treatise of Horses),* written by *Yu Benyuan* and *Yu Benheng* in 1608. It is composed of *Hou Po* (Magnolia), *Qing Pi* (Citrus), *Chen Pi* (Citrus), *Dang Gui* (Angelica), *Bai Zhi* (Angelica), *Bing Lang* (Areca), *Rou Gui* (Cinnamon) and *Xiao Hui Xiang* (Foeniculum). It is commonly used for acute onset of colic in horses, cattle, and dogs.

Ban Xia Hou Po Tang (Pinellia and Magnolia) 半夏厚朴汤

The formula is named for its first two primary herbs of the formula: *Ban Xia* (Pinellia) and *Hou Po* (Magnolia). *Tang* is decoction, the form of herbal administration.

Source: *Jin Gui Yao Lue Fang Lun (Synopsis of Prescription from the Golden Cabinet)*, written by *Zhang Zhongjing* and published in 220 CE

Ingredients: This formula was originally prepared as a decoction. *Ban Xia Hou Po Tang* contains 12g *Ban Xia* (Pinellia), 9g *Hou Po* (Magnolia), 12g *Fu Ling* (Poria), 15g *Sheng Jiang* (Zingiberis), and 6g *Zi Su Ye* (Perilla) (Table 24.9).

Preparation:
1. Powder or capsule method: Herbs are ground into a fine powder. Powder can be encapsulated.
2. Decoction or teapill method: Raw herbs are mixed together and decocted. Herbal water extract (decoction) can be concentrated as granules or teapills.

Actions: Promote the movement of *Qi*, resolve Phlegm, dissipate lumps, and direct rebellious *Qi* downward

Indications: Constant swallowing or gagging as if something is obstructing the throat with no physical evidence of obstruction; thoracic resistance to compression; cough; possible vomiting; white, greasy tongue coating; and a wiry, slippery pulse[2–4]

Table 24.9. Ingredients and actions of *Ban Xia Hou Po Tang.*

%	English Name	Chinese *Pin-Yin*	Actions
22	Pinellia	*Ban Xia*	Transform Phlegm, calm Rebellious *Qi*
17	Magnolia	*Hou Po*	Transform Damp, regulate *Qi*
22	Poria	*Fu Ling*	Drain Damp
28	Zingiberis	*Sheng Jiang*	Harmonize Stomach, calm Rebellious *Qi*
11	Perilla	*Zi Su Ye*	Move *Qi*, Resolve Food Toxicity

Dosage and Usage:
Horses and Cattle: 15–60g, twice daily
Camels: 30–75g, twice daily
Llamas, Alpacas, Goats, Sheep, and Pigs: 10–15g, twice daily
Dogs: 0.5–5g (or 0.1g per kg body weight), twice daily
Cats and Rabbits: 0.2–0.5g (or 0.1g per kg body weight), twice daily
Birds: 0.1–0.2g per kg body weight, twice daily
Use 1–3 weeks until primary clinical signs resolve.

Analysis of Formula: This formula was developed for psychological or *Shen* disturbance leading to *Qi* Stagnation and either substantial or insubstantial Phlegm in the throat. The King herb, *Ban Xia* (Pinellia), transforms Phlegm, stops vomiting and directs Stomach *Qi* downward. The Minister herbs *Hou Po* (Magnolia) and *Fu Ling* (Poria) reinforce the King herb by regulating Stomach *Qi* and transforming and draining Dampness and Phlegm. The Adjuvant herb, *Sheng Jiang* (Zingiberis), harmonizes the Stomach, reduces and redirects rebellious Stomach *Qi*. The Messenger herb, *Zi Su Ye* (Perilla), directs the formula to the throat where the *Qi* Stagnation and Phlegm manifest.[5,6]

Cautions and Contraindications: This formula is contraindicated in cases of body fluid Deficiency or Heat from *Yin* Deficiency.

Dr. Xie's Comments: *Ban Xia Hou Po Tang* is designed for the wet cough due to accumulation of Damp-Phlegm in horses, cats, and dogs.

Hou Po Wen Zhong Tang (Magnolia for Warming the Middle) 厚朴温中汤

The formula name refers to both the King ingredient *Hou Po* (Magnolia) and the primary function (*Wen Zhong*) of this formula. *Hou Po* is Magnolia. *Wen* means warming. *Zhong* refers to middle, or Middle Burner (Spleen and Stomach). *Tang* is decoction, the form of original herbal administration.

Source: *Nei Wai Shang Bian Huo Lun* (*Clarifying Doubts about Injury from Internal and External Causes*), written by *Li Ao* and published in 1247 CE

Ingredients: The original formula was created by grinding the ingredients into powder and taking them in fluid with 3g of *Sheng Jiang* (Zingiberis) before meals. *Hou Po Wen Zhong Tang* contains 30g *Hou Po* (Magnolia), 15g *Cao Dou Kou* (Alpinia), 30g *Chen Pi* (Citrus), 15g

Table 24.10. Ingredients and actions of *Hou Po Wen Zhong Tang.*

%	English Name	Chinese *Pin-Yin*	Actions
24	Magnolia	*Hou Po*	Transform Damp, regulate *Qi*
12	Alpinia	*Cao Dou Kou*	Dry Damp, Warm the Middle
24	Citrus	*Chen Pi*	Regulate *Qi*
12	Saussurea	*Mu Xiang*	Regulate *Qi*
12	Poria	*Fu Ling*	Drain Damp
12	Glycyrrhiza	*Gan Cao*	Harmonize, tonify *Qi*
2.4	Zingiberis	*Gan Jiang*	Dispel Interior Cold
1.6	Zingiberis	*Sheng Jiang*	Harmonize Stomach

Mu Xiang (Saussurea), 2g *Gan Jiang* (Zingiberis), 15g *Fu Ling* (Poria), and 15g *Gan Cao* (Glycyrrhiza) (Table 24.10).[2]

Preparation:

1. Powder or capsule method: Herbs are ground into a fine powder. Powder can be encapsulated.
2. Decoction or teapill method: Raw herbs are mixed together and decocted. Herbal water extract (decoction) can be concentrated as granules or teapills.

Actions: Warm the Middle Burner, dispel Cold, move *Qi*, dry Dampness and relieve abdominal distension

Indications: Epigastric and abdominal distension and resistance to compression; loss of appetite; muscular weakness and fatigue; diarrhea; white, moist tongue coating; and a slippery pulse[2–4]

Dosage and Usage:

Horses and Cattle: 15–60g, twice daily
Camels: 30–75g, twice daily
Llamas, Alpacas, Goats, Sheep, and Pigs: 10–15g, twice daily
Dogs: 0.5–5g (or 0.1g per kg body weight), twice daily
Cats and Rabbits: 0.2–0.5g (or 0.1g per kg body weight), twice daily
Birds: 0.1–0.2g per kg body weight, twice daily
Use 1–3 weeks until primary clinical signs resolve.

Analysis of Formula: This formula is constructed to treat Damp and Cold pathogens that are injuring the Spleen and Stomach. The King herb, *Hou Po* (Magnolia), is warm, transforms Damp, and regulates Middle Burner *Qi*. The Minister herb, *Cao Dou Kou* (Alpinia), supports the King herb by warming the Middle Burner and transforming Dampness. The following four Adjuvant herbs all reinforce the actions of the King herb in varying degrees. *Chen Pi* (Citrus) and *Mu Xiang* (Saussurea) regulate and promote normal downward motion of Middle Burner *Qi* as well as reduce pain. The fresh and dried *Sheng Jiang and Gan Jiang* (Zingiberis) both warm and harmonize the Middle Burner while expelling Cold. *Fu Ling* (Poria) assists in draining Dampness from the Middle Burner while mildly supporting Spleen *Qi*. *Gan Cao* (Glycyrrhiza) harmonizes and serves as a Messenger herb to direct the actions of the formula to the Middle Burner.[5,6]

Cautions and Contraindications: None known

Dr. Xie's Comments: *Hou Po Wen Zhong Tang* is used for the treatment of abdominal pain, vomiting, or anorexia due to accumulation of Damp-Cold at the Middle Burner in cats and dogs.

Jin Ling Zi San (Melia Powder) 金铃子散

This formula is simply named for the primary ingredient, *Jin Ling Zi* or Melia. *San* is powder, the form of original medication.

Source: *Tai Ping Sheng Hui Fang* (*Peaceful Holy Benevolent Prescriptions*), written by *Wang Huai-Yin* and published in 992 (CE)

Ingredients: The original formula was made by grinding the herbal ingredients into fine powder and was taken with a liquid carrier. *Jin Ling Zi San* contains 30g *Chuan Lian Zi* (Melia) and 30g *Yan Hu Suo* (Corydalis) (Table 24.11).[2]

Preparation:

1. Powder or capsule method: Herbs are ground into a fine powder. Powder can be encapsulated.
2. Decoction or teapill method: Raw herbs are mixed together and decocted. Herbal water extract (decoction) can be concentrated as granules or teapills.

Actions: Spread Liver *Qi*, clear Heat, promote Blood circulation, relieve pain

Indications: Intermittent epigastric, costochondral and hypochondriac pain; irritability; pain that is worsened by ingestion of hot food and fluids; a red tongue with a yellow coating; and a wiry and/or rapid pulse[2–4]

Table 24.11. Ingredients and actions of *Jin Ling Zi San.*

%	English Name	Chinese *Pin-Yin*	Actions
50	Melia	*Chuan Lian Zi*	Move *Qi*, stop pain
50	Corydalis	*Yan Hu Suo*	Invigorate Blood and *Qi*, alleviate pain

Dosage and Usage:
Horses and Cattle: 15–60 g, twice daily
Camels: 30–75 g, twice daily
Llamas, Alpacas, Goats, Sheep, and Pigs: 10–15 g, twice daily
Dogs: 0.5–5 g (or 0.1 g per kg body weight), twice daily
Cats and Rabbits: 0.2–0.5 g (or 0.1 g per kg body weight), twice daily
Birds: 0.1–0.2 g per kg body weight, twice daily
Use 1–3 weeks until primary clinical signs resolve.

Analysis of Formula: This formula is designed to treat Liver *Qi* Stagnation with Heat. The King herb, *Chuan Lian Zi* (Melia), promotes the movement of *Qi* and stops pain associated with Liver *Qi* Stagnation. The Cold nature of *Chuan Lian Zi* (Melia) also clears Heat from Liver *Qi* Stagnation. The Adjuvant herb, *Yan Hu Suo* (Corydalis), invigorates both *Qi* and Blood, thus giving it broad spectrum in relieving many types of pain.[5,6]

Cautions and Contraindications: Use this formula with caution during pregnancy.

Dr. Xie's Comments: *Jin Ling Zi San* is used for the treatment of intermittent abdominal pain due to Liver *Qi* Stagnation with Heat in horses, cats, and dogs.

Nuan Gan Jian (Warming the Liver) 暖肝煎

Nuan means warming. *Gan* is the Liver. *Jian* here means decoction, the form of original medication. This formula is named for its primary action of treating Cold in the Liver channel, especially in the genital region.

Source: *Jing Yue Quan Shu* (*Collected Treatises of Zhang Jing-Yue*), written by *Zhang Jie-Bing* and published in 1624 CE

Ingredients: This formula was originally made as a decoction to be taken warm. *Nuan Gan Jian* contains 9 g *Dang Gui* (Angelica), 9 g *Gou Qi Zi* (Lycium), 6 g *Xiao Hui Xiang* (Foeniculum), 6 g *Rou Gui* (Cinnamomum), 6 g *Wu Yao* (Lindera), 3 g *Chen Xiang* (Aquilaria), 6 g *Fu Ling* (Poria), and 3 g *Sheng Jiang* (Zingiberis) (Table 24.12).[2]

Preparation:
1. Powder or capsule method: Herbs are ground into a fine powder. Powder can be encapsulated.
2. Decoction or teapill method: Raw herbs are mixed together and decocted. Herbal water extract (decoction) can be concentrated as granules or teapills.

Actions: Warm the Kidney *Yang* and Liver, move *Qi*, alleviate pain

Table 24.12. Ingredients and actions of *Nuan Gan Jian*.

%	English Name	Chinese *Pin-Yin*	Actions
18.8	Angelica	*Dang Gui*	Tonify and invigorate Blood
18.8	Lycium	*Gou Qi Zi*	Nourish Blood
12.5	Foeniculum	*Xiao Hui Xiang*	Regulate Liver and Middle *Jiao Qi*
12.5	Cinnamomum	*Rou Gui*	Warm Interior, dispel Cold
12.5	Lindera	*Wu Yao*	Move *Qi*, alleviate Pain
6.2	Aquilaria	*Chen Xiang*	Move *Qi*, alleviate Pain
12.5	Poria	*Fu Ling*	Drain Damp
6.2	Zingiberis	*Sheng Jiang*	Harmonize the Stomach

Indications: Lower abdominal, genital, reproductive or hernial pain that is aggravated by Cold; pale and/or purple tongue; and a deep, tight pulse[2–4]

Dosage and Usage:
Horses and Cattle: 15–60 g, twice daily
Camels: 30–75 g, twice daily
Llamas, Alpacas, Goats, Sheep, and Pigs: 10–15 g, twice daily
Dogs: 0.5–5 g (or 0.1 g per kg body weight), twice daily
Cats and Rabbits: 0.2–0.5 g (or 0.1 g per kg body weight), twice daily
Birds: 0.1–0.2 g per kg body weight, twice daily
Use 1–3 weeks until primary clinical signs resolve.

Analysis of Formula: This formula is designed to treat Cold hernial disorder from Kidney *Yang* and Liver Deficiency. The King herb, *Xiao Hui Xiang* (Foeniculum), warms the Kidneys and dispels internal Cold. The Minister herbs, *Wu Yao* (Lindera) and *Chen Xiang* (Aquilaria), both move *Qi* and alleviate pain in the Lower *Jiao*. There are four Adjuvant herbs: *Rou Gui* (Cinnamomum) warms the Kidneys and expels Cold; *Gou Qi Zi* (Lycium) nourishes Kidney and Liver Blood and *Yin*, the material basis of *Yang*; *Fu Ling* (Poria) drains Dampness and strengthens the Spleen to support the upright *Qi*; and *Dang Gui* (Angelica) nourishes and invigorates Liver Blood to mildly warm and supplement the Liver while relieving pain. The Messenger *Sheng Jiang* (Zingiberis) harmonizes the Stomach and warms the Middle Burner.[5,6]

Cautions and Contraindications: This formula is contraindicated for scrotal Damp-Heat with signs such as Heat, erythema, pain and swelling.

Dr. Xie's Comments: *Luan Gan Jian* is used for the treatment of hernia, prostate enlargement, scrotal swelling due to Liver *Qi* Stagnation, and Kidney *Yang*/*Qi* Deficiency in horses, cats and, dogs.

REFERENCES

1. Qiao Y. The Traditional Chinese Medicine Formula Study Guide, Peter Holmes (ed). Boulder, CO: Snow Lotus Press, 2000.
2. Bensky D, Barolet R. Chinese Herbal Medicine, Formulas and Strategies. Seattle, WA: Eastland Press, Inc., 1990.
3. Zong LX. Pocket Handbook of Chinese Herbal Prescriptions. Miami: Waclion International, Inc., 2001.
4. Ehling D. The Chinese Herbalist's Handbook. Twin Lakes, WI: Lotus Press, 2002.
5. Bensky D, Gamble A. Chinese Herbal Medicine Materia Medica. Seattle, WA: Eastland Press, Inc., 1993.
6. Zong LX. Pocket Handbook of Chinese Herbal Medicine. Miami: Waclion International, Inc., 2000.
7. Chang JS, Wang DC, Liu HW, Chen MC, Chiang LC, Lin CC. Sho-saiko-to (*Xiao-Chai-Hu-Tang*) and crude saikosaponins inhibit hepatitis B virus in a stable HBV-producing cell line. American Journal of Chinese Medicine 2007;35(2):341–351.
8. Chen MH, Chen JC, Tsai CC, Wang WC, Chang DC, Lin CC, Haieh HY. Sho-saiko-to prevents liver fibrosis induced by bile duct ligation in rats. American Journal of Chinese Medicine 2004;32(2):195–207.
9. Iizuka A, Iijima OT, Yoshie F, Makino B, Amagaya S, Komatsu Y, Kondo K, Matsumoto A, Itakura H. Inhibitory effects of Dai-saiko-to (*Da-Chai-Hu-Tang*) on the progression of atherosclerotic lesions in Kurosawa and Kusanagi-hypercholesterolemic rabbits. Journal of Ethnopharmacology 1998;63(3):209–218. Erratum in: Journal of Ethnopharmacology 1999;65(1):79.
10. Zhang L, Dong Y, Sun Y, Chen T, Xu Q. Role of four major components in the effect of Si-Ni-San, a traditional Chinese prescription, against contact sensitivity in mice. Journal of Pharmaceutical Pharmacology 2006;58(9):1257–1264.
11. Jiang J, Zhou C, Xu Q. Alleviating effects of Si-Ni-San, a traditional Chinese prescription, on experimental liver injury and its mechanisms. Biological Pharmaceutical Bulletin 2003;26(8):1089–1094.
12. Ninomiya Fumino. Clinical evaluation of perspiration reducing effects of a kampo formula, Shigyaku-san, on palmoplantar hidrosis. Evidence Based Complementary Alternative Medicine 2007;10.1093/ecam/nem008.
13. Kobayashi Hiromi, Takahashi Kuniaki, Mizuno Nobuyuki, Kutsuna Haruo, Ishii Masamitsu. An alternative approach to atopic dermatitis: Part I—Case-Series Presentation. Evidence Based Complementary Alternative Medicine 2004; 1:49–62.
14. Bensoussan A. Treatment of irritable bowel syndrome with Chinese herbal medicine, A randomized controlled trial. JAMA. 1998;280:1585–1589.
15. Bian Z. Effectiveness of the Chinese herbal formula *Tong Xie Yao Fang* for irritable bowel syndrome: A systematic review. Journal of Alternative Complementary Medicine 2006;12(4):401–407.

25 Herbal Formulas to Relieve Food Stagnation 消食剂

Bruce Ferguson

The formulas in this chapter are used to treat dysfunctions of the Spleen and Stomach that lead to a Stagnation and accumulation of food and drink contents in the stomach and/or intestines. Food Stagnation is a true accumulation disharmony that may also be due to simply acute or chronic overeating. Companion animals may develop Food Stagnation by eating biologically inappropriate diets as well (e.g., excess refined carbohydrates/kibbled diets for carnivores).

Primary symptoms of Food Stagnation Patterns are Excess in nature. A patient may exhibit epigastric and abdominal distension, bloating, or abdominal fullness and pain. They may have acid regurgitation in those species that may safely physiologically regurgitate. There may be fetid belching or nausea and vomiting. Appetite loss is common and there may be diarrhea, sometimes accompanied by undigested food particles. Sometimes the accumulation may be in the large bowel leading to constipation. The tongue tends to have a thick, greasy coating and the pulse may have a slippery quality or rapid rate if Stagnation is transforming to Heat, or be wiry if pain is dominant.

Etiological factors involved in Food Stagnation may be both exogenous and endogenous. Exogenous factors include constitution- or species-inappropriate diet, or excesses and irregularities in diet. Endogenous factors. such as emotional overeating or herd/flock/group feeding stimulation that leads to excessive social facilitation of ingestive behavior, may be the root cause. Constitutional *Zang-Fu* organ weakness in the gastrointestinal system is also a common basis for Food Stagnation.

The pathogenesis of Food Stagnation is due to disruption of the pivotal role of the Spleen's ascending and Stomach's descending function in the Middle Burner. The Spleen is also responsible for transformation and transportation of ingested food and drink. Disruption of this function may lead to the pathogenic accumulation termed Food Stagnation.

TCVM treatment principles for Food Stagnation are to improve digestion, reduce Food Stagnation, and resolve accumulation. TCVM formulas to relieve Food Stagnation tend to use herbs that promote digestion as King or chief ingredients. Minister and Adjuvant ingredients include *Qi* Regulators, *Qi* Tonics, Damp-Draining, and Heat-clearing herbs.[1]

Western research into TCVM Food Stagnation formulas tend to note the digestion-promoting, enzyme-containing, and promotility agents included in the formula. Heat-clearing herbs found in some Food Stagnation formulas have been found to have antimicrobial properties that may inhibit the intestinal dysbiosis found in Food Stagnation disorders.

In TCVM we should observe the general cautions and contraindications that dispersing herbs have. They may injure and disperse the *Qi*, so they should be discontinued as soon as the accumulation is resolved. Because of Spleen *Qi* weakness as a common root of this disharmony and the potential injury by dispersion of the *Qi*, Spleen *Qi* tonics are commonly either a part of the following formulas or may be added as separate formulas. Table 25.1 provides an overview of formulas to relieve Food Stagnation.

Bao He Wan (Preserving Harmony) 保和丸

Bao means preserving and *He* means harmony. *Wan* is pill, the form of original herbal administration. When the digestive organs function well and harmoniously with one another, there is health. This formula consists of relatively mild harmonizing herbs rather than harsh draining ones. The name, *Bao He*, implies both harmonizing the gastrointestinal system and harmonious herbs working together.

Source: *Dan Xi Xin Fa* (*Teachings of Dan-Xi*), written by *Zhu Dan-Xi* and published in 1481 CE

Table 25.1. Overview of Food Stagnation-Relieving formulas.

Formula Name	Common Signs	Diagnosis	Differentiating Signs	Indications
Bao He Wan	Focal abdominal distension, reduced food intake	Acute, mild conditions with no underlying Deficiency	Acute onset, fetid belching, acid regurgitation, nausea/vomiting	Slippery pulse, with a yellow, greasy tongue coating
Mu Xiang Bing Lang Wan	Focal abdominal distension, reduced food intake	Severe Stagnation and food accumulation	Painful distension, constipation or foul diarrhea	Full and tight pulse with a yellow, greasy tongue coating
Jian Pi Wan	Focal abdominal distension, reduced food intake	Spleen *Qi* Deficiency with mild heat signs	Loose or watery diarrhea	Thin yellow greasy tongue coating with weak, thin pulse
Zhi Zhu Wan	Focal abdominal distension, reduced food intake	Mild Middle Burner Deficiency with Stagnation	Mild abdominal pain	Normal or white tongue coating with weak and/or slippery pulse
Zhi Shi Xiao Pi Wan	Focal abdominal distension, reduced food intake	Spleen *Qi* Deficiency with cold/heat due to *Qi* Stagnation	Cranial abdominal distension, lack of thirst or appetite, fatigue, irregular bowel movements	Pale tongue with thin yellow coat and slippery pulse

Table 25.2. Ingredients and actions of *Bao He Wan*.

%	English Name	Chinese *Pin-Yin*	Actions
35.3	Crataegus	*Shan Zha*	Relieve Food Stagnation
11.8	Massa Fermentata	*Shen Qu*	Relieve Food Stagnation
5.9	Raphanus	*Lai Fu Zi*	Relieve Food Stagnation
5.9	Citrus	*Chen Pi*	Regulate *Qi*
17.6	Pinellia	*Ban Xia*	Transform Phlegm
17.6	Poria	*Fu Ling*	Drain Damp, strengthen Spleen
5.9	Forsythia	*Lian Qiao*	Clear Heat, relieve toxicity

Ingredients: The original formula for *Bao He Wan* (Table 25.2) was made by grinding the ingredients into powder and forming pills by moistening with water. *Bao He Wan* is composed of 180 g *Shan Zha* (Crataegus), 60 g *Shen Qu* (Massa Fermentata), 30 g *Lai Fu Zi* (Raphanus), 30 g *Chen Pi* (Citrus), 90 g *Ban Xia* (Pinellia), 90 g *Fu Ling* (Poria), and 30 g *Lian Qiao* (Forsythia).[2]

Preparation:

1. Powder or capsule method: Herbs are ground into a fine powder. Powder can be encapsulated.
2. Decoction or teapill method: Raw herbs are mixed together and decocted. Herbal water extract (decoction) can be concentrated as granules or teapills.

Actions: Reduce Food Stagnation and harmonize the Stomach

Indications: Food Stagnation, abdominal distension with or without pain, malodorous belching, regurgitation, nausea and vomiting, yellow and/or greasy tongue coating, and a slippery pulse[2–4]

Dosage and Usage:

Horses and Cattle: 15–60 g, twice daily
Camels: 30–75 g, twice daily
Llamas, Alpacas, Goats, Sheep, and Pigs: 10–15 g, twice daily
Dogs: 0.5–5 g (or 0.1 g per kg body weight), twice daily
Cats and Rabbits: 0.2–0.5 g (or 0.1 g per kg body weight), twice daily
Birds: 0.1–0.2 g per kg body weight, twice daily
Use 1–6 weeks until primary clinical signs resolve.

Analysis of Formula: *Bao He Wan* is the fundamental formula for reducing Food Stagnation. Sour, sweet, and slightly warm *Shan Zha* (Crataegus) is the King herb because it reduces all types of Food Stagnation, especially from protein and fats. The Minister herbs are sweet, acrid, and warm *Shen Qu* (Massa Fermentata), which reduces Food Stagnation from starchy foods, and sweet, acrid, and slightly warm *Lai Fu Zi* (Raphanus), which reduces Food Stagnation and Phlegm from stagnant grains. *Lai Fu Zi* (Raphanus) also has a mild *Qi*-descending effect. Acrid and warm *Ban Xia* (Pinellia) and acrid, bitter, warm, and aromatic *Chen Pi* (Citrus) are Adjuvant herbs, which promote the descending movement of *Qi* and transform Stagnation to stop rebellious Stomach *Qi*, nausea, and vomiting. Sweet, bland, and neutral *Fu Ling* (Poria) acts as another Adjuvant herb by strengthening the Spleen and leaching out Dampness. The last Adjuvant herb, bitter, slightly acrid, and cool *Lian Qiao* (Forsythia), clears the Heat generated from unresolved Food Stagnation in the Stomach.[5,6]

Cautions and Contraindications: This formula is contraindicated in patients with Spleen *Qi* Deficiency Patterns.

Dr. Xie's Comments: *Bao He Wan* is used in treating Food Stagnation, which can be caused by Spleen *Qi* Deficiency, Damp, or excessive food intake (especially highly greasy and rich foods). Thus, a balanced dietary program is needed. After Food Stagnation is reduced or eliminated, Spleen *Qi* tonics or formulas to eliminate Damp may be needed to treat the underlying cause.

Mu Xiang Bing Lang Wan (Saussurea and Areca) 木香槟榔丸

This formula is named for the two King ingredients, *Mu Xiang* (Saussurea) and *Bing Lang* (Areca). *Wan* is pill, the form of original herbal administration. Thus, *Mu Xiang Bing Lang* translates directly to Saussurea and Areca.

Source: *Ru Men Shi Qin* (*Confucians Duties to Their Parents*), written by *Zhang Cong-Zheng* and published in 1228 CE

Ingredients: The original formula for *Mu Xiang Bing Lang Wan* (Table 25.3) was made by grinding the ingredients into a fine powder and forming into pills with water. *Mu Xiang Bing Lang Wan* is composed of 30 g *Mu Xiang* (Saussurea), 30 g *Bing Lang* (Areca), 90 g *Da Huang* (Rheum), 120 g *Qian Niu Zi* (Pharbitis), 30 g *Qing Pi* (Citrus), 30 g *Chen Pi* (Citrus), 120 g *Xiang Fu* (Cyperus), 30 g *E Zhu* (Zedoaria), 30 g *Huang Lian* (Coptis), and 90 g *Huang Bai* (Phellodendron).[2]

Preparation:

1. Powder or capsule method: Herbs are ground into a fine powder. Powder can be encapsulated.
2. Decoction or teapill method: Raw herbs are mixed together and decocted. Herbal water extract (decoction) can be concentrated as granules or teapills.

Actions: Promote the movement of *Qi*, guide Stagnation out, purge accumulation, drain Heat

Indications: Focal or generalized distension, pain and fullness in the abdomen with constipation or malodorous diarrhea. The patient usually has a reddish tongue with a greasy, yellow coating, and a slippery, full or rapid pulse.[2–4]

Table 25.3. Ingredients and actions of *Mu Xiang Bing Lang Wan*.

%	English Name	Chinese *Pin-Yin*	Actions
5	Saussurea	*Mu Xiang*	Regulate *Qi*
5	Areca	*Bing Lang*	Expel Parasites/Regulate *Qi*
15	Rheum	*Da Huang*	Purgative
20	Pharbitis	*Qian Niu Zi*	Harsh Expellent
5	Citrus	*Qing Pi*	Regulate *Qi*
5	Citrus	*Chen Pi*	Regulate *Qi*
20	Cyperus	*Xiang Fu*	Regulate *Qi*
5	Zedoaria	*E Zhu*	Invigorate Blood
5	Coptis	*Huang Lian*	Clear Heat, dry Damp
15	Phellodendron	*Huang Bai*	Clear Heat, dry Damp

Dosage and Usage:

Horses and Cattle: 15–60 g, twice daily
Camels: 30–75 g, twice daily
Llamas, Alpacas, Goats, Sheep, and Pigs: 10–15 g, twice daily
Dogs: 0.5–5 g (or 0.1 g per kg body weight), twice daily
Cats and Rabbits: 0.2–0.5 g (or 0.1 g per kg body weight), twice daily
Birds: 0.1–0.2 g per kg body weight, twice daily
Use 2–6 weeks until primary clinical signs resolve.

Analysis of Formula: The King herbs, *Mu Xiang* (Saussurea) and *Bing Lang* (Areca), are powerful *Qi* regulators that transform Stagnation in all three *Jiaos*. The Minister herbs, *Da Huang* (Rheum) and *Qian Niu Zi* (Pharbitis), strongly purge accumulation, guide Stagnation downward, and drain Heat caused by Stagnation. Additional Minister herbs, *Chen Pi* (Citrus) (aged) and *Qing Pi* (Citrus) (immature), act to reinforce the *Qi* regulating effects of the King herbs. The last group of Minister herbs, *Xiang Fu* (Cyperus) and *E Zhu* (Zedoaria), relieve Liver *Qi* Stagnation and Blood Stagnation. Finally, serving as the Adjuvant herbs, *Huang Lian* (Coptis) and *Huang Bai* (Phellodendron), clear Heat and dry Damp in the gastrointestinal system, which may result from enduring Stagnation and cause hot and painful diarrhea.[5,6]

Cautions and Contraindications: This formula is contraindicated in cases of Deficiency and pregnancy.

Dr. Xie's Comments: *Mu Xiang Bing Lang Wan* is effective for the treatment of acute onset of colitis or dysentery due to Damp-Heat in the gastrointestinal tract in horses, dogs, and cats.

Jian Pi Wan (Strengthening the Spleen) 健脾丸

Jian means strengthening, *Pi* is the Spleen, and *Wan* is pill for the form of original herbal administration. This formula has a dual effect: it strengthens the Spleen, and it reduces Food Stagnation that may occur because of a weak Spleen or may further injure the Spleen.

Source: *Zheng Zhi Zhun Sheng* (*Standards of Patterns and Treatments*), written by *Wang Ken-Tang* and published in 1602 CE

Ingredients: The original formula of *Jian Pi Wan* (Table 25.4) was made by grinding the ingredients into powder and forming into pills with water. *Jian Pi Wan* is composed of 75 g *Bai Zhu* (Atractylodes), 60 g *Fu Ling* (Poria), 45 g *Ren Shen* (Ginseng), 30 g *Shan Yao* (Dioscorea), 30 g

Table 25.4. Ingredients and actions of *Jian Pi Wan*.

%	English Name	Chinese *Pin-Yin*	Actions
16.4	Atractylodes	*Bai Zhu*	Tonify *Qi*
13	Poria	*Fu Ling*	Drain Damp
9.7	Ginseng	*Ren Shen*	Tonify *Qi*
6.6	Dioscorea	*Shan Yao*	Tonify *Qi*
6.6	Myristica	*Rou Dou Kou*	Warm the Middle Burner
6.6	Crataegus	*Shan Zha*	Reduce Food Stagnation
6.6	Massa Fermentata	*Shen Qu*	Reduce Food Stagnation
6.6	Hordeum	*Mai Ya*	Reduce Food Stagnation
4.9	Saussurea	*Mu Xiang*	Regulate *Qi*
6.6	Citrus	*Chen Pi*	Regulate *Qi*
6.6	Amomum	*Sha Ren*	Aromatically transform Damp
4.9	Coptis	*Huang Lian*	Clear Heat, dry Damp
4.9	Glycyrrhiza	*Gan Cao*	Tonify *Qi* and harmonize

Rou Dou Kou (Myristica), 30 g *Shan Zha* (Crataegus), 30 g *Shen Qu* (Massa Fermentata), 30 g *Mai Ya* (Hordeum), 22.5 g of *Mu Xiang* (Saussurea), 30 g *Chen Pi* (Citrus), 30 g *Sha Ren* (Amomum), 22.5 g *Huang Lian* (Coptis), and 22.5 g of *Gan Cao* (Glycyrrhiza).[2]

Preparation:

1. Powder or capsule method: Herbs are ground into a fine powder. Powder can be encapsulated.
2. Decoction or teapill method: Raw herbs are mixed together and decocted. Herbal water extract (decoction) can be concentrated as granules or teapills.

Actions: Strengthen the Spleen and harmonize the Stomach, reduce Food Stagnation and stop diarrhea

Indications: Reduction in appetite with impaired digestion, bloating and focal abdominal distension with loose or watery diarrhea. The patient usually has a pale or pink tongue with a slightly yellow, greasy coating and a thin or deficient pulse.[2–4]

Dosage and Usage:

Horses and Cattle: 15–60 g, twice daily
Camels: 30–75 g, twice daily
Llamas, Alpacas, Goats, Sheep, and Pigs: 10–15 g, twice daily
Dogs: 0.5–5 g (or 0.1 g per kg body weight), twice daily
Cats and Rabbits: 0.2–0.5 g (or 0.1 g per kg body weight), twice daily
Birds: 0.1–0.2 g per kg body weight, twice daily
Use 4–8 weeks until primary clinical signs resolve.

Analysis of Formula: *Jian Pi Wan* is constructed to address the branch (*Biao*) of Food Stagnation that has its root (*Ben*) in Spleen Deficiency. The King herbs are *Bai Zhu* (Atractylodes), which strengthens Spleen *Qi* while drying Dampness; *Fu Ling* (Poria), which mildly tonifies Spleen *Qi* while leaching out Dampness; *Ren Shen* (Ginseng), which strongly tonifies Spleen *Qi*; and *Gan Cao* (Glycyrrhiza) which tonifies Spleen *Qi* and harmonizes the formula. When used as a separate formula, these four herbs together are the fundamental Spleen *Qi* tonic called *Si Jun Zi Tang*, or Four Gentlemen Decoction. There are eight Minister herbs. *Shan Yao* (Dioscorea) tonifies the Spleen and Stomach, and *Rou Dou Kou* (Myristica), warms the Middle Burner and astringes the bowels to stop diarrhea. Three other Minister herbs, *Shan Zha* (Crataegus), *Shen Qu* (Massa Fermentata), and *Mai Ya* (Hordeum), are used to reduce Food Stagnation from protein, fats, and carbohydrates. The last three Minister herbs, *Mu Xiang* (Saussurea), *Chen Pi* (Citrus), and *Sha Ren* (Amomum), serve to regulate *Qi* and harmonize the Stomach. Serving as the Adjuvant herb, *Huang Lian* (Coptis) is used to clear Heat that may be generated from Stagnation and to dry Dampness. *Gan Cao* (Glycyrrhiza) has the additional role of Messenger herb to guide the herbal formula actions to the Middle Burner.[5,6]

Cautions and Contraindications: This formula is contraindicated in acute cases of Food Stagnation due to ingestion of contaminated food or due to excessive intake of food or fluids.

Dr. Xie's Comments: *Jian Pi Wan* is often used successfully in treating chronic colitis, poor digestion, inflammatory bowel disease due to Spleen *Qi* Deficiency, and Damp or Food Stagnation in dogs, cats, and horses.

Zhi Zhu Wan (Aurantium and Atractylodes) 枳术丸

This formula is named for the two ingredients *Zhi Shi* (Aurantium) and *Bai Zhu* (Atractylodes). *Wan* is pill, the form of original herbal administration. Thus, *Zhi Zhu Wan* translates literally to Aurantium and Atractylodes Pill.

Source: *Nei Wai Shang Bian Huo Lun* (*Clarifying Doubts about Injury from Internal and External Causes*), written by *Li Ao* and published in 1247 CE

Ingredients: The original formula for *Zhi Zhu Wan* (Table 25.5) was made by grinding the ingredients into powder and forming into pills with rice fried in *He Ye* (Nelumbo). *Zhi Zhu Wan* is composed of 60 g *Bai Zhu* (Atractylodes), and 30 g *Zhi Shi* (Aurantium).[2]

Preparation:

1. Powder or capsule method: Herbs are ground into a fine powder. Powder can be encapsulated.

Table 25.5. Ingredients and actions of *Zhi Zhu Wan.*

%	English Name	Chinese *Pin-Yin*	Actions
67	Atractylodes	*Bai Zhu*	Tonify *Qi*
33	Aurantium	*Zhi Shi*	Regulate *Qi*

2. Decoction or teapill method: Raw herbs are mixed together and decocted. Herbal water extract (decoction) can be concentrated as granules or teapills.

Actions: Tonify the Spleen and reduce abdominal distension

Indications: Reduction of appetite with focal abdominal distension. There may be a normal or white tongue coating with a weak or tight pulse.[2–4]

Dosage and Usage:
Horses and Cattle: 15–60 g, twice daily
Camels: 30–75 g, twice daily
Llamas, Alpacas, Goats, Sheep, and Pigs: 10–15 g, twice daily
Dogs: 0.5–5 g (or 0.1 g per kg body weight), twice daily
Cats and Rabbits: 0.2–0.5 g (or 0.1 g per kg body weight), twice daily
Birds: 0.1–0.2 g per kg body weight, twice daily
Use 4–12 weeks until primary clinical signs resolve.

Analysis of Formula: This is a very simple yet elegant formula, which both tonifies deficient Spleen *Qi* and regulates stagnant *Qi* and descends it downward. The King herb *Bai Zhu* (Atractylodes) both tonifies Spleen *Qi* and reduces Dampness that may have accumulated due to weak Spleen *Qi*. The Minister herb *Zhi Shi* (Aurantium) breaks up stagnant *Qi* and reduces accumulation, while directing the *Qi* downward.[5,6]

Cautions and Contraindications: None known

Dr. Xie's Comments: Both *Zhi Zhu Wan* and *Jian Pi Wan* are used in treating Spleen *Qi* Deficiency with Food Stagnation. However, *Zhi Zhu Wan* is a much milder herbal formula, and often used for maintenance. In addition, *Jian Pi Wan* can clear Damp Heat and stop diarrhea; thus, it is often used in treating diarrhea and poor digestion due to Spleen *Qi* Deficiency with Damp-Heat.

Zhi Shi Xiao Pi Wan (Aurantium to Reduce Distension) 枳实消痞丸

This formula is named for its King herb, *Zhi Shi* (Aurantium) and its primary effect of reducing focal abdominal distention. *Wan* is pill, the form of original herbal administration.

Table 25.6. Ingredients and actions of *Zhi Shi Xiao Pi Wan.*

%	English Name	Chinese *Pin-Yin*	Actions
17.3	Aurantium	*Zhi Shi*	Regulate *Qi*
13.8	Magnolia	*Hou Po*	Move *Qi*, transform Damp
17.3	Coptis	*Huang Lian*	Clear Heat, dry Damp
10.3	Pinellia	*Ban Xia*	Resolve Phlegm
10.3	Ginseng	*Ren Shen*	Tonify *Qi*
6.9	Atractylodes	*Bai Zhu*	Tonify *Qi*
6.9	Poria	*Fu Ling*	Drain Damp
6.9	Hordeum	*Mai Ya*	Reduce Food Stagnation
3.4	Zingiberis	*Gan Jiang*	Warm the Middle, expel cold
6.9	Glycyrrhiza	*Gan Cao*	Tonify *Qi*, harmonize

Source: *Lan Shi Mi Cang* (*Secrets from the Orchid Pavilion*), written by *Li Ao* and published in 1336 CE

Ingredients: The original formula for *Zhi Shi Xiao Pi Wan* (Table 25.6) was made by grinding the ingredients into powder and rolling into small pills. *Zhi Shi Xiao Pi Wan* is composed of 15 g *Zhi Shi* (Aurantium), 12 g *Hou Po* (Magnolia), 15 g *Huang Lian* (Coptis), 9 g *Ban Xia* (Pinellia), 9 g *Ren Shen* (Ginseng), 6 g *Bai Zhu* (Atractylodes), 6 g *Fu Ling* (Poria), 6 g *Mai Ya* (Hordeum), 3 g *Gan Jiang* (Zingiberis), and 6 g *Gan Cao* (Glycyrrhiza).[2]

Preparation:
1. Powder or capsule method: Herbs are ground into a fine powder. Powder can be encapsulated.
2. Decoction or teapill method: Raw herbs are mixed together and decocted. Herbal water extract (decoction) can be concentrated as granules or teapills.

Actions: Reduce focal abdominal distension, eliminate fullness, tonify the Spleen and harmonize the Stomach

Indications: Focal distension and fullness in the cranial abdomen, reduced appetite and/or thirst, fatigue and weakness. Stools may vary from loose to firm, the tongue usually is pale with a central purple area, and the pulse tight to wiry.[2–4]

Dosage and Usage:
Horses and Cattle: 15–60 g, twice daily
Camels: 30–75 g, twice daily
Llamas, Alpacas, Goats, Sheep, and Pigs: 10–15 g, twice daily
Dogs: 0.5–5 g (or 0.1 g per kg body weight), twice daily
Cats and Rabbits: 0.2–0.5 g (or 0.1 g per kg body weight), twice daily
Birds: 0.1–0.2 g per kg body weight, twice daily
Use 3–8 weeks until primary clinical signs resolve.

Analysis of Formula: In contradistinction to prior Food Stagnation formulas, *Zhi Shi Xiao Pi Wan* is designed with a primary emphasis on reducing focal abdominal distension and secondarily strengthening the Spleen and harmonizing the Stomach. The King herb *Zhi Shi* (Aurantium) promotes the movement of *Qi* downward and reduces focal distension of the cranial abdomen. *Hou Po* (Magnolia) promotes *Qi* movement and eliminates fullness and thus reinforces the effect of the King herb. *Huang Lian* (Coptis) clears Heat and dries Dampness; *Ban Xia* (Pinellia) descends rebellious *Qi* and transforms Phlegm. *Ren Shen* (Ginseng) tonifies the Spleen and supports the *Zhong Qi*, which might be damaged by the prior herbs. *Bai Zhu* (Atractylodes) and *Fu Ling* (Poria) strengthen the Spleen and dry Dampness. These six herbs are all Minister herbs. *Mai Ya* (Hordeum) reduces Food Stagnation and harmonizes the Stomach. *Gan Jiang* (Zingiberis) disperses Cold in the Middle Burner. These two herbs are the Adjuvant herbs that treat the Cold obstruction unique to the Pattern addressed by this formula. *Gan Cao* (Glycyrrhiza), serving as the Messenger herb, harmonizes the other herbs and strengthens Spleen *Qi*.[5,6]

Cautions and Contraindications: Use this formula with caution in cases of excess fullness Patterns of Food Stagnation.

Dr. Xie's Comments: *Zhi Shi Xiao Pi Wan* is also called *Shi Xiao Wan* (Loss of Happy Face). It is designed for the *Pi* syndrome (focal distention/fullness and pain around the chest and diaphragm). When the *Pi* syndrome occurs, patients feel discomfort and pain, resulting in no more happy face; hence, the formula to treat this condition is named *Shi Xiao Wan*. Spleen *Qi* Deficiency leads to generation of Damp and *Qi* Stagnation, which can transform into Heat. Damp further attracts Cold. A combination of *Qi* Deficiency and *Qi* Stagnation, with Cold and Heat, eventually leads to the *Pi* syndrome around the chest and diaphragm.

REFERENCES

1. Qiao Y. The Traditional Chinese Medicine Formula Study Guide, Peter Holmes (ed). Boulder, CO: Snow Lotus Press, 2000.
2. Bensky D, Barolet R. Chinese Herbal Medicine, Formulas and Strategies. Seattle WA: Eastland Press, 1990.
3. Zong LX. Pocket Handbook of Chinese Herbal Prescriptions. Miami, FL: Waclion International, Inc., 2001.
4. Ehling D. The Chinese Herbalist's Handbook. Twin Lakes, WI: Lotus Press, 2002.
5. Bensky D, Gamble A. Chinese Herbal Medicine Materia Medica. Seattle, WA: Eastland Press, Inc., 1993.
6. Zong Lan Xu. Pocket Handbook of Chinese Herbal Medicine. Miami, FL: Waclion International Inc., 2000.

26 Herbal Formulas to Stop Bleeding 止血剂

Bruce Ferguson

The formulas in this chapter are used to counteract the Blood leaving the Blood vessels. Signs of bleeding vary with body region or tissue origin but may include nasal bleeding, coughing of Blood, vomiting of Blood, hemafecia, hematuria, uterine or vaginal bleeding, intraabdominal bleeding, and subcutaneous hemorrhage such as pettechiae and echymoses. TCVM *Bian Zheng* or Pattern Differentiation of bleeding may involve *Zang-Fu* organ(s), Heat and Cold, Deficiency and Excess, and acute and chronic nature of the Blood loss.[1]

Etiological factors involved in Bleeding Patterns are both exogenous and endogenous. Exogenous factors include invasion of *Liu Qi* or exogenous pathogens, especially Hot and Cold, excessive training, parturition, chronic overconsumption of hot/spicy foods, and various forms of trauma. Endogenous factors such as global *Qi* Deficiency, Spleen *Qi* Deficiency, *Qi* Stagnation, and Blood Stagnation may be involved in Bleeding Patterns.

The pathogenesis of Bleeding Patterns is variable and may arise from Excess, Deficient, Interior, or Exterior Patterns. Direct invasion by any of the six pathogenic factors (including Wind, Cold, Heat, Dryness, Damp, and Summer Heat) into the Lung, Large Intestine, or Uterus may cause bleeding. Internally, any disharmony leading to Heat may accelerate and disrupt the flow of Blood in the vessels and lead to bleeding. Blood Heat or Blood Stasis may force the Blood out of the vessels and cause bleeding. Spleen *Qi* Deficiency, from constitution (species)-inappropriate diet or overtraining for example, may impair the Spleen's function of holding Blood in the vessels. Chronic and/or febrile diseases, which consume and damage the *Yin*, and Body Fluids may also damage the Blood vessels and lead to bleeding.

TCVM treatment principles for bleeding are to stop the overt bleeding and treat the underlying disharmony (Table 26.1). In acute bleeding, stopping Blood loss and restoring Body Fluids and Blood takes precedence. In cases of chronic, non–life-threatening bleeding, both the branch (*Biao*) of bleeding and the root (*Ben*) cause of the bleeding may be treated simultaneously.

Western biomedical viewpoints on the herbal formulas used to treat bleeding disorders are still evolving. To date, it appears that many of the herbs influence the absolute numbers and functions of various Blood cells, including leukocytes, erythrocytes, thrombocytes, and mast cells. The herbs also appear to modify vascular permeability and adhesion factors. Future research should further clarify many of these important functions.

In TCVM we should observe the general cautions and contraindications that are true for herbal formulas used to treat acute bleeding. Generally, these formulas should be discontinued when the bleeding disharmony has resolved. At that point the underlying Ben or Root disharmony should be addressed.

The bitter, Cold herbs may damage the Spleen and are to be used with caution in cases of Spleen *Qi* Deficiency. Warming and tonifying herbs should be used with caution in full Heat conditions because they may exacerbate the Heat. Herbs that have a raising and diaphoretic quality should be used with caution in Upper *Jiao* bleeding. Descending and purgative herbs should be used with caution when treating bleeding from the Lower *Jiao*.

Shi Hui San (Ten Ash Powder) 十灰散

This formula is named for the original method of preparation of the ten ingredients, which was to partially char each of the herbs in the formula. *Shi* means ten or ten ingredients. *Hui* is ash and *San* is powder, the form of original herbal administration.

Source: *Shi Yao Shen Shu* (*Miraculous Book of Ten Remedies*), written by *Ge Qian-Sun* and published in 1348 CE

Table 26.1. Differentiation of bleeding signs.

TCVM Pattern	Heat in the Zang-Fu	Blood Heat	*Qi* Deficiency	*Yin* Deficiency
Pathoetiology	External pathogenic invasion, overconsumption of hot foods, chronic species-inappropriate diet, emotional Stagnation	Invasion of pathogenic Heat	Chronic overexertion, chronic debilitation, Cold or Damp foods	Chronic overexertion, chronic consumptive disease or fever leading to dryness
Location	Lung, Large Intestine, Stomach, Liver, Genitourinary	Blood (*Xue*) Level	Spleen	*Yin* and Body Fluids
Type	Acute bleeding of bright red Blood, may occasionally be purple	Acute and excessive bleeding of fresh red or dark purple Blood	Chronic bleeding of pale and/or thin Blood	Bleeding of small amounts of pink or fresh red Blood
Clinical Signs	Epistaxis, coughing or vomiting Blood, hematuria, hemafecia, genitourinary bleeding with full Heat signs such as irritability, increased thirst	Echymosis, petechiae, genitourinary bleeding with intense Heat signs such as fever, irritability, thirst	Bleeding may be from anywhere with concurrent signs of fatigue	Bleeding may be from anywhere with concurrent dryness, thirst and low-grade fever
Tongue	Red	Bright red	Pale, moist	Red, dry
Pulse	Rapid	Rapid and full	Weak, forceless, thin	Rapid and thin or tight
Treatment in addition to Stop Bleeding	Clear Heat from affected *Zang-Fu*	Cool Blood and clear Heat, replenish fluids if damaged	Tonify Spleen *Qi*, nourish Blood	Nourish *Yin*, moisten dryness

Table 26.2. Ingredients and actions of *Shi Hui San*.

%	English Name	Chinese *Pin-Yin*	Actions
7.5	Cirsium	*Da Ji*	Stop bleeding, cool Blood
12.5	Cephalanoplus	*Xiao Ji*	Stop bleeding
7.5	Nelumbo	*He Ye*	Stop bleeding
7.5	Biota	*Ce Bai Ye*	Stop bleeding, cool Blood
25	Imperata	*Bai Mao Gen*	Stop bleeding, cool Blood
10	Rubia	*Qian Cao*	Stop bleeding, cool Blood, dispel Blood Stasis
10	Gardenia	*Zhi Zi*	Drain Fire from *San Jiao*, cool Blood, stop Bleeding
7.5	Rheum	*Da Huang*	Purge Heat, reduce Blood Stasis
7.5	Moutan	*Mu Dan Pi*	Clear Heat, cool Blood, dispel Blood Stasis
5	Trachycarpus	*Zong Lu*	Astringe and stop bleeding

Ingredients: The original formula for *Shi Hui San* was made by partially charring equal amounts of the herbs and grinding them into a fine powder. A dosage of 9–15 grams of the powder was mixed with either lotus root juice or Japanese radish. *Shi Hui San* is composed of 9g *Da Ji* (Cirsium), 15g *Xiao Ji* (Cephalanoplus), 9g *He Ye* (Nelumbo), 9g *Ce Bai Ye* (Biota), 30g *Bai Mao Gen* (Imperata), 12g *Qian Cao* (Rubia), 12g *Zhi Zi* (Gardenia), 9g *Da Huang* (Rheum), 9g *Mu Dan Pi* (Moutan), and 6g *Zong Lu* (Trachycarpus) (Table 26.2).[2]

Preparation:

1. Powder or capsule method: Herbs are ground into a fine powder. Powder can be encapsulated.
2. Decoction or teapill method: Raw herbs are mixed together and decocted. Herbal water extract (decoction) can be concentrated as granules or teapills.

Actions: Cool Blood, stop bleeding

Indications: Epistaxis, hematemesis, hemoptysis. Commonly there is a dry mouth and throat; a dark red tongue with a yellow coat; and a rapid, tight to wiry, forceful pulse.[2–4]

Dosage and Usage:

Horses and Cattle: 15–60g, twice daily
Camels: 30–75g, twice daily
Llamas, Alpacas, Goats, Sheep, and Pigs: 10–15g, twice daily
Dogs: 0.5–5g (or 0.1g per kg body weight), twice daily
Cats and Rabbits: 0.2–0.5g (or 0.1g per kg body weight), twice daily
Birds: 0.1–0.2g per kg body weight, twice daily
Use 1–4 weeks until primary clinical signs resolve.

Analysis of Formula: This formula is used for fire disharmonies in the Upper and Middle Burners, which injure the Blood vessels and induce the movement of hot, reckless Blood out of the vessels. The primary thrust of this formula is accomplished by *Da Ji* (Cirsium), *Xiao Ji* (Cephalanoplus), *He Ye* (Nelumbo), *Ce Bai Ye* (Biota), *Bai Mao Gen* (Imperata), and *Qian Cao* (Rubia), which, as a group, are the King herbs and serve to cool Blood and stop bleeding. Heat may leave the body by direct radiation, vomiting, sweating, urination, and defecation. *Zhi Zi* (Gardenia) serves as the Minister herb to drain Heat downward through all three burners and out through the urine. Working as the Adjuvant herbs, *Mu Dan Pi* (Moutan) and *Da Huang* (Rheum) both act to cool the Blood and dispel Blood Stasis that may be caused by the original disharmony or may arise as the King herbs successfully stop bleeding.[2,5,6]

Cautions and Contraindications: This formula is contraindicated for treating bleeding that results from Deficiency and/or Cold disorders.

Dr. Xie's Comments: In veterinary classical texts, this formula is referred to as *Shi Hei San* (Ten Black Powder). *Shi* means ten. *Hei* means black. *San* is powder. Ingredients and actions of *Shi Hei San* are the same ones as *Shi Hui San* (Ten Ash Powder). In Five Element theory, the black color (Water) controls the red color (Fire). Therefore, the ashed herbs (black) are capable of stopping bleeding (red).

Clinical and Pharmacological Studies: Emodin (1, 3, 8-trihydroxy-6-methyl-anthraquinone) is an anthraquinone derivative from the roots of Rheum officinale Baill, a Chinese herb widely and traditionally used for wound healing. The objectives of this study were to determine whether topically applied emodin enhanced repair of rats' excisional wounds, and define its possible mechanism. Wounds were treated with either topical emodin (100, 200, and 400 μg/ml), recombinant human epidermal growth factor (rhEGF, 10 μg/ml), or vehicle for 7 or 14 days, consecutively. At day 5 postinjury, wounds receiving emodin (400 μg/ml) were significantly smaller than those treated with the vehicle. Emodin treatments had markedly more hydroxyproline content in day 7 wounds and tensile strength in day 14 wounds than that of the vehicle control. The level of transforming growth factor-beta(1) [TGF-beta(1)] in wound tissues assessed by immunohistochemistry and reverse transcription polymerase chain reaction (RT-PCR) showed a dose-dependent increase in emodin-treated wounds compared with the vehicle-treated wounds. Western immunoblotting analysis of wound tissues for Smad 2, 3, 4, 7 protein expression showed an increase in Smad 2, 3 in the emodin-treated wounds compared with the vehicle. By contrast, a reduction of Smad 7 was observed in emodin-treated wounds compared with the vehicle, and there was no change of Smad 4. In summary, the results showed that emodin promoted repair of rats' excisional wounds via a complex mechanism involving stimulation of tissue regeneration and regulating Smads-mediated TGF-beta(1) signaling pathway.[7]

Cirsium japonicum De Candole is widely used in traditional herbal medicine for the treatment of hemorrhage, hypertension, or Blood circulation in Korea. In this work, the vasorelaxant activity of an aqueous extract of C. japonicum whole plant (CjEx), and its possible mechanism in isolated rat thoracic aortic rings constricted with norepinephrine (NE; 300 nmol/l), was evaluated. CjEx elicited an acute relaxation in endothelium-intact rings in a concentration-dependent manner (0.1–1.0 mg/ml). This relaxation was eliminated by the removal of the endothelium and pretreatment with N(G)-nitro-L-arginine (10 μmol/l), methylene blue (1 μmol/l), or diphenylhydramine (10 μmol/l), but indomethacin (10 μmol/l) atropine (100 nmol/l), [D-Pro(2), D-Trp(7,9)] substance P (5 μmol/l), or HOE-140 (10 nmol/l) did not affect the relaxation. The results indicate that the response to CjEx involves enhancement of the nitric oxide-cyclic guanosine monophosphate system and that it occurs via histamine H(1)-receptor. These findings may contribute to better understanding of the potential link between the clinical use of CjEx and its beneficial effects on vascular health[8]

Huai Hua San (Sophora Powder) 槐花散

This formula is named for the King ingredient, *Huai Hua* (Sophora). *San* is powder, the form of the original of herbal medication. Thus, *Huai Hua San* translates literally to Sophora Powder.

Source: *Pu Ji Ben Shi Fang* (*Formulas of Universal Benefit*), written by *Xu Shu-Wei* and published in 1132 CE

Ingredients: The original formula was made by grinding equal amounts of the separate herbs into powder and taking with boiled water or thin rice gruel on an empty stomach. *Huai Hua San* is composed of 9–30 g *Huai Hua* (Sophora), 9–15 g *Ce Bai Ye* (Biota), 6–9 g *Jing Jie* (Schizonepeta), and 6–9 g *Zhi Ke* (Aurantium) (Table 26.3).[2]

Preparation:

1. Powder or capsule method: Herbs are ground into a fine powder. Powder can be encapsulated.
2. Decoction or teapill method: Raw herbs are mixed together and decocted. Herbal water extract (decoction) can be concentrated as granules or teapills.

Actions: Clear Heat toxin from the intestines, stop bleeding, dispel Wind, promote the normal directional movement of *Qi*

Table 26.3. Ingredients and actions of *Huai Hua San*.

%	English Name	Chinese *Pin-Yin*	Actions
48	Sophora	*Huai Hua*	Stop bleeding, cool Blood
24	Biota	*Ce Bai Ye*	Stop bleeding, cool Blood
14	Schizonepeta	*Jing Jie*	Stop bleeding
14	Aurantium	*Zhi Ke*	Regulate *Qi*

Indications: Bright-red bleeding from the rectum either preceding, accompanying, or following defecation; hemorrhoids; and/or dark red or bright red Blood in the stools. There is usually a red tongue and wiry, rapid pulse.[2–4]

Dosage and Usage:
Horses and Cattle: 15–60 g, twice daily
Camels: 30–75 g, twice daily
Llamas, Alpacas, Goats, Sheep, and Pigs: 10–15 g, twice daily
Dogs: 0.5–5 g (or 0.1 g per kg body weight), twice daily
Cats and Rabbits: 0.2–0.5 g (or 0.1 g per kg body weight), twice daily
Birds: 0.1–0.2 g per kg body weight, twice daily
Use 1–4 weeks until primary clinical signs resolve.

Analysis of Formula: This formula is constructed to treat either Wind-Heat or Damp-Heat in the bowels. *Huai Hua* (Sophora), the King herb, clears Damp-Heat from the bowels, cools Blood, stops bleeding and relieves toxicity. Serving as the Minister herb, *Ce Bai Ye* (Biota) assists the King by astringing bleeding and cooling the Blood. *Jing Jie* (Schizonepeta) is the Adjuvant herb, which dispels Wind and is an auxiliary herb to stop bleeding. *Zhi Ke* (Aurantium) is used as the Messenger herb to rectify the flow of *Qi* in the bowels. This action normalizes *Qi* flow, thereby reducing pain, and reduces the propensity of the other herbs, which stop bleeding, to actually cause Blood Stagnation.[2,5,6]

Cautions and Contraindications: Do not use long-term, as the Cold-natured herbs may damage the Spleen. Do not use for bleeding in the absence of Heat and Damp-Heat.

Dr. Xie's Comments: *Huai Hua San* is used for bloody stool due to Wind-Heat or Damp-Heat accumulated in the intestines. It is often used for the acute onset of bloody diarrhea in colitis or inflammatory bowel disease in horses and dogs.

Xiao Ji Yin Zi (Cephalanoplos Decoction)
小蓟饮子

This formula is named for the King ingredient, *Xiao Ji* or Cephalanoplus. *Yin Zi* refers to decoction, the original form of herbal medication. *Xiao Ji Yin Zi* therefore translates to Cephalanoplus Decoction.

Source: *Ji Sheng Fang* (*Formulas to Aid the Living*), written by *Yan Yong-He* and published in 1253 CE

Ingredients: The original formula was made by coarsely grinding the ingredient herbs and taking in a suspension. *Xiao Ji Yin Zi* is composed of 15 g *Xiao Ji* (Cephalanoplos), 15 g *Ou Jie* (Nelumbo), 15 g *Pu Huang* (Typhae), 120 g *Sheng Di Huang* (Rehmannia), 15 g *Hua Shi* (Talcum), 15 g *Mu Tong* (Akebia), 15 g *Dan Zhu Ye* (Lophatherum), 15 g *Zhi Zi* (Gardenia), 15 g *Dang Gui* (Angelica), and 15 g *Gan Cao* (Glycyrrhiza) (Table 26.4).[2]

Table 26.4. Ingredients and actions of *Xiao Ji Yin Zi*.

%	English Name	Chinese *Pin-Yin*	Actions
5.9	Cephalanoplos	*Xiao Ji*	Cool Blood, stop bleeding
5.9	Nelumbo	*Ou Jie*	Stop bleeding, astringe, break Blood Stasis
5.9	Typha	*Pu Huang*	Stop bleeding, dispel Blood Stasis
47	Rehmannia	*Sheng Di Huang*	Cool Blood, generate fluids
5.9	Talcum	*Hua Shi*	Promote Urination, drain Heat from Bladder
5.9	Akebia	*Mu Tong*	Promote urination, drain Heat, relieve dysuria
5.9	Lophatherum	*Dan Zhu Ye*	Promote urination, clear Damp Heat
5.9	Gardenia	*Zhi Zi*	Clear Heat from *San Jiao*, cool Blood, Stop Bleeding
5.9	Angelica	*Dang Gui*	Nourish Blood, invigorate Blood
5.8	Glycyrrhiza	*Gan Cao*	Harmonize

Preparation:
1. Powder or capsule method: Herbs are ground into a fine powder. Powder can be encapsulated.
2. Decoction or teapill method: Raw herbs are mixed together and decocted. Herbal water extract (decoction) can be concentrated as granules or teapills.

Actions: Cool Blood, stop bleeding, promote urination, resolve painful urinary dysfunction

Indications: Bloody, painful urination with pollakiuria, stranguria, dysuria, or Blood in the urine; signs of Heat in the body such as increased thirst, irritability, a red tongue with/without a yellow coating, and a rapid, strong pulse[2–4]

Dosage and Usage:
Horses and Cattle: 15–60 g, twice daily
Camels: 30–75 g, twice daily
Llamas, Alpacas, Goats, Sheep, and Pigs: 10–15 g, twice daily
Dogs: 0.5–5 g (or 0.1 g per kg body weight), twice daily
Cats and Rabbits: 0.2–0.5 g (or 0.1 g per kg body weight), twice daily
Birds: 0.1–0.2 g per kg body weight, twice daily
Use 1–4 weeks until primary clinical signs resolve.

Analysis of Formula: This formula is constructed to treat Heat accumulation in the Lower Burner and urinary bladder that injures the blood vessels and collaterals and causes Blood to drain downward into the bladder. The King herb, *Xiao Ji* (Cephalanoplos), and its two Minister herbs, *Ou Jie* (Nelumbo) and *Pu Huang* (Typha), cool the Blood, stop bleeding, and dispel Blood Stasis. *Sheng Di Huang* (Rehmannia) serves to nourish *Yin* and clear Heat, while secondarily cooling the Blood and stopping bleeding. *Hua Shi* (Talcum) clears Heat and promotes urination, thereby reducing stranguria/dysuria and allowing the pathogenic Heat to exit the body. *Mu Tong* (Akebia) and *Dan Zhu Ye* (Lophatherum) clear Heat and drain Damp-Heat downward. *Zhi Zi* (Gardenia) clears Heat and Fire from the Triple Burner (*San Jiao*) and mildly promotes urination. *Dang Gui* (Angelica) nourishes and invigorates Blood, helping to replace lost Blood as well as reducing Blood Stasis from the herbs that work to stop bleeding. These six ingredients are the Adjuvant herbs. Serving as the Messenger herb, *Gan Cao* (Glycyrrhiza) both reduces painful spasm and harmonizes the formula.[2,5,6]

Cautions and Contraindications: This formula is contraindicated for painful, bloody urinary dysfunction from Deficiency. It is also cautioned for patients with weak Spleen and Stomach. It is not intended for long-term use.

Dr. Xie's Comments: *Xiao Ji Yin Zi* is used for bloody urination due to Damp-Heat accumulated in the Lower Burner (primarily in Bladder). It is often used for the acute onset of bloody urine in cystitis and urinary tract infection in dogs, cats, and horses.

Huang Tu Tang (Yellow Earth) 黄土汤

This formula is named for its main ingredient, *Fu Long Gan* (Terra Flava), which has a similar appearance to yellow earth (soil). *Huang* means yellow and *Tu* is soil, dirt, or earth. *Tang* is decoction, the form of the original administration.

Source: *Jin Gui Yao Lue Fang Lun* (*Synopsis of Prescriptions from the Golden Cabinet*), written by *Zhang Zhong-Jing* and published in 220 CE

Ingredients: The original formula was made by decocting the *Fu Long Gan* (Terra Flava) for 30 minutes before adding the other herbs to the decoction. *E Jiao* (Gelatinum) was dissolved separately in boiling water and then added to the decoction. *Huang Tu Tang* is composed of 18 g *Fu Long Gan* (Terra Flava), 9 g *Sheng Di Huang* (Rehmannia), 9 g *E Jiao* (Gelatinum), 9 g *Bai Zhu* (Atractylodes), 9 g *Gan Cao* (Glycyrrhiza), 9 g *Fu Zi* (Aconite), and 9 g *Huang Qin* (Scutellaria) (Table 26.5).[2]

Preparation:

1. Powder or capsule method: Herbs are ground into a fine powder. Powder can be encapsulated.
2. Decoction or teapill method: Raw herbs are mixed together and decocted. Herbal water extract (decoction) can be concentrated as granules or teapills.

Table 26.5. Ingredients and actions of *Huang Tu Tang*.

%	English Name	Chinese *Pin-Yin*	Actions
25	Terra Flava	*Fu Long Gan*	Warm Middle Burner, stop bleeding
12.5	Rehmannia	*Sheng Di Huang*	Cool Blood, generate fluids
12.5	Gelatinum	*E Jiao*	Nourish Blood and *Yin*, stop bleeding
12.5	Atractylodes	*Bai Zhu*	Strengthen the Spleen, dry Damp
12.5	Glycyrrhiza	*Gan Cao*	Tonify Spleen *Qi*, harmonize
12.5	Aconite	*Fu Zi*	Warm *Yang*, tonify the Spleen and Kidney
12.5	Scutellaria	*Huang Qin*	Clear Heat, stop bleeding

Actions: Warm the Spleen *Yang*, strengthen the Spleen *Qi*, nourish Blood, stop bleeding

Indications: Blood in the stool or urine, epistaxis, hematemesis, abnormal uterine bleeding; the color of the bleeding is pale-red with Cold signs such as Cold extremities, pale tongue with white coating, and a deep, thin, feeble pulse.[2–4]

Dosage and Usage:

Horses and Cattle: 15–60 g, twice daily
Camels: 30–75 g, twice daily
Llamas, Alpacas, Goats, Sheep, and Pigs: 10–15 g, twice daily
Dogs: 0.5–5 g (or 0.1 g per kg body weight), twice daily
Cats and Rabbits: 0.2–0.5 g (or 0.1 g per kg body weight), twice daily
Birds: 0.1–0.2 g per kg body weight, twice daily
Use 4–8 weeks until primary clinical signs resolve.

Analysis of Formula: This formula is constructed to treat Spleen *Yang* Deficiency, which is manifested in systemic Cold signs and failure of the Spleen *Qi* to hold the Blood in the vessels. *Fu Long Gan* (Terra Flava), the King ingredient, warms the Blood and stops bleeding caused by Deficiency of the Middle Burner, while harmonizing the Stomach. The Minister herbs *Bai Zhu* (Atractylodes) and *Fu Zi* (Aconite) warm and strengthen the Spleen in order to facilitate its ability to hold the Blood in the vessels. Serving as the Adjuvant herbs, *Sheng Di Huang* (Rehmannia) and *E Jiao* (Gelatinum) nourish Blood and *Yin*, while mildly inhibiting bleeding; *Huang Qin* (Scutellaria) is used to balance their warming, drying, and invigorating nature. *Gan Cao*

(Glycyrrhiza) harmonizes the formula and strengthens the Middle Burner, working as the Messenger herb.[2,5,6]

Cautions and Contraindications: This formula is contraindicated for bleeding from full-Heat Patterns

Dr. Xie's Comments: *Huang Tu Tang* is good at tonifying Spleen *Qi* to stop bleeding. Hence, it is often used for chronic hemorrhage in the gastrointestinal tract when deficient *Qi* fails to hold Blood inside the blood vessels.

Yunnan Bai Yao (*Yunnan* White Medicine) 云南白药

This formula is named for its Chinese province of origin, *Yunnan*, and the color of the final product, White (*Bai*). *Yao* means medicine.

Source: *Qu Huangzhang* in 1902

Ingredients: The main ingredients are steamed and raw *Sanqi* (Tienchi ginseng, Notoginseng roots of Panax pseudoginseng)—used to normalize Blood flow, enhance poor circulation, and heal internal bleeding in injuries and bleeding ulcers—and Rhizoma Dioscoreae. The two tienchi ginsengs are combined with astringent herbs that absorb excess bleeding, invigorate the Blood, and enhance healing, including Myrrh and "Dragon's Blood," another resinous herb for internal bleeding. The exact formula is a closely guarded secret. The company website mentions that progesterone has been analyzed from the formula, as well as several saponins, alkaloids, and the pharmacologically active compound calcium phosphate. However, the progesterone may not exist as such in the herbal product, provided that the formula is still the traditional formula, because Dioscorea requires laboratory alteration to become progesterone. The separate herbal ingredients are reportedly made up by 13 separate teams, none of whom have any knowledge of the ingredients the other teams are mixing (Table 26.6).

Table 26.6. Ingredients and actions of *Yunnan Bai Yao*.

%	English Name	Chinese *Pin-Yin*	Actions
40	Notoginseng	*San Qi*	Stops bleeding, transforms Stasis, reduces swelling, alleviates pain
13.3	Dioscorea	*Huan Shan Yao*	Tonify *Qi*
6	Dioscorea Parviflora	*Ku Liang Jiang*	Resolve Stagnation
11.5	Dioscorea Nipponica	*Chuan Shan Long*	Invigorate Blood and unblocks the channels
5	Inulae Cappae	*Bai Niu Dan*	Clear Heat, remove toxins
17	Ajuga Forrestii	*San Yu Cao*	Resolve Stagnation
7.2	Geranii	*Lao He Cao*	Resolve Stagnation

Preparation: Capsule method: Herbs are ground into a fine powder and encapsulated.

Actions: Stop bleeding and invigorate Blood Stasis

Indications: Blood in the stool or urine, epistaxis, hematemesis, abnormal uterine bleeding, excessive bleeding from surgical trauma, and bleeding from most tumor types such as hemangiosarcoma

Dosage and Usage:

Horses and Cattle: 15–60 g, twice daily
Camels: 30–75 g, twice daily
Llamas, Alpacas, Goats, Sheep, and Pigs: 10–15 g, twice daily
Dogs: 0.5–5 g (or 0.1 g per kg body weight), twice daily
Cats and Rabbits: 0.2–0.5 g (or 0.1 g per kg body weight), twice daily
Birds: 0.1–0.2 g per kg body weight, twice daily

Use 1–2 weeks until primary clinical signs resolve.

Analysis of Formula: This formula is constructed to stop bleeding from any cause. It has the added action of invigorating Blood so that it does not cause Blood Stasis while it works to stop bleeding.

Cautions and Contraindications: This formula is not intended for long-term use. The underlying cause of the bleeding should always be addressed. The formula may cause gastrointestinal upset.

Dr. Xie's Comments: *Yunnan Bai Yao* is one of the few emergency herbal formulas herbalists carry all the time. It can be used topically and orally for any types of bleeding. However, it treats the symptom (hemorrhage) and should be followed by the herbal formula(s) to treat the underlying cause(s) as soon as the hemorrhage is under control. Even though it may upset the stomach and damage Spleen *Qi*, and is often recommended short-term, it can be used long-term (with lower dosage) for the treatment and prevention of hemangiosarcoma in dogs.

Clinical and Pharmacological studies: Ginsenoside Rb1 (Rb1), ginsenoside Rg1 (Rg1), and notoginsenoside R1 (R1) are major active components of Panax notoginseng, a Chinese herb that is widely used in traditional Chinese medicine to enhance Blood circulation and dissipate Blood Stasis. To evaluate the effect of these saponins on microcirculatory disturbance induced by lipopolysaccharide (LPS), vascular hemodynamics in rat mesentery was observed continuously during their administration using an inverted microscope and a high-speed video camera system. LPS administration decreased red Blood cell velocity but Rb1, Rg1, and R1 attenuated this effect. LPS administration caused leukocyte adhesion to the venular wall, mast cell degranulation, and the release of cytokines. Rb1, Rg1, and R1 reduced the number of adherent leukocytes and inhibited mast cell degranulation and cytokine elevation. In vitro experiments using flow cytometry further demonstrated that 1) the LPS-enhanced expression of CD11b/CD18 by neutrophils was significantly depressed by Rb1 and R1, and 2) hydrogen peroxide (H_2O_2) release from neutrophils in response to LPS stimulation was inhibited by treatment with Rg1 and R1. These results suggest that the protective effect of Rb1 and R1 against leukocyte adhesion elicited by LPS may be associated with the suppressive action of Rb1 and R1 on the expression of CD11b/CD18 by neutrophils. The protective effect against mast cell degranulation by Rb1 and R1, and the blunting of H_2O_2 release from neutrophils by Rg1 and R1, suggest mechanistic diversity in the effects of Panax notoginseng saponins in the attenuation of microcirculatory disturbance induced by LPS.[9]

REFERENCES

1. Qiao Y. The Traditional Chinese Medicine Formula Study Guide, Peter Holmes (ed). Boulder, CO: Snow Lotus Press, 2000.
2. Bensky D, Barolet R. Chinese Herbal Medicine, Formulas and Strategies. Reddick, FL: Eastland Press, 1990.
3. Zong LX. Pocket Handbook of Chinese Herbal Prescriptions. Miami, FL: Waclion International, Inc., 2001.
4. Ehling D. The Chinese Herbalist's Handbook. Twin Lakes, WI: Lotus Press, 2002.
5. Bensky D, Gamble A. Chinese Herbal Medicine Materia Medica. Seattle, WA: Eastland Press, Inc., 1993.
6. Zong Lan Xu. Pocket Handbook of Chinese Herbal Medicine. Miami, FL: Waclion International Inc., 2000.
7. Tang T, Yin L, Yang J, Shan G. Emodin. An anthraquinone derivative from Rheum officinale Baill, enhances cutaneous wound healing in rats. European Journal of Pharmacology 2007;Feb 27.
8. Kim EY, Jho HK, Kim DI, Rhyu MR. Cirsium japonicum elicits endothelium-dependent relaxation via histamine H(1)-receptor in rat thoracic aorta. Journal of Ethnopharmacology 2007; Nov 12.
9. Sun K, Wang CS, Guo J, Horie Y, Fang SP, Wang F, Liu YY, Liu LY, Yang JY, Fan JY, Han JY. Protective effects of ginsenoside Rb1, ginsenoside Rg1, and notoginsenoside R1 on lipopolysaccharide-induced microcirculatory disturbance in rat mesentery. Life Science 2007;81(6):509–518. Epub 2007 Jun 28.

27 Herbal Formulas to Invigorate Blood and Break Blood Stasis 活血化瘀消瘤剂

Bruce Ferguson

Blood Stagnation refers to two primary disharmonies in Traditional Chinese Veterinary Medicine (TCVM). First and simplest, Blood Stagnation describes Blood that has extravasated into body cavities or areas. Second, Blood Stagnation Patterns involve the accumulation of *Xue*/Blood due to obstruction of the natural flow in the Channels, collaterals, and *Zang-Fu* organs. The reader should remember that TCVM *Xue* or Blood overlaps but is not completely inclusive of Western blood. Blood Stagnation Patterns of disharmony are noteworthy for the presence of distinct/focal pain or palpable masses.[1]

Blood Stagnation Patterns may be classified based upon the degree and progression of the blockage of Blood flow in the organs and Channels. The milder condition of slowed and impaired Blood flow in the *Jing-Luo* is termed Blood Stagnation. The more severe condition of complete loss of normal flow of Blood, which leads to cessation of circulation, is termed Blood Stasis. Blood Stasis Patterns tend to have firmer, fixed masses and/or more severe pain associated with them than Blood Stagnation Patterns.[2]

Blood Stagnation Patterns generally give rise to pain that is sharp and focal. Blood Stagnation and Stasis pain is not relieved by topical application of warmth or cold and is, like most Excess Patterns, worse with pressure. There may be purple mucous membranes, tissues, or lesions. There may also be bleeding that is deep or dark purple and easily clots, and a darkening of normally light tissues such as lips and sclera. The epidermis may be thickened (parakeratosis and hyperkeratosis) and dry. There may be firm masses, particularly intraabdominal benign and malignant tumors. The tongue body tends to be purple or dark with congested, dark, and tortuous sublingual veins. The pulse may vary from thin, if Blood deficiency predominates, to choppy, if Blood Stagnation is more prominent. The degree of choppy found in the pulse may be directly correlated to the severity of Blood Stagnation in the Channels and collaterals, or with parenchymal tissue damage in the *Zang-Fu* organs.

Various etiological agents may be responsible for Blood Stagnation Patterns. *Qi* deficiency may lead to Blood Stagnation because the *Qi* "commands" the Blood and is responsible for its ability to adequately circulate. *Qi* stagnation may also directly lead to Blood Stagnation through similar mechanisms. Either endogenous or exogenous Cold may congeal, slow, or otherwise lead to an impairment in Blood circulation. Heat may consume *Yin* fluids and ultimately "dry" the Blood and increase its tendency to stagnate. Heat in the Blood drives the Blood out of the vessels, possibly creating Blood pooling and, consequently, localized areas of Blood Stagnation. Finally, birth trauma and other traumatic physical events such as surgery, accidents, and sporting injuries may all lead to varying degrees of Blood Stagnation.

The general heteropathic principle for treating Blood Stagnation Patterns is to invigorate the Blood and dispel Blood Stasis. However, invigorating the Blood addresses only the *Biao* or branch. In order to prevent reoccurrence, the Ben or root cause of the Blood Stagnation Pattern should also be addressed. In acute conditions, the *Biao* or branch should be addressed and root treatment may be delayed until a later time.

The cautions and contraindications related to treating Blood Stagnation Patterns are based upon the very strong moving and invigorating properties of the herbs and formulas. A strategy of invigorating the Blood also tends to consume the Blood and *Qi*, so the following formulas should be used cautiously in deficiency conditions and the debilitated and elderly. Because a fetus is an intraabdominal "mass," Blood Stagnation formulas are contraindicated in pregnancy. Finally, Blood Stagnation formulas are generally contraindicated in patients with current or recent bleeding diatheses or tendencies.[3,4]

Western biomedical research has revealed some interesting observations of the mechanisms of Blood

Table 27.1. Differentiation of Blood Stagnation by location.

Location	Clinical Signs
Channels and collaterals	Localized pain in muscles, tendons, ligaments, and joints Lavender tongue; tight to wiry, choppy pulse
Integument	Purpura; ecchymoses; dry, thickened skin; pruritis; self-trauma Pale lavender tongue; thin, tight to wiry, choppy pulse
Heart	Pain on thoracic compression; pain when extending fore limbs in quadrupeds; lavender tongue; wiry, hesitant pulse
Lung	Pain on thoracic compression, hemoptysis, cough, exercise intolerance Lavender tongue tip, tight to wiry pulse
Bowels	Hematemesis, hematochezia, palpable abdominal masses Lavender tongue base; tight to wiry, choppy pulse
Liver	Hypochondriac and chondriac pain, resistance to compression Palpable abdominal mass; lavender tongue edges; wiry, choppy pulse
Uterus	Abnormal estrus cycle, dark and clotted bloody discharge Lavender tongue base, choppy pulse

Stasis formulas (Table 27.1).[1] Some play a role of removing Blood Stasis and promoting cellular regeneration through improving hematopoietic function by means of increasing the number and enhancing the function of premature hematopoietic stem cells. Others may partly protect against atherogenesis by an inhibition of expression of adhesion molecules. References related to specific formulas in the following text delineate more mechanisms, and the astute reader will realize that future scientific studies will likely provide evidence that further supports the efficacy of these formulas.[5,6]

Tao He Cheng Qi Tang (Persica for Purgation) 桃核承气汤

Tao He, or *Tao Ren* is Persica, the King ingredient of this formula. *Cheng Qi* refers to purgation. *Tang* is decoction, the form of original herbal administration. The formula is very potent to break up Blood Stasis by purging the Interior.

Source: *Shang Han Za Bing Lun* (*Treatise on Cold-Induced Disorders and Miscellaneous Diseases*), written by *Zhang Zhong-Jing* and published in 220 CE

Ingredients: The original formula for *Tao He Cheng Qi Tang* (Table 27.2) was made by boiling the ingredients together as a decoction.[2–4] *Tao He Cheng Qi Tang* is composed of 12–15 g *Tao Ren* (Persica), 12 g *Da Huang* (Rheum), 6 g *Gui Zhi* (Cinnamomum), 6 g *Mang Xiao* (Mirabilite), and 6 g *Gan Cao* (Glycyrrhiza).

Table 27.2. Ingredients and actions of *Tao He Cheng Qi Tang*.

%	English Name	Chinese *Pin-Yin*	Actions
29	Persica	*Tao Ren*	Break Blood Stasis, unblock the bowels
29	Rheum	*Da Huang*	Drain Heat, drain Damp-Heat, invigorate the Blood
14	Cinnamomum	*Gui Zhi*	Unblock vessels and circulate blood
14	Mirabilite	*Mang Xiao*	Guide accumulation out, clear Heat
14	Glycyrrhiza	*Gan Cao*	Reduce pain, harmonize

Preparation:

1. Powder or capsule method: Herbs are ground into a fine powder. Powder can be encapsulated.
2. Decoction or teapill method: Raw herbs are mixed together and decocted. Herbal water extract (decoction) can be concentrated as granules or teapills.

Actions: Drain Heat and break up Blood Stasis

Indications: Acute onset caudal abdominal pain that is worse with pressure; urinary incontinence with Heat signs such as constipation with dark feces, irritability, restlessness, and thirst; a red or purple dry tongue; and a deep, forceful, wiry to choppy pulse. Females may have painful or early estrus.

Dosage and Usage:

Horses and Cattle: 15–60 g, twice daily
Camels: 30–75 g, twice daily
Llamas, Alpacas, Goats, Sheep, and Pigs: 10–15 g, twice daily
Dogs: 0.5–5 g (or about 0.1 g per kg body weight), twice daily
Cats and Rabbits: 0.2–0.5 g (or about 0.1 g per kg body weight), twice daily
Birds: 0.1–0.2 g per kg body weight, twice daily

Use 1–3 weeks until primary clinical signs resolve. Do not use for extended duration.

Analysis of Formula: *Tao He Cheng Qi Tang*'s two King ingredients separately yet synergistically accomplish the primary actions of draining Heat and breaking up Blood Stasis. *Tao Ren* (Persica) breaks up Blood Stasis and moistens the intestines to unblock the bowels. *Da Huang* (Rheum) purges accumulation, clears pathogenic Heat, and assists *Tao Ren* (Persica) in breaking up Blood Stasis. The Minister herb *Gui Zhi* (Cinnamomum) unblocks the vessels and facilitates Blood flow in the Lower Burner. The Adjuvant herb *Mang Xiao* (Mirabilite) is cold and bitter, softens hardness, and mildly guides out accumulation, thus facilitating the actions of *Da Huang* (Rheum).

The Messenger herb *Gan Cao* (Glycerrhiza) protects the Middle Burner from the strong herbs in the formula while mildly alleviating pain.

Cautions and Contraindications: This formula is contraindicated during pregnancy. When the patient has an Exterior disharmony, the Exterior should be released before using *Tao He Cheng Qi Tang*.

Dr. Xie's Comments: *Tao He Cheng Qi Tang* is often used in treating retained placenta, intestinal obstruction, and acute onset of endometritis due to Heat and Blood Stagnation in the Lower Burner in cows and horses.

Xue Fu Zhu Yu Tang (Stasis in the Mansion of Blood) 血府逐瘀汤

Xue is Blood. *Fu* means mansion or house. *Zhu* means eliminating. *Yu* means stasis or stagnation. *Tang* is decoction, the form of original herbal administration. *Xue Fu* together refers to the "mansion of Blood," which is the area above the diaphragm that Wang Qing-Ren found commonly to be full of Blood in his postmortem examinations. This formula is constructed to drive out stasis of Blood, particularly but not exclusively, above the diaphragm.

Source: *Yi Lin Gai Cuo* (*Corrections of Errors among Physicians*), written by *Wang Qing-Ren* and published in 1830 CE

Ingredients: The original formula for *Xue Fu Zhu Yu Tang* (Table 27.3) was made by boiling the ingredients together as a decoction.[2–4] *Xue Fu Zhu Yu Tang* is composed of 12 g *Tao Ren* (Persica), 9 g *Hong Hua* (Carthamus), 9 g *Dang Gui* (Angelica), 4.5 g *Chuan Xiong* (Ligusticum), 6 g *Chi Shao Yao* (Paeonia), 9 g *Niu Xi* (Cyathula), 3 g *Chai Hu* (Bupleurum), 4.5 g *Jie Geng* (Platycodon), 6 g *Zhi Ke* (Aurantium), 9 g *Sheng Di Huang* (Rehmannia), and 3 g *Gan Cao* (Glycyrrhiza).

Preparation:
1. Powder or capsule method: Herbs are ground into a fine powder. Powder can be encapsulated.
2. Decoction or teapill method: Raw herbs are mixed together and decocted. Herbal water extract (decoction) can be concentrated as granules or teapills.

Actions: Invigorate the Blood, dispel Blood Stasis, disperse Liver *Qi*, unblock the Channels and relieve pain

Indications: Chest pain evidenced by pain and resistance to thoracic compression; vomiting; depression; arrhythmias or cardiac murmurs; dark colored, benign, or malignant masses; insomnia; irritability; moodiness; a dark red tongue with lavender hue, or tortuous and lavender sublingual veins; and a choppy or wiry pulse

Table 27.3. Ingredients and actions of *Xue Fu Zhu Yu Tang*.

%	English Name	Chinese *Pin-Yin*	Actions
16	Persica	*Tao Ren*	Break Blood Stasis
12	Carthamus	*Hong Hua*	Invigorate Blood, dispel Blood Stasis and pain in chest
12	Angelica	*Dang Gui*	Nourish Blood, invigorate Blood
6	Ligusticum	*Chuan Xiong*	Invigorate *Qi* and Blood, relieve pain
8	Paeonia	*Chi Shao Yao*	Invigorate Blood, clear Heat and cool Blood
12	Cyathula	*Niu Xi*	Invigorate Blood and dispel Blood Stasis
4	Bupleurum	*Chai Hu*	Invigorate Liver *Qi*, relieve constraint
6	Platycodon	*Jie Geng*	Guide to upper *Jiao*, benefit throat and lungs
8	Aurantium	*Zhi Ke*	Move *Qi* and reduce distension
12	Rehmannia	*Sheng Di Huang*	Cool Blood, nourish Blood
4	Glycyrrhiza	*Gan Cao*	Reduce pain, harmonize

Dosage and Usage:
Horses and Cattle: 15–60 g, twice daily
Camels: 30–75 g, twice daily
Llamas, Alpacas, Goats, Sheep, and Pigs: 10–15 g, twice daily
Dogs: 0.5–5 g (or about 0.1 g per kg body weight), twice daily
Cats and Rabbits: 0.2–0.5 g (or about 0.1 g per kg body weight), twice daily
Birds: 0.1–0.2 g per kg body weight, twice daily

Use 3–6 weeks until primary clinical signs resolve. May be used for an extended duration if the disharmony persists.

Analysis of Formula: The King herbs in *Xue Fu Zhu Yu Tang* work together to invigorate the Blood and dispel Blood Stasis. *Tao Ren* (Persica), *Hong Hua* (Carthamus), and *Chuan Xiong* (Ligusticum) accomplish this. *Hong Hua* (Carthamus) has the added benefit of acting specifically in the chest. *Chuan Xiong* (Ligusticum) invigorates the Blood in any Pattern of Blood Stasis and, in particular, relieves headaches. *Niu Xi* (Cyathula) guides Blood Stasis downward from the Upper Burner; *Dang Gui* (Angelica) generates new Blood; and *Chi Shao Yao* (Paeonia) cools Blood that may be heated by chronic stasis. These three are the Minister herbs, which assist the King ingredients in invigorating the Blood. The Adjuvant herbs are *Sheng Di Huang* (Rehmannia), which cools and nourishes Blood; *Chai Hu* (Bupleurum), which relaxes constrained Liver *Qi*; *Jie Geng* (Platycodon), which expands the chest and acts as a Messenger herb to the Upper Burner; and *Zhi Ke* (Aurantium), which moves *Qi* and reduces distension. When distension is relieved, Blood is more easily invigorated. *Gan Cao* (Glycyrrhiza) is also a Messenger herb and acts to regulate and harmonize the other herbs in the formula while mildly relieving pain.

Cautions and Contraindications: Like many Blood-invigorating formulas, *Xue Fu Zhu Yu Tang* is contraindicated during pregnancy and for any disharmonies with bleeding diatheses.

Dr. Xie's Comments: In modern veterinary practice, *Xue Fu Zhu Yu Tang* is considered one of the main herbal formulas to move Blood and resolve stagnation. It is often used in treating general *Qi*-blood stagnation in the chest including endocarditis, pericarditis, vasculitis, valvular diseases, and heart failure. It can serve as the transporter herb to treat the metastatic or primary cancer in the chest together with other herbal formula(s) to break up Blood Stasis to shrink the tumor mass.

Clinical and Pharmacological Studies: The purpose of this study was to evaluate the cardioprotective effects of purified Salvia miltiorrhiza extract (PSME) on myocardial ischemia/reperfusion injury in isolated rat hearts. Hearts were excised and perfused at constant flow (7–9 ml/min(−1)) via the aorta. Non-recirculating perfusion with Krebs-Henseleit (KH) solution was maintained at 37°C and continuously gassed with 95% O_2 and 5% CO_2. KH solution with or without PSME (100 mg per liter solution) was used after 30 minutes of zero-flow ischemia for the PSME and control group, respectively. Left ventricular (LV) developed pressure, its derivatives, diastolic pressure, and so on were continuously recorded via a pressure transducer attached to a polyvinylchloride balloon that was placed in the left ventricle through an incision in the left atrium. PSME-treated hearts showed significant postischemic contractile function recovery (developed pressure recovered to 44.2 ± 4.9% versus 17.1 ± 5.7%, $P < 0.05$; maximum contraction recovered to 57.2 ± 5.9% versus 15.1 ± 6.3%, $P < 0.001$; maximum relaxation restored to 69.3 ± 7.3% versus 15.4 ± 6.3%, $P < 0.001$ in the PSME and control group, respectively). Significant elevation in end-diastolic pressure, which indicated LV stiffening in PSME hearts, might have resulted from the excessively high dose of PSME used. Further study will be conducted on the potential therapeutic value with a lower dose of PSME on prevention of ischemic heart disease.[7] Another study's objective was to investigate the effect of *Xue Fu Zhu Yu* Decoction (XFZYD) on the number, phenotype, cell cycle, and colony formation of bone marrow hematopoietic stem cells (HSC) in mice. Kunming mice were randomly divided into four groups: the control group, and the low- (3.25 g/kg), middle- (6.5 g/kg), and high-dose (13.0 g/kg) XFZYD groups. After they were medicated by gastrogavage with saline or corresponding dose of XFZYD for 7 days, their bone marrow HSC were separated and counted. The phenotype Sca and cell cycle of HSC were detected by flow cytometer, and the colony formation was determined with semisolid methyl media culture. The results showed that no obvious difference in the number of mononuclear-cell, suspended-cell, and colony production was found among all the groups ($P > 0.05$); the expression of CD34 and Sca-1 increased in the low-dose XFZYD group; but in the middle-dose XFZYD group increase showed only in Sca-1 expression.

CONCLUSION: XFZYD plays a role in removing Blood Stasis and promoting regeneration through improving hematopoietic function by means of increasing the number and enhancing the function of premature HSC.[8]

Ge Xia Zhu Yu Tang (Stasis below the Diaphragm) 膈下逐瘀汤

Ge means diaphragm. *Xia* means below. *Zhu* means eliminating. *Yu* means stasis or stagnation. and *Tang* is decoction, the form of original herbal administration. *Ge Xia Zhu Yu Tang* is a derivation of *Xue Fu Xue Yu Yang* that has its focus on driving out Blood Stasis directly below the diaphragm in the area commonly associated with the liver.

Source *Yi Lin Gai Cuo* (*Corrections of Errors Among Physicians*), written by *Wang Qing-Ren* and published in 1830 CE

Ingredients: The original formula for *Ge Xia Zhu Yu Tang* (Table 27.4) was made by boiling the ingredients together as a decoction.[2–4] *Ge Xia Zhu Yu Tang* is composed of 9 g *Wu Ling Zhi* (Trogopterus), 9 g *Dang Gui* (Angelica), 6 g *Chuan Xiong* (Ligusticum), 9 g *Tao Ren* (Persica), 6 g *Mu Dan Pi* (Moutan), 6 g *Chi Shao Yao* (Paeonia), 9 g *Wu Yao* (Lindera), 3 g *Yan Hu Suo* (Corydalis), 9 g *Gan Cao* (Glycerrhiza), 4.5 g *Xiang Fu* (Cyperus), 9 g *Hong Hua* (Carthamus), and 4.5 g *Zhi Ke* (Aurantium).

Preparation:

1. Powder or capsule method: Herbs are ground into a fine powder. Powder can be encapsulated.
2. Decoction or teapill method: Raw herbs are mixed together and decocted. Herbal water extract (decoction) can be concentrated as granules or teapills.

Actions: Invigorate Blood and *Qi*, dispel Blood Stasis, alleviate pain

Indications: Blood Stasis and Liver *Qi* stagnation leading to resistance and pain upon costal compression; palpable abdominal masses; fixed pain that is

Table 27.4. Ingredients and actions of *Ge Xia Zhu Yu Tang.*

%	English Name	Chinese *Pin-Yin*	Actions
10.7	Trogopterus	*Wu Ling Zhi*	Invigorate Blood
10.7	Angelica	*Dang Gui*	Nourish Blood, invigorate Blood
7.1	Ligusticum	*Chuan Xiong*	Invigorate *Qi* and Blood, relieve pain
10.7	Persica	*Tao Ren*	Break Blood Stasis
7.1	Moutan	*Mu Dan Pi*	Clear Heat, cool Blood, dispel Blood Stasis
7.1	Paeonia	*Chi Shao Yao*	Invigorate Blood, clear Heat and cool Blood
10.7	Lindera	*Wu Yao*	Move *Qi* and alleviate pain, warm and disperse *Qi* Stagnation
3.7	Corydalis	*Yan Hu Suo*	Invigorate Blood and *Qi*, alleviate pain
10.7	Glycyrrhiza	*Gan Cao*	Reduce pain, harmonize
5.4	Cyperus	*Xiang Fu*	Spread and regulate Liver *Qi*, reduce pain
10.7	Carthamus	*Hong Hua*	Invigorate Blood, dispel Blood Stasis
5.4	Aurantium	*Zhi Ke*	Move *Qi* and reduce distension

worse with pressure; a purple tongue center or sides; wiry or choppy pulse.

Dosage and Usage:
Horses and Cattle: 15 ± 60 g, twice daily
Camels: 30 ± 75 g, twice daily
Llamas, Alpacas, Goats, Sheep, and Pigs: 10 ± 15 g, twice daily
Dogs: 0.5 ± 5 g (or about 0.1 g per kg body weight), twice daily
Cats and Rabbits: 0.2 ± 0.5 g (or about 0.1 g per kg body weight), twice daily
Birds: 0.1 ± 0.2 g per kg body weight, twice daily

Use 3 ± 6 weeks until primary clinical signs resolve. May be used for an extended duration if the disharmony persists.

Analysis of Formula: The King ingredients to dispel Blood Stasis in the abdomen are *Wu Ling Zhi* (Trogopterus) and *Yan Hu Suo* (Corydalis). *Tao Ren* (Persica) and *Hong Hua* (Carthamus) are the Minister herbs to break up Blood Stasis. These four ingredients synergistically work to invigorate Blood and alleviate pain. Three Adjuvant herbs, *Chuan Xiong* (Ligusticum), *Zhi Ke* (Aurantium), and *Xiang Fu* (Cyperus), reduce pain and hypochondriac distention by moving and dispersing stagnant Liver *Qi*. Two more Adjuvant herbs, *Mu Dan Pi* (Moutan) and *Chi Shao Yao* (Paeonia), cool the Blood that is heated by constraint and further invigorate the Blood to remove Blood Stasis. The last two Adjuvant herbs are *Dang Gui* (Angelica) and *Wu Yao* (Lindera). *Dang Gui* (Angelica) nourishes Blood to replace Blood damaged by Heat, and *Wu Yao* (Lindera) activates and warms the Channels to disperse Blood Stasis and counteract the cooling tendencies of *Mu Dan Pi* (Moutan) and *Chi Shao Yao* (Paeonia). *Gan Cao* (Glycerrhiza) serves as the Messenger herb to coordinate all other herbs.

Cautions and Contraindications: Like many Blood-invigorating formulas, *Ge Xia Zhu Yu Tang* is contraindicated during pregnancy and for any disharmonies with bleeding diatheses.

Dr. Xie's Comments: In modern veterinary practice, *Ge Xia Zhu Yu Tang* is often used as the transporter to treat tumor masses around the diaphragm.

Shao Fu Zhu Yu Tang (Stasis in the Lower Abdomen) 少腹逐瘀汤

Shao means lower. *Fu* here is abdomen. *Zhu* means eliminating. *Yu* means stasis or stagnation. *Tang* is decoction, the form of original herbal administration. *Shao Fu Zhu Yu Tang* is a derivation of *Xue Fu Xue Yu Yang* that has its focus on driving out Blood Stasis from the lower abdomen, particularly around the uterus and prostate.

Source: *Yi Lin Gai Cuo* (*Corrections of Errors among Physicians*), written by *Wang Qing-Ren* and published in 1830 CE

Ingredients: The original formula for *Shao Fu Zhu Yu Tang* (Table 27.5) was made by boiling the ingredients together as a decoction.[2–4] *Shao Fu Zhu Yu Tang* is composed of 1.5 g *Xiao Hui Xiang* (Foeniculum), 0.6 g *Gan Jiang* (Zingiberis), 3 g *Yan Hu Suo* (Corydalis), 9 g *Dang Gui* (Angelica), 3 g *Chuan Xiong* (Ligusticum), 3 g *Mo Yao* (Myrrh), 3 g *Rou Gui* (Cinnamomum), 6 g *Chi Shao Yao* (Paeonia), 9 g *Pu Huang* (Typha), and 6 g *Wu Ling Zhi* (Trogopterus).

Preparation:
1. Powder or capsule method: Herbs are ground into a fine powder. Powder can be encapsulated.
2. Decoction or teapill method: Raw herbs are mixed together and decocted. Herbal water extract (decoction) can be concentrated as granules or teapills.

Actions: Invigorate Blood, dispel Blood Stasis, warm the Channels and alleviate pain

Indications: Blood Stasis in the caudal abdomen that results in either 1) palpable masses that may or may not be painful, or 2) caudal abdominal pain without palpable masses. There may caudal abdominal and

Table 27.5. Ingredients and actions of *Shao Fu Zhu Yu Tang.*

%	English Name	Chinese *Pin-Yin*	Actions
3	Foeniculum	*Xiao Hui Xiang*	Spread Liver *Qi*, regulate Middle *Jiao Qi*
1	Zingiberis	*Gan Jiang*	Warm Middle *Jiao*, warm channels and stop bleeding
7	Corydalis	*Yan Hu Suo*	Invigorate Blood and *Qi* and alleviate pain
20	Angelica	*Dang Gui*	Nourish Blood, invigorate Blood
7	Ligusticum	*Chuan Xiong*	Invigorate *Qi* and Blood, relieve pain
7	Myrrh	*Mo Yao*	Invigorate Blood and dispel Blood Stasis
7	Cinnamomum	*Rou Gui*	Warm the Middle *Jiao*, dry dampness
14	Paeonia	*Chi Shao Yao*	Invigorate Blood, clear Heat and cool Blood
20	Typha	*Pu Huang*	Stop Bleeding, invigorate Blood and dispel Blood Stasis
14	Trogopterus	*Wu Ling Zhi*	Disperse Blood Stasis, alleviate pain, stop bleeding

lumbar pain during estrus, abnormally frequent estrous cycles, or excessive Blood loss during estrus. There will commonly be a purple tongue and a tight to wiry pulse.

Dosage and Usage:

Horses and Cattle: 15–60 g, twice daily
Camels: 30–75 g, twice daily
Llamas, Alpacas, Goats, Sheep, and Pigs: 10–15 g, twice daily
Dogs: 0.5–5 g (or about 0.1 g per kg body weight), twice daily
Cats and Rabbits: 0.2–0.5 g (or about 0.1 g per kg body weight), twice daily
Birds: 0.1–0.2 g per kg body weight, twice daily

Use 1–3 weeks until primary clinical signs resolve. Do not use for extended duration.

Analysis of Formula: The herbs in this formula invigorate the Blood to dispel Blood Stasis but also function to warm the uterus and lower abdomen and stop excessive estrous Blood loss. The King herbs, serving to dispel Blood Stasis, are *Yan Hu Suo* (Corydalis), which dispels Blood Stasis in the abdomen and alleviates pain; *Chuan Xiong* (Ligusticum), which invigorates both *Qi* and Blood to relieve pain; and *Mo Yao* (Myrrh), which dispels Blood Stasis from abdominal masses. There are three Minister herbs: *Xiao Hui Xiang* (Foeniculum) helps spread Liver *Qi* while warming the Middle and Lower Burner; *Chi Shao Yao* (Paeonia) invigorates Blood, clears Heat, and cools Blood; and *Dang Gui* (Angelica) invigorates Blood and promotes the generation of new Blood. The other four herbs in this formula are Adjuvant herbs. *Gan Jiang* (Zingiberis) stops bleeding and *Rou Gui* (Cinnamomum) dries Dampness. These two Adjuvant herbs also serve to further warm the Middle and Lower Burners. *Pu Huang* (Typha) and *Wu Ling Zhi* (Trogopterus) further dispel Blood Stasis while acting to stop bleeding.

Cautions and Contraindications: Like many Blood-invigorating formulas, *Shao Fu Zhu Yu Tang* is contraindicated during pregnancy and any disharmonies with bleeding diatheses.

Dr. Xie's Comments: In modern veterinary practice, *Shao Fu Zhu Yu Tang* is often used as the transporter to treat tumor masses around the small intestines, uterus, prostate, adrenal gland, and kidney.

Tao Hong Si Wu Tang (Persica and Carthamus) 桃红四物汤

This formula is simply named for the modification of *Si Wu Tang* (Four Substances) with the pair of Blood invigorating herbs ***Tao*** *Ren* (Persica) and ***Hong*** *Hua* (Carthamus). *Tang* is decoction, the form of the original administration.

Source: *Yi Zong Jin Jian* (*Golden Mirror of the Medical Tradition*), written by *Wu Qian* et al. and published in 1742 CE

Ingredients: The original formula for *Tao Hong Si Wu Tang* (Table 27.6) was made by boiling the ingredients together as a decoction.[2–4] *Tao Hong Si Wu Tang* is composed of 3 g *Chuan Xiong* (Ligusticum), 6 g *Dang Gui* (Angelica), 6 g *Bai Shao Yao* (Paeonia), 6 g *Shu Di Huang* (Rehmannia), 6 g *Tao Ren* (Persica), and 3 g *Hong Hua* (Carthamus).

Preparation:

1. Powder or capsule method: Herbs are ground into a fine powder. Powder can be encapsulated.

Table 27.6. Ingredients and actions of *Tao Hong Si Wu Tang.*

%	English Name	Chinese *Pin-Yin*	Actions
10	Ligusticum	*Chuan Xiong*	Invigorate *Qi* and Blood, relieve pain
20	Angelica	*Dang Gui*	Nourish Blood, invigorate Blood
20	Paeonia	*Bai Shao Yao*	Nourish Blood
20	Rehmannia	*Shu Di Huang*	Tonify Blood, nourish *Yin*
20	Persica	*Tao Ren*	Break up Blood Stasis
10	Carthamus	*Hong Hua*	Invigorate Blood, dispel Blood Stasis

2. Decoction or teapill method: Raw herbs are mixed together and decocted. Herbal water extract (decoction) can be concentrated as granules or teapills.

Actions: Nourish Blood, invigorate Blood, dispel Blood Stasis

Indications: Blood deficiency with mild Blood Stagnation leading to a deranged or shortened estrous cycle with excessive bleeding of dark, tenacious Blood with or without clots. This formula may also be used for trauma with concurrent Blood deficiency. Typically these patients present with a pale-purple tongue and thin, wiry pulse.

Dosage and Usage:
Horses and Cattle: 15–60 g, twice daily
Camels: 30–75 g, twice daily
Llamas, Alpacas, Goats, Sheep, and Pigs: 10–15 g, twice daily
Dogs: 0.5–5 g (or about 0.1 g per kg body weight), twice daily
Cats and Rabbits: 0.2–0.5 g (or about 0.1 g per kg body weight), twice daily
Birds: 0.1–0.2 g per kg body weight, twice daily

Use 1–3 weeks until primary clinical signs resolve. May be used for a more extended duration if signs of blood deficiency and mild stagnation persist.

Analysis of Formula: This formula is *Si Wu Tang* or Four Substances (Chapter 18), modified with two Blood-invigorating herbs. Serving as the King herbs, *Shu Di Huang* (Rehmannia) and *Bai Shao Yao* (Paeonia), work together to nourish Blood and *Yin*. The Minister herb, *Dang Gui* (Angelica), nourishes and invigorates Blood, thus countering the potential Blood-stagnating effect of the King herbs. *Chuan Xiong* (Ligusticum) invigorates both *Qi* and Blood and relieves pain. The pair of Blood-invigorating herbs, *Tao Ren* (Persica) and *Hong Hua* (Carthamus), both serve to dispel Blood Stasis and relieve pain. The last three ingredients are the Adjuvant and Messenger herbs.

Cautions and Contraindications: This formula is contraindicated during pregnancy.

Dr. Xie's Comments: In modern veterinary practice, *Tao Hong Si Wu Tang* is often used in treating poor performance or postparturition syndrome due to Blood Deficiency with Blood Stagnation.

Shen Tong Zhu Yu Tang (Body Sore) 身痛逐瘀汤

Shen means the body. *Tong* is pain or soreness. *Zhu* means eliminating. *Yu* means stasis or stagnation. *Tang* is decoction, the form of original herbal administration. *Shen Tong Zhu Yu Tang* is a derivation of *Xue Fu Xue Yu Yang*, which has its focus on driving out Blood Stasis from the Channels and collaterals of the entire body.

Source: *Yi Lin Gai Cuo* (*Corrections of Errors among Physicians*), written by *Wang Qing-Ren* and published in 1830 CE

Ingredients: The original formula for *Shen Tong Zhu Yu Tang* (Table 27.7) was made by boiling the ingredients together as a decoction.[2–4] *Shen Tong Zhu Yu Tang* is composed of 3 g *Qin Jiao* (Gentiana), 6 g *Chuan Xiong* (Ligusticum), 9 g *Tao Ren* (Persica), 12 g *Hong Hua* (Carthamus), 6 g *Gan Cao* (Glycyrrhiza), 3 g *Qiang Huo* (Notopterygium), 6 g *Mo Yao* (Myrrh), 9 g *Dang Gui* (Angelica), 6 g *Wu Ling Zhi* (Trogopterus), 3 g *Xiang Fu* (Cyperus), 9 g *Chuan Niu Zi* (Cyathula), and 6 g *Di Long* (Pheretima).

Preparation:
1. Powder or capsule method: Herbs are ground into a fine powder. Powder can be encapsulated.
2. Decoction or teapill method: Raw herbs are mixed together and decocted. Herbal water extract (decoction) can be concentrated as granules or teapills.

Actions: Invigorate Blood and *Qi*, dispel Blood Stasis, unblock the Channels and collaterals, unblock painful obstruction and relieve pain

Table 27.7. Ingredients and actions of *Shen Tong Zhu Yu Tang*.

%	English Name	Chinese *Pin-Yin*	Actions
4	Gentiana	*Qin Jiao*	Dispel wind-damp, relax sinews, relieve pain
8	Ligusticum	*Chuan Xiong*	Invigorate *Qi* and Blood, relieve pain
12	Persica	*Tao Ren*	Break up Blood Stasis
12	Carthamus	*Hong Hua*	Invigorate Blood, dispel Blood Stasis
8	Glycyrrhiza	*Gan Cao*	Reduce pain, harmonize
4	Notopterygium	*Qiang Huo*	Unblock painful obstruction and alleviate pain
8	Myrrh	*Mo Yao*	Invigorate Blood and dispel Blood Stasis
12	Angelica	*Dang Gui*	Nourish Blood, invigorate Blood
8	Trogopterus	*Wu Ling Zhi*	Disperse Blood Stasis, alleviate pain
4	Cyperus	*Xiang Fu*	Spread and regulate Liver *Qi*, reduce pain
12	Cyathula	*Chuan Niu Zi*	Expel Wind-Damp and relieve pain
8	Pheretima	*Di Long*	Promote movement in the channels and collaterals

Indications: Stagnation of Blood and *Qi* in the Channels and collaterals leading to clinical signs of pain in both the appendicular and axial musculoskeletal system. This is the most commonly used herbal formula for arthralgia accompanied by a purple tongue and tight or wiry pulse.

Dosage and Usage:
Horses and Cattle: 15–60g, twice daily
Camels: 30–75g, twice daily
Llamas, Alpacas, Goats, Sheep, and Pigs: 10–15g, twice daily
Dogs: 0.5–5g (or about 0.1g per kg body weight), twice daily
Cats and Rabbits: 0.2–0.5g (or about 0.1g per kg body weight), twice daily
Birds: 0.1–0.2g per kg body weight, twice daily

Use 1–3 months until primary clinical signs resolve. May be used for extended duration of 6–12 months for unremitting Blood Stagnation pain.

Analysis of Formula: The King herbs in this formula invigorate Blood and dispel Blood Stasis. These include *Tao Ren* (Persica), *Hong Hua* (Carthamus), *Mo Yao* (Myrrh), and *Wu Ling Zhi* (Trogopterus), which all work together synergistically to dispel Blood Stasis and alleviate pain. The Minister herbs, *Chuan Xiong* (Ligusticum) and *Xiang Fu* (Cyperus), both further serve to alleviate pain by invigorating *Qi* stagnation. The Adjuvant herbs *Qin Jiao* (Gentiana), *Qiang Huo* (Notopterygium), and *Chuan Niu Zi* (Cyathula) expel Wind-Damp from the Channels, unblock the sinews, and relieve pain. *Dang Gui* (Angelica), a fourth Adjuvant herb, assists by both generating new Blood and mildly invigorating Blood Stasis. The first Messenger herb, *Di Long* (Pheretima), serves to transport the remainder of the herbs into the Channels and collaterals. The second Messenger herb, *Gan Cao* (Glycyrrhiza), both harmonizes the formula and mildly relieves pain.

Cautions and Contraindications: Like many Blood-invigorating formulas, *Shen Tong Zhu Yu Tang* is contraindicated during pregnancy and for any disharmonies with bleeding diatheses.

Dr. Xie's Comments: In modern veterinary practice, *Shen Tong Zhu Yu Tang* is often used in treating generalized back soreness and pain in muscles and joints due to *Qi*-Blood Stagnation.

Yan Hu Suo Tang (Corydalis Decoction) 延胡索汤

This formula is named for its powerful King ingredient, *Yan Hu Suo*, or Corydalis. *Tang* is decoction, the form of original herbal medication. Thus, *Yan Hu Suo Tang* translates literally to Corydalis Decoction.

Source: *Ji Sheng Fang* (*Formulas to Aid the Living*), written by *Yan Yong-He* and published in 1253 CE

Ingredients: The original formula for *Yan Hu Suo Tang* (Table 27.8) was made by grinding the ingredients together as a coarse powder and drinking the liquid off of the dregs.[2–4] *Yan Hu Suo Tang* is composed of 45g *Yan Hu Suo* (Corydalis), 15g *Pu Huang* (Typha), 15g *Chi Shao Yao* (Paeonia), 15g *Dang Gui* (Angelica), 15g *Rou Gui* (Cinnamomum), 90g *Jiang Huang* (Curcuma), 90g *Ru Xiang* (Olibanum), 90g *Mo Yao* (Myrrh), 90g *Mu Xiang* (Saussurea), and 7.5g *Gan Cao* (Glycerrhiza).

Preparation:
1. Powder or capsule method: Herbs are ground into a fine powder. Powder can be encapsulated.
2. Decoction or teapill method: Raw herbs are mixed together and decocted. Herbal water extract (decoction) can be concentrated as granules or teapills.

Actions: Invigorate *Qi* and Blood, dispel Blood Stasis, alleviate pain

Indications: Stagnation of Blood and *Qi* due to cold invasion or emotional lability that leads to epigastric or abdominal pain; lumbar pain; reproductive organ pain and/or irregular estrous with dark, clotted Blood; a purple tongue; a tight to wiry pulse

Dosage and Usage:
Horses and Cattle: 15–60g, twice daily
Camels: 30–75g, twice daily
Llamas, Alpacas, Goats, Sheep, and Pigs: 10–15g, twice daily

Table 27.8. Ingredients and actions of *Yan Hu Suo Tang*.

%	English Name	Chinese *Pin-Yin*	Actions
10	Corydalis	*Yan Hu Suo*	Invigorate Blood and *Qi* and alleviate pain
3	Typha	*Pu Huang*	Stop Bleeding, invigorate Blood and dispel Blood Stasis
3	Paeonia	*Chi Shao Yao*	Invigorate Blood, clear Heat and cool Blood
3	Angelica	*Dang Gui*	Nourish Blood, invigorate Blood
3	Cinnamomum	*Rou Gui*	Warm the Middle *Jiao*, dry dampness
19	Curcuma	*Jiang Huang*	Invigorate Blood and *Qi*, expel Wind-Damp, alleviate pain
19	Olibanum	*Ru Xiang*	Invigorate Blood and *Qi*, reduce swelling
19	Myrrh	*Mo Yao*	Invigorate Blood and dispel Blood Stasis
19	Saussurea	*Mu Xiang*	Move *Qi*, alleviate pain
2	Glycerrhiza	*Gan Cao*	Reduce pain, harmonize

Dogs: 0.5–5 g (or about 0.1 g per kg body weight), twice daily
Cats and Rabbits: 0.2–0.5 g (or about 0.1 g per kg body weight), twice daily
Birds: 0.1–0.2 g per kg body weight, twice daily
Use 2–6 weeks until primary clinical signs resolve. Do not use for extended duration.

Analysis of Formula: The King ingredient, *Yan Hu Suo* (Corydalis), is the premier herb in the TCVM Materia Medica to alleviate pain by invigorating *Qi* and Blood, particularly in the reproductive organs. The formula has two groups of Minister herbs. The first group, *Ru Xiang* (Olibanum) and *Mo Yao* (Myrrh), invigorates Blood and dispels Blood Stasis. The second group of Minister herbs, *Mu Xiang* (Saussurea) and *Jiang Huang* (Curcuma), moves *Qi* and alleviates pain. Together these four herbs increase the Blood-invigorating and *Qi*-moving effect of the King herb. There are three Adjuvant herbs: *Dang Gui* (Angelica) serves to nourish Blood to counteract Blood loss and mildly invigorate the Blood; *Chi Shao Yao* (Paeonia) cools the Blood, which tends to become hot when it is Stagnant, clears Heat, and further invigorates Blood; and *Pu Huang* (Typha) stops excessive bleeding caused by stagnant, hot Blood leaving the vessels and invigorates Blood to dispel Blood Stasis. There are two Messenger herbs: *Rou Gui* (Cinnamomum) serves to guide the formula into the Middle and Lower Burner as well as warm the Channels. *Gan Cao* (Glycyrrhiza) harmonizes the formula and mildly relieves pain while protecting the stomach.

Cautions and Contraindications: This formula is contraindicated during pregnancy.

Dr. Xie's Comments: *Yan Hu Suo Tang* is useful in treating colic due to Blood Stagnation in the abdomen.

Bu Yang Huan Wu Tang (Tonifying *Yang* to Restore Five-Tenths) 补阳还五汤

Bu means tonifying. *Huan* means restore. *Wu* refers to five out of ten. *Tang* is decoction, the form of original herbal medication. Wang Qing-Ren noted that five-tenths (or one-half) of the body's true *Qi* was injured or lost when suffering from a disharmony, which induced hemiparesis or hemiplegia. The name, *Bu Yang Huan Wu Tang*, or Tonifying *Yang* to Restore Five-Tenths Decoction reflects that observation.

Source: *Yi Lin Gai Cuo* (*Corrections of Errors among Physicians*), written by *Wang Qing-Ren* and published in 1830 CE

Ingredients: The original formula for *Bu Yang Huan Wu Tang* (Table 27.9) was made by grinding the ingredients together as a coarse powder and drinking the liquid off of the dregs.[2–4] *Bu Yang Huan Wu Tang* is composed of 120 g *Huang Qi* (Astragalus), 6 g *Dang Gui* (Angelica), 3 g *Chuan Xiong* (Ligusticum), 4.5 g *Chi Shao Yao* (Paeonia), 3 g *Tao Ren* (Persica), 3 g *Hong Hua* (Carthamus), and 3 g *Di Long* (Pheretima).

Table 27.9. Ingredients and actions of *Bu Yang Huan Wu Tang*.

%	English Name	Chinese *Pin-Yin*	Actions
84.2	Astragalus	*Huang Qi*	Tonify *Qi* and Blood, raise the *Yang Qi*
4.2	Angelica	*Dang Gui*	Nourish Blood, invigorate Blood
2.1	Ligusticum	*Chuan Xiong*	Invigorate *Qi* and Blood, relieve pain
3.2	Paeonia	*Chi Shao Yao*	Invigorate Blood, clear Heat and cool Blood
2.1	Persica	*Tao Ren*	Break up Blood Stasis
2.1	Carthamus	*Hong Hua*	Invigorate Blood, dispel Blood Stasis
2.1	Pheretima	*Di Long*	Promote movement in the channels and collaterals

Preparation:
1. Powder or capsule method: Herbs are ground into a fine powder. Powder can be encapsulated.
2. Decoction or teapill method: Raw herbs are mixed together and decocted. Herbal water extract (decoction) can be concentrated as granules or teapills.

Actions: Tonify *Qi*, invigorate Blood, dispel Blood Stasis, unblock Channels

Indications: *Qi* deficiency with Blood Stasis blocking the Channels with signs of hemiparesis or hemiparalysis such as atrophy and weakness of the hind limbs; circling to one side; urinary and occasionally fecal incontinence; pale purple tongue with a thin clear or white coat and a slow, weak, or frail pulse

Dosage and Usage:
Horses and Cattle: 15–60 g, twice daily
Camels: 30–75 g, twice daily
Llamas, Alpacas, Goats, Sheep, and Pigs: 10–15 g, twice daily
Dogs: 0.5–5 g (or about 0.1 g per kg body weight), twice daily
Cats and Rabbits: 0.2–0.5 g (or about 0.1 g per kg body weight), twice daily
Birds: 0.1–0.2 g per kg body weight, twice daily
Use 4–8 weeks until all clinical signs and any *Qi* deficiency resolve.

Analysis of Formula: The King ingredient, *Huang Qi* (Astragalus), tonifies *Qi*, mildly tonifies Blood, and raises the *Yang Qi*. A large dose is used in this formula to treat severe *Qi* deficiency. The Minister herbs, *Dang Gui* (Angelica), *Chuan Xiong* (Ligusticum), and *Chi Shao Yao* (Paeonia), invigorate and nourish the Blood and alleviate pain. The Adjuvant herbs, *Tao Ren* (Persica) and *Hong Hua* (Carthamus), further serve to invigorate the Blood and dispel Blood Stasis. *Di Long* (Pheretima) acts as both an Adjuvant herb in moving stagnant *Qi* and invigorating the Channels, and as a Messenger herb to direct the formula into the Channels.

Cautions and Contraindications: This formula breaks Blood Stasis and should be used only when there are no indications of active hemorrhage. Because it so strongly tonifies deficiency, *Bu Yang Huan Wu Tang* should not be used for excess conditions evidenced by a strong pulse. It should also be avoided when there is Liver Wind or *Yin* deficiency. This formula is contraindicated during pregnancy.

Dr. Xie's Comment: *Bu Yang Huan Wu Tang* is used very effectively in treating rear weakness, paresis, and paralysis when it is combined with acupuncture. One-half of the clinical effect is achieved from acupuncture and the other half (50%) comes from this herbal medication. Thus, it is called *Huan Wu* (restoring the functions by 50% or five-tenths).

Fu Yuan Huo Xue Tang (Restoring Health by Invigoration) 复元活血汤

Fu means restore or revive. *Yuan* means original (normal), healthy status. *Huo* means activating or invigoration. *Xue* is Blood. *Tang* is decoction, the form of original herbal medication. When Blood Stasis occurs, health is devitalized. This formula restores health by invigorating Blood Stasis.

Source: *Yi Xue Fa Ming* (*Medical Innovations*), written by *Li Ao* and published during the *Jian* Dynasty (from 1115 to 1234 CE).

Ingredients: The original formula for *Fu Yuan Huo Xue Tang* (Table 27.10) was made by grinding the ingredients together as a coarse powder and drinking the liquid off of the dregs.[2–4] *Fu Yuan Huo Xue Tang* is composed of 9g *Dang Gui* (Angelica), 9g *Tao Ren* (Persica), 6g *Hong Hua* (Carthamus), 6g *Chuan Shan Jia* (Manitis) (in modern practice, substitute *Wang Bu Liu Xing*, (Vaccaria) for Manitis, 30g *Da Huang* (Rheum), 9g *Tian Hua Fen* (Trichosanthes), 15g *Chai Hu* (Bupleurum), and 6g *Gan Cao* (Glycyrrhiza).

Table 27.10. Ingredients and actions of *Fu Yuan Huo Xue Tang*.

%	English Name	Chinese *Pin-Yin*	Actions
10	Angelica	*Dang Gui*	Nourish Blood, invigorate Blood
10	Persica	*Tao Ren*	Break up Blood Stasis
7	Carthamus	*Hong Hua*	Invigorate Blood, dispel Blood Stasis
7	Manitis*	*Chuan Shan Jia*	Dispel Blood Stasis, reduce swelling, expel Wind-Dampness from channels
33	Rheum	*Da Huang*	Drain Heat, drain Damp-Heat, invigorate the Blood
10	Trichosanthes	*Tian Hua Fen*	Drain Heat, generate fluids and flesh, relieve toxicity and expel purulent material
16	Bupleurum	*Chai Hu*	Invigorate Liver *Qi*, relieve constraint
7	Glycyrrhiza	*Gan Cao*	Reduce pain, harmonize

*Manitis is substituted with Vaccaria (*Wang Bu Liu Xing*) in modern practice.

Preparation:

1. Powder or capsule method: Herbs are ground into a fine powder. Powder can be encapsulated.
2. Decoction or teapill method: Raw herbs are mixed together and decocted. Herbal water extract (decoction) can be concentrated as granules or teapills.

Actions: Promote Blood circulation, dispel Blood Stasis, move Liver *Qi*, unblock Channels

Indications: Blood Stasis and *Qi* stagnation in the chest, hypochondriac area, and lateral thorax and abdomen from traumatic injury. The pain is commonly localized and severe, is worse with pressure, may be accompanied by bruising and swelling, and is accompanied by a purple tongue and a wiry pulse.

Dosage and Usage:

Horses and Cattle: 15–60g, twice daily
Camels: 30–75g, twice daily
Llamas, Alpacas, Goats, Sheep, and Pigs: 10–15g, twice daily
Dogs: 0.5–5g (or about 0.1g per kg body weight), twice daily
Cats and Rabbits: 0.2–0.5g (or about 0.1g per kg body weight), twice daily
Birds: 0.1–0.2g per kg body weight, twice daily
Use 1–3 weeks until primary clinical signs resolve.

Analysis of Formula: The wine-prepared *Da Huang* (Rheum) is the King herb, which invigorates Blood, dispels Blood Stasis, and directs the stagnant Upper Burner *Qi* downward. The Minister herbs include *Dang Gui* (Angelica), which generates new Blood; *Tao Ren*

(Persica), *Hong Hua* (Carthamus), and *Chuan Shan Jia* (Mantis) which reduce painful swelling in the chest; and *Tian Hua Fen* (Trichosanthes), which drains Heat from stagnation and generates new flesh. The King and Minister ingredients work synergistically to invigorate Blood, dispel Blood Stasis, and reduce swelling. The Adjuvant herb *Chai Hu* (Bupleurum) moves stagnant Liver *Qi* and acts as a Messenger herb to direct the formula into the lateral and ventral thoracic Liver Channel. *Gan Cao* (Glycyrrhiza) is also a Messenger herb, working to both harmonize the formula and mildly relieve pain.

Cautions and Contraindications: This formula is contraindicated in pregnancy and weak patients.

Dr. Xie's Comments: In TCVM theory, "new blood will not be generated until the old (stagnant) blood is removed." Thus, *Fu Yuan Huo Xue Tang* is like hemo-acupuncture therapy, which also works on the principle that new blood will be generated and will circulate as soon as the old blood (stagnation) is removed from the body. Because it is a very potent blood mover, the dosage of *Fu Yuan Huo Xue Tang* should be decreased or the formula discontinued as soon as pain (stagnation) is reduced or relieved.

Qi Li San (Seven-Thousandths) 七厘散

This formula is named for the original dosage to be taken. *Qi* means seven. *Li* is a measurement unit for weight in ancient China. *Liang* is the basic measure, about 31 grams. 1 *liang* = 1000 *li*. Thus, *Li* is one-thousandth (1/1000) and means a very small amount. *Qi Li* means seven-thousandths.

Source: *Liang Fang Ji Ye (Small Collection of Fine Formulas)*, written by *Xie Yuan-Qing*, 1842 CE 良方集腋

Ingredients: The original formula for *Qi Li San* (Table 27.11) was made by grinding the ingredients together as a fine powder and taking 0.25–1.5 g with yellow wine or water.[2–4] *Qi Li San* is composed of 30 g *Xue Jie* (Draconis), 4.5 g *Hong Hua* (Carthamus), 4.5 g *Ru Xiang* (Olibanum), 4.5 g *Mo Yao* (Myrrh), 0.36 g *She Xiang* (Moschus), 0.36 g *Bing Pian* (Borneol), 7.5 g *Er Cha* (Acacia), and 3.6 g *Zhu Sha* (Cinnabaris). (Listed for historical accuracy. Cinnabaris (*Zhu Sha*) is considered too toxic to ingest; please omit).

Preparation:

1. Powder or capsule method: Herbs are ground into a fine powder. Powder can be encapsulated.
2. Decoction or teapill method: Raw herbs are mixed together and decocted. Herbal water extract (decoction) can be concentrated as granules or teapills.

Table 27.11. Ingredients and actions of *Qi Li San*.

%	English Name	Chinese *Pin-Yin*	Actions
54	Sanguis Draconis	*Xue Jie*	Dispel Blood Stasis, alleviate pain, stop bleeding
8.1	Carthamus	*Hong Hua*	Invigorate Blood, dispel Blood Stasis
8.1	Olibanum	*Ru Xiang*	Invigorate Blood and *Qi*, reduce swelling
8	Myrrh	*Mo Yao*	Invigorate Blood and dispel Blood Stasis
0.65	Moschus	*She Xiang*	Invigorate Blood, reduce swelling, alleviate pain
0.65	Borneol	*Bing Pian*	Clear Heat, alleviate pain, dissipate nodules
14	Acacia	*Er Cha*	Drain Damp, absorb seepage
6.5	Cinnabaris*	*Zhu Sha*	Clear Heat, relieve toxicity

*Cinnabaris is listed for historical accuracy. Cinnabaris (*Zhu Sha*) is considered too toxic to ingest; please omit.

Actions: Invigorate Blood, dispel Blood Stasis, reduce swelling, stop bleeding and alleviate pain

Indications: Traumatic injuries that manifest either externally or internally with pain, bruises, lacerations, tissue swelling, fractures, burns and abrasions, and bleeding

Dosage and Usage: Use topical application only if the ingredients contain Cinnabaris (*Zhu Sha*). If there is no Cinnabaris, this formula may be used orally for 1–3 weeks until primary clinical signs resolve. Do not use for extended duration.

Analysis of Formula: The King ingredient, *Xue Jie* (Sanguis Draconis), alleviates pain and is one of only a few herbs that can simultaneously dispel Blood Stasis and stop bleeding. The Minister herb, *Hong Hua* (Carthamus), dispels Blood Stasis from wounds and other trauma, and invigorates Blood. *Ru Xiang* (Olibanum) and *Mo Yao* (Myrrh) invigorate Blood, dispel Blood Stasis, and promote healing of injured tissues when used topically, by reducing swelling and generating flesh. *She Xiang* (Moschus) and *Bing Pian* (Borneol) are aromatic herbs that assist in invigorating Blood, clearing the Channels of stagnation, and regenerating flesh when applied topically. *Er Cha* (Acacia) clears Heat and Damp from the injuries and helps reduce bleeding. These last five herbs are the Adjuvant herbs.

Cautions and Contraindications: This formula is contraindicated during pregnancy.

Dr. Xie's Comment: *Qi Li San* was originally designed for topical application. It is very toxic when taken orally, because one ingredient, *Zhu Sha* (Cinnabaris), contains the heavy metal mercury. Even ancient practitioners recognized this toxicity because only "seven-thousandths" was used if it was necessary to use orally. Today, *Zhu Sha* (Cinnabaris) is no longer used and the formula can be taken orally or applied topically.

Die Da Wan (Trauma Pill) 跌打丸

Die means falling down. *Da* means traumatic injuries from being punched, kicked or bit, or being in a crash. *Wan* is pill, the form of herbal administration. This formula is simply named for its efficacy and primary intended usage, to treat trauma-induced soft tissue injury.

Source: *Quan Guo Zhong Cheng Yao Chu Fang Ji* (*National Collection of Chinese Herbal Prepared Medicines*). Its authors are unknown and it was published in post-1949 China.

Ingredients: The original formula for *Die Da Wan* (Table 27.12) was made by grinding the ingredients together as a fine powder and forming into pills with honey.[2–4] *Die Dan Wan* is composed of 30g *Dang Gui* (Angelica), 30g *Chuan Xiong* (Ligusticum), 60g *Ru Xiang* (Olibinum), 30g *Mo Yao* (Myrrh), 30g *Xue Jie* (Sanguis Draconis), 30g *Tu Bie Chong* (Eupolyphaga), 60g *Ma Huang* (Ephedra), and 30g *Zi Ran Tong* (Pyritum).

Table 27.12. Ingredients and actions of *Die Da Wan*.

%	English Name	Chinese *Pin-Yin*	Actions
10	Angelica	*Dang Gui*	Nourish Blood, invigorate Blood
10	Ligusticum	*Chuan Xiong*	Invigorate *Qi* and Blood, relieve pain
20	Olibinum	*Ru Xiang*	Invigorate Blood and *Qi*, reduce swelling
10	Myrhh	*Mo Yao*	Invigorate Blood and dispel Blood Stasis
10	Sanguis Draconis	*Xue Jie*	Dispel Blood Stasis, alleviate pain, stop bleeding
10	Eupolyphaga	*Tu Bie Chong*	Break up and drive out blood Stasis, renew sinews and join bones
20	Ephedra	*Ma Huang*	Envoy to the muscles and exterior
10	Pyritum	*Zi Ran Tong*	Dispel Blood Stasis and promote healing of bones and sinews

Preparation:

1. Powder or capsule method: Herbs are ground into a fine powder. Powder can be encapsulated.
2. Decoction or teapill method: Raw herbs are mixed together and decocted. Herbal water extract (decoction) can be concentrated as granules or teapills.

Actions: Invigorate Blood, transform Blood Stasis, reduce swelling, alleviate pain

Indications: Traumatic injuries that are not particularly severe and tend to be lodged in more exterior areas of the body such as sprains, strains, swelling, and fixed or distending pain around an area of injury

Dosage and Usage:

Horses and Cattle: 15–60g, twice daily
Camels: 30–75g, twice daily
Llamas, Alpacas, Goats, Sheep, and Pigs: 10–15g, twice daily
Dogs: 0.5–5g (or about 0.1g per kg body weight), twice daily
Cats and Rabbits: 0.2–0.5g (or about 0.1g per kg body weight), twice daily
Birds: 0.1–0.2g per kg body weight, twice daily

Use 1–3 weeks until primary clinical signs resolve. Do not use for extended duration.

Analysis of Formula: The King ingredients *Dang Gui* (Angelica), *Xue Jie* (Sanguis Draconis), and *Chuan Xiong* (Ligusticum) work together to invigorate Blood, dispel Blood Stasis, and alleviate pain. Additionally, *Dang Gui* (Angelica) generates new Blood, *Chuan Xiong* (Ligusticum) invigorates stagnant *Qi* to drive the Blood Stasis, and *Xui Jie* (Sanguis Draconis) stops bleeding. *Ru Xiang* (Olibanum) and *Mo Yao* (Myrrh) help to move Blood, reduce swelling, and regenerate new tissue, working as the Minister herbs. Serving as the Adjuvant herbs, *Tu Bie Chong* (Eupolyphaga) and *Zi Ran Tong* (Pyritum), drive out Blood Stasis and regenerate injured sinews and fractured bones. *Ma Huang* (Ephedra) serves as a Messenger herb to guide the formula to the skin and muscles.

Cautions and Contraindications: This formula is contraindicated during pregnancy.

Dr. Xie's Comments: In modern veterinary practice, *Die Da Wan* is often used in treating general *Qi*-Blood Stagnation (pain and stiffness) due to any traumatic injuries.

Huo Luo Xiao Ling Dan (Effective to Activate the Channels) 活络效灵丹

Huo means activating. *Luo* is Channels or Meridians. *Xiao* here means effective. *Ling* means "it works all the

Table 27.13. Ingredients and actions of *Huo Luo Xiao Ling Dan*.

%	English Name	Chinese *Pin-Yin*	Actions
25	Angelica	*Dang Gui*	Nourish Blood, invigorate Blood
25	Salvia	*Dan Shen*	Invigorate Blood
25	Olibinum	*Ru Xiang*	Invigorate Blood and *Qi*, reduce swelling
25	Myrhh	*Mo Yao*	Invigorate Blood and dispel Blood Stasis, relieve swelling

time." This formula is named for its originator's belief that it was very effective at invigorating and activating the Channels and collaterals.

Source: *Yi Xue Zhong Zhong Can Xi Lu* (*Records of Heartfelt Experiences in Medicine with Reference to the West*), written by *Zhang Xi-Chun* and published in 1918 CE

Ingredients: The original formula for *Huo Luo Xiao Ling Dan* (Table 27.13) was made by grinding the ingredients together as a fine powder and taking with water.[2–4] *Huo Luo Xiao Ling Dan* is composed of 15 g *Dang Gui* (Angelica), 15 g *Dan Shen* (Salvia), 15 g *Ru Xiang* (Olibinum), and 15 g *Mo Yao* (Myrrh).

Preparation:

1. Powder or capsule method: Herbs are ground into a fine powder. Powder can be encapsulated.
2. Decoction or teapill method: Raw herbs are mixed together and decocted. Herbal water extract (decoction) can be concentrated as granules or teapills.

Actions: Invigorate Blood, dispel Blood Stasis, unblock the Channels and collaterals, alleviate pain

Indications: Internal or external Blood Stagnation Patterns due to trauma or other causes of fixed pain, including internal masses and external or internal tissue wounds or ulcerations. Blood Stagnation treated by this formula may be in various areas of the body including the musculoskeletal system and internal organs, and patients will usually present with a dark or purple tongue and a tight to wiry pulse.

Dosage and Usage:

Horses and Cattle: 15–60 g, twice daily
Camels: 30–75 g, twice daily
Llamas, Alpacas, Goats, Sheep, and Pigs: 10–15 g, twice daily
Dogs: 0.5–5 g (or about 0.1 g per kg body weight), twice daily
Cats and Rabbits: 0.2–0.5 g (or about 0.1 g per kg body weight), twice daily
Birds: 0.1–0.2 g per kg body weight, twice daily
Use 2–4 weeks or until Blood Stagnation signs resolve.

Analysis of Formula: This is a simple and elegant formula that invigorates Blood and dispels Blood Stasis from the Channels and, especially, the collaterals and small, injured, and static Blood vessels. *Dang Gui* (Angelica) is the King herb, which invigorates Blood, nourishes Blood, and alleviates pain. The Minister herb, *Dan Shen* (Salvia), invigorates Blood and dispels Blood Stasis, alleviates pain, clears Heat from Blood Stagnation, and soothes the irritated patient. *Ru Xiang* (Olibanum) and *Mo Yao* (Myrrh) are two Adjuvant herbs that work together to further invigorate the Blood, dispel Blood Stasis, and reduce pain associated with Blood Stasis and swelling.

Cautions and Contraindications: This formula is contraindicated during pregnancy.

Dr. Xie's Comments: *Huo Luo Xiao Ling Dan* can be used as a basic *Qi*-Blood mover and modified for the treatment of any *Qi*-Blood Stagnation.

REFERENCES

1. Qiao Y. The Traditional Chinese Medicine Formula Study Guide, Peter Holmes (ed). Boulder, CO: Snow Lotus Press, 2000.
2. Bensky D, Barolet R. Chinese Herbal Medicine, Formulas and Strategies. Seattle, WA: Eastland Press, Inc., 1990.
3. Zong LX. Pocket Handbook of Chinese Herbal Prescriptions. Miami, FL: Waclion International, Inc., 2001.
4. Ehling D. The Chinese Herbalist's Handbook. Twin Lakes, WI: Lotus Press, 2002.
5. Bensky D, Gamble A. Chinese Herbal Medicine Materia Medica. Seattle, WA: Eastland Press, Inc., 1993.
6. Zong Lan Xu. Pocket Handbook of Chinese Herbal Medicine. Miami, Florida: Waclion International Inc., 2000.
7. Chang PN, Mao JC, Huang SH, Ning L, Wang ZJ, On T, Duan W, Zhu YZ. Analysis of cardioprotective effects using purified Salvia miltiorrhiza extract on isolated rat hearts. Journal of Pharmacological Science 2006;101(3):245–249.
8. Gao D, Lin JM, Zheng LP. Experimental study on effect of *Xue Fu Zhu Yu* decoction on bone marrow hematopoietic stem cells of mice. [Article in Chinese] Zhongguo Zhong Xi Yi Jie He Za Zhi 2007;27(6):527–530.

28 Herbal Formulas to Stabilize and Bind (Astringents) 固涩收敛剂

Sara Jane Skiwski

The formulas discussed in this chapter stabilize and bind (*Gu Se Ji*). This idea was first discussed in the book *Su Wen* (*Basic Questions*, Chapter 74): "For dispersion, retain" and "Astringents can stabilize abandonment." The term abandonment (*Tuo*) refers to a condition in which there is external draining of the body's fundamental substances. This is a serious condition that requires immediate and strong intervention.[1]

The formulas that stabilize and bind are used to control and stop various types of abnormal Body Fluid leakage. Astringent herbs stabilize the Essence, Body Fluids, and *Qi*. They treat excessive loss of the essential substances from the body through sweating, vomiting, urination, spermatorrhea, and diarrhea. These formulas also treat a depletion of the *Qi* from excessive coughing, shortness of breath, asthma, and palpitations. They are occasionally used to stabilize the structure of organs to keep them from slipping from their proper positions, such as seen in prolapse of the rectum or uterus due to *Qi* Deficiency.

In Traditional Chinese Veterinary Medicine (TCVM), improper loss or leakage of Body Fluids and other substances can be due to Excess or Deficiency. Body Fluids and other substances can be forced out by Excess Heat, associated with Exterior Wind-Heat, Phlegm-Heat in the Lung, Blood Heat, or Damp-Heat in the Lower Burner (*Xia Jiao*). In a Deficiency, the processes that normally hold in the Body Fluids and other substances are weakened and cause excessive loss and instability. Formulas that stabilize and bind are used only for Deficiency Pattern diseases with excessive leakage and loss and are contraindicated in Excess Patterns.

The formulas that stabilize and bind combine tonifying substances that strengthen the Deficiency and astringent substances that stabilize the processes to prevent abnormal leakage. If these formulas are used in Excess conditions, patients may actually worsen because pathogens can become trapped and remain much longer than if left untreated.[1,3,5,6]

Qi Deficiency causes an abnormal loss of essential substances. When the internal organs are very weak, the *Qi* is not strong enough to retain the Essence and Body Fluids or keep the organs in their proper position. Geriatric patients and patients with a chronic disease or weak constitution are most likely to have loss of Essence, Body Fluids, and prolapse. Deficiency can also arise from the misuse of purgatives and dispersing herbs or formulas.

Herbal formulas that stabilize abnormal loss of the essential substances treat only the signs, but they have little influence on the organ itself, so once the signs are controlled, they may be combined with formulas that treat the underlying root cause.[1,3,5,6]

Most of the herbs that stabilize the *Qi*, Essence, and Body Fluids are sour or astringent. Sourness has a contracting ability and an "inward-moving" tendency. Herbs with an astringent property are able to prevent or reverse the abnormal loss and leakage of the *Qi*, Essence, and Body Fluids. Of these herbal formulas, some particularly stabilize the Lung *Qi*, and others are effective at stabilizing the Heart *Qi* or the Kidney Essence, or binding up the Intestines.[1,5,6]

Deficiencies of specific organs result in specific types of leakage, and herbal formulas are available for each. There are four major categories of formulas that stabilize and bind: those that stabilize the Exterior and the Lung (for sweating and coughing), those that restrain leakage from the Intestines (for diarrhea), those that stabilize the Kidneys and astringe the Essence (for spermatorrhea and incontinence), and those that restrain flooding (for uterine bleeding or vaginal discharge). To treat chronic conditions, astringent herbs should be used with herbs and formulas that tonify the *Qi* in order to treat the Deficiency completely. In acute conditions such as excessive sweating and diarrhea, the astringent herbs can be used alone initially, but when the condition is stabilized, the appropriate tonifying herbs or formula are prescribed.[1,5]

The astringent herbs should be used for Deficiency Patterns only and are prohibited for use in Excess Patterns or Patterns in which both Deficiency and Excess Patterns occur, because they hold Pathogens in the body.

There are many factors that can cause abnormal loss of the Body Fluids and Essence; therefore, correct differentiation of the Pattern is required. Astringent herbs are prohibited for use in the following clinical presentations: diarrhea caused by Damp Heat in the intestines, excessive urination or spermatorrhea caused by Damp Heat in the Lower Burner (*Xia Jiao*), shortness of breath due to accumulation of Phlegm, or excessive sweating due to Excessive or Deficient-Heat in the body.[1–3]

Mu Li San (Oyster Powder) 牡蛎散

There are many formulas by this name; the formula described here is the most common. *Mu Li San* is named after the King ingredient in the formula, *Mu Li* (Oyster); and *San* means powder, the form of original medication.

Source: *Tai Ping Hui Min He Ji Ju Fang (Imperial Grace Formulary of Tai Ping Era)* by *Chen Shi-Wen* et al. and published by the *Song* Dynasty government in 1078 CE

Ingredients: *Mu Li San* consists of 30g *Mu Li* (Ostrea), 30g *Huang Qi* (Astragalus), 30g *Ma Huang Gen* (Ephedra), and 30g *Fu Xiao Mai* (Triticum) (Table 28.1).

Preparation:
1. Capsule method: Herbs are ground into a fine powder and encapsulated.
2. Teapill method: Raw herbs are mixed together, decocted, and formed into firm teapills.
3. Granular extract method: Raw herbs are mixed together, decocted, sprayed onto inert materials, and dried.

Table 28.1. Ingredients and actions of *Mu Li San.*

%	English Name	Chinese *Pin-Yin*	Actions
25	Ostrea	*Mu Li*	Astringe, stop perspiration, constrain *Yin*, subdue *Yang*
25	Astragalus	*Huang Qi*	Supplement *Qi*, stabilize the Exterior, stop perspiration
25	Ephedra	*Ma Huang Gen*	Stop perspiration, replete the Exterior, secure defensive *Qi*
25	Triticum	*Fu Xiao Mai*	Astringe, clear Heat, supplement *Qi*, nourish Heart, secure the Exterior

Actions: Inhibit/astringe sweating and stabilize the Exterior, tonify *Qi*, consolidate the Exterior, anchor the *Yang* and nourish the Heart

Indications: Heart *Qi* and *Yin* Deficiencies that lead to an unstable Exterior and spontaneous sweating (unassociated with exercise), worse at night, as well as palpitations; being easily startled; irritability; debility; shortness of breath; and lethargy with a pale tongue and a thin, frail pulse; Spontaneous sweating is due to unstable *Wei Qi* (Defensive *Qi*). Sweat is the Body Fluid of the Heart, and prolonged and inappropriate sweating injures Heart *Yin* and *Yin* deficiency.[1,5]

Dosage and Usage:

Horses and Cattle: 15–60g, twice daily
Camels: 30–75g, twice daily
Llamas, Alpacas, Goats, Sheep, and Pigs: 10–15g, twice daily
Dogs: 0.5–5g (or 0.1g per kg body weight), twice daily
Cats and Rabbits: 0.2–0.5g (or 0.1g per kg body weight), twice daily
Birds: 0.1–0.2g per kg body weight, twice daily

Use for 1–3 weeks until the primary clinical signs have resolved.[8]

Analysis of Formula: The King herb of this formula is Ostrea *Mu Li*, which benefits the *Yin*, anchors the floating *Yang*, inhibits sweating, and relieves irritability. The Minister herb, *Huang Qi* (Astragalus), strongly tonifies the Lung *Qi*, is beneficial to the *Wei Qi* (Defense *Qi*), strengthens the *Wei Qi* (Defensive *Qi*), and stabilizes the Exterior. *Huang Qi* (Astragalus) treats shortness of breath and fatigue. The Adjuvant herb, *Ma Huang Gen* (Ephedra), similar to *Mu Li* (Ostrea), augments Heart *Qi*, restrains sweat, and stabilizes the Exterior. *Fu Xiao Mei* (Triticum), the Messenger herb, mildly nourishes the Heart *Yin* and clears Heat from the Heart. Together these ingredients stabilize the Exterior, nourish the *Yin*, and stop excessive sweating. When this has been accomplished, the normal *Qi* returns.[1,2,5] *Fu Xiao Mai* (Triticum) and *Huang Qi* (Astragalus), combined, work synergistically to supplement the *Qi* and nourish the Heart, clear Heat, secure the Exterior, and stop perspiration. For spontaneous perspiration, *Huang Qi* (Astragalus) treats the root—Exterior vacuity—while *Fu Xiao Mai* (Triticum) treats the branch by astringing the perspiration. *Fu Xiao Mai* (Triticum) and *Huang Qi* (Astragalus) are both light. *Fu Xiao Mai* (Triticum) is floating in nature and directed at the Exterior to stop perspiration, while *Huang Qi* (Astragalus) travels toward the Exterior and pores of the skin to supplement *Wei Qi (*Defensive *Qi*). *Ma Huang Gen* (Ephedra) and *Fu Xiao Mai* (Triticum) work synergistically to supplement the *Qi*, nourish the Heart, and secure the Exterior, as well as clear Heat and stop perspiration. This combination of herbs is also used to address spontaneous sweating due to *Qi* and *Yin* Deficiency (vacuity).[1,2,5]

Cautions and Contraindications: *Mu Li San* should be used with caution and is contraindicated for treating profuse, oily sweating with cold limbs and a weak pulse commonly found with exhaustion *Yang* or night sweating due to *Yin* vacuity with flaring Fire.[1]

Dr. Xie's Comments: *Mu Li San* is useful for treating restlessness or panting (in dogs) or spontaneous sweating (in horses) after surgery or parturition due to *Qi* and *Yin* Deficiency.

Wu Mei San (Mume Powder) 乌梅散

Wu Mei San was named after the main ingredient in the formula, *Wu Mei* (Mume) and *San* means powder, the original form of herbal administration.

Source: *Yuan Heng Liao Ma Ji* (*Yuan-Heng's Therapeutic Treatise of Horses*) by *Yu Benyuan* and *Yu Benheng* and published in 1608

Ingredients: The ingredients of *Wu Mei San* are 45 g *Wu Mei* (Mume), 45 g *Huang Lian* (Coptis), 45 g *Jiang Huang* (Curcuma), and 45 g *He Zi* (Chebula) (Table 28.2).

Preparation:

1. Capsule method: Herbs are ground into a fine powder and encapsulated.
2. Teapill method: Raw herbs are mixed together, decocted, and formed into firm teapills.
3. Granular extract method: Raw herbs are mixed together, decocted, sprayed onto inert materials, and dried.

Actions: Clear Heat, detoxify and astringently stop diarrhea[8]

Indications: Diarrhea in foals or other young animals due to bacteria, viruses, parasites, and other factors

Dosage and Usage:

Horses and Cattle: 15–60 g, twice daily
Camels: 30–75 g, twice daily

Table 28.2. Ingredients and actions of *Wu Mei San*.

%	English Name	Chinese *Pin-Yin*	Actions
25	Mume	*Wu Mei*	Astringently stop diarrhea, eliminate ascaris
25	Coptis	*Huang Lian*	Clear Heat, detoxify
25	Curcuma	*Jiang Huang*	Move Blood, relieve pain
25	Chebula	*He Zi*	Bind the intestines to stop diarrhea

Llamas, Alpacas, Goats, Sheep, and Pigs: 10–15 g, twice daily
Dogs: 0.5–5 g (or 0.1 g per kg body weight), twice daily
Cats and Rabbits: 0.2–0.5 g (or 0.1 g per kg body weight), twice daily
Birds: 0.1–0.2 g per kg body weight, twice daily

Use for 1–4 weeks until the primary clinical signs have resolved.[8]

Analysis of Formula: The King herb, *Huang Lian* (Coptis), expels the pathogenic influences and relieves toxicity. The Minister herb, *Wu Mei* (Mume), is sour and astringent and stops diarrhea. *Jiang Huang* (Curcuma), the Adjuvant herb, is pungent and bitter in nature and acts on the Liver and Spleen, activating Blood and relieving pain. The Messenger and guiding herb, *He Zi* (Chebula) is bitter, sour, and neutral, and is very useful for binding the intestines and stopping diarrhea. *He Zi* (Chebula)can be used in both Hot or Cold Patterns and combines well with *Wu Mei* to treat chronic dysenteric problems.[8]

Cautions and Contraindications: *Wu Mei San* should be used with caution in patients with Spleen *Qi* Deficiency.

Dr. Xie's Comments: *Wu Mei San* is a classical veterinary herbal formula to treat any diarrhea in foals, calves, and young goats and sheep.

Clinical and Pharmacological studies: *Wu Mei San* has been used to treat diarrhea in foals. In one study, after two daily treatments, all foals recovered.[9,10]

Zhen Ren Yang Zang Tang (True Man to Nourish the Organs) 真人养脏汤

Zhen means true, *Ren* means man, *Yang* means nourish and *Zang* is internal organs. *Tang* is decoction, the original form of herbal administration. Therefore, *Zhen Ren Yang Zang* can be translated as True Man to Nourish the Organs.

Source: *Tai Ping Hui Min He Ji Ju Fang* (*Imperial Grace Formulary of Tai Ping Era*) by *Chen Shi-Wen* et al. and published by the *Song* Dynasty government in 1078 CE

Ingredients: *Zhen Ren Yang Zang Tang* consists of 18 g *Ren Shen* (Ginseng), 18 g *Bai Zhu* (Atractylodes), 24 g *Rou Gui* (Cinnamomum), 15 g *Rou Dou Kou* (Myristica), 36 g *He Zi* (Chebula), 108 g *Ying Su Ke* (Papaver), 48 g *Bai Shao* (Paeonia), 18 g (6–12 g) *Dang Gui* (Angelica), 42 g (6–9 g) *Mu Xiang* (Sassurea), 24 g (3–9 g), and *Gan Cao* (Glycerrhiza) (Table 28.3).

Preparation:

1. Capsule method: Herbs are ground into a fine powder and encapsulated.

Table 28.3. Ingredients and actions of *Zhen Ren Yang Zang Tang*.

%	English Name	Chinese *Pin-Yin*	Actions
5	Ginseng	*Ren Shen*	Tonify *Yuan* (Source) *Qi*, Spleen *Qi*, Stomach *Qi*
5	Atractylodes	*Bai Zhu*	Dry Damp and tonify *Spleen*
7	Cinnamomum	*Rou Gui*	Warm Kidney, strengthen *Yang*, dispel Cold, warm Spleen, alleviate pain
4	Myristica	*Rou Dou Kou*	Warm and tonify Spleen, astringe the intestines, stop diarrhea, move *Qi*, alleviate pain
10	Chebula	*He Zi*	Astringe intestines, stop diarrhea
31	Papaver	*Ying Su Ke*	Astringe intestines, stabilize Lower Burner (*Xia Jiao*), alleviate pain
14	Paeonia	*Bai Shao*	Nourish Blood, alleviate pain, astringe *Yin*
5	Angelica	*Dang Gui*	Tonify and invigorate Blood, nourish Heart Blood, alleviate pain
12	Sassurea	*Mu Xiang*	Revive Spleen, regulate *Qi*, prevent Stagnation, eliminate tenesmus
7	Glycerrhiza	*Gan Cao*	Harmonize and tonify *Qi* and Middle Burner (*Zhong Jiao*)

2. Teapill method: Raw herbs are mixed together, decocted, and formed into firm teapills.
3. Granular extract method: Raw herbs are mixed together, decocted, sprayed onto inert materials, and dried.

Actions: Warm and tonify Spleen and Kidney *Yang*, restrain leakage from the Intestine, stop diarrhea

Indications: Chronic diarrhea or dysenteric disorders with fecal incontinence and, in severe cases, a prolapsed rectum characterized by abdominal pain, alleviated by warmth and pressure; listlessness; lassitude; sore lower back with cold limbs; reduced appetite; pale tongue with a white coat and deep, weak, and slow pulse[1,3,5,7]

Dosage and Usage:
Horses and Cattle: 15–60g, twice daily
Camels: 30–75g, twice daily
Llamas, Alpacas, Goats, Sheep, and Pigs: 10–15g, twice daily
Dogs: 0.5–5g (or 0.1g per kg body weight), twice daily
Cats and Rabbits: 0.2–0.5g (or 0.1g per kg body weight), twice daily
Birds: 0.1–0.2g per kg body weight, twice daily

Use for 3–6 weeks until the primary clinical signs have resolved. *Zhen Ren Yang Zang Tang* may be used for an extended duration if the disharmony persists.[8]

Analysis of Formula: The main effect of *Zhen Ren Yang Zang Tang* is to warm the middle and tonify Deficiency. The King ingredients, *Ren Shen* (Ginseng) and *Bai Zhu* (Atractylodes) strengthen the Spleen and augment the middle *Qi* especially when combined. There are two sets of Minister herbs in this formula. *Rou Gui* (Cinnamomum) and *Rou Dou Kou* (Myristica) warm the Kidney *Yang* and Spleen to dispel Cold and strengthen the Spleen. *Rou Gui* is the stronger of the two. *He Zi* (Chebula) and *Ying Su Ke* (Papaver), also Minister herbs, bind the intestines and stop diarrhea. Chronic diarrhea depletes the Body Fluids that in turn exhaust the *Yin* and Blood. Two Adjuvant herbs, *Bai Shao* (Paeonia) and *Dang Gui* (Angelica), tonify the *Yin* and Blood. The other Adjuvant, *Mu Xiang* (Sassurea), revives the Spleen, regulates *Qi*, and alleviates tenesmus. It prevents the astringent binding properties of the other herbs from causing Stagnation. The Messenger, *Gan Cao* (Glycerrhiza), helps the *Ren Shen* (Ginseng) and *Bai Zhu* (Atractylodes) tonify the Middle Burner (*Zhong Jiao*) and harmonizes the action of the other herbs. With *Bai Shao* (Paeonia), *Gan Cao* (Glycerrhiza) also alleviates abdominal pain.[1,4,5,7] The diarrhea may contain pus and Blood and there may also be tenesmus. In severe cases Spleen *Qi* becomes so deficient that the intestines can lose their stability and capacity to absorb nutrients. This results in unrelenting diarrhea to the point of incontinence. There may also be a prolapse of the rectum due to the sinking of the Spleen *Qi*. Long-term diarrhea not only leads to Deficiency of the Spleen *Qi* and *Yang*, but also invariably involves the Kidney. This aggravates the diarrhea, which further injures the Spleen and Kidney, and a viscous cycle results.[1,3,5,7]

Cautions and Contraindications: *Zhen Ren Yang Zang Tang* should never be used to treat disorders of Excess or when Stagnation or Damp-Heat are present. *Zhen Ren Yang Zang* should not be used in initial stages of dysentery and diarrhea when Interior toxic Heat is present. Patients taking this formula should avoid wheat, cold raw foods, fish, and greasy foods.[1,5]

Dr. Xie's Comments: *Zhen Ren Yang Zang Tang* is useful for chronic severe colitis in horses and dogs due to Spleen and Kidney *Yang* Deficiency.

Jin Suo Gu Jing Wan (Metal Lock to Consolidate Essence) 金锁固精丸

Jin means metal or gold, *Suo* means lock, *Gu* means consolidate, and *Jing* means Essence. *Wan* means pill, the original form of the herbal medication. Thus, *Jin Suo Gu Jing* is translated as Metal Lock to Consolidate

Table 28.4. Ingredients and actions of *Jin Suo Gu Jing Wan.*

%	English Name	Chinese *Pin-Yin*	Actions
25	Astragalus	*Sha Yuan Zi*	Tonify *Kidney Qi*, astringe
25	Euryale	*Qian Shi*	Astringe urine, tonify Kidney and Spleen *Qi*, consolidate *Jing*
25	Nelumbo	*Lian Xu*	Strengthen *Qi*, astringently consolidate Lower Burner (*Xia Jiao*), nourish *Jing*
12.5	Draconis	*Long Gu*	Astringe, calm *Shen*, tranquilize, anchor and prevent floating *Yang*, consolidate *Jing*
12.5	Ostrea	*Mu Li*	Astringe, calm *Shen*, tranquilize, anchor floating *Yang*, consolidate *Jing*

Essence. This formula stabilizes the Essence, locking it in the body as effectively as a metal lock keeps a chest closed.

Source: *Yi Fang Ji Jie* (*Analytic Collection of Medical Formulas*), written by *Wang Ang* in 1682.

Ingredients: *Jin Suo Gu Jing Wan* consists of 60g *Sha Yuan Zi* (Astragalus), 60g *Qian Shi* (Euryale), 60g *Lian Xu* (Nelumbo), 30g *Long Gu* (Draconis), 30g *Mu Li* (Ostrea), and 60g *Lian Xu* (Nelumbo) (Table 28.4).

Preparation:
1. Capsule method: Herbs are ground into a fine powder and encapsulated.
2. Teapill method: Raw herbs are mixed together, decocted, and formed into firm teapills.
3. Granular extract method: Raw herbs are mixed together, decocted, sprayed onto inert materials, and dried.

Actions: Tonify Kidney and astringe Essence

Indications: Chronic spermatorrhea, impotence, fatigue and weakness, sore and weak limbs, lower back pain, tinnitus, a pale tongue with a white coating and a thin frail pulse; also used to treat enuresis and insomnia with excessive dreaming due to neurasthenia[1,4,5,7]

Dosage and Usage:
Horses and Cattle: 15–60g, twice daily
Camels: 30–75g, twice daily
Llamas, Alpacas, Goats, Sheep, and Pigs: 10–15g, twice daily
Dogs: 0.5–5g (or 0.1g per kg body weight), twice daily
Cats and Rabbits: 0.2–0.5g (or 0.1g per kg body weight), twice daily
Birds: 0.1–0.2g per kg body weight, twice daily

Use for 3–6 weeks until the primary clinical signs have resolved; it may be used for a longer duration if the disharmony persists.[8]

Analysis of Formula: The Kidney stores the Essence of all the organs, and the Liver governs the free-flowing or spreading functions of the body. When the Kidneys are deficient they cannot store Essence, and the gate of the Essence becomes destabilized and spermatorrhea and urinary incontinence can result. The King ingredient, *Sha Yuan Zi* (Astragalus), tonifies the Kidneys and benefits the Essence, to stop leakage and stabilize the gate of the Essence. The Minister herb, *Qian Shi* (Euryale), assists *Sha Yuan Zi* (Astragalus) to stabilize the gate of the Essence. The Adjuvant ingredients, *Long Gu* (Draconis) and *Mu Li* (Ostrea), are powerful restraining substances that suppress blazing Fire and assist in preventing spermatorrhea. The Messenger, *Lian Xu* (Nelumbo), binds the Kidney *Jing* to stop leakage. This formula can treat any problem due to the loss of Essence. Because the effects of this formula are to stabilize and astringe, Kidney tonics should be added when leakage ceases in order to treat the underlying Deficiency. This formula can also be used to treat pediatric enuresis.[1,4,5,7]

Cautions and Contraindications: Since the herbs in this formula are primarily astringent and restraining in nature, *Jin Suo Gu Jing Wan* is contraindicated in cases of Damp Heat in the Lower Burner (*Xia Jiao*) and should be modified if used for spermatorrhea at night due to blazing Fire from Deficiency.[1]

Dr. Xie's Comments: *Jin Suo Gu Jing Wan* is effective for the treatment of chronic urinary incontinence due to Kidney *Qi* Deficiency in dogs, cats, and horses.

Jiu Xian San (Nine Immortals) 九仙散

Jiu means nine or nine ingredients, *Xian* means immortals, and *San* means powder, the original form of the herbal medication. This formula contains nine ingredients and is said to be so effective that it must have been devised by immortals—hence, the name Nine Immortals.

Source: *Yi Xue Zheng Chuan* (*True Lineage of Medicine*), written by *Yu Tuan* in 1515 during the *Ming* Dynasty

Ingredients: *Jiu Xian San* consists of 9g *Ren Shen* (Ginseng), 9g *Ying Su Ke* (Papaver), 15g *Wu Mei* (Mume), 9g *Wu Wei Zi* (Schisandra), 12g *E Jiao* (Asinum), 12g *Kuan Dong Huan* (Tussilago), 9g *Zhe Bei Mu* (Fritillaria), 9g *Jie Geng* (Platycodon), and 15g *Sang Bai Pi* (Morus) (Table 28.5).

Table 28.5. Ingredients and actions of *Jiu Xian San*.

%	English Name	Chinese *Pin-Yin*	Actions
7	Ginseng	*Ren Shen*	Tonify *Qi*
25.5	Papaver	*Ying Su Ke*	Astringe intestines, stabilize Lower Burner (*Xia Jiao*), alleviate pain
25.5	Mume	*Wu Mei*	Astringently stop diarrhea, eliminate ascaris
7	Schisandra	*Wu Wei Zi*	Consolidate Kidney and Spleen, stop diarrhea, astringe and consolidate Large Intestine
7	Asinum	*E Jiao*	Tonify Blood, replenish *Yin*
7	Tussilago	*Kuan Dong Huan*	Treat rebellious Lung *Qi*
7	Fritillaria	*Zhe Bei Mu*	Remove Heat, dispel accumulation
7	Platycodon	*Jie Geng*	Tonify Lung *Qi*
7	Morus	*Sang Bai Pi*	Relieve Lung Heat, relieve asthma

Preparation:

1. Capsule method: Herbs are ground into a fine powder and encapsulated.
2. Teapill method: Raw herbs are mixed together, decocted, and formed into firm teapills.
3. Granular extract method: Raw herbs are mixed together, decocted, sprayed onto inert materials, and dried.

Actions: Astringe the Lung, stop coughing, augment the *Qi* and nourish the *Yin*

Indications: Chronic unremitting cough with wheezing and shortness of breath, spontaneous sweating and a Deficient rapid pulse. Chronic coughing will exhaust the *Qi* and *Yin* of the Lung that causes further coughing.[1,5,7]

Dosage and Usage:

Horses and Cattle: 15–60 g, twice daily
Camels: 30–75 g, twice daily
Llamas, Alpacas, Goats, Sheep, and Pigs: 10–15 g, twice daily
Dogs: 0.5–5 g (or 0.1 g per kg body weight), twice daily
Cats and Rabbits: 0.2–0.5 g (or 0.1 g per kg body weight), twice daily
Birds: 0.1–0.2 g per kg body weight, twice daily

Use for 3–6 weeks until the primary clinical signs have resolved; it may be used for a longer time if the disharmony persists.[8]

Analysis of Formula: One of the King herbs, *Ren Shen* (Ginseng), is a very effective herb for tonifying and augmenting the *Qi*. The other King herb, *Ying Su Ke* (Papaver), is very effective for restraining the Lung and stopping coughs. *Wu Wei Zi* (Schisandra) and *Wu Mei* (Mume), Minister herbs, assist *Ying Su Ke* (Papaver) in restraining the Lung and stopping coughing. *Wu Wei Zi* (Schisandra) also assists *Ren Shen* (Ginseng) in augmenting Lung *Qi*. The last Minister, *E Jiao* (Asinum), nourishes the Lung *Yin* and has a minor astringent effect. Adjuvant herbs, *Zhe Bei Mu* (Fritillaria) and *Kuan Dong Huan* (Tussilago), stop coughing, transform Phlegm, and direct rebellious *Qi* downward to calm wheezing. *Jie Geng* (Platycodon) is both an Adjuvant and Messenger herb, and it directs the effects of all the other ingredients to the Lung. *Sang Bai Pi* (Morus), another Messenger herb, is effective for coughs and wheezing, especially from *Yin* Deficiency. *Sheng Jiang* (Zingiberis) and *Da Zao* (Jujube) may be added to the formula as Adjuvants to regulate the interaction between *Ying Qi* (Nutritive *Qi*) and (*Wei Qi*) (Defensive *Qi*) and thus reinforce the Lung and enable it to recover more quickly.

Deficiency of Lung *Qi* causes wheezing, shortness of breath, and a deficient pulse. The Lung governs the skin and the Exterior of the body, and weak Lung *Qi* results in open pores and spontaneous sweating. Injury to Lung *Yin* results in a nonproductive cough and rapid pulse.[1,4,5,7]

Cautions and Contraindications: Because *Jiu Xian San* restrains the Lung and stops coughing, it should not be used for patients with Phlegm or a concurrent Exterior condition, unless modified, even if a long-term unremitting cough and other typical clinical signs are present.[1,5,7]

Dr. Xie's Comments: *Jiu Xian San* is effective for the treatment of severe chronic cough due to Lung *Qi* and *Yin* Deficiency in horses, dogs, and cats.

Suo Quan Wan (Stopping Waterfall) 缩泉丸

Suo means reduce or stop and *Quan* means waterfall, which symbolizes urinary dribbling, thus translated as Stopping Waterfall. This formula can stop frequent urination due to loss of bladder control.

Source: *Fu Ren Liang Fang* (*Fine Formulas for Women*), written by *Chen Zi-Ming* in 1237 during the *Song* Dynasty

Ingredients: *Suo Quan Wan* consists of 9–12 g *Yi Zhi Ren* (Alpinia), and 9–12 g *Wu Yao* (Lindera) (Table 28.6).

Preparation:

1. Traditional method: Herbs are ground into a fine powder and mixed with the paste of *Shan Yao* (Dioscorea) to be made as small pills.
2. Teapill method: Raw herbs are mixed together, decocted, and formed into firm teapills.

Table 28.6. Ingredients and actions of *Suo Quan Wan*.

%	English Name	Chinese *Pin-Yin*	Actions
50	Alpinia	*Yi Zhi Ren*	Warm the Spleen and Kidney, stabilize and bind urine
50	Lindera	*Wu Yao*	Consolidate *Kidney Qi*, disperse Cold in the Lower Burner (*Xiao Jiao*)

3. Granular extract method: Raw herbs are mixed together, decocted, sprayed onto inert materials, and dried.

Actions: Warm and consolidate the Kidneys and astringe the urination to reduce urinary frequency and stop incontinence

Indications: Deficiency of the Kidney *Qi* and *Yang* with Deficient Cold in the Bladder characterized by frequent clear and prolonged urination or enuresis, accompanied by a pale tongue with a white coating and a submerged, frail, or slow pulse[1,5]

Dosage and Usage:
Horses and Cattle: 15–60g, twice daily
Camels: 30–75g, twice daily
Llamas, Alpacas, Goats, Sheep, and Pigs: 10–15g, twice daily
Dogs: 0.5–5 g (or 0.1g per kg body weight), twice daily
Cats and Rabbits: 0.2–0.5g (or 0.1g per kg body weight), twice daily
Birds: 0.1–0.2g per kg body weight, twice daily

Use for 3–6 weeks until the primary clinical signs have resolved; it may be used for a longer period if the disharmony persists.[8]

Analysis of Formula: The Bladder stores and discharges urine, and its functions are dependent on the Kidney. When Kidney *Qi* is deficient, it fails to transform Bladder *Qi* and diminished Bladder function results. This condition is often due to Cold associated with Kidney *Yang* Deficiency, and the Bladder loses its restraint and frequent clear, prolonged urination or enuresis occurs. The King herb, *Yi Zhi Ren* (Alpinia), warms the Kidney and helps it grasp the Bladder *Qi* and warms the Spleen to govern the Body Fluids and hold urine in the bladder. By tonifying the postnatal *Qi* it indirectly strengthens the prenatal *Qi*. *Yi Zhi Ren* (Alpinia) also directly stabilizes and binds the urine. The Minister herb, *Wu Yao* (Lindera), disperses Excess or Deficient Cold from the Lower Burner (*Xia Jiao*) and transforms Bladder *Qi* to restrain urine. *Wu Yao* (Lindera) effectively disperses the *Qi* between the Kidney and Bladder. Within traditional preparation, the Adjuvant herb, Dioscorea *Shan Yao*, strengthens the Spleen, tonifies the Kidneys, and binds the Essence, supporting the actions of the King herb.[1,2,5]

Cautions and Contraindications: None known

Dr. Xie's Comments: I have effectively used *Suo Quan Wan* to treat urinary dribbling or incontinence in young puppies and kittens.

Si Shen Wan (Four Immortals) 四神丸

Si means four or four ingredients, *Shen* means immortal, and *Wan* means pill, the original form of the herbal formula. These four ingredients of *Si Shen Wan* work so quickly that it appears to be a miracle from the Immortals, and thus it is called Four Immortals.

Source: *Zheng Zhi Zhun Sheng* (*Standards of Patterns and Treatments*), written by *Wang Ken-Tang* in 1602

Ingredients: *Si Shen Wan* consists of 120g *Bu Gu Zhi* (Psoralea), 30g *Wu Zhu Yu* (Evodia), 60g *Wu Wei Zi* (Schisandra), and 60g *Rou Dou Kou* (Myristica). Sometimes, *Gan Jiang* (Zingiberis) and *Da Zao* (Jujube) are added to the decoction (Table 28.7).

Preparation:
1. Decoction: *Si Shen Wan* may be prepared as a decoction.[1,5]
2. Capsule method: Herbs are ground into a fine powder and encapsulated.
3. Teapill method: Raw herbs are mixed together, decocted, and formed into firm teapills.
4. Granular extract method: Raw herbs are mixed together, decocted, sprayed onto inert materials, and dried.

Table 28.7. Ingredients and actions of *Si Shen Wan*.

%	English Name	Chinese *Pin-Yin*	Actions
30	Psoralea	*Bu Gu Zhi*	Warm and tonify Kidney *Yang*, stop diarrhea
15	Evodia	*Wu Zhu Yu*	Warm and tonify Kidney and Spleen *Yang*, dry Damp
10	Schisandra	*Wu Wei Zi*	Consolidate Kidney and Spleen, stop diarrhea, astringe and consolidate Large Intestine
15	Myristica	*Rou Dou Kou*	Warm and tonify Spleen, astringe the intestines, stop diarrhea
15	Zingiberis	*Gan Jiang*	Warm Middle Burner (*Zhong Jiao*), harmonize
15	Jujube	*Da Zao*	Strengthen Spleen, tonify *Qi*, harmonize

Actions: Warm and tonify the Spleen and Kidney, bind up the intestine, stop diarrhea

Indications: Spleen and Kidney *Yang* Deficiency with False Cold (vacuity cold) characterized by diarrhea that occurs daily just before sunrise (*Wu Geng Xie* or "cock-crow" diarrhea); anorexia; inability to digest what is eaten; lower back pain; cold limbs; fatigue; lethargy; a pale tongue with a thin white coating; a submerged, slow, forceless pulse.[1,3,5,7]

Dosage and Usage:
Horses and Cattle: 15–60g, twice daily
Camels: 30–75g, twice daily
Llamas, Alpacas, Goats, Sheep, and Pigs: 10–15g, twice daily
Dogs: 0.5–5g (or 0.1g per kg body weight), twice daily
Cats and Rabbits: 0.2–0.5g (or 0.1g per kg body weight), twice daily
Birds: 0.1–0.2g per kg body weight, twice daily

Use for 3–6 weeks until the primary clinical signs have resolved; it may be used longer if the disharmony persists.[8]

Analysis of Formula: Diarrhea just before sunrise is significant because it is the time of day when *Yin* is at its peak. If the source *Yang* (Kidney) is weak, the *Yang* will not rise and the *Yin* will suddenly descend causing diarrhea. When the *Yang* of the Spleen and Kidney are weak, there is no interest in food because the Spleen cannot decompose food and what is eaten is not digested. Pain results from Cold in the abdomen. When the Spleen and Kidney are warmed, the Large Intestine is stabilized. *Bu Gu Zhi* (Psoralea), the King herb, tonifies the gate of vitality and benefits the Earth (Spleen) by fortifying this aspect of Fire. The Messenger herb, *Rou Dou Kou* (Myristica), warms the Spleen and Kidney, binds up the Intestines, and works synergistically with *Bu Gu Zhi* (Psoralea) to focus its action on the Intestines. The Minister herb, *Wu Zhu Yu* (Evodia), disperses Cold in the Middle Burner (*Zhong Qi*) and thereby complements the action of *Bu Gu Zhi* (Psoralea) by warming the source of the postnatal *Qi*. *Wu Wei Zi* (Schisandra), an Adjuvent herb, is strong, warm, and astringent and strengthens the ability of *Rou Dou Kou* (Myristica) to bind up the Intestines. *Gan Jiang* (Zingiberis) and *Da Zao* (Jujube), Messenger herbs, are added to the decoction and removed before the pills are made. They disperse Cold and activate the metabolism of water, and *Da Zao* (Jujube) also nourishes the Spleen and Stomach.[1,2,3,5,7]

Cautions and Contraindications: Without modification *Si Shen Wan* should not be used if there is an accumulation or Stagnation in the Stomach or Intestines.

Dr. Xie's Comments: *Si Shen Wan* is useful in treating chronic diarrhea due to Kidney *Yang* Deficiency.

Yu Ping Feng San (Jade Wind Screen) 玉屏风散

Yu means jade, *Ping* means screen, and *Feng* means wind. Thus, *Yu Ping Feng* is translated as Jade Wind Screen. *San* is powder, the original form of the herbal administration.

Source: *Shi Yi De Xiao Fang* (*Effective Prescriptions for Generations*), written by *Wei Li-Yin* in 1337 during the *Yuan* Dynasty; also mentioned in *Dan Xi Xin Fan* (*Teaching of [Zhu] Dan Xi*), written by *Zhu Dan-Xi* in 1481

Ingredients: *Yu Ping Feng San* is composed of 30g *Huang Qi* (Astragalus), 60g *Bai Zhu* (Atractylodes), and 60g *Fang Feng* (Ledebouriella) (Table 28.8).

Preparation:
1. Decoction: For acute conditions it can be prepared as a decoction.[1,5]
2. Capsule method: Herbs are ground into a fine powder and encapsulated.
3. Teapill method: Raw herbs are mixed together, decocted, and formed into firm teapills.
4. Granular extract method: Raw herbs are mixed together, decocted, sprayed onto inert materials, and dried.

Actions: Augment the *Qi*, stabilize the Exterior and stop sweating, strengthen the Spleen and Lung, clear Heat, consolidate the Exterior

Indications: Deficiency of *Wei Qi* (defensive *Qi*) or an Exterior Deficiency characterized by an aversion to drafts, spontaneous sweating, recurrent colds, a pale tongue with a white coating, a floating deficient and soft pulse.1,4,5,7

Dosage and Usage:
Horses and Cattle: 15–60g, twice daily
Camels: 30–75g, twice daily

Table 28.8. Ingredients and actions of *Yu Ping Feng San*.

%	English Name	Chinese *Pin-Yin*	Actions
20	Astragalus	*Huang Qi*	Spleen and Lung *Qi* tonic, supplement *Qi*, stabilize the Exterior, stop perspiration
40	Atractylodes	*Bai Zhu*	Remove Damp, dispel Wind, tonify Spleen
40	Ledebouriella	*Fang Feng*	Release the Exterior

Llamas, Alpacas, Goats, Sheep, and Pigs: 10–15 g, twice daily
Dogs: 0.5–5 g (or 0.1 g per kg body weight), twice daily
Cats and Rabbits: 0.2–0.5 g (or 0.1 g per kg body weight), twice daily
Birds: 0.1–0.2 g per kg body weight, twice daily

Use for 3–6 weeks until the primary clinical signs have resolved; it may be used longer if the disharmony persists.[8]

Analysis of Formula: The Lung governs the *Qi*, skin, and body hair. Together with the *Wei Qi* (Defensive *Qi*), these guard the Exterior of the body and ward off External Pathogens. Part of the protective mechanism is to regulate the opening and closing of the pores. When the pores are not working properly, spontaneous sweating and aversions to drafts occur as well as increased susceptibility to External Pathogens. The King herb, *Huang Qi* (Astragalus), is a powerful substance for strengthening the *Qi* and stabilizing the Exterior. It tonifies the Exterior or superficial aspects of the Lung and Spleen and is well suited to treat External Deficiency Patterns. The Minister herb, *Bai Zhu* (Atractylodes) strengthens the Spleen and augments the *Qi*. It reinforces the actions of the *Huang Qi* (Astragalus) and strengthens the Metal (Lung) by cultivating the Earth (Spleen). The combination of these herbs generates *Qi* by tonifying the Spleen that is the source of *Qi* and Blood. The Messenger herb, *Fang Feng* (Ledebouriella), circulates in the Exterior of the body, where it expels Wind. Wind is the major External Pathogen to which the other pathogens attach to invade the body. In concert with *Fang Feng* (Ledebouriella), *Huang Qi* (Astragalus) stabilizes the Exterior without causing the Pathogens to linger and can expel Pathogens without harming the normal *Qi*.[1,2,4,5,7]

Cautions and Contraindications: None known

Dr. Xie's Comments: I have often used *Yu Ping Feng San* to prevent respiratory infections, particularly in horses, dogs, and cats that suffer from recurrent respiratory infections.

Gao Lin San (Turbid Dribbling) 膏淋散

This formula is named after one of the *Lin* syndromes. *Gao lin* means turbid dribbling, and this formula is used to treat turbid dribbling.

Source: *Chinese Veterinary Herbal Handbook*, composed by *Dr. Huisheng Xie* and published and distributed by the Chi Institute of Chinese Medicine in 2004

Ingredients: *Gao Lin San* consists of *Bai Shao Yao* (Paeonia), *Dang Shen* (Codonopsis), *Long Gu* (Draconis), *Mu Li* (Ostrea), *Qian Shi* (Euryale), *Shan Yao* (Dioscorea), *Sheng Di Huang* (Rehmannia), and *Wu Wei Zi* (Schisandra)(Table 28.9).

Table 28.9. Ingredients and actions of *Gao Lin San*.

%	English Name	Chinese *Pin-Yin*	Actions
10	Paeonia	*Bai Shao Yao*	Nourish the Blood, soothe Liver *Yang*
15	Codonopsis	*Dang Shen*	Tonify *Qi*
10	Draconis	*Long Gu*	Astringe, soothe Liver *Yang*, calm *Shen*
10	Ostrea	*Mu Li*	Astringe, soothe Liver *Yang*, calm *Shen*
15	Euryale	*Qian Shi*	Astringently consolidate urine
15	Dioscorea	*Shan Yao*	Tonify *Qi*
15	Rehmannia	*Sheng Di Huang*	Cool Blood, clear Heat, nourish *Yin*
10	Schisandra	*Wu Wei Zi*	Astringently consolidate urine

Preparation:

1. Capsule method: Herbs are ground into a fine powder and encapsulated.
2. Teapill method: Raw herbs are mixed together, decocted, and formed into firm teapills.
3. Granular extract method: Raw herbs are mixed together, decocted, sprayed onto inert materials, and dried.

Actions: Tonify *Yin* and *Qi*, hold urination, secure the *Jing*

Indications: Urinary dribbling, turbid urination with mucus or white flocculent materials due to Kidney *Yin* and *Qi* Deficiency, with a pale or red tongue and fast or weak pulse

Dosage and Usage:
Horses and Cattle: 15–60 g, twice daily
Camels: 30–75 g, twice daily
Llamas, Alpacas, Goats, Sheep, and Pigs: 10–15 g, twice daily
Dogs: 0.5–5 g (or 0.1 g per kg body weight), twice daily
Cats and Rabbits: 0.2–0.5 g (or 0.1 g per kg body weight), twice daily
Birds: 0.1–0.2 g per kg body weight, twice daily

Use for 3–6 weeks until the primary clinical signs have resolved; it may be used longer if the disharmony persists.[8]

Analysis of Formula: The King herbs, *Sheng Di Huang* (Rehmannia) and *Bai Shao Yao* (Paeonia), nourish and constrain the *Yin*. The Minister herbs, *Dang Shen* (Codonopsis) and *Shan Yao* (Dioscorea), tonify the *Qi*, and *Wu Wei Zi* (Schisandra) nourishes the Kidney and secures the Essence (*Jing*). *Long Gu* (Draconis) is astringent and, along with *Mu Li* (Ostrea), also secures the Essence, calms the Liver and *Shen*, and subdues the *Yang*. *Long Gu* (Draconis) and *Mu Li* (Ostrea) are the Adjuvant herbs; they mutually reinforce each other and are very effective at holding and astringing. The Messenger herb, *Qian Shi* (Euryale), secures the Essence to hold urination and stop dribbling, tonifies the Spleen and Kidney, and resolves turbidity of the urine. This formula is a balanced combination of clearing, astringing, and nourishing. *Dang Shen* (Codonopsis) and *Bai Shao Yao* (Paeonia) supplement and nourish the Middle Burner (*Zhong Jiao*) to help protect it against the astringing qualities of the herbs.[2,8]

Cautions and Contraindications: None known

Dr. Xie's Comments: *Gao Lin San* is useful for treating urinary incontinence or turbid urinations due to Kidney *Yin* Deficiency with *Qi* Deficiency.

Wu Bi Shan Yao Fang (Matchless Dioscorea) 无比山药方

Wu means no, *Bi* here means comparable or match, *Shan Yao* refers to Dioscorea, the King ingredient of the formula, and *Fang* means formulation. *Wu Bi Shan Yao Fang*, which infers there is no match for Dioscorea, is then translated as Matchless Dioscorea.

Source: *Chinese Veterinary Herbal Handbook*, written by *Dr. Huisheng Xie* and published and distributed by the Chi Institute of Chinese Medicine in 2004

Ingredients: The ingredients of *Wu Bi Shan Yan Fang* are 15 g *Shan Yao* (Dioscorea), 9 g *Rou Cong Rong* (Cistanche), 9 g *Shu Di Huang* (Rehmannia), 6 g *Shan Zhu Yu* (Cornus), 6 g *Fu Ling* (Poria), 9 g *Tu Si Zi* (Cuscuta), 4.5 g *Wu Wei Zi* (Schisandra), 6 g *Ba Ji Tian* (Morinda), 6 g *Ze Xie* (Alisma), 6 g *Du Zhong* (Eucommia), and 6 g *Niu Xi* (Achyranthes) (Table 28.10).

Table 28.10. Ingredients and actions of *Wu Bi Shan Yao Fang*.

%	English	Chinese *Pin Yin*	Actions
12	Dioscorea	*Shan Yao*	Tonify *Qi*
8	Cistanche	*Rou Cong Rong*	Tonify *Yin* and *Yang*
10	Rehmannia	*Shu Di Huang*	Tonify *Yin*
8	Cornus	*Shan Zhu Yu*	Tonify *Yin*
10	Poria	*Fu Ling*	Resolve Damp, transporter to the Bladder and Kidney
8	Cuscuta	*Tu Si Zi*	Tonify *Yang*
10	Schisandra	*Wu Wei Zi*	Astringe
10	Morinda	*Ba Ji Tian*	Tonify *Yang*
8	Alisma	*Ze Xie*	Resolve Damp, transporter to the Bladder and Kidney
8	Eucommia	*Du Zhong*	Tonify *Yang*
8	Achyranthes	*Niu Xi*	Tonify *Yang*

Preparation:

1. Capsule method: Herbs are ground into a fine powder and encapsulated.
2. Teapill method: Raw herbs are mixed together, decocted, and formed into firm teapills.
3. Granular extract method: Raw herbs are mixed together, decocted, sprayed onto inert materials, and dried.

Actions: Warm the Kidney *Yang*, strengthen the Spleen, benefit urination, tonify Spleen and Kidney *Qi*

Indications: Chronic dribbling due to Kidney *Qi* and *Yang* Deficiency characterized by dribbling worse after work or exertion, weakness and pain of the lower back and pelvic limbs, a pale tongue, weak pulse[8]

Dosage and Usage:

Horses and Cattle: 15–60 g, twice daily
Camels: 30–75 g, twice daily
Llamas, Alpacas, Goats, Sheep, and Pigs: 10–15 g, twice daily
Dogs: 0.5–5 g (or 0.1 g per kg body weight), twice daily
Cats and Rabbits: 0.2–0.5 g (or 0.1 g per kg body weight), twice daily
Birds: 0.1–0.2 g per kg body weight, twice daily

Use for 3–6 weeks until the primary clinical signs have resolved; it may be used longer if the disharmony persists.[8]

Analysis of Formula: *Wu Bi Shan Yan Fang* is used for chronic urinary incontinence due to Kidney *Qi* or *Yang* Deficiency. *Shan Yao* (Dioscorea), the King Herb, tonifies *Qi* and *Jing*. The Minister herbs, *Rou Cong Rong* (Cistanche), *Tu Si Zi* (Cuscuta), *Ba Ji Tian* (Morinda), *Du Zhong* (Eucommia), and *Niu Xi* (Achyranthes), tonify the Kidney *Yang* and strengthen the back and bones. The Adjuvant herbs, *Shu Di Huang* (Rehmannia), *Shan Zhu Yu* (Cornus), and *Wu Wei Zi* (Schisandra) tonify *Yin*, secure the Essence to hold urine, and stop incontinence. The Messenger herbs, *Fu Ling* (Poria) and *Ze Xie* (Alisma), resolve Damp and are the transporters to the Bladder and Kidney.

Cautions and Contraindications: None known

Dr. Xie's Comments: *Wu Bi Shan Yao Fang*, *Gao Lin San*, *Jin Suo Gu Jing Wan*, and *Suo Quan Wan* can be used for urinary dribbling or incontinence. *Wu Bi Shan*

Yao Fang is often used for urinary incontinence due to Kidney *Qi* or *Yang* Deficiency secondary to chronic back injuries or intervertebral disk disease (IVDD). *Gao Lin San* is often used for urinary dribbling or turbid urination with mucus or white flocculent materials due to Kidney *Yin* and *Qi* Deficiency. *Jin Suo Gu Jing Wan* is used to treat chronic urinary incontinence due to Kidney *Qi* Deficiency in geriatric patients. *Suo Quan Wan* is used to treat urinary dribbling or mild incontinence in young animals.

REFERENCES

1. Bensky D, Barolet R. Chinese Herbal Medicine, Formulas and Strategies. Seattle, WA: Eastland Press, Inc., 1990.
2. Bensky D, Gamble A. Chinese Herbal Medicine Materia Medica. Seattle, WA: Eastland Press, Inc., 1993.
3. Flaws B. Seventy Essential TCM Formulas for Beginners. Boulder, CO: Blue Poppy Press, 1994.
4. Flaws B. 160 Essential Chinese Ready-Made Medicines. Boulder CO: Blue Poppy Press, 2005.
5. Liu C, Tseng A. Chinese Herbal Medicine: Modern Applications of Traditional Formulas. Boca Raton, FL: CRC Press LLC, 2005.
6. Wicke R. Traditional Chinese Herbal Studies: Computer TCM Database. Rocky Mountain Herbal Institute, RMH Publications Trust, 1999–2003.
7. Zong LX. Pocket Handbook of Chinese Herbal Prescriptions. Miami: Waclion International, Inc., 2001.
8. Xie HS. Chinese Veterinary Herbal Handbook. Reddick, FL: Chi Institute of Chinese Medicine, 2004.
9. Liu GC. Treatment according to Pattern differentiation for animal diarrhea. Journal of Traditional Chinese Veterinary Medicine 1983;2:33–35. (In Chinese)
10. Zhang CS. Herbal treatment of diarrhea in 180 foals. In: The Complete Works of Secret Recipe of Chinese Veterinary Medicine, Yu Chuan and Zhang Liqun (editors-in-chief). Shanxi, China: Shanxi Science & Technology Press, 1992:165. (In Chinese)

29 Herbal Formulas to Calm *Shen* 安神剂

Sara Jane Skiwski

The formulas discussed in this chapter are used to treat *Shen* Disturbances (Disturbances of the Spirit or behavior problems), which result from Excess or Deficiency Patterns of the Heart and Liver. The treatment strategy for a *Shen* disturbance is to sedate and calm the *Shen*. The clinical signs of *Shen* disturbances are usually complex and may involve aspects of both Deficiency and Excess. Therefore, it may be necessary to sedate the *Shen*, reduce Fire, direct the Liver *Yang* to descend, and tonify the Blood and *Yin*. A combination of strategies is utilized in most cases.[1]

The herbal formulas that sedate the *Shen* and calm the Mind are designed to treat restlessness, anxiety, palpitations, irritability, insomnia, and emotional distress. The clinical signs are directly caused by a disturbance of the Heart, which is the residence of the *Shen* and determines the emotional, mental, and spiritual features of the individual. The syndrome of Heart *Shen* disturbance can be associated with Excess Heat and Blood/*Yin* Deficiency Patterns.[1–5] In an Excess Heat Pattern, the clinical signs include acting stressed, manic behavior, bad temper, and agitation. Rage and stress can quickly occur owing to Liver *Qi* Stagnation and Liver Fire Blazing Upwards (Liver *Yang* rising) affecting the Heart.

The Heart *Yin* can be directly injured by Heat in infectious or febrile diseases. Chronic diseases often consume the Heart *Yin* also. All these factors cause the Heart Fire to blaze upward, which disturbs the *Shen* and leads to anxiety, irritability, palpitations, insomnia, and dream-disturbed sleep.

In Blood Deficiency Patterns, the clinical signs are milder and more chronic. Since sufficient Blood is necessary for a balanced Heart *Shen*, Blood Deficiency causes restlessness and fear for no reason, emotional distress, palpitations with anxiety, forgetfulness, disorientation, dream-disturbed sleep, and frequent awakening at night or insomnia. The tongue body is usually pale or delicate red with a thin white coating and the pulse is often thready, weak, and restless. The treatment strategy is to nourish and enrich the Heart Blood and *Yin*.[1,5]

The herbal formulas that sedate the *Shen* and calm the Mind can be divided into two groups. The first group focuses on sedating the *Shen*, and these substances rapidly control the clinical signs as in acute Excess Patterns. The second group of formulas is used for chronic or mild *Shen* disturbances and treats the underlying Deficiency or root cause. They tonify the Blood and *Yin* to reduce Heart Heat and calm the Mind.[5,6]

Each of the five *Zang* organs is connected with one or more of seven emotions. Restlessness with anxiety, palpitations, and difficulty falling asleep are associated with Heart disturbances. Irritability, insomnia, and dream-disturbed sleep are associated with Liver disturbances. Restlessness and fear with anxiety are associated with Kidney disturbances. Most of the herbal formulas that sedate the *Shen* and calm the Mind enter the Heart, Liver, and Kidney Channels and control disorders from these three different aspects.[5,6]

Mineral substances are often contained in formulas to calm *Shen*. They are considered to have a descending nature in Traditional Chinese Veterinary Medicine (TCVM) because they are heavier in weight and more solid than the plant-based herbs. Heaviness can sedate the *Shen*, descend the *Yang* and Fire, and control fear. Minerals are often parts of formulas that treat acute Excess Patterns.

Most of the formulas to calm *Shen* are cold and salty. In acute *Shen* disturbances, caused by Excess or Deficient Fire, a cold and salty substance is able to reduce and purge the Fire and protect the *Yin*.

Sweetness can moderate, tonify, and moisten; some formula ingredients used for acute and severe *Shen* disturbances are also sweet. Sweet herbs moderate the conflict and reduce the speed of the pathological progress of the disorder. In chronic or mild cases, the sweet herbs are often used to tonify Heart and Liver Blood and moisten the Dryness caused by *Yin* and *Blood* Deficiency.[5,6]

The mineral substances control only the clinical signs of the disorder rather than treat the underlying cause, so they should not be used for a prolonged period of time. Once the clinical signs have improved, a formula to treat the underlying cause should be used.

Mineral substances negatively affect the Stomach and the gastrointestinal tract and cause indigestion, stomach pain, and constipation. Since the mineral substances have a descending tendency, they should be used with caution and should not be used during pregnancy. Some minerals or other heavy substances are toxic and accumulate in the Liver, Kidney, Nervous System, and bones, causing serious chronic health problems if used improperly or for long periods of time. Mineral substances should be broken up, and when used in decoctions they are generally cooked for 30–60 minutes before adding the other ingredients.

Since psychological factors play a very important role in *Shen* disturbances, these must be taken into consideration during treatment as well.[5]

Tian Wang Bu Xin Dan (Emperor's Pill to Tonify the Heart) 天王补心丹

Tian means heaven, *Wang* means King or emperor, *Bu* means tonifying and *Xin* means Heart. *Dan* is pill, the original form of herbal administration. *Tian Wang Bu Xin Dan* is literally translated as Emperor's Pill to Tonify Heart. It is said that this formula came in a dream from the emperor of heaven.

Source: *She Sheng Mi Pou* (*Secret Investigations into Obtaining Health*) by *Hong Ji* in 1638 during the *Ming* Dynasty

Ingredients: *Tian Wang Bu Xin Dan* consists of 120 g *Sheng Di Huang* (Rehmannia), 15 g *Ren Shen* (Ginseng), 30 g *Tian Men Dong* (Asparagus), 30 g *Mai Men Dong* (Ophiopogon), 15 g *Xuan Shen* (Scrophularia), 15 g *Dan Shen* (Salvia), 15 g *Fu Ling* (Poria), 15 g *Yuan Zhi* (Polygala), 30 g *Dang Gui* (Angelica), 30 g *Wu Wei Zi* (Schisandra), 30 g *Bai Zi Ren* (Biota), 30 g *Suan Zao Ren* (Ziziphus), 15 g *Jie Geng* (Platycodon), and 15 g *Zhu Sha* (Cinnabaris) (Table 29.1).

Preparation:

1. Capsule method: Herbs are ground into a fine powder and encapsulated.
2. Teapill method: Raw herbs are mixed together, decocted, and formed into firm teapills.
3. Granular extract method: Raw herbs are mixed together, decocted, sprayed onto inert materials, and dried.

Table 29.1. Ingredients and actions of *Tian Wang Bu Xin Dan.*

%	English	Chinese *Pin-Yin*	Actions
10	Rehmannia	*Sheng Di Huang*	Cool Blood, clear Heat, nourish *Yin*
8	Ginseng	*Ren Shen*	Tonify Heart *Qi* and calm *Shen*
8	Asparagus	*Tian Men Dong*	Nourish Heart *Yin*
8	Ophiopogon	*Mai Men Dong*	Nourish Heart *Yin*, clear Heart
8	Scrophularia	*Xuan Shen*	Cool Blood Heat, enrich *Yin*
8	Salvia	*Dan Shen*	Invigorate Blood, dispel Stasis, cool and nourishes Blood
8	Poria	*Fu Ling*	Calm *Shen*, strengthen Spleen, pacify Heart
8	Polygala	*Yuan Zhi*	Calm *Shen*, sedate Heart, open channels between Heart and Kidney
8	Angelica	*Dang Gui*	Tonify and Invigorate Blood, nourish Heart Blood
8	Schisandra	*Wu wei Zi*	Consolidate and astringe, tonify *Qi* and Kidney *Jing*, calm *Shen*
5	Biota	*Bai Zi Ren*	Calm *Shen*, nourish Heart and Kidney, astringe *Yin* deficiency perspiration
5	Ziziphus	*Suan Zao Ren*	Calm *Shen*, nourish Heart *Yin*, augment Liver Blood, astringe sweat
5	Platycodon	*Jie Geng*	Tonifiy Lung *Qi*, direct formulas upward
3	Cinnabaris	*Zhu Sha*	Tranquilize the Mind and clear Heat and toxin, anchor and calm *Shen*

Actions: Enrich the *Yin*, clear deficient Heat, the Blood, tonify the Heart Blood and *Qi* and calm the *Shen*.

Indications: *Yin* and Blood Deficiency of the Heart and Kidney with Deficient Fire flaring up disturbing the *Shen* characterized by irritability, insomnia, palpitations, forgetfulness, mental fatigue, ulcerations of the mouth and tongue, dry stool, red tongue, scanty tongue coating and a thin rapid pulse.[1,2,4–7]

Dosage and Usage:

Horses and Cattle: 15–60 g, twice daily
Camels: 30–75 g, twice daily
Llamas, Alpacas, Goats, Sheep, and Pigs: 10–15 g, twice daily
Dogs: 0.5–5 g (or 0.1 g per kg body weight), twice daily
Cats and Rabbits: 0.2–0.5 g (or 0.1 g per kg body weight), twice daily
Birds: 0.1–0.2 g per kg body weight, twice daily

Use for 1–3 weeks until the primary clinical signs have resolved.[8]

Analysis of Formula: This formula is for a *Yin* Deficiency of the Heart and Kidney. The Heart governs the Blood and stores the *Shen*, and its Fire normally descends to meet the Kidney. The Kidney stores the Essence and Will, and Kidney Water normally rises to meet the Heart. When the Heart and Kidney communicate harmoniously, Fire and Water balance each other and the Essence and Heart are sufficient. Under such circumstances, the *Shen* and Will are calm and settled. *Sheng Di Huang* (Rehmannia) is the King herb, which nourishes the *Yin* and clears Heat. It enriches the Kidney *Yin* (Water), which is then able to control the disturbance of the *Shen* due to Fire. *Sheng Di Huang* (Rehmannia) also nourishes the Blood. There are three groups of the Minister herbs. In the first group, *Dan Shen* (Salvia) and *Dang Gui* (Angelica) tonify and move the Blood to nourish the Heart without causing Stasis. *Bai Zi Ren* (Biota) and *Yuan Zhi* (Polygala) calm the *Shen*, and *Ren Shen* (Ginseng) and *Fu Ling* (Poria) assist the Heart *Qi*. There are two groups of Adjuvant herbs. The first group, *Tian Men Dong* (Asparagus), *Mai Men Dong* (Ophiopogon), and *Xuan Shen* (Scrophularia) enrich the *Yin* and clear Heat from Deficiency. The second group includes *Wu Wei Zi* (Schisandra) and *Suan Zao Ren* (Ziziphus) to prevent leakage of Heart *Qi*, and *Zhu Sha* (Cinnabaris) that anchors and calms the wayward *Shen*. The Messenger herb, *Jie Geng* (Platycodon), conducts the actions of the other herbs upward toward the Upper Burner (*Shang Jiao*), the House of the *Shen*.[1,2,4–7]

Cautions and Contraindications: *Tian Wang Bu Xin Dan* should not be overdosed, administered long-term, or used during pregnancy. Use with caution in patients with weak digestive systems.

Dr. Xie's Comments: *Tian Wang Bu Xin Dan* is one of the very popular classical herbal formulas to treat *Shen* Disturbance due to Heart *Yin* Deficiency and/or Blood Deficiency, but it traditionally contains *Zhu Sha* (Cinnabaris), which is very toxic because of its mercury content. Thus, only short-term use is usually recommended.

Zhen Xin San (Tranquilizing the Heart) 镇心散

Zhen means tranquilizing, *Xin* means the Heart so *Zhen Xin* translates as Tranquilizing the Heart. *San* means powder, the original form of herbal medication.

Source: *Yan Heng Ciao Ma Ji* (*Yaun-Heng's Therapeutic Treatise of Horses*), written by *Yu Ben Yuan & Yu Benheng* and published in 1608

Ingredients: The ingredients of *Zhen Xin San* are 30 g *Dang Shen* (Codonopsis), 30 g *Fang Feng* (Ledebouriella), 30 g *Fu Ling* (Poria), 30 g *Huang Lian* (Coptis), 30 g *Huang Qin* (Scutellaria), 30 g *Yu Jin* (Curcuma), 30 g *Yuan Zhi* (Polygala), 30 g *Zhi Zi* (Gardenia) with 10 g *Zhu Sha* (Cinnabaris), 20 g *Ma Huang* (Ephedra), and 20 g *Gan Cao* (Glycyrrhiza) (Table 29.2).

Table 29.2. Ingredients and actions of *Zhen Xin San*.

%	English	Chinese *Pin-Yin*	Actions
10	Coptis	*Huang Lian*	Clear Heart Heat, detoxify
11	Scutellaria	*Huang Qin*	Clear Heart Heat, detoxify
11	Curcuma	*Yu Jin*	Cool Blood, cool Heat
11	Gardenia	*Zhi Zi*	Clear Heat from the Triple Burners (*San Jiao*), detoxify
11	Codonopsis	*Dang Shen*	Tonify *Qi* and calm *Shen*
10	Poria	*Fu Ling*	Drain Damp and calm *Shen*
10	Polygala	*Yuan Zhi*	Calm *Shen*, nourish the Heart
3	Cinnabaris	*Zhu Sha*	Tranquilize the Mind, clear Heat and toxins
10	Ledebouriella	*Fang Feng*	Eliminate Wind to relieve the Exterior
6	Ephedra	*Ma Huang*	Stop perspiration, replete the Exterior, secure *Wei Qi*
7	Glycyrrhiza	*Gan Cao*	Harmonize and tonify *Qi* and the Middle Burner (*Zhong Jiao*)

Preparation:

1. Capsule method: Herbs are ground into a fine powder and encapsulated.
2. Teapill method: Raw herbs are mixed together, decocted, and formed into firm teapills.
3. Granular extract method: Raw herbs are mixed together, decocted, sprayed onto inert materials, and dried.

Actions: Eliminate the Heat, Fire, and Phlegm from the Heart; calm the Heart Mind and open the orifices

Indications: Uneasiness of the Mind due to extreme Heat of the Heart characterized by fright, panic, aimless running; muscle tremors of the whole body, biting at the trunk or foot, quickly eating and then immediately stopping; aggressively attacking other animals or humans; a deep red mouth and tongue with yellow and greasy coating; a slippery, forceful, rapid pulse

Dosage and Usage:

Horses and Cattle: 15–60 g, twice daily
Camels: 30–75 g, twice daily
Llamas, Alpacas, Goats, Sheep, and Pigs: 10–15 g, twice daily
Dogs: 0.5–5 g (or 0.1 g per kg body weight), twice daily

Cats and Rabbits: 0.2–0.5 g (or 0.1 g per kg body weight), twice daily
Birds: 0.1–0.2 g per kg body weight, twice daily

Use for 30–60 days weeks until the primary clinical signs have resolved.[8]

Analysis of Formula: This herbal formula is used to treat *Shen* disturbances due to extreme Heart Heat with Phlegm. *Huang Lian* (Coptis) is used to clear the excessive Fire and Heat from the Heart, serving as the King herb of this formula. *Huang Qin* (Scutellaria), *Zhi Zi* (Gardenia), and *Yu Jin* (Curcuma) are the three Minister herbs, which clear Heat, cool Blood, and remove Toxins. Extreme Heat boils the Body Fluids and transforms them into Phlegm, which can further mist the Mind (*Shen*). Therefore, *Dang Shen* (Codonopsis) and *Fu Ling* (Poria) strengthen the Spleen *Qi* and resolve Damp, the source of Phlegm. Working as the Adjuvant herbs, *Yuan Zhi* (Polygala) nourishes the Heart and tranquilizes the Mind, *Zhu Sha* (Cinnabaris) tranquilizes the Mind, and *Fang Feng* (Ledebouriella) and *Ma Huang* (Ephedra) dispel Wind and relieve the Exterior to force the Pathogens out of the body. *Gan Cao* (Glycyrrhiza) is the Messenger herb to harmonize all other herbs' actions. When used, *Feng Mai* (Honey) and eggs are also used to harmonize and detoxify the body along with *Gan Cao* (Glycyrrhiza).

Cautions and Contraindications: Be careful not to overdose *Zhen Xin San* and do not use long-term or during pregnancy.

Dr. Xie's Comments: *Zhen Xin San* is one of the very popular veterinary classical herbal formulas to treat *Shen* Disturbance due to extreme Heart Fire with Phlegm. It can be used to treat aggressive behavior, stall anxiety, and separation anxiety due to excessive Heart Fire combined with Phlegm.

Suan Zao Ren Tang (Jujube Decoction) 酸枣仁汤

Suan Zao Ren is Ziziphus or Jujube, the King ingredient of the formula and *Tang* means decoction, the original form of herbal medication.

Source: *Jin Gui Yao Lue* (*Synopsis of Prescriptions from the Golden Cabinet*), written by *Zhang Zhong-Jing* and published in 220 CE

Ingredients: *Suan Zao Ren Tang* contains 15–18 g *Suan Zao Ren* (Ziziphus), 6 g *Fu Ling* (Poria), 6 g *Zhi Mu* (Anemarrhena), 6 g *Chuan Xiang* (Ligusticum), 3 g *Gan Cao* (Glycerrhiza) (Table 29.3).

Table 29.3. Ingredients and actions of *Suan Zao Ren Tang*.

%	English	Chinese *Pin-Yin*	Actions
46	Ziziphus	*Suan Zao Ren*	Nourish Liver Blood and Heart *Yin*
15	Poria	*Fu Ling*	Calm *Shen*, strengthen the Spleen
15	Anemarrhena	*Zhi Mu*	Nourish *Yin*, clear Heat
15	Ligusticum	*Chuan Xiang*	Move *Qi* and Blood, soothe Liver
9	Glycyrrhiza	*Gan Cao*	Harmonize and tonify *Qi* and the Middle Burner (*Zhong Jiao*)

Preparation:

1. Traditional method: Decoct *Suan Zao Ren* first and then decoct with the rest of the ingredients and divide into three doses; administer the decoction warm.
2. Capsule method: Herbs are ground into a fine powder and encapsulated.
3. Teapill method: Raw herbs are mixed together, decocted, and formed into firm teapills.
4. Granular extract method: Raw herbs are mixed together, decocted, sprayed onto inert materials, and dried.

Actions: Nourish the Blood, calm the *Shen*, clear Heat, soothe Liver *Qi* to eliminate irritability, vexation, restlessness[1,3–7]

Indications: *Shen* Disturbances due to *Yin* and Blood deficiency characterized by muscle spasms during sleep; insomnia, panic, and nervousness at night; night sweats (or panting); poor memory; dizziness or vertigo; dry throat and mouth; a dry red tongue; a wiry thin rapid pulse[1,3–7]

Dosage and Usage:
Horses and Cattle: 15–60 g, twice daily
Camels: 30–75 g, twice daily
Llamas, Alpacas, Goats, Sheep, and Pigs: 10–15 g, twice daily
Dogs: 0.5–5 g (or 0.1 g per kg body weight), twice daily
Cats and Rabbits: 0.2–0.5 g (or 0.1 g per kg body weight), twice daily
Birds: 0.1–0.2 g per kg body weight, twice daily

Use for up to 4 months as needed until the primary clinical signs have resolved.[8]

Analysis of Formula: *Suan Zao Ren Tang* is used for a form of consumption due to Liver Blood Deficiency together with Heat due to *Yin* Deficiency. When the Liver is deficient in Blood, there is not enough Blood to nourish the Heart. The lack of nourishment is accompanied by Liver Fire from Deficiency that moves upward into the chest and disturbs the Heart. This causes irritability, inability to sleep, palpitations, night sweats, and a dry mouth. The deficient Liver Blood cannot restrain the *Yang*, which rises and manifests as dizziness and vertigo. *Yin* and Blood Deficiency fail to nourish the Heart, and Deficient Fire disturbs the Mind. The effect of *Suan Zao Ren Tang* is more to nourish the Heart and calm the *Shen* than to clear Heat. The King herb, *Suan Zao Ren* (Ziziphus) nourishes the Heart and Liver while calming the *Shen*. *Chuan Xiang* (Ligusticum), one of the Minister herbs, regulates Liver Blood by encouraging it to flow freely. This combination of one astringent herb and one dispersing herb is very effective to nourish and regulate the Liver while calming the *Shen*. The other Minister herb, *Fu Ling* (Poria), tonifies the Spleen and Stomach and also calms the *Shen* along with the Adjuvant herb, *Zhi Mu* (Anemarrhena). *Zhi Mu* (Anemarrhena) enriches the *Yin*, clears Heat and moistens internal dryness, and moderates the drying properties of *Fu Ling* (Poria). This formula tonifies and drains mildly.[1,3–8]

Cautions and Contraindications: Stop administration immediately if the patient develops diarrhea, vomiting, or other unusual signs.

Dr. Xie's Comments: *Suan Zao Ren Tang* can be used to treat any nervousness due to *Yin* Deficiency and floating *Yang*, especially nighttime restlessness.

An Shen Fang (*Shen* Calmer) 安神方

An means pacifying or calming. *An Shen* can be translated as *Shen* Calmer. *Fang* refers to formulation.

Source: *Chinese Veterinary Herbal Handbook* by *Huisheng Xie* published by the Chi Institute of Chinese Medicine, 2004

Ingredients: The ingredients of *An Shen Fang* are *Bai Shao* (Paeonia), *Bai Zi Ren* (Biota), *Chai Hu* (Bupleurum), *Dan Shen* (Salvia), *Dang Gui* (Angelica), *Fu Shen* (Poria), *Mai Men Dong* (Ophiopogon), *Mu Li* (Ostrea), *Qing Pi* (Citrus), *Suan Zao Ren* (Ziziphus), *Tian Men Dong* (Asparagus), *Wu Wei Zi* (Schisandra), *Xiang Fu* (Cyperus), *Xuan Shen* (Scrophularia), *Ye Jiao Teng* (Polygonum) and *Yuan Zhi* (Polygala) (Table 29.4).

Preparation:

1. Capsule method: Herbs are ground into a fine powder and encapsulated.
2. Teapill method: Raw herbs are mixed together, decocted, and formed into firm teapills.
3. Granular extract method: Raw herbs are mixed together, decocted, sprayed onto inert materials, and dried.

Actions: Nourish Heart *Yin* and Blood, calm *Shen*, soothe Liver *Qi*

Table 29.4. Ingredients and actions of *An Shen Fang*.

%	English	Chinese *Pin-Yin*	Actions
7	Paeonia	*Bai Shao*	Smooth Liver *Qi*, nourish Blood
7	Biota	*Bai Zi Ren*	Calm *Shen*, nourish the Heart
5	Bupleurum	*Chai Hu*	Regulate Liver *Qi*, relieve stress
5	Salvia	*Dan Shen*	Invigorate Blood, dispel Stasis
7	Angelica	*Dang Gui*	Tonify and invigorate Blood, nourish Heart Blood
5	Poria	*Fu Shen*	Calm *Shen*
7	Ophiopogon	*Mai Men Dong*	Nourish Heart *Yin*
11	Ostrea	*Mu Li*	Calm *Shen*, subdue Liver *Yang*
4	Citrus	*Qing Pi*	Smooth Liver *Qi*, move *Qi*, relax costal tension
7	Ziziphus	*Suan Zao Ren*	Calm *Shen*, nourish Heart
7	Asparagus	*Tian Men Dong*	Nourish Heart *Yin*
4	Schisandra	*Wu Wei Zi*	Consolidate and astringe
7	Cyperus	*Xiang Fu*	Smooth Liver *Qi*
5	Scrophularia	*Xuan Shen*	Cool Blood Heat
5	Polygonum	*Ye Jiao Teng*	Calm *Shen*, nourish Heart
7	Polygala	*Yuan Zhi*	Calm *Shen*, nourish Heart

Indications: Heart *Yin* and Blood Deficiency characterized by anxiety, nervousness, restlessness, insomnia; a red dry tongue; a thin fast pulse[8]

Dosage and Usage:

Horses and Cattle: 15–60 g, twice daily
Camels: 30–75 g, twice daily
Llamas, Alpacas, Goats, Sheep, and Pigs: 10–15 g, twice daily
Dogs: 0.5 5 g (or 0.1 g per kg body weight), twice daily
Cats and Rabbits: 0.2–0.5 g (or 0.1 g per kg body weight), twice daily
Birds: 0.1–0.2 g per kg body weight, twice daily

Use for up to 4 months or until the primary clinical signs have resolved.[8]

Analysis of Formula: Stress easily causes Liver *Qi* Stagnation, and long-term Liver *Qi* Stagnation will transform into Fire that tends to consume Heart *Yin* and disturb *Shen*. The patient can show anxiety, nervousness, predisposition toward stress, a lack of focus on the rider (in horses), restlessness, poor performance, and madness. The treatment strategy is to nourish Heart *Yin*, cool Fire, and soothe Liver *Qi*. Therefore, *Bai Shao* (Paeonia) is the King herb of this formula and is used to smooth Liver *Qi* and nourish the Blood. It also reinforces the *Yin* and suppresses the Liver *Yang*. The eight Minister herbs are *Bai Zi Ren* (Biota), *Suan Zao Ren* (Ziziphus), *Tian Men Dong* (Asparagus), *Wu Wie Zi* (Schisandra), *Xuan Shen* (Scrophularia), *Ye Jiao Teng* (Polygonum),

Yuan Zhi (Polygala), and *Mu Li* (Ostrea). *Bai Zi Ren* (Biota) nourishes the Heart to calm the *Shen*. *Suan Zao Ren* (Ziziphus) helps nourish the Heart and tranquilize the Mind. *Tian Men Dong* (Asparagus) nourishes the *Yin*, especially in the Heart. *Wu Wie Zi* (Schisandra) astringes and nourishes the Kidney and helps to tranquilize the Mind. *Xuan Shen* (Scrophularia) counteracts toxicity, clears pathogenic Heat, and quenches Fire in the Blood. *Ye Jiao Teng* (Polygonum) and *Yuan Zhi* (Polygala) nourish Heart Blood and tranquilize the Mind. *Mu Li* (Ostrea) soothes the Liver and suppresses hyperactivity of Liver *Yang*, dissipates Stagnation, and is an astringent. *Xiang Fu* (Cyperus), *Chai Hu* (Bupleurum), *Dan Shen* (Salvia), *Dang Gui* (Angelica), and *Qing Pi* (Citrus) are the Adjuvant herbs. *Xiang Fu* (Cyperus) regulates the flow of *Qi* and soothes the Liver. *Chai Hu* (Bupleurum) also regulates the Liver *Qi* and relieves constraint to help relieve stress. *Dan Shen* (Salvia) invigorates the Blood to dispel Stasis, nourishes the Blood, and helps to tranquilize the Mind. *Dang Gui* (Angelica) also nourishes the Blood, and *Qing Pi* (Citrus) normalizes the function of the Spleen and Stomach, dries Damp, and resolves Phlegm. *Fu Shen* (Poria) and *Mai Men Dong* (Ophiopogon) are the Messengers and guiding herbs. *Fu Shen* (Poria) calms the Mind. *Mai Men Dong* (Ophiopogon) clears Heat from the Heart and nourishes *Yin*.

Cautions and Contraindications: *An Shen Fang* should be used with caution in patients with Spleen *Qi* Deficiency.

Dr. Xie's Comments: *An Shen Fang* is often used for anxiety, thunderstorm phobia, loss of focus, excessive grooming, or any other behavior problems due to Liver *Qi* Stagnation, Heart *Yin*, and/or Blood Deficiency in horses, dogs, and cats. The unique thing about this formula is that it is safe because it contains no toxic heavy metals. The majority of the classical formulas to calm the *Shen* contain *Zhu Sha* (Cinnabaris), which is very toxic because of its high mercury content.

Zhu Sha An Shen Wan (Cinnabaris to Calm *Shen*) 朱砂安神丸

Zhu Sha refers to Cinnabaris, the King ingredient of the formula, *An* means to calm or pacify and *Wan* means pill, the original form of medication. The author of this formula is a famous physician of the *Jin-Tartar* period, *Li Dong-Yuan*. Variations of the formula appear in different books attributed to him.[1]

Source: *Nei Wai Shang Bian Huo Lun* (*Clarifying Doubts about Injury from Internal & External Causes*), written by *Li Dong-Yuan* and published in 1231 during the *Song* Dynasty and also *Lan Shi Mi Cang (Secret Record of the Chamber of Orchids)* by *Li Dong-Yuan* published in 1249

Table 29.5. Ingredients and actions of *Zhu Sha An Shen Wan*.

%	English	Chinese *Pin-Yin*	Actions
23	Cinnabaris	*Zhu Sha*	Tranquilize the Mind, clear Heat and toxins
28	Coptis	*Huang Lian*	Clear Heat, detoxify
12	Angelica	*Dang Gui*	Tonify and invigorate Blood, nourish Heart Blood
12	Rehmannia	*Sheng Di Huang*	Cool Blood, clear Heat, nourish *Yin*
25	Glycyrrhiza	*Gan Cao*	Harmonize and tonify *Qi* and the Middle Burner (*Zhong Jiao*)

Ingredients: The ingredients of *Zhu Sha An Shen Wan* are 15 g *Zhu Sha* (Cinnabaris), 18 g *Huang Lian* (Coptis), 7.5 g *Dang Gui* (Angelica), 7.5 g *Sheng Di Huang* (Rehmannia), 16.5 g *Gan Cao* (Glycerrhiza) (Table 29.5).

Preparation:

1. Capsule method: Herbs are ground into a fine powder and encapsulated.
2. Teapill method: Raw herbs are mixed together, decocted, and formed into firm teapills.
3. Granular extract method: Raw herbs are mixed together, decocted, sprayed onto inert materials, and dried.

Actions: Sedate the Heart; calm the *Shen*; drain Fire; nourish *Yin* and Blood and anchor the Heart so that insomnia, agitation, restlessness, and other clinical signs can be resolved[1,4,5,7]

Indications: Heart Fire flaring up with insufficient Heart Blood and *Yin* (Heart *Yin* Deficiency with hyperactive Heart *Yang*) characterized by insomnia or dream-disturbed sleep, restlessness, continuous palpitations, irritability, Heat in the chest, nausea, and forgetfulness with a red tongue that may be ulcerated at the tip and a thin rapid pulse

Dosage and Usage:

Horses and Cattle: 15–60 g, twice daily
Camels: 30–75 g, twice daily
Llamas, Alpacas, Goats, Sheep, and Pigs: 10–15 g, twice daily
Dogs: 0.5–5 g (or 0.1 g per kg body weight), twice daily
Cats and Rabbits: 0.2–0.5 g (or 0.1 g per kg body weight), twice daily
Birds: 0.1–0.2 g per kg body weight, twice daily

Use for 1–3 weeks until the primary clinical signs have resolved.

Analysis of Formula: *Zhu Sha An Shen Wan* nourishes Heart *Yin* and clears Heart Fire, balancing *Yin* and *Yang*. When vigorous Heart Fire injures the Blood and *Yin*, the scorching from Heart Fire depletes the Blood and *Yin*, which in turn deprives the Heart of nourishment. The combination of Heat and Deficiency disturbs the serenity of the *Shen* that manifests as insomnia and continuous palpitations. This Heart Fire also prevents the Heart from rooting in the Kidney, which is necessary to house the *Shen*. The *Shen* therefore has no place to reside during the *Yin* time (the nighttime), so insomnia results. The primary effect of this formula is to drain Fire and clear the Heart. The King herb, *Zhu Sha* (Cinnabaris) has a sedating and slightly cold nature. It calms the *Shen* and also clears Fire from the Heart. The Minister herb, *Huang Lian* (Coptis) strongly drains Fire from the Heart and works synergistically with the *Zhu Sha* (Cinnabaris). Together they address both the manifestation and root of the *Shen* Disturbance. The two Adjuvant herbs, *Dang Gui* (Angelica) and *Sheng Di Huang* (Rehmannia), nourish the Blood and replenish the *Yin* to tonify aspects of the body that have been injured by the Heart Fire as well as prevent further injury. *Sheng Di Huang* (Rehmannia) also helps drain Fire. The Messenger herb, *Gan Cao* (Glycerrhiza) harmonizes the actions of the other ingredients while protecting the Stomach from the harsh effects of *Zhu Sha* (Cinnabaris) and *Huang Lian* (Coptis). This formula is used to treat insomnia due to a deficient type of excitation in patients with neurasthenia.[1,4,5,7]

Cautions and Contraindications: *Zhu Sha* (Cinnabaris) should not be taken in large doses or used for a long period of time.

Dr. Xie's Comments: *Zhu Sha An Shen Wan* contains *Zhu Sha* (Cinnabaris), which is very toxic because of its mercury content; it should not be used for more than 5 days.

REFERENCES

1. Bensky D, Barolet R. Chinese Herbal Medicine Formulas and Strategies. Seattle, WA: Eastland Press, Inc., 1990.
2. Bensky D, Gamble A. Chinese Herbal Medicine Materia Medica. Seattle, WA: Eastland Press, Inc., 1993.
3. Flaws B. Seventy Essential TCM Formulas for Beginners. Boulder CO: Blue Poppy Press, 1994.
4. Flaws B. 106 Essential Chinese Ready-Made Medicines. Boulder CO: Blue Poppy Press, 2005.
5. Liu C, Tseng A. Chinese Herbal Medicine: Modern Applications of Traditional Formulas. Boca Raton, FL: CRC Press LLC, 2005.
6. Wicke R. Traditional Chinese Herbal Studies: Computer TCM Database. Rocky Mountain Herbal Institute, RMH Publications Trust, 1999–2003.
7. Zong LX. Pocket Handbook of Chinese Herbal Prescriptions. Miami: Waclion International, Inc., 2001.
8. Xie HS. Chinese Veterinary Herbal Handbook. Reddick, FL: Chi Institute of Chinese Medicine, 2004.

30 Herbal Formulas to Open the Orifices (Senses) 开窍剂

Sara Jane Skiwski

The herbal formulas discussed in this chapter aromatically open the orifices and sense organs or *Shen*. Formulas that open the orifices are used for unconsciousness or coma due to Excess factors.

Loss of consciousness may be due to either Excess or Deficiency. When the problem is one of Excess, it is known as a Closed Syndrome (*Bi Zheng*) in which the pathogenic *Qi* obstructs the sensory orifices. When the problem is one of Deficiency, it is called the Collapsing Syndrome (*Tuo Zheng*) that manifests as loss of consciousness with excessive sweating, cold extremities, bowel and urinary incontinence, flaccidity, open mouth and eyes, and a frail or faint pulse.[1–4]

A Closed Syndrome can develop from severe disease. In severe acute conditions it is also called a Locked Up Syndrome. The pathological change is a sudden disturbance of *Qi* and Blood, with blockage of the sensory orifices and internal organ associations by Rebellious *Qi*, Blood, Phlegm, or Rising *Yang*. Clinical signs in this syndrome show blockage of the orifices and a locked-up body, such as loss of consciousness, clenched jaw, flexed paws, rigid limbs, and a lack of urination and bowel movements. A Closed Syndrome can be divided into Hot or Cold Closed Syndromes. The Hot Closed Syndrome is due to pathogenic Heat or Heat Toxin penetrating into the Pericardium. The animal is presented with a high fever; irritability; panting; warm limbs; a yellow, thick tongue coating; and a rapid, slippery, forceful pulse. The Hot Closed Syndrome is treated by clearing the Heat to open the orifices.

A Cold Closed Syndrome is due to pathogenic Cold and constrained *Qi* generating turbid Phlegm, which obstructs the orifices of the Heart. Clinical signs include cold limbs; a white, thick tongue coating; and a deep, wiry pulse. A Cold Closed Syndrome is treated by warming the Cold and unblocking the *Qi* to open the orifices.[4,5]

In clinical practice, Closed Syndromes can be associated with a severe infection, cerebrovascular accident, hepatic coma, uremia, sunstroke, syncope, lightning strikes, drowning, and hysteria. Since these patients may have lost consciousness, it is important to determine whether it is a Hot or Cold Closed Syndrome so that the correct treatment is given.

A Locked Up Syndrome is a severe form of the Closed Syndrome due to either an acute Excess Hot or Cold Pattern. The orifices are "locked up" by a disturbance of the *Qi* and Blood, which are complicated with Phlegm, Heat, or Cold, and uprising *Yang*. The clinical signs can include loss of consciousness; clenched jaw; flexed paws; rigid limbs; and a wiry, slippery, and forceful pulse. The Locked Up Syndrome is seen mainly in cerebrovascular accidents, epilepsy, sunstroke, hysteria, severe pain, anaphylaxis, syncope, hepatic coma, and uremia. The treatment strategy is to open the orifices, expel Phlegm, either clear Heat or warm the internal Cold depending on the Pattern, and harmonize the *Qi* and Blood.[4,5]

Collapsing Syndrome (*Tuo Zheng*) is a Deficiency Syndrome. It is caused by disharmony of the *Yin*, *Yang*, *Qi* and Blood when the *Yang* and *Qi* are too weak to hold the *Yin* and Blood and carry on the functions of the internal organs. In this syndrome patients lose consciousness gradually and they have shallow respiration, shortness of breath, cold limbs, profuse sweating, and incontinence of urine. The pulse is very deep and weak. The Collapsing syndrome (*Tuo Zheng*) occurs in conditions where patients lose a large amount of blood, in severe dehydration, in myocardial infarction, and in severe infections. The treatment strategy for the collapsing Syndrome is to strongly strengthen the *Qi* and to rescue the *Yang*.[3] The herbal formulas to resuscitate *Yang* are discussed in Chapter 22.

The herbal formulas that open the orifices are used for treating both Closed and Locked Up Syndromes (Excess Syndromes) but not Collapsing Syndromes. The herbs are very pungent, have strong aromatic smells, move quickly, and are able to penetrate the body, break up blockage, and revive the *Shen*. If combined with other herbs that expel Phlegm and eliminate Heat-Toxin or Cold turbidity, they can rapidly open the orifices. These herbal formulas are able to stimulate the central nervous system, the peripheral nervous system and the heart, and to irritate the respiratory mucosa and smooth the muscles.[1,4]

When using formulas to open the orifices it must be determined whether the reduced consciousness or coma is due to a Deficiency or an Excess. These formulas are used only if Excess pathogens predominate, and clinical signs include reduced consciousness or coma with a clenched jaw, flexed paws, rigid limbs, and a forceful pulse. These formulas should be used only short term for treating the acute clinical signs. If used long term their dispersing properties can easily injure the normal *Qi*.[3]

The aromatic components of the formulas needed to open the orifices are easily destroyed by high temperatures during cooking, so the formulas must be prepared at a low temperature. Formulas to open the orifices are often combined with other herbs to eliminate Phlegm, reduce Toxins, and harmonize *Qi* and Blood. Some of their ingredients, such as *She Xiang* (Moschus) and *Niu Huang* (Bovis Calculus), can be substituted with synthetic versions.

Although necessary for acute conditions, the aromatic substances must be used with caution. They can open the blocked orifices and stimulate *Yin*, *Yang*, *Qi*, and Blood, but scatter and weaken the *Qi*, so they are used only for a short time. After the acute treatment, the treatment strategy will change depending on the underlying Pattern. Formulas that open the orifices should not be used during pregnancy, in conditions of heavy bleeding, or during comas associated with the Collapsing Syndrome.[2,4]

An Gong Niu Huang Wan (Pacifying the Pericardium) 安宫牛黄丸

An means pacifying or calming, and *Gong* means the Palace, the place where the emperor resides. *Gong* here is a metaphor for the Pericardium, which surrounds and shields the Heart (the Emperor) in the same manner as a palace surrounds and protects the ruler. Thus, the translation of Pacifying the Pericardium. The formula clears Heat from the Pericardium and thereby calms the *Shen*.

Source: *Weng Bing Tiao Bian* (*Systematic Differentiation of Warm Diseases*), written by *Wu Ju-Tong* and published in 1798

Ingredients: The ingredients of *An Gong Niu Huang Wan* are 30 g *Niu Huang* (Bovis Calculus), 30 g *Xi Jiao* (Rhinoceros), 7.5 g *She Xiang* (Moschus), 30 g *Huang Lian* (Coptis), 30 g *Huan Qin* (Scutellaria), 30 g *Zhi Zi* (Gardenia), 30 g *Xiong Huang* (Realgar), 7.5 g *Bing Pian* (Borneol), 30 g *Yu Jin* (Curcuma), 30 g *Zhu Sha* (Cinnabaris), and 15 g *Zhen Zhu* (Margarita) (Table 30.1). *Jin Bo* (Gold Foil) and *Feng Mi* (Honey) may be added in a traditional preparation method.

Preparation:

1. Traditional method: Grind all ingredients except *Jin Bo* into an extremely fine powder. Mix with honey and form into balls, 3 g each, coat with *Jin Bo*, and protect with wax.[2]
2. Capsule method: Herbs are ground into a fine powder and encapsulated.
3. Teapill method: Raw herbs are mixed together, decocted, and formed into firm teapills.
4. Granular extract method: Raw herbs are mixed together, decocted, sprayed onto inert materials, and dried.[7]

Table 30.1. Ingredients and actions of *An Gong Niu Huang Wan*.

%	English Name	Chinese *Pin Yin*	Actions
11	Bovis Calculus	*Niu Huang*	Clear pathogenic Heat, relieve convulsions by settling Internal Wind, restore consciousness
11	Rhinoceros	*Xi Jiao*	Clear Heat, relieve Fire toxicity, cool the Blood, arrest tremors
3	Moschus	*She Xiang*	Open the orifice to restore consciousness, enter all 12 channels to revive *Shen*
11	Coptis	*Huang Lian*	Clear Heat, detoxify
11	Scutellaria	*Huang Qin*	Clear Heat and Damp, purge Fire, remove toxins
11	Gardenia	*Zhi Zi*	Reduce pathogenic Fire, relieve irritability, clear pathogenic Heat from Blood
11	Realgar	*Xiong Huang*	Remove toxins, dislodge Phlegm to open the orifice and drain turbid Phlegm
3	Borneol	*Bing Pian*	Open the orifice to restore consciousness, relieve pain, revive the *Shen*, Clear Heat
11	Curcuma	*Yu Jin*	Clear Heat from the Heart and Pericardium, promote *Qi* flow to relieve depression
11	Cinnabaris	*Zhu Sha*	Tranquilize the Mind, clear Heat and toxins
6	Margarita	*Zhen Zhu*	Sedate the Heart and settle tremors and palpitations, clear Heart and Liver Fire

Actions: Clear Heat, relieve toxicity, open the orifices, calm *Shen*, sweep away Phlegm and remove Toxins

Indications: Heat that attacks the Pericardium with Phlegm obstructing the orifices characterized by high fever, delirium, irritability, agitation, stroke, coma, neonatal convulsions, a dark red dry tongue, and a rapid pulse[3]

Dosage and Usage:
Horses and Cattle: 15–60 g, twice daily
Camels: 30–75 g, twice daily
Llamas, Alpacas, Goats, Sheep, and Pigs: 10–15 g, twice daily
Dogs: 0.5–5 g (or 0.1 g per kg body weight), twice daily
Cats and Rabbits: 0.2–0.5 g (or 0.1 g per kg body weight), twice daily
Birds: 0.1–0.2 g per kg body weight, twice daily
Use for 1–3 weeks until the primary clinical signs have resolved.[7]

Analysis of Formula: This formula is used when both Phlegm and Heat are very strong. If turbid Phlegm is not eliminated, it will be very difficult to clear the Heat. *An Gong Niu Huang Wan* combines ingredients for clearing Heat with herbs that dislodge and drain turbid Phlegm. *Niu Huang* (Bovis Calculus), one of the King herbs, is very effective at clearing Heat from both the Liver and Heart. Its aromatic properties clear Heat via the Pericardium. *Niu Huang* (Bovis Calculus) also relieves toxicity and dislodges Phlegm to open the orifices, extinguish Wind, and stop spasms and convulsions. *Niu Huang* (Bovis Calculus) therefore addresses all the major aspects of a Hot Closed Syndrome. The other King herb, *Xi Jiao* (Rhinoceros), enters the *Ying* (nutritive) and *Xue* (Blood) levels to clear Fire and Heat from the Heart, Liver, and Stomach. *Xi Jiao* (Rhinoceros) clears Heat from the Heart, calms the *Shen*, cools the Blood, and relieves toxicity. *Xi Jiao* (Rhinoceros) will also clear Heat via the Pericardium. The Minister herb, *She Xiang* (Moschus) aromatically opens the orifices and revives the *Shen*, because it penetrates all 12 channels. Its aromatic and strong nature is an essential treatment when Phlegm obstructs the orifices. The Adjuvant herbs, *Huang Lian* (Coptis), *Huan Qin* (Scutellaria), and *Zhi Zi* (Gardenia), conduct the Heat downward, helping *Niu Huang* (Bovis Calculus) and *Xi Jiao* (Rhinoceros) clear and drain Heat toxin from the Pericardium. *Xiong Huang* (Realgar) dislodges Phlegm and relieves toxicity to help open the orifice by draining the turbid Phlegm. The Messenger herbs, *Bing Pian* (Borneol) and *Yu Jin* (Curcuma), aromatically unblock the orifice and disperse Heat from constraint, thereby helping to vent Heat through the Pericardium. Both of the other Adjuvant herbs, *Zhu Sha* (Cinnabaris) and *Zhen Zhu* (Margarita), sedate the Heart and Liver. When used, *Feng Mi* (Honey) is also a Messenger serving to harmonize the Stomach and regulate the Middle Burner (*Zhong Jiao*). Gold coating (*Jin Bo*) on the pills is also a Messenger that calms the *Shen*.[1,3–5]

Cautions and Contraindications: *An Gong Niu Huang Wan* should not be used during pregnancy, at high doses, or long term and should not be heated. *An Gong Niu Huang Wan* is contraindicated in patients with coma due to Cold Phlegm.

Dr. Xie's Comments: *An Gong Niu Huang Wan* is useful to treat an acute onset of epidemic meningitis and encephalitis with clinical signs of fever, irritability, agitation, and seizures with a purple or red tongue and a wiry or fast pulse.

Zi Xue Dan (Purple Snow Pill) 紫雪丹

Zi means purple, *Xue* means snow and *Dan* means pill. The name *Zi Xue Dan* is derived from its appearance because it looks like purple colored frost; thus, it is translated as Purple Snow Pill.

Source: *Wai Tai Mi Yao* (*Arcane Essentials from the Imperial Library*), written by *Wang Tao* and published in 752

Ingredients: *Zi Xue Dan* is composed of 1500 g *Shi Gao* (Gypsum), 1500 g *Han Shui Shi* (Calcite), 1500 g *Hua Shi* (Talcum), 150 g *Xi Jiao* (Rhinoceros), 150 g *Ling Yang Jiao* (Antelopis), 37.5 g *She Xiang* (Moschus), 500 g *Xuan Shen* (Scrophularia), 1500 g *Ci Shi* (Magnetite), 500 g *Sheng Ma* (Cimicifuga), 240 g *Gan Cao* (Glycyrrhiza), 150 g *Qing Mu Xiang* (Aristolochia), 150 g *Chen Xiang* (Aquilaria), 30 g *Ding Xiang* (Caryophyllum), 90 g *Zhu Sha* (Cinnabaris), 5000 g *Mang Xiao* (Mirabilitum), 96 g *Xiao Shi* (Niter), and 3000 g *Huang Jin* (Gold) (Table 30.2).

Preparation:
1. Capsule method: Herbs are ground into a fine powder and encapsulated.
2. Teapill method: Raw herbs are mixed together, decocted, and formed into firm teapills.
3. Granular extract method: Raw herbs are mixed together, decocted, sprayed onto inert materials, and dried[7]

Actions: Control spasms and convulsions, open the orifices, clear Heat, relieve toxicity, and calm the *Shen* while extinguishing Wind

Indications: Internal and External Excess Heat with high fever, irritability, restlessness, delirium, impaired consciousness, syncope, twitching, spasms, convulsions, increased thirst, dry mouth, dark urine, severe

Table 30.2. Ingredients and actions of *Zi Xue Dan*.

%	English Name	Chinese *Pin Yin*	Actions
9	Gypsum	*Shi Gao*	Clear Heat, quell Fire, relieve thirst and restlessness
9	Calcite	*Han Shui Shi*	Clear Heat, drain Fire
9	Talcum	*Hua Shi*	Clear Summer Heat
1	Rhinocerus	*Xi Jiao*	Clear Heat, relieve Fire toxicity, cool the Blood, arrest tremors
1	Antelopis	*Ling Yang Jiao*	Soothe Liver to stop Wind, clear Liver Heat, remove toxins
1	Moschus	*She Xiang*	Open the orifice to restore consciousness, enter all 12 channels to revive *Shen*
3	Scrophularia	*Xuan Shen*	Cool Blood Heat
9	Magnetite	*Ci Shi*	Settle *Yang* to tranquilize Mind, improve sensory function, improve *Qi* receiving function
3	Cimicifuga	*Sheng Ma*	Clear Heat, clear Toxins
1	Glycerrhiza	*Gan Cao*	Harmonize and tonify *Qi* and Middle Burner (*Zhong Jiao*)
1	Aristolochia	*Qing Mu Xiang*	Promote *Qi*, relieve pain, reduce swelling
1	Aquilaria	*Chen Xiang*	Promote *Qi* flow, relieve pain, normalize function of the Stomach, warm the Kidney
1	Caryophyllum	*Ding Xiang*	Warm the Middle Burner (*Zhong Jiao*), redirect rebellious Stomach *Qi*, warm Kidneys, aid *Yang*
1	Cinnabaris	*Zhu Sha*	Tranquilize the Mind, clear Heat and toxins
30	Mirabilitum	*Mang Xiao*	Clear Heat and toxins
1	Niter	*Xiao Shi*	Drain Heat
19	Gold	*Huang Jin*	Weigh upon and sedate the *Shen*

constipation, a dark red tongue with no coating, a rapid forceful pulse

Dosage and Usage:

Horses and Cattle: 15–60 g, twice daily

Camels: 30–75 g, twice daily

Llamas, Alpacas, Goats, Sheep, and Pigs: 10–15 g, twice daily

Dogs: 0.5–5 g (or 0.1 g per kg body weight), twice daily

Cats and Rabbits: 0.2–0.5 g (or 0.1 g per kg body weight), twice daily

Birds: 0.1–0.2 g per kg body weight, twice daily

Use for 1–3 weeks until the primary clinical signs have resolved.[7]

Analysis of Formula: *Zi Xue Dan* is very effective to clear Heat, open the orifices, calm the *Shen*, and extinguish Wind, when Heat attacks the Pericardium and sends blazing Heat into both *Qi* and Blood Levels. This formula contains ingredients that clear Heat and are sweet and cold instead of bitter and cold to avoid injury to the Body Fluids. *Zi Xue Dan* is recommended to treat Patterns of vigorous Heat and injury to Body Fluids, which manifest as spasms and convulsions.[3] There are 2 groups of King herbs. The first consists of *Shi Gao* (Gypsum), *Han Shui Shi* (Calcite) and *Hua Shi* (Talcum). *Shi Gao* (Gypsum) is an important substance to clear Fire and Heat from the *Qi* level. It causes the Heat to recede and encourages Body Fluid production, thereby eliminating irritability and increased thirst. *Han Shui Shi* (Calcite) also clears Heat and drains Fire to eliminate irritability and increased thirst. *Hua Shi* (Talcum) enables the formula to conduct Heat downward so that it can be eliminated through the urine. The second group of King herbs are *Xi Jiao* (Rhinoceros), *Ling Yang Jiao* (Antelopis) and *She Xiang* (Moschus). *Xi Jiao* (Rhinoceros) is cool and aromatic and ascends and disperses. It enters the *Ying* (nutritive) and *Xue* (Blood) Levels and is an important substance to clear Fire and Heat from the Heart and Liver channels. Clearing Heat from the *Ying* (nutritive) Level, it cools the Blood and relieves toxicity. Because of its active nature it can be cold without retarding movement, making it useful for venting Heat through the Pericardium. *Ling Yang Jiao* (Antelopis) is particularly useful to drain Liver Fire and is an important herb for cooling the Liver and extinguishing Wind. Together *Xi Jiao* (Rhinoceros) and *Ling Yang Jiao* (Antelopis) treat the Heat in the Heart and Liver, and effectively resolve spasms, convulsions and impaired consciousness. *She Xiang* (Moschus) is an intense aromatic substance that opens the orifice of the Heart and restores consciousness. One of the Minister herbs, *Xuan Shen* (Scrophularia) conducts the Fire downward, enriches the *Yin* and eliminates agitation. *Xuan Shen* (Scrophularia) is combined with another Minister, *Sheng Ma* (Cimicifuga), to strengthen its ability to clear Heat and relieve toxicity. The Adjuvant herbs, *Qing Mu Xiang* (Aristolochia), *Chen Xiang* (Aquilaria) and *Ding Xiang* (Caryophyllum) promote the movement of *Qi* and assist the *She Xiang* (Moschus) to open the orifices. The other Adjuvant herbs, *Zhu Sha* (Cinnabaris) and *Ci Shi* (Magnetite) sedate the Heart and calm the *Shen*, which strengthens the formula's ability to eliminate irritability. The Messenger herbs, *Mang Xiao* (Mirabilitum) and *Xiao Shi* (Niter) also drain Heat and dissipate clumps especially when combined with *Xuan Shen* (Scrophularia). This strong combination of ingredients is called "removing the firewood from under the cauldron." The last Messenger ingredients are *Huang Jin* (Gold) that weighs upon and sedates the *Shen* and *Gan Cao* (Glycyrrhiza) that relieves toxicity, harmonizes the Stomach, and protects the Stomach from injury by the heavy mineral ingredients.[1,4,6]

Cautions and Contraindications: Do not overdose *Zi Xue Dan*, or use it long term or during pregnancy. Overuse can impair *Yuan Qi* (Source *Qi*) and exhaust the *Yin*. To avoid mercury poisoning, *Zhu Sha* (Cinnabaris) should not be taken in large doses or used for a long time.[3,4]

Dr. Xie's Comments: *Zi Xue Dan* is useful to treat Liver Wind due to extreme Heat characterized by an acute onset of seizures or convulsions after a high fever, and irritability, with a purple or red tongue and a wiry or fast pulse.

Zhi Bao Dan (Greatest Treasure) 至宝丹

Zhi means greatest, *Bao* means treasure, and *Dan* means pill, the form of formula. *Zhi Bao* translates as Greatest Treasure because it is highly efficacious and expensive.

Source: *Tai Ping Hui Min He Ji Ju Fang* (*Imperial Grace Formulary of Tai Ping Era*), written by *Chen Shi-Wen* et al. in 1078

Ingredients: The ingredients of *Zhi Bao Dan* are 30 g *Xi Jiao* (Rhinoceros), 15 g *Niu Huang* (Bovis Calculus), 30 g *Dai Mao* (Eretmochelydis), 0.3 g *Bing Pian* (Borneol), 0.3 g *She Xiang* (Moschus), 45 g *An Xi Xiang* (Benzoin), 30 g *Zhu Sha* (Cinnabaris), 30 g *Hu Po* (Succinum), and 30 g *Xiong Huang* (Realgar) (Table 30.3).

Preparation:
1. Capsule method: Herbs are ground into a fine powder and encapsulated.
2. Teapill method: Raw herbs are mixed together, decocted, and formed into firm teapills.
3. Granular extract method: Raw herbs are mixed together, decocted, sprayed onto inert materials, and dried.[7]

Actions: Clear Heat, open the sensory orifices, transform turbidity, relieve toxicity

Indications: Closed disorder from Heat Phlegm characterized by fever; irritability; restlessness; delirium; impaired consciousness; coma; copious amounts of saliva with labored and raspy breathing; spasms; convulsions and a red tongue with thick greasy, yellow coating; a slippery, rapid pulse.

Dosage and Usage:
Horses and Cattle: 15–60 g, twice daily
Camels: 30–75 g, twice daily
Llamas, Alpacas, Goats, Sheep, and Pigs: 10–15 g, twice daily

Table 30.3. Ingredients and actions of *Zhi Bao Dan*.

%	English Name	Chinese *Pin Yin*	Actions
14	Rhinocerus	*Xi Jiao*	Clear Heat, relieve Fire toxicity, cool the Blood, arrest tremors
7	Bovis Calculus	*Niu Huang*	Clear pathogenic Heat, relieve convulsions by settling Internal Wind, restore consciousness
14	Eretmochelydis	*Dai Mao*	Sedate the Heart, calm the Liver, clear Heat, relieve toxicity
1	Borneol	*Bing Pian*	Open the orifice to restore consciousness, relieve pain, revive the *Shen*, Clear Heat
1	Moschus	*She Xiang*	Open the orifice to restore consciousness, relieve pain
21	Benzoin	*An Xi Xiang*	Open the orifice, promote the movement of *Qi*, Invigorate Blood
14	Cinnabaris	*Zhu Sha*	Tranquilize the Mind and clear Heat and toxins.
14	Succinum	*Hu Po*	Calm the *Shen*, tranquilize the mind
14	Realgar	*Xiong Huang*	Remove toxins, antihelminthic

Dogs: 0.5–5 g (or 0.1 g per kg body weight), twice daily
Cats and Rabbits: 0.2–0.5 g (or 0.1 g per kg body weight), twice daily
Birds: 0.1–0.2 g per kg body weight, twice daily

Use for 1–3 weeks until the primary clinical signs have resolved.[7]

Analysis of Formula: The primary actions of *Zhi Bao Dan* are to transform Phlegm and open the orifices, rather than to clear Heat. Since the ability of the formula to open the orifices is stronger than its ability to clear Heat, it may be combined with other cool or cold decoctions to open up Closed Syndromes with intense Heat and to revive the *Shen*.[3] The King ingredient, *Xi Jiao* (Rhinoceros), clears Heat from the *Ying* (nutritive) Level and cools the Blood. Its cool, aromatic properties make it useful for treating Heat that affects the Pericardium. Because Phlegm and Heat influence each other, it will be difficult to clear the Heat unless the turbid Phlegm is eliminated. The Minister ingredient, *Niu Huang* (Bovis Calculus), clears Heat, relieves toxicity, clears Phlegm, and opens the orifices, so it is used to eliminate the Phlegm Heat that obstructs the orifices of the Heart. Another Minister ingredient, *Dai Mao* (Eretmochelydis), enters both the Heart and Liver channels. Its sweet and cold properties sedate the Heart, calm the Liver, clear

Heat, and relieve toxicity. *Dai Mao* (Eretmochelydis) is particularly useful to cool the Liver, extinguish Wind, and stop spasms and convulsions. Because the Heart stores the *Shen* and the Liver stores the *Hun* (Soul), clearing Heat from these two channels serves to calm both the *Shen* and *Hun*. The Adjuvant ingredients, *Bing Pian* (Borneol), *She Xing* (Moschus), and *An Xi Xiang* (Benzoin), are all very aromatic, and they break up turbid Phlegm and open the orifices, thus eliminating the internal obstruction. The Messenger ingredients, *Zhu Sha* (Cinnabaris) and *Hu Po* (Succinum), sedate the Heart and calm the *Shen*, resolving irritability and the impairment of consciousness. The last Messenger ingredient, *Xiong Huang* (Realgar), eliminates Phlegm, relieves toxicity, and strengthens the actions of *Niu Huang* (Bovis Calculus) to break up Phlegm and open the orifices.[1,4,6]

Cautions and Contraindications: Do not overdose *Zhi Bao Dan* or use long term or during pregnancy. Overuse of this formula can impair *Yuan* (Source) *Qi* and exhaust the *Yin*. To avoid mercury poisoning, *Zhu Sha* (Cinnabaris) should not be taken in large doses or used for a long period of time.

Dr. Xie's Comments: *Zhi Bao Dan* is useful to treat a Closed Syndrome (*Bi Zheng*) due to Phlegm-Heat or head trauma with clinical signs of fever, irritability, restlessness, hypersalivation, impaired consciousness to the point of coma, a deep red tongue, and a slippery or fast pulse.

REFERENCES

1. Bensky D, Barolet R. Chinese Herbal Medicine Formulas and Strategies. Seattle, WA: Eastland Press, Inc., 1990.
2. Bensky D, Gamble A. Chinese Herbal Medicine Materia Medica. Seattle, WA: Eastland Press, Inc., 1993.
3. Flaws B. Seventy Essential TCM Formulas for Beginners. Boulder, CO: Blue Poppy Press, 1994.
4. Liu C, Tseng A. Chinese Herbal Medicine: Modern Applications of Traditional Formulas. Boca Raton, FL: CRC Press LLC, 2005.
5. Wicke R. Traditional Chinese Herbal Studies: Computer TCM Database. Rocky Mountain Herbal Institute, RMH Publications Trust, 1999–2003.
6. Zong LX. Pocket Handbook of Chinese Herbal Prescriptions. Miami: Waclion International, Inc., 2001.
7. Xie HS. Chinese Veterinary Herbal Handbook. Reddick, FL: Chi Institute of Chinese Medicine, 2004.

31 Herbal Formulas to Expel Wind 祛风镇痉剂

Chaoying Luo, Huisheng Xie, Kelly Chandler

The formulas in this chapter are used to treat patients with a *Feng Zheng* or Wind Pattern, which includes exogenous and endogenous Wind Patterns. In patients with exogenous Wind Patterns, *Feng Xie* (pathogenic Wind) invades the body and stays at the skin, channel, muscle, and bone levels but does not reach the deep level of the internal organs. The typical clinical signs of these Patterns include head-pressing or shaking, upper respiratory signs, fever, aversion to wind, pruritus, dermatitis, stiffness of neck and limbs, shifting joint aches and pains, facial distortion, and opisthotonos. The treatment strategy for this condition is to dispel Wind. Exogenous Wind often combines with Cold, Heat, or Damp to cause disease, leading to *Feng Han* (Wind-Cold Pattern), *Feng Re* (Wind-Heat Pattern), or *Feng Shi* (Wind-Damp Pattern). These Patterns are treated with formulas that expel Wind and dissipate Cold, dispel Wind and clear Heat, and dispel Wind while dissipating Damp, respectively.

Endogenous Wind Patterns, or Internal Wind, are commonly caused by pathology of internal organs: 1) Liver *Yang* Rising leading to Liver Wind (*Gan Feng Nei Dong*), 2) Extreme Heat causing Internal Wind (*Re Ji Sheng Feng*), 3) Blood Deficiency leading to Internal Wind (*Xue Xu Sheng Feng*), and 4) *Yin* Deficiency generating Wind (*Yin Xu Sheng Feng*). The typical clinical signs of the endogenous Wind Patterns include seizures, tremors, muscle twitches, neck rigidity, opisthotonos, paresis or paralysis, facial distortion, and an inability to stand. The treatment strategy for these Patterns is to subdue the Internal Wind to stop tremors.

The formulas in this chapter are divided into formulas for dispelling exogenous Wind and those for subduing endogenous Wind. When applying this group of formulas it is essential to differentiate between exogenous and endogenous Wind, between Cold and Heat Patterns, as well as between Deficiency and Excess Patterns. Exogenous Wind should be dispelled, while endogenous Wind needs to be subdued. If Wind is complicated with pathogenic Cold, Heat, Damp, or Phlegm, it is necessary to add herbs that expel cold, clear Heat, induce diuresis, or eliminate Phlegm, respectively. In addition, in case of exogenous Wind occurring concomitantly with endogenous Wind, it is necessary to differentiate the primary cause from the secondary cause in order to select the appropriate herbal formula. The herbal formulas to dispel exogenous Wind are mainly made of pungent and dispersing herbs with the effect of dispelling pathogenic Wind. These are used for treating diseases resulting from the attack on muscles, meridians and Collaterals, and tendons and joints by exogenous Wind. The formulas to subdue endogenous Wind consist chiefly of herbs that balance Liver *Yang* to stop endogenous Wind. These are used for diseases caused by Liver Wind disturbing normal metabolic functions.

Chuan Xiong Cha Tiao San (Ligusticum Powder) 川芎茶调散

Chuan Xiong is Ligusticum, the King ingredient of this formulation. *Cha Tiao* refers to taking with tea. *San* refers to powder, the original form of herbal administration.

Source: *Tai Ping Hui Min He Ji Ju Fang* (*Imperial Grace Formulary of the Tai Ping Era*), written by *Chen Shi-Wen* et al. and published by the *Song* Dynasty government in 1078 CE

Ingredients: The original formula (Table 31.1) is composed of 120 g *Chuan Xiong* (Ligusticum), 120 g *Jing Jie* (Schizonepeta), 60 g *Bai Zhi* (Angelica), 60 g *Qiang Huo* (Notopterygium), 60 g *Gan Cao* (Glycyrrhiza), 30 g *Xi Xin* (Asarum), 45 g *Fang Feng* (Ledebouriella), and 240 g *Bo He* (Mentha).

Table 31.1. Ingredients and actions of *Chuan Xiong Cha Tiao San.*

%	English Name	Chinese *Pin-Yin*	Actions
16.3	Ligusticum	*Chuan Xiong*	Expel Wind, move Blood to resolve Stagnation
16.3	Schizonepeta	*Jing Jie*	Expel Wind-Cold
8.2	Angelica	*Bai Zhi*	Expel Wind-Cold and relieve pain
8.2	Notopterygium	*Qiang Huo*	Expel Wind and resolve Stagnation
8.2	Glycyrrhiza	*Gan Cao*	Mediate the properties of other herbs
4.1	Asarum	*Xi Xin*	Expel Wind-Cold
6.1	Ledebouriella	*Fang Feng*	Expel Wind-Cold
32.6	Mentha	*Bo He*	Expel Wind and clear Heat

Preparation:

1. Powder or capsule method: Herbs are ground into a fine powder. Powder can be encapsulated.
2. Decoction or teapill method: Raw herbs are mixed together and decocted. Herbal water extract (decoction) can be concentrated as granules or teapills.

Actions: Dispel Wind to relieve pain.

Indications: This formula is indicated for Exogenous Wind Invasion, marked by aversion to Wind or Cold, with fever, nasal congestion, headache (head-shaking, or very sensitive to palpation of head), thin white coating of the tongue, and a superficial pulse.

Dosage and Usage:

Horses and Cattle: 15–30 g, twice daily
Camels: 30–45 g, twice daily
Llamas, Alpacas, Goats, Sheep, and Pigs: 5–10 g, twice daily
Dogs: 0.5–5 g (or 0.05 g per kg body weight), twice daily
Cats and Rabbits: 0.1–0.5 g (or 0.05 g per kg body weight), twice daily
Birds: 0.05 g per kg body weight, twice daily
Use 1–3 weeks until primary clinical signs resolve.

Analysis of Formula: When exogenous Wind invades the head and obstructs the *Yang-Qi*, it leads to local Stagnation and headache or head-shaking. The treatment is to dispel Wind and resolve Stagnation. The combination of Ligusticum (*Chuan Xiong*), Angelica (*Bai Zhi*), and Notopterygium (*Qiang Huo*) has the strong effect of expelling Wind and resolving Stagnation in the head. Ligusticum (*Chuan Xiong*) moves *Qi* and Blood, and resolves Stagnation in the *Shaoyang* meridian (Gallbladder and Triple Heater Channels). Notopterygium (*Qiang Huo*) is effective for removing Stagnation in the *Taiyang* Meridian (Bladder and Small Intestine Channels). Angelica (*Bai Zhi*) is good for resolving Stagnation along the *Yangming* Meridian (Stomach and Large Intestine Channels). These three herbs supplement one another in their effects and functions, acting as King herbs. Asarum (*Xi Xin*) dispels Cold, and Mentha (*Bo He*) expels Wind and opens the mind, acting as Minister herbs. Schizonepeta (*Jing Jie*) and Ledebouriella (*Fang Feng*) strengthen the effect of both King and Minister herbs in dispelling Wind and are used as Adjuvant herbs. Glycyrrhiza (*Gan Cao*) is the Messenger herb, which mediates the properties of other herbs.

Cautions and Contraindications: Do not use in patients with *Qi* Deficiency, Blood Deficiency, and headache caused by Liver Wind or Liver *Yang* Rising.

Dr. Xie's Comments: *Chuan Xiong Cha Tiao San* means Ligusticum Powder Taken with Tea. Historically, the herbal water extract or powder was taken with a cup of green tea. Since most ingredients are warm or dry with an expelling effect, the tea is used to prevent damage of body fluids and consumption of *Qi* since tea is cold and bitter in nature and has a descending effect. This makes the formula warm but not dry, maintains ascending and descending effects, and expels pathogenic factors without impairing healthy *Qi*. For veterinary use, this formula can be taken without the tea. I have used *Chuan Xiong Cha Tiao San* for acute onset of head-shaking in horses.

Clinical and Pharmacological Studies: One animal study in which the effects of *Chuan Xiong Cha Tiao San* were evaluated involved applying heat, acetic acid, or dimethylbenzene to mice. The researchers found the herbal formula to be beneficial in several ways: It provided pain relief; reduced fever; decreased vasodilation and permeability of celiac and endodermic capillaries; produced a strong antiinflammatory effect; was sedating; and improved respiratory function.[1]

Mei and *Liang* summarized and reported that *Chuan Xiong Cha Tiao San* was effective for the treatment of facial paralysis, trigeminal neuralgia, nasal polyp, cervical spondylosis, headache or migraine, rheumatic arthritis, infraorbital neuralgia, acute frontal sinusitis, bronchitis in children, cerebrovascular disease, allergic coryza urticaria, and other illnesses.[2–4]

Chuan Xiong Cha Tiao San was used for the treatment of 60 cases of neck pain and cervical spondylosis with a history of 6 months to more than 10 years. The results were that 27 cases were cured, 9 cases were significantly improved, 17 cases were improved, and 7 cases were not improved. The cases associated with nerve root and sympathetic nerve diseases were found to have a better response rate.[5] One patient with rheumatic arthritis lasting more than 2 years who didn't respond to prednisone and indomethacin, was treated with *Chuan*

Xiong Cha Tiao San at a dose of 6 g twice daily. A significant therapeutic result was seen after 18 days of herbal therapy and the patient was still healthy at the 6-month follow-up visit.[6] In another clinical study, 12 cases with acute frontal sinusitis were treated with *Chuan Xiong Cha Tiao San*; 11 were cured, and one case improved.[7]

Ju Hua Cha Tiao San (Chrysanthemum Powder) 菊花茶调散

Ju Hua means Chrysanthemum, the King ingredient of the formula. *Cha Tiao* refers to taking with tea. *San* refers to powder, the original form of herbal administration.

Source: *Dan Xi Xin Fa Fu Yu* (*Additions to Teachings of Zhu Dan-Xi*), written by *Fang Guang-Lei* and published in 1536 CE

Ingredients: *Ju Hua Cha Tiao San* is *Chuan Xiong Cha Tiao San* plus two more ingredients. It includes 60 g *Ju Hua* (Chrysanthemum) and 15 g *Jiang Can* (Bombyx), in addition to the ingredients of *Chuan Xiong Cha Tiao San*, which are: 60 g *Chuan Xiong* (Ligusticum), 60 g *Jing Jie* (Schizonepeta), 60 g *Bai Zhi* (Angelica), 60 g *Qiang Huo* (Notopterygium), 60 g *Gan Cao* (Glycyrrhiza), 30 g *Xi Xin* (Asarum), 45 g *Fang Feng* (Ledebouriella), and 15 g Bo He (Mentha).

Preparation:

1. Powder or capsule method: Herbs are ground into a fine powder. Powder can be encapsulated.
2. Decoction or teapill method: Raw herbs are mixed together and decocted. Herbal water extract (decoction) can be concentrated as granules or teapills.

Actions: Expel Wind and stop head-pressing and head-shaking, clear Heat and ease mental anxiety

Indications: This formula is indicated for Exogenous Wind-Heat Invasion to the head and neck. The main signs include ataxia, circling, general head pain or sensitivity to palpation of the head, head-pressing or head-shaking, fever, pain on swallowing, a red tongue, and a superficial and fast pulse.

Dosage and Usage:

Horses and Cattle: 15–30 g, twice daily
Camels: 30–45 g, twice daily
Llamas, Alpacas, Goats, Sheep, and Pigs: 5–10 g, twice daily
Dogs: 0.5–5 g (or 0.05 g per kg body weight), twice daily
Cats and Rabbits: 0.2–0.5 g (or 0.05 g per kg body weight), twice daily
Birds: 0.05 g per kg body weight, twice daily
Use 1–3 weeks until primary clinical signs resolve.

Analysis of Formula: *Ju Hua Cha Tiao San* is composed of *Chuan Xiong Cha Tiao San* plus *Ju Hua* (Chrysanthemum) and *Jiang Can* (Bombyx). *Chuan Xiong Cha Tiao San* expels Wind to resolve Stagnation and is used for the treatment of head-pressing or head-shaking due to exogenous Wind. *Ju Hua* (Chrysanthemum) is Cold and clears Wind-Heat, removes toxins, brightens the eyes, and works to ease anxiety. *Jiang Can* (Bombyx) extinguishes endogenous Wind to stop spasm, and expels exogenous Wind to stop pain. Therefore, *Ju Hua Cha Tiao San* is good at clearing Wind-Heat, and resolving Stagnation to stop head pain. It is often used for pain or head-shaking due to Wind-Heat.

Cautions and Contraindications: Do not use in patients with *Qi* Deficiency.

Dr. Xie's Comments: The title of *Ju Hua Cha Tiao San* means Chrysanthemum Powder Taken with Tea. Traditionally, the herbal powder is taken orally with a cup of tea. However, powder or capsule without the tea is more practical in veterinary patients. I have used *Ju Hua Cha Tiao San* for seasonal head-shaking in horses due to Stagnation at the head.

Cang Er Zi San (Xanthium Powder) 苍耳子散

Cang Er Zi refers to Xanthium, the King ingredient of the formula. *San* means powder, the form of the herbal administration. *Cang Er Zi San* means Xanthium Powder.

Source: *Ji Sheng Fang* (*Formulas to Aid the Living*), written by *Yan Yong-He* and published in 1253 CE

Ingredients: The ingredients of *Cang Er Zi San* (Table 31.2) are 15 g *Xin Yi Hua* (Magnolia), 8 g *Cang Er Zi* (Xanthium), 30 g *Bai Zhi* (Angelica), and 10 g *Bo He* (Mentha).

Preparation:

1. Powder or capsule method: Herbs are ground into a fine powder. Powder can be encapsulated.

Table 31.2. Ingredients and actions of *Cang Er Zi San*.

%	English Name	Chinese *Pin-Yin*	Actions
23.8	Magnolia	*Xin Yi Hua*	Clear Wind-Cold and open congested nose
12.7	Xanthium	*Cang Er Zi*	Clear Wind-Cold and open congested nose
47.6	Angelica	*Bai Zhi*	Dispel Wind-Cold, move *Qi* to stop pain
15.9	Mentha	*Bo He*	Clear Wind-Heat

2. Decoction or teapill method: Raw herbs are mixed together and decocted. Herbal water extract (decoction) can be concentrated as granules or teapills.

Actions: Clear Wind-Cold and open congested nose to stop pain

Indications: Nasal congestion or sinusitis due to Wind-Cold. The main signs include sneezing, nasal congestion, a pale tongue with a white and greasy coating, and a superficial and tight pulse.

Dosage and Usage:
Horses and Cattle: 15–30 g, twice daily
Camels: 30–45 g, twice daily
Llamas, Alpacas, Goats, Sheep, and Pigs: 5–10 g, twice daily
Dogs: 0.5–5 g (or 0.05 g per kg body weight), twice daily
Cats and Rabbits: 0.2–0.5 g (or 0.05 g per kg body weight), twice daily
Birds: 0.05 g per kg body weight, twice daily
Use 1–4 weeks until primary clinical signs resolve.

Analysis of Formula: *Cang Er Zi* (Xanthium) works as the King herb to clear Wind, dispel Cold, and open congested nasal passages. Serving as the Minister herbs, *Xin Yi Hua* (Magnolia) and *Bai Zhi* (Angelica) dispel Wind-Cold, clear congested nasal passages, and move *Qi* to stop pain. *Bo He* (Mentha) clears Wind Heat and soothes Liver *Qi* to resolve Stagnation, thereby acting as Adjuvant and Messenger herb.

Cautions and Contraindications: This formula should be used with caution with Wind-Heat.

Dr. Xie's Comments: I have used *Cang Er Zi San* for sinusitis, nasal congestion and general head pain due to Wind-Cold.

Xiao Feng San (Dispersing Wind) 消风散

Xiao means disperse. *Feng* means Wind. *San* refers to powder, the form of the original herbal administration method. *Xiao Feng San* means Dispersing Wind Powder.

Source: *Wai Ke Zheng Zong* (*The True Lineage of External Medicine*), written by *Chen Shi-Gong* and published in 1617 CE

Ingredients: The original formula (Table 31.3) is composed of 3 g Schizonepeta (*Jing Jie*), 3 g Ledebouriella (*Fang Feng*), 3 g Arctium (*Niu Bang Zi*), 3 g Cicada (*Chan Tui*), 3 g Atractylodes (*Cang Zhu*), 3 g Sophora (*Ku Shen*), 3 g Sesame (*Hei Zhi Ma*), 3 g Rehmannia (*Sheng Di Huang*), 3 g Anemarrhena (*Zhi Mu*), 3 g Angelica (*Dang Gui*), 3 g Gypsum (*Shi Gao*), 1.5 g Glycyrrhiza (*Gan Cao*), and 1.5 g Akebia (*Mu Tong*).

Table 31.3. Ingredients and actions of *Xiao Feng San*.

%	English Name	Chinese *Pin-Yin*	Actions
8.33	Schizonepeta	*Jing Jie*	Expel Wind, promote sweat, relieve the Exterior
8.33	Ledebouriella	*Fang Feng*	Expel Wind
8.33	Arctium	*Niu Bang Zi*	Expel Wind, benefit the throat, relieve the Exterior
8.33	Cicada	*Chan Tui*	Expel Wind and diaphoretic, relieve the Exterior
8.33	Atractylodes	*Cang Zhu*	Expel Wind and dry up Dampness
8.33	Sophora	*Ku Shen*	Expel Wind and clear Heat
8.33	Sesame	*Hei Zhi Ma*	Increase *Yin* and moisturize dryness
8.33	Rehmannia	*Sheng Di Huang*	Increase *Yin* and moisturize dryness
8.33	Anemarrhena	*Zhi Mu*	Clear Heat
8.33	Angelica	*Dang Gui*	Nourish Blood and promote Blood flow
8.3	Gypsum	*Shi Gao*	Clear Heat and purge pathogenic Fire
4.2	Akebia	*Mu Tong*	Benefit urination, drain Damp-Heat, clear Heat
4.2	Glycyrrhiza	*Gan Cao*	Mediate the properties of other herbs

Preparation:
1. Powder or capsule method: Herbs are ground into a fine powder. Powder can be encapsulated.
2. Decoction or teapill method: Raw herbs are mixed together and decocted. Herbal water extract (decoction) can be concentrated as granules or teapills.

Actions: Dispel Wind and nourish Blood, clear Heat and remove Damp

Indications: This formula is indicated for pruritus due to Wind-Heat marked with red skin rash, moist, exudative dermatitis, a red tongue with white or yellow coating, and a superficial and rapid pulse. It is applicable to urticaria, allergic dermatitis, pododermatitis, and other dermatopathies that are characterized by red skin rashes with pruritus and are caused by pathogenic Wind-Heat.

In case of fever and thirst due to Wind-heat, add *Jin Yin Hua* (Lonicera) and *Lian Qiao* (Forsythia) to dispel Wind and clear Heat; in case of Damp Heat with moist dermatitis on the abdomen and rear limbs, and a thick and greasy tongue coating, add *Di Fu Zi* (Kochia), *Che Qian Zi* (Plantago), and *Zhi Zi* (Gardenia) to clear Heat and induce diuresis. In case of excessive Heat in Blood with open ulcerations, (e.g., Lupus), and red or deep-red tongue, add *Chi Shao* (Paeonia), *Mu Dan Pi* (Moutan), and *Zi Cao* (Lithospermum) to clear Heat from Blood and cool the Blood.

Dosage and Usage:

Horses and Cattle: 15–30g, twice daily
Camels: 30–45g, twice daily
Llamas, Alpacas, Goats, Sheep, and Pigs: 5–10g, twice daily
Dogs: 0.5–5g (or 0.05g per kg body weight), twice daily
Cats and Rabbits: 0.1–0.3g (or 0.05g per kg body weight), twice daily
Birds: 0.05g per kg body weight, twice daily

Use 2–6 weeks until primary clinical signs resolve.

Analysis of Formula: Wind-Heat or Wind-Damp in the skin and subcutaneous space should be treated by dispelling Wind and nourishing Blood, as well as clearing Heat and draining Damp. *Jing Jie* (Schizonepeta), *Fang Feng* (Ledebouriella), *Niu Bang Zi* (Arctium), and *Chan Tui* (Cicada) are the King herbs in the formula, which can dispel Wind from the Exterior and relieve itching. *Cang Zhu* (Atractylodes) has the function of expelling Wind and Damp, and *Ku Shen* (Sophora) clears Heat and eliminates Damp. *Mu Tong* (Akebia) clears Damp-Heat by promoting a diuretic effect. *Zhi Mu* (Anemarrhena) and *Shi Gao* (Gypsum) clear Heat and purge Fire. Together these five ingredients eliminate Damp-Heat and function as Minister herbs. *Dang Gui* (Angelica), *Sheng Di Huang* (Rehmannia), and *Hei Zhi Ma* (Sesame) serve as Adjuvant herbs to nourish Blood and promote Blood circulation. Not only can they prevent Wind from impairing Blood, but they also can prevent herbs with a bitter and dry nature from impairing *Yin* and consuming Blood. *Gan Cao* (Glycyrrhiza) can clear Fire and mediate the properties of all other herbs, thereby playing the role of Messenger and guiding herb.

Cautions and Contraindications: None known

Dr. Xie's Comments: I have used *Xiao Feng San* for pruritus due to Wind Heat in dogs and horses.

Clinical and Pharmacological Studies: Animal studies indicate that *Xiao Feng San* has a significant antiallergenic effect and prevents hypersensitivity reactions in mice.[8] Effects of *Xiao Feng San* on hypersensitivity induced by 2,4-dinitroflurobenzene (DNFB) was investigated in mice. The results showed that *Xiao Feng San* inhibited ear swelling and the activity of interleukins 1, 2, and 4 in the affected skin tissues. *Xiao Feng San* also influenced the immune functions through its regulatory effects on T and B lymphocytes, and its inhibitory effects on cytokine production.[9,10]

Another study on *Xiao Feng San* on acute inflammatory responses was conducted in mice and rats. The results showed that this herbal medicine inhibited allergic edema induced by carrageenan in rear paws of rats and ear edema caused by xylol in mice. The study found that *Xiao Feng San* increased the activity of superoxide dismutase-1 (SOD-1), and decreased the activity of thromboxane A_2 (TXA_2) and the ratio of TXA_2/prostaglandin I_2 (PGI_2). These results indicated that *Xiao Feng San* reduced acute inflammation and this antiinflammatory mechanism may be related to increasing the activity of SOD-1 and adjusting the ratio of TXA_2/PGI_2.[11]

A *Xiao Feng San* modification was used for the treatment of 45 people with eczema. The added ingredients of this modified herbal formula were: 30g *Bai Fan* (Alum), 20g *Bai Xian Pi* (Dictamnus), 20g *Di Fu Zi* (Kochia), and 20g *She Chuang Zi* (Cnidium). Herbs were mixed and decocted. The herbal water extract, mixed with 50g *Hong Tang* (brown sugar), was given orally. This clinical trial showed that 38 out of 45 cases were healed and had not had a recurrence during the 2-year follow-up period, and 7 cases showed significant improvement.[12] *Lin Han-Fang* treated 38 cases of psoriasis using *Xiao Feng San* as the basic ingredients. In cases of Excessive Heat in Blood phase with dermal ulcerations, warm or sweaty feet, and red or deep-red tongue, subtract Angelica (*Dang Gui*) and add *Jin Yin Hua* (Lonicera) and *Tu Fu Ling* (Smilax). In cases of dryness and Blood Deficiency, subtract *Cang Zhu* (Atractylodes) and add *Bai Shao* (Paeonia) and *Mai Men Dong* (Ophiopogon). In cases of Blood Stagnation, add *Dan Shen* (Salvia) and *Chi Shao* (Paeonia). In cases of severe pruritus, add *Di Fu Zi* (Kochia) and *Bai Xian Pi* (Dictamnus). In cases of Dampness, add *Che Qian Zi* (Plantago) and *Ze Xie* (Alisma), In cases of diarrhea after taking medicine, add *Bai Zhu* (Atractylodes). In cases of nausea or vomiting after taking medicine, add *Shen Qu* (Massa) and *Mai Ya* (Hordeum). Twenty-three out of thirty-eight cases (60.53%) were clinically cured (all the symptoms including red maculae disappeared and did not return in 2 years); 12 cases improved (over 50% of the skin lesions disappeared); and 3 cases were not improved.[13] *Wang Yue* treated 68 human cases of allergic dermatitis caused by Ampicillin with *Xiao Feng San*. In cases of Wind-Heat, add 6g *Lian Qiao* (Forsythia). In cases of Damp-Heat, subtract *Cang Zhu* (Atractylodes) and add 6g *Che Qian Zi* (Plantago). In cases of Blood Heat, add 9g *Chi Shao* (Paeonia). In cases of Excessive Heat Toxin, add 6g *Da Huang* (Rheum).[14]

A combination of *Xiao Feng San* and *Si Wu Tang* was used for the treatment of 11 human cases of allergic dermatitis associated with ampicillin. Herbs were decocted in water and water extract was given orally, one dose, twice daily for 7 days. Another 11 cases (control group) were randomly selected and treated with 10ml 10% glucobiogen, 1g vitamin C, 5mg Decaesadril and 20ml 25% Amylaceum, by intravenous injection, once daily for 7 days. Eight of 11 patients (73%) who received the herbal formula healed completely, and 3 others improved. In the control group, only 4 of 11 healed completely, and 5 others showed improvement.[15]

From March 2003 to March 2005, 30 cases of cough due to pharyngitis were treated with *Xiao Feng San* modification. In cases of cough with white and watery Phlegm, subtract *Shi Gao* (Gypsum) and *Zhi Mu* (Anemarrhena) and add 10 g *Ban Xia* (Pinellia) and 20 g *Che Qian Zi* (Plantago). In cases of angina, add 20 g *Jin Yin Hua* (Lonicera) and 15 g *Lian Qiao* (Forsythia). In cases of a paroxysm of coughing, add 9 g *Chai Hu* (Bupleurum) and 10 g *Huang Qin* (Scutellaria). Herbs were decocted in water for oral dose, one dose daily for 7 days. Another 30 cases (control group) were treated with antibiotics (0.25 g Azithromycin collocystis), twice daily for 7 days; 26 of 30 patients who took the herbal formula improved (86.6%), and only 16 of 30 (53.3%) in the Azithromycin group showed improvement. The herbal treatment was significantly more effective than the antibiotic therapy ($P < 0.05$).[16]

Xiao Feng San modification and polyinosinic acid were used for the treatment of 40 cases of herpes. In case of Excessive Heat (hot, red, or bloody skin lesions), subtract *Cang Zhu* (Atractylodes) and *Ku Shen* (Sophora), and add *Jin Yin Hua* (Lonicera), *Da Qing Ye* (Isatis), *Pu Gong Ying* (Taraxacum), *Dan Pi* (Moutan), and *Chi Shao* (Paeonia). In cases of more Damp (oozing skin lesions, less painful or loose stool), subtract *Shi Gao* (Gypsum), *Zhi Mu* (Anemarrhena), *Huo Ma Ren* (Cannabis), *Niu Bang Zi* (Arctium), and *Sheng Di Huang* (Rehmannia) and add *Bai Zhu* (Atractylodes), *Fu Ling* (Poria), *Ze Xie* (Alisma), *Bai Xian Pi* (Dictamnus), and *Ban Lan Gen* (Isatis). In cases of Blood Stagnation (local painful swelling), subtract *Cang Zhu* (Atractylodes), *Niu Bang Zi* (Arctium), *Huo Ma Ren* (Cannabis), and add *Ji Xue Teng* (Millettia), *Tao Ren* (Persica), *Hong Hua* (Carthamus) and *Mu Xiang* (Saussurea). In cases of chronic pain after skin exudation disappeared, add *Pu Huang* (Typha), *Wu Ling Zhi* (Trogopterus), and *Si Gua Luo* (Luffa). In cases of facial herpes, add *Ju Hua* (Chrysanthemum) and *Quan Xie* (Buthus). In cases of herpes on lower limbs, add *Huang Bai* (Phellodendron) and *Niu Xi* (Achyranthes). Herbs were decocted in water for oral dose, one dose daily for 10 days. Simultaneously, 2 mg polyinosinic acid was injected intramuscularly once every other day for 10 days. In addition, calamine lotion was topically applied on the skin lesions. After the treatment, 29 out of 40 cases (72.5%) were clinically healed; another 10 cases (25%) were significantly improved. The longest period of treatment was 12 days, the shortest was 6 days, and the average was 9 days.[17] *Xiao Feng San* was used as a basic formulation for the treatment of 48 cases of conjunctivitis. In cases of conjunctivitis of limbus corneae, add 12 g *Huang Qin* (Scutellaria) and 12 g *Bai Ji Li* (Tribulus). In cases of conjunctival conjunctivitis, add 15 g *Shi Gao* (Gypsum) and 10 g *Lian Qiao* (Forsythia). In cases of a mixed Pattern, add 10 g *Chi Shao* (Paeonia). In cases of severe pruritus, add 3 g *Xi Xin* (Asarum) and 10 g *Bai Ju Hua* (White Chrysanthemum). In cases of redness and Heat signs, subtract *Huo Xiang* (Pogostemon) and *Fu Ling* (Poria) and add 12 g *Sheng Di Huang* (Rehmannia) and 12 g *Mu Dan Pi* (Moutan). In cases of filiform secretion, add 12 g *Pu Gong Ying* (Taraxacum). In cases of gelatinous secretion, add 12 g *Xia Ku Cao* (Prunella). In cases of constipation, add 6 g *Da Huang* (Rheum). In cases of dyspepsia, add 6 g *Shan Zha* (Crataegus) and 6 g *Shen Qu* (Massa). In cases of weakness or prolonged illness, add 15 g *Huang Qi* (Astragalus) and 10 g *Bai Zhu* (Atractylodes)l In cases of concurrent allergic rhinitis, add 12 g *Cang Er Zi* (Xanthium) and *Bai Zhi* (*Angelica*). Herbs were decocted in water for oral dose, one dose daily for 15 days. The period of treatment was 12 days to 3 months. After the treatment, 34 out of 48 (70.83%) were clinically cured.[18]

Xiao Huo Luo Dan (Few Ingredients Activating the Channels) 小活络丹

Xiao means minor or small, and in this instance refers to few ingredients. *Huo* means activating, or moving. *Luo* means the Meridians or Channels. *Dan* is the teapill, the original method of administration. *Xiao Huo Luo Dan* means Few Ingredients Activating the Channels.

Source: *Tai Ping Hui Min He Ji Ju Fang* (*Imperial Grace Formulary of the Tai Ping Era*), written by *Chen Shi-Wen* et al. and published by the *Song* Dynasty government in 1078 CE

Ingredients: The original formula (Table 31.4) is composed of 180 g *Chuan Wu* (Aconite), 180 g *Cao Wu* (Aconite), 180 g *Di Long* (Pheretima), 180 g *Tian Nan Xing* (Arisaema), 66 g *Ru Xiang* (Olibanum), and 66 g *Mo Yao* (Myrrh).

Preparation:

1. Powder or capsule method: Herbs are ground into a fine powder. Powder can be encapsulated.
2. Decoction or teapill method: Raw herbs are mixed together and decocted. Herbal water extract (decoction) can be concentrated as granules or teapills.

Actions: Dispel Wind-Damp, remove Phlegm and activate the Collaterals, promote Blood circulation and relieve pain

Indications: This formula is indicated for *Bi* syndrome due to Wind-Cold-Damp marked with pain in joints or back; stiffness and decreased range of motion of joints; aversion to cold and preference for warmth; a pale or

Table 31.4. Ingredients and actions of *Xiao Huo Luo Dan.*

%	English Name	Chinese *Pin-Yin*	Actions
21.1	Aconite	*Chuan Wu*	Dispel Wind, Cold, and Damp; warm Meridians and relieve pain
21.1	Aconite	*Cao Wu*	Dispel Wind, Cold, and Damp; warm Meridians and relieve pain
21.1	Pheretima	*Di Long*	Activate the Meridians and Collaterals and lead other herbs to the Collaterals to eliminate pathogenic factors
21.1	Arisaema	*Tian Nan Xing*	Dry up Damp, resolve Phlegm, expel Wind, activate the Meridians and Collaterals
7.8	Olibanum	*Ru Xiang*	Adjuvant herb to promote the circulation of *Qi* and Blood and alleviate pain
7.8	Myrrh	*Mo Yao*	Adjuvant herb to promote the circulation of *Qi* and Blood and alleviate pain

purple tongue with a white coating; and a deep, thready pulse. It is used for osteoarthritis, degenerative joint disease (DJD), intervertebral disc disease (IVDD), and immune-mediated polyarthritis. In case of long-term illness occurring concomitantly with Liver Blood and Kidney *Qi* deficiency, *Du Huo Ji Sheng Tang* can be used simultaneously.

Dosage and Usage:

Horses and Cattle: 15–30g, twice daily
Camels: 30–45g, twice daily
Llamas, Alpacas, Goats, Sheep, and Pigs: 5–10g, twice daily
Dogs: 0.3–3g (or 0.05g per kg body weight), twice daily
Cats and Rabbits: 0.1–0.3g (or 0.05g per kg body weight), twice daily
Birds: 0.05g per kg body weight, twice daily

Use 2–4 weeks until primary clinical signs resolve.

Analysis of Formula: When Wind, Cold, and Damp stay in the Meridians and Collaterals for so long that *Qi* and Blood fail to circulate normally, Phlegm and Blood Stasis are generated. The key treatment is to eliminate Wind, Cold, and Damp, remove Phlegm and Blood Stasis, and activate the Meridians and Collaterals. *Chuan Wu* (Aconite) and *Cao Wu* (Aconite) act as King herbs to dispel Wind, Cold, and Damp; warm Meridians; and relieve pain. *Tian Nan Xing* (Arisaema) can dry Damp, resolve Phlegm, expel Wind, and activate the Meridians and Collaterals, acting as the Minister herb. *Ru Xiang* (Olibanum) and *Mo Yao* (Myrrh) are used as Adjuvant herbs to promote the circulation of *Qi* and Blood to alleviate pain. *Di Long* (Pheretima) has the function of activating the Meridians and Collaterals and leading other herbs to the Collaterals to eliminate pathogenic factors; and *Di Long* plays the part of Messenger and guiding herb.

Cautions and Contraindications: This formula is used in patients with a strong constitution and excess Pattern. It cannot be used in patients with Heat Pattern due to *Yin* Deficiency or in pregnant animals.

Dr. Xie's Comments: I have used *Xiao Huo Luo Dan* with great success for severe back pain associated with IVDD and painful DJD due to Wind-Cold-Damp in dogs.

Clinical and Pharmacological Studies: Animal studies in mice indicated that *Xiao Huo Luo Dan* had a pharmacological effect of immunosuppression, antiinflammation, analgesia, and antioxidation.[19]

Chui treated 32 human cases of sciatica using *Xiao Huo Luo Dan*: 9g *Cao Wu* (Aconite), 9g *Chuan Wu* (Aconite), 9g *Tian Nan Xing* (Arisaema), 9g *Ru Xiang* (Olibanum), 9g *Mo Yao* (Myrrh), and 15g *Di Long* (Pheretima). Herbs were decocted and water extract was given orally, twice a day for 20 days. The courses of sciatica were 7 days to 2.5 years. Diagnosis of sciatica was based on clinical symptoms and radiographs, which were used to rule out other causes of pain, including tumor, tuberculosis, and fracture. Among 32 cases of sciatica, 20 cases were cured clinically, 7 cases were significantly improved, 3 cases were noticeably improved, and 2 cases were unchanged.[20] Veterinary patients with hind limb weakness and pain without radiographic evidence of an explanation might benefit from this formula.

Xue used a combination of *Xiao Huo Luo Dan* and *Du Huo Ji Sheng Tang* for the treatment of 32 cases of chronic DJD and osteoarthritis in horses, cattle, and buffalo. The combined ingredients of the herbal medicine were 30g each of *Cao Wu* (Aconite), *Chuan Wu* (Aconite), *Ru Xiang* (Olibanum), *Mo Yao* (Myrrh), *Dang Gui* (Angelica), *Chuan Xiong* (Ligusticum), *Bai Zhi* (Angelica), *Qiang Huo* (Notopterygium), *Sang Ji Sheng* (Loranthus), *Du Zhong* (Eucommia), *Niu Xi* (Achyranthes), *Xu Duan* (Dipsacus), and *Rou Gui* (Cinnamomum); 24g each of *Tian Nan Xing* (Arisaema) and *Chen Pi* (Citrus); 15g each of *Di Long* (Pheretima) and *Hou Po* (Magnolia); 12g *Gan Cao* (Glycyrrhiza); and 6g *Xi Xin* (Asarum). Herbs were decocted four times in water, and water extract was given orally, twice daily for 2 to 4 days. Among 32 cases, 30 cases were significantly improved (93.7%).[21]

Paralysis due to disc diseases and rheumatic arthritis in pigs was also successfully treated with *Xiao Huo Luo Dan* and *Du Luo Ji Sheng Tang*. The ingredients of this herbal combination are 30g *Cao Wu* (Aconite), 30g *Chuan Wu* (Aconite), 25g Tian Nan Xing (Arisaema), 15g *Di Long* (Pheretima), 30g *Ru Xiang* (Olibanum), 30g *Mo Yao* (Myrrh), 30g *Dang Gui* (Angelica), 30g *Chuan Xiong* (Ligusticum), 30g *Qiang Huo* (Notopterygium), 30g *Sang Ji Sheng* (Loranthus), 30g *Du Zhong* (Eucommia), 30g *Niu Xi* (Achyranthes), 30g *Xu Duan* (Dipsacus), 30g *Rou Gui* (Cinnamomum), 10g *Xi Xin* (Asarum), 25g *Chen Pi* (Citrus), 15g *Hou Po* (Magnolia), and 25g *Gan Cao* (Glycyrrhiza). Herbs were decocted three times in water; water extract was given orally, one dose daily for 3 days. Additionally, an intramuscular injection of *Yan Hu Suo* (Corydalis) was administered twice a day for 3 days. Twenty-eight out of 29 paralyzed pigs were able to walk and run after the herbal treatment (96.55%).[22] *Xiao Huo Luo Dan* was used for the treatment of 49 cases of duodenal Stasis, taken orally after meals, 1 pill, 2 to 3 times daily for 5 to 10 days. This clinical study showed that 37 cases were clinically cured and 8 cases were improved after herbal treatment.[23] *Xiao Huo Luo Dan* was also used in treating 18 cases of calcaneus pain for a duration of 3 months to 5.5 years. After 7–14 daily herbal treatments, 11 cases were clinically cured and 5 cases improved.[23]

Da Huo Luo Dan (Many Ingredients Activating the Channels) 大活络丹

Da is big or large, and in this instance refers to the large number of ingredients. *Huo* means activating or moving. *Luo* is the Meridians or Channels. *Dan* is the teapill, the original method of administration. *Da Huo Luo Dan* means Many Ingredients Activating the Channels.

Source: *Lan Tai Gui Fan* (*The Examples of Lan Tai*), written by *Xu Da-chun* and published in 1764 CE

Ingredients: The original formula (Table 31.5) is composed of 60g *Bai Hua She* (Agkistrodon), 60g *Wu Shao She* (Zaocys), 60g *Wei Ling Xian* (Clematis), 60g *Liang Tou Jian* (Anemone), 60g *Cao Wu* (Aconite), 60g *Tian Ma* (Gastrodia), 60g *Quan Xie* (Buthus), 60g *He Shou Wu* (Polygonam), 60g *Gui Ban* (Testudinis), 60g *Ma Huang* (Ephedra), 60g *Guan Zhong* (Dryopteris), 60g *Gan Cao* (Glycyrrhiza), 60g *Qiang Huo* (Notopterygium), 60g *Rou Gui* (Cinnamomum), 60g *Huo Xiang* (Pogostemon), 60g *Wu Yao* (Lindera), 60g *Huang Lian* (Coptis), 60g *Shu Di Huang* (Rehmannia), 60g *Da Huang* (Rheum), 60g *Mu Xiang* (Saussurea), 60g *Chen Xiang* (Aquilaria), 30g *Xi Xin* (Asarum), 30g *Chi Shao* (Paeonia), 30g *Ding Xiang* (Caryophylli), 30g *Ru Xiang* (Olibanum), 30g *Jiang Can* (Bombyx), 30g *Tian Nan Xin* (Arisaema), 30g *Qing Pi* (Citrus), 30g *Gu Sui Bu* (Drynaria), 30g *Bai Dou Kou* (Cardamon), 30g *An Xi Xiang* (Benzoin), 30g *Fu Zi* (Aconite), 30g *Huang Qin* (Scutellaria), 30g *Fu Ling* (Poria), 30g *Xiang Fu* (Cyperus), 30g *Xuan Shen* (Scrophularia), 30g *Bai Zhu* (Atractylodes), 75g *Fang Feng* (Ledebouriella), 45g *Ge Gen* (Pueraria), 45g *Hu Gu* (Tigris [swine bones are now substituted for the tiger bone in the original formula]), 45g *Dang Gui* (Angelica), 21g *Xue Jie* (Draconis), 15g *Di Long* (Pheretima), 45g *Shui Niu Jiao* (Bubali cornu), 15g *She Xiang* (Moschus), 15g *Song Zhi* (Colophonium), 4.5g *Niu Huang* (Bovis), 4.5g *Bing Pian* (Borneol), and 90g *Ren Shen* (Ginseng).

Preparation:

1. Powder or capsule method: Herbs are ground into a fine powder. Powder can be encapsulated.
2. Decoction or teapill method: Raw herbs are mixed together and decocted. Herbal water extract (decoction) can be concentrated as granules or teapills.

Actions: Clear Wind-Damp, Tonify *Qi* and Blood, activate the Meridians to relieve pain

Indications: This formula is indicated for paralysis or severe paresis due to Stagnation of Wind-Damp or Phlegm in the Meridians and Channels. It can be used for IVDD; degenerative myelopathy; spondylosis; and the sequelae of cerebral thrombosis, cerebral embolism, and cerebral hemorrhage. Tongue is pale or purple, with a weak or wiry pulse.

Dosage and Usage:

Horses and Cattle: 15–30g, twice daily
Camels: 30–45g, twice daily
Llamas, Alpacas, Goats, Sheep, and Pigs: 5–10g, twice daily
Dogs: 0.5–5g (or 0.05g per kg body weight), twice daily
Cats and Rabbits: 0.2–0.5g (or 0.05g per kg body weight), twice daily
Birds: 0.05g per kg body weight, twice daily

Use 2–4 weeks until primary clinical signs resolve.

Analysis of Formula: The actions of *Da Huo Luo Dan* are similar to *Xiao Huo Luo Dan*. The main difference is that *Da Huo Luo Dan* can tonify *Qi* and *Yang* and nourish Blood and *Yin* in addition to clearing Wind-Damp. Thus, it can be used for the treatment of excessive Wind-Damp combined with *Qi* and Blood Deficiency. On the other hand, *Xiao Huo Luo Dan* is used only for Excess Pattern of *Bi* syndrome due to Wind-Cold-Damp.

Cautions and Contraindications: It cannot be used in patients with Heat Pattern due to *Yin* Deficiency or in pregnant animals.

Dr. Xie's Comments: I have successfully used *Da Huo Luo Dan* for paralysis or paresis associated with IVDD

Table 31.5. Ingredients and actions of *Da Huo Luo Dan.*

%	English Name	Chinese *Pin-Yin*	Actions	%	English Name	Chinese *Pin-Yin*	Actions
2.8	Agkistrodon	*Bai Hua She*	Subdue Wind and remove obstruction in the Meridians	1.4	Bombyx	*Jiang Can*	Subdue Wind and stop convulsion
2.8	Zaocys	*Wu Shao She*	Dispel Wind and stop convulsion, activate Collaterals	1.4	Arisaema	*Tian Nan Xin*	Dry up Damp and eliminate Phlegm, expel endogenous Wind to relieve convulsion
2.8	Clematis	*Wei Ling Xian*	Dissolve Damp and resolve Stagnation of Collaterals	1.4	Citrus	*Qing Pi*	Sooth the Liver *Qi*, resolve Stagnation
2.8	Anemone	*Liang Tou Jian*	Dissolve Wind and eliminate Damp	1.4	Drynaria	*Gu Sui Bu*	Tonify the Kidney and strengthen bone and muscle
2.8	Aconite	*Cao Wu*	Dispel Wind to relieve pain	1.4	Cardamon	*Bai Dou Kou*	Dispel Damp and strengthen the Spleen, stop vomiting
2.8	Gastrodia	*Tian Ma*	Soothe the Liver to stop Wind and convulsions	1.4	Benzoin	*An Xi Xiang*	Promote *Qi* flow to relieve pain
2.8	Buthus	*Quan Xie*	Subdue Wind, dispel Wind to relieve spasm	1.4	Aconite	*Fu Zi*	Dispel Cold to relieve pain, warm Kidney *Yang*
2.8	Polygonum	*He Shou Wu*	Nourish Liver, Kidney, and Blood	1.4	Scutellaria	*Huang Qin*	Dispel Damp and clear Heat, cool Blood
2.8	Testudines	*Gui Ban*	Nourish *Yin* to suppress *Yang*				
2.8	Ephedra	*Ma Huang*	Dispel Cold and eliminate Damp	1.4	Poria	*Fu Ling*	Excrete Damp and strengthen Spleen
2.8	Dryopteris	*Guan Zhong*	Clear Heat and relieve the Exterior	1.4	Cyperus	*Xiang Fu*	Soothe the Liver and regulate *Qi*, eliminate Stagnation
2.8	Glycyrrhiza	*Gan Cao*	Coordinate all other herbs' actions	1.4	Scrophularia	*Xuan Shen*	Nourish *Yin*, cool Blood, soften lumps
2.8	Notopterygium	*Qiang Huo*	Expel Wind, remove Cold to stop pain	1.4	Atractylodes	*Bai Zhu*	Strengthen the Spleen and eliminate Damp
2.8	Cinnamomum	*Rou Gui*	Warm the Kidney and Spleen and dispel Cold	3.4	Ledebouriella	*Fang Feng*	Expel Wind, eliminate Damp, relieve convulsion
2.8	Pogostemon	*Huo Xiang*	Dissolve Damp and Summer-Heat, stop vomiting	2	Pueraria	*Ge Gen*	Relax the muscles and other soft tissues
2.8	Lindera	*Wu Yao*	Warm the Kidney, move *Qi* to stop pain	2	Tigris*	*Hu Gu*	Dispel Wind, activate Collaterals, strengthen the bones
2.8	Coptis	*Huang Lian*	Clear Heat and eliminate Damp, detoxify				
2.8	Rehmannia	*Shu Di Huang*	Tonify Blood and nourish *Yin*	2	Angelica	*Dang Gui*	Nourish Blood, eliminate Stagnation to relieve pain
2.8	Rheum	*Da Huang*	Clear Heat, activate Blood and remove Stasis	0.9	Draconis	*Xue Jie*	Eliminate Stagnation to relieve pain, regenerate tissues to heal wounds
2.8	Saussurea	*Mu Xiang*	Promote *Qi* flow to relieve pain	0.7	Pheretima	*Di Long*	Clear Heat, relieve convulsion, dispel Wind and remove obstruction in the Meridians
2.8	Aquilaria	*Chen Xiang*	Dispel Cold to relieve pain				
1.4	Asarum	*Xi Xin*	Relieve the Exterior, dispel Wind-Cold to relieve pain	2	Bubali cornu	*Shui Niu Jiao*	Clear Heat, calm the mind and stop convulsion
1.4	Paeonia	*Chi Shao*	Cool Blood to clear Heat, move Blood to remove Stasis	0.7	Moschus	*She Xiang*	Subside swelling, relieve pain
1.4	Caryophylli	*Ding Xiang*	Warm the Middle Burner to descend rebellious Stomach *Qi*	0.7	Colophonium	*Song Zhi*	Eliminate Damp, dispel Wind, remove toxins
				0.2	Bovis	*Niu Huang*	Clear Heat, calm the mind and stop convulsion
1.4	Olibanum	*Ru Xiang*	Move *Qi* to relieve pain and relax and activate the tendons	0.2	Borneol	*Bing Pian*	Clear Heat, stop pain
				4	Ginseng	*Ren Shen*	Tonify *Qi*

*Swine bones are now substituted for the tiger bone in the original formula.

and spondylosis due to Wind-Damp and general *Qi*-Blood Deficiency in dogs.

Clinical and Pharmacological Studies: Eleven minerals, including zinc (Zn), manganese (Mg), potassium (K), and Chromium (Cr), were found in *Da Huo Luo Dan*. The concentration of these minerals from the water extract of *Da Huo Luo Dan* is much lower than the pills made of the powder. The concentration of Cr, Zn, K, and Mg from herbal powder was 0.147, 2.792,

2.997, and 678.3 μg/g, respectively. The effect of *Da Huo Luo Dan* on hemiplegia due to stroke may be related to the fact that *Da Huo Luo Dan* can correct underlying mineral deficiencies, including Cr, Zn, K, and Mg, in stroke patients.[24]

Antiepileptic effects of *Da Huo Luo Dan* were studied in comparison to Phenytoin sodium. The Scale for the Assessment of Positive Symptoms (SAPS), the Treatment Emergent Symptom Scale (TESS), and the Clinical Global Impression Scale (CGIS) were used to evaluate clinical observations. The results were that the difference in antiepileptic effects of the two groups was not remarkable ($P > 0.05$), but the side effect of behavior disorder from Phenytoin sodium was remarkable; in the *Da Huo Luo Dan* group, this side effect was not noticed.[25]

Da Hao Luo Dan was combined with *Qu Feng Jie Du Tang* for the treatment of 31 cases of polyneuritis. *Qu Feng Jie Du Tang* is composed of 10 g *Xu Chang Qing* (Cynanchum), 15 g *Xi Xian Cao* (Siegesbeckia), 15 g *Luo Shi Teng* (Trachelospermi), 10 g *Wu Shao She* (Zaocys), 15 g *Ban Lan Gen* (Isatis), 15 g *Ju Hua* (Chrysanthemum), and 15 g *Jin Yin Hua* (Lonicera). In case of intense Damp Heat, *Huang Bai* (Phellodendron), *Cang Zhu* (Atractylodes), and *Yi Yi Ren* (Coix) were added. In case of long-term illness occurring concomitantly with heavy pain and ecchymosis or petechiae on the tongue, *San Qi* (Notoginseng), *Dang Gui* (Angelica), and *Ji Xue Teng* (Millettia) were added. In case of *Yin* deficiency, *Bie Jia* (Trionycis), *Shi Hu* (Dendobium), and *Xuan Shen* (Scrophularia) were added. Herbs were decocted three times in water; the herbal extract of *Qu Feng Jie Du Tang* was given twice a day. Twelve grams of *Da Hao Luo Dan* were taken twice daily. After a 3-month herbal treatment, all 31 cases were clinically cured and did not recur in 1 year.[26] Several clinical trials were performed on the effectiveness of *Da Hao Luo Dan*.[27] In one study, 42 cases of gastrocnemius muscle atrophy and pain were treated with *Da Hao Luo Dan*; 31 cases were clinically cured, and 8 cases were significantly improved. In another study, 26 cases of epilepsy caused by internal Phlegm were treated with *Da Hao Luo Dan*, 12 grams, taken twice daily for 30 days. After 3–4 months of herbal treatments, 7 cases were clinically seizure free, and 15 cases had fewer and less-severe seizure activity.[27]

Ban Xia Bai Zhu Tian Ma San (Pinellia and Atractylodes with Gastroida) 半夏白术天麻散

Ban Xia Bai Zhu Tian Ma refers to the three main ingredients of this herbal formula: *Ban Xia* is Pinellia, *Tian Ma* refers to Gastrodia, and *Bai Zhu* is Atractylodes. San is the powder form of herbal administration.

Source: *Yi Xue Xin Wu* (*Medical Revelations*), written by *Cheng Guo-Peng* and published in 1732 CE

Table 31.6. Ingredients and actions of *Ban Xia Bai Zhu Tian Ma San*.

%	English Name	Chinese *Pin-Yin*	Actions
16.4	Pinellia	*Ban Xia*	Dry up Damp to eliminate Phlegm, reduce swelling
27.3	Atractylodes	*Bai Zhu*	Strengthen the Spleen to eliminate Damp
10.9	Gastrodia	*Tian Ma*	Calm the Liver to stop Wind and convulsions
10.9	Citrus	*Chen Pi*	Dry up Damp to eliminate Phlegm, move *Qi*
10.9	Poria	*Fu Ling*	Induce diuresis to drain Damp
7.3	Glycyrrhiza	*Zhi Gan Cao*	Coordinate the other herbs' actions
5.5	Zingiberis	*Sheng Jiang*	Expel Wind-Cold, warm the Stomach to stop vomiting
10.8	Jujube	*Da Zao*	Mildly tonify the Spleen *Qi*, harmonize all other herbs

Ingredients: The original formula (Table 31.6) is composed of 9 g *Ban Xia* (Pinellia), 15 g *Bai Zhu* (Atractylodes), 6 g *Tian Ma* (Gastrodia), 6 g *Chen Pi* (Citrus), 6 g *Fu Ling* (Poria), 4 g *Zhi Gan Cao* (Glycyrrhiza), 3 g *Sheng Jiang* (Zingiberis), and 6 g *Da Zao* (Jujube).

Preparation:

1. Powder or capsule method: Herbs are ground into a fine powder. Powder can be encapsulated.
2. Decoction or teapill method: Raw herbs are mixed together and decocted. Herbal water extract (decoction) can be concentrated as granules or teapills.

Actions: Dry up Damp to eliminate Phlegm, calm the Liver to stop Wind

Indications: This formula is indicated for Phlegm-Damp Patterns marked by seizures; loss of balance; head-pressing or head-shaking; excessive salivation; nausea and vomiting; soft or mucoid stools; a white, greasy tongue coating and a soft, wiry pulse.

Dosage and Usage:

Horses and Cattle: 15–30 g, twice daily
Camels: 30–45 g, twice daily
Llamas, Alpacas, Goats, Sheep, and Pigs: 5–10 g, twice daily
Dogs: 0.5–5 g (or 0.05 g per kg body weight), twice daily
Cats and Rabbits: 0.2–0.5 g (or 0.05 g per kg body weight), twice daily
Birds: 0.05 g per kg body weight, twice daily

Use 4–12 weeks until primary clinical signs resolve.

Analysis of Formula: Loss of balance accompanied by signs of head pain, nausea, and vomiting, and a white and greasy tongue coating are the effect of Phlegm caused by Spleen Deficiency and Liver Wind stirring. The key treatment is to transform Phlegm, subdue Wind, strengthen the Spleen, and dry up Damp. *Ban Xia* (Pinellia) and *Tian Ma* (Gastrodia) are the King herbs, which dry up Damp, eliminate Phlegm, and subdue Wind to stop signs of dizziness. *Bai Zhu* (Atractylodes) acts as the Minister herb to strengthen the Spleen and eliminate Damp; it has a stronger effect on dissolving Damp to dissipate Phlegm when combined with *Ban Xia* (Pinellia) and *Tian Ma* (Gastrodia). *Chen Pi* (Citrus) regulates *Qi* to eliminate Phlegm. *Sheng Jiang* (Zingiberis) and *Da Zao* (Jujube) harmonize the Spleen and Stomach. *Chen Pi*, *Sheng Jiang*, and *Da Zao* play the part of Adjunct herbs. *Gan Cao* (Glycyrrhiza) regulates the Middle Burner and plays the part of Messenger herb. Together they can subdue Wind, eliminate Phlegm, and treat loss of balance or other signs of dizziness.

Cautions and Contradictions: This formula is contraindicated in cases showing Dryness due to *Yin* Deficiency.

Dr. Xie's Comments: I have used *Ban Xia Bai Zhu Tian Ma San* for seizure cases with Spleen *Qi* Deficiency (loose stool, or excessive salivation) in dogs.

Clinical and Pharmacological Studies: *Ban Xia Bai Zhu Tian Ma San* modification was used for the treatment of primary hypertension, cardiovascular and cerebrovascular diseases, diabetes mellitus, hyperlipidemia, and cardiopulmonary syndromes. There were 102 cases in total: 46 cases of hypertension, 30 cases of the sequelae of brain infarction, 10 cases of diabetes mellitus, 9 cases of coronary artery disease, and 7 cases of other diseases. In the herbal group, 62 cases were treated with both conventional medicines and *Ban Xia Bai Zhu Tian Ma San* modification, which contained the following ingredients: *Ban Xia* (Pinellia), *Bai Zhu* (Atractylodes), *Tian Ma* (Gastrodia), *Fu Ling* (Poria), *Chen Pi* (Citrus), *Dan Shen* (Salvia), *Dang Gui* (Angelica), *Shi Chang Pu* (Acorus), *Dan Nan Xing* (Arisaema), *Tian Qi* (Notoginseng), and *Chi Shao* (Paeonia). In the control group, 40 cases were treated only with conventional medicines. Standard conventional medicines included antihypertensive agents, hypoglycemic agents, and anticoagulants. After 1 to 2 courses of combined conventional and herbal treatment in the herbal group, 44 cases were clinically cured (all the clinical symptoms disappeared), and 15 cases were improved. In the control group, 21 cases were clinically cured, and 12 cases were improved after 1 to 2 courses of treatment. The difference between the herbal and control groups was significant ($P < 0.01$).[28]

In 2004, *Li* and *Lu* observed the influence of *Ban Xia Bai Zhu Tian Ma San* and *Yu Ping Feng San* on the state of immunity disequilibrium in 120 cases of hypertension. The formula was composed of 12 g *Ban Xia* (Pinellia), 12 g *Bai Zhu* (Atractylodes), 6 g *Tian Ma* (Gastrodia), 20 g *Fu Ling* (Poria), 6 g *Chen Pi* (Citrus), and 5 g *Gan Cao* (Glycyrrhiza). A total of 120 cases was randomly divided into 3 groups, i.e., Traditional Chinese Medicine (TCM) group, Western Medicine (WM) group, and TCM + WM group. The TCM group used a combination of *Ban Xia Bai Zhu Tian Ma San* and *Yu Ping Feng San*. The WM group used 10 mg Nifedipine orally 3 times per day, and the TCM + WM group used TCM and WM medicines on the same dosage schedule as the WM group. The treatment period was 8 weeks; 40 healthy patients were in the control group. The results showed the following:

1. *Ban Xia Bai Zhu Tian Ma San* and *Yu Ping Feng San* significantly improved the clinical symptoms, including vertigo, headache, dyspnea, abdominal distension, insomnia, poor appetite, vomiting, and sputum. By comparison, Nifedipine could markedly improve vertigo only and did not have a remarkable effect on other symptoms.
2. *Ban Xia Bai Zhu Tian Ma San* and *Yu Ping Feng San* could regulate both humoral and cellular immunity, whereas Nifedipine had no remarkable action on regulating immunity.[29]

Li treated 82 cases of Cervical Spondylosis with a combination of *Ban Xia Bai Zhu Tian Ma San* and *Zhi Mi Fu Ling Wan*. The combined formula was composed of 15 g *Ban Xia* (Pinellia), 15 g *Tian Ma* (Gastrodia), 10 g *Bai Zhu* (Atractylodes), 10 g *Ju Hong* (Citrus), 10 g *Fu Zi* (Aconite), 10 g *Zhi Shi* (Aurantium), 10 g *Dan Nan Xing* (Arisaema), 10 g *Gan Cao* (Glycyrrhiza), 20 g *Fu Ling* (Poria). In case of shoulder pain, 30 g *Ge Gen* (Pueraria) and 10 g *Jiang Huang* (Curcuma) were added; in case of brachialgia and upper extremity numbness, 10 g *Quan Xie* (Buthus) and 15 g *Sang Zhi* (Morus) were added; in case of nausea and vomiting, 10 g *Zhu Ru* (Bambusa) and 30 g *Dai Zhe Shi* (Hematite) were added. Herbs were decocted twice in water. The water extract was taken orally once daily. After 10–20 days of herbal treatments, 43 cases were clinically cured (52.43%), and 29 cases were improved.[30] *Ban Xia Bai Zhu Tian Ma San* modification was also successfully used to treat headache (head-shaking).[31] A *Ban Xia Bai Zhu Tian Ma San* modification was used for the treatment of 45 cases of Meniere's syndrome (similar to Vestibular syndrome). The formula was composed of 10 g *Ban Xia* (Pinellia), 10 g *Che Qian Zi* (Plantago), 10 g *Shi Chang Pu* (Acorus), 10 g *Di Long* (Pheretima), 15 g *Tian Ma* (Gastrodia), 15 g *Bai Zhu* (Atractylodes), 15 g *Chuan Xiong* (Ligusticum), 20 g *Fu Ling* (Poria), 20 g *Ze Xie* (Alisma), 30 g *Dan Shen* (Salvia), and 8 g *Chen Pi*

(Citrus). In case of serious vomiting, 15 g *Xuan Fu Hua* (Inula) and 20 g *Dai Zhe Shi* (Hematite) were added. In cases of *Qi* deficiency and hemoptysis, 30 g *Huang Qi* (Astragalus) and 10 g *Dang Gui* (Angelica) were added; in case of Kidney deficiency, 10 g *Dong Chong Xia Zao* (Cordyceps) and 15 g *Tu Si Zi* (Cuscuta) were added; in case of a bitter taste in the mouth and yellow tongue coating, 12 g *Huang Qin* (Scutellaria) and 10 g *Xia Ku Cao* (Prunella) were added. Herbs were decocted twice in water, and water extract was given once daily. After 7–14 day herbal treatments, 32 cases were clinically cured (symptoms and signs disappeared), and 10 cases were improved (symptoms and signs lessened but did not disappear).[32]

From 1996 to 2000, *Zhang* treated 106 cases of stroke with *Ban Xia Bai Zhu Tian Ma San*. The basic ingredients of this formula were 10 to 15 g *Ban Xia* (Pinellia), 10 to 15 g *Bai Zhu* (Atractylodes), 15 to 20 g *Tian Ma* (Gastrodia), 15 to 20 g *Ju Hua* (Chrysanthemum), 20 g *Fu Ling* (Poria), 15 g *Chen Pi* (Citrus), 6 to 10 g *Shui Zhi* (Hirudo), 30 to 45 g *Niu Xi* (Achyranthes), and 5 g *Gan Cao* (Glycyrrhiza). In cases of Liver *Yang* hyperactivity, 30 g *Shi Jue Ming* (Haliotis), 30 g *Zhen Zhu Mu* (Margarita), and 20 g *Xia Ku Cao* (Prunella) were added. In cases of Liver and Kidney *Yin* deficiency, 10 g *Gou Qi Zi* (Lycium) and 20 g Gui Ban (Testudinis) were added. In case of *Qi* deficiency, 30 to 60 g *Huang Qi* (Astragalus) was added. In cases of phlegmatic hydrosis, 20 g *Shi Chang Pu* (Acorus) and 10 g *Cang Zhu* (Atractylodes) were added. In cases of Phlegm and Heat, 15 g *Zhe Bei Mu* (Fritillaria), 10 g *Dan Nan Xing* (Arisaema), and 20 to 30 g *Zhu Li* (Fresh Bamboo Juice) were added; in case of Blood Stasis, 10 to 15 g *Chuan Xiong* (Ligusticum), 9 g *Hong Hua* (Carthamus), and 30 g *Ji Xue Teng* (Millettia) were added. Herbs were decocted twice in water for oral use twice per day, and the complications were treated with symptomatic treatment at the same time. After herbal treatments, 68 cases were clinically cured (all symptoms and signs disappeared, and no recurrence in 2 years), and 34 cases were improved (symptoms and signs disappeared, but had recurrence in 2 years).[33]

He treated 24 cases of trigeminal neuralgia with a *Ban Xia Bai Zhu Tian Ma San* modification. The shortest course of disease was half a year and the longest was 7 years, the average being 3.4 years. The formula was composed of 15 g *Ban Xia* (Pinellia), 30 g *Bai Zhu* (Atractylodes), 15 g *Tian Ma* (Gastrodia), 30 g *Fu Ling* (Poria), 10 g *Quan Xie* (Buthus), 20 g *Jiang Can* (Bombyx), 10 g *Chan Tui* (Cicada), 10 g *Ku Shen* (Sophora), 15 g *Ju Hua* (Chrysanthemum), 30 g *Chuan Xiong* (Ligusticum), and 5 g *Gan Cao* (Glycyrrhiza). In cases of Wind Stagnation in the Meridians and Collaterals, 15 g *Qiang Huo* (Notopterygium) and 30 g *Bai Zhi* (Angelica) were added. In cases of *Qi* and Blood Deficiency, 20 g *Bai Shao* (Paeonia) was added. In cases of Liver Wind and Liver *Yang* rising, 10 g *Huang Qin* (Scutellaria), 30 g *Zhen Zhu Mu* (Margarita), and 30 g *Gou Teng* (Uncaria) were added. Herbs were decocted twice in water for oral use, and the dose was taken once every 2 days for 30 days. After herbal treatments, 5 cases were clinically cured (all symptoms and signs disappeared, and no recurrence in 6 months), 14 cases were significantly improved (all symptoms and signs disappeared, with no recurrence in 3 months), and 4 cases were remarkably improved (all symptoms and signs improved remarkably with some recurrence in 1 month).[34]

Ding Xian Wan (Stopping Seizure) 定痫丸

Ding refers to stopping. *Xian* means seizure. *Wan* is pill, the form of original herbal administration. Ding Xian Wan, therefore, means Stopping Seizure Pill.

Source: *Yi Xue Xin Wu* (*Medical Revelations*), written by *Cheng Guo-Peng* and published in 1732 CE

Ingredients: The original formula for *Ding Xian Wan* (Table 31.7) is composed of 30 g *Tian Ma* (Gastrodia), 30 g *Chuan Bei Mu* (Fritillaria), 30 g *Ban Xia* (Pinellia), 30 g *Fu Ling* (Poria), 30 g *Fu Shen* (Poria), 15 g *Dan Nan Xing* (Arisaema), 15 g *Shi Chang Pu* (Acorus), 15 g *Quan Xie* (Buthus), 15 g *Gan Cao* (Glycyrrhiza), 15 g *Jiang Can* (Bombyx), 15 g *Hu Po* (Succinum), 15 g *Deng Xin Cao* (Juncus), 20 g *Chen Pi* (Citrus), 20 g *Yuan Zhi* (Polygala), 60 g *Dan Shen* (Salvia), 60 g *Mai Men Dong* (Ophiopogon), and 9 g *Zhu Sha* (Cinnabaris).

Preparation:

1. Powder or capsule method: Herbs are ground into a fine powder. Powder can be encapsulated.
2. Decoction or teapill method: Raw herbs are mixed together and decocted. Herbal water extract (decoction) can be concentrated as granules or teapills.

Actions: Transform Phlegm and subdue Wind to stop seizure

Indications: This formula is indicated for epilepsy or seizure due to internal Phlegm and Heat.

Dosage and Usage:

Horses and Cattle: 15–30 g, twice daily
Camels: 30–45 g, twice daily
Llamas, Alpacas, Goats, Sheep, and Pigs: 5–10 g, twice daily
Dogs: 0.5–5 g (or 0.05 g per kg body weight), twice daily
Cats and Rabbits: 0.2–0.5 g (or 0.05 g per kg body weight), twice daily
Birds: 0.05 g per kg body weight, twice daily

Use 2–6 weeks until primary clinical signs resolve.

Table 31.7. Ingredients and actions of *Ding Xian Wan.*

%	English Name	Chinese *Pin-Yin*	Actions
7.1	Gastrodia	*Tian Ma*	Calm the Liver to stop Wind and convulsions
7.1	Fritillaria	*Chuan Bei Mu*	Transform Phlegm, clear Heat
7.1	Pinellia	*Ban Xia*	Dry up Damp to eliminate Phlegm, reduce swelling
7.1	Poria	*Fu Ling*	Induce diuresis to drain Damp
7.1	Poria	*Fu Shen*	Strengthen the Spleen, calm the mind
3.5	Arisaema	*Dan Nan Xing*	Eliminate Phlegm, subdue Wind and stop spasm
3.5	Buthus	*Quan Xie*	Dispel Wind and stop spasm
3.5	Acorus	*Shi Chang Pu*	Transform Phlegm, dissipate Damp
3.5	Glycyrrhiza	*Gan Cao*	Coordinate all other herbs' actions
3.5	Bombyx	*Jiang Can*	Subdue Wind and relieve convulsion
3.5	Succinum	*Hu Po*	Relieve convulsion
3.5	Juncus	*Deng Xin Cao*	Induce diuresis and clear Heart Heat
4.7	Citrus	*Chen Pi*	Dry up Damp to eliminate Phlegm, move *Qi*
4.7	Polygala	*Yuan Zhi*	Calm the mind, expel Phlegm
14.2	Salvia	*Dan Shen*	Activate Blood to remove Stasis, cool Blood
14.2	Ophiopogon	*Mai Men Dong*	Tonify *Yin*, promote body fluid production
2.2	Cinnabaris*	*Zhu Sha*	Relieve convulsion and decrease swelling

*Because it contains the toxic heavy metal mercury (Hg), *Zhu Sha* (Cinnabaris) is not used in the modern formulation.

Analysis of Formula: Seizure or epilepsy can be caused by Stagnation of Phlegm in the Interior, or by Liver Heat. The main treatment strategy is to transform Phlegm and subdue the Internal Wind. Serving as the King herb, *Dan Nan Xing* (Arisaema) transforms Phlegm by cooling and treats epilepsy. *Ban Xia* (Pinellia), *Quan Xie* (Buthus), *Jiang Can* (Bombyx), *Chuan Bei Mu* (Fritillaria), and *Tian Ma* (Gastrodia) synergistically work as the Minister herbs to transform Phlegm to relieve convulsion and spasm and subdue Internal Wind to stop seizures. *Chen Pi* (Citrus), *Fu Ling* (Poria), *Dan Shen* (Salvia), and *Shi Chang Pu* (Acorus) move *Qi*, drain Damp, and move Blood to resolve Stagnation. *Zhu Sha* (Cinnabaris), *Hu Po* (Succinum), *Yuan Zhi* (Polygala), *Deng Xin Cao* (Juncus), and *Fu Shen* (Poria) are the Adjunct herbs to calm the Mind and relieve seizures. *Gan Cao* (Glycyrrhiza) coordinates the other herbs' actions, eliminates Phlegm, and serves as the Messenger herb.

Epileptic seizures may be mild or severe, with a long or short course. Initially, the treatment should emphasize clearing Phlegm and subduing Wind to alleviate the symptoms. After the symptoms (seizures) are under control, the treatment should focus on treating the underlying causes by strengthening the Spleen, nourishing the Heart, reinforcing the Liver to benefit the Kidney, and/or invigorating *Qi* and nourishing Blood.

Cautions and Contraindications: It should be used cautiously with *Yin* Deficiency or Blood Deficiency.

Dr. Xie's Comments: *Ding Xian Wan* is effectively used for control of seizure symptoms. As soon as the seizure is under control (seizure free for 2 months), other herbal formula(s) should be combined to treat the underlying causes, including Liver *Yin* Deficiency and Liver Blood Deficiency. I have successfully used *Ding Xian Wan* with a combination of other herbals to control seizure activity in dogs.

Clinical and Pharmacological Studies: A *Ding Xian Wan* modification was used to treat 27 human cases of epilepsy: 25 cases with primary epilepsy and 2 cases with secondary causes. The course of disease was 1 to 5 years (5 cases), 6 to 10 years (9 cases), 11 to 20 years (10 cases), 21 to 30 years (2 cases), and 1 case was more than 30 years duration. The average course of epilepsy was 13.9 years. The formula was composed of 0.5 g *Niu Huang* (Bovis), 15 g *Tian Ma* (Gastrodia), 30 g *Ci Shi* (Magnetite), 10 g *Qing Dai* (Indigo), 10 g *Zhi Zi* (Gardenia), 12 g *Yu Jin* (Curcuma), and 15 g *Tian Zhu Huang* (Bambusa). Herbs were ground into a fine powder and made into a small pill with honey (6 g per pill). The herbal pill was given as 1 pill twice daily with yellow rice wine or warm boiled water. After 3 months of herbal treatment, 12 cases had excellent results (seizures reduced by 76 to 100%), 10 cases had good results (seizures reduced by 51 to 75%), and 3 cases were slightly improved (seizures reduced by 26 to 50%).[35]

From 1999 to 2001, *Huang* and *Li* treated 118 human cases of refractory epilepsy with a combination of Lamotrigine and *Ding Xian Wan*. Lamotrigine was given 50 mg once daily for adults and 2 mg per kg body weight per day for children. After 2 weeks of the lower dosage, Lamotrigine was given orally 50 mg, twice daily for adults and 5 mg per kg body weight per day for children. The herbal formula *Ding Xian Wan* was given orally, twice daily; 65 cases were male, and 53 cases were female. The patients were 5 to 63 years old. The shortest course of disease was 1 year, and the longest was 20 years. After 12 weeks of herbal treatment, 55 cases had excellent results (seizures reduced by more than 50%) and 29 cases improved (seizures reduced by 26 to 49%).[36]

A *Ding Xian Wan* modification was used for 30 cases of seizure. This herbal modification consisted of 60g *Shen Qu* (Massa), 60g *Mai Ya* (Hordeum), 60g *Sha Zha* (Crataegus), 30g *Dai Zhe Shi* (Hematite), 15g *Da Huang* (Rheum), 15g *Zhu Ru* (Bambusa), 15g *Long Gu* (Draconis), 15g *Mu Li* (Ostrea), 10g *Chen Pi* (Citrus), and 10g *Jiang Can* (Bombyx). Herbs were ground into a fine powder and made into a small pill (6g pill) with honey. In cases with opisthotonos and obvious convulsion, *Quan Xie* (Buthus), *Tian Ma* (Gastrodia), *Gou Teng* (Uncaria), and *Bai Fu Zi* (Typhonium) were added. In cases with Phlegm in the throat and greasy coating of the tongue, Meng Shi (Lapis), *Tian Ma* (Gastrodia), *Ban Xia* (Pinellia), and *Dan Nan Xing* (Arisaema) were added. In cases with dry and hard stools, stomatitis, gingivitis, and a red tongue, *Zi Shi Ying* (Fluorite), *Shi Gao* (Gypsum), *Zhi Zi* (Gardenia), and *Huang Lian* (Coptis) were added. The added herbs were decocted as water extract for oral use and were taken as herbal pills. The conventional drugs were reduced by 1/3 after 10 days of herbal medication and then completely discontinued after 30 days of herbal medication. The dosage was 1 pill for 3- to 7-year-old patients, 3 times daily; 2 pills twice daily for 8- to 14-year-old patients, 2 pills 3 times daily for patients older than 14 years. Herbal treatments lasted 3–6 months; 15 cases were clinically cured (seizures disappeared, and there was no recurrence in 1 year; 6 cases took 3 months of treatment; 5 cases took 4 months of treatments; and 4 cases took 6 months of treatments). Another 15 cases had good results (there was recurrence in 1 year, but the seizures and the symptoms were remarkably reduced).[37]

From 1992 to 2003, *Zhang* treated 69 cases of seizure secondary to stroke with a *Ding Xian Wan* modification, which was composed of *Lu Rong* (Cervus), *Quan Xie* (Buthus), *Chan Tui* (Cicada), *Shui Zhi* (Hirudo), *Ma Huang* (Ephedra), *Ma Qian Zi* (Strychnos), *Bing Pian* (Borneol), 10g *Tian Ma* (Gastrodia), 10g *Jiang Can* (Bombyx), 10g *Shi Chang Pu* (Acorus), 10g *Dan Nan Xing* (Arisaema), 10g *Jiang Ban Xia* (Pinellia), and 50g *Huang Qi* (Astragalus). In cases with frequent seizures, 2g *Zhen Zhu* (Margarita) was added. In cases of Heart-Spleen Deficiency, 10 to 20g *Bai Zhu* (Atractylodes) and *Fu Shen* (Poria) were added. In cases of manic behavior, 20ml *Zhu Ru* (Bambusa) was added. In cases of Liver-Kidney deficiency, 20g *Shan Zhu Yu* (Cornus) was added. Herbs were decocted twice in water, and the herbal water extract was given twice daily after meals. After 1–3 herbal treatments, 52 cases were cured (no recurrence in 1 year), and 17 cases improved (symptoms were remarkably reduced).[38]

Di Tan Tang (Cleansing Phlegm) 涤痰汤

Di refers to cleansing. *Tan* means Phlegm. *Tang* is decoction, the original form of herbal administration. *Di Tan Tang* means Cleansing Phlegm Decoction.

Source: *Ji Sheng Fang* (*Formulas to Aid the Living*), written by *Yan Yong-He* and published in 1253 CE

Ingredients: The original formula (Table 31.8) is composed of 8g *Ban Xia* (Pinellia), 8g *Dan Nan Xing* (Arisaema), 6g *Ju Hong* (Citrus), 6g *Zhi Shi* (Aurantium), 6g *Fu Ling* (Poria), 3g *Ren Shen* (Ginseng), 3g *Shi Chang Pu* (Acorus), 2g *Zhu Ru* (Bambusa), and 2g *Gan Cao* (Glycyrrhiza).

Preparation:

1. Powder or capsule method: Herbs are ground into a fine powder. Powder can be encapsulated.
2. Decoction or teapill method: Raw herbs are mixed together and decocted. Herbal water extract (decoction) can be concentrated as granules or teapills.

Table 31.8. Ingredients and actions of *Di Tan Tang*.

%	English Name	Chinese *Pin-Yin*	Actions
18.2	Pinellia	*Ban Xia*	Dry up Damp to eliminate Phlegm, descend *Qi* and stop vomiting
13.6	Citrus	*Ju Hong*	Dry up Damp to eliminate Phlegm, regulate *Qi* to relax Intestines
13.6	Poria	*Fu Ling*	Induce diuresis to alleviate edema, strengthen Spleen, and calm the nerves
4.6	Bambusa	*Zhu Ru*	Promote the circulation of *Qi* to relieve pain, relax and activate the tendons
6.8	Acorus	*Shi Chang Pu*	Dispel Phlegm, promote *Qi* and dissipate Damp
18.2	Arisaema	*Dan Nan Xing*	Eliminate Phlegm, spasmolytic, subdue Wind
13.6	Aurantium	*Zhi Shi*	Move *Qi*, and dispel Food Stagnation, descend *Qi*, purgative
6.8	Ginseng	*Ren Shen*	Tonify *Qi* for emergency treatment of collapse, invigorate the Spleen, body fluid regeneration, nourish the Heart
4.6	Glycyrrhiza	*Gan Cao*	Regulate the Middle Burner, coordinate the actions of other herbs

Actions: Transform Phlegm, dry up Damp and stop seizure

Indications: This formula is indicated for seizure and/or mental confusion accompanied by a pale or purple tongue and wiry or deep pulse.

Dosage and Usage:

Horses and Cattle: 15–30g, twice daily

Camels: 30–45g, twice daily

Llamas, Alpacas, Goats, Sheep, and Pigs: 5–10g, twice daily

Dogs: 0.5–5g (or 0.05g per kg body weight), twice daily

Cats and Rabbits: 0.2–0.5g (or 0.05g per kg body weight), twice daily

Birds: 0.05g per kg body weight, twice daily

Use 4–12 weeks until primary clinical signs resolve.

Analysis of Formula: *Ban Xia* (Pinellia), *Ju Hong* (Citrus), *Fu Ling* (Poria) and *Zhu Ru* (Bambusa) are the King herbs in the formula, which can dry up Damp and eliminate Phlegm. *Shi Chang Pu* (Acorus) and *Dan Nan Xing* (Arisaema) have the function of transforming Phlegm for resuscitation, and they serve as the Minister herbs. Being the Adjuvant herbs, *Ren Shen* (Ginseng) tonifies *Qi*, and *Zhi Shi* (Aurantium) descends *Qi*. *Gan Cao* (Glycyrrhiza) harmonizes all other herbs and is the Messenger herb.

Cautions and Contraindications: It should be used cautiously with *Yin* Deficiency.

Dr. Xie's Comments: I have used *Di Tan Tang* for the treatment of seizures in dogs and cats.

Clinical and Pharmacological Studies: A *Di Tan Tang* modification was used for the treatment of two cases of stiffness of the tongue. This herbal modification consisted of 10g *Chen Pi* (Citrus), 15g *Ban Xia* (Pinellia), 30g *Fu Ling* (Poria), 10g *Gan Cao* (Glycyrrhiza), 9g *Zhi Shi* (Aurantium), 15g *Zhu Ru* (Bambusa), 9g *Dan Nan Xing* (Arisaema), 15g *Shi Chang Pu* (Acorus), 15g *Yuan Zhi* (Polygala), 20g *Dang Shen* (Codonopsis), 10g *Qiang Huo* (Notopterygium), 10g *Fang Feng* (Ledebouriella), 10g *Bai Fu Zi* (Typhonium), 15g *Tian Ma* (Gastrodia), 0.6g *Ling Yang Jiao* (Antelope Horn), 30g *Dan Shen* (Salvia), and 6g *Quan Xie* (Buthus). Herbs were decocted and the water extract given orally twice daily. After the initial 3 days of herbal treatments, the tongue could start to move better, but its movement was still stiff. After 3 more daily treatments, the tongue could move spontaneously. After another 3 days of treatment, these two patients were normal and had no recurrence of this problem in 5 years.[39]

From 2000 to 2002, *Meng Fan-xia*, *Wang Ai-yu*, and *Wang Gui-qing* treated 103 cases of stroke with a *Di Tan Tang* modification; 65 cases were male, 53 were female, the patients were 34 to 82 years old, and the average was 63.2 years. The course of disease was less than 1 week in 52 cases, 1 to 3 weeks in 31 cases, 3 to 6 weeks in 6 cases, and more than 6 weeks in 4 cases. These cases were complicated by other medical conditions: 38 cases had hypertension, 17 cases had coronary artery disease, 18 cases had high Blood viscosity, and 30 cases had hyperlipidemia. The herbal modification was composed of 12g *Ban Xia* (Pinellia), 12g *Ju Hong* (Citrus), 12g *Fu Ling* (Poria), 6g *Gan Cao* (Glycyrrhiza), 10g *Dan Nan Xing* (Arisaema), 10g *Zhu Ru* (Bambusa), 10g *Zhi Ke* (Aurantium), 10g *Tao Ren* (Persica), 10g *Hong Hua* (Carthamus), 15g *Dan Shen* (Salvia), and 2g *Wu Gong* (Scolopendra). In cases of dry stool, 6g *Sheng Di Huang* (Rehmannia) was added. In cases of loss of *Shen*, 10g *Yuan Zhi* (Polygala), 10g *Yu Jin* (Curcuma), and 10g *Shi Chang Pu* (Acorus) were added. Herbal water extract was taken twice daily. Another 39 cases of stroke with hypertension were used as the control group. The treatment for the control group was 250ml 0.9% physiological saline and 0.4g *San Qi* (Notoginseng) administered intravenously. After 20 days of herbal treatments in the herbal group, 24 cases were significantly improved and 75 cases were somewhat improved. In the control group, 4 cases were significantly improved and 30 cases were somewhat improved. The difference in clinical results was significant between the two groups ($P < 0.05$).[40]

A total of 13 human cases of mental depression were treated with a *Di Tan Tang* modification: 5 cases male, 8 cases female, and ages ranged from 22 to 51 years old. The shortest course of disease was 1 month, and the longest was 3 months. All of the cases were in line with CCMD (Chinese Classification and Diagnostic Criteria of Mental Disorders)-II-12, and the total score of Hamilton depression rating scale–20. The formula modification was composed of 12g *Ban Xia* (Pinellia), 12g *Dan Nan Xing* (Arisaema), 15g *Zhi Shi* (Aurantium), 15g *Fu Ling* (Poria), 12g *Shi Chang Pu* (Acorus), 15g *Zhu Ru* (Bambusa), 10g *Gan Cao* (Glycyrrhiza), 5g *Sheng Jiang* (Zingiberis), 5 *Da Zao* (Jujube), and 9g *Ren Shen* (Ginseng). In cases with Liver *Qi* Stagnation, 6g *Chai Hu* (Bupleurum), 10g *Xiang Fu* (Cyperus) and 12g *Yu Jin* (Curcuma) were added. In cases with excess Heat, 6g *Long Dan Cao* (Gentiana) and 10g *Zhi Zi* (Gardenia) were added. In cases with anxiety and restlessness, 15g *He Huan Hua* (Albizzia), 15g *Long Gu* (Draconis), and 15g *Mu Li* (Ostrea) were added. In cases with poor appetite, 10g *Chen Pi* (Citrus), 15g *Mai Ya* (Hordeum), 15g *Shen Qu* (Massa), and 15g *Shan Zha* (Crataegi) were added. In cases with dry stool, 10g *Sheng Di Huang* (Rehmannia) was added. Herbal water extract was taken twice daily. After 10 days of herbal treatments, 7 cases had significant results (symptoms disappeared), and 5 cases were improved.[41]

From 1994 to 2000, *Tang* and *Li* treated 72 cases of cough due to acute tracheitis and bronchitis with *Di Tan Tang* modification. The cases consisted of 30 males and 42 females. Their ages ranged 6 to 82 years old: 10 cases were less than 30 years old, 15 were 30 to 39 years old, 18 were 40 to 49 years old, 19 were 50 to 59 years old, and 10 were more than 60 years old. The shortest course of disease was 3 days, and the longest was 20 days. The formula was composed of 12g *Dang Gui* (Angelica), 10g *Chuan Bei Mu* (Fritillaria), 9g *Chen Pi* (Citrus), 9g *Ban Xia* (Pinellia), 10g *Fu Ling* (Poria), 6g *Zhi Shi* (Aurantium), 10g *Zhu Ru* (Bambusa), 6g *Dan Nan Xing* (Arisaema), 9g *Shi Chang Pu* (Acorus), and 6g *Gan Cao* (Glycyrrhiza). In cases with Wind and Heat invasion of the Lung, 12g *Jin Yin Hua* (Lonicera) and 10g *Sang Bai Pi* (Morus) were added. In cases with Wind-Cold invasion of the Lung, 3g *Xi Xin* (Asarum) and 6g *Gan Jiang* (Zingiberis) were added. In cases with persistent coughing, 10g *Wu Wei Zi* (Schisandra) and 12g *Bai Bu* (Stemona) were added. Herbs were decocted with 300ml water and taken twice daily. After the treatment, 38 cases were clinically cured (cough disappeared, and the hemogram and thoracic radiography were normal); 22 cases had excellent results (cough almost disappeared, and the hemogram and thoracic radiography were normal); and 9 cases improved (cough reduced, and the hemogram and thoracic radiography improved remarkably).[42]

From 1998 to 2004, *Zhang* treated 38 cases of sequelae of carbon monoxide poisoning with a *Di Tan Tang* modification: 26 cases were outpatient treatments, and 12 cases were hospitalized; 23 cases were male, 15 were female; the patients were 25 to 66 years old, and the average was 48 years old. The course of the disease was 10 days to 1 month for 20 cases, 1 to 2 months for 10 cases, and more than 1 year for 8 cases. The basic ingredients were 12g *Ban Xia* (Pinellia), 10g *Dan Nan Xing* (Arisaema), 12g *Ju Hong* (Citrus), 10g *Zhi Shi* (Aurantium), 12g *Fu Ling* (Poria), 15g *Shi Chang Pu* (Acorus), 12g *Zhu Ru* (Bambusa), 12g *Gui Ban* (Testudinis), 12g *Zhi Zi* (Gardenia), 3g *Gan Cao* (Glycyrrhiza), and 9g *Ren Shen* (Ginseng). In cases with sputum obstructing the throat and airway, *Chuan Bei Mu* (Fritillaria) was added. In cases of restlessness, *Hou Po* (Magnolia) and *Zhen Zhu Mu* (Margarita) were added. In cases of insomnia due to excessive Heat, *Huang Qin* (Scutellaria) and *Zhi Zi* (Gardenia) were added. Herbal water extract was taken twice daily; 21 cases were clinically cured, 8 cases had excellent results, and 5 cases improved.[43]

The modified *Di Tan Tang* was used in treating hyperlipidemia with 105 cases, which were randomly divided in the treatment group and the control group: 60 cases were in the treatment group and treated with the modified *Di Tan Tang*; 45 cases were the control group, which were treated with an herbal product called *Dong Ang Jiang Zhi Ling Pian*. The formula of modified *Di Tan Tang* was composed of 30g *Shan Zha* (Crataegus), 20g *He Shou Wu* (Polygonum), 20g *Dan Shen* (Salvia), 20g *Fu Ling* (Poria), 15g *Bai Zhu* (Atractylodes), 15g *Ze Xie* (Alisma), 15g *Chen Pi* (Citrus), 15g *Ji Nei Jin* (Gallus), 15g *E Zhu* (Zedoaria), 15g *Ban Xia* (Pinellia), 5g *San Qi* (Notoginseng), and 10g *Jue Ming Zi* (Cassia). In cases with Spleen *Qi* Deficiency and greasy coating of the tongue, 5g *Bai Jie Zi* (Sinapis) was added. In cases with Spleen *Qi* Deficiency and loose stool, 5g *He Zi* (Chebula) and 5g *Gan Jiang* (Zingiberis) were added. Herbal water extract was taken orally twice daily. After 3 months of herbal treatments, the total effectiveness rate of the treatment group was 94.9% and of the control group it was 71.1%. There was a remarkable difference in reducing blood fat level between them ($P < 0.01$).[44]

Yang Jiao Gou Teng Tang (Horn and Uncaria) 羊角钩藤汤

Yang Jiao is goat horn. *Gou Teng* refers to Uncaria stem. Both are the King herbs of this herbal formula. *Tang* is decoction, the original form of the herbal administration. *Yang Jiao Gou Teng Tang* means Decoction of Goat Horn and Uncaria Stem.

Source: *Tong Su Shang Han Lun* (*Popular Guide to Discussion of Cold-Induced Disorders*), written by *Yu Gen-Chu* and published in 1650 CE. The original formula's name was *Ling Yang Gou Teng Tang* (Decoction of Antelope's Horn and Uncaria Stem). Since Antelope is a protected species, its horn is now replaced with goat's horn, and the formula is called *Yang Jiao Gou Teng Tang* (Decoction of Goat's Horn and Uncaria Stem).

Ingredients: The original formula (Table 31.9) is composed of 5g *Shan Yang Jiao* (Capra), 9g *Gou Teng* (Uncaria), 6g *Sang Ye* (Morus), 9g *Chuan Bei Mu* (Fritillaria), 10g *Zhu Ru* (Bambusa), 15g *Sheng Di Huang* (Rehmannia), 9g *Ju Hua* (Chrysanthemum), 12g *Bai Shao* (Paeonia), 10g *Fu Shen* (Poria), and 3g *Gan Cao* (Glycyrrhiza).

Preparation:
1. Powder or capsule method: Herbs are ground into a fine powder. Powder can be encapsulated.
2. Decoction or teapill method: Raw herbs are mixed together and decocted. Herbal water extract (decoction) can be concentrated as granules or teapills.

Actions: Calm the Liver to stop Wind, clear Heat and stop convulsions

Indications: This formula is indicated for Internal Wind due to excessive Liver Heat marked with tremors,

Table 31.9. Ingredients and actions of *Yang Jiao Gou Teng Tang.*

%	English Name	Chinese *Pin-Yin*	Actions
5.7	Capra*	*Shan Yang Jiao*	Soothe the Liver to stop Internal Wind, clear the Liver to improve eyesight
10.2	Uncaria	*Gou Teng*	Subdue Wind, calm the Liver and subdue *Yang*
6.8	Morus	*Sang Ye*	Expel Wind and clear Heat, clear the Liver to improve eyesight, relieve sore throat and moisturize the Lung
10.2	Fritillaria	*Chuan Bei Mu*	Dissipate Phlegm to stop coughing, clear Heat and eliminate Stagnation
11.4	Bambusa	*Zhu Ru*	Clear Lung and dissipate Phlegm, stop vomiting, cool Blood to stop bleeding
17.1	Rehmannia	*Sheng Di Huang*	Cool Blood to stop bleeding, nourish *Yin* and regenerate body fluids
10.2	Chrysanthemum	*Ju Hua*	Expel Wind and clear Heat, clear the Liver to improve eyesight, detoxify, clear the Liver to subdue Wind
13.6	Paeonia	*Bai Shao*	Clear the Liver and nourish Blood, relax tendons and activate Blood circulation to relieve pain
11.4	Poria	*Fu Shen*	Pacify Liver, calm the mind
3.4	Glycyrrhiza	*Gan Cao*	Mediate the properties of other herbs

*Originally, *Ling Yang Jiao* (Antelope) was used, but now *Shan Yang Jiao* (Capra) is substituted because antelope is an endangered species and use of *Ling Yang Jiao* is prohibited.

spasm, or seizures; fever; irritability and restlessness; tetany and even coma; a dark red, dry tongue; and a wiry and fast pulse. This formula can also be used for signs of head pain, loss of balance or disorientation, and hypertension caused by Liver *Yang* rising.

Dosage and Usage:

Horses and Cattle: 15–30 g, twice daily
Camels: 30–45 g, twice daily
Llamas, Alpacas, Goats, Sheep, and Pigs: 5–10 g, twice daily
Dogs: 0.5–5 g (or 0.05 g per kg body weight), twice daily
Cats and Rabbits: 0.2–0.5 g (or 0.05 g per kg body weight), twice daily
Birds: 0.05 g per kg body weight, twice daily
Use 2–4 weeks until primary clinical signs resolve.

Analysis of Formula: Internal Wind due to excessive Liver Heat should be treated by tranquilizing the Liver to stop the Internal Wind, and to clear Heat to relieve convulsions. In the formula, *Shan Yang Jiao* (Capra) and *Gou Teng* (Uncaria) are the King herbs, which tranquilize the Liver to stop Internal Wind, and clear Heat to relieve convulsions and spasm. *Sang Ye* (Morus) and *Ju Hua* (Chrysanthemum) are the Minister herbs and help the King herbs clear Heat and subdue Wind. Body fluid can easily be consumed and damaged because of febrile disease complicated by Wind, so *Bai Shao* (Paeonia) and *Sheng Di Huang* (Rehmannia) are used for nourishing *Yin* and regenerating body fluids to nourish the Liver and to relax the tendons. Excessive Heat can easily scorch and boil the body fluids into Phlegm, so *Chuan Bei Mu* (Fritillaria) and *Zhu Ru* (Bambusa) are used for transforming and eliminating Phlegm. Excessive Heat can disturb the Heart-*Shen*, so *Fu Shen* (Poria) is used as an Adjunct herb for pacifying the Heart and calming the mind. *Bai Shao, Chuan Bei Mu, Zhu Ru,* and *Fu Shen* are the Adjuvant herbs. *Gan Cao* (Glycyrrhiza) can mediate the properties of other herbs and is a Messenger herb. Combined with *Bai Shao* (Paeonia), it nourishes *Yin*, relaxes the tendons, and relieves spasm. This formula also can be used for headache, dizziness, and tremor caused by Liver *Yang* rising.

Cautions and Contraindications: This formula is contraindicated with Internal Wind due to Liver Blood Deficiency.

Dr. Xie's Comments: I have used *Yang Jiao Gou Teng Tang* in dogs to treat seizures due to Blood Stagnation in the brain after injury or encephalitis in dogs.

Clinical and Pharmacological Studies: Modified *Yang Jiao Gou Teng Tang* was used for the treatment of cerebroventricular hemorrhage diagnosed by cranium computerized tomography (CT) or MRI (magnetic resonance imaging). A total of 59 cases of cerebroventricular hemorrhage were randomly divided into an herbal group (35 cases) and a control group (24 cases). Based on the volume of brain ventricle hemorrhage, brain ventricle paracentesis was applied in 13 out of 59 cases, 15 received craniotomy to clear the hematoma, and 19 cases were also assisted with lumbar puncture to release cerebrospinal fluid based on the pathogenic condition. In addition, the treatment group was given the herbal medication of modified *Yang Jiao Gou Teng Tang*, which was composed of 3 g *Ling Yang Jiao* (Antelope Horn), 20 g *Gou Teng* (Uncaria), 6 g *Sang Ye* (Morus), 20 to 20 g *Sheng Di Huang* (Rehmannia), 10 to 15 g *Tian Ma* (Gastrodia), 15 g *Chuan Bei Mu* (Fritillaria), 20 to 30 g *Fu Ling* (Poria), 9 g *San Qi* (Notoginseng), 10 to 30 g *Ju Hua* (Chrysanthemum), 15 to 30 g *Dan Shen* (Salvia), 15 to 25 g *Jiang Can* (Bombyx), and 20 to 30 g *Sang Ji Sheng* (Loranthus). Herbs were decocted twice in water for oral dosing, one dose daily. If unable to take orally, patients took the medicine via a nasogastric feeding tube. In case of convulsion, 6g *Ling Yang Jiao* (Antelope Horn), 30g *Di Long* (Pheretima), and 12g *Chan Tui* (Cicada) were added. In cases of disoriented consciousness, 12g *Shi Chang Pu* (Acorus) and 0.5g *Niu Huang* (Bovis) were added. In cases of severe headache, 30g *Shi Jue Ming* (Haliotis), 30g *Zhen Zhu Mu* (Margarita), and 15g *Xia Ku Cao* (Prunella) were added. In cases of alimentary tract hemorrhage, 9g *Da Huang* (Rheum) was added. The treatment for the control group was use of drugs with intracranial pressure control and blood pressure adjustment in the period of onset of cerebral hemorrhage. The drugs were 1g cytidine diphosphate choline and 500ml 5% glucose in normal saline, administered by intravenous injection. In the herbal group, 20 of the 35 cases were clinically cured (consciousness was clear, intellect remained intact, the functions of limbs and language were normal, and patients were able to take care of their activities of daily living); 9 cases were significantly improved (consciousness was clear, intellect remained intact, the functions of limbs were almost normal, and patients were able to take care of their activities of daily living partially and do simple language exchange, but had some persistant neurological signs); 5 cases were improved (consciousness, intelligence, and the functions of limbs and oral communication had gotten better, but patients were unable to perform their activities of daily living). In the control group, 6 of 24 cases were clinically cured, 7 cases were significantly improved, and 6 cases were improved. The difference in improvement between the two groups was significant ($P < 0.05$).[45]

From 1981 to 1985, *Zhuang* treated 72 cases of encephalitis B in children with a combination of herbal and Western medicines. Another 45 cases were used as the control group using only Western medicine. Western medicines included a small dose of Aminopyrine by intramuscular injection or 0.5 to 1mg/kg Chlorpromazine and 0.5 to 1mg/kg Promethazine by intramuscular injection, once every 4 to 6 hours, as needed for up to 3 days. In case of convulsion, 0.1 to 0.3mg/kg Diazepam and 5 to 8mg/kg Phenobarbital were used by intramuscular injection. In case of increased intracranial pressure, 1 to 2g/kg 20% Mannitol was administered by intravenous injection, once every 4 to 6 hours. Dexamethasone was given as an intravenous injection, 5mg, twice daily for patients younger than 5 years old, or 5mg, 3 to 4 times daily for 5- to 10-year-olds, used as needed for up to 5 days. In case of respiratory failure, 0.15 to 0.2mg/kg Lobelin or 5 to 10mg/kg Nikethamide and 10% glucose solution were used as an intravenous drip, as needed to improve respiration. Acid-based equilibrium of the body was maintained with fluid therapy (50 to 80ml/kg/d). In addition to the above Western medicines, the patients in the herbal group received modified *Ling Yang Gou Teng Tang* which consisted of 2g *Ling Yang Jiao* (Antelope Horn), 6g *Gou Teng* (Uncaria), 6g *Chuan Bei Mu* (Fritillaria), 6g *Bai Shao* (Paeonia), 6g *Jin Yin Hua* (Lonicera), 6g *Sheng Di Huang* (Rehmannia), 6g *Sang Ye* (Morus) and 3g *Gan Cao* (Glycyrrhiza). Herbs were decocted twice in water for oral dose, one dose daily divided 4 to 6 times. In cases of coma, it was administered via nasogastric feeding tube. In cases of drowsiness, 10g *Shi Chang Pu* (Acorus) was added. In cases of Phlegm Stagnation in the larynx, 3g *Tian Zhu Huang* (Bambusa) and 3g *Dan Nan Xing* (Arisaema) were added. In cases of continuing high fever, 50g *Shi Gao* (Gypsum) was added. In cases of frequent convulsions, 3g *Quan Xie* (Buthus) and 3g *Jiang Can* (Bombyx) were added. In the herbal group, 66 out of the 72 cases were clinically cured (the symptoms at the acute stage disappeared in 10 to 14 days, and the symptoms and signs at the stationary phase disappeared in 6 months); 3 cases were improved (the symptoms at the acute stage disappeared, and the symptoms and signs at stationary phase improved, but some sequelae were left); the total effectiveness rate was 95.8%. In the control group, 23 out of the 45 cases of the control group were clinically cured; 5 cases were improved, and the total effectiveness rate was 62.0%. The effectiveness rate was significantly different between the two groups ($P < 0.01$).[46] This study result indicates that modified, *Ling Yang Gou Teng Tang* may be useful in treating encephalitis in birds, swine, horses, and lizards.

Yang Yi-Ping also found *Yang Jiao Gou Teng Tang* improved the patients with poststroke symptoms, including consciousness disorder, drowsiness, dizziness, numbness of the limbs, hemiplegia, strong convulsions and contracture of limbs, constipation, red or purple-red tongue, yellow and greasy coating of the tongue, and a wiry and fast pulse.[47]

Zhen Gan Xi Feng Tang (Tranquilizing Liver to Extinguish Wind) 镇肝熄风汤

Zhen means tranquilize. Gan means the Liver. *Xi* refers to extinguish. *Feng* means Wind. *Tang* is decoction.

Source: *Yi Xue Zhong Zhong Can Xi Lu* (*Discourses on Integrated Traditional Chinese and Western Medicine*), written by *Zhang Xi-chun* and published in 1918 to 1934 CE

Ingredients: The original formula (Table 31.10) is composed of 30g *Niu Xi* (Achyranthes), 30g *Dai Zhe Shi* (Hematite), 10g *Long Gu* (Draconis), 15g *Mu Li* (Ostrea), 15g *Gui Ban* (Testudinis), 15g *Bai Shao* (Paeonia), 15g *Xuan Shen* (Scrophularia), 15g *Tian Men Dong* (Asparagus), 6g *Chuan Lian Zi* (Melia), 6g *Mai Ya* (Hordeum), 6g *Yin Chen Hao* (Artemisia), and 5g *Gan Cao* (Glycyrrhiza).

Table 31.10. Ingredients and actions of *Zhen Gan Xi Feng Tang*.

%	English Name	Chinese *Pin-Yin*	Actions
17.9	Achyranthes	*Niu Xi*	Activate Blood, ensure proper downward flow of *Qi*
17.9	Hematite	*Dai Zhe Shi*	Tranquilize the Liver and subdue *Yang*
6.0	Draconis	*Long Gu*	Tranquilize the Liver and subdue *Yang*, relieve convulsion
8.9	Ostrea	*Mu Li*	Nourish *Yin* to suppress *Yang*
8.9	Testudinis	*Gui Ban*	Nourish *Yin* to suppress *Yang*
8.9	Paeonia	*Bai Shao*	Clear the Liver and nourish Blood, relax tendons and activate Blood circulation to relieve pain
8.9	Scrophularia	*Xuan Shen*	Nourish *Yin* to lessen Fire, cool Blood to remove pathogenic Heat
8.9	Asparagus	*Tian Men Dong*	Eliminate Heat and moisturize Lung by nourishing *Yin*, body fluid regeneration
3.6	Melia	*Chuan Lian Zi*	Promote *Qi* circulation to relieve pain, clear Heat and promote diuresis
3.6	Hordeum	*Mai Ya*	Strengthen Spleen to promote digestion
3.6	Artemisia	*Yin Chen Hao*	Clear Heat and dissipate Damp
2.9	Glycyrrhiza	*Gan Cao*	Mediate the properties of other herbs

Preparation:

1. Powder or capsule method: Herbs are ground into a fine powder. Powder can be encapsulated.
2. Decoction or teapill method: Raw herbs are mixed together and decocted. Herbal water extract (decoction) can be concentrated as granules or teapills.

Actions: Tranquilize the Liver to stop the Wind, nourish *Yin* to resolve seizures

Indications: This formula is indicated for Internal Wind due to *Yin* deficiency and Liver *Yang* Rising with seizure; loss of balance or disorientation; increased intraocular pressure; pain and hot sensation on palpation of the head; restlessness; frequent belching or vomiting; slowly progressive paresis of limbs; a dry mouth with a red, dry tongue; and a wiry and forceful pulse. It is also applicable to hypertension and signs of head pain due to Liver and Kidney *Yin* Deficiency and Liver *Yang* Excess. In case of excessive Phlegm, *Dan Nan Xing* (Arisaema) and *Chuan Bei Mu* (Fritillaria) can be added to dissipate Phlegm; in case of severe *Yin* deficiency, *Shu Di Huang* (Rehmannia) and *Shan Zhu Yu* (Cornus) are added to reinforce the Liver and Kidney. In cases of intense headache and increased intraocular pressure, *Xia Ku Cao* (Prunella), *Gou Teng* (Uncaria), and *Ju Hua* (Chrysanthemum) are added to clear Liver-Heat. In cases of extreme Heat in the Heart, *Shi Gao* (Gypsum) is added to clear Heat.

Dosage and Usage:

Horses and Cattle: 15–30g, twice daily
Camels: 30–45g, twice daily
Llamas, Alpacas, Goats, Sheep, and Pigs: 5–10g, twice daily
Dogs: 0.5–5g (or 0.05g per kg body weight), twice daily
Cats and Rabbits: 0.2–0.5g (or 0.05g per kg body weight), twice daily
Birds: 0.05g per kg body weight, twice daily
Use 2–4 weeks until primary clinical signs resolve.

Analysis of Formula: *Yin* Deficiency leads to Liver *Yang* Rising, resulting in seizure and Internal Wind. This Internal Wind Pattern should be treated by expelling endogenous Wind from the Liver, nourishing *Yin* and suppressing hyperactive *Yang*. The large proportion of *Tu Niu Xi* (Achyranthes) functions as the King herb to lead Blood downward and nourish the Liver and Kidney. *Dai Zhe Shi* (Hematite), *Long Gu* (Draconis) and *Mu Li* (Ostrea) descend *Qi*, suppress hyperactive *Yang*, and expel endogenous Wind; they are used as Minister herbs. *Gui Ban* (Testudinis), *Bai Shao* (Paeonia), *Xuan Shen* (Scrophularia), and *Tian Men Dong* (Asparagus) can nourish *Yin* and clear Heat to suppress the hyperactive *Yang*, while *Chuan Lian Zi* (Melia), *Mai Ya* (Hordeum), and *Yin Chen Hao* (Artemisia) can clear Heat from the Liver and regulate Liver-*Qi*; these are Adjuvant herbs. Working as the Messenger herb, *Gan Cao* (Glycyrrhiza) can mediate the properties of other herbs and regulate the Stomach. Combined with *Mai Ya* (Hordeum), *Gan Cao* (Glycyrrhiza) can prevent *Dai Zhe Shi* (Hematite) from impairing the Stomach.

Cautions and Contraindications: This formula has drastic effects of expelling endogenous Wind and suppressing hyperactive *Yang*; thus, it can be applied only to severe Patterns with hyperactive Liver *Yang* Rising (seizure).

Dr. Xie's Comments: *Zhen Gan Xi Feng Tang* is often used for seizure, hypertension, and hyperactive behavior due to Liver *Yang* Rising and *Yin* Deficiency in cats and dogs.

Clinical and Pharmacological Studies: *Zhen Gan Xi Feng Tang* was used for the treatment of 68 cases of facial paralysis in combination with *Dang Gui Bu Xue Tang*, *Qian Zheng San*, and *Bu Yang Huan Wu Tang*: 96% of the patients had a positive outcome.[48] A perimenopausal syndrome was also successfully treated with *Zhen Gan Xi Feng Tang*. All clinical signs, including anger or vexation, irritability, dizziness and tinnitus, were significantly improved after the herbal treatment.[49] Veterinary patients with Deficient Heat and Liver *Qi* Stagnation in Cushing's disease might similarly benefit from this formula. From 2005 to 2006, 80 cases of hypertensive intracerebral hemorrhage (HICH) with Stereotaxis Intracerebral Hematoma Evacuate (SIHE) were selected and treated with modified *Zhen Gan Xi Feng Tang*. Three days after experiencing SIHE, the patients begun to take *Zhen Gan Xi Feng Tang* orally or via a nasogastric feeding tube. The formula was composed of 30g *Dai Zhe Shi* (Hematite), 15g *Mu Li* (Ostrea), 15g *Gui Ban* (Testudinis), 30g *Tu Niu Xi* (Achyranthes), 15g *Long Gu* (Draconis), 15g *Tian Men Dong* (Asparagus), 15g *Xuan Shen* (Scrophularia), 15g *Bai Shao* (Paeonia), 5g *Chuan Lian Zi* (Melia), 5g *Mai Ya* (Hordeum), 5g *Yin Chen Hao* (Artemisia), and 5g *Gan Cao* (Glycyrrhiza). Herbs were decocted in water for oral dose, and the herbal water extract was taken twice daily for 10 days. During the 3-month follow-up, 12 cases (15%) died, no case was in the vegetative state, 14 cases (17.5%) had severe disability, 31 cases (38.5%) had moderate disability, and 23 cases (28.75%) recovered well. This result was better than the existing fatality rate of HICH, which is greater than 50% and with about 75% of living patients left with some degree of disability.[50]

A study was conducted on the effect of *Zhen Gan Xi Feng Tang* on the expression of Intercellular Adhesion Molecule-1 (ICAM-1) and nuclear factor–kappa B (NF-$_{\kappa}$B) protein in cerebral tissue after focal cerebral ischemia—reperfusion injury model in rats. The results indicated that subjects given this herbal formula resisted pathologic inflammatory injury after focal cerebral ischemia and reperfusion in rats.[51]

Jiang treated 37 cases of refractory insomnia with the modified *Zhen Gan Xi Feng Tang*: 16 cases were male, 21 were female; patients were 26 to 73 years old, and the average was 52 years old. The longest course of disease was 7 years, and the shortest was 3 months; the average was 2 years and 7 months. All laboratory tests of 37 cases had no abnormalities. The formula used in this study was composed of 30g *Tu Niu Xi* (Achyranthes), 30g *Dai Zhe Shi* (Hematite), 15g *Long Gu* (Draconis), 15g *Mu Li* (Ostrea), 15g *Gui Ban* (Testudinis), 15g *Bai Shao* (Paeonia), 15g *Xuan Shen* (Scrophularia), 15g *Tian Men Dong* (Asparagus), 6g *Chuan Lian Zi* (Melia), 6g *Mai Ya* (Hordeum), 6g *Yin Chen Hao* (Artemisia), and 5g *Gan Cao* (Glycyrrhiza). Herbal water extract was given twice daily for 15 to 45 days. After administration of the 15- to 45-day herbal treatments, 21 out of 37 cases were clinically cured (sleeping was normal and the symptoms disappeared), and 9 cases were improved (sleeping time lengthened and the symptoms improved).[52]

Li used 60 cases of hyperlipidemia as the herbal group treated with *Zhen Gan Xi Feng Tang* modification. Another 60 cases of hyperlipidemia were used as the control group. Among all 120 cases, cholesterol was more than 6.1 mmol/L, and triglycerides more than 1.6 mmol/L. The herbal formula was composed of 30g *Tu Niu Xi* (Achyranthes), 30g *Dai Zhe Shi* (Hematite, decocted first), 30g *Long Gu* (Draconis), 30g *Mu Li* (Ostrea), 10g *Gui Ban* (Testudinis), 10g *Di Long* (Pheretima), 15g *Chi Shao* (Paeonia), 30g *Bai Shao* (Paeonia), 10g *Chuan Niu Xi* (Cyathula), 10g *Chuan Lian Zi* (Melia), 15g *Mai Ya* (Hordeum), 10g *Gan Cao* (Glycyrrhiza), 45g *Jue Ming Zi* (Cassia), and 30g *Sha Zha* (Crataegus). In case of obesity, 10g each of *Fu Ling* (Poria), *Ze Xie* (Alisma), and *Dan Shen* (Salvia) were added. In cases of Liver/Kidney *Yin* deficiency, 30g *Sheng Di Huang* (Rehmannia), 30g *Nü Zhen Zi*(Ligustrum), and 30g *Dan Shen* (Salvia) were added. Herbs were soaked with 1000ml of water for 30 minutes and decocted by simmering for 30 minutes after boiling, resulting in a 200ml water extract. Herbs were then decocted again with 500ml water to produce a 150ml water extract. The two water extracts were mixed and taken orally twice a day for 30 days. In the herbal group, hyperlipidemia in all 60 cases was improved significantly.[53]

Tian Ma Gou Teng Yin (Gastrodia and Uncaria Decoction) 天麻钩藤汤

Tian Ma is Gastrodia, and *Gou Teng* is Uncaria. Both are the King herbs of this formula. *Yin* refers to decoction here.

Source: *Za Bing Zheng Zhi Xin Yi* (*New Concepts for Diagnosis and Treatment in Miscellaneous Diseases*), written by *Hu Guang-ci* and published in 1958

Ingredients: The original formula (Table 31.11) is composed of 9g *Tian Ma* (Gastrodia), 12g *Gou Teng* (Uncaria) 18g *Shi Jue Ming* (Haliotis), 9g *Zhi Zi* (Gardenia), 9g *Huang Qin* (Scutellaria), 12g *Chuan Niu Xi* (Cyathula), 9g *Du Zhong* (Eucommia), 9g *Yi Mu Cao* (Leonurus), 9g *Sang Ji Sheng* (Loranthus), 9g *Ye Jiao Teng* (Polygonum), and 9g *Fu Shen* (Poria).

Preparation:

1. Powder or capsule method: Herbs are ground into a fine powder. Powder can be encapsulated.
2. Decoction or teapill method: Raw herbs are mixed together and decocted. Herbal water extract (decoction) can be concentrated as granules or teapills.

Actions: Tranquilize the Liver to stop Internal Wind, clear Heat and activate Blood circulation

Table 31.11. Ingredients and actions of *Tian Ma Gou Teng Yin*.

%	English Name	Chinese *Pin-Yin*	Actions
7.9	Gastrodia	*Tian Ma*	Relieve convulsion and spasm, calm the Liver and subdue *Yang*
10.5	Uncaria	*Gou Teng*	Clear Heat and pacify Liver, relieve convulsion and spasm
15.8	Haliotis	*Shi Jue Ming*	Calm the Liver and subdue *Yang*, clear Liver and improve eyesight
7.9	Gardenia	*Zhi Zi*	Clear Heat and promote diuresis, cool Blood, reduce Fire
7.9	Scutellaria	*Huang Qin*	Clear Heat, eliminate Damp, purge Fire to remove toxin and soothe fetus
10.5	Cyathula	*Chuan Niu Xi*	Activate Blood and remove Stasis, nourish Kidney and Liver, induce diuresis for treating stranguria, ensure proper downward flow of Blood
7.9	Eucommia	*Du Zhong*	Nourish Kidney and Liver, soothe fetus
7.9	Leonurus	*Yi Mu Cao*	Activate Blood and remove Stasis, induce diuresis to reduce edema
7.9	Loranthus	*Sang Ji Sheng*	Dispel Wind and eliminate Damp, nourish Kidney and Liver, soothe fetus
7.9	Polygonum	*Ye Jiao Teng*	Calm the mind and nourish the Heart
7.9	Poria	*Fu Shen*	Calm the mind

Indications: This formula is indicated for Internal Wind or hypertension due to excessive Liver *Yang* Rising, marked with head-pressing, head-shaking, or other signs of head pain, disorientation, loss of balance, insomnia, a red tongue with yellow coating, and a wiry pulse. In case of severe head pain and disorientation, *Shan Yang Jiao* (Goat horn) and *Dai Zhe Shi* (Hematite) can be added to strengthen the effect of suppressing the hyperactive *Yang* and expelling endogenous Wind.

Dosage and Usage:

Horses and Cattle: 15–30 g, twice daily
Camels: 30–45 g, twice daily
Llamas, Alpacas, Goats, Sheep, and Pigs: 5–10 g, twice daily
Dogs: 0.5–5 g (or 0.05 g per kg body weight), twice daily
Cats and Rabbits: 0.2–0.5 g (or 0.05 g per kg body weight), twice daily
Birds: 0.05 g per kg body weight, twice daily

Use 4–12 weeks until primary clinical signs resolve.

Analysis of Formula: Liver *Yang* Rising leads to Internal Wind, disorientation, head pain, and hypertension. Liver *Yang* Rising can also generate Heat, which can disturb Shen and cause Blood Stagnation. The key treatment principles are to tranquilize the Liver to stop Internal Wind, clear Heat, and activate Blood circulation. *Tian Ma* (Gastrodia) and *Gou Teng* (Uncaria) work synergistically as the King herbs to tranquilize the Liver to stop the Wind. *Shi Jue Ming* (Haliotis), *Zhi Zi* (Gardenia), and *Huang Qin* (Scutellaria) clear Liver Heat and subdue the excessive Liver *Yang*, so they act as the Minister herbs. The rest of the ingredients serve as Adjuvant herbs: *Yi Mu Cao* (Leonurus) activates Blood circulation and eliminates water retention, *Chuan Niu Xi* (Cyathula) ensures the proper downward flow of Blood, *Sang Ji Sheng* (Loranthus) strengthens the Liver and tonifies the Kidney, and *Ye Jiao Teng* (Polygonum) and *Fu Shen* (Poria) calm the mind.

Cautions and Contraindications: It should be used with caution in Spleen *Qi* Deficiency.

Dr. Xie's Comments: I have used *Tian Ma Gou Teng Yin* for the treatment of seizures due to *Yin* Deficiency in dogs and cats.

Clinical and Pharmacological Studies: *Tian Ma Gou Teng Yin* modification was used for 32 patients with mild to moderate primary hypertension due to Liver *Yang* Rising (vertigo, headache, red face, irritability, restlessness, tantrum, bitter taste in mouth, thirst, red tongue, and wiry pulse). The formula was composed of 9 g *Tian Ma* (Gastrodia), 12 g *Gou Teng* (Uncaria), 18 g *Shi Jue Ming* (Haliotis), 9 g *Zhi Zi* (Gardenia), 9 g *Huang Qin* (Scutellaris), 12 g *Chuan Niu Xi* (Cyathula), 9 g *Du Zhong* (Eucommia), 9 g *Yi Mu Cao* (Leonurus), 9 g *Sang Ji Sheng* (Loranthus), and 9 g *Ye Jiao Teng* (Polygonum). Herbal water extract was orally given, one dose daily. After 4 weeks of herbal medication, all 32 patients' blood pressures decreased notably, especially in the daytime; the heart rates did not change.[54] Modified *Tian Ma Gou Teng Yin* was found to be more effective in controlling blood pressure for hypertension cases associated with pregnancy. A total of 22 patients were selected as the herbal group and treated with Nifedipine and *Tian Ma Gou Teng Yin*. Another 22 patients were used as the control group and treated only with Nifedipine. A dose of 10 mg Nifedipine was taken orally three times daily in both groups. *Tian Ma Gou Teng Yin* was composed of 12 g *Tian Ma* (Gastrodia), 12 g *Gou Teng* (Uncaria) 12 g *Huang Qin* (Scutellaria), 12 g *Dan Shen* (Salvia), 12 g *Fu Shen* (Poria), 12 g *Du Zhong* (Eucommia), 12 g *Sheng Di Huang* (Rehmannia), 12 g *Mai Men Dong* (Ophiopogon), 12 g *Sang Ji Sheng* (Loranthus), 12 g *He Shou Wu* (Polygonum), 12 g *Bai Zhu* (Atractylodes), 15 g *Shi Jue Ming* (Haliotis), 15 g

Huang Qi (Astragalus), 10g *Bai Shao* (Paeonia), and 10g *Mu Dan Pi* (Moutan). Herbs were decocted in water for oral use, one dose 3 times a day in concurrence with Nifedipine. After the 2-week treatment, 14 cases in the herbal group had normal blood pressure, and 7 cases were significantly improved. In the control group, 10 cases had normal blood pressure, and 8 cases were significantly improved.[55]

The modified *Tian Ma Gou Teng Yin* was used for the treatment of 40 cases of chronic migraine. The formula was composed of 15g *Tian Ma* (Gastrodia), 12g *Gou Teng* (Uncaria), 12g *Shi Jue Ming* (Haliotis), 12g *Huang Qin* (Scutellaris), 15g *Sang Ji Sheng* (Loranthus), 15g *Du Zhong* (Eucommia), 20g *Chuan Niu Xi* (Cyathula), 20g *Yi Mu Cao* (Leonurus), 30g *Dan Shen* (Salvia), 10g *Chuan Xiong* (Ligusticum), 12g *Chao Da Zao* (Jujube), 10g *Fu Shen* (Poria), 12g *Ge Gen* (Pueraria), 12g *Yan Hu Suo* (Corydalis), 10g *Gan Cao* (Glycyrrhiza). Herbs were decocted in water for oral use, one dose twice daily on an empty stomach: 8 cases were cured clinically (the clinical symptoms of migraine disappeared, and there was no recurrence 1 month after the herb withdrawal); 16 cases were significantly improved (the score of migraine symptoms was reduced by more than 50% after treatment); and 9 cases were improved (the score of migraine was reduced by 21% to 50% after treatment).[56]

The protective effects of *Tian Ma Gou Teng Yin* were investigated on the human umbilical vein endothelin cells (HUVECs) induced by angiotensin II (Ang II). HUVECs were cultured in vitro by collagenase digestive method. HUVECs were randomly divided into three groups: control group, Ang II group, and Ang II + *Tian Ma Gou Teng Yin* group. The morphology and density of HUVECs were observed with an inverted microscope. The results showed that *Tian Ma Gou Teng Yin* could inhibit the injury of HUVECs induced by Ang II.[57] Ménière's disease is a disorder of the inner ear that can affect hearing and balance. *Wang* treated 140 cases of Liver *Yang* Rising of Meniere's diseases with *Tian Ma Gou Teng Yin* modification. Herbs were decocted in water for oral dose, one dose daily; 124 out of 140 cases were clinically cured (all symptoms including dizziness, nausea, vomiting and headache, etc., disappeared), 16 cases were significantly improved.[58] *Yang* also found that *Tian Ma Gou Teng Yin* was effective for the treatment of migraine and seizures.[59]

Da Ding Feng Zhu (Great Wind Stopper) 大定风珠

Da refers to large or great. *Ding* means stop. *Feng* refers to Wind. *Zhu* means pill.

Source: *Wen Bing Tiao Bian* (*Treatise on Differentiation and Treatment of Seasonal Febrile Diseases*), written by *Wu Ju-tong* and published in 1798 CE

Table 31.12. Ingredients and actions of *Da Ding Feng Zhu*.

%	English Name	Chinese *Pin-Yin*	Actions
14.6	Paeonia	*Bai Shao*	Cool the Liver and nourish the Blood
7.3	Asinum	*E Jiao*	Tonify the Blood, nourish *Yin*
9.8	Testudinis	*Gui Ban*	Nourish *Yin* to suppress *Yang*
14.6	Rehmannia	*Sheng Di Huang*	Clear Heat to cool the Blood, nourish *Yin* and Blood
4.9	Cannabis	*Huo Ma Ren*	Moisten the Interior to relieve Dryness
4.9	Schisandra	*Wu Wei Zi*	Astringently nourish *Yin*, tranquilize *Yang*
9.8	Ostrea	*Mu Li*	Nourish *Yin* to suppress *Yang*
14.6	Ophiopogon	*Mai Men Dong*	Nourish *Yin*, promote body fluid regeneration
9.7	Glycyrrhiza	*Zhi Gan Cao*	Mediate the properties and actions of other herbs
9.8	Amyda	*Bie Jia*	Nourish *Yin* to suppress *Yang*

Ingredients: The original formula (Table 31.12) is composed of 18g *Bai Shao* (Paeonia), 9g *E Jiao* (Asinum), 12g *Gui Ban* (Testudinis), 18g *Sheng Di Huang* (Rehmannia), 6g *Huo Ma Ren* (Cannabis), 6g *Wu Wei Zi* (Schisandra), 12g *Mu Li* (Ostrea), 18g *Mai Men Dong* (Ophiopogon), 12g *Zhi Gan Cao* (Glycyrrhiza), and 12g *Bie Jia* (Amyda).

Preparation:

1. Traditional Method: The first 10 ingredients are ground and mixed with water and 2 pieces of chicken egg yolk (*Ji Zi Huang*) and made into a pill.
2. Powder or capsule method: All ingredients are ground into a fine powder. Powder can be encapsulated.
3. Decoction or teapill method: Raw herbs are mixed together and decocted. Herbal water extract (decoction) can be concentrated as granules or teapills.

Actions: Nourish *Yin* to extinguish Wind

Indications: This formula is indicated for Internal Wind due to *Yin* Deficiency marked with cool-seeking behavior, red and dry tongue, and thin and fast pulse. It also is applicable to epidemic encephalitis B, epidemic cerebrospinal meningitis, and other diseases related to the severe impairment of body fluids leading to *Yin* Deficiency and seizures. In case of wheezing and shortness of breath, add *Ren Shen* (Ginseng). In case of spontaneous perspiration, add *Long Gu* (Draconis), *Ren Shen* (Ginseng), and *Fu Xiao Mai* (Triticum).

Dosage and Usage:
Horses and Cattle: 15–30 g, twice daily
Camels: 30–45 g, twice daily
Llamas, Alpacas, Goats, Sheep, and Pigs: 5–10 g, twice daily
Dogs: 0.5–5 g (or 0.05 g per kg body weight), twice daily
Cats and Rabbits: 0.2–0.5 g (or 0.05 g per kg body weight), twice daily
Birds: 0.05 g per kg body weight, twice daily
Use 4–8 weeks until primary clinical signs resolve.

Analysis of Formula: Impairment of body fluids and *Yin* leads to *Yin* Deficiency, which allows *Yang* to rise and generate seizure activity. This Pattern should be treated by nourishing *Yin* and subduing Wind. Acting as the King herbs, *Sheng Di Huang* (Rehmannia), *Mai Men Dong* (Ophiopogon), and *Bai Shao* (Paeonia) nourish *Yin*, cool the Liver, and subdue the excessive Liver *Yang*. *E Jiao* (Asinum), *Gui Ban* (Testudinis), *Bie Jia* (Amyda), and *Ji Zi Huang* (chicken egg yolk), if used, nourish *Yin* and Blood and suppress *Yang* to expel endogenous Wind. They are the Minister herbs. Both King and Minister herbs, strong in flavor and greasy in nature, are used for nourishing *Yin*, suppressing *Yang*, and dispelling Wind. Acting as the Adjuvant herbs, *Huo Ma Ren* (Cannabis) nourishes *Yin* and moistens dryness; *Mu Li* (Ostrea) subdues Wind and suppresses *Yang*; while *Wu Wei Zi* (Schisandra), in combination with *Zhi Gan Cao* (Glycyrrhiza), are sour and sweet in nature and increase *Yin*, thereby strengthening the effects of nourishing *Yin* and subduing Wind. *Zhi Gan Cao* (Glycyrrhiza) also serves as a guiding herb to mediate the properties of other herbs.

This formula is derived from *Jia Jian Fu Mai Tang* of *Wenbing Tiao Bian*. *Jia Jian Fu Mai Tang* is composed of *Zhi Gan Cao* (Glycyrrhiza), *Sheng Di Huang* (Rehmannia), *Bai Shao* (Paeonia), *Mai Men Dong* (Ophiopogon), *E Jiao* (Asinum), and *Huo Ma Ren* (Cannabis). It is used in case of impairment of *Yin* caused by chronic febrile diseases. In the formulation of *Da Ding Feng Zhu*, *Wu Wei Zi* (Schisandra), *Gui Ban* (Testudinis), *Bie Jia* (Amyda), and *Mu Li* (Ostrea) are added to reinforce *Yin* tonification and subdue the excessive *Yang* Rising to extinguish Wind.

Cautions and Contraindications: This formula aims to replenish *Yin*; thus, it is contraindicated for Excess Heat.

Dr. Xie's Comments: *Da Ding Feng Zhu* is often used for seizure, urticaria, and encephalitis due to *Yin* Deficiency with False Heat in cats, dogs, and horses.

Clinical and Pharmacological Studies: Modified *Da Ding Feng Zhu* was used for the treatment of Liver Fibrosis: 56 patients with Liver Fibrosis due to chronic hepatitis B were randomly divided into an herbal group (30 cases) and a control group (26 cases). The patients in the herbal group were treated with modified *Da Ding Feng Zhu*, which was composed of 15 g *Bie Jia* (Amyda), 15 g *Gui Ban* (Testudinis), 20 g *Mu Li* (Ostrea), 20 g *Bai Shao* (Paeonia), 5 g *Huo Ma Ren* (Cannabis), 20 g *Sheng Di Huang* (Rehmannia), 10 g *Mai Men Dong* (Ophiopogon), 6 g *Wu Wei Zi* (Schisandra), 10 g *E Jiao* (Asinum), 12 g *Zhi Gan Cao* (Glycyrrhiza), and 2 egg yolks (*Ji Zi Huang*.) All ingredients except the yolks were decocted in water. After the residue was removed, yolks were added to the decoction. Half of the mixture was administered twice daily for 3 months. The patients in the control group took colchicine tablets orally (1 mg/tablet, produced by Kunming Pharmaceutical Company, Yunnan, China), 1 tablet once a day for 3 months. The serum levels of hyaluronic acid (HA), procollagen III (PC-III), IV collagen IV-C), and Laminin (LN) of the patients were determined, compared, and analyzed before treatment and after a 3-month treatment in both groups. The results showed that in the herbal group, the levels of HA, PC-III, IV-C, and LN after the 3-month treatment were significantly lower than those before treatment ($P < 0.01$). In the control group, only the HA level was significantly lower ($P < 0.05$). There was a significant difference ($P < 0.05$) in PC-III and IV-C and a very significant difference ($P < 0.01$) in HA after treatment between the two groups. The researchers therefore concluded that *Da Ding Feng Zhu* decoction can lower serum indexes of Liver Fibrosis. [60]

It was reported that bone mineral metabolism disorder was improved with *Da Ding Feng Zhu* for Internal Wind due to *Yin* Deficiency in Chronic Renal Insufficiency (CRI) cases. Internal Wind due to *Yin* Deficiency was marked by convulsion; weakness and pain in the back, waist, and knees; pruritis; burning sensation of the palms and feet; red tongue with no coating; and deep, thin, and weak pulse. A total of 30 cases of Internal Wind due to *Yin* Deficiency in CRI were randomly divided into an herbal group ($n = 15$) and a control group ($n = 15$). The herbal group was treated with *Da Ding Feng Zhu*, which was composed of 18 g *Bai Shao Yao* (Paeonia), 18 g *Shu Di Huang* (Rehmannia), 9 g *E Jiao* (Asinum), 12 g *Gui Ban* (Testudinis), 6 g *Huo Ma Ren* (Cannabis), 6 g *Wu Wei Zi* (Schisandra), 24 g *Mu Li* (Ostrea), 18 g *Mai Men Dong* (Ophiopogon), 12 g *Zhi Gan Cao* (Glycyrrhiza), 2 *Ji Zi Huang* (chicken egg yolks), and 12 g *Sheng Bie Jia* (Amyda). All the herbs, except *Ji Zi Huang*, were decocted twice; and 300 ml herbal water extract was administered orally 3 to 4 times after mixing with 1 to 2 yolks, one dose daily, for 3 months. The second group was treated with soft gelatin capsules of calcitriol (1, 25 $(OH)_2$ D_3 0.25 μg/tablet, produced by Roche, Switzerland, taken orally, 1 tablet once a day for 3 months). After comparing the serum calcium, serum phosphorus, bone gla-protein, C-parathyroid hormone, bone mineral content (g/cm), bone width (cm), and clinical symptoms before and after treatment, the researchers found that there was a remarkable disorder of mineral metabolism in all 30 cases of CRI. *Da Ding Feng Zhu* not only improved the mineral metabolism disorder, but also improved ($P < 0.05$) serum calcium, serum phosphorus, and anemia. The soft gelatin capsules of calcitriol did not induce a remarkable effect ($P > 0.05$) on serum calcium, serum phosphorus, and anemia.[61]

From 1995 to 1999, *Ni Xiao-chou* treated 31 cases of urticaria with *Da Ding Feng Zhu* modification; 17 out of 31 cases were male, and 14 cases were female; the age was 21 to 65 years, and the average was 41.9 years; the course of disease was 2 to 23 years, and the average was 7 years. The formula is composed of 12 g *Bai Shao* (Paeonia), 12 g *Sheng Di Huang* (Rehmannia), 12 g *Mai Men Dong* (Ophiopogon), 10 g *E Jiao* (Asinum), 15 g *Gui Ban* (Testudinis), 15 g *Bie Jia* (Amyda), 15 g *Mu Li* (Ostrea), 10 g *Zhi Gan Cao* (Glycyrrhiza), 8 g *Huo Ma Ren* (Cannabis), 10 g *Wu Wei Zi* (Schisandra), 10 g *Da Zao* (Jujube), 3 pieces (diameter 15–20 mm, 1–2 mm thick) of *Sheng Jiang* (Zingiberis), and 1 *Ji Zi Huang* (chicken egg yolk–Gallus). All of the herbs were decocted in water for oral use, one dose daily for 3 days (1 egg yolk/day, mixed with water decoction). The researchers note that because they are expensive, *Gui Ban* (Testudinis) and *Bie Jia* (Amyda) may be replaced by *Zhen Zhu Mu* (Margarita) and *Long Gu* (Draconis). In case of severe itching, *Bai Xian Pi* (Dictamnus) and *Di Fu Zi* (Kochia) were added. All 31 cases had positive results: 8 out of 31 cases were clinically cured in 10 days, 23 cases were clinically cured in 14 days, and 1 case recurred in 2 years.[62] *Da Ding Feng Zhu* was also used successfully for the treatment of depression and chorea syndromes due to Liver *Yin* Deficiency in humans.[63,64]

REFERENCES

1. Deng ZW. The pharmacology study of *Chuan Xiong Cha Tiao San*, Pharmacology and Clinics of Chinese Materia Medica 1992;8(1):11. (In Chinese)
2. Mei QX, Liang B. The clinical new uses of *Chuan Xiong Cha Tiao San* (powder preparation for infusion). Journal of Medicinal Materials of Chinese Drugs 2001;24(12):911–912. (In Chinese)
3. Mei QX. The Clinical New Application of Patent Medicines of TCM. Beijing: People's Medical Publishing House, 2001:68. (In Chinese)
4. Wu JQ. The clinical new application of *Chuan Xiong Cha Tiao San*. Journal of Traditional Chinese Medicine 1991;5:21.
5. Wang ZS. Analysis of 60 cases of cervical spondylosis were treated with *Chuan Xiong Cha Tiao San* (a prepared pill). patent medicines of TCM 1991;13(1):23.
6. Miao HQ. The clinical new application of *Chuan Xiong Cha Tiao San*. Zhejiang Journal of Traditional Chinese Medicine 1993;28(4):184.
7. Jiang YC. 12 cases of acute frontal sinusitis were treated with *Chuan Xiong Cha Tiao San*. Zhejiang Journal of Traditional Chinese Medicine 1993;28(4):184.
8. Liang XY, Guang HQ. Effects of *Xiao Feng San* on ultrastructure of skin in delayed hypersensitivity. Journal of Liaoning University of TCM 2007;9(2):29–30.
9. Li GZ, Zheng YQ. The immunoregulatory effects and mechanism of *Xiao Fengsan* granules. Chinese Journal of Experimental Traditional Medical Formulae 2004;10(4):39–42.
10. Zheng YQ, Dai M, Chen GL. Study of the anti-allergy and mechanism of *Xiao Feng San* granules. Chinese Journal of Experimental Traditional Medical Formulae 2002;8(6):26–28.
11. Zheng YQ, Cheng GL, Dai M. The anti-inflammation and mechanism of *Xiao Feng San* granules. Primary Journal of Chinese Materia Medicine 2002;16(5):7–8.
12. Huo H. The clinical observation on treating 45 cases of eczema with modified *Xiao Feng San*. Chinese Magazine of Clinical Medicinal Professional Research 2006;12(5):658–659.
13. Lin HF. Treating 38 cases of psoriasis with a plus formula of *Xiao Feng San*. Hebei Journal of TCM 2002;24(3):185.
14. Wang Y. Treatment of drug eruption due to ampicillin with *Xiao Feng San*. Journal of Sichuan Traditional Chinese Medicine 1993;11(4):34.
15. Wang LH, Wang YZ. Treating 22 cases of drug eruption due to ampicillin with *Si Wu Xiao Feng San*. Chinese Research Journal of Practical Medicine 2003;2(3):354.
16. Tu QN, Wan BJ. Treating 30 cases of cough due to pharyngitis with a modified *Xiao Feng San*. Tianjin Journal of Traditional Chinese Medicine 2005;22(6):470.
17. Yang WQ, Zheng TF. Treatment of 40 cases of herpes with *Xiao Feng San* and polyinosinic acid. Journal of Sichuan Traditional Chinese Medicine 2002;20(9):65.
18. Zhang ZJ, Kou N. 48 cases of conjunctivitis were treated with *Xiao Feng San*. Journal of Shaanxi College of Traditional Chinese Medicine 2001;5(9):41.
19. Pan JQ, Xiao LY, Zhang D. Immunosuppresive, antioxidative, anti-inflammatory analgesic effect of *Xia Huo Luo* pills. Chinese Journal of Clinical Rehabilitation 2006;10(47):183–188.
20. Chui WS. 32 cases of sciatica were treated with *Xiao Huo Luo Dan*. Inner Mongolia Journal of Traditional Chinese Medicine 1993;28(4):184. (In Chinese)
21. Xue TB. Chronic *Bi* syndrome in horses, cattle and buffalo was successfully treated with *Xiao Huo Luo Dan* and *Du Huo Ji Sheng Tang*. Journal of Traditional Chinese Veterinary Medicine 2005;24(3):49. (In Chinese)
22. Li CQ. Paralysis in pigs was treated with *Xiao Huo Luo Dan* and *Du Luo Ji Sheng Tang*. Journal of Traditional Chinese Veterinary Medicine 2001;20(5):25. (In Chinese)
23. Mei QX. A new application of *Xiao Huo Luo Dan*. Family and Traditional Chinese Medicine 2003;1:43. (In Chinese)
24. Yuan BY. Studies on metallic elements in the boiling water extracts of *Da Hao Luo Dan*. Studies on Microelement and Health 1997;14(3):37–39.
25. Liu WG, Wang WA, Zhou RL. The clinical studies on treatment of mental disorders of epilepsy with *Da Hao Luo Dan*. Nervous Diseases and Mental Hygiene 2003;3(2):141–142. (In Chinese)
26. Qi JH. 31 cases of acute infectious polyneuritis were treated with *Qu Feng Jie Du Tang* and *Da Huo Luo Dan*. Jiangsu Journal of Traditional Chinese Medicine 1998;19(4):22. (In Chinese)
27. Niu GK, Niu XQ. The new usages of *Da Huo Luo Dan*. Traditional Chinese Medicine of family 2005;2:49. (In Chinese)
28. Chen SJ, Qiu Y. Influences of *Ban Xia Bai Zhu Tian Ma San* on hemorheology of hyperviscousemia. Practical Journal of Internal Medicine of TCM 2003;17(5):407. (In Chinese)
29. Li XB, Lu JM. Influences of *Ban Xia Bai Zhu*, *Tian Ma San* and *Yu Ping Feng San* on immunity disequilibrium state of hypertensive disease. China Journal of Chinese Materia Medica 2005;30(12):949–951. (In Chinese)

30. Li XL. Vertebral artery type of cervical spondylosis was treated with *Ban Xia Bai Zhu, Tian Ma San* and *Zhi Mi Fu Ling Wan*. Sichuan Journal of Traditional Chinese Medicine 2004; 22(7):82. (In Chinese)
31. Zhao YG. 68 cases of tension headache were treated with *Ban Xia Bai Zhu Tian Ma San*. Acta Chinese Medicine and Pharmacology 1999;20(3):27–28. (In Chinese)
32. Huang W. 45 cases of Meniere's Syndrome were treated with *Ban Xia Bai Zhu Tian Ma San*. Traditional Chinese Medicine of *Ji Lin* 2000;4:39. (In Chinese)
33. Zhang WC. 106 cases of apoplexy aura were treated with *Ban Xia Bai Zhu Tian Ma San*. Traditional Chinese Medicine of *Gan Su* 2001;14(6):28–29. (In Chinese)
34. He HX. 24 cases of trigeminal neuralgia were treated with *Ban Xia Bai Zhu Tian Ma San*. Chinese Medical Research & Clinic 2007;15(4):74–75. (In Chinese)
35. Ma XQ, Ma SH, Geng X. 27 cases of epilepsy were treated with *Ding Xian Wan*. Beijing Journal of Traditional Chinese Medicine 1993;4:29–30. (In Chinese)
36. Huang YJ, Li YY. Clinical observation of 118 cases of treatment of refractory epilepsy combined with Traditional Chinese Medicine and Western Medicine. Jiangxi Journal of Traditional Chinese Medicine 2003;3:20. (In Chinese)
37. Wang MY, Jin T, Yao JX. Epilepsy with *Fu Fang San Xian Ding Xian Wan*. New Journal of Traditional Chinese Medicine 1994;24(10):26. (In Chinese)
38. Zhang WL. 69 cases of secondary epilepsy from apoplexy were treated with *Ling Yi San* and *Ding Xian Wan*. Zhejiang Journal of Traditional Chinese Medicine 2004;14(9):587. (In Chinese)
39. Zhang SH. Stiffness of the tongue was treated with *Di Tan Tang* and *Jie Yu Dan*. Hebei Journal of Traditional Chinese Medicine 2003;25(2):121.
40. Meng FX, Wang AY, Wang GQ. 103 cases of apoplexy treated with a modified *Di Tan Tang*. Shandong Journal of Traditional Chinese Medicine 2002;21(9):531–532.
41. Jia AM, Wen X. 13 cases of depression were treated with modified *Di Tan Tang*. Henan Traditional Chinese Medicine 2003;23(9):23.
42. Tang ZL, Li JM. 72 cases of acute tracheitis and bronchitis were treated with modified *Di Tan Tang*. Heilongjiang Journal of Traditional Chinese Medicine 2001;No. 4:15.
43. Zhang LM. 38 cases of sequelae of carbon monoxide poisoning treated with *Di Tan Tang*. Hebei Journal of Traditional Chinese Medicine 2005;27(9):678.
44. Shao M, Yang J, Liu WH. Clinical observation on hyperlipidemia treated with *Jiang Zhi Di Tan Tang*. Liaoning Journal of Traditional Chinese Medicine 2005;32(9):926.
45. Sha SH. Observation and treatment 59 cases of cerebroventricular hemorrhage. Henan Journal of Traditional Chinese Medicine 1999;14(2):25–26. (In Chinese)
46. Zhuang YY. Clinical observation on 72 cases of encephalitis B treated with integrated TCM and Western medicine. Hunan Journal of Traditional Chinese Medicine 1998;14(6):8–9. (In Chinese)
47. Yang YP. Clinical observation on 37 cases of poststroke syndrome. Hunan Journal of Traditional Chinese Medicine 2003;19(1):7–9. (In Chinese)
48. Zhang LS, Shen WH. Clinical analysis on the treatment of facial paralysis by Traditional Chinese Medicine. World Journal of Acupuncture-Moxibustion 2005;15(1):46–51.
49. Li Q, Shu YQ, Lai HH. Clinical observation of *Zhen Gan Xi Feng* decoction in treating peri-menopausal syndrome. Chinese Journal of Integrative Medicine 2003;9(1):63–66.
50. Fang YJ, Li B, Hu YL. 80 cases of hypertensive intracerebral hemorrhage (HICH) were treated with Stereotaxis Intracerebral Hematoma Evacuate (SIHE) and *Zhen Gan Xi Feng Tang*. Journal of Shaanxi College of Traditional Chinese Medicine 2007;30(4):16–17. (In Chinese)
51. HU JP, Wang J, Wu L. The dynamic study of the influence of 3 Chinese herbal formulas on the expression of ICAM-1 and NF-$_{\kappa}$B protein in cerebral tissue after focal cerebral ischemia-reperfusion in rats. Journal of Emergencies of Traditional Chinese Medicine 2007;16(5):571–573.
52. Jiang ZQ. 37 cases of refractory insomnia were treated with *Zhen Gan Xi Feng Tang*. Chinese Journal of Guangming Traditional Chinese Medicine 2005;20(3):61–62.
53. LI XZ. 60 cases of hyperlipidemia were treated with *Zhen Gan Xi Feng Tang* modification. Chinese Journal of Guangming Traditional Chinese Medicine 2000;15(5):50–51.
54. Zhou H, Xing ZH, Liu WP. Analysis of the effects of *Tian Ma Gou Teng* decoction on ambulatory blood pressure. Journal of Traditional Chinese Medicine University of Hunan 2005; 25(4):40–41.
55. Wang WH, Qin AM. Observation on curative effect of integrated TCM-WM on pregnancy-hypertension syndrome. Lishizhen Medicine and Materia Medica Research 2004; 15(9):626. (In Chinese)
56. Li H, Li SG. Observations on the curative effect of *Tian Ma Gou Teng Yin* on 40 cases of migraine. Chinese Technology of Traditional Chinese Medicine 2007;14(1):7. (In Chinese)
57. Meng YH, Tu X, Tu JW. Protective effects of *Tian Ma Gou Teng Yin* on the injury of human umbilical vein endothelin cells. Chinese Journal of Experimental Traditional Medical Formula 2007;13(1):26–28.
58. Wang HY. 140 cases of Meniere's Diseases were treated with *Tian Ma Gou Teng Yin*. Forum on Traditional Chinese Medicine 2005;20(5):30–31. (In Chinese)
59. Yang LB. 68 cases of migraine were treated with *Tian Ma Gou Teng Yin*. Traditional Chinese Medicine of Jiangxi 2006; 37(4):39. (In Chinese)
60. Li WL, Wang CD, Zhang JL. Effects of *Da Ding Feng Zhu* Decoction in 30 cases of liver fibrosis. Journal of Traditional Chinese Medicine 2003;23(4):251–254.
61. Wu YS, Li SL, Li JH. Mineral metabolism disorder of bone was improved with *Da Ding Feng Zhu* in patients with Chronic Renal Insufficiency (CRF) with the syndrome of Wind stirring due to *Yin* deficiency. Pharmacology and Clinic of Traditional Chinese Medicine 1999;15(1):39–40. (In Chinese)
62. Ni XC. 31 cases of urticaria were treated with *Da Ding Feng Zhu*. Chinese folk therapeutics 2000;8(8):30–31. (In Chinese)
63. Li YP. Observation on curative effect on 38 cases of postpartum depression treated with *Da Ding Feng Zhu*. Chinese Archives of Traditional Chinese Medicine 2005;23(8):1491. (In Chinese)
64. Jiang ZZ, Yu HJ, Wang GJ. Treatment of 12 cases of Chorea Minor with *Da Ding Feng Zhu*. Information on Traditional Chinese Medicine 1996;13(4):38. (In Chinese)

32 Purgative Herbal Formulas 泻下剂

Chaoying Luo, Michael Bartholomew, Huisheng Xie

The formulas in this chapter are used to treat patients with an Interior Excess Pattern (*Li Shi Zheng*). Interior Excess Patterns can be differentiated by their clinical signs, including accumulation of Heat, accumulation of Cold, fluid-consuming constipation, and accumulation of water or fluids. These signs are usually accompanied by a forceful pulse and a red or purple tongue. The signs are based on the etiological factors and different presenting conditions. There are five kinds of purgative therapy, including purgation by cooling, purgation by warming, lubricant laxation, elimination of excess fluid, and simultaneous application of purging and tonifying.

As previously stated, purgative herbal formulas are used for Interior Excess Patterns. If the Interior Excess exists simultaneously with an Exterior Pattern (*Biao Zheng*), the treatment should be first directed at the Exterior and later at the Interior Pattern. Treatment can also be based on the severity or degree of the Interior Pattern. In a case of constipation in aged, weak, or postpartum patients, the constipation itself is the Interior Excess. However, it is caused by the underlying Deficiency of *Yin*, *Qi*, or Blood. Thus, the treatment in this case should not only involve purging, but also address the Deficiency, which is the root of the problem. This can be accomplished by treating the Deficiency after purging, or by simultaneously purging the Excess and tonifying the Deficiency. Drastic purgatives should be used cautiously in pregnant animals. Because purgative herbal formulas can easily consume and injure Stomach *Qi*, their application should be stopped as soon as the curative effect appears, in order to avoid any negative side effects from a purge. To prevent any damage of Stomach *Qi*, fatty foods and foods that are difficult to digest should not be reintroduced too early.

Da Cheng Qi Tang (Drastic Purgation) 大承气汤

Da means large, big, or drastic. *Cheng Qi* refers to purgative. *Tang* is decoction, the original form of herbal administration. *Da Cheng Qi* can be literally translated as Drastic Purgative.

Source: *Shang Han Lun* (*Treatise on Exogenous Febrile Diseases*), written by *Zhang Zhong-jing* in 220 CE

Ingredients: The original formula for *Da Cheng Qi Tang* (Table 32.1) is composed of 12 g *Da Huang* (Rheum), 15 g *Hou Pu* (Magnolia), 12 g *Zhi Shi* (Aurantium), and 9 g *Mang Xiao* (Mirabilite).

Preparation:

1. Herbs are ground into a fine powder and mixed with water, or the first three herbs are decocted with water and then taken orally with *Mang Xiao* (Mirabilite).
2. Powder or capsule method: Herbs are ground into a fine powder. Powder can be encapsulated.
3. Decoction or teapill method: Raw herbs are mixed together and decocted. Herbal water extract (decoction) can be concentrated as granules or teapills.

Actions: Drastic purgation for eliminating accumulated Heat

Indications: This formula is indicated for Excess-Heat Patterns of *Yangming-Fu* organs (Large Intestine, Stomach), which are marked by constipation, abdominal pain with tenderness, afternoon fever, thirst with great desire to drink, red tongue with dry yellow coating, and deep and forceful pulse. It can be applied

Table 32.1. Ingredients and actions of *Da Cheng Qi Tang*.

%	English Name	Chinese *Pin-Yin*	Actions
25.0	Rheum	*Da Huang*	Purge the Large Intestines to remove Food Stasis, clear Heat and activate Blood
31.3	Magnolia	*Hou Po*	Promote *Qi* flow, eliminate dampness, remove food retention
25.0	Aurantium	*Zhi Shi*	Move *Qi* and remove food retention, stop colic
18.7	Mirabilitum	*Mang Xiao*	Purge the Large Intestines, soften hard mass, clear Heat

to an acute onset of impaction, or Interior Excess Heat in the course of febrile diseases. In the case of consumption of *Qi* due to Excess Heat with lassitude, add *Dang Shen* (Codonopsis) to replenish *Qi* and prevent exhaustion of *Qi* induced by drastic purgation. If the accumulating Heat impairs *Yin* by manifesting in extreme thirst with great desire to drink and a dry, red tongue with little coating, add *Xuan Shen* (Scrophularia) and *Sheng Di Huang* (Rehmannia) to nourish *Yin* to aid in the production of body fluid, and to moisten Dryness for relieving constipation.

Dosage and Usage:

Horses and Cattle: 15–30 g, twice daily
Camels: 30–45 g, twice daily
Llamas, Alpacas, Goats, Sheep, and Pigs: 5–10 g, twice daily
Dogs: 0.3–3 g (or 0.05 g per kg body weight), twice daily
Cats and Rabbits: 0.1–0.3 g (or 0.05 g per kg body weight), twice daily
Birds: 0.05 g per kg body weight, twice daily
Use 3–10 days until primary clinical signs resolve.

Analysis of Formula: Patterns that can benefit from this formula typically result from pathogenic Heat accumulating in the large intestine, leading to obstructed *Qi* flow of *Yang* organs (*Fu-Qi*), Food Stagnation, and constipation. This should be treated by eliminating Heat to promote the bowel movement. *Da Huang* (Rheum) acts as the King herb to eliminate Heat, stagnated food, and stool in the gastrointestinal tract, thereby relieving constipation. *Mang Xiao* (Mirabilite) possesses the effect of moistening Dryness and softening masses, and it is used as Minister herb to reinforce the effect of the King herb. Both *Zhi Shi* (Aurantium) and *Hou Po* (Magnolia) are Adjuvant herbs, capable of promoting the flow of *Qi*, relieving fullness, and helping the King and Minister herbs remove the stagnated food and stool. These actions accelerate the discharge of Heat and mass. Working together, these four herbs are highly efficacious in purging Heat and mass.

Cautions and Contraindications: This formula is used only for Excess Patterns of *Yangming-Fu* organs (including Stomach and Large Intestine) with excessive Heat or Food Stagnation. It must be applied with great care to patients without Excess Heat, or those with a constitutional Deficiency of *Qi* and *Yin*. Stop using the formula as soon as the curative effect appears.

Dr. Xie's Comments: I have used *Da Cheng Qi Tang* for impaction due to Excess Heat and Food Stagnation in horses.

Clinical and Pharmacological Studies: In 2001, a study demonstrated that *Da Cheng Qi Tang* protected brain tissues from injuries during the acute stages of cerebral hemorrhage.[1] 23 cases of omasal blockage were treated with injections of modified *Da Cheng Qi Tang* decoction into the omasum of cattle. The modified formula was composed of 250 g *Sheng Huang Qi* (Astragalus), 250 g *Dang Gui* (Angelica), 60 g *Da Huang* (Rheum), 30 g *Zhi Shi* (Aurantium), 30 g *Hou Po* (Magnolia), 30 g *Huang Lian* (Coptis), 30 g *Fan Xie Ye* (Senna), 30 g *Tao Ren* (Persica), 120 g *San Leng* (Sparganium), 120 g *E Zhu* (Zedoaria), 120 g *Huo Ma Ren* (Cannabis), 120 g *Yu Li Ren* (Prunus), and 300 g *Mang Xiao* (Mirabilite). Herbs except *Mang Xiao* (Mirabilitum) were decocted twice with 2500 ml water. Then, *Mang Xiao* (Mirabilitum) was added into the herbal water extract, dissolved, and then filtered. 500 ml of warmed saline was injected into the omasum first, the herbal water extract followed, and 2000 ml of warmed saline was injected again. A large quantity of loose, soft stool was usually discharged in 12–32 hours. 20 of 23 cases recovered clinically. This is an effective rate of 87%.[2]

In 2006, Tian and Ding reviewed the clinical and pharmaceutical research of *Da Cheng Qi*. It was found that the application and research of *Da Cheng Qi Tang* gained more attention; therefore, the depth and range of the research has increased significantly for the past 30 years. All of the diseases that were treated with *Da Cheng Qi Tang* are related to Interior Excess-Heat Patterns. Interior Excess Heat can be caused by intestinal obstruction, acute pancreatitis, infection of biliary tract, appendicitis, abdominal cramps, ascariasis of biliary tract, postoperative complications of abdomen, cerebral infarction, heatstroke, intracranial hypertension, hypertensive cerebral hemorrhage, hepatic encephalopathy, subarachnoid hemorrhage, headache, congestive heart failure of cor pulmonale, dizziness, tetanus, depression, hysteria, psychosis, eclampsia, acute kidney failure, lobar pneumonia, asthma, pulmonary infection, gouty arthritis, acute eczema, hives, burns, stress ulcer. Thus, modified *Da Cheng Qi Tang* can be used to treat many different diseases.[3]

Xiao Cheng Qi Tang (Mild Purgative) 小承气汤

Xiao means small, or mild. *Cheng Qi* refers to purgative. *Tang* is decoction, the original form of the herbal administration. *Xiao Cheng Qi* can be literally translated as Mild Purgative.

Source: *Shang Han Lun* (*Treatise on Exogenous Febrile Diseases*), written by *Zhang Zhong-jing* in 220 CE

Ingredients: The original formula of *Xiao Cheng Qi Tang* is composed of 12 g *Da Huang* (Rheum), 6 g *Hou Po* (Magnolia), and 9 g *Zhi Shi* (Aurantium). This formula is *Da Cheng Qi Tang* minus *Mang Xiao* (Mirabilitum), and has a mild purgative effect.

Preparation:
1. Powder or capsule method: Herbs are ground into a fine powder. Powder can be encapsulated.
2. Decoction or teapill method: Raw herbs are mixed together and decocted. Herbal water extract (decoction) can be concentrated as granules or teapills.

Actions: Mildly purge large intestines and clear Heat accumulation

Indications: This formula is indicated for Excess-Heat Patterns of *Yangming-Fu* organs with mild Food Stagnation. The main clinical signs are high fever, constipation or dysentery, abdominal pain or distention, yellow coating of the tongue, and a slippery and fast pulse.

Dosage and Usage:
Horses and Cattle: 15–30 g, twice daily
Camels: 30–45 g, twice daily
Llamas, Alpacas, Goats, Sheep, and Pigs: 5–10 g, twice daily
Dogs: 0.3–3 g (or 0.05 g per kg body weight), twice daily
Cats and Rabbits: 0.1–0.3 g (or 0.05 g per kg body weight), twice daily
Birds: 0.05 g per kg body weight, twice daily
Use 3–14 days until primary clinical signs resolve.

Analysis of Formula: *Da Huang* (Rheum) acts as the King herb to eliminate Heat, eliminate stagnated food and stool in the gastrointestinal tract, and relieve constipation. Both *Zhi Shi* (Aurantium) and *Hou Po* (Magnolia) are the Adjuvant and Messenger herbs, which move *Qi* and relieve abdominal distention and pain.

Cautions and Contraindications: This formula is contraindicated in cases with Spleen *Qi* Deficiency.

Dr. Xie's Comments: *Xiao Cheng Qi Tang* has similar actions to *Da Cheng Qi Tang* except with a milder purgative effect. Therefore, it is often used in treating Heat in the gastrointestinal tract with mild constipation or impaction.

Tiao Wei Cheng Qi Tang (Regulating the Stomach for Purgative) 调胃承气汤

Tiao means harmonizing or regulating. *Wei* is the Stomach. *Cheng Qi* refers to purgative. Tang is decoction, the form of herbal administration. Therefore *Tiao Wei Cheng Qi Tang* translates to Purgative That Regulates the Stomach.

Source: *Shang Han Lun* (*Treatise on Exogenous Febrile Diseases*), written by *Zhang Zhong-jing* in 220 CE

Ingredients: *Tiao Wei Cheng Qi Tang* is composed of 12 g *Da Huang* (Rheum), 6 g *Zhi Gan Cao* (Glycyrrhiza), and 9 g *Mang Xiao* (Mirabilite). This formula is again similar to *Da Cheng Qi Tang*, but now *Zhi Shi* (Aurantium) and *Hou Po* (Magnolia) are replaced with *Gan Cao* (Glycyrrhiza).

Preparation:
1. Powder or capsule method: Herbs are ground into a fine powder. Powder can be encapsulated.
2. Decoction or teapill method: Raw herbs are mixed together and decocted. Herbal water extract (decoction) can be concentrated as granules or teapills.

Actions: Slowly purge the large intestines and clear Heat accumulation

Indications: This formula is indicated for Dry-Heat Patterns of *Yangming-Fu* organs, (Stomach and Large Intestine). The main clinical signs are retention of feces, thirst, high fever, full abdomen, red tongue with yellow coating, and slippery and full pulse.

Dosage and Usage:
Horses and Cattle: 15–30 g, twice daily
Camels: 30–45 g, twice daily
Llamas, Alpacas, Goats, Sheep, and Pigs: 5–10 g, twice daily
Dogs: 0.3–3 g (or 0.05 g per kg body weight), twice daily
Cats and Rabbits: 0.1–0.3 g (or 0.05 g per kg body weight), twice daily
Birds: 0.05 g per kg body weight, twice daily
Use 3–10 days until primary clinical signs resolve.

Analysis of Formula: *Da Huang* (Rheum) acts as the King herb to eliminate Heat, Food Stagnation, and stool in the gastrointestinal tract, and to relieve constipation. *Mang Xiao* (Mirabilite) possesses the effect of moistening Dryness and softening masses, and it is used as the Minister herb to reinforce the effect of the King herb. Glycyrrhiza harmonizes other herbs while serving as the Messenger herb.

Cautions and Contraindications: This formula should be used cautiously in patients with Spleen *Qi* Deficiency.

Dr. Xie's Comments: *Tiao Wei Cheng Qi Tang* is often used for mild constipation or impaction, or chronic constipation in elderly patients.

Da Huang Fu Zi Tang (Rheum and Aconite) 大黄附子汤

Da Huang is Rheum and *Fu Zi* is Aconite. Both are the King herbs of this formulation. *Tang* is decoction, the original form of the herbal administration. *Da Huang Fu Zi Tang* translates to Rheum and Aconite Decoction.

Source: *Jin Gui Yao Lue* (*Synopsis of Prescriptions from the Golden Cabinet*), written by *Zhang Zhong-jing* in 220 CE

Ingredients: The original formula for *Da Huang Fu Zi Tang* (Table 32.2) is composed of 9 g *Da Huang* (Rheum), 9 g *Fu Zi* (Aconite), and 3 g *Xi Xin* (Asarum).

Preparation:
1. Powder or capsule method: Herbs are ground into a fine powder. Powder can be encapsulated.
2. Decoction or teapill method: Raw herbs are mixed together and decocted. Herbal water extract (decoction) can be concentrated as granules or teapills.

Actions: Warm *Yang* to dispel Cold, purge blockage to resolve stagnant *Qi*

Indications: This formula is indicated for blockage and Interior Excess Pattern, which is marked by abdominal pain and constipation, fever, a white and greasy tongue coating, and a stringy and tight pulse. It is applicable to diseases of the Gallbladder and chronic dysentery due to Cold accumulation in the Interior. In case of severe abdominal pain, add *Hou Po* (Magnolia) and *Zhi Shi* (Aurantium) to promote the flow of *Qi* and relieve the pain. In case of abdominal distention and fullness, with a thick greasy coating of the tongue, which is indicative of an Excess Cold Pattern, add *Rou Gui* (Cinnamomum) to warm the Interior and dispel Cold.

Table 32.2. Ingredients and actions of *Da Huang Fu Zi Tang*.

%	English Name	Chinese *Pin-Yin*	Actions
42.9	Rheum	*Da Huang*	Purge the Large Intestines to remove Food Stasis, clear Heat and activate Blood
42.9	Aconite (Prepared)	*Fu Zi*	Warm *Yang* to dispel Cold
14.2	Asarum	*Xi Xin*	Dispel Cold to stop colic

Dosage and Usage:
Horses and Cattle: 15–30 g, twice daily
Camels: 30–45 g, twice daily
Llamas, Alpacas, Goats, Sheep, and Pigs: 5–10 g, twice daily
Dogs: 0.3–3 g (or 0.05 g per kg body weight), twice daily
Cats and Rabbits: 0.1–0.3 g (or 0.05 g per kg body weight), twice daily
Birds: 0.05 g per kg body weight, twice daily
Use 3–10 days until primary clinical signs resolve.

Analysis of Formula: This formula treats Patterns that arise from accumulated Cold leading to a functional disorder of *Yang-Qi* as well as the obstructed flow of *Qi*. Therefore, treat by dispelling Cold and relieving pain. *Da Huang* (Rheum) and *Fu Zi* (Aconite, Prepared) act as the King herbs. *Da Huang* is capable of removing pathogenic accumulation to relieve constipation, while *Fu Zi* warms the interior to dispel Cold. *Xi Xin* (Asarum) functions as a Minister and Adjuvant herb to help *Fu Zi* dispel the Interior Cold. The Cold nature of *Da Huang* (Rheum) can be mitigated when combined with the other herbs that are pungent and hot in nature. However, the purgative function remains well preserved.

Cautions and Contraindications: When this herbal formula is used, the percentage of ingredient herbs with a warm nature must be larger than that of *Da Huang* (Rheum), which has a Cold nature. It is contraindicated for patients with Deficient Cold (False Cold) due to *Yang* Deficiency. Stop using as soon as the curative effect appears.

Dr. Xie's Comments: *Da Huang Fu Zi Tang Tang* can be useful for the treatment of acute abdominal pain due to accumulation of Excess Cold in horses.

Clinical and Pharmacological Studies: In 2007, Zhang reported that acute abdomens, such as acute pancreatitis, intestinal obstruction, acute appendicitis, acute cholecystitis, biliary ascariasis, etc., were treated with a variety of *Da Huang Fu Zi Tang* modifications: 1) The modified formula for acute pancreatitis was composed of 15 g *Da Huang* (Rheum, decocted later), 15 g *Yin Chen*

Hao (Artemisia), 6g *Fu Zi* (Aconite), 6g *Huang Lian* (Coptis), 3g *Xi Xin* (Asarum), 30g *Gua Lou* (Trichosanthes), 15g *Ban Xia* (Pinellia), 15g *Zhi Shi* (Aurantium), 15g *Yan Hu Suo* (Corydalis), 15g *Hou Po* (Magnolia), and 15g Yu Jin (Curcuma). Abdominal pain was remarkably reduced and vomiting stopped after 2 doses. All of the symptoms were diminished and the hemogram, urinary amylase, and white cell count returned to normal after 5 doses. Following an additional month of treatment, the pancreas, monitored by ultrasound, was shown to be normal and there was no reoccurrence of symptoms. 2) The formula for intestinal obstruction was composed of 15g *Da Huang* (Rheum, decocted later), 15g *Fu Zi* (Aconite), 6g *Xi Xin* (Asarum), 15g *Lai Fu Zi* (Raphanus), 10g *Zhi Shi* (Aurantium), and 10g *Hou Po* (Magnolia). Herbs were decocted with water for oral dosing. Abdominal pain was remarkably decreased and a bowel movement was seen in an average of 4 hours after the herbal administration. Abdominal pain was eliminated, and there was no vomiting. 3) The formula for acute appendicitis was composed of 15g *Da Huang* (Rheum, decocted later), 9g *Xi Xin* (Asarum), 6g *Fu Zi* (Aconite), 30g *Yi Yi Ren* (Coix), and 15g *Mu Dan Pi* (Moutan). Herbs were decocted with water for an oral dose. After 5 doses, the body temperature was almost normal, the WBC was 10.1 × 10/L (normal range: 0.33 to 0.67), abdominal pain was sometimes noted, and urine and stool were normal. All abnormal clinical signs returned to normal after another 4 doses. 4) The formula for acute cholecystitis was composed of 15g *Da Huang* (Rheum, decocted later), 10g *Fu Zi* (Aconite), 6g *Xi Xin* (Asarum), 15g *Jin Qian Cao* (Lysimachia), 15g *Yu Jin* (Curcuma), 10g *Zhi Shi* (Aurantium), 15g *Ji Nei Jin* (Gallus) 15g *Yan Hu Suo* (Corydalis), 10g *Hou Po* (Magnolia), and 10g *Gan Cao* (Glycyrrhiza). Herbs were decocted with water for oral dosing. After 2 doses, patients defecated and the abdominal pain subsided. After 15g *Ze Xie* (Alisma) and 15g *Yin Chen Hao* (Artemisia) were added to the formula and it was taken for 15 days, the abdominal pain disappeared, the jaundice faded, and the blood biochemical indicators and indices were nearly normal.[4]

In 1997, Chen treated 32 cases of biliary calculi with a *Da Huang Fu Zi Tang* modification. The formula was composed of 10–20g *Da Huang* (Rheum, decocted later), 6–10g *Fu Zi* (Aconite), 6–10g *Xi Xin* (Asarum), 6–10g *Ji Nei Jin* (Gallus), 10–20g *Wei Ling Xian* (Clematis), and 10–15g *San Leng* (Sparganium). In patients with yellow eyes, yellow body, and yellow urine, 30g *Yin Chen Hao* (Artemisia), 10g *Chuan Lian Zi* (Melia), and 15g *Mai Ya* (Hordeum) were added. In case of a severe infection, antibiotics and maintenance therapy was used during the course of the disease. Seventeen additional cases with biliary calculi were used as a control group. The treatment period was 1 month long and patients usually underwent 1–2 periods of treatment. 23 of the 32 cases of the treatment group were clinically cured (symptoms and clinical signs disappeared), and 8 cases showed improvement.[5]

From 1998 to 1999, Peng and Li treated 21 cases of uremia with *Da Huang Fu Zi Tang*. The formula was composed of 10–15g *Da Huang* (Rheum, decocted later), 15g *Fu Zi* (Aconite), 30g *Mu Li* (Ostrea), 15g *Pu Gong Ying* (Taraxacum), 15g *Zhi Zi* (Gardenia), and 6g *Gan Cao* (Glycyrrhiza). In cases with shortness of breath and lethargy, 30g *Dang Shen* (Codonopsis) 15g *Huang Qi* (Astragalus) were added. In cases with nausea and vomiting, 15g *Shan Yao* (Dioscorea), 10g *Ban Xia* (Prepared Pinellia), 6g *Chen Pi* (Citrus), 6g *Sha Ren* (Amomum), and 5g *Sheng Jiang* (Zingiberis) were added. In cases of severe edema, 20–30g *Fu Ling* (Poria), 15g *Ze Xie* (Alisma), and 15g *Che Qian Zi* (Plantago) were added. In cases with dizziness and headache associated with hypertensive disease, 15g *Gou Teng* (Uncaria) and 30g *Shi Jue Ming* (Haliotis) were added. In case of Blood Stagnation, 9g *Chuan Xiong* (Ligusticum), 15g *Dan Shen* (Salvia), and 3g *Hong Hua* (Carthamus) were added. Herbs were decocted twice with water and taken twice a day; the period of treatment was 6 weeks. An additional 24 cases were treated with Western medicine as a control group. In cases with slight edema and oliguresis, furosemide tablets were administered orally. In cases with severe edema and oliguresis with uremia, phentolamine, dopamine (light concentration), and furosemide were administered intravenously. Lotensin and furazosin were used together only for pressure release. Sodium hydrogen carbonate was taken orally or intravenously to correct acidosis. After a 6-week course of treatment, BUN, Scr, Hb, and CO_2CP in the herbal treatment group decreased remarkably ($P < 0.05$), with a positive response seen in 80.9% of patients. This was significantly better (37.5%) than that of the control group ($P < 0.05$).[6]

In 2002, 30 cases of diabetic nephropathy were treated with *Da Huang Fu Zi Tang*.[7] 18 of the 30 total cases were male and 12 cases were female. Ages ranged from 35–68 years, with the average age being 46 years. The course of disease ranged from 2–12 years. All of the cases had type II diabetes and were complicated by diabetic retinopathy. 15 cases were complicated by hypertension, 10 cases were complicated by coronary heart disease, and 8 cases were complicated by renal insufficiency. The herbal formula was composed of 9g *Da Huang* (Rheum, decocted later), 9g *Fu Zi* (Prepared Aconite), 30g *Huang Qi* (Astragalus), 6g *Zhu Ru* (Bambusa), 60g *Yi Mu Cao* (Leonurus), 30g *Che Qian Zi* (Plantago, decocted in a wrapped condition), 15g *Bai Zhu* (Atractylodes), 15g *Dan Shen* (Salvia), 12g *Dang Gui* (Angelica), 12g *Chuan Xiong* (Ligusticum), 15g *Ba Ji Tian* (Morinda), 15g *Rou Cong Rong* (Cistanche), 12g *Gou Qi Zi* (Lycium), 12g *Jiang Can* (Bombyx), 9g *Chan Tui* (Cicada), 15g *Huang Lian*

(Coptis), and 12 g *Shan Zhu Yu* (Cornus). Herbs were decocted once with water for oral dosing and taken twice daily. In cases of severe vomiting, 12 g *Huo Xiang* (Pogostemon) and 12 g *Ban Xia* (Prepared Pinellia) were added. In cases with abdominal distension, 6 g *Chen Xiang* (Aquilaria) and 12 g *Chen Pi* (Citrus) were added. In case of severe Blood Stasis, *Tao Ren* (Persica) and 3 g *Hong Hua* (Carthamus) were added. In conjunction with the herbal treatment, the patient's diet was controlled. In cases of renal insufficiency, a low phosphorus and low protein diet was included in the program. Protein intake was 0.5 g/kg body weight daily. The period of treatment was 1 month. 9 cases showed excellent improvement (nephrotic symptoms decreased within 24 hours; the quantity of urine protein decreased by more than 40%; fasting blood sugar, urea nitrogen, creatinine, and the clearance of endogenous creatinine decreased remarkably). 18 cases showed improvement (the symptoms continued to improve remarkably; the quantity of urine protein decreased by 10–40% at 24 hours; and fasting blood sugar, urea nitrogen, creatinine, and the clearance of endogenous creatinine all decreased), with 90% of patients showing a positive response.[7]

Ma Zi Ren Wan (Cannabis Pill) 麻子仁丸

Ma Zi Ren is the cannabis seed, which is the King herb of this formulation. *Wan* is pill, the original form of the herbal administration. Thus, *Ma Zi Ren Wan* means Cannabis Pill.

Source: *Shang Han Lun* (*Treatise on Exogenous Febrile Diseases*), written by *Zhang Zhong-jing* in 220 CE

Ingredients: The original formula for *Ma Zi Ren Wan* (Table 32.3) is composed of 500 g *Ma Zi Ren* (Cannabis), 250 g *Bai Shao Yao* (Paeonia), 250 g *Zhi Shi* (Aurantium), 500 g *Da Huang* (Rheum), 250 g *Hou Po* (Magnolia), and 250 g *Xing Ren* (Armeniaca).

Table 32.3. Ingredients and actions of *Ma Zi Ren Wan*.

%	English Name	Chinese *Pin-Yin*	Actions
25.0	Cannabis	*Ma Zi Ren*	Loosen bowel to relieve constipation
12.5	Paeonia	*Bai Shao Yao*	Nourish Blood and retain *Yin*
12.5	Aurantium	*Zhi Shi*	Move *Qi*, remove food retention, stop colic
25.0	Rheum	*Da Huang*	Purge the Large Intestines, remove Food Stasis
12.5	Magnolia	*Hou Po*	Move *Qi*, eliminate dampness, remove food retention
12.5	Armeniaca	*Xing Ren*	Loosen the bowel to relieve constipation

Preparation:

1. Powder or capsule method: Herbs are ground into a fine powder. Powder can be encapsulated.
2. Decoction or teapill method: Raw herbs are mixed together and decocted. Herbal water extract (decoction) can be concentrated as granules or teapills.

Actions: Loosen bowel to purge Heat, promote *Qi* flow to relieve constipation

Indications: This formula is indicated for constipation due to intestinal Dryness, which is marked by dry stool, frequent urination, dry mouth, and slight yellow coating of the tongue. In the absence of Excess Dryness and Heat, subtract the ingredients *Zhi Shi* (Aurantium) and *Hou Po* (Magnolia) and lessen the dosage of the ingredient *Da Huang* (Rheum).

Dosage and Usage:

Horses and Cattle: 15–30 g, twice daily
Camels: 30–45 g, twice daily
Llamas, Alpacas, Goats, Sheep, and Pigs: 5–10 g, twice daily
Dogs: 0.5–5 g (or 0.1 g per kg body weight), twice daily
Cats and Rabbits: 0.2–0.5 g (or 0.1 g per kg body weight), twice daily
Birds: 0.05 g per kg body weight, twice daily
Use 1–4 weeks until primary clinical signs resolve.

Analysis of Formula: This formula is used to treat Patterns caused by gastrointestinal Dryness and Heat, Deficiency of body fluid, and lack of lubrication in the intestines. It should be treated by moistening the bowels to purge Heat and promoting the flow of *Qi* to relieve constipation. *Ma Zi Ren* (Cannabis), which is mild in nature and abundant in lipids, functions as the King herb to moisten the large intestine, thus relieving constipation. *Da Huang* (Rheum), *Xing Ren* (Armeniaca), and *Bai Shao Yao* (Paeonia) act as Minister herbs to purge Heat and Dryness from the stomach and intestine, to descend *Qi* and relax the bowels, to nourish *Yin*, and to help the King herb carry out its actions. *Zhi Shi* (Aurantium) and *Hou Po* (Magnolia) serve as Adjuvant herbs to promote the flow of *Qi*, dissolve masses, and enhance the effect of *Da Huang* (Rheum).

This formula is made by taking *Xiao Cheng Qi Tang* and adding *Ma Zi Ren* (Cannabis), *Xing Ren* (Armeniaca), *Bai Shao Yao* (Paeonia), and *Feng Mi* (honey). It has the actions of purging Heat, Dryness, and dyspeptic disease from the stomach and intestine, similar to *Xiao Cheng Qi Tang*. However, its dosage is smaller and it uses the greasy agents of *Ma Zi Ren* (Cannabis), *Xing Ren* (Armeniaca), *Bai Shao Yao* (Paeonia) and *Feng Mi* (honey) to nourish *Yin* and increase body fluids to loosen the bowels to relieve constipation. Also, their sweet flavor and moisturizing nature can tone down the vigorous actions of *Xiao Cheng Qi Tang* and can purge without damaging healthy *Qi*. Therefore, this formula is mostly indicated for chronic constipation or Dryness of the intestines in senior or weak patients.

Cautions and Contraindications: Use with caution in patients who exhibit constipation without Dryness and Internal Heat. Stop using as soon as the curative effect appears.

Dr. Xie's Comments: I have used *Ma Zi Ren Wan* with great success for chronic constipation in dogs and megacolon in cats.

Clinical and Pharmacological Studies: The influence of *Ma Zi Ren Wan* on fasting blood sugar, fasting blood fat, fasting serum creatinine, and fasting serum urea nitrogen was evaluated in diabetic rat models.[8] After *Ma Zi Ren Wan* was taken orally for 30 days, the levels of the above parameters were remarkably improved ($P < 0.01$ or $P < 0.05$). The results showed that *Ma Zi Ren Wan* could regulate a glycometabolism disorder, control hyperglycemia of diabetes, regulate lipid disorders, and control diabetic hyperlipemia. *Ma Zi Ren Wan* also improved kidney function in STZ rats, and could especially lower the levels of blood serum creatinine and blood urea nitrogen.[8]

In 1991, Wu and Tong reported that 300 cases of Spleen *Qi* Stagnation (*Pi Yu Zheng*), in pigs were treated with *Ma Zi Ren Wan*. *Pi Yu Zheng* is a common disease of pigs and is marked by frequent urination, dry and hard stools, poor appetite, weight loss, etc. The formula was composed of 15 g *Ma Zi Ren* (Cannabis), 9 g *Bai Shao Yao* (Paeonia), 9 g *Da Huang* (Rheum), 9 g *Hou Po* (Magnolia), 9 g *Xing Ren* (Armeniaca), 9 g *Mai Ya* (Hordeum), 9 g *Shen Qu* (Massa), 9 g *Shan Zha* (Crataegus), and 50 g *Feng Mi* (honey). All of the herbs were ground into a fine powder, mixed with the honey, and fed to pigs orally via mixing with food. One dose was administered every other day for a total of 3 doses. This dosage was for 40–80 kg pigs; smaller pigs received a reduced dose based on their body weight. All 300 cases were clinically cured.[9] Purulent meningitis, schizophrenia, and acute bronchitis were also successfully treated with the modified *Ma Zi Ren Wan*: 1) The formula for purulent meningitis was composed of 10 g *Ma Zi Ren* (Cannabis), 6 g *Tao Ren* (Persica), 6 g *Xing Ren* (Armeniaca), 6 g *Da Huang* (Rheum), 10 g *Zhi Shi* (Aurantium), 9 g *Hou Po* (Magnolia), 10 g *Xuan Shen* (Scrophularia), 10 g *Sheng Di* (Rehmannia), 10 g *Mai Men Dong* (Hordeum), and 6 g *Ju Hua* (Chrysanthemum). 2) The formula for schizophrenia was composed of 15 g *Da Huang* (Rheum, decocted later), 30 *Sheng Long Gu* (Draconis, decocted first), 30 g *Sheng Mu Li* (Ostrea, decocted first), 12 g *Zhi Shi* (Aurantium), 12 g *Hou Po* (Magnolia), 15 g *Ma Zi Ren* (Cannabis), 10 g *Xing Ren* (Armeniaca), and 10 g *Tao Ren* (Persica). 3) The formula for acute bronchitis was composed of 10 g *Ma Zi Ren* (Cannabis), 10 g *Xing Ren* (Armeniaca), 10 g *Bai Shao* (Paeonia), 8 g *Da Huang* (Rheum, decocted later), 10 g *Zhi Shi* (Aurantium), 10 g *Hou Po* (Magnolia), 10 g *Chuan Mu Bei* (Fritillaria), and 20 g *Yu Xing Cao* (Houttuynia).[10]

Run Chang Wan (Moistening the Intestines) 润肠丸

Run means moistening. *Chang* is the intestines. *Wan* refers to pill, the original form of the herbal administration. Therefore, *Run Chang* means Moistening the Intestines.

Source: *Run Chang Wan* was recorded in *Pi Wei Lun* (*Discussion of Spleen and Stomach*), written by *Li Dongyuan* in 1249 CE

Ingredients: The ingredients are 15 g *Da Huang* (Rheum), 15 g *Dang Gui* (Angelica), 15 g *Qiang Huo* (Notopterygium), 30 g *Tao Ren* (Persica), and 38 g *Ma Zi Ren* (Cannabis).

Preparation:

1. Powder or capsule method: Herbs are ground into a fine powder. Powder can be encapsulated.
2. Decoction or teapill method: Raw herbs are mixed together and decocted. Herbal water extract (decoction) can be concentrated as granules or teapills.

Actions: Moisten the intestines, benefit defecation

Indications: This formula is indicated for constipation due to Heat with *Yin* Deficiency. The main signs include constipation or impaction, obesity, dry skin, dry and red tongue, and a fast pulse.

Dosage and Usage:

Horses and Cattle: 15–30 g, twice daily
Camels: 30–45 g, twice daily
Llamas, Alpacas, Goats, Sheep, and Pigs: 5–10 g, twice daily
Dogs: 0.5–5 g (or 0.1 g per kg body weight), twice daily
Cats and Rabbits: 0.2–0.5 g (or 0.1 g per kg body weight), twice daily
Birds: 0.05 g per kg body weight, twice daily

Use 1–4 weeks until primary clinical signs resolve.

Analysis of Formula: *Da Huang* (Rheum) is the King herb, which clears Heat and purges the intestines. Working as the Minister herbs, *Ma Zi Ren* (Cannabis) and *Dang Gui* (Angelica) moisten the intestines to promote defecation. *Zhi Ke* (Aurantium) and *Tao Ren* (Persica) are the Adjuvant and Messenger herbs that move *Qi* and Blood in order to relieve abdominal pain.

Cautions and Contraindications: Use cautiously in patients with Spleen *Qi* Deficiency

Dr. Xie's Comments: *Run Chang Wan* is useful for treating chronic constipation due to Excess Heat or *Yin* Deficiency in geriatric horses and dogs.

Wu Ren Wan (Five Seeds) 五仁丸

Wu means five. *Ren* is the seed. *Wan* refers to pill, the original form of the herbal administration. *Wu Ren* refers to the fact that the first five ingredients of the formula are seeds.

Source: *Wu Ren Wan* was recorded in *Shi Yi Xiao Fang* (*Effective Formulas from Generations of Physicians*), written by *Wei Yi-lin* in 1345 CE

Ingredients: The ingredients are 15 g *Tao Ren* (Persica), 30 g *Xing Ren* (Armeniaca), 4 g *Bai Zi Ren* (Biota), 3 g *Yu Li Ren* (Prunus), 3 g *Song Zi Ren* (Pinus), and 120 g *Chen Pi* (Citrus).

Preparation:

1. Five seeds (the first five ingredients) are ground into a powder and made into a paste, added and mixed with powdered *Chen Pi* (Citrus), and finally formed into small pills with honey.
2. Powder or capsule method: Herbs are ground into a fine powder. Powder can be encapsulated.
3. Decoction or teapill method: Raw herbs are mixed together and decocted. Herbal water extract (decoction) can be concentrated as granules or teapills.

Actions: Moisten the intestines, promote defecation

Indications: This formula is indicated for constipation due to intestinal Dryness caused by consumption of body fluids or Blood Deficiency. The main signs are chronic constipation, difficult defecation, dry and pale tongue, and a thin and weak pulse.

Dosage and Usage:

Horses and Cattle: 15–30 g, twice daily
Camels: 30–45 g, twice daily
Llamas, Alpacas, Goats, Sheep, and Pigs: 5–10 g, twice daily
Dogs: 0.5–5 g (or 0.1 g per kg body weight), twice daily
Cats and Rabbits: 0.2–0.5 g (or 0.1 g per kg body weight), twice daily
Birds: 0.05 g per kg body weight, twice daily
Use 1–4 weeks until primary clinical signs resolve.

Analysis of Formula: *Tao Ren* (Persica) and *Xing Ren* (Armeniaca) are the King herbs to lubricate the intestines and promote defecation. Working as the Minister herbs, *Bai Zi Ren* (Biota), *Yu Li Ren* (Prunus) and *Song Zi Ren* (Pinus) enhance the King herbs to moisten the intestines and benefit defecation. *Chen Pi* (Citrus) serves as the Adjuvant herb to move *Qi* to resolve Stagnation.

Cautions and Contraindications: Use cautiously in patients with Spleen *Qi* Deficiency

Dr. Xie's Comments: *Wu Ren San* moistens Interior Dryness to lubricate the intestines without purging Excess or Heat. Therefore, it is often used in treating constipation in elderly patients who do not have any Excess conditions.

Zeng Ye Cheng Qi Tang (Increasing Body Fluids for Purgative) 增液承气汤

Zeng means to increase. *Ye* refers to body fluids. *Cheng Qi* refers to purgative. *Tang* is decoction, the original form of the herbal administration. Literally *Zeng Ye Cheng Qi* can be translated as Increasing Body Fluids for Purgative.

Source: *Wen Bing Tiao Bian* (*Treatise on Differentiation and Treatment of Seasonal Febrile Diseases*), written by *Wu Ju-tong* and published in 1798 CE

Ingredients: The original formula for *Zeng Ye Cheng Qi Tang* (Table 32.4) is composed of 30 g *Xuan Shen* (Scrophularia), 25 g *Mai Men Dong* (Ophiopogon), 25 g *Sheng Di Huang* (Rehmannia), 9 g *Da Huang* (Rheum), and 5 g *Mang Xiao* (Mirabilite).

Preparation:

1. Herbs are ground into a fine powder and taken orally with water, or the first four ingredients are decocted

Table 32.4. Ingredients and actions of *Zeng Ye Cheng Qi Tang*.

%	English Name	Chinese *Pin-Yin*	Actions
31.9	Scrophularia	*Xuan Shen*	Nourish yin to lessen fire, cool Blood
26.6	Ophiopogon	*Mai Men Dong*	Moisturize the Lung and nourish *Yin*, benefit body fluid
26.6	Rehmannia	*Sheng Di Huang*	Cool Blood, nourish *Yin* and body fluid
9.6	Rheum	*Da Huang*	Purge the intestines to remove Food Stasis, clear Heat
5.3	Mirabilitum	*Mang Xiao*	Purge the Large Intestine, soften hard mass, clear Heat

in water; then *Mang Xiao* (Mirabilitum) is dissolved in the decoction after the residue is removed.
2. Powder or capsule method: Herbs are ground into a fine powder. Powder can be encapsulated.
3. Decoction or teapill method: Raw herbs are mixed together and decocted. Herbal water extract (decoction) can be concentrated as granules or teapills.

Actions: Nourish *Yin* to increase fluid, purge Heat and induce defecation

Indications: This formula is indicated for constipation due to accumulation of Heat and *Yin* Deficiency, which is marked by fever; constipation; abdominal distention and fullness; dry mouth and lips; a red tongue with a yellow coating; and a thready, rapid pulse. It can be modified to treat high fever with constipation from acute infectious diseases and dry stool, which is caused by retained Heat and impairment of *Yin* fluids with the chief symptom being constipation. It can also be used for the fluid-consuming constipation due to a chronic illness. The dosage of *Da Huang* (Rheum) and *Mang Xiao* (Mirabilite) should be lessened accordingly if the accumulated Heat is not so excessive.

Dosage and Usage:
Horses and Cattle: 15–30 g, twice daily
Camels: 30–45 g, twice daily
Llamas, Alpacas, Goats, Sheep, and Pigs: 5–10 g, twice daily
Dogs: 0.5–5 g (or 0.1 g per kg body weight), twice daily
Cats and Rabbits: 0.2–0.5 g (or 0.1 g per kg body weight), twice daily
Birds: 0.05 g per kg body weight, twice daily
Use 1–2 weeks until primary clinical signs resolve.

Analysis of Formula: This formula is used for constipation or impaction caused by accumulated Heat in the stomach, which burns body fluid and causes it to fail to moisten the intestines. This Pattern should be treated by relieving constipation by purgation and producing body fluid by nourishing *Yin*. *Xuan Shen* (Scrophularia) is the King herb, which acts to nourish *Yin* for production of body fluid and purge Heat for relieving constipation. *Mai Men Dong* (Ophiopogon) and *Sheng Di* Huang (Rehmannia) can enhance the effects of the King herb and function as the Minister herbs. *Da Huang* (Rheum) and *Mang Xiao* (Mirabilite) soften and moisten hard masses as Adjuvant herbs. All of the herbs combined can restore *Yin* fluid and eliminate hard masses in order to clear all symptoms.

Cautions and Contraindications: This formula should be applied with great caution to patients with Spleen *Qi* Deficiency.

Dr. Xie's Comments: I have used *Zeng Ye Cheng Qi Tang* for impaction, constipation, and megacolon due to *Yin* Deficiency with Heat in elderly or weak horses, cats, and dogs.

Clinical and Pharmacological Studies: In 2006, Niu and Yang reported that 86 cases of lingering hyperpyrexia were treated with *Zeng Ye Cheng Qi Tang* in animals, including dairy cows and cattle. The basic formula was composed of 30 g *Da Huang* (Rheum), 250 g *Mang Xiao* (Mirabilitum), 30 g *Zhi Shi* (Aurantium), 30 g *Hou Po* (Magnolia), 30 g *Xuan Shen* (Scrophularia), 30 g *Mai Men Dong* (Ophiopogon), and 30 g *Sheng Di Huang* (Rehmannia). The herbs were ground into a fine powder and taken orally with water. In cases of hyperpyrexia, the dosage of *Da Huang* (Rheum) was increased, and *Huang Lian* (Coptis), *Huang Qin* (Scutellaria), *Zhu Ye* (Bambusa), *Lu Gen* (Phragmites), *Jin Yin Hua* (Lonicera), *Lian Qiao* (Forsythia), and *Ban Lan Gen* (Isatis) were added to increase the action of relieving fever. In cases of abdominal distension, *Qing Pi* (Citrus), *Xiang Fu* (Cyperus), *Mu Xiang* (Saussurea), and *Lai Fu Zi* (Raphanus) were added to promote *Qi* circulation for the relief of abdominal fullness. In cases of night sweats, *Fu Xiao Mai* (Triticum), *Long Gu* (Draconis), and *Mu Li* (Ostrea) were added to regenerate body fluid. In cases of dry, small stools, *Dang Gui* (Angelica, fried), *Rou Cong Rong* (Cistanche, fried), *Fan Xie Ye* (Senna), and *Bing Lang* (Areca) were added to loosen bowels and relieve constipation. In cases with hematuria and pollakiuria, *Zhu Ling* (Polyporous), *Fu Ling* (Poria), *Ze Xie* (Alisma), and *Mu Tong* (Akebia) were added to eliminate dampness and benefit urination. 9 out of 86 cases showed no remarkable effects but the others were clinically cured, with a recovery rate of 89.5%.[11]

In 2004, Guo reported that 55 cases of refractory anorexia were treated with *Zeng Ye Cheng Qi Tang* in sows. The clinical manifestations were depression, poor or no appetite, exercise intolerance, excessive sleep, constipation, dry mouth, and normal or a slightly increased body temperature. The formula was composed of 20 g *Da Huang* (Rheum), 10 g *Hou Po* (Magnolia), 10 g *Zhi Ke* (Aurantium), 15 g *Mang Xiao* (Mirabilite), 20 g *Xuan Shen* (Scrophularia), 15 g *Mai Men Dong* (Ophiopogon), 15 g *Sheng Di Huang* (Rehmannia), 20 g *Dang Gui* (Angelica), 10 g *Ma Ren* (Hemp Fruit), and 10 g *Fan Xie Ye* (Senna). In cases of antepartum anorexia with constipation, *Mang Xiao* (Mirabilite) was substituted with *Huang Qin* (Scutellaria) and *Bai Zhu* (Atractylodes) to clear Heat and reduce fire to prevent miscarriage. In cases of postpartum anorexia with constipation, *Sheng Di Huang* (Rehmannia) was substituted with *Shu Di* (Rehmannia) and *Bai Shao* (Paeonia). In cases of *Qi* Deficiency and general weakness, *Huang Qi* (Astragalus), *Bai Zhu* (Atractylodes), and *Dang Shen* (Codonopsis) were added. In cases of refractory anorexia with constipation of the open sow postbreeding, *Zhi Ke* (Aurantium) was substituted with *Zhi Shi* (Aurantium) and *Da Huang* (Rheum). Herbs were decocted with water for oral dosing once a day. All of the cases were clinically cured, with 42 cases being clinically cured in only 1 dose. The remaining 13 cases were clinically cured in 2 doses.[12]

In 2007, Chen reported that 39 cases of severe acute pancreatitis (SAP) were treated with *Zeng Ye Cheng Qi Tang* combined with Western medicine. 76 cases of SAP were randomly divided into 39 cases in the herbal group and 37 cases in the control group. The control group was treated only with the conventional therapy of standard Western medicine, including antibiotics and pharmaceutical drugs to inhibit pancreatic and gastric acid secretion. The herbal group was treated with *Zeng Ye Cheng Qi Tang* combined with the standard Western medicine. The herbal formula was composed of 15 g *Xuan Shen* (Scrophularia), 20 g *Mai Men Dong* (Ophiopogon), 20 g *Da Huang* (Rheum), 20 g *Sheng Di Huang* (Rehmannia), 10 g *Hou Po* (Magnolia), and 20 g *Mang Xiao* (Mirabilite). Herbs were decocted with water for oral dosing, with 1 dose being administered 4 times daily via a gastric tube. In the herbal group, abdominal distension disappeared in 4 days and all other clinical signs disappeared within 10 days. The death rates in the herbal group were significantly less than that of the control group ($P < 0.05$).[13]

From 1998 to 2005, Chen treated type II diabetes with *Zeng Ye Cheng Qi Tang* combined with Western medicine. 120 Cases of type II diabetes, diagnosed with the diabetes standard procedure of the American Diabetes Association, were randomly divided between the herbal group and control group, respectively. The control group ($n = 60$) was treated with 5mg meibida, 3 times daily before meals, and 0.25 g melbine, 3 times daily with meals. The herbal group ($n = 60$) was treated with *Zeng Ye Cheng Qi Tang* combined with the above Western medicine. The formula was composed of 10 g *Da Huang* (Rheum), 3 g *Mang Xiao* (Mirabilite), 15 g *Sheng Di Huang* (Rehmannia), 10 g *Mai Men Dong* (Ophiopogon), 15 g *Xuan Shen* (Scrophularia), 12 g *Ze Xie* (Alisma), 15 g *Niu Xi* (Achyranthes), 15 g *Ge Gen* (Pueraria), 15 g *Tian Hua Fen* (Trichosanthes), 6 g *Huang Lian* (Coptis), 30 g *Huai Shan Yao* (Dioscorea), 10 g *Shan Zhu Yu* (Cornus), 15 g *Fu Ling* (Poria), and 15 g *Dan Shen* (Salvia). Herbs were decocted with water for oral dosing with 1 dose administered daily. A 2-month period of treatment ensued. At the same time, all patients were asked to adhere to a diabetic diet and exercise program. 47 cases of the herbal group showed significant improvement, and 11 cases were moderately improved. Compared with the herbal group, 31 cases of the control group were significantly improved and 18 cases were moderately improved. The herbal group was remarkably better than the control group ($P < 0.05$).[14]

Cheng Qi Yang Ying Tang (Purgative with Nourishing *Ying*) 承气养营汤

Cheng Qi refers to purgative. *Yang* here means nourishing or increasing. *Ying* refers to the deeper level of the Interior. *Tang* is decoction, the original form of herbal administration.

Source: *Cheng Qi Yang Ying Tang* was recorded in *Wen Yi Lun (Discussion of Epidemic Warm Diseases)*, written by *Wu You-xing* in 1642 CE

Ingredients: *Cheng Qi Yang Ying Tang* is composed of 9 g *Zhi Mu* (Anemarrhena), 6 g *Dang Gui* (Angelica), 12 g *Sheng Di Huang* (Rehmannia), 12 g *Da Huang* (Rheum), 9 g *Zhi Shi* (Aurantium), 9 g *Hou Po* (Magnolia), and 12 g *Bai Shao Yao* (Paeonia).

Preparation:

1. Powder or capsule method: Herbs are ground into a fine powder. Powder can be encapsulated.
2. Decoction or teapill method: Raw herbs are mixed together and decocted. Herbal water extract (decoction) can be concentrated as granules or teapills.

Actions: Nourish Blood and moisten the Interior, move *Qi* to relieve pain

Indications: This formula is indicated for constipation due to *Ying* and Blood Deficiency. The clinical signs are dehydration, dry skin, desiccated lips with fissure, dry throat, thirst, persistent general fever, constipation or impaction, abdominal distention and fullness, colic, pale and dry tongue, and a thin and weak pulse.

Dosage and Usage:

Horses and Cattle: 15–30 g, twice daily
Camels: 30–45 g, twice daily
Llamas, Alpacas, Goats, Sheep, and Pigs: 5–10 g, twice daily
Dogs: 0.5–5 g (or 0.1 g per kg body weight), twice daily
Cats and Rabbits: 0.2–0.5 g (or 0.1 g per kg body weight), twice daily
Birds: 0.05 g per kg body weight, twice daily

Use 1–4 weeks until primary clinical signs resolve.

Analysis of Formula: *Dang Gui* (Angelica) and *Sheng Di Huang* (Rehmannia) are the King herbs, which nourish Blood and moisten the Interior to release constipation. Working as the Minister herbs, *Zhi Mu* (Anemarrhena) and *Bai Shao Yao* (Paeonia) enhance the effects of the King herbs to nourish Blood and *Yin*. *Da Huang* (Rheum), *Zhi Shi* (Aurantium), and *Hou Po* (Magnolia) purge the large intestine, clear Heat, and move *Qi* to relieve pain.

Cautions and Contraindications: Contraindicated in cases with Spleen *Qi* Deficiency.

Dr. Xie's Comments: *Zeng Ye Cheng Qi Tang* and *Cheng Qi Yang Ying Tang* purge Heat, nourish *Yin*, moisten Dryness, and promote defecation. They are both used in treating constipation due to Interior Dryness. *Cheng Qi Yang Ying Tang* is made by adding *Xiao Cheng Qi Tang* to *Si Wu Tang* [*Dang Gui* (Angelica), *Chuan Xiong* (Ligusticum), *Bai Shao* (Paeonia), *and Sheng Di Huang* (Rehmannia)] and substituting *Chuan Xiong* (Ligusticum) with *Zhi Mu* (Anemarrhena). It is an herbal formula that combines a purgative with a Blood tonic; hence, it is often used in treating constipation or impaction due to Blood Deficiency. On the other hand, *Zeng Ye Cheng Qi Tang* is made by adding *Zeng Ye Tang* (*Xuan Shen* [Scrophularia], *Mai Men Dong* [Ophiopogon], and *Sheng Di Huang* [Rehmannia]) to *Tiao Wei Cheng Qi Tang*. Therefore, *Zeng Ye Cheng Qi Tang* is good at nourishing *Yin* to increase body fluid, and is often used for the treatment of constipation or impaction due to *Yin* Deficiency.

Ma Jia Wan (Cost of a Horse) 马价丸

Ma is horse. *Jia* refers to cost, or money. *Wan* is pill, the original form of herbal administration. *Ma Jia* can be translated literally as the Cost of a Horse. This formula got its name from the fact that it can save (cost) a life of a horse.

Source: *Yuan Heng Liao Ma Ji* (*Yuan-Heng's Therapeutic Treatise of Horses*), written by *Yu Ben-yuan* and *Yu Ben-heng* and published in 1608 CE

Ingredients: The original formula for *Ma Jia Wan* (Table 32.5) is composed of 20 g *Mu Xiang* (Saussurea), 20 g *Bing Lang* (Areca), 25 g *Qing Pi* (Citrus), 60 g *Da Huang* (Rheum), 120 g *Mang Xiao* (Mirabilite), 60 g *Qian Niu Zi* (Pharbitis), 30 g *San Leng* (Sparganium), 15 g *Mu Tong* (Akebia), and 30 g *Yu Li Ren* (Prunus).

Table 32.5. Ingredients and actions of *Ma Jia Wan*.

%	English Name	Chinese *Pin-Yin*	Actions
5.3	Saussurea	*Mu Xiang*	Promote *Qi* flow, regulate the Middle *Jiao* to relieve pain
5.3	Areca	*Bing Lang*	Promote *Qi* flow, remove food retention, benefit urination to alleviate water retention, expel parasites
6.6	Citrus	*Qing Pi*	Soothe the Liver *Qi* to Stagnation
15.8	Rheum	*Da Huang*	Purge the Large Intestine to remove Food Stasis, clear Heat and activate Blood
31.6	Mirabilitum	*Mang Xiao*	Purge the Large Intestine, soften hard mass, clear Heat
15.8	Pharbitis	*Qian Niu Zi*	Purge the Large Intestine, eliminate excessive fluid,
7.9	Sparganium	*San Leng*	Remove Blood Stasis, promote *Qi* flow to relieve pain
3.9	Akebia	*Mu Tong*	Promote diuresis, drain Damp-Heat
7.9	Prunus	*Yu Li Ren*	Loosen bowels to relieve constipation

Preparation:

1. Horses: Herbs are ground into a fine powder, 1 with hot water, and taken with a few segments of *Cong Bai* (Onion Bulb).
2. Powder or capsule method: Herbs are ground into a fine powder. Powder can be encapsulated.
3. Decoction or teapill method: Raw herbs are mixed together and decocted. Herbal water extract (decoction) can be concentrated as granules or teapills.

Actions: Clear Heat, loosen the bowels to remove food retention, promote *Qi* flow to stop colic

Indications: This formula is indicated for impaction or constipation of the equine colon. In cases of secondary abdominal distension, add *Lai Fu Zi* (Raphanus), *Hou Po* (Magnolia), and *Sha Ren* (Amomum) to regulate *Qi* and dissolve Stagnation. In cases of generalized *Qi*-Blood Deficiency typical of chronic disease, add *Dang Shen* (Codonopsis), *Dang Gui* (Angelica), *Gan Cao* (Glycyrrhiza), and *Da Zao* (Jujube) to tonify *Qi* and Blood. In cases of severe body fluid consumption typically seen in dehydrated patients, add *Xuan Shen* (Scrophularia), *Mai Men Dong* (Ophiopogon), and *Sheng Di Huang* (Rehmannia) to nourish *Yin* and to moisten Dryness.

Dosage and Usage:

Horses and Cattle: 15–30 g, twice daily
Camels: 30–45 g, twice daily
Llamas, Alpacas, Goats, Sheep, and Pigs: 5–10 g, twice daily
Dogs: 0.5–5 g (or 0.1 g per kg body weight), twice daily
Cats and Rabbits: 0.2–0.5 g (or 0.1 g per kg body weight), twice daily
Birds: 0.05 g per kg body weight, twice daily
Use 1–2 weeks until primary clinical signs resolve.

Analysis of Formula: Patterns that benefit from this formula are caused by *Qi* Stagnation and accumulated Heat in the gastrointestinal tract. Treat by promoting *Qi*, removing food retention, and expelling pathogenic Heat in order to loosen the bowels. *Da*

Huang (Rheum) and *Mang Xiao* (Mirabilite) are the King herbs used to purge Heat and promote bowel movement. *Qian Niu Zi* (Pharbitis) and *Bing Lang* (Areca) can help bring about the effects of the King herbs to purge the intestinal tract, and they function as the Minister herbs. *Mu Xiang* (Saussurea), *Qing Pi* (Citrus), and *San Leng* (Sparganium) have the functions of regulating *Qi* and activating Blood circulation, and they can help expel Food Stagnation and relieve pain. *Yu Li Ren* (Prunus) can lubricate the intestines. When used, *Cong Bai* (Onion Bulb) moves *Qi* and Blood to resolve Stagnation. All of them work together as the Adjuvant herbs. *Mu Tong* (Akebia), which promotes urination and leads all other herbs downward, is the Messenger herb. These herbals combined engage in the action of promoting *Qi*, removing food retention, and expelling pathogenic Heat to loosen the bowels.

Cautions and Contraindications: Because this formula has moderate actions and safely treats equine impaction or constipation, this formula is commonly used in the equine clinic.

Dr. Xie's Comments: I have used *Ma Jia Wan* for the treatment of impaction in horses. It can also be used in small animals and farm animals.

Clinical and Pharmacological Studies: In 2004, Wang studied the effects of *Ma Jia Wan* on gastrointestinal motility of the intestinal tract in mice. The formula *Ma Jia Wan* was composed of 4g *Da Huang* (Rheum), 5g *Mang Xiao* (Mirabilitum), 3g *Qian Niu Zi* (Pharbitis), 4g *Bing Lang* (Areca), 1.5g *Mu Xiang* (Saussurea), 1.5g *Qing Pi* (Citrus), 1g *San Leng* (Sparganium), 1ml *Bai Jiu* (white wine), 2g *Yu Li Ren* (Prunus), and 2g *Mu Tong* (Akebia). All herbs except *Da Huang* (Rheum) and *Mang Xiao* (Mirabilite) were decocted twice with water. The first decoction lasted 40 minutes, and the second boiled for 30 minutes. The two herbal water extracts were collected into a container; then *Da Huang* (Rheum) was put into the container and decocted again for 10 minutes. Continuing the process, *Mang Xiao* (Mirabilite), *Bai Jiu* (white wine), and 10ml of a 1% suspension of liquid activated charcoal (serving as the experimental marker) were added and mixed. The results showed that *Ma Jia Wan* could remarkably increase gastrointestinal motility.[15]

Wen Pi Tong Jie San (Warming the Spleen to Purge Stagnation) 温脾通结散

Wen refers to warm. *Pi* is the Spleen. *Tong* refers to purge. *Jie* is Stagnation. *San* is powder, the original form of herbal administration. Thus, *Wen Pi Tong Jie* means Warming the Spleen to Purge Stagnation.

Source: *Zhong Shou Yi Xue* (*Traditional Chinese Veterinary Medicine*), editor-in-chief *Yu Chuan*, and published in 1979.

Ingredients: The original formula for *Wen Pi Tong Jie San* (Table 32.6) is composed of 60g *Gan Jiang* (Zingiberis), 30g *Rou Gui* (Cinnamomum), 30g *Wu Zhu Yu* (Evodia), 30g *Wu Yao* (Lindera), 30g *Hou Po* (Magnolia), 30g *Chen Pi* (Citrus), 15g *Bing Lang* (Areca), 25g *Mu Xiang* (Saussurea), 30g *Cang Zhu* (Atractylodes), 30g *Cao Dou Kou* (Alpinia), 60g *Qian Niu Zi* (Pharbitis), 30g *Xu Sui Zi* (Euphorbia), and 30g *Da Huang* (Rheum).

Table 32.6. Ingredients and actions of *Wen Pi Tong Jie San*.

%	English Name	Chinese *Pin-Yin*	Actions
13.9	Zingiberis	*Gan Jiang*	Warm the Spleen and Stomach to dispel Cold
7.0	Cinnamomum	*Rou Gui*	Warm the Kidney and Spleen, eliminate Cold to stop pain
7.0	Evodia	*Wu Zhu Yu*	Eliminate Cold to stop pain, soothe the Liver *Qi*
7.0	Lindera	*Wu Yao*	Promote *Qi* flow to relieve pain, warm the Kidney to eliminate Cold
7.0	Magnolia	*Hou Po*	Promote *Qi* flow to stop pain, remove food retention
7.0	Citrus	*Chen Pi*	Regulate the Spleen-Stomach, transform Phlegm
3.4	Areca	*Bing Lang*	Promote *Qi* flow, remove food retention
5.8	Saussurea	*Mu Xiang*	Move *Qi* to stop colic, regulate the Spleen and Stomach
7.0	Atractylodes	*Cang Zhu*	Eliminate dampness, strengthen the Spleen
7.0	Alpinia	*Cao Dou Kou*	Eliminate dampness, warm the Spleen and Stomach
13.9	Pharbitis	*Qian Niu Zi*	Purge the Large Intestines, eliminate excessive fluid, remove food retention
7.0	Euphorbia	*Xu Sui Zi*	Eliminate excessive fluids to reduce swelling, move Blood to eliminate abdominal mass
7.0	Rheum	*Da Huang*	Purge the Large Intestine to resolve constipation, activate Blood to remove Stasis

Preparation:

1. Powder or capsule method: Herbs are ground into a fine powder. Powder can be encapsulated.
2. Decoction or teapill method: Raw herbs are mixed together and decocted. Herbal water extract (decoction) can be concentrated as granules or teapills.

Actions: Warm Spleen and Stomach to eliminate Cold, purge the Large Intestine and relieve constipation, and eliminate excessive fluid

Indications: This formula is indicated for retention of body fluids, Phlegm Stagnation in the Interior or constipation, purple tongue, deep or slow pulse.

Dosage and Usage:

Horses and Cattle: 15–30 g, twice daily
Camels: 30–45 g, twice daily
Llamas, Alpacas, Goats, Sheep, and Pigs: 5–10 g, twice daily
Dogs: 0.5–5 g (or 0.1 g per kg body weight), twice daily
Cats and Rabbits: 0.2–0.5 g (or 0.1 g per kg body weight), twice daily
Birds: 0.05 g per kg body weight, twice daily
Use 1–4 weeks until primary clinical signs resolve.

Analysis of Formula: Certain foods or environmental factors encourage chronic Cold-Damp to invade the body and damage the Spleen *Qi* and *Yang*, leading to retention of fluid in the Interior or Phlegm Stagnation in the body. *Gan Jiang* (Zingiberis), *Rou Gui* (Cinnamomum), and *Wu Zhu Yu* (Evodia) are used to warm and tonify Spleen *Yang* to dispel Cold and are therefore the King herbs. *Cao Dou Kou* (Alpinia), *Hou Po* (Magnolia), and *Cang Zhu* (Atractylodes) can warm the Spleen and Stomach and eliminate Dampness, thereby helping the King herbs to strengthen the Spleen and to dispel Cold. They act as the Minister herbs. *Qian Niu Zi* (Pharbitis), *Da Huang* (Rheum), *Xu Sui Zi* (Euphorbia), and *Bing Lang* (Areca) purge and eliminate excess fluid, and they act as the Adjuvant herbs. *Chen Pi* (Citrus), *Mu Xiang* (Saussurea), and *Wu Yao* (Lindera) promote *Qi* flow to harmonize the Middle *Jiao*, and they function as the Messenger herbs.

Cautions And Contraindications: Use cautiously in patients with Spleen *Qi* Deficiency

Dr. Xie's Comments: This herbal formula is useful for constipation or water retention due to Cold-Damp. It causes a drastic purgative effect in *Qi* deficient patients. In cases with *Qi* Deficiency, subtract *Qian Niu Zi* (Pharbitis), *Xu Sui Zi* (Euphorbia), *Da Huang* (Rheum), and *Bing Lang* (Areca), and add *Dang Shen* (Codonopsis), *Bai Zhu* (Atractylodes), *Shan Yao* (Dioscorea), and *Sha Ren* (Amomum) to strengthen Spleen and tonify *Qi*.

Dang Gui Cong Rong Tang (Angelica and Cistanche) 当归苁蓉汤

Dang Gui is Angelica, and *Cong Rong* is Cistanche. They are the King herbs of this formula. *Tang* is decoction, the original form of herbal administration. *Dang Gui Cong Rong Tang* literally means Angelica and Cistanche Decoction.

Source: *Zhong Shou Yi Zhi Liao Jin Yan (Volume 2)* (*Experienced Collection of Traditional Chinese Veterinary Medicine on Diagnosis and Treatment*), written by *Pei Yao-qing* and published in 1956.

Ingredients: The original formula for *Dang Gui Cong Rong Tang* (Table 32.7) is composed of 200 g *Dang Gui* (Angelica), 100 g *Rou Cong Rong* (Cistanche), 60 g *Fan Xie Ye* (Senna), 15 g *Mu Xiang* (Saussurea), 30 g *Hou Po* (Magnolia), 30 g *Zhi Ke* (Aurantium), 30 g *Xiang Fu* (Cyperus), 15 g *Qu Mai* (Dianthus), 10 g *Tong Cao* (Tetrapanax), and 30 g *Shen Qu* (Massa Fermentata).

Preparation:

1. Horses: Herbs are ground into a fine powder and taken orally with water and 250–500 g *Ma You* (Sesame Oil). Or decoct the above herbs in water with dosages in proportion to the original formula and mix the herbal water extract and 250–500 g *Mu You* (Sesame Oil).
2. Powder or capsule method: Herbs are ground into a fine powder. Powder can be encapsulated.

Table 32.7. Ingredients and actions of *Dang Gui Cong Rong Tang*.

%	English Name	Chinese *Pin-Yin*	Actions
38.5	Angelica	*Dang Gui*	Nourish Blood, activate Blood, moisturize the intestines
19.2	Cistanche	*Rou Cong Rong*	Reinforce the Kidney, loosen bowel to relieve constipation
11.5	Senna	*Fan Xie Ye*	Purge the Large Intestine to dredge Food Stasis
2.9	Saussurea	*Mu Xiang*	Move *Qi* to relieve pain
5.8	Magnolia	*Hou Po*	Move *Qi* to relieve pain, remove food retention
5.8	Aurantium	*Zhi Ke*	Promote *Qi* flow to alleviate Middle *Jiao*
5.8	Cyperus	*Xiang Fu*	Soothe the Liver *Qi* to relieve pain
2.9	Dianthus	*Qu Mai*	Promote diuresis to drain Damp-Heat
1.9	Tetrapanax	*Tong Cao*	Drain Damp-Heat
5.8	Massa Fermentata	*Shen Qu*	Promote digestion and regulate the Stomach

3. Decoction or teapill method: Raw herbs are mixed together and decocted. Herbal water extract (decoction) can be concentrated as granules or teapills.

Actions: Moisten the Dryness and purge the Large Intestine to remove Food Stasis, regulate *Qi* to stop pain

Indications: This formula is indicated for chronic constipation of frail, elderly, pregnant, or generally weak animals. In cases with severe *Qi* Deficiency, add *Huang Qi* (Astragalus); in pregnancy, substitute *Qu Mai* (Dianthus) and *Tong Cao* (Tetrapanax) with *Bai Shao Yao* (Paeonia).

Dosage and Usage:
Horses and Cattle: 15–30 g, twice daily
Camels: 30–45 g, twice daily
Llamas, Alpacas, Goats, Sheep, and Pigs: 5–10 g, twice daily
Dogs: 0.5–5 g (or 0.1 g per kg body weight), twice daily
Cats and Rabbits: 0.2–0.5 g (or 0.1 g per kg body weight), twice daily
Birds: 0.05 g per kg body weight, twice daily
Use 2–6 weeks until primary clinical signs resolve.

Analysis of Formula: Chronic constipation or impaction is caused by *Qi* Deficiency and Dryness of the intestines in older and weaker animals. Thus, it should be treated by moistening the Dryness, regulating *Qi* to loosen the bowels, and purging the bowels. *Dang Gui* (Angelica) can nourish Blood and moisten the intestines, and *Rou Cong Rong* (Cistanche) can tonify the Kidney and moisten the intestines. Together they are the King herbs. *Fan Xie Ye* (Senna) loosens the bowels, and *Ma You* (Sesame Oil) moistens the intestines. They act as the Minister herbs. *Mu Xiang* (Saussurea), *Xiang Fu* (Cyperus), *Hou Po* (Magnolia), *Zhi Ke* (Aurantium), and *Shen Qu* (Massa Fermentata) promote *Qi* to remove food retention and help the King herbs to regulate *Qi* to loosen the bowels. *Qu Mai* (Dianthus) and *Tong Cao* (Tetrapanax) can drain Heat. As a group, these last seven herbs function as Adjuvant herbs.

Cautions and Contraindications: None known

Dr. Xie's Comments: I have used *Dang Gui Cong Rong Tang* for the treatment of chronic constipation in geriatric cats, dogs, and horses with a great success. It is safe to use during pregnancy.

Clinical and Pharmacological Studies: In 1998, Xue reported that 300 cases of disease of the proventriculus were treated with *Dang Gui Cong Rong Tang* in cattle. The basic formula was composed of 125–250 g *Dang Gui* (Angelica), 60–120 g *Rou Cong Rong* (Cistanche), 30–60 g *Fan Xie Ye* (Senna), 40 g *Mu Xiang* (Saussurea), 40 g *Hou Po* (Magnolia), 30–60 g *Zhi Ke* (Aurantium), 30–60 g *Xiang Fu* (Cyperus), 40 g *Qu Mai* (Dianthus), 30–60 g *Shen Qu* (Massa Fermentata), 40 g *Tong Cao* (Tetrapanax), 60 g *Ma Zi Ren* (Cannabis), 60 g *Qian Niu Zi* (Pharbitis), and 500 ml *Ma You* (Sesame Oil). In cases of chronic ruminal impaction, *San Leng* (Sparganium) and *E Zhu* (Zedoaria) were added. In cases of ruminal atony, *Bing Lang* (Areca) was added. In cases of ruminal atony with weak patients and a wet and pale tongue, *Cang Zhu* (Atractylodes), *Rou Dou Kou* (Myristica), and *Ban Xia* (Pinellia) were added. In cases of ruminal atony with loose and watery stool, *Fu Ling* (Poria), *Bai Zhu* (Atractylodes), *Qing Pi* (Citrus), and *Mu Tong* (Akebia) were substituted for *Ma Zi Ren* (Cannabis) and *Ma You* (Sesame Oil). In cases of ruminal atony with mucus and bleeding stool, *Huang Qin* (Scutellaria) and *Huang Bai* (Phellodendron) were added. In cases with too much saliva, *Cang Zhu* (Atractylodes) and *Cao Dou Kou* (Alpinia) were added. In cases with general Spleen *Qi* Deficiency, *Bai Zhu* (Atractylodes), *Fu Ling* (Poria), *Qing Pi* (Citrus), *Dang Shen* (Codonopsis), and *Huang Qi* (Astragalus) were added. 95% of patients had a positive response.[16]

Wang reported that 45 cases of abomasal blockage were treated with modified *Dang Gui Cong Rong Tang* in cattle. The formula was composed of 200–300 g *Dang Gui* (Angelica), 120–200 g *Rou Cong Rong* (Cistanche), 50–100 g *Fan Xie Ye* (Senna), 20–30 g *Mu Xiang* (Saussurea), 100–200 g *Zhi Ke* (Aurantium), 100–200 g *Jin Yin Hua* (Lonicera), 20–30 g *Qu Mai* (Dianthus), 20–30 g *Tong Cao* (Tetrapanax), 60–100 g *Lai Fu Zi* (Raphanus), 60–100 g *Hou Po* (Magnolia), 60–100 g *Xiang Fu* (Cyperus), and 1000–2000 ml *Ma You* (Sesame Oil). First, gastric lavage was performed to reduce endogastric strain before the herbs were administered via a gastric tube. 38 out of 45 cases were clinically cured.[17]

Wen Pi Tang (Warming the Spleen) 温脾汤

Wen refers to warm. *Pi* is the Spleen. *Tang* is decoction, the original form of herbal administration. *Wen Pi Tang* translates directly to Warming the Spleen Decoction.

Source: *Qian Jin Yao Fang* (Thousand Ducat Formulas), written by *Sun Si-miao* and published in 652 CE

Ingredients: The original formula for *Wen Pi Tang* (Table 32.8) is composed of 12 g *Da Huang* (Rheum), 9 g *Fu Zi* (Aconite), 6 g *Gan Jiang* (Zingiberis), 9 g *Ren Shen* (Ginseng), and 3 g *Gan Cao* (Glycyrrhiza).

Preparation:
1. Powder or capsule method: Herbs are ground into a fine powder. Powder can be encapsulated.

Table 32.8. Ingredients and actions of *Wen Pi Tang*.

%	English Name	Chinese *Pin-Yin*	Actions
30.8	Rheum (decocted later)	*Da Huang*	Purge the Large Intestine to remove Food Stasis, clear Heat and activate Blood
23.1	Aconite (Prepared)	*Fu Zi*	Warm and tonify the Kidney *Yang*, dispel Cold to stop pain
15.3	Zingiberis	*Gan Jiang*	Warm the Spleen *Yang* to dispel Cold in the Middle *Jiao*
23.1	Ginseng	*Ren Shen*	Tonify *Qi*
7.7	Glycyrrhiza	*Gan Cao*	Mediate the properties of other herbs

2. Decoction or teapill method: Raw herbs are mixed together and decocted. Herbal water extract (decoction) can be concentrated as granules or teapills.

Actions: Tonify the Spleen to warm *Yang*, purge accumulation of pathogenic Cold

Indications: This formula is indicated for Spleen *Yang* Deficiency with accumulation and Stagnation of Internal Cold, which is marked by constipation, chronic dysentery, abdominal pain, chilly limbs, and deep pulse—all typical of the accumulation of pathogenic Cold. This formula is a derivative of *Da Huang Fu Zi Tang*, made by subtracting *Xi Xin* (Asarum) and adding *Gan Jiang* (Zingiberis), *Ren Shen* (Ginseng), and *Gan Cao* (Glycyrrhiza). *Da Huang Fu Zi Tang* was originally formulated by Zhang Zhong-Jing in his text *Jin Gui Yao Lue Fang Lun* (*Synopsis of Prescriptions from the Golden Cabinet*) published in 220 AD. Clinically, it is utilized more for the accumulation of pathogenic Cold without *Qi* Deficiency. *Wen Pi Tang* is also similar to *Si Ni Tang* (also from *Jin Gui Yao Lue Fang Lun*); *Ren Shen* (Ginseng) and *Da Huang* (Rheum) are added to *Si Ni Tang* to make *Wen Pi Tang*. *Si Ni Tang* tonifies *Yang* for resuscitation. *Wen Pi Tang* is a warm purgation and also treats lingering dysentery with *Qi* Deficiency.

Dosage and Usage:

Horses and Cattle: 15–30 g, twice daily
Camels: 30–45 g, twice daily
Llamas, Alpacas, Goats, Sheep, and Pigs: 5–10 g, twice daily
Dogs: 0.5–5 g (or 0.1 g per kg body weight), twice daily
Cats and Rabbits: 0.2–0.5 g (or 0.1 g per kg body weight), twice daily
Birds: 0.05 g per kg body weight, twice daily

Use 1–4 weeks until primary clinical signs resolve.

Analysis of Formula: *Yang* Deficiency and Cold leading to an accumulation of Food Stagnation in the Middle Burner. If treated only by tonifying and warming the Spleen *Yang*, the inner pathogenic Cold may be eliminated, but the Food Stagnation will not be removed. Conversely, if only purgation is used as a method of treatment, Spleen *Yang* would be harmed and the accumulation of pathogenic Cold would not removed. So, successful treatment must tonify and warm the Spleen *Yang* and purge the accumulation of pathogenic Cold. In the formula, *Fu Zi* (Aconite) and *Gan Jiang* (Zingiberis) warm *Yang* in order to dispel Cold and also serve as the King herbs. *Ren Shen* (Ginseng) tonifies *Qi* and strengthens the Spleen, and it functions as the Minister herb. *Da Huang* (Rheum) clears accumulation, balances the hot nature of *Fu Zi*, and works as the Adjuvant herb. *Gan Cao* (Glycyrrhiza) harmonizes all other herbs and serves as the Messenger herb. The combination of these herbs works synergistically to dispel the pathogenic Cold, dissipate accumulation of food, and help tonify Spleen *Yang*.

Cautions and Contraindications: This formula should be used with great caution in patients with *Yin* Deficiency or excessive Heat.

Dr. Xie's Comments: *Wen Pi Tang* is useful for the treatment of Food Stagnation due to Cold accumulation secondary to Spleen *Yang* Deficiency.

Clinical and Pharmacological Studies: In 2007, Zhao reported that 29 cases of chronic renal insufficiency were treated with *Wen Pi Tang*. The formula was composed of 5–10 g *Ren Shen* (Ginseng), 10 g *Fu Zi* (Aconite, decocted first), 6 g *Gan Jiang* (Zingiberis), 5–10 g *Da Huang* (Rheum), 10 g *Mu Gua* (Chaenomeles), 30 g *Ren Shen* (Ginseng), 10 g *Chuan Xiong* (Ligusticum), and 20–30 g *Ze Lan* (Lycopus). Herbs were decocted with water for oral dosing, and administered once daily. After 3 months of treatment, 11 of 29 cases showed significant improvement (creatinine was decreased by more than 50 μmol/L, and blood urea nitrogen was decreased by more than 5 mmol/L). 16 cases showed a positive effect (creatinine was decreased by more than 10–50 μmol/L, and blood urea nitrogen was decreased by more than 1–5 mmol/L). Overall, 93.1% of patients responded well to treatment.[18]

In 2001, Jiang reported that 60 cases of chronic nonspecific colitis were treated with Modified *Wen Pi Tang*. The formula was composed of 5–10 g *Ren Shen* (Ginseng), 12 g *Fu Zi* (Aconite, decocted first), 12 g *Gan Jiang* (Zingiberis), 9 g *Rou Gui* (Cinnamomum), 9 g *Mu Xiang* (Saussurea), *Bing Lang* (Areca), 6 g *Hou Po* (Magnolia), *Bai Zhu* (Atractylodes), *Bai Shao* (Paeonia), 6 g *Gan Cao* (Glycyrrhiza), 20 g *Huang Qi* (Astragalus), and 12 g *Da Huang* (Rheum, decocted first). In cases of severe Damp-Heat, 15 g *Bai Jiang Cao* (Patrinia) and 20 g *Bai Tou Wong* (Pulsatilla) were added. In cases of remarkable *Qi-Yin* Deficiency, *Huang Qi* (Astragalus) was increased to 30 g and 15 g of *Shi Hu* (Dendobium) was added. In cases of excessive Liver overcontrolling the Spleen, 8 g *Chai hu* (Bupleurum) and 8 g *Chen Pi* (Citrus) were added. In cases of insufficiency of Spleen-*Yang*, 9 g *Wei Ge Gen* (Pueraria, roasted) and 9 g *Qiang Huo* (Notopterygium) were added. At the same time, another 60 cases of chronic nonspecific colitis were used as the control group. They were treated with 1 g Azosulfasalazine tablets, taken orally 4 times daily, 10mg prednisone tablets, taken orally 3 times daily, 0.5 g pipemidic acid tablets, taken orally 3 times daily, and 0.4 g metronidazole tablets, taken orally 3 times daily. After the pathogenic condition was stabilized, 0.5 g azosulfasalazine tablets were taken orally twice daily. After 1 month of herbal treatment, 25 of 60 cases from the herbal group were clinically cured (clinical symptoms and signs disappeared, the results of fecal tests were all normal, and the results of the colonoscopy and radiographs were also normal), and 30 cases were improved (clinical symptoms and signs disappeared partially or the chief symptoms were improved, fecal tests were normal, and results of colonoscopy were improved). After 1 month of conventional treatment, 15 of 60 cases from the control group were clinically cured, and 31 cases were improved. The results from the herbal group were remarkably better than the control group ($P < 0.05$).[19]

The effects of *Wen Pi Tang* were evaluated in vitro. Glomerular mesangial cells were divided and cultured successfully in vitro. LPS was used to induce proliferation of mesangial cells. Changes in mesangial cell proliferation and cell cycle were detected. The results were that mesangial cells showed a proliferation trend after stimulation by LPS in different concentrations, and cells in LPS group 3 (1 μg/m1) had the strongest trend. After adding both *Wen Pi Tang* pharmacologic serum in high concentration and LPS into the medium, a significant inhibitory function on the proliferation of mesangial cells was noted. Further research showed that the percent of cells in the Gl cycle was increased, and the percent of cells in the S cycle was decreased. The results showed that *Wen Pi Tang* pharmacologic serum can partially inhibit the proliferation of mesangial cells induced by LPS.[20]

Another study focused on the influence of different decocting processes on the content of aconitine from *Fu Zi* (Aconite), one ingredient of *Wen Pi Tang*. Using the *Wen Pi Tang* as a base formula, different prescriptions were made and different decocting processes were adopted. Then the content of aconitine was determined with UV-spectrophotometry. The results were that combining *Fu Zi* (Aconite) with *Gan Jiang* (Zingiberis) can increase the content of aconitine; combining Aconite with *Da Huang* (Rheum) and *Gan Cao* (Glycyrrhiza) can decrease the content of aconitine; and combining Aconite with *Ren Shen* (Ginseng) had no remarkable influence on the content of aconitine. The results showed that *Da Huang* (Rheum) and *Gan Cao* (Glycyrrhiza) can decrease the toxicity of Aconite in *Wen Pi Tang*, and *Gan Jiang* (Zingiberis) can promote the effect of Aconite to warm the interior in *Wen Pi Tang*.[21]

Shi Zao Tang (Ten Jujube Decoction) 十枣汤

Shi is ten. *Zao* refers to *Da Zao*, or jujube (dates). *Tang* is decoction, the original form of the herbal administration. *Shi Zao Tang* translates to Ten Jujube Decoction.

Source: *Shang Han Lun* (*Treatise on Exogenous Febrile Diseases*), written by *Zhang Zhong-jing* in 220 CE

Ingredients: The original formula for *Shi Zao Tang* (Table 32.9) is composed of 0.3 g *Yuan Hua* (Genkwa), 0.3 g *Gan Sui* (Euphorbia), 0.3 g *Da Ji* (Euphorbia), and 10 pieces of *Da Zao* (Jujube).

Preparation:

1. 10 pieces of *Da Zao* (Jujube) are decocted with water to obtain water extract. Remaining herbs are ground into a fine powder or encapsulated and are taken orally with the jujube water extract each time, once daily, in the morning, on an empty stomach.
2. Powder or capsule method: Herbs are ground into a fine powder. Powder can be encapsulated.
3. Decoction or teapill method: Raw herbs are mixed together and decocted. Herbal water extract (decoction) can be concentrated as granules or teapills.

Actions: Drastic purgation of the Large Intestine for eliminating retention of fluid in the body

Indications: This formula is indicated for 1) *Xuan Yin* (retention of fluid in the thoracic cavity), marked by cough with thoracic and cranial abdominal pain, fullness and splinting of the anterior abdomen, vomiting,

Table 32.9. Ingredients and actions of *Shi Zao Tang*.

%	English Name	Chinese *Pin-Yin*	Actions
33.3	Genkwa	*Yuan Hua*	Purge water retention in the body, expel parasites
33.3	Euphorbia	*Gan Sui*	Eliminate excessive fluid and reduce swelling
33.3	Euphorbia	*Da Ji*	Purge the retained fluids in the body
10 pieces	Jujube	*Da Zao*	Tonify the Spleen and Stomach, coordinate the other herbs' actions

dyspnea and tachypnea, signs of head pain, loss of balance or disorientation, wet pale or purple tongue, and a deep or wiry pulse; 2) *Shi Shui* (substantial edema), marked by severe edema, particularly in the distal extremities, ascites, dyspnea, dysuria, and constipation. This formula is used to treat pleural effusion, edema secondary to renal failure, and excessive fluid retention in a strong body condition or a strong constitution. In case of a weak patient with edema or retention of fluids, *Shi Zao Tang* must be combined with Spleen *Qi* tonic such as *Shen Ling Bai Zhu San* or *Si Jun Zi Tang*.

Dosage and Usage:

Horses and Cattle: 5–10 g, twice daily
Camels: 10–20 g, twice daily
Llamas, Alpacas, Goats, Sheep, and Pigs: 1–5 g, twice daily
Dogs: 0.1–1 g, twice daily
Cats and Rabbits: 0.05–0.1 g , twice daily
Birds: 0.05 g, twice daily

Use 2–5 days until primary clinical signs resolve.

Analysis of Formula: When excessive fluid is retained in the Interior, treatment must include elimination of retained fluid by purgation. *Yuan Hua* (Genkwa) can remove fluid and Phlegm from the chest and anterior abdomen, *Gan Sui* (Euphorbia) excels in eliminating retention of fluid and Dampness from the meridians, and *Da Ji* (Euphorbia) is good at eliminating Damp and Phlegm from the *Zang-Fu* organs, particularly the Intestines and Stomach. These three ingredients have their respective advantages and, when combined, can enhance the effect of eliminating retained fluid and relieving edema and fullness. However, they are drastic and toxic in nature and may impair *Zheng Qi*. *Da Zao* (Jujube) is therefore used to reinforce the Spleen and Stomach to reduce the toxic and drastic properties of these herbs. Together they can achieve the desired purgative result without damaging the Zheng *Qi*.

Cautions and Contraindications: Contraindicated for pregnant animals due to its drastic efficacy.

Dr. Xie's Comments: *Shi Zao Tang* is useful for the treatment of severe ascites in dogs.

Clinical and Pharmacological Studies: A modified *Shi Zao Tang* was used in 38 cases of viral pneumonia in children. The formula was composed of equal proportions of *Da Ji* (Euphorbia), *Gan Sui* (Euphorbia), and *Yuan Hua* (Genkwa). The herbs were decocted with vinegar for 10–15 minutes, open-air dried, and ground into a fine powder or encapsulated for storage. The dosage of powdered herbs was 0.75 g for children 0.5–1 year old, 1 g for 1–1.5 years old, 1.5 g for 1.5–3 years old, and 1.5–2.0 g for children over 4 years old. Additionally, 10 *Da Zao* (Jujubes) were decocted with water, which yielded about 50 ml water extract. The powder (or capsules) was taken orally with the *Da Zao* water extract, once daily for 2 days. At the same time in the control group, another 30 cases of viral pneumonia in children were treated with 15 mg/kg body weight/day ribovirin (intravenously). In more severe cases, or if there was a poor response to treatment, a compound formula of *folium isatidis* for intramuscular injection was added, or *Radix Isatidis* granules were taken orally. The results indicated that *Shi Zao Tang* remarkably reduced all clinical signs and induced a more significant positive result when compared with the ribovirin group ($P < 0.01$).[22]

In 2007, Li reported on the treatment of 30 cases of hepatic cirrhosis and ascites with modified *Shi Zao Tang*. 21 cases were male and 9 cases were female. The youngest was 45 years old and the oldest was 73 years old, with the courses of disease ranging from 1–8 years. 12 cases presented with recurrent ascites, 24 cases were caused by a previous hepatitis B infection, 5 cases were alcoholic cirrhosis ascites, and 1 case was blood fluke cirrhosis ascites. The basic formula was composed of 60 g *Zhi Huang Qi* (honey-fried Astragalus), 60 g *Sheng Bai Zhu* (Raw Atractylodes), 9 g *Gan Sui* (Euphorbia), 9 g *Da Ji* (Euphorbia), 9 g *Yuan Hua* (Genkwa), 10 g *Da Zao* (Jujube), 9 g *Chen Pi* (Citrus), and 30 g *Yi Yi Ren* (Coix). In cases with severe jaundice, *Yin Chen Hao* (Artemisia) and *Jin Qian Cao* (Lysimachia) were added. In cases with excess ascites, *Fu Shui Cao* (veronicastrum herb), *Qian Niu Zi* (Pharbitis), and *Chen Hu Lu* (Lagenaria) were added. In cases with hemorrhagic tendencies, *Xian He Cao* (Agrimony) and *Ce Bai Tan* (Biota) were added. Herbs were decocted twice daily with water for oral dosing. The period of treatment was 70 days. At the same time, patients were asked to observe bed rest; maintain a low salt and low protein diet; and refrain from smoking, drinking alcohol, and eating fatty or spicy food. 7 out of 30 cases were clinically cured (ascites disappeared and general conditions were good), and 15 cases were significantly improved (ascites was reduced by more than 50%).[23]

From 2000 to 2005, Lu treated 52 cases of hydrothorax with *Shi Zao Tang*. 38 cases were male and 14 cases were female, the oldest being 69 years old and the youngest being 16 years old. The average age was 41.5 years old. The longest period of disease was 90 days and the shortest was 7 days. All of them were diagnosed by thoracic radiographs and type-B ultrasound. 39 cases were exudative pleurisy and hydrothorax, 10 cases were pleurisy with tuberculum and hydrothorax, 1 case was lung cancer with hydrothorax, and 3 cases were encapsulated effusion. Most patients had clinical manifestations of dyspnea, chest pain, cough with shortness of breath, restlessness, fever, and irritability. Chest pain was more severe with coughing. Dyspnea was worse when inhaling. The formula was composed of equivalent portions of *Gan Sui* (Euphorbia), *Da Ji* (Euphorbia), and *Yuan Hua* (Genkwa). The dose for strong patients was 3 g, and the dose for the weak patients was 2 g each time. The formula was given orally once daily in the morning, on an empty stomach, with a decoction of 10 pieces of *Da Zao* (Jujubes). In cases of weak patients, this formula and *Gui Pi Wan* were used alternately. Each period of treatment was 2 days, which was based on the dose and elimination of hydrothorax. Treatment was discontinued as soon as the hydrothorax resolved. After 2–5 periods of treatment, 40 out of 52 cases were clinically cured (clinical symptoms, such as cough, chest pain, etc., were in complete remission, and hydrothorax, detected by thoracic radiographs and type-B ultrasound, was completely resolved), and 7 cases showed improvement (the symptoms lessened remarkably and the hydrothorax was reduced, but it did not completely disappear).[24]

In 1994, Han reported three methods of clinical use of *Shi Zao Tang*: 1) *Gan Sui* (Euphorbia), *Da Ji* (Euphorbia), and *Yuan Hua* (Genkwa) are ground and mixed into a fine powder. 15 pieces of *Da Zao* (Jujube) are decocted with water, resulting in about 300 ml of water extract. Half of the jujube water extract is taken to protect Stomach *Qi*. Then the mixed herbal powder is taken with the other half of the jujube water extract 10 minutes later. The actions of this herbal medication for purgation and elimination of excess fluid are potent; thus, it is indicated only for thoracic fluid retention in strong patients. It is important that it is used carefully. 2) 15 pieces of *Da Zao* (Jujube) are first steamed and mashed. Equivalent portions of *Gan Sui* (Euphorbia), *Da Ji* (Euphorbia), and *Yuan Hua* (Genkwa) are ground and mixed into a fine powder and made into pills with the mashed jujube. Then another 15 pieces of *Da Zao* (Jujube) are decocted with water; the pills are taken with this water extract. This method has a less intense effect and can be used 2–5 times. 3) First, 1 piece of *Da Zao* (Jujube) is decocted with water to obtain about 200 ml of water extract. Equivalent amounts of *Gan Sui* (Euphorbia), *Da Ji* (Euphorbia), and *Yuan Hua* (Genkwa) are ground into a fine powder and mixed with the jujube water extract. This is taken orally on an empty stomach in the morning. This method has the most potent actions for purgation and eliminating excess fluid. Thus, it has more adverse effects and can be used only 1 or 2 times, with great caution.[25]

Kong Xian Dan (Controlling Salivation) 控涎丹

Kong means controlling. *Xian* is salivation or mucus. *Dan* refers to pill, the form of the herbal administration. Thus, *Kong Xian* means Controlling Salivation.

Source: *San Yin Ji Yi Bing Zheng Fang Lun* (*Treatise on Three Categories of Pathogenic Factors in Disease*), written by *Chen Yan* and published in 1174 CE 三阴极一病症方论

Ingredients: *Kong Xian Dan* is composed of 12 g of *Gan Sui* (Euphorbia), *Da Ji* (Euphorbia), and *Bai Jie Zi* (Sinapsis). It is made by eliminating *Yuan Hua* (Genkwa) and *Da Zao* (Jujube) from *Shi Zao Tang* and adding *Bai Jie Zi* (Sinapsis).

Preparation:
1. Powder or capsule method: Herbs are ground into a fine powder. Powder can be encapsulated.
2. Decoction or teapill method: Raw herbs are mixed together and decocted. Herbal water extract (decoction) can be concentrated as granules or teapills.

Actions: Eliminate Phlegm and expel congested fluids

Indications: This formula is indicated for the accumulation of Phlegm and congested fluids in the chest. The main clinical signs are pain of the chest, back, neck, lumbar area, and hips; referred pain of bones and muscles; shifting lameness or pain; paresis of limbs; signs of marked head pain such as head-pressing or shaking, or restricted movement of the head and neck; coma and drowsiness; hypersalivation; wheezing with copious saliva in the throat and larynx; greasy coating of the tongue; and a slippery or weak pulse.

Dosage and Usage:
Horses and Cattle: 15–30 g, twice daily
Camels: 30–45 g, twice daily
Llamas, Alpacas, Goats, Sheep, and Pigs: 5–10 g, twice daily
Dogs: 0.5–5 g (or 0.1 g per kg body weight), twice daily
Cats and Rabbits: 0.2–0.5 g (or 0.1 g per kg body weight), twice daily
Birds: 0.05 g per kg body weight, twice daily
Use 2–5 days until primary clinical signs resolve.

Analysis of Formula: Working as the King herb, *Gan Sui* (Euphorbia) eliminates retention of fluid and Dampness to expel Phlegm. *Da Ji* (Euphorbia) is the Minister herb, which eliminates Damp and Phlegm from the *Zang-Fu* organs, intestines, and Stomach. Working as the Adjuvant and Messenger herb, *Bai Jie Zi* (Sinapsis) is good for dispelling Phlegm and sputum between the chest and diaphragm.

Cautions and Contraindications: Use cautiously in patients with a weak constitution and in pregnancy

Dr. Xie's Comments: *Kong Xian Dan* and *Shi Zao Tang* are both drastic and toxic in nature and may impair

Zheng Qi. Therefore, they are used only for a short period. *Kong Xian Dan* is good at resolving congested fluids in the chest, and *Shi Zao Tang* is often used in treating both ascites and pleural effusions

Fan Xie Ye San (Senna) 番泻叶散

Fan Xie Ye is Senna, the only ingredient of this formula.

Source: *Chinese Veterinary Herbal Handbook*, written by *Dr. Hui-sheng Xie* and published and distributed by the Chi Institute of Chinese Medicine in 2002

Ingredients: *Fan Xie Ye San* is composed of the single herb *Fan Xie Ye* Senna (Table 32.10).

Preparation:

1. Powder or capsule method: Herbs are ground into a fine powder. Powder can be encapsulated.
2. Decoction or teapill method: Raw herbs are mixed together and decocted. Herbal water extract (decoction) can be concentrated as granules or teapills.

Actions: Purge Large Intestine, resolve Food Stasis

Indications: Food Stagnation in the Large Intestine. The main signs are abdominal fullness, focal distention, colic, impaction, constipation, red or pale tongue, and strong or weak pulse.

Dosage and Usage:

Horses and Cattle: 15–30g, twice daily
Camels: 30–45g, twice daily
Llamas, Alpacas, Goats, Sheep, and Pigs: 5–10g, twice daily
Dogs: 0.5–5g (or 0.1g per kg body weight), twice daily
Cats and Rabbits: 0.2–0.5g (or 0.1g per kg body weight), twice daily
Birds: 0.05g per kg body weight, twice daily
Use 4–8 weeks until primary clinical signs resolve.

Analysis of Formula: *Fan Xie Ye San* is used for the Food Stasis accumulated in the gastrointestinal tract. The only ingredient of this formula, *Fan Xie Ye* (Senna), can purge the Large Intestine, to resolve food stasis.

Table 32.10. Ingredients and actions of *Fan Xie Ye San*.

English Name	Chinese *Pin-Yin*	Actions
Senna	*Fan Xie Ye*	Purge the Large Intestines and eliminate dyspeptic disease

Cautions and Contraindications: Caution with Spleen *Qi* Deficiency.

Dr. Xie's Comments: *Fan Xie Ye San* is effective for chronic constipation in dogs and megacolon in cats.

Clinical and Pharmacological Studies: In 2002, Wang reported that 3 cases of constipation in animals (2 pigs and 1 dog), due to accumulation of Heat, were treated with *Fan Xie Ye* (Senna).[26]

Case one: A pig of 50kg was ill for 8 days and was treated with penicillin and aminopyrine. The fever broke, but the patient still had symptoms of abdominal distention and constipation. The pig's stool was small and hard. Its body temperature was 38.5°C. 10g *Fan Xie Ye* (Senna) was soaked, boiled with 300ml of water, cooled, and then administered orally twice daily (in the morning and evening). After 3 days of treatment, the pig was cured clinically.

Case two: 12 piglets of 15–20kg were vaccinated with the hog cholera vaccine and were ill later. At first, the body temperatures ranged from 40.5–41.6°C, but after treatments with penicillin, gentamicin, and analgin, the temperatures normalized. However, 8 piglets displayed significant distention of the abdomen, constipation, depression, and polydipsia. Their stool was very hard and small. 30ml of vegetable oil was mixed with a little water and this was given via a gastric tube to each piglet. Then, 6g *Fan Xie Ye* (Senna) was soaked and boiled with 1000ml of water and taken orally twice daily after cooling. After 3 days of herbal treatment, all 8 piglets had normal bowel movements and stool.

Case three: A 3kg dog had chronic constipation and anorexia. Sometimes the dog had to be seen at the clinic for manual removal of stool. The body temperature and other parameters were normal. 1g *Fan Xie Ye* (Senna) was soaked and boiled with 200ml of water, and the herbal water extract was taken orally twice daily (in the morning and evening) after cooling. After 2 days of treatment, the dog had a normal stool and bowel movement.

REFERENCES

1. Wang JQ, Zhou XY, Yang WQ. Research on *Da Cheng Qi Tang* protecting cerebral hemorrhage brain tissue. Modem Rehabilitation 2001;5(9):47–48. (In Chinese)
2. Meng ZJ, Wang JG, Liu P. 23 cases of omasum blockage were treated with omasum injections of *Da Cheng Qi Tang* decoction in cattle. Journal of Traditional Chinese Veterinary Medicine 2006;23(5):53–54. (In Chinese)
3. Tian YQ, Ding P. Overview on clinical and pharmaceutical research of *Da Cheng Qi Tang*. Chinese Archives of Traditional Chinese Medicine 2006;24(11):2134–2135. (In Chinese)
4. Zhang L. On treatment of acute abdomen with modified *Da Huang Fu Zi Tang* from *Jin Gui Yao Lue*. Jiangxi Journal of Traditional Chinese Medicine 2007;38(5):50–51. (In Chinese)

5. Chen RL. 32 cases of biliary calculi were treated with modified *Da Huang Fu Zi Tang*. Hunan Journal of Traditional Chinese Medicine 1998;14(5):57–58. (In Chinese)
6. Peng B, Li XG. Observation on clinical curative effect of *Da Huang Fu Zi Tang* on uremia. Chinese Nephrosis Journal of Integrated TCM-WM 2000;1(2):106–107. (In Chinese)
7. Lv HY, Zhu WJ and An L. 30 Cases of diabetic nephropathy were treated with *Da Huang Fu Zi Tang*. Chinese Folk Therapeutics 2002;10(8):41–42. (In Chinese)
8. Li GL, Zhang WG, Wang DP. Experimental studies on influences of *Ma Zi Ren Wan* on diabetes model in rats. Jilin Traditional Chinese Medicine 2007;27(7): 59–60. (In Chinese)
9. Wu ZP, Tong XL. *Pi Yu Zheng* was treated with *Ma Zi Ren Wan* in pigs. Journal of Traditional Chinese Veterinary Medicine 1991;9(1):26–27. (In Chinese)
10. Wu Z, Zhang YZ, Zhang JR. A new clinical application of *Ma Zi Ren Wan* form *Jin Gui Yao Lue*. Guangming Traditional Chinese Medicine 2000;15(5):23–24. (In Chinese)
11. Niu YB, Yang YS. Lingering hyperpyrexia was treated with *Zengye Cheng Qi Tang* in animals. Village Technology 2006;12:58. (In Chinese)
12. Guo YZ. Refractory anorexia was treated with *Zengye Cheng Qi Tang* in sows. Journal of Animal Science and Veterinary Medicine 2004;23(4):29. (In Chinese)
13. Chen J. Severe acute pancreatitis (SAP) was treated with integrated TCM-WM. Modern Medical Science 2007;23(8):1204–1205. (In Chinese)
14. Chen H. 60 cases of diabetes type II were treated with integrated TCM-WM. Zhejiang Journal of Integrated TCM-WM 2006;16(4):235–236. (In Chinese)
15. Wang XM. The accelerated effects of *Ma Jia Wan* on gastrointestinal motility in white rats. Chinese Journal of Traditional Veterinary Medicine 2004;4:6–7. (In Chinese)
16. Xue YL. Diseases of proventriculus were treated with *Dang Gui Chong Rong Tang* in cattle. Dairy Cow Science of Sichuan 1998;1: 27–28. (In Chinese)
17. Wang JB. Treatment of abomasums blockage. Journal of Yellow Cattle Science 2005;31(6):93–96. (In Chinese)
18. Zhao L. Chronic kidney insufficiency was treated with *Wen Pi Tang*. Zhejiang Journal of Integrated TCM-WM 2007; 17(9):531–533. (In Chinese)
19. Jiang SG. Clinical observation of 60 cases with chronic non-specific colitis with modified spleen-warming decoction. Hunan Guiding Journal of TCMP 2001;7(7):367,378. (In Chinese)
20. Li Y, Zhang HM, Li J. Effects of Wenpitang-contained serum on LPS-induced proliferation of mesangial cells in vitro. Chinese Journal of Basic Medicine in Traditional Chinese Medicine 2005;11(2):125–127. (In Chinese)
21. Cheng MJ, Feng GY, Huang QH. Influence of different composed herbs and decocting processes on the content of aconitine in *Wen Pi Tang*. Heilongjiang Medicine Journal 2005;18(4):249–250. (In Chinese)
22. Xu CL, Qin XH, Wang MF. Clinical report on 38 cases of viral pneumonia in children with *Shi Zao Tang*. Journal of Linyi medical technical school 1996;18(2):179–180. (In Chinese)
23. Li W. 30 Cases of hepatic cirrhosis ascites treated with *Qi Zhu Shi Zao Tang*. Chinese Journal of Clinical Medicine Research 2007;13(3):382–383. (In Chinese)
24. Lu ZL. 52 cases of hydrothorax were treated with *Shi Zao Tang*. China and Foreign Medical Journal 2006;4(7):68–69. (In Chinese)
25. Han MD. Development of decoction of *Shi Zao Tang*. Shanxi Traditional Chinese Medicine 1994;10(2):42–43. (In Chinese)
26. Wang HZ. Constipation due to accumulation of Heat was treated with *Fan Xie Ye* (Senna) in animals. Inner Mongolia Journal of Animal Sciences 2002;3:31. (In Chinese)

33 Herbal Formulas to Expel Parasites 驱虫剂

Chaoying Luo, Huisheng Xie, Michael Bartholomew

The formulas in this chapter are chiefly composed of parasite repellents and are mainly used for the treatment of internal parasites including roundworms, tapeworms, and hookworms, and external parasites including mites and fleas. In general, the herbal formulas are chosen based on an overall Pattern analysis of the illness and the patient's condition. Alone, they may not be as effective as modern anthelminthic drugs. However, a better curative effect can be achieved for each patient when the herbal formulas and modern parasiticides are combined. Modern anthelminthics have a strong, rapid mode of action to kill parasites; herbal medicine is able to address underlying pathology such as tonifying Deficiency or resolving Excess in the body. For example, in the formula *Hua Chong Tang* (see formula #2 below), some of the herbs are used to expel parasites in the intestinal tract while others warm the Spleen and Stomach to dispel Cold, purge intestinal Stagnation, promote *Qi* flow to relieve abdominal pain, and regulate the Middle Burner.

When considering using herbal formulas to expel parasites, the practitioner needs to consider the following:

1. Greasy or fatty foods should not be fed with the formulas.
2. At first it is best to take the formulas on an empty stomach.
3. Because of the potential for toxicity, one must be cautious when dosing, because a dose that is too high can be toxic, but a dose that is too low will not be effective.
4. Because some herbals have a purgative function, they should be used carefully, or not used at all, in aged, weak, or pregnant patients.
5. In case of weakness of the Spleen and Stomach, the Spleen and Stomach should be tonified and regulated.

Wan Ying San (Always Responsive to Parasites) 万应散

Wan refers to ten thousand or always. *Ying* means responsive. *Wan Ying* means Always Responsive. *San* is powder, the original form of herbal administration. Thus, *Wan Ying San* can be read as Always Responsive (to Parasites) Powder.

Source: *Yi Xue Zheng Zhuan* (*True Lineage of Medicine*), written by *Yu Tian-Min* and published in 1515 CE

Ingredients: The original formula for *Wan Ying San* (Table 33.1) is composed of 30 g *Bing Lang* (Areca), 30 g *Da Huang* (Rheum), 30 g *Zao Jiao Ci* (Gleditsia), 30 g *Ku Lian Pi* (Melia), 30 g *Qian Niu Zi* (Pharbitis), 20 g *Lei Wan* (Omphalia), 10 g *Chen Xiang* (Aquilaria), and 15 g *Mu Xiang* (Saussurea).

Preparation:
1. Powder or capsule method: Herbs are ground into a fine powder. Powder can be encapsulated.
2. Decoction or teapill method: Raw herbs are mixed together and decocted. Herbal water extract (decoction) can be concentrated as granules or teapills.

Actions: Expel parasites and purge the intestines

Indications: This formula is indicated for intestinal parasitism including roundworms, hookworms, and tapeworms.

Dosage and Usage:
Horses and Cattle: 15–60 g, twice daily
Camels: 30–75 g, twice daily
Llamas, Alpacas, Pigs, and Sheep: 5–15 g, twice daily
Dogs: 0.5–5 g (or 0.1 g per kg body weight), twice daily
Cats/Rabbits: 0.2–0.5 g (or 0.1 g per kg body weight), twice daily

Table 33.1. Ingredients and actions of *Wan Ying San*.

%	English Name	Chinese *Pin-Yin*	Actions
15.4	Areca	*Bing Lang*	Promote *Qi* flow, remove food retention
15.4	Rheum	*Da Huang*	Purge the Large Intestine and relieve constipation, clear Heat and reduce Fire, activate Blood to remove Stasis
15.4	Gleditsea	*Zao Jiao Ci*	Transform Phlegm
15.4	Melia	*Ku Lian Pi*	Kill and expel parasites
15.4	Pharbitis	*Qian Niu Zi*	Purge the Intestines to remove food retention, expel parasites
10.3	Omphalia	*Lei Wan*	Expel parasites
7.7	Aquilaria	*Chen Xiang*	Promote *Qi* flow to relieve pain
5.0	Saussurea	*Mu Xiang*	Promote *Qi* flow to relieve pain, regulate the Spleen and Stomach

Birds: 0.1–0.2 g per kg body weight, twice daily

Use 3–4 weeks until primary clinical signs resolve.

Analysis of Formula: Gastrointestinal parasites including roundworms, hookworms, and tapeworms should be treated by herbals that chiefly expel parasites. Consideration should also be given to the generalized impairment of the body caused by the parasites. *Lei Wan* (Omphalia) and *Ku Lian Pi* (Melia) expel common worms from the gastrointestinal tract and act as the King herbs. *Qian Niu Zi* (Pharbitis), *Da Huang* (Rheum), *Bing Lang* (Areca), and *Zao Jiao Ci* (Gleditsia) can purge and expel parasites and are the Minister herbs. *Mu Xiang* (Saussurea) and *Chen Xiang* (Aquilaria) can promote *Qi*, warm the Spleen and Stomach, and function as Adjuvant herbs. All of them work together synergistically to expel parasites in the gastrointestinal tract.

Cautions and Contraindications: This formula must be used carefully in pregnant animals due to its drastic purgative effect. It should be used cautiously in patients with Spleen *Qi* Deficiency because it may cause diarrhea.

Dr. Xie's Comments: *Wan Ying San* is useful for the treatment and prevention of general gastrointestinal parasites, including roundworms, hookworms, and tapeworms in horses and dogs.

Clinical and Pharmacological Studies: In 2006, Chen reported that three cases of ascariasis were treated with *Wan Ying San* in domestic animals.[1]

Case One: A male, intact calf, 90 days old, had a consistently poor appetite, abdominal pain, loss of body weight, and smelled bad. The calf's body temperature was normal. Its respiratory rate was 37 breaths per minute, and the heart rate was 79 beats per minute. Many roundworm eggs were found in the stool by the saturated brine flotation method. The herbal water extract of modified *Wan Ying San* was given via a gastric tube. The formula was composed of 40 g *Da Huang* (Rheum), 30 g *Bing Lang* (Areca), 30 g *Qian Niu Zi* (Pharbitis), 30 g *Shi Jun Zi* (Quisqualis), 30 g *Ku Lian Pi* (Melia), 25 g *Lei Wan* (Omphalia), 25 g *Zao Jiao Ci* (Gleditsia), and 20 g *Mu Xiang* (Saussurea). The next morning after one dose of the herbal medicine, the calf's appetite was improved, the abdominal pain had disappeared, and more than 100 roundworms were ejected in diarrhea. The formula was modified: *Lei Wan* (Omphalia), *Zao Jiao* Ci (Gleditsia), *Da Huang* (Rheum), and *Qian Niu Zi* (Pharbitis) were subtracted and 50 g *Huang Qi* (Astragalus), 30 g *Dang Shen* (Codonopsis), 30 g *Bai Zhu* (Atractylodes), 25 g *Fu Ling* (Poria), 20 g *Zhi Gan Cao* (Glycyrrhiza), 20 g *Wu Mei* (Mume), and 10 pieces of *Da Zao* (Jujube) were added. After receiving another three doses (one dose daily), the diarrhea stopped and the calf began to gain weight and thrive.

Case Two: A 4-month-old black mule foal showed chronic inappetence, occasional cough, poor growth, progressive weight loss, a pale tongue, alternating loose and dry stools, and abdominal pain. Its body temperature was 39.5°C, its respiratory rate was 14 breaths per minute, its heart rate was 42 beats per minute, and many roundworms eggs were found in the stool by the saturated brine flotation method. The foal was treated with a modified *Wan Ying San* formula, composed of 40 g *Da Huang* (Rheum), 40 g *Bai Bu* (Stemona), 30 g *Shi Jun Zi* (Quisqualis), 30 g *Ku Lian Pi* (Melia), 25 g *Bing Lang* (Areca), 25 g *Mu Xiang* (Saussurea), 25 g *Qian Niu Zi* (Pharbitis), 25 g *Zao Jiao Ci* (Gleditsia), 25 g *Nan Gua Zi* (Curcubita), and 20 g *Lei Wan* (Omphalia). Herbs were decocted twice with water for oral dosing, and the herbal water extract was mixed with 150 ml vegetable oil. The mule was first drenched with 200 ml vinegar, followed by the water extract of the modified *Wan Ying San* formula, via a gastric tube. By the next morning, the foal's abdominal pain was remarkably reduced, the stool was normal, and more than 20 roundworms of 20–30 cm length were ejected. 30 g *He Shi* (Carpesium), 25 g *Shi Liu Pi* (Punica), 25 g *Mai Ya* (Hordeum), and 25 g *Sha Zha* (Crataegus) were added to the formula. One dose was administered daily for 3 days. The foal's appetite improved remarkably, a large number of roundworms were ejected, and it was clinically cured by the end of the dosage regimen. At the return visit a month later the foal had a normal body score and was strong and in good health.

Case Three: A 5-month-old female, intact, white pig had a poor appetite; was fatigued, weak, drowsy, too lethargic to move; and sometimes had stools with roundworms. She was diagnosed with ascariasis and was treated with *Wan Ying San*. The formula was composed of 30g *Shi Jun Zi* (Quisqualis), 30g *Ku Lian Pi* (Melia), 30g *Da Huang* (Rheum), 25g *Qian Niu Zi* (Pharbitis), 25g *Bing Lang* (Areca), 25g *Guan Zhong* (Dryopteris), 25g *Bai Bu* (Stemona), 20g *Lei Wan* (Omphalia), 25g *Zao Jiao Ci* (Gleditsia), 25g *Mu Xiang* (Saussurea), 25g *Lian Zi* (Nelumbo), 20g *Suan Zao Ren* (Ziziphus), 20g *Fu Shen* (Poria), and *Bai Zhu* (Atractylodes). The herbs were ground into a fine powder and administered orally. One dose was administered daily for 3 days. Many worms were ejected and the pig was clinically normal by the 4th day.

Hua Chong Tang (Dissolving Parasites) 化虫汤

Hua is dissolve or resolve. *Chong* is parasite. *Tang* is decoction, the original form of herbal administration. Thus, *Hua Chong Tang* can be read as Dissolving Parasites Decoction.

Source: *Zhong Shou Yi Yao Fang Ji Zhen Jiu (The Formulas and Acupuncture of Traditional Chinese Veterinary Medicine)*, written by *Qinghai* Institute of Animal Science and Veterinary Medicine and published in 1972

Ingredients: The original formula for *Hua Chong Tang* (Table 33.2) is composed of 30g *He Shi* (Carpesium), 30g *Shi Jun Zi* (Quisqualis), 30g *Bing Lang* (Areca), 30g *Wu Yi* (Ulmus), 30g *Lei Wan* (Omphalia), 30g *Guan Zhong* (Dryopteris), 30g *Wu Mei* (Mume), 30g *Bai Bu* (Stemona), 30g *He Zi* (Chebula), 30g *Da Huang* (Rheum), 30g *Fei Zi* (Torreya), 15g *Gan Jiang* (Dried Zingiberis), 15g *Fu Zi* (Prepared Aconite), and 15g *Mu Xiang* (Saussurea).

Preparation:

1. Powder or capsule method: Herbs are ground into a fine powder. Powder can be encapsulated.
2. Decoction or teapill method: Raw herbs are mixed together and decocted. Herbal water extract (decoction) can be concentrated as granules or teapills.

Actions: Expel parasites

Indications: This formula is indicated for patients with intestinal parasites and secondary *Qi* Stagnation.

Dosage and Usage:

Horses and Cattle: 15–60g, twice daily
Camels: 30–75g, twice daily
Llamas, Alpacas, Pigs, and Sheep: 5–15g, twice daily
Dogs: 0.5–5g (or 0.1g per kg body weight), twice daily
Cats/Rabbits: 0.2–0.5g (or 0.1g per kg body weight), twice daily
Birds: 0.1–0.2g per kg body weight, twice daily
Use 3–4 weeks until primary clinical signs resolve.

Table 33.2. Ingredients and actions of *Hua Chong Tang*.

%	English Name	Chinese *Pin-Yin*	Actions
8.0	Carpesium	*He Shi*	Expel parasites and relieve pain
8.0	Quisqualis	*Shi Jun Zi*	Expel parasites and eliminate food retention
8.0	Areca	*Bing Lang*	Promote *Qi* flow, eliminate food retention, alleviate water retention
8.0	Ulmus	*Wu Yi*	Expel parasites and eliminate food retention
8.0	Omphalia	*Lei Wan*	Kill and expel parasites
8.0	Dryopteris	*Guan Zhong*	Expel parasites, clear Heat and detoxify, promote hemostasis
8.0	Mume	*Wu Mei*	Astringently consolidate the Lung, relieve diarrhea, numb the intestinal parasites
8.0	Stemona	*Bai Bu*	Moisten the Lung to arrest cough, expel parasites
8.0	Chebula	*He Zi*	Astringently consolidate the Intestines to relieve diarrhea
8.0	Rheum	*Da Huang*	Purge the Large Intestine to eliminate Food Stasis
8.0	Torreya	*Fei Zi*	Kill and expel parasites
4.0	Aconite (Prepared)	*Fu Zi*	Warm the Kidney to strengthen *Yang*, eliminate cold to stop pain
4.0	Dried Zingiberis	*Gan Jiang*	Warm the Spleen
4.0	Saussurea	*Mu Xiang*	Promote *Qi* flow to relieve pain

Analysis of Formula: Parasites accumulated in the intestinal tract lead to Stagnation of *Qi* and Food Stasis, resulting in abdominal pain and vomiting. This condition should be treated chiefly by expelling parasites in the intestinal tract. *He Shi* (Carpesium), *Shi Jun Zi* (Quisqualis), *Bing Lang* (Areca), *Wu Yi* (Ulmus), *Lei Wan* (Omphalia), *Guan Zhong* (Dryopteris), *Wu Mei* (Mume), *Bai Bu* (Stemona), and *Fei Zi* (Torreya) are the King herbs in the formula and serve to kill and expel parasites from the intestinal tract. *Gan Jiang* (Dried Zingiberis), *Fu Zi* (Prepared Aconite), and *He Zi* (Chebula) act as the Minister herbs to warm the Spleen and gastrointestinal tract. *Da Huang* (Rheum) purges, *Mu Xiang* (Saussurea) promotes *Qi* flow to relieve pain, and *Feng Mi* (Honey) moistens the Middle Burner. The last three herbs together are Adjuvant and Messenger herbs.

Cautions and Contraindications: Use with caution in pregnant animals due to its drastic purgative effect.

Dr. Xie's Comments: There is a similar formulation called *Hua Chong Wan,* which was recorded in *Tai Ping Hui Min He Ji Ju Fang (Imperial Grace Formulary of the Tai Ping Era)*, written by *Chen Shi-Wen* et al. and published by the *Song* Dynasty government in 1078 CE. Its ingredients are 1500g *He Shi* (Carpesium), 1500g *Ku Lian Pi* (Melia), 1500g *Bing Lang* (Areca), 1500g *Ku Fan* (Dried Alum), and 1500g *Qian Fen* (Lead Carbonate). All the ingredients are ground into a fine powder mixed with water to make small, 1g balls. They are taken on an empty stomach, 0.5g per 5–10kg body weight twice daily for dogs and cats. The formula is indicated for parasites in the intestinal tract. Another formulation also similar to *Hua Chong Tang, Yi Fang Ji Jie Hua Chong Wan*, was recorded in *Yi Fang Ji Jie (Explain Collection of Medical Formulas*, written by *Wang Ang* in 1682). Its ingredients are *He Shi* (Carpesium), *Ku Lian Pi* (Melia), *Bing Lang* (Areca), *Ku Fan* (Dried Alum), *Qian Fen* (Lead Carbonate), *Shi Jun Zi* (Quisqualis), and *Wu Yi* (Ulmus). The therapeutic principles and actions are similar to *Hua Chong Wan*, but this formula has a stronger action. These two formulas contain lead carbonate; therefore, *Hua Chong Tang* is listed.

Clinical and Pharmacological Studies: *Hua Chong Wan* combined with *Si Miao Wan* was used for the treatment of 58 human cases of trichomonas vaginitis. The youngest was 19 years old, and the oldest was 56 years old; the shortest period of disease was 1 week, and the longest was 3 years; much yellow morbid leucorrhea with odor was found by gynecological examination in 51 cases, with vaginal wall hyperemia in 37 cases, cervical erosion in 4 cases, and red and white morbid leucorrhea in 3 cases. Examination of vaginal secretions found that all cases were *Trichomonas vaginalis* positive. Eight cases were complicated by ulceration of the vulva; 3 cases had uterine prolapse (1st degree); 4 cases had endometritis; 7 cases had cervicitis; and 3 cases had pelvic inflammatory disease. The formula was composed of 10g *Huang Bai* (Phellodendron), 10g *Cang Zhu* (Atractylodes), 10g *Chuan Niu Xi* (Cyathula), 10g *Yi Yi Ren* (Coix), 10g *He Shi* (Carpesium), 10g *Shi Jun Zi* (Quisqualis), 10g *Da Fu Pi* (Areca), 10g *Wu Yi* (Ulmus), and 10g *Ku Lian Pi* (Melia). Herbs were decocted with water for 30 minutes, with one dose administered orally daily for 7 days. In cases of vaginal itching, *Bai Xian Pi* (Dictamnus), *Di Fu Zi* (Kochia), and *Ku Shen* (Sophora) were added. In cases of copious red and white morbid leucorrhea, *Qian Shi* (Euryale), *Duan Long Gu* (calcined Draconis), and *Duan Mu Li* (calcined Ostrea) were added. In cases complicated by ulceration of the vulva or cervical erosion, *Tu Fu Ling* (Smilax), *Bai Zhi* (Angelica), *Bai Jiang Cao* (Patrinia), and *Yu Xing Cao* (Houttuynia) were added. In cases of uterine prolapse, *Sheng Ma* (Cimicifuga), *Huang Qi* (Astragalus), and *Chai Hu* (Bupleurum) were added. In cases of cervictis or endometritis, *Jin Yin Hua* (Lonicera), and *Hong Teng* (Sargentodoxa) were added. In cases of pelvic inflammatory disease, *Hua Shi* (Talcum), *Che Qian Zi* (Plantago), *Qu Mai* (Dianthus), and *Shi Wei* (Pyrrosia) were added. In cases with vaginal wall hyperemia, *Mu Dan Pi* (Moutan), *Sheng Di Huang* (Rehmannia), and *Chi Shao* (Paeonia) were added. In cases of red swelling of the vulva, *Qing Dai* (Indigo) and *Jin Yin Hua* (Lonicera) were added. By the end of the treatment cycle, 26 of the 58 cases were clinically cured, 16 cases showed significant improvement, and 9 cases were improved.[2]

Gan Zhi San (Liver Fluke) 肝蛭散

Gan is the Liver. *Zhi* refers to the fluke. *Gan Zhi* refers to the Liver fluke, or Fasciola hepatica. *San* is the powder, the form of the original administration. Thus, *Gan Zhi San* means Liver Fluke Powder.

Source: *Zhong Shou Yi Yao Fang Ji Zhen Jiu (The Formulas and Acupuncture of Traditional Chinese Veterinary Medicine*), written by *Qinghai* Institute of Animal Science and Veterinary Medicine and published in 1972

Ingredients: The original formula for *Gan Zhi San* (Table 33.3) is composed of 30g *Su Mu* (Sappan), 20g *Rou Dou Kou* (Myristica), 30g *Fu Ling* (Poria), 45g *Guan Zhong* (Dryopteris), 30g *Long Dan Cao* (Gentiana), 20g *Mu Tong* (Akebia), 20g *Gan Cao* (Glycyrrhiza), 20g *Hou Po* (Magnolia), 20g *Ze Xie* (Alisma), and 30g *Bing Lang* (Areca).

Table 33.3. Ingredients and actions of *Gan Zhi San.*

%	English Name	Chinese *Pin-Yin*	Actions
11.3	Sappan	*Su Mu*	Activate Blood to remove Stasis and relieve pain
7.6	Myristica	*Rou Dou Kou*	Warm the Middle Burner and move *Qi*
11.3	Poria	*Fu Ling*	Drain Damp and promote dieresis, strengthen the Spleen
17.0	Dryopteris	*Guan Zhong*	Expel parasites, clear heat and detoxify
11.3	Gentiana	*Long Dan Cao*	Clear Heat and eliminate Damp
7.6	Akebia	*Mu Tong*	Drain Damp and clear Heat
7.6	Glycyrrhiza	*Gan Cao*	Mediate the properties of other herbs
7.5	Magnolia	*Hou Po*	Promote *Qi* flow, eliminate Damp, eliminate food retention
7.5	Alisma	*Ze Xie*	Drain Damp and promote dieresis
11.3	Areca	*Bing Lang*	Promote *Qi* flow, eliminate food retention

Preparation:

1. Powder or capsule method: Herbs are ground into a fine powder. Powder can be encapsulated.
2. Decoction or teapill method: Raw herbs are mixed together and decocted. Herbal water extract (decoction) can be concentrated as granules or teapills.

Actions: Expel parasites, drain Damp to alleviate water retention, move *Qi* and strengthen the Spleen

Indications: This formula is designed to treat fascioliasis hepatica.

Dosage and Usage:

Horses and Cattle: 15–60 g, twice daily
Camels: 30–75 g, twice daily
Llamas, Alpacas, Pigs, and Sheep: 5–15 g, twice daily
Dogs: 0.5–5 g (or 0.1 g per kg body weight), twice daily
Cats/Rabbits: 0.2–0.5 g (or 0.1 g per kg body weight), twice daily
Birds: 0.1–0.2 g per kg body weight, twice daily
Use 3–4 weeks until primary clinical signs resolve.

Analysis of Formula: Parasites migrate to the Liver, leading to Damp-Heat in the Liver. Treat by expelling parasites and clearing Liver Damp-Heat. *Guan Zhong* (Dryopteris) and *Bing Lang* (Areca) are the King herbs and expel parasites. *Long Dan Cao* (Gentiana), *Mu Tong* (Akebia), *Ze Xie* (Alisma), and *Fu Ling* (Poria) work synergistically as the Minister herbs to drain Damp Heat. Serving as the Adjuvant herbs, *Su Mu* (Sappan), *Hou Po* (Magnolia), and *Rou Dou Kou* (Myristica) move *Qi* and Blood and resolve Stagnation to relieve pain. *Gan Cao* (Glycyrrhiza) harmonizes all other herbs and works as the Messenger herb.

Cautions and Contraindications: Use with caution in pregnant animals due to the formula's drastic purgative effect.

Dr. Xie's Comments: *Gan Zhi San* is useful for the treatment and prevention of fascioliasis hepatica in ruminant animals.

Clinical and Pharmacological Studies: A clinical study on fascioliasis hepatica in goats was conducted with the treatment of *Gan Zhi San*. Seventy-six natural cases of fascioliasis hepatica in goats were divided into a *Gan Zhi San* group, a nitroclofene group, a Trichlorobenzene Eusaprim group, and a bromofenofos group at random. Each group had 19 cases. The formula of *Gan Zhi San* was composed of 15 g *Guan Zhong* (Dryopteris), 15 g *Bing Lang* (Areca), 12 g *Su Mu* (Sappan), 10 g *Rou Dou Kou* (Myristica), 12 g *Fu Ling* (Poria), 15 g *Long Dan Cao* (Gentiana), 6 g *Mu Tong* (Akebia), 15 g *Ze Xie* (Alisma), 10 g *Hou Po* (Magnolia), and 10 g *Gan Cao* (Glycyrrhiza). Herbs were ground into a fine powder and administered with warm water in the morning, and half of a dosage was given to goats younger than 1 year old. Nitroclofene was administered by deep intramuscular injection at a dose of 1 mg/kg. Trichlorobenzene Eusaprim was given orally at a dose of 12 mg/kg. Bromofenofos was given orally at a dose of 16 mg/kg. Fifteen days after the treatments, the *Gan Zhi San* group, the Nitroclofene group, the Trichlorobenzene Eusaprim group, and the Bromofenofos group had feces that were 100%, 60%, 100% and 80% clear of parasite eggs, respectively. Seven goats from the Nitroclofene group died, and all goats of the other groups were in good health.[3] In 2004, Zhou and Han reported that two cases of fascioliasis hepatica in cattle were treated with *Gan Zhi San*. The formula was composed of 50 g *Guan Zhong* (Dryopteris), 40 g *Ku Shen* (Sophora), 40 g *Bing Lang* (Areca), 40 g *Ku Lian Pi* (Melia), 40 g *Long Dan Cao* (Gentiana), 30 g *Da Huang* (Rheum), 50 g *Fu Ling* (Poria), 30 g *Ze Xie* (Alisma), 30 g *Hou Po* (Magnolia), 20 g *Su Mu* (Sappan), and 20 g *Rou Dou Kou* (Myristica). Herbs were decocted with water, and then the herbal extract was mixed with 250 g *Feng Mi* (honey). Both cases were clinically normal after the herbal treatment (given orally one dose daily for 15 days) of *Gan Zhi San*. The clinical symptoms all disappeared, the egg examination 15 days later was negative, and both patients were in good health at a return visit 2 months later.[1]

Guan Zhong San (Dryopteris Powder) 贯众煎

Guan Zhong is Dryopteris, the King ingredient of this herbal formulation. *San* is powder, the original form of herbal administration. *Guan Zhong San* literally translates as Dryopteris Powder.

Source: *Zhong Shou Yi Zhi Liao Xue* (*Therapeutics of Traditional Chinese Veterinary Medicine*), written by the Institute of Traditional Chinese Veterinary Medicine, Chinese Academy of Agricultural Science, and published in 1963

Ingredients: *Guan Zhong San* (Table 33.4) is composed of 60 g *Guan Zhong* (Dryopteris), 30 g *Shi Jun Zi* (Quisqualis), 30 g *Bing Lang* (Areca), 30 g *He Shi* (Carpesium), 30 g *Wu Yi* (Ulmus), 40 g *Da Huang* (Rheum), and 15 g *Ku Lian Pi* (Melia).

Preparation:

1. Powder or capsule method: Herbs are ground into a fine powder. Powder can be encapsulated.
2. Decoction or teapill method: Raw herbs are mixed together and decocted. Herbal water extract (decoction) can be concentrated as granules or teapills.

Actions: Expel parasites

Table 33.4. Ingredients and actions of *Guan Zhong San.*

%	English Name	Chinese *Pin-Yin*	Actions
25.5	Dryopteris	*Guan Zhong*	Expel parasites, clear Heat
12.8	Quisqualis	*Shi Jun Zi*	Expel parasites and eliminate food retention
12.8	Areca	*Bing Lang*	Promote *Qi flow*, eliminate food retention
12.8	Carpesium	*He Shi*	Expel parasites and relieve pain
12.8	Ulmus	*Wu Yi*	Expel parasites and eliminate food retention
17.0	Rheum	*Da Huang*	Purge the Intestines to relieve constipation, remove food Stasis
6.3	Melia	*Ku Lian Pi*	Kill and expel parasites

Indications: This formula is used to treat gastrointestinal worms.

Dosage and Usage:
Horses and Cattle: 15–60 g, twice daily
Camels: 30–75 g, twice daily
Llamas, Alpacas, Pigs, and Sheep: 5–15 g, twice daily
Dogs: 0.5–5 g (or 0.1 g per kg body weight), twice daily
Cats/Rabbits: 0.2–0.5 g (or 0.1 g per kg body weight), twice daily
Birds: 0.1–0.2 g per kg body weight, twice daily
Use 3–4 weeks until primary clinical signs resolve.

Analysis of Formula: *Guan Zhong* (Dryopteris) is the King herb to expel the parasites. *He Shi* (Carpesium), *Ku Lian Pi* (Melia), and *Wu Yi* (Ulmus) are the Minister herbs, which expel parasites from the gastrointestinal tract. *Shi Jun Zi* (Quisqualis), *Bing Lang* (Areca), and *Da Huang* (Rheum) act as the Adjuvant and Messenger herbs. *Shi Jun Zi* (Quisqualis) expels parasites, enhances transportation and transformation of the Spleen, and relieves food retention. *Bing Lang* (Areca) expels parasites, moves *Qi* in a descending manner, and eliminates dyspeptic retention. *Da Huang* (Rheum) purges the Intestines and moves Stagnation.

Cautions and Contraindications: Use cautiously in pregnant animals due to its drastic purgative effect.

Dr. Xie's Comments: I have used *Guan Zhong San* for the treatment and prevention of general gastrointestinal worms in horses and dogs. Another *Guan Zhong San* was recorded in *Xin Bian Ji Cheng Ma Yi Fang Niu Yi Fang* (*New Integrated Prescriptions for Equine and Bovine Diseases*) written in 1399 and published in 1633. The ingredients of this *Guan Zhong San* are 60 g *Guan Zhong* (Dryopteris), 30 g *Zao Jiao Ci* (Gleditsia), and 125 g *Huo Ma Ren* (Cannabis). This formula has a milder action to expel parasites and can be used for weak and geriatric patients.

Ku Shen Tang (Sophora Decoction) 苦参汤

Ku Shen is Sophora, the King herb of this formula. *Tang* is decoction, the original form of herbal administration. Thus, *Ku Shen Tang* translates literally to Sophora Decoction.

Source: *Zhong Shou Yi Zhen Liao Shou Ce* (*Handbook of Diagnosis and Treatment of Traditional Chinese Veterinary Medicine*), editor-in-chief *Zheng Ji-fang*, and published in 2006

Ingredients: The original formula for *Ku Shen Tang* (Table 33.5) is composed of 60 g *Ku Shen* (Sophora), 40 g *She Chuang Zi* (Cnidium), 30 g *Bai Zhi* (Angelica), 30 g *Jin Yin Hua* (Lonicera), 30 g *Ju Hua* (Chrysanthemum), 40 g *Huang Bai* (Phellodendron), 40 g *Di Fu Zi* (Kochia), and 30 g *Shi Chang Pu* (Acorus).

Preparation:
1. Powder or capsule method: Herbs are ground into a fine powder. Powder can be encapsulated.
2. Decoction or teapill method: Raw herbs are mixed together and decocted. Herbal water extract (decoction) can be concentrated as granules or teapills.

Actions: Clear Heat and desiccate, kill parasites to relieve itching

Table 33.5. Ingredients and actions of *Ku Shen Tang.*

%	English Name	Chinese *Pin-Yin*	Actions
20	Sophora	*Ku Shen*	Clear Heat and eliminate Damp, dispel Wind to stop itching
13.4	Cnidium	*She Chuang Zi*	Kill fungus and stop itching
10	Angelica	*Bai Zhi*	Dispel Wind and eliminate Damp, resolve swelling
10	Lonicera	*Jin Yin Hua*	Clear Heat and remove toxins
10	Chrysanthemum	*Ju Hua*	Expel Wind and clear Heat, detoxify
13.3	Phellodendron	*Huang Bai*	Clear Heat and eliminate Damp, remove toxin
13.3	Kochia	*Di Fu Zi*	Clear Heat, expel parasites and alleviate itching
10.	Acorus	*Shi Chang Pu*	Clear Damp

Indications: This formula is used to treat mange and moist, red skin lesions due to Damp-Heat pathogens, marked by pruritus, alopecia, scabbing, severe itching, and erosion.

Dosage and Usage: Topical washing for 1 to 2 weeks until primary clinical signs resolve.

Analysis of Formula: Mites, pollen, pathogenic Wind, Heat, and Damp invade the body, leading to Damp-Heat in the skin. *Ku Shen* (Sophora) is the King herb and clears Damp-Heat in both the Interior and Exterior (the skin). *She Chuang Zi* (Cnidium) and *Di Fu Zi* (Kochia) expel parasites, clear Heat, eliminate Damp, alleviate itching, and act as the Minister herbs. Serving as the Adjuvant herbs, *Huang Bai* (Phellodendron), *Shi Chang Pu* (Acorus), *Ju Hua* (Chrysanthemum), and *Jin Yin Hua* (Lonicera) clear Heat, resolve Damp, detoxify, and expel superficial pathogens. *Bai Zhi* (Angelica) with *Di Fu Zi* (Kochia), acting as transporters to the skin, relieve the Exterior and stop itching. Together, they work synergistically to clear Heat, resolve Damp, and kill parasites to relieve itching.

Cautions and Contraindications: None known

Dr. Xie's Comments: *Ku Shen Tang* is a very useful topical herbal formula for any infectious and inflammatory skin conditions due to Damp-Heat in dogs, horses, and fish.

Qing Hao San (Artemisia Powder) 青蒿散

Qing Hao is Artemisia. *San* refers to powder, the form of herbal administration. Thus, *Qing Hao San* means Artemisia Powder.

Source: *Chinese Veterinary Herbal Handbook*, written by *Huisheng Xie* and published by the Chi Institute of Chinese Medicine in 2004

Ingredients: The ingredients and their actions of *Qing Hao San* are listed in Table 33.6.

Preparation:
1. Powder or capsule method: Herbs are ground into a fine powder. Powder can be encapsulated.
2. Decoction or teapill method: Raw herbs are mixed together and decocted. Herbal water extract (decoction) can be concentrated as granules or teapills.

Actions: Tonify *Qi*, enhance *Zheng-Qi*, kill parasites

Indications: This formula is used for *Qi* Deficiency with parasites in the Blood. The main signs are anemia or fever, lameness or ataxia, rear weakness, pale tongue, and weak pulse.

Table 33.6. Ingredients and actions of *Qing Hao San*.

%	English Name	Chinese *Pin-Yin*	Actions
13	Artemisia	*Qing Hao*	Kill and expel Blood-mediated parasites
12	Areca	*Bing Lang*	Expel Gastrointestinal worms and parasites
12	Dryopteris	*Guan Zhong*	Kill parasites
12	Quisqualia	*Shi Jun Zi*	Kill Gastrointestinal worms
12	Omphalia	*Lei Wan*	Kill internal and external worms
11	Condonopsis	*Dang Shen*	Tonify *Qi* and strengthen *Zheng Qi*
11	Atractylodes	*Bai Zhu*	Tonify *Qi* and strengthen Spleen
12	Astragalus	*Huang Qi*	Tonify *Qi* and enhance immune functions
5	Glycyrrhiza	*Gan Cao*	Harmonize

Dosage and Usage:
Horses and Cattle: 15–60 g, twice daily
Camels: 30–75 g, twice daily
Llamas, Alpacas, Pigs, and Sheep: 5–15 g, twice daily
Dogs: 0.5–5 g (or 0.1 g per kg body weight), twice daily
Cats/Rabbits: 0.2–0.5 g (or 0.1 g per kg body weight), twice daily
Birds: 0.1–0.2 g per kg body weight, twice daily
Use 3–4 weeks until primary clinical signs resolve.

Analysis of Formula: Equine protozoal myeloencephalitis (EPM) is a common neurological disease of horses in the U.S. that often causes an asymmetrical gait deficit. Weakness of *Zheng Qi* permits the invasion, development, and growth of parasites. Thus, the key to treating this condition is to both strengthen *Zheng Qi* and expel the internal parasites. *Qing Hao* (Artemisia) is the King herb to expel the parasites in the deep level of the body including Blood. Serving as the Minister herbs, *Guan Zhong* (Dryopteris), *Shi Jun Zi* (Quisqualia), *Lei Wan* (Omphalia), and *Bing Lang* (Areca) kill and expel the parasites. *Dang Shen* (Codonopsis), *Bai Zhu* (Atractylodes), and *Huang Qi* (Astragalus) tonify *Qi*, strengthen the Spleen, and enhance immune functions, acting as the Adjuvant herbs. *Gan Cao* (Glycyrrhiza) harmonizes and acts as the Messenger herb. Together, these herbs work synergistically to eliminate parasites, tonify *Qi*, and enhance immune function.

Cautions and Contraindications: None known

Dr. Xie's Comments: I have used *Qing Hao San* for the treatment and prevention of Equine Protozoal Myeloencephalitis (EPM) in horses.

Clinical and Pharmacological Studies: Wen and Meng reviewed the research progression on the pharmaco-effects of artemisinin and its derivatives. The results showed that artemisinin and its derivatives are not only antimalarial, but are also antineoplastic, antiarrhythmic, anti-Bilharzia worm, and can regulate functions of the immune system.[5]

Tao Chong Fang (Tapeworm Formula) 绦虫方

Tao Chong refers to tapeworms. *Fang* refers to Formula.

Source: *Chinese Veterinary Herbal Handbook,* by *Huisheng Xie* and published by Chi Institute of Chinese Medicine in 2004

Ingredients: The ingredients and actions are listed in Table 33.7.

Table 33.7. Ingredients and actions of *Tao Chong Fang.*

%	English Name	Chinese *Pin-Yin*	Actions
25	Areca	*Bing Lang*	Strengthen Spleen and kill tapeworms
25	Allium	*Da Suan*	Warm the Middle Jiao and expel tapeworms
25	Omphalia	*Lei Wan*	Expel and kill tapeworms
25	Curcubita	*Nan Gua Zi*	Expel tapeworms

Preparation:

1. Powder or capsule method: Herbs are ground into a fine powder. Powder can be encapsulated.
2. Decoction or teapill method: Raw herbs are mixed together and decocted. Herbal water extract (decoction) can be concentrated as granules or teapills.

Actions: Kill tapeworms and strengthen Spleen/Stomach

Indications: This formula is used for tapeworms.

Dosage and Usage:

Horses and Cattle: 15–60 g, twice daily
Camels: 30–75 g, twice daily
Llamas, Alpacas, Pigs, and Sheep: 5–15 g, twice daily
Dogs: 0.5–5 g (or 0.1 g per kg body weight), twice daily
Cats/Rabbits: 0.2–0.5 g (or 0.1 g per kg body weight), twice daily
Birds: 0.1–0.2 g per kg body weight, twice daily
Use 3–4 weeks until primary clinical signs resolve.

Analysis of Formula: *Lei Wan* (Omphalia) expels and kills tapeworms and functions as the King herb. Serving as the Minister herbs, *Nan Gua Zi* (Curcubita) and *Bing Lang* (Areca) expel and kill parasites and strengthen the Spleen. *Da Suan* (Allium) warms the Middle Burner and expels tapeworms, and it functions as the Adjuvant and Messenger herb. The formula's functions for expelling and killing tapeworms may be milder than conventional medications, but its clinical curative effect, especially when combined with conventional medication, may be better than that of conventional medication alone because the formula strengthens the Spleen and warms the Middle Burner to treat the underlying the constitutional imbalance.

Cautions and Contraindications: None known

Dr. Xie's Comments: I have used *Tao Chong Fang* for the treatment of tapeworms in dogs.

REFERENCES

1. Chen XD. Ascariasis was treated with *Wan Ying San* in domestic animals. Chinese Journal of Traditional Veterinary Medicine 2007;13(3):382–383. (In Chinese)
2. Dong ZL, Wu LM, Liang JZ. 58 Cases of trichomonas vaginitis were treated with *Hua Chong Wan* combined with *Si Miao Wan*. Jiangsu Journal of Traditional Chinese Medicine 1997; 18(9):20–21. (In Chinese)
3. Liu XL, Liu WP. A clinical research on Fascioliasis Hepatica treatment with *Gan Zhi San* in goats. Chinese Journal of Traditional Veterinary Medicine 2007;2:5–7. (In Chinese)
4. Zhou DZ, Han ZQ. Fascioliasis Hepatica was treated with *Gan Zhi San* in cattle. Guizhou Animal and Veterinary Sciences 2004;18(5):18. (In Chinese)
5. Wen Y, Meng DS. Research progression on pharmaco-effects of artemisinin and its derivatives. Herald of Medicine 2007;26(10):1193–1195. (In Chinese)

34 Herbal Formulas for External Application 外用方

Chaoying Luo, Michael Bartholomew, Huisheng Xie

Based on the TCVM Pattern diagnosis and the patient's condition, open wounds, sores, and ulcerations can be divided into *Yin* Pattern (Deficiency) and *Yang* Pattern (Excess) of sores/ulceration. The *Yin* Pattern should be treated with a reinforcing method, and the *Yang* Pattern should be treated with a reducing method. According to the TCVM Pattern of sores/ulcerations and the patient's condition, there are different treatments, such as removing Heat to cool Blood, reducing swelling to relieve pain, removing the necrotic tissue, astringing sores/ulcerations and promoting tissue regeneration, reuniting bone, and killing parasites to relieve itching. Oral formulas can be given concurrently with the topical formulas for refractory conditions.

Ru Yi Jin Huang San (Golden Yellow Powder) 如意金黄散

Ru Yi refers to luck, or one who easily achieves one's goal. *Jin* is golden or gold. *Huang* means yellow. *San* refers to powder, the form of herbal medication. Thus, this formula can be translated as Golden Yellow Powder that Will Bring Healing.

Source: *Wai Ke Zheng Zhong* (*True Lineage of External Medicine*), written by *Chen Shi-gong* and published in 1617 CE

Ingredients: The original formula for *Ru Yi Jin Huang San* (Table 34.1) is composed of 300 g *Tian Hua Fen* (Trichosanthes), 150 g *Huang Bai* (Phellodendron), 150 g *Da Huang* (Rheum), 150 g *Bai Zhi* (Angelica), 150 g *Jiang Huang* (Curcuma), 60 g *Tian Nan Xing* (Arisaema), 60 g *Cang Zhu* (Atractylodes), 60 g *Hou Po* (Magnolia), 60 g *Chen Pi* (Citrus), and 60 g *Gan Cao* (Glycyrrhiza).

Preparation:

1. Herbs are ground into a fine powder for topical application only.
2. Traditional method: All ingredients are ground into powder and then mixed with honey or vinegar to form a paste for application.

Actions: Clear Damp-Heat, clear Heat-toxin, activate Blood and relieve pain

Indications: This formula is used for open wounds or sores due to Heat toxin or localized Damp Heat marked by redness, swelling and distension, Heat, and severe pain. It is also used for acute inflammatory conditions accompanied by Heat, swelling and pain, open wounds, skin ulcers, founder/laminitis, torn ligaments, bowed tendons, bucked shins, bruises, splints, stress fractures, and other acute injuries. Typically, the tongue is red and the pulse is fast and forceful.

Dosage and Usage:

Horses: Apply topically on and around open wounds or sores. Spread the herbal powder directly on the wound or sore. Bandage normally if applicable, leave on for 12 hours, then remove residual powder and bandage, and leave uncovered for 12 hours. Repeat the cycle as needed up to 14 days. Discontinue immediately if blistering or skin irritation occurs.

Dogs and cats: Topical application, 1 to 3 times daily for 3 to 5 days.

Analysis of Formula: Mechanical trauma causes wounds or open sores with local inflammation or infection. Heat Toxin, or Damp-Heat accumulates in the Interior, spreads to the body surface, burns and boils the muscles, and leads to open sores or ulcerations on the skin, such as systemic lupus erythematosis skin lesions. The treatment strategy is to clear Heat, detoxify, drain Damp, and resolve local Stagnation to relieve pain. Therefore, *Tian Hua Fen* (Trichosanthes) is used as the King herb to clear Heat and reduce swelling. *Huang Bai* (Phellodendron), *Jiang Huang* (Curcuma),

Table 34.1. Ingredients and actions of *Ru Yi Jin Huang San.*

%	English Name	Chinese *Pin-Yin*	Actions
25.0	Trichosanthes	*Tian Hua Fen*	Clear Heat to reduce swelling
12.5	Phellodendron	*Huang Bai*	Clear Heat and eliminate Damp, purge fire to remove toxin, reduce Deficient Heat
12.5	Rheum	*Da Huang*	Purge the Large Intestine to remove Food Stasis
12.5	Angelica	*Bai Zhi*	Dispel Wind and remove Damp, relieve pain
12.5	Curcuma	*Jiang Huang*	Move Blood and promote *Qi* flow to relieve pain
5.0	Arisaema	*Tian Nan Xing*	Dry up Damp to eliminate Phlegm, dispel Wind to stop convulsion
5.0	Atractylodes	*Cang Zhu*	Eliminate Damp and strengthen the Spleen, dispel Wind and Damp
5.0	Magnolia	*Hou Po*	Promote *Qi* flow, eliminate damp, remove food retention
5.0	Citrus	*Chen Pi*	Regulate the Middle Burner, dry up Damp to eliminate Phlegm
5.0	Glycyrrhiza	*Gan Cao*	Coordinate the herb actions of this whole formulation

and *Da Huang* (Rheum) are used as the Minister herbs to clear Heat, detoxify, purge Fire, remove toxins, and dispel swelling. *Tian Nan Xing* (Arisaema), *Cang Zhu* (Atractylodes), *Hou Po* (Magnolia), *Chen Pi* (Citrus), and *Bai Zhi* (Angelica) are the Adjuvant herbs and activate Blood circulation and promote the flow of *Qi*, thereby reducing swelling and relieving pain. *Gan Cao* (Glycyrrhiza), vinegar, and honey clear Heat, remove toxins, harmonize all other herbs, and function as the Messenger herbs. Together, these herbs clear Heat, remove toxins, dispel swelling, and relieve pain.

Cautions and Contraindications: This formula is for topical use only.

Dr. Xie's Comments: I have used *Ru Yi Jin Huang San* for the treatment of inflamed and infected wounds due to Heat Toxin or Damp-Heat in horses and dogs.

Clinical and Pharmacological Studies: In 2005, *Li* reported that 120 human cases of traumatic injuries were treated topically with *Ru Yi Jin Huang San*; 84 cases were male and 36 cases were female; the youngest was 2 years old and the oldest was 72 years old; 81 cases were closed fractures, 39 cases were collateral ligament injuries of the knee or ankle joint, and 6 of these were collateral ligament injuries of the left ankle joint combined with tarsal fractures. The formula was composed of 20g *Tian Hua Fen* (Trichosanthes), 15g *Huang Bai* (Phellodendron), 10g *Jiang Huang* (Curcuma), 5g *Bai Zhi* (Angelica), 5g *Da Huang* (Rheum), 10g *Tian Nan Xing* (Arisaema), 10g *Cang Zhu* (Atractylodes), 10g *Hou Po* (Magnolia), 10g *Chen Pi* (Citrus), and 2g *Bing Pian* (Borneol). Herbs were ground into a fine powder and placed in a bottle for topical application. The herbal powder was mixed into a paste with honey and then was applied around the injury site(s), once daily. At the same time, the injured bones were externally fixed with small splints. If the fracture was combined with collateral ligament injury, the small splints were replaced by plaster casts. Patients were asked to do permissive functional exercises. All 120 cases showed positive clinical results. The shortest time of complete pain relief was 2 hours and the longest time was 72 hours, with an average of 24 hours. The shortest time of swelling and distension elimination was 36 hours, and the longest time was 7 days, with an average of 3 days. The herbal treatment was the only medication.[1]

Twenty cases of sclerosis caused by intramuscular injection and phlebitis were treated with *Ru Yi Jin Huang San*. Twelve of the cases were sclerosis caused by intramuscular injection and eight cases were due to phlebitis. The formula was composed of 150g *Da Huang* (Rheum),150g *Huang Bai* (Phellodendron), 150g *Jiang Huang* (Curcuma), 150g *Bai Zhi* (Angelica), 60g *Dan or Tian Nan Xing* (Arisaema), 60g *Chen Pi* (Citrus), 60g *Cang Zhu* (Atractylodes), 60g *Hou Po* (Magnolia), 60g *Gan Cao* (Glycyrrhiza), and 300g *Tian Hua Fen* (Trichosanthes). Herbs were ground into a fine powder and placed in a bottle for topical application. The powder was mixed into a paste with rice vinegar. Then it was applied twice daily around the affected area and was covered first with carbasus and then with plastic. Eight cases were clinically cured in 2 days, seven cases were clinically cured in 3 to 4 days, and three cases were clinically cured in 5 or more days.[2]

Bing Peng San (Borneol and Borax) 冰硼散

Bing refers to *Bing Pian* or Borneol. *Peng* refers to *Peng Sha* or Borax. Both are the main ingredients of this formulation. *San* is powder, the form of herbal administration. Thus, *Bing Peng San* means Borneal and Borax Powder.

Source: *Wai Ke Zheng Zhong* (*True Lineage of External Medicine*), written by *Chen Shi-gong* and published in 1617 CE.

Ingredients: The original formula for *Bing Peng San* (Table 34.2) is composed of 50g *Bing Pian* (Borneol),

Table 34.2. Ingredients and actions of *Bing Peng San*.

%	English Name	Chinese *Pin-Yin*	Actions
4.5	Borneol	*Bing Pian*	Reduce swelling and relieve pain
5.4	Cinnabaris*	*Zhu Sha*	Detoxify to treat sores
45.0	Borax	*Peng Sha*	Detoxify and have an antiseptic effect
45.0	Alum	*Ming Fan*	Clear Heat and reduce swelling

**Zhu Sha* (Cinnabaris) contains the heavy metal mercury. It is not used in the modern formulation.

60 g *Zhu Sha* (Cinnabaris), 500 g *Peng Sha* (Borax), and 500 g *Ming Fan* (Alum).

Preparation: Herbs are ground into a fine powder and stored in a brown bottle for topical use only.

Actions: Clear Heat and detoxify, reduce swelling, relieve pain

Indications: This formula is used for swelling; pain or ulceration of the tongue, gums, and throat; gingivitis; stomatitis; and open sores or ulcerations in the oral cavity.

Dosage and Usage: Powder is applied topically directly to the sore or ulceration of the tongue and gums, 2–3 times daily for 2 to 7 days.

Analysis of Formula: Heat Toxin burns or boils the muscles and local tissues, leading to ulcerations, open sores, swelling, and pain. Serving as the King ingredients, *Bing Pian* (Borneol) and *Peng Sha* (Borax) clear Heat and reduce swelling. *Ming Fan* (Alum) is the Minister ingredient used to clear Heat and reduce swelling to relieve pain. Together, they can clear Heat, detoxify, reduce swelling, and relieve pain.

Cautions and Contraindications: This formula is for topical use in the oral cavity. It can be ingested.

Dr. Xie's Comments: I have used *Bing Peng San* (mixed with baby toothpaste) for the treatment of stomatitis or gingivitis due to Heat toxin or Damp Heat in cats and dogs.

Clinical and Pharmacological Studies: *Feng* reported a good response to treatment of laryngotracheitis with *Bing Peng San* in chickens. 0.05 to 0.1 g Chinese patent medicine of *Bing Peng San* was sprinkled into the throat with a paper tube through the chickens' mouths 2 to 3 times daily for 2 to 4 days. The clinical cure rate was 95.3%.[3] *Yuan* reported that 10 cases of endometritis in cows were treated with *Bing Peng San*. The formula was composed of 50 g *Bing Pian* (Borneol), 60 g *Zhu Sha* (Cinnabaris), 500 g *Peng Sha* (Borax), and 500 g *Ming Fan* (Alum). The herbs were ground into a fine powder and filled in a brown bottle. The cows were restrained in a standing position and the uterus of each cow was flushed with 5 to 10 liters of warm 1% saline until the drainage was clear. Then the powder was infused into the uterus once or twice daily for 5 to 7 days. The dosage of *Bing Peng San* for each cow was 300 to 500 g. After a treatment of 5 to 7 days, 9 of 10 cases were clinically cured and later conceived.[4] Ecthyma contagiosum is a highly contagious, zoonotic, viral skin disease that affects sheep, goats, and some other domesticated and wild ruminants. The skin lesions often occur on the mouth and muzzle and are so painful they can cause anorexia or starvation. In one clinical trial in 2003, 198 cases of Ecthyma contagiosum in goats were treated with *Bing Peng San*. The composition and preparation were the same as above. *Bing Peng San* was topically applied around the skin lesions, 2 or 3 times daily. The attitude of the goats gradually improved and they started to eat some fresh grass 3 days after the initial treatment. The blisters and the pustules started healing 5 days later, and all goats were clinically cured in 12 to 15 days.[5]

Fang Feng Tang (Ledebouriella Decoction) 防风汤

Fang Feng is Ledebouriella, the King herb of this formulation. *Tang* is the decoction, the form of herbal administration. *Fang Feng Tang* translates literally to Ledebouriella Decoction.

Source: *Yuan Heng Liao Ma Ji* (*Yuan-Heng's Therapeutic Treatise of Horses*), written by *Yu Ben-yuan and Yu Ben-heng* in 1608 CE

Ingredients: The original formula for *Fang Feng Tang* (Table 34.3) is composed of equivalent portions of *Fang Feng* (Ledebouriella), *Jing Jie* (Schizonepeta), *Hua Jiao* (Zanthoxylum), *Bo He* (Mentha), *Ku Shen* (Sophora), and *Huang Bai* (Phellodendron).

Preparation: Herbs are decocted twice; the herbal water extract is then used for topical washing.

Actions: Clear Heat, remove toxins, reduce swelling, top itching

Indications: This formula is used for swelling, open sores and skin diseases, or infections.

Dosage and Usage: Topically wash the local lesions 1–3 times daily for 3 to 7 days.

Table 34.3. Ingredients and actions of *Fang Feng Tang*.

%	English Name	Chinese *Pin-Yin*	Actions
16.7	Ledebouriella	*Fang Feng*	Expel Wind, eliminate Damp, relieve spasms and Exterior Pattern
16.7	Schizonepeta	*Jing Jie*	Clear Wind to stop itching
16.6	Zanthoxylum	*Hua Jiao*	Dispel Cold to relieve pain, dry Damp, destroy parasites
16.7	Mentha	*Bo He*	Dispel Wind and Heat, expel Wind to improve visual acuity
16.7	Sophora	*Ku Shen*	Clear Heat and eliminate Damp, dispel Wind and expel parasites
16.6	Phellodendron	*Huang Bai*	Clear Heat and eliminate Damp, purge Fire and remove toxin

Analysis of Formula: This formula is applied topically to treat open sores or infections, and to treat pruritis. *Fang Feng* (Ledebouriella) is the King herb and clears Wind to stop itching. Serving as the Minister herbs, *Jing Jie* (Schizonepeta), *Bo He* (Mentha), and *Hua Jiao* (Zanthoxylum) clear Wind to stop itching, disperse Blood Stasis, and reduce swelling. *Huang Bai* (Phellodendron) and *Ku Shen* (Sophora) clear Heat, eliminate Damp, detoxify, and function as the Adjuvant and Messenger herbs. Combined, they clear Wind to stop itching, clear Heat to remove toxins, and move Blood to reduce swelling.

Cautions and Contraindications: This formula is for topical use only.

Dr. Xie's Comments: I have used *Fang Feng Tang* as an herbal bath for the treatment of skin infections in fish.

Sheng Ji San (Granulation Regeneration) 生肌散

Sheng refers to generate. *Ji* is muscle. *Sheng Ji* refers to generation of granulation tissue. *San* is the powder form of administration.

Source: *Wai Ke Zheng Zong* (*True Lineage of External Medicine*), written by *Chen Shi-Gong* in 1617 CE

Ingredients: The original formula for *Sheng Ji San* (Table 34.4) is composed of 500 g *Shi Gao* (Gypsum), 500 g *Qing Fen* (Calomel), 500 g *Chi Shi Zhi* (Halloysite), 100 g *Huang Dan* (Yellow Lead), 150 g *Long Gu* (Draconis), 150 g *Xue Jie* (Draconis), 150 g *Ru Xiang* (Olibanum), and 150 g *Bing Pian* (Borneol).

Table 34.4. Ingredients and actions of *Sheng Ji San*.

%	English Name	Chinese *Pin-Yin*	Actions
22.8	Gypsum	*Shi Gao*	Dry Damp to destroy parasites, promote granulation
22.7	Calomel	*Qing Fen*	Kill parasites to relieve itching, counteract toxic substances and treat sores
22.8	Halloysite	*Chi Shi Zhi*	Consolidate the tissues and promote wound healing
4.5	Yellow Lead	*Huang Dan*	Detoxify and promote granulation
6.8	Draconis	*Long Gu*	Consolidate the tissues and promote wound healing
6.8	Draconis	*Xue Jie*	Remove Blood Stasis to relieve pain, promote granulation
6.8	Olibanum	*Ru Xiang*	Promote *Qi* flow to relieve pain, relax and activate the tendons
6.8	Borneol	*Bing Pian*	Reduce swelling and relieve pain

Preparation: All ingredients are ground into a fine powder and stored in a brown bottle for topical use only.

Actions: Remove the necrotic tissue, promote granulation and healing

Indications: This formula is used for nonhealing wounds, including surgical incisions, other open ulcerations, and sores.

Dosage and Usage: The herbal powder is sprinkled over the affected area(s), 1–2 times daily for 3–7 days.

Analysis of Formula: This formula is indicated for nonhealing wounds and chronic open sores. Serving as the King ingredients, *Xue Jie* (Draconis) and *Ru Xiang* (Olibanum) activate Blood circulation, relieve pain, and promote the healing process. *Shi Gao* (Gypsum), *Long Gu* (Draconis), and *Chi Shi Zhi* (Halloysite) function as the Minister herbs to consolidate the tissues and promote wound healing and closure. *Qing Fen* (Calomel), *Huang Dan* (Yellow Lead), and *Bing Pian* (Borneol) work as the Adjuvant and Messenger ingredients to clear Heat, reduce swelling, and penetrate the skin to relieve pain.

Cautions and Contraindications: It is for topical use only and cannot be taken orally.

Dr. Xie's Comments: This formula contains lead and is used topically only. Therefore, a bandage in horses or E-collar in dogs and cats must be used to prevent oral ingestion.

Clinical and Pharmacological Studies: Wang reported that 6 cases of fistulas were treated with *Sheng Ji San* (produced by Beijing Chinese Herbal Medicine Manufactory) and benzylpenicillin. After using 0.2% potassium permanganate or 3% hydrogen peroxide to clean the wound and remove any foreign bodies and necrotic tissue, the wound cavity was packed with *Sheng Ji San* and benzylpenicillin. This was performed once daily for 3 to 10 days. All 6 cases healed within 20 days.[6]

Tao Hua San (Peach Flower) 桃花散

Tao refers to peach. *Hua* is flower. *Tao Hua* refers to peach flower. *San* is powder, the form of medication. *Tao Hua* is named because the color of this formulation is like peach flowers (*Tao Hua*).

Source: *Yi Zong Jin Jian* (*Golden Mirror of the Medical Tradition*), written by *Wu Qian* et al. and published in 1742 CE

Ingredients: The original formula for *Tao Hua San* (Table 34.5) is composed of 500 g *Chen Shi Hui* (Slaked lime) and 90 g *Da Huang* (Rheum).

Preparation: *Chen Shi Hui* (Slaked lime) and *Da Huang* (Rheum) are ground separately into fine powders and then mixed, becoming pink like the color of a peach flower (*Tao Hua*). The powder is stored in a brown bottle for topical use only.

Actions: Consolidate the surface to stop bleeding and promote healing

Indications: This formula is used for bleeding associated with a new wound.

Dosage and Usage: The herbal powder is sprinkled over the affected areas, 1–2 times daily for 3–7 days.

Analysis of Formula: This formula is indicated for bleeding associated with a new wound. *Chen Shi Hui* (Slaked lime) can astringe and consolidate the wound and stop bleeding. *Da Huang* (Rheum) can astringe the wound and cool the Blood. Together, these two herbs work synergistically to stop hemorrhage and promote healing.

Table 34.5. Ingredients and actions of *Tao Hua San.*

%	English Name	Chinese *Pin-Yin*	Actions
84.7	Slaked lime	*Chen Shi Hui*	Hemostasis and promote granulation, dry Damp to destroy parasites
15.3	Rheum	*Da Huang*	Activate Blood, remove Stasis, clear Heat, detoxify

Cautions and Contraindications: It is for topical use only and cannot be taken orally.

Dr. Xie's Comments: This formula is useful for a new traumatic wound with bleeding.

Qing Dai San (Indigo Powder) 青黛散

Qing Dai is Indigo, the King herb in this formula. *San* is the powder form of medication.

Source: *Yuan Heng Liao Ma Ji* (*Yuan-Heng's Therapeutic Treatise of Horses*), written by *Yu Ben-yuan* and *Yu Ben-heng* and published in 1608 CE

Ingredients: The original formula for *Qing Dai San* (Table 34.6) is composed of equivalent portions of *Qing Dai* (Indigo), *Huang Lian* (Coptis), *Huang Bai* (Phellodendron), *Bo He* (Mentha), *Jie Geng* (Platycodon), and *Er Cha* (Acacia).

Preparation: All ingredients are ground into a fine powder and stored in a brown bottle for topical use.

Actions: Clear Heat, detoxify, reduce swelling, relieve pain

Indications: This formula is used for stomatitis, gingivitis, open sores, and sore throat.

Dosage and Usage: The herbal powder is sprinkled over the affected area(s) 1–2 times daily for 3–7 days.

Table 34.6. Ingredients and actions of *Qing Dai San.*

%	English Name	Chinese *Pin-Yin*	Actions
16.7	Indigo	*Qing Dai*	Antipyretic, detoxify, cool Blood, and eliminate purpura
16.7	Coptis	*Huang Lian*	Clear Heat and eliminate Damp, purge Fire to remove toxins, remove Heat to cool Blood
16.7	Phellodendron	*Huang Bai*	Antipyretic, dry Damp, purge Fire for removing toxins
16.7	Mentha	*Bo He*	Remove throat and chest Heat, expel Wind and clear Heat
16.6	Platycodon	*Jie Geng*	Transform Phlegm
16.6	Acacia	*Er Cha*	Clear Heat and dissipate Phlegm, astringe to stop diarrhea and bleeding, regenerate tissue to heal wound

Analysis of Formula: Heat Toxin accumulated in the Interior flares up and burns the local tissues leading to open sores, ulceration, stomatitis, swelling, and pain. *Qing Dai* (Indigo) functions as the King herb to clear Heat, detoxify, remove toxins, and resolve Stagnation to relieve pain. Serving as the Minister herbs, *Huang Lian* (Coptis) and *Huang Bai* (Phellodendron) clear Heat and detoxify. *Er Cha* (Acacia) and *Bo He* (Mentha) clear Heat to relieve sore throat, astringe wounds to promote healing, and serve as the Adjuvant herbs. *Jie Geng* (Platycodon) relieves sore throat, is the transporter to the Upper *Jiao*, and functions as the Messenger herb. As a group, these herbs are antipyretic, detoxifying, and can reduce swelling and produce analgesia.

Cautions and Contraindications: This formula is for topical use only.

Dr. Xie's Comments: This formula is mixed with baby toothpaste for the treatment of stomatitis and gingivitis in dogs and cats. This paste can be ingested, but it may cause vomiting.

Clinical and Pharmacological Studies: Zhang reported that 362 cases of infectious stomatitis in sheep were treated with a modified *Qing Dai San*. The formula was composed of 10g *Qing Dai* (Indigo), 10g *Bo He* (Mentha), 10g *Huang Lian* (Coptis), 10g *Huang Qin* (Scutellaria), 10g *Huang Bai* (Phellodendron), 6g *Jie Geng* (Platycodon), 6g *Zhi Zi* (Gardenia), 6g *Er Cha* (Acacia), 3g *Bing Pian* (Borneol), 3g *Ming Fan* (Alum), and 5g Sulfaguanidine. All the ingredients were ground into a fine powder and placed in a brown bottle for use. After flushing the mouths of the sheep, *Qing Dai San* was sprinkled all over the oral cavity. This was done 3 times daily for 3–7 days; 168 of 362 cases were clinically cured in 3–7 days; 36 of 362 cases were clinically cured within 8–14 days; 142 cases were clinically cured in 15 or more days; 16 cases died from other diseases.[7] *Liu* reported that there was a curative effect when treating ulceration of the tongue when *Qing Dai San* was administered along with oral doses of *Huang Lian Jie Du Tang*, which consists of *Huang Lian* (Coptis), *Huang Qin* (Scutellaria), *Huang Bai* (Phellodendron), and *Zhi Zi* (Gardenia).[8]

Fang Fu Sheng Ji San (Antiseptic and Promoting Granulation) 防腐生肌散

Fang Fu refers to antiseptic. *Sheng* means regeneration. *Ji* refers to granulation tissue. *San* means powder.

Source: *Zhong Shou Yi Zhen Liao (Diagnosis and Treatment of Traditional Chinese Veterinary Medicine)*, written by *Li Fu-ji* and published in 1972

Ingredients: The original formula for *Fang Fu Sheng Ji San* (Table 34.7) is composed of 500g *Ku Fan* (Dried alum), 500g *Chen Shi Hui* (Slaked lime), 400g *Shi Gao* (Gypsum), 400g *Mo Yao* (Myrrh), 250g *Xue Jie* (Draconis), 250g *Ru Xiang* (Olibanum), 50g *Huang Dan* (Yellow Lead), 50g *Bing Pian* (Borneol), and 50g *Qing Fen* (Calomel).

Table 34.7. Ingredients and actions of *Fang Fu Sheng Ji San*.

%	English Name	Chinese *Pin-Yin*	Actions
20.4	Dried Alum	*Ku Fan*	Expel parasites and alleviate itching
20.4	Slaked lime	*Chen Shi Hui*	Promote granulation, dry up Damp, expel parasites
16.3	Gypsum	*Shi Gao*	Dry up Damp, promote granulation
16.3	Myrrh	*Mo Yao*	Remove Blood Stasis to relieve pain, reduce swelling
10.2	Draconis	*Xue Jie*	Remove Blood Stasis to relieve pain, promote granulation
10.2	Olibanum	*Ru Xiang*	Promote *Qi* flow to relieve pain, relax the tendons and ligaments
2.1	Yellow lead	*Huang Dan*	Detoxify and promote granulation
2.1	Borneol	*Bing Pian*	Reduce swelling and relieve pain
2.0	Calomel	*Qing Fen*	Kill parasites to relieve itching

Preparation: All ingredients are ground into a fine powder and stored in a brown bottle for topical use only.

Actions: Prevent sepsis, absorb moisture, promote granulation, close wounds

Indications: This formula is used to treat deep folliculitis and pyoderma, sores and ulcerations, wounds, and bleeding wounds.

Dosage and Usage: The herbal powder is sprinkled over the affected area(s), 1–2 times daily for 3–7 days.

Analysis of Formula: This formula is indicated for deep folliculitis or pyoderma and nonhealing wounds or sores, which are caused by Dampness and toxins. *Ku Fan* (Dried alum), and *Chen Shi Hui* (Slaked lime) function as the King ingredients to dry up Dampness and absorb moisture to promote wound healing. Serving as the Minister herbs, *Shi Gao* (Gypsum), *Huang Dan* (Yellow Lead), and *Qing Fen* (Calomel) clear Heat, prevent sepsis, absorb moisture, and promote granulation. *Mo Yao* (Myrrh), *Xue Jie* (Draconis), and *Ru Xiang* (Olibanum) reduce swelling and relieve pain, and work as the Adjuvant herbs. Functioning as the transporter and Messenger ingredient, *Bing Pian* (Borneol) clears Heat to relieve pain and penetrate the skin.

Cautions and Contraindications: It is for topical use only. Do not take orally.

Dr. Xie's Comments: This formula is used topically only. Therefore, a bandage or e-collar has to be used to prevent oral ingestion.

Clinical and Pharmacological Studies: *Jiang* and *Wang* reported that external injury wounds were treated with modified *Fang Fu Sheng Ji San* in dogs and cats. The formula was composed of 50g *Ku Fan* (Dried alum), 50g *Chen Shi Hui* (Slaked lime), 40g *Shi Gao* (Gypsum), 40g *Mo Yao* (Myrrh), 25g *Xue Jie* (Draconis), 25g *Ru Xiang* (Olibanum), 5g *Huang Dan* (Yellow Lead), 5g *Bing Pian* (Borneol), and 5g *Qing Fen* (Calomel). The wound was completely healed after 15 daily topical applications of *Fang Fu Sheng Ji San*.[9] Qu reported that 63 cases of refractory sores in animals were clinically healed with *Nei Tuo Sheng Ji San* (modified *Fang Fu Sheng Ji San* for oral medication). The formula was composed of 60g *Huang Qi* (Astragalus), 30g *Dan Shen* (Salvia), 40g *Bai Shao* (Paeonia), 40g *Tian Hua Fen* (Trichosanthes), 30g *Ru Xiang* (Olibanum), 30g *Mo Yao* (Myrrh), and 20g *Gan Cao* (Glycyrrhiza). Herbs were decocted with water for oral dosing. The herbal water extract was administered orally once a day. The open sores in all 63 cases were healed in 10 days.[10]

Tang Huo San (Scalds and Burns) 烫火散

Tang Huo refers to scald or burns (due to fire or chemicals). *San* is the powder form of the medication.

Source: *Zhong Hua Ren Min Gong He Guo Yao Dian* (*Pharmacopoeias of the People's Republic of China*), written by the Pharmacopeia Committee of the Ministry of Health, China, and published in 1977

Ingredients: The original formula for *Tang Huo San*, (Table 34.8), is composed of 500g *Di Yu* (Sanguisorba), 250g *Huang Bai* (Phellodendron), 250g *Shi Gao* (Gypsum), 125g *Da Huang* (Rheum), and 125g *Han Shui Shi* (Calcite).

Preparation:

1. All ingredients are ground into a fine powder and stored in a brown bottle for topical use only.
2. Traditional method: All ingredients are ground into powder and mixed with *Ma You* (sesame oil) into paste.

Actions: Clear Heat, cool Blood and detoxify

Indications: This formula is used to treat burns or scalds.

Dosage and Usage: The herbal powder is sprinkled over the affected area(s) 1–2 times daily for 3–7 days.

Table 34.8. Ingredients and actions of *Tang Huo San*.

%	English Name	Chinese *Pin-Yin*	Actions
40.0	Sanguisorba	*Di Yu*	Cool Blood to stop bleeding, reduce fire
20.0	Phellodendron	*Huang Bai*	Clear Damp-Heat, purge Fire to remove toxin
20.0	Gypsum	*Shi Gao*	Clear Heat
10.0	Rheum	*Da Huang*	Activate Blood to remove Stasis, cool Blood, detoxify
10.0	Calcite	*Han Shui Shi*	Clear Heat and reduce Fire

Analysis of Formula: This formula is indicated for burns or scalds, which are often caused by Heat Toxin. *Di Yu* (Sanguisorba) and *Da Huang* (Rheum) cool Blood to stop bleeding and remove toxins, and they function as the King herbs. Serving as the Minister herbs, *Huang Bai* (Phellodendron) clears Heat and reduces swelling, and *Sheng Shi Gao* (Gypsum) and *Han Shui Shi* (Calcite) clear Heat and reduce fire. *Ma You* (sesame oil) moistens the muscles and skin and works as the Adjuvant and Messenger.

Cautions and Contraindications: This formula is for topical use only.

Dr. Xie's Comments: I have used *Tang Huo San* for the treatment of scalds and burns in horses and dogs.

Clinical and Pharmacological Studies: A combination of *Tang Huo San* and *Zi Cao You* was used for the treatment of 126 human cases of burns and scalds; 88 of 126 cases were male and 38 cases were female; the youngest was 1 year old and the oldest was 62 years old. A total of 76 cases were treated within 12 hours after skin burning, 11 cases were treated within 12 to 24 hours, 25 cases were treated within 24 to 48 hours, and 14 cases were treated after 48 hours. The wound surfaces of 104 cases were not infected and 22 cases were infected. The burn surface area of 92 cases was less than 9%, of 18 cases was 9% to 18%, and of 10 cases was 18% to 27%; 3 cases had a burn surface area of more than 27%. The depth of the burn in 120 cases was less than deep second degree burns, and the remaining 6 cases had deep second degree burns. The formula of *Zi Cao You* was composed of 100g *Zi Cao* (Lithospermum), *Bing Pian* (Borneol), and 1000ml vegetable oil. *Zi Cao* (Lithospermum) was fried on a low fire in warm vegetable oil until the oil became purple red. The residue was discarded, and the oil was filtered and added to finely ground *Bing Pian* (Borneol). After cooling, it was placed in a bottle for use. *Tang Huo San* was a Chinese patent medicine (ingredients, preparation, and processing based on the above-mentioned procedures). First, the burn surface was thoroughly cleaned with saline. Large blisters were drained and the water on the wound surface was lightly blotted with a dry, sterile swab. Infected wounds were carefully cleaned, and the pus or transudate removed. *Tang Huo San* was uniformly applied on wound surfaces after being mixed with *Zi Cao You*. It was applied 2 to 3 times daily with enough medicine to cover the wound. During treatment, the wound was not bandaged and was left exposed to air. Uncomplicated wounds usually healed in 7 days; wound surfaces that had secondary infections healed in about 2 weeks. Ninety-seven percent of patients showed a positive response. In all cases, there was no scar formation and no complications were noted. Children had a better clinical result.[11]

Zhi Tong Gao (Relief Salve) 止痛膏

Zhi is stop. *Tong* means pain. *Zhi Tong* refers relief of pain. *Gao* is the salve form of the medication.

Source: *Chinese Veterinary Herbal Handbook*, by *Huisheng Xie* and published by the Chi Institute of Chinese Medicine in 2004

Ingredients: The ingredients and actions of this formula are listed in Table 34.9.

Table 34.9. Ingredients and actions of *Zhi Tong Gao*.

%	English Name	Chinese *Pin-Yin*	Actions
8.0	Clematis	*Wei Ling Xian*	Clear Wind-Damp, move *Qi* and relieve pain
9.0	Olibanum	*Ru Xiang*	Invigorate Blood, relieve pain, repair tissues
9.0	Myrrh	*Mo Yao*	Invigorate Blood, relieve pain, repair tissues
3.5	Draconis	*Xue Jie*	Dissipate Stagnation, relieve pain, promote healing
9.0	Angelica	*Dang Gui*	Invigorate Blood and relieve pain
8	Angelica	*Bai Zhi*	Clear the surface, relieve pain, promote healing
9.0	Corydalis	*Yan Hu Suo*	Invigorate Blood and relieve pain
9.0	Rheum	*Da Huang*	Break down Stasis, dissipate swelling, cool Blood
8.0	Momordica	*Mu Bie Zi*	Dissipate swelling and nodules, relieve pain
3.5	Carthamus	*Hong Hua*	Move Blood, disperse swelling
9.0	Gardenia	*Zhi Zi*	Clear Heat, detoxify, cool blood, dissipate Stagnation
8.0	Erythinia	*Hai Tong Pi*	Dispel Damp and invigorate Channels
7.0	Zanthoxylum	*Hua Jiao*	Warm the Middle, dispel Cold, relieve pain, dry up Damp
4.7	Camphora	*Zhang Nao*	Open the orifice, kill parasites, relieve pain
3.1	Borneol	*Bing Pian*	Open the orifice, dissipate Stagnation, clear Heat, relieve pain

Preparation: The 15 ingredients are ground into a fine powder and then mixed with beeswax and olive oil, making a paste. Store in a container for topical use only.

Actions: Invigorate Blood, move *Qi*, relieve pain, dissipate swelling

Indications: This formula is used to treat acute or chronic pain or discomfort due to traumatic injuries of soft tissues, including tendons, ligaments, muscles, and fascia. Typically, the tongue is purple and the pulse is fast.

Dosage and Usage:

Horses: Apply topically to painful locations. Spread the salve on a clean gauze pad, apply directly to the injured area, and then bandage normally. Leave on for 12 hours then remove the residue herbs and bandage, and leave uncovered for 12 hours. Repeat the cycle as needed up to 1 month.

Dog/Cat: Topical application. Rub and massage around the areas of pain, muscle spasm, or joints for 5 minutes, twice daily for 5 to 10 days.

Analysis of Formula: Traumatic injury causes local *Qi*-blood Stagnation, leading to pain and swelling. Serving as the King herbs, *Ru Xiang* (Olibanum), *Mo Yao* (Myrrh), *Dang Gui* (Angelica), and *Yan Hu Suo* (Corydalis) invigorate Blood and relieve pain. *Hong Hua* (Carthamus), *Xue Jie* (Draconis), *Mu Bie Zi* (Momordica), and *Bai Zhi* (Angelica) move *Qi* and Blood to relieve pain, resolve Stagnation to reduce swelling, and function as the Minister herbs. *Da Huang* (Rheum) and *Zhi Zi* (Gardenia) clear Heat and resolve Stagnation. *Hai Tong Pi* (Erythrinia), *Wei Ling Xian* (Clematis), and *Hua Jiao* (Zanthoxylum) dispel Damp and invigorate the channels to relieve pain. These last five herbs work together as the Adjuvant herbs. Serving as the Transporter and Messenger herbs, *Zhang Nao* (Camphora) and *Bing Pian* (Borneol) penetrate the skin and relieve pain. *Feng La* (Beeswax) and *Zhi Wu You* (Olive Oil) are carriers.

Cautions and Contraindications: This formula is for topical use only. Do not apply to the lumbar spine during pregnancy, do not apply to open wounds, and discontinue if blistering or skin irritation occurs.

Dr. Xie's Comments: I have used *Zhi Tong Gao* for the treatment of acute or chronic pain due to traumatic injuries of soft tissues including tendons, ligaments, muscles, and fascia in horses and dogs.

Si Sheng Gao (Four Herbs Salve) 四生膏

Si means four. *Sheng* means raw, or fresh. *Si Sheng* refers to four raw herbs that make up this formula. *Gao* is the salve form of the medication.

Source: *Chinese Veterinary Herbal Handbook*, written by *Huisheng Xie* and published by the Chi Institute of Chinese Medicine in 2004

Ingredients: The ingredients and actions are listed in Table 34.10.

Preparation: The first four ingredients are ground into a fine powder and then mixed with beeswax and olive oil to make a paste and stored in a container for topical use.

Actions: Transform Phlegm, resolve Stagnation, move *Qi*, relieve pain

Indications: This formula is used to treat severe pain due to acute musculoskeletal injury, hoof soreness, joint pain, navicular disease or laminitis, purple tongue, and wiry pulse.

Dosage and Usage: Horses: Apply topically to painful locations. Spread the salve on a clean gauze pad, apply directly to the injured area, and then bandage normally. Leave on for 12 hours and then remove bandage and residue ointment, and leave uncovered for 12 hours. Repeat the cycle as needed up to 14 days. Discontinue immediately if blistering or skin irritation occurs.

Analysis of Formula: *Chuan Wu* (Aconite) functions as the King herb and is very potent for clearing Wind-Damp, moving *Qi*, and blocking pain. *Cao Wu* (Aconite) is the Minister herb and moves *Qi* and relieves pain. *Ban Xia* (Pinellia) and *Tian Nan Xing* (Arisaema) transform Phlegm and resolve Stagnation to relieve pain and serve as the Adjuvant herbs. *Feng La* (Beeswax) and *Zhi Wu You* (Olive Oil) are carriers.

Cautions and Contraindications: This formula is for topical use only. **Oral ingestion is toxic to the Kidney.** Use for 14 days or less. It is contraindicated during pregnancy. Do not apply to open wounds (use Golden Yellow Salve instead). Dogs and cats can be very sensitive to this topical formulation.

Dr. Xie's Comments: I have used *Si Sheng Gao* for the treatment of severe foot pain due to laminitis or navicular disease in horses.

Table 34.10. Ingredients and actions of *Si Sheng Gao*.

%	English Name	Chinese *Pin-Yin*	Actions
25	Pinellia	*Ban Xia*	Transform Phlegm, resolve Stagnation
25	Aconite	*Chuan Wu*	Move *Qi*, relieve pain
25	Aconite	*Cao Wu*	Move *Qi*, relieve pain
25	Arisaema	*Tian Nan Xing*	Transform Phlegm, resolve Stagnation

Di Er You (Ear Drop) 滴耳油

Di means drop. *Er* refers to ear. *You* means ointment, the form of medication.

Source: *Chinese Veterinary Herbal Handbook*, by *Huisheng Xie* and published by the Chi Institute of Chinese Medicine in 2004

Ingredients: The ingredients and actions of this formula are listed in Table 34.11.

Preparation: First, 240 g of *Huang Lian* (Coptis) are boiled three times, and 1,000 ml of herbal water extract are obtained. This water extract is mixed with 90 g *Bai Fan* (Alum) and 1.2 g *Bing Pian* (Borneal), which have been ground into a fine powder. Finally, these three are mixed with 1000 ml Glycerol as a carrier. This mixture is stored in a brown container for topical use only.

Actions: Clear Heat, dry up Damp, relieve itching, dissipate swelling

Indications: This formula is used for acute or chronic canine otitis due to excess heat, red tongue, and forceful pulse.

Dosage and Usage: Apply topically in the external ear canal. Use 2 to 7 drops 5 to 8 times a day as needed for up to 1 month.

Analysis of Formula: Damp-Heat leads to local redness, Heat, swelling, and pain. *Huang Lian* (Coptis) clears Heat, dries up Damp, detoxifies, and is the King herb. *Bai Fan* (Alum) dries up Damp, transforms Phlegm, stops bleeding, relieves itching, and is the Minister

Table 34.11. Ingredients and actions of *Di Er You*.

%	English Name	Chinese *Pin-Yin*	Actions
83.3	Coptis	*Huang Lian*	Clear heat, detoxify
16.5	Alum	*Bai Fan*	Dry up Damp, transform Phlegm, stop bleeding, relieve itching
0.2	Borneol	*Bing Pian*	Clear Heat, relieve pain, dissipate swelling

herb. *Bing Pian* (Borneol) clears Heat, relieves pain, opens the orifices, dissipates swelling, and is the Adjuvant herb. *Gan You* (Glycerol) acts as a carrier and is the Messenger herb.

Cautions and Contraindications: This formula is for topical use in the ear canal only. It should be cautioned if the tympanic membrane is ruptured.

Dr. Xie's Comments: I have used *Di Er You* for the treatment of otitis externa in dogs.

Pi Jie Gao (Dermo-Paste) 皮疥膏

Pi is skin. *Jie* is mange or skin parasite. *Gao* refers to paste, the form of the medication. *Pi Jie Gao* translates to Paste for Skin Parasites.

Source: *Chinese Veterinary Herbal Handbook*, by *Huisheng Xie* and published by the Chi Institute of Chinese Medicine in 2004

Ingredients: The ingredients and actions of this formula are listed in Table 34.12.

Preparation: The first seven ingredients are ground into a fine powder and then mixed with beeswax and olive oil to make a paste that is stored in a container for topical use.

Actions: Clear Wind to stop itching, dry up Damp, kill parasites and fungi

Indications: This formula is used for skin itching and fungal skin infections due to Damp-Heat. Typically, the tongue is red with a greasy coating and the pulse is fast and forceful.

Dosage and Usage: Apply topically directly on the skin lesion(s) 5 to 8 times a day as needed up to 1 month.

Table 34.12. Ingredients and actions of *Pi Jie Gao*.

%	English Name	Chinese Pin-Yin	Actions
17	Dictamnus	*Bai Xian Pi*	Clear Wind, dry up Damp, clear Heat, detoxify
17	Kochia	*Di Fu Zi*	Clear Heat, drain Damp, stop itching
13.4	Stemona	*Bai Bu*	Kill parasites, moisten the Lung and stop cough
17	Sophora	*Ku Shen*	Clear Heat, dry up Damp, clear Wind, kill parasites
17	Alum	*Bai Fan*	Dry up Damp, transform Phlegm, relieve itching
1.6	Zanthoxylum	*Hua Jiao*	Warm the Middle, move *Qi*, relieve pain, dry damp
17	Pseudolarix	*Tu Jing Pi*	Kill and inhibit fungi

Analysis of Formula: *Bai Bu* (Stemona) and *Tu Jing Pi* (Pseudolarix) kill and inhibit fungi or parasites and are the King herbs. *Bai Xian Pi* (Dictamnus), *Di Fu Zi* (Kochia), *Ku Shen* (Sophora), and *Bai Fan* (Alum) dry up Damp, transform Phlegm, and relieve itching, and are the Minister herbs. *Hua Jiao* (Zanthoxylum) can warm the Middle, move *Qi*, relieve pain, dry up Damp, and is the Adjuvant herb. *Gan Lan You* (Olive oil) and *Feng La* (Beeswax) act as carriers and are the Messenger herbs.

Cautions and Contraindications: This formula is for topical use only.

Dr. Xie's Comments: I have used *Pi Jie Gao* for the treatment of fungal skin infections in horses and dogs.

Yu He Gao (Healing Salve) 愈合膏

Yu He refers to healing. *Gao* is the salve, the form of the medication. Literally, *Yu He Gao* means Healing Salve.

Source: *Chinese Veterinary Herbal Handbook*, written by *Huisheng Xie* and published by the Chi Institute of Chinese Medicine in 2004

Ingredients: Ingredients and actions of this formula are listed in Table 34.13.

Preparation: The first eight ingredients are ground into a fine powder, mixed with beeswax and olive oil to make a paste, and then stored in a container for topical use.

Actions: Invigorate Blood, dissipate swelling, relieve pain, astringently consolidate wound, promote healing

Table 34.13. Ingredients and actions of *Yu He Gao*.

%	English Name	Chinese Pin-Yin	Actions
5.5	Borneol	*Bing Pian*	Clear Heat, relieve pain, dissipate swelling
10.9	Draconis	*Xue Jie*	Dissipate Stagnation, relieve pain, promote healing
10.9	Olibanum	*Ru Xiang*	Invigorate Blood, relieve pain, repair tissues
18.2	Gypsum	*Shi Gao*	Astringently consolidate wound, promote healing
10.9	Draconis	*Long Gu*	Astringently consolidate wound, promote healing
10.9	Myrrh	*Mo Yao*	Invigorate Blood, relieve pain, repair tissues
10.9	Angelica	*Bai Zhi*	Clear the surface, relieve pain, promote healing
10.9	Rheum	*Da Huang*	Break down Stasis, dissipate swelling, cool Blood
10.9	Alum	*Ming Fan*	Dry Damp, promote healing

Indications: This formula is used for slow-healing wounds (including abscesses and ulcers).

Dosage and Usage:

Horse: Apply topically directly on the skin lesion. Spread the salve on a clean gauze pad, apply directly to the wound, and bandage normally. Leave on for 12 hours and then remove the bandage for 12 hours. Repeat the cycle as needed for up to 1 month until the wound is healed.

Dog/Cat: Apply topically directly on the skin lesion, 2 to 4 times daily for 5 to 10 days.

Analysis of Formula: This formula is indicated for nonhealing wounds due to *Qi* Stagnation and Dampness. Serving as the King herbs, *Xue Jie* (Draconis), *Mo Yao* (Myrrh), and *Ru Xiang* (Olibanum) move *Qi* and Blood to relieve pain and promote granulation and the healing process. *Shi Gao* (Gypsum), *Long Gu* (Draconis), *Ming Fan* (Alum), and *Bai Zhi* (Angelica) function as the Minister herbs to astringently consolidate the local tissues, promote granulation and healing, and close wounds. Serving as the Adjuvant herbs, *Da Huang* (Rheum) breaks down Stasis, dissipates swelling, and cools the Blood; *Bing Pian* (Borneol) clears Heat and reduces swelling. *Gan Lan You* (Olive oil) and *Feng La* (Beeswax) are carriers and work as Messenger herbs.

Cautions and Contraindications: This formula is for topical use only. Accidental oral ingestion must be prevented in pregnant animals. In cats, topical application might induce vomiting if the cat licks the wound.

Dr. Xie's Comments: I have used *Yu He Gao* for the treatment of chronic nonhealing wounds in horses and dogs.

Bo Yun San (Clearing the Opacity) 拨云散

Bo means clearing. *Yun* refers to opacity, or nebula. *San* is the powder form of the medication. Thus, *Bo Yun* means Clearing the Opacity.

Source: *Chinese Veterinary Herbal Handbook*, written by *Huisheng Xie* and published by the Chi Institute of Chinese Medicine in 2004

Ingredients: The ingredients and actions of this formula are listed in Table 34.14.

Preparation: All ingredients are ground into a fine powder and stored in a container for topical use.

Actions: Clear Heat, detoxify, brighten eyes, resolve swelling, resolve nebula

Table 34.14. Ingredients and actions of *Bo Yun San*.

%	English Name	*Pin Yin*	Actions
33	Borneol	*Bing Pian*	Clear Heat, resolve swelling, stop pain
33	Borax	*Peng Sha*	Clear Heat, detoxify
17	Calamina	*Lu Gan Shi*	Detoxify, brighten eyes, stop itching
17	Cinnabaris	Zhu Sha	Detoxify to treat sores

Indications: This formula is used to treat various ocular conditions: Keratoconjunctivitis Sicca, chronic conjunctivitis, keratitis, uveitis, Equine Recurrent Uveitis due to Liver Heat/Fire with local Stagnation, swollen eyelids, ocular discharge, opacity of the cornea, miosis, photophobia, grey or blue nebula (turbidity of the cornea), red or purple tongue, and surging and fast (or weak) pulse.

Dosage and Usage: Apply topically directly inside the eyelids. Dust the tip of a cotton ball, place it adjacent to the eye(s), and gently blow the powder into the eye(s) 2 to 4 times a day, as needed, for up to 5 days. You will achieve better results if you use the oral medicaton *Jue Ming San* concurrently.

Analysis of Formula: This formula is indicated for inflammatory eye conditions due to Liver Heat or Fire with local Stagnation. Serving as the King herb, *Lu Gan Shi* (Calamina) clears Heat, detoxifies, brightens eyes, and stops itching. *Peng Sha* (Borax) and *Zhu Sha* (Cinnabaris) are the Minister ingredients that clear excess Heat and detoxify. *Bing Pian* (Borneol) clears Heat and reduces swelling and serves as the Adjuvant and Messenger herbs.

Cautions and Contraindications: This formula is for topical use only.

Dr. Xie's Comments: I have used *Bo Yun San* for the treatment of inflammatory ocular conditions, including Keratoconjunctivitis Sicca (KCS) in dogs and Equine Recurrent Uveitis (ERU) in horses.

REFERENCES

1. Li Q. 120 cases of fractures were treated with *Ru Yi Jin Huang San*. Liaoning Journal of Traditional Chinese Medicine 2005;32(12):1286–1287. (In Chinese)
2. Zhang HF, Zheng JP, Qin HW. 20 Cases of sclerosis caused by intramuscular and phlebitis were treated with *Ruyi Jinhuang San*. Heilongjiang Journal of Nursing 1996;2(1):50. (In Chinese)
3. Feng GM. *Bing Peng San* for the treatment of laryngotracheitis in chicken. Sandong Traditional Chinese Medicine 2007;9:26. (In Chinese)

4. Yuan JZ. Chronic endometritis was treated with *Bing Peng San* in cows. Chinese Journal of Traditional Veterinary Medicine 2006;2:46–47. (In Chinese)
5. Ren Z, Lu AF, Lu Y. Ecthyma Contagiosa was treated with *Bing Peng San* in goats. Guizhou Animal and Veterinary Sciences 2003;27(5):24. (In Chinese)
6. Wang GL. Fistula was treated with *Sheng Ji San*. Liaoning Animal and Veterinary Sciences 2004;5:16. (In Chinese)
7. Zhang SK. Stomatitis was treated with *Qing Dai San* in sheep. Qinghai Journal of Animal and Veterinary Sciences. 2005; 35(5):28. (In Chinese)
8. Liu XL. Diagnosis and treatment on the basis of an overall analysis of the illness and the patient's condition on ulceration of the tongue. Chinese Journal of Veterinary Medicine 2005;41(2):59–60. (In Chinese)
9. Jiang XG, Wang J. Application of *Fang Fu Sheng Ji San* in wounds in small animals. Journal of Traditional Chinese Veterinary Medicine 2005;24(5):43. (In Chinese)
10. Qu CL. Application of *Nei Tuo Shengji San* in veterinary clinic. Journal of Traditional Chinese Veterinary Medicine 2005; 24(5):51–52. (In Chinese)
11. Wang TP, Wang LJ, Wang JD. 126 Cases of burns and scalds were treated with a combination of *Zi Cao You* and *Tang Huo San*. Journal of Chinese Fold Medicine 1995;10(5):32. (In Chinese)

Part 3 Clinical Application of Chinese Veterinary Herbology
中药学在临床上的应用

35 How to Integrate Chinese Herbal Medicine into Veterinary Practice
中药临床应用须知

Tiffany Rimar

"Only when one refines the old and learns from the new can one become a real doctor."

—*Huang Di Nei Jing*
(Yellow Emperor's Classic of Internal Medicine)

At first, the process of integrating herbal medicine into your veterinary practice can be intimidating, but with determination you can easily make the transition. A clear understanding of Traditional Chinese Veterinary Medicine (TCVM) tenets and diagnoses creates the foundation of your practice. Herbal preparations, energetics, properties, and methods of administration need to be understood. Knowledge of common mistakes and their prevention can build confidence and enhance clinical results. Examples of commonly used formulas can help start an herbal pharmacy. Knowledge of other medications or modalities being used is also an important consideration because this might alter an herbal plan.

When a patient presents for preventative medicine, an energetic imbalance, or a clinical disease manifestation, a Pattern diagnosis must be made based on TCVM tenets. The evaluation of the entire animal is represented by the patient's pertinent medical history, including conventional diagnostics, appetite, thirst, urination, defecation, constitution, environmental preference, signalment, and thorough physical exam. When these variables have been assessed, a TCVM diagnostic Pattern can be developed. This Pattern is formed by incorporating some or all of the following tenets: Eight Principles, *Zang-Fu* disharmonies, Six channels, Four stages, *San Jiao* Patterns, Pathogen Patterns, *Qi*, Blood and Body Fluid Patterns, and Meridian Patterns. When a Pattern has been identified, one can select a single herb or combination herbal formula appropriate for the Pattern or action desired, as well as an appropriate means of administration.

HOW TO START

History

A complete history is needed to determine the patient's overall physiological and constitutional personality state. This information helps the practitioner develop a TCVM Pattern and appropriate herbal plan. The history includes any clinical presentation, diagnostic information, or a confirmed medical diagnosis. It is also important to know whether medications have been used and the clinical or physiologic responses to that medication. When establishing an herbal treatment plan, it is also very important to discern the patient's appetite, thirst, urination, defecation, and constitution (personality), in addition to its preference for Heat or Cold, hard or soft surfaces, and busy, loud, or quiet environments.

Conventional Western medical presentation and diagnostics are the cornerstones on which to build any additional modality, including herbal medicine, into practice. The more information we can gather as scientists, the better we can treat our patients. Knowledge of any conventional disease processes, medications used, and their energetics is important when selecting an herbal plan. If a patient has an Excess Heat condition such as a bacterial infection, the cooling nature of antibiotics can help balance the entire animal. If a Deficient condition exists, such as Kidney *Qi* Deficiency, the warming nature of short-term corticosteroids may be of some benefit. However, if an animal has a Cold *Bi* Syndrome and is given cooling medication, such as NSAIDS, the *Bi* Syndrome may worsen. Even in conventional Western medicine, we are still using herbal energetic properties to treat our patients. Having knowledge of a conventional diagnosis and/or medications used can be of utmost importance when developing an herbal treatment strategy.

In addition to conventional diagnostics, the importance of an animal's appetite, thirst, bodily function, constitution, and environmental preference can help develop a TCM Pattern. For example, animals with Stomach Heat are more likely to develop polydipsia, polyphagia, coprophagia, or pica, and a *Qi* or *Yang* Deficient animal is more likely to exhibit anorexia. A pet may have an Excess Heat condition if the urine or feces has too strong an odor or if a fecal evaluation or urinalysis shows a bacterial infection. In contrast, *Qi* or *Yang* Deficiency can manifest as polyuria, hyposthenuria, isosthenuria, or loose feces. Personality and environmental factors are important to determine the constitution of the animal as Wood, Fire, Earth, Metal, or Water and can help determine an Excess or Deficient state. An Excess animal will more likely prefer a Cold or soft substrate with a quiet environment, and a Deficient animal may need to be near Heat or may prefer to lean on walls or furniture and prefer an active or loud environment. Any historic information can be useful to determine a TCVM Pattern diagnosis and herbal medications needed for that Pattern.

Signalment

The species, age, gender, reproductive status, and age of castration, if applicable, are important data to help determine the treatment plan.

The animal species can dictate the form in which the herb should be used. For example, equine patients typically consume powders better than capsules, and topical preparations are usually well tolerated. Feline patients usually prefer teapills or incorporating raw herbs or food therapy for their treatment, and they usually do not prefer topical treatments. Birds and ferrets are more easily treated with liquids and not topical preparations. Dogs are independent—some prefer powders, capsules, teapills, or raw herbs cooked in food, and some even prefer topical preparations.

Age is also a consideration. Very young or very old animals should be medicated gently because herbs that are too strong (too Hot, too Cold, too moving) may not be well tolerated. Gender considerations are relative to breeding or pregnant animals and should be treated with gentler herbs than their castrated counterparts. The exception to this occurs when specific herbs are needed for breeding or gestational disorders. Age of castration can also have an influence because animals that are altered too young may have concurrent *Jing* Deficiency manifesting or compounding of an existing condition. These animals may need a *Jing* tonic such as *Yin Yang Huo San* (Chapter 18) in addition to other herbal preparations.

Physical Exam

A TCVM physical exam includes a conventional exam with auscultation, ophthalmoscopic, and otoscopic exam, as well as evaluation using sight, smell, touch, temperature, tongue, and pulse diagnosis.

Sight This is a visual interpretation of the animal's overall presentation, including general appearance, *Shen* mental status, tongue (color, shape, moisture, and coating), skin and hair/fur coat, physical conformation, and mobility.

What is the overall general body appearance including *Shen* (spirit, mental attitude, or acuity)? A healthy animal should present with a strong demeanor, head held high, and bright eyes searching for environmental cues. If an animal presents too strong—for example, immediately trying to dominate the room or stall with hard eyes—an Excess Pattern or Heat Pattern may be present. If an animal presents with weakness, emaciation, head down, cloudy eyes, or without interest in the surrounding environment, a Deficient or Cold Pattern may exist. This may also indicate a decline in *Shen*, the manifestation of the body's psychological or emotional standpoint. For example, if an animal presents with a hot head, is easily frustrated, and displays Excessive dominating behavior, Liver *Qi* Stagnation might be present and an herbal formula is indicated to soothe stagnant Liver *Qi*. In contrast, if an animal presents with Deficient signs, such as with his head down or a depressed *Shen*, perhaps a *Yang* tonic is indicated.

How does the tongue look? Evaluation of the tongue should include the color, shape, moisture content, and coating. Due to the nature of this herbal book, tongue evaluation will be a simple overview and can be referenced in depth in *Traditional Chinese Veterinary Medicine-Fundamental Principles*.[1] The normal tongue is bright pink and full with adequate moisture. An Excess condition may be determined by a tongue that is colored dark red, yellow, or lavender, and is thin and dry with longitudinal crack lines or a thick coating. An animal with a Deficient condition may have a tongue that is pale, thick, or excessively wet. For example, if an animal presents as *Yin* Deficient with Heat signs and has a dark red tongue with deep longitudinal cracks, perhaps a *Yin* tonic could be used. How does the skin or hair/fur coat look? A healthy animal should have supple skin with a lustrous, well-groomed hair/fur coat. The exception to this includes reptiles, which should have dry skin or scales, and birds, which should have ample, well-groomed feather coverage. The TCM *Zang-Fu* Lung controls the outer body surface; therefore, disharmony can manifest as a dermatologic condition. For example, if a patient presents with a "hot spot," a clearly demarcated, erythematous, ulcerative lesion radiating Heat with a burned fur coat, an Excess Pattern of Lung Heat or Damp Heat would be indicated. If a patient presents with a dry crusting planum nasale, dandruff, and dry footpads or cracked hooves, a Blood Deficiency may be indicated and an herbal formula can be given as a Blood tonic.

How does the animal stand and move? A healthy animal should stand strong and have definitive, fluid movement with normal gait, range of motion, and conscious proprioception. The TCM *Zang-Fu* Kidney governs bone and the back end, so a Kidney disharmony can manifest as an orthopedic condition. For example, if a patient presents with a hunched or guarded posture, stilted gait, decreased or painful range of motion, and difficult or painful ambulation, an Excess condition such as intervertebral disk disease may be present. In this case, an herbal formulation can help clear Blood and *Qi* Stagnation and can be used as a transporter to the spine. If an animal presents with difficulty rising, inability to stand for long periods of time, ataxic movement, or conscious proprioceptive deficits, a Deficient condition such as Kidney *Qi* or *Yang* Deficiency may be present. Moxibustion may be indicated as a *Qi* or *Yang* tonic.

Hearing This is an audible investigation of the patient's vocalization, chewing ability, cardiac, respiratory, and gastrointestinal function.

How does your patient vocalize? A healthy animal should have a strong species-appropriate sound at appropriate times of alerting the herd, calling for a mate, or showing excitement. The voice is controlled by *Zhong-Qi*; therefore, disharmony can be associated with *Zang-Fu* Lung or Heart and can affect the strength or frequency of vocalization. A strong coarse voice or a frequent need to be heard can exemplify an Excess condition such as Lung Heat. A weak or inaudible voice can be associated with a Deficient condition such as Heart Blood Deficiency.

How is the patient chewing? A healthy pet should chew rhythmically on both sides of the mouth when eating. The Kidney governs the bones, including those of mastication. If a patient chews too delicately or makes too much noise while eating, perhaps an Excess condition of Stomach Heat or periodontal disease is present. A Deficient condition, such as Kidney *Qi* Deficiency manifesting as tooth or bone decay, may require dental care as the treatment of choice. If a large animal is chewing without food, perhaps Stomach *Qi* Stagnation is present and *Ju Pi San* (Chapter 24) can be helpful.

How does the heart sound? The cardiac sound can be appreciated by auscultation with a stethoscope or by simply placing your ear on the chest of the patient. A healthy animal will have an appropriate strength, rate, and rhythm associated with the heartbeat. Cardiac abnormalities, such as irregular rhythm, in an Excess patient can be created by a Heart *Qi* Stagnation condition, such as hypertrophic cardiomyopathy. The same irregular rhythm in a Heart *Qi* Deficient patient may be associated with functional abnormalities, such as dilated cardiomyopathy secondary to mitral valve insufficiency; and an herbal formula can be incorporated into the diet as a Blood or Heart tonic.

How is the patient breathing? Does it wheeze or cough? A healthy patient, assuming no nasal, palate, laryngeal, or other genetic defect (which would fall under the category of *Jing* Deficiency), should not cough. A balanced patient should not make Excessive noise when breathing or exhibit shortness of breath manifested as exercise intolerance. If a patient presents with a forceful, loud, hacking cough, an Excess condition such as Lung Heat may be indicated and *Qing Fei San* (Chapter 21) may be used to clear Lung Heat. If a patient presents weak with a prolonged cough or wheezing, a Deficient condition such as Lung *Yin* Deficiency may be associated and *Bai He Gu Jin Tang* (Chapter 18) may be used.

How are the patient's borborygmi? Intestinal gas motility can be appreciated by auscultation with a stethoscope or by placing your ear on the flank of a patient. A healthy animal should exhibit audible peristaltic contractions every few seconds. Increased intestinal sound or rate of contraction could be due to Heat or Cold invasion. A decreased sound or rate of peristaltic contractions could be due to Stomach *Qi* Stagnation, and ginger root can help to move the *Qi*. If constipation is present due to *Yin* or Blood Deficiency, *Dang Gui Cong Rong Tang* (Chapter 32) may be incorporated into the diet as a *Yin* or Blood tonic.

Smell This diagnostic method differentiates change of odor of the entire animal, including the outer surface, any orifice, and even the smell of urine or feces. If a patient presents with an offensive, foul odor, especially if accompanied by a discolored exudate, Heat or Damp Heat is usually present and *Long Dan Xie Gan Tang* (Chapter 21) may be indicated, or herbal food therapy may be instituted to drain Heat and Dampness. In contrast, if a patient presents dehydrated with urine that has no odor or is clear in color, further investigation of a Kidney Deficiency may be in order.

Touch Palpation is a diagnostic method used to determine energetic imbalance or pathological disease states by using the sense of touch. This diagnostic method is used to determine temperature (*Yang*), imbalance in any Meridian systems, including acupoints (*Qi*), Body Fluid content (*Yin*), range of motion or pain (*Qi*/Blood), and pulse diagnosis.

Temperature (*Yang*) is determined by using a four-finger ear technique on the concave aspect of pinna as well as using the back of the hand to evaluate the entire body. A practitioner can wrap the hand around the ear with the fingertips longitudinally equidistant on the inner pinna, the concave surface. In a healthy animal, the two fingertips closest to the head should be warm, the third finger out should be cooler, and the fingertip closest to the eartip should be the coolest. A Heat condition exists if the eartip is as warm as the base, and a Deficient or Cold condition exists if the base of the ear is as cool as the tip. The back of the practitioner's hand is used to determine the overall temperature of the animal's body as well as to determine specific areas of Heat or Cold. Body temperature is used to determine the presence of *Yang* energy and its Excess or Deficiency. If a patient presents with *Yang* Deficiency, this would be *Qi* Deficiency with Cold signs, and moxabustion can be used to warm the body and generate and move *Qi*.

To determine an imbalance in the Meridian system, a practitioner can palpate the Meridian pathways, *Shu* points (back association point) or *Mu* points (front alarm points). Palpation can determine whether there is a bulge or sensitivity as an Excess condition versus a depression for a Deficient condition. Each *Shu* point or *Mu* point corresponds to a *Zang-Fu* organ dysfunction or local issue such as *Qi* Stagnation. For example, an animal that has a depression at BL-13 or LU-1 may have Lung *Qi* or *Yin* Deficiency, where sensitivity at BL-18 or LIV-14 can indicate Liver Heat or disharmony. This diagnostic technique has no parallels in conventional medicine but is incredibly useful in TCVM diagnostics and herbal treatments.

Body Fluid content (*Yin*) can be determined by visualizing swelling or dander or by palpating edema or dryness of the patient's skin. An animal with normal *Yin* will have soft skin with appropriate elasticity. A *Yang* Deficient/*Yin* Excess animal may have pitting edema or be stocked up. In contrast, a *Yin* or Blood Deficient animal will have small or large flake dander, respectively. The exception to this is when evaluating birds and reptiles, because they should be dry and flaky naturally. Frogs and salamanders should be moist and plump with no Dry signs. Based on these Patterns and species considerations, a practitioner can select an appropriate herb or formula to drain Excess fluid, such as *Wu Ling San* (Chapter 23), to nourish *Yin*, such as *Zeng Ye Tang* (Chapter 18), or to nourish Blood, such as *Si Wu Tang* (Chapter 18).

Range of motion or pain (*Qi*/Blood Stagnation) can be assessed by a general orthopedic exam. A palpable orthopedic exam should yield appropriate range of motion without pain or weakness. If there is mild pain elicited with significant palpable pressure, *Qi* Stagnation at the Channels is indicated and *Huo Luo Xiao Ling Dan* (Chapter 27) may be helpful. If very mild digital pressure or general range of motion evokes a significant pain response, Blood Stagnation is indicated and *Shen Tong Zhu Yu Tang* (Chapter 27) can be used to help clear this Stagnation. If an animal exhibits hind-end weakness upon palpation, Kidney *Qi* Deficiency may be diagnosed, and *Bu Yang Huan Wu Tang* (Chapter 27) may be helpful.

Pulse diagnosis is one of the most important palpable characteristics for Pattern differentiation. Due to the nature of this herbal book, pulse diagnosis will be a simple overview and can be referenced in depth in *Traditional Chinese Veterinary Medicine-Fundamental Principles*.[1] The location of the pulse used for pulse diagnosis varies among species. Dogs, cats, pigs, and reptiles are palpated at the femoral artery; horses and turtles at the carotid or maxillary; cows at the median caudal; and birds at the axillary. A three-finger palpation, using fingertips only, is preferable to appreciate the Upper *Jiao*, Middle *Jiao*, and Lower *Jiao* signified by the index, middle, and ring finger, respectively. The left side of the animal relative to the Upper, Middle, and Lower *Jiao* reflects the energetics of the Heart, Liver, and Kidney *Yin*/Blood, respectively. The right side of the animal relative to the Upper, Middle, and Lower Burners (*Jiao*) reflects the energetics of the Lung, Spleen, and Kidney *Qi*/*Yang*, respectively. If a practitioner can just appreciate a difference of the right versus the left side pulse, a relative Pattern can be differentiated. For example, if a 6-year-old castrated, male Boxer presents for episodes of exercise intolerance, syncope, and has an audible heart murmur and pulses weaker on the left than the right, Heart *Qi* Deficiency may be diagnosed and *Yang Xin Tang* (Chapter 18) may be indicated.

A good history, signalment, and physical exam are the most important tools to create an appropriate herbal treatment course for bodily imbalances. Noticing details of patients' presentation and environmental preference is necessary to see the patient as a whole and not just as a clinical disease. When all variables are seen, a proper diagnosis can be made and appropriate herbal treatment can be implemented.

TRADITIONAL CHINESE VETERINARY MEDICINE—PATTERN DIFFERENTIATION

Pattern differentiation for diagnostic purposes, known as *Bian Zheng*, allows the practitioner to appropriately select a treatment method for each individual patient. *Bian Zheng* includes the following: Eight Principles, *Zang-Fu* disharmonies, Six channels, Four stages, *San Jiao* Patterns, Pathogen Patterns, *Qi*, Blood and Body Fluid Patterns, and Meridian Patterns. Only the most basic and common diagnostic Patterns will be reviewed herein. Further Patterns and greater in-depth information relative to *Bian Zheng* can be researched in other TCVM texts.

Eight Principles/Six Roots

The Eight principles encompass the six roots of Interior/Exterior, Cold/Heat, and Deficiency/Excess within the super-category of *Yin* and *Yang*. *Yin* implies Interior, Cold and Deficiency, while *Yang* implies Exterior, Heat, and Excess.

Yin*/*Yang The *Yin*/*Yang* Pattern is used to summarize the three pairs of principles as well as an individual Pattern. *Yin* refers to Interior, Deficiency, and Cold but also as chronic illness, inactivity, weakness, depression, the downward or inward nature of pathology due to *Zheng-Qi* (antipathogenic *Qi*) Deficiency, or *Xie Qi* (pathogenic *Qi*) retention. *Yang* refers to Exterior, Excess, and Heat, as well as acute disease, fever, hyperactive, hypermetabolic states, the upward or outward nature of pathology due to hyperactivity of *Yang Qi* and Excess pathogenic Heat.

Interior/Exterior Pattern The Interior/Exterior Pattern determines the location or depth of pathology. The Exterior includes the skin, hair, muscle, fascia, and everything among them, as well as the superficial aspects of the Meridians and their collaterals. The Exterior is then further subdivided into Exterior Heat, Exterior Cold, Exterior Excess, and Exterior Deficiency. The Interior includes the *Zang-Fu* organs, vessels, lymphatics, bone, and the nervous system. This could be analogous to the difference between an acute and a chronic disease.

Cold/Heat Pattern The Cold/Heat Pattern determines the nature of the pathogen. The Cold Pattern can be Interior or Exterior, Excess or Deficient Cold. Excess Cold is usually due to pathogenic invasion by itself or accompanied by Wind. The Heat Pattern can be Interior or Exterior. Interior Heat can be Excess or Deficient Heat, and external Heat is usually caused by the invasion of Wind-Heat, Summer-Heat, or Dryness. Excess Heat can arise from severe Wind-Cold invasion.

Deficiency/Excess Pattern The Deficiency/Excess Pattern determines the strength of *Zheng Qi* (antipathogenic *Qi*) and *Xie Qi* (pathogenic *Qi*). Deficiency Patterns usually arise from chronic disease, overwork, or Body Fluid loss and encompass *Yin*, *Yang*, *Qi*, and Blood. Excess Patterns are usually due to exogenous pathogens that override the body's immune system. Excess pathogens include Wind, Cold, Heat, Dampness, Summer Heat, and Dryness. Excess can also be secondary to Stagnation of *Qi*, Blood, Phlegm, and Food.

Examples

1. "Miss Sally," a 12-year-old intact, female, quarter horse presented for pitting edema of her hind legs from flank to fetlock, a condition that waxed and waned several times per year during the past 3 years. Her tongue was pale and wet, pulses were weaker on the right side, and temperature was cool on ears, limbs, and back. Her *Shen* was mildly depressed. Miss Sally was diagnosed as a Kidney *Yang* Deficiency, an Interior, Cold, Deficiency Pattern. The herbal treatment was moxabustion along her Governing Vessel Meridian 3 times daily to warm her internally and added *Shen Qi Wan* (Chapter 18) to warm and tonify her Kidney *Yang*.
2. "Max," a 7-year-old castrated, male Doberman presented for a behavioral issue of attacking any dog in his path. Mood-altering medications and behavior modification were unsuccessful. His tongue was lavender-red and ear temperature was warm, but the top of his head and his body were radiating Heat, his pulses were bounding and fast, and his nose and footpads had become depigmented. Max was diagnosed with Interior Heat and treated with *Xi Xin San* (Chapter 21) to clear the Interior Heat from the Heart.

Zang-Fu Pattern

This means of Pattern differentiation is in terms of pathological manifestation and physiological function of *Zang-Fu* organs. It denotes the location, nature, and Pattern of disharmony or pathology. *Zang-Fu* Pattern differentiation dates back to the Warring States period (475–221 BC) when the Yellow Emperor's Canon on Internal Medicine was published. The *Zang-Fu* systems are usually described as the *Yin* organ relative to the Five Elements. The *Zang-Fu* Five Elements describe the location of disharmony relative to the Liver, Heart, Spleen, Lung, and Kidney systems. When diagnosing a Pattern, an exact organ should be identified as affected, and then the Eight Principles can further describe how that organ is affected. This is the core of TCVM diagnosis. For example, if a patient presents for thunderstorm phobia, the pathology is associated with the Heart. This phobia can manifest from an Interior, Excess condition such as Heart Heat or *Yin* Deficient False Heat. It can also manifest from an Interior, Cold, Deficiency Pattern such as Blood Deficiency.

Four Stages or Four Levels

The Four stages or Four levels, known as *Wei*, *Qi*, *Ying*, and *Xue* are used to describe the depth and development of acute febrile diseases. The disease is typically induced by Excess Heat and is able to flourish because *Zheng Qi* (antipathogenic *Qi*) is too weak to defend the strong *Xie Qi* (pathogenic *Qi*). These are important levels to differentiate so that practitioners can appreciate which level to treat and which herbal application should be used. The *Wei* stage is easily treated with diet or antibiotics and the *Ying* or *Xue* stage is best treated with herbal medications:

1. The *Wei* stage is the defensive stage at the superficial level of the body. This includes the outer body surface, skin, muscles, and joints.
2. The *Qi* stage includes internal organs as well as Lung, Stomach, and Large Intestines.
3. The *Ying* stage is the nutrient level, including the nervous system as well as the Heart, Pericardium, and *Shen*.
4. The *Xue* stage is the deepest stage at the level of Blood.

Pathogen Patterns

Many Patterns exist to describe pathogenic invasion of the body. Six major pathogens are most commonly used when integrating TCVM into a conventional practice. Other pathogen Patterns can be referenced in TCM textbooks. The six most common pathogenic Patterns are Wind, Cold, Heat, Summer-Heat, Damp, and Dry:

1. **Wind** is the master pathogen because it can invade and move anywhere. This pathogen includes pruritus and seizures.
2. **Cold** is considered a *Yin* pathogen, obstructs *Qi* and Blood flow, and can lead to Stagnation and therefore pain or stiffness.
3. **Heat** can be internal, external, acute, or chronic.
4. **Summer-Heat** usually occurs in the summer and is associated with extreme Heat. This pathogen can combine with Damp-Heat or Damp-Cold.
5. **Damp** is a pathogen that is heavy and obstructs *Qi* or Blood flow and can yield Stagnation. It can manifest as masses or cancer.
6. **Dry** usually occurs during times or geographic locations of extremely low humidity. This pathogen consumes Body Fluid. It can manifest as dermatologic conditions, asthma, or even epilepsy.

Qi, Blood, and Body Fluid Patterns

Qi, Blood, and Body Fluid are imperative substances for the physiologic functions of the body. These substances are produced by *Gu Qi* (food essence), distributed by the Meridian system to the *Zang-Fu* organs. Disharmony in any of the systems can lead to pathological conditions:

1. ***Qi*** is the vital energetic force of the entire body. Pathology can be described in terms of Deficiency, Stagnation, rebellious, or sinking.
2. **Blood** nourishes Body Fluid associated with Spleen, Kidney, Heart, and Liver. The Spleen and Kidney make the Blood (Spleen *Qi* also holds the Blood in the vessels), the Heart moves the Blood, and the Liver stores the Blood. Pathology can be described as Deficiency, Heat, Cold, or hemorrhage.
3. **Body Fluid** nourishes the body and is associated with Spleen, Lung, Stomach, Small Intestine, Kidney, Bladder and *San-Jiao*. The associated organs or levels separate clear fluid (to nourish the body) from turbid fluid (to be excreted from the body). Pathology can include Internal Dryness, Edema, or Phlegm.

Now that you have all the tools to make an accurate TCVM diagnosis, herbal formulas, preparations, energetics, and properties need to be understood to treat these pathologies. Once you select an herbal formula to balance the TCVM Pattern, you are ready to go. An important aspect when incorporating many modalities of healing and medicine is to know everything the animal is being treated with so far. This allows the practitioner to appropriately select a balanced treatment plan for the pathology or imbalance at hand.

For example, a patient presents with a *Jing* Deficiency leading to Liver *Qi* Stagnation, which causes clinical gastrointestinal disorder (Spleen and Stomach) signs including intermittent anorexia, vomiting, and diarrhea. All laboratory tests and radiographs are unremarkable; the patient has been living on famotidine and metronidazole for over 1 year and still having breakthrough events. In this example, the medications have been addressing only the clinical manifestation and not the root problem. The medications are cooling and will therefore work symptomatically, but they will not solve the root problem. Initially, the treatment should be to clear Liver *Qi* Stagnation and harmonize the Spleen and Stomach with *Xiao Yao San* (Chapter 24). After the GI disorders are under control, the *Jing* Deficiency (the underlying problem) needs to be addressed further with *Yin Yang Huo San* (Chapter 18).

HERBAL ADMINISTRATION

When integrating herbal medicine into practice, appreciating various administration forms and techniques is essential. Administering herbal medicine, much like the tenets of TCVM, is a very unique process for each individual patient. It is the job of the practitioner to evaluate the patient, the environment, and the humans associated in order to implement an appropriate herbal strategy. A variety of herbal forms offers the practitioner the artistic liberty to create and change herbal medicine to best suit all needs. The most common forms of herbal administration are powders, capsules, tablets, teapills, liquids, tinctures, flavored compounds, raw herbs, pastes, and moxibustion.[2–8]

Powders

Powders are a very common form of herbal medicine because they are very versatile. Orally, they are readily absorbed from the GI tract, and rectally they are absorbed to a lesser extent. Some herbal formulas are very bitter and may not be as palatable as others.

Powders can be refrigerated to cut down the taste and dust, mixed with honey or molasses for palatability, or encapsulated for pilling. They can also be mixed with various liquids, such as chicken broth, tuna juice, or fruit juice to entice the patient. Powders can also be mixed with water, aloe, vitamin E, or even vinegar and used topically. Herbs that have a very bitter taste can be perfect for topical treatments because animals are less likely to lick them off, therefore enabling a longer contact time.

Capsules, Tablets, and Teapills

Capsules, tablets, and teapills are very convenient because owners can disguise them in food or just pill the medication into the animal.

Teapills tend to be the easiest form of pill because they are sweet and round; they glide down the throat easily and leave a sweet aftertaste. They can also be dissolved in warm water and syringed to the uncooperative patient. This form is very convenient for the feline or very small dog patient.

Liquids, Tinctures, and Flavored Compounds

Liquids, tinctures, and flavored compounds can be used to syringe medications orally. Some liquids are made with honey or royal jelly, and the sweet flavor is palatable to most animals. Tinctures are usually made with alcohol or purified water. Alcohol preparations may not be palatable or appropriate for some animals. Purified water tinctures may taste better and do not have the adversity of alcohol, but they do not have the same shelf-life longevity. Flavored compounds can be made from the powders into any flavor imaginable.

Raw Herbs

Raw herbs can be made into decoctions or mixed with home-cooked food preparations. Some raw herbs can also be given directly as a medicated treat. For example, dried Crataegus (*Sha Zha*, Chapter 9) can be soaked, and the sweet, flavorful fruit can be given to any patient with cardiac issues or one that may need a gentle Blood tonic. Dogs and horses love this little treat and it also nourishes the human-animal bond.

Pastes

Pastes are primarily used topically. Some pastes are purchased prepared, and others can be made based on the needs of the patient. For example, a practitioner can purchase the paste form of *Ru Yi Jin Huang San* (Chapter 34) to use as an antimicrobial wound dressing or mix its powder form with organic honey for enhanced granulation. Coptis (*Huang Lian*, Chapter 4) powder can be used topically on an open wound, such as a lick granuloma, to clear Heat. It also has such a horrific taste that most animals will not try to lick it off more than once. If they like to lick it off, it can be mixed with vinegar to enhance the bitter taste and applied to fully intact skin (contraindicated on ulcerated skin). If they still lick it off, they are probably self medicating, and a small amount can be added to the food as well used topically.

Moxibustion

Moxibustion is considered a topical herb made from ground mugwort and is burned atop an acupuncture needle or above the skin and transdermally absorbed. The herb is available as a loose powder, in small and large sticks. This herbal treatment is used to promote the flow of *Qi* and Blood; relieve Stagnation, swelling, and pain; and enhance humoral and cell-mediated immunity. Moxibustion treatments are well tolerated by most animals, but they should not be used in a closed space if an animal has a respiratory condition, because the smoke can be a respiratory irritant. This treatment should be used cautiously with birds, reptiles, and amphibians because it may be too warming or drying for these animals.

Having a firm knowledge of herbal forms and means of administration can help make a practitioner successful with a complete herbal pharmacy. Sometimes practitioners get overwhelmed trying to incorporate the herbal medicine into their practice. Having an awareness of some common mistakes and how to avoid them can help to enhance the practitioner's clinical results and decrease the anxiety about getting started.

FIVE MOST COMMON MISTAKES

Treating Symptoms and Not the TCVM Pattern

While this may alleviate the clinical symptoms at hand for a short time, it will not solve the problem. It is appropriate to use herbs to relieve acute clinical manifestations as long as the majority of the formula plan addresses the root imbalance.

Using Too Many Herbs at One Time

Select three or less formulas to treat the primary Pattern. This would include moxabustion because it can be a strong means of treatment. Other topical herbal preparations can be used in conjunction with up to three oral formulas.

Trying to Treat Too Many Conditions

Pick the primary problem and Pattern seen at the time of examination. Do not treat the history of clinical symptoms the owner is observing. Treat what you see in the present moment.

Expecting Herbal Medicine to Work as Quickly as Western Medication

The goal of herbal medicine is to address the root cause of imbalance, not treat the symptoms; therefore, this can take time. Herbal medicine is much gentler than Western medications and can take longer for a physiochemical response.

Tunnel Vision

It is tempting to get entangled following a specific pathophysiologic disease and to focus on clearing the symptoms. However, it is important to look at the entire animal, including its environment and emotional standpoint.

TOP 10 HERBS TO START AN HERBAL PHARMACY

Starting an herbal pharmacy can be overwhelming. This is because most practitioners are unsure of the most common herbal medicines used in an integrative or complete TCVM practice. The most common herbal medicines used are based on the most common Patterns seen in practice. The top 5 are "must have" herbal formulas; 6–10 are "should have" formulas. These categories are divided into both small-animal and large-animal medications. Most of the large-animal formulas are primarily for horses, but they are also applicable to farm animals. The author believes the top 10 are all "must have" formulas!

Small-Animal "Must Have" Herbal Formulas

1. *Sheng Tong Zhu Yu Tang* (Chapter 27)—musculoskeletal pain, *Qi* and Blood Stagnation
2. *Long Dan Xie Gan Tang* (Chapter 21)—dermatitis, otitis, Liver Damp Heat
3. *Du Huo Ji Sheng Tang* (Chapter 23)—arthritis, Bony *Bi* Syndrome
4. *Xiang Shan Liu Jun Zi Tang* (Chapter 18)—vomiting, poor appetite, body weight loss, chronic inflammatory bowel disease (IBD)
5. *Yunnan Bai Yao* (Chapter 26)—helps stop hemorrhage, Stagnation, and pain (topical/oral)

Small-Animal "Should Have" Herbal Formulas

6. *Liu Wei Di Huang Wan* (Chapter 18)—renal failure, Cushing's disease due to *Yin* Deficiency
7. *An Shen Fang* (Chapter 29)—behavioral anxiety, aggression due to Heart *Yin* and Blood *Yin* Deficiency with Liver *Qi* Stagnation
8. *Ba Zheng San* (Chapter 23)—urinary tract infection (UTI), hematuria, or urinary crystals
9. *Shen Ling Bai Zhu San* (Chapter 18)—chronic diarrhea due to Spleen *Qi* Deficiency
10. *Ru Yi Jin Huang San* (Chapter 34)—any open infectious wound due to Damp Heat (topical)

Large-Animal "Must Have" Herbal Formulas

1. *Sheng Tong Zhu Yu Tang* (Chapter 27)—musculoskeletal pain, *Qi* and Blood Stagnation
2. *Wu Shen San* (Chapter 18)—skin itching, hair loss due to Blood or/and *Yin* Deficiency with Heat
3. *An Shen Fang* (Chapter 29)—stall anxiety, aggression due to Heart *Yin* and Blood *Yin* Deficiency with Liver *Qi* Stagnation
4. *Chai Hu Shu Gan San* (Chapter 24)—liver problems or behavioral aggression due to Liver *Qi* Stagnation
5. *Qi Sai Fang* (Chapter 18)—poor performance due to *Qi* Deficiency with Stagnation

Large-Animal "Should Have" Herbal Formulas

6. *Hu Xi Cang* (Chapter 18)—recurrent airway obstruction, heaves, or chronic obstructive pulmonary disease due to Lung *Qi* Deficiency with Heat
7. *Yin Qiao San* (Chapter 19)—upper airway infection, Wind-Heat
8. *Du Huo Ji Sheng Tang* (Chapter 23)—arthritis, Bony *Bi* Syndrome
9. *Bai He Gu Jin Tang* (Chapter 18)—chronic cough due to Lung *Qi* Deficiency
10. *Jue Ming San* (Chapter 21)—Equine recurrent uveitis due to Liver Heat and Stagnation

Many other herbal formulas exist and are commonly used in practice. These are the most common herbs the author uses on a daily basis. Some of these can be used both orally and topically. The combinational uses are listed; otherwise, the formula is assumed as oral use. Do not let this inhibit the imagination from devising new topical applications from oral herbal formulas. The only limitations we have are those we put on ourselves.

OTHER TIPS TO HELP BEGINNERS START AN HERBAL PHARMACY AND HERBAL PRACTICE

Top Five Raw Herbs to Incorporate into any Herbal Pharmacy, Small or Large Animal

Having a few raw herbs in any herbal pharmacy is imperative. This enables the practitioner to enhance formulas already chosen or to use them independently. Raw herbs can be decocted and used as a broth over feed, through a tube, or with a syringe, or used when making a home-cooked diet. They can also be used for gentle treatment if a strong formula is not needed but a single herbal action is appropriate. These are the top five raw herbs the author uses most commonly:

1. *Chen Pi* (Citrus) (Chapter 8)—bitter, regulates *Qi*, transforms Phlegm
2. *Da Zao* (Jujube) (Chapter 1)—sweet, tonifies Blood, strengthens middle Jiao
3. *Fu Ling* (Poria) (Chapter 7)—neutral, drains Damp, harmonizes the mind
4. *Shan Zha* (Crataegus) (Chapter 9)—sour, reduces food or Blood Stagnation, dissolves masses
5. *Yi Yi Ren* (Coix) (Chapter 7)—sweet, promotes urination, strengthens Spleen

Incorporate Different Herbal Forms

Every animal is unique and individual, so if one form of herbal treatment is challenging, simply modify that form or try a new one. For example, if an animal will not eat the powder on food try to refrigerate it and mix it with a flavored broth, molasses, honey, or fruit preserves. If that does not work, try capsules or teapills. If the owners are unable to pill the patient, they can decoct some raw herbs and slowly introduce the broth into the diet.

Incorporate Different Herbal Preparations

Sometimes an animal may need different oral or topical preparations. These can be used concurrently or in different combinations relative to the pathological transformation. For example, a severely arthritic animal may need oral formulas, raw herbs as a treat with a very subtle property (such as *Sha Zha*), topical analgesics daily (such as *Zhen Gu Shui*, or commercial tincture) and moxabustion several times per week. Some of these may taper as the animal improves.

Knowledge of Other Medications Used When Starting Herbal Therapy

Do not use pharmaceutical and herbal medications with the same properties concurrently for too long. Starting Western pharmaceuticals and Chinese herbal formulas together is appropriate because Chinese herbs take a longer time before serum concentration yields an onset of action. Keeping a patient on both for too long may be detrimental. Overmedicating with a specific action can manifest a completely different problem. For example, a patient presents with acute cardiogenic pulmonary edema and dyspnea. Pulses are weak, especially on the right side, the tongue is thick and pale with a thick white coating, and temperature is cool. Heart *Qi* and *Yang* Deficiency is diagnosed. *Yang Xin Tang* (Chapter 18) and Poria (*Fu Ling*) (Chapter 7) may be used with cardiac medications, such as ACE inhibitors and diuretics, until clinical signs resolve. When the emergency becomes a chronic condition, pharmaceuticals can be weaned off and herbs can be continued. When the patient becomes more balanced through acupuncture and diet, the herbal medications can be reduced or eliminated as well.

GENERAL EXAMPLES OF HOW TO INTEGRATE HERBAL MEDICINE INTO PRACTICE

Example 1

"Roxanne," a 5-year-old, spayed, female, American Staffordshire Terrier presented for behavioral aggression. She primarily exhibited intermittent, unprovoked, severe bouts of death defying aggression toward one of her housemates. Roxanne's owner could usually snap her out of these attacks if she was near. If she was not present to control the situation, Roxanne has gone so far as to completely destroy a metal crate to get out of it and attack the housemate. Interestingly, she has caused only minor injury to her geriatric, arthritic housemate, whom she could kill quite easily. This housemate was usually the boss of the house in a very passive yet definitive way. Roxanne obviously wanted to be the top dog, second in command to the human. Roxanne is one of the sweetest, happiest, loving dogs I have ever had the pleasure of meeting; she just goes crazy sometimes as though in an uncontrollable trance. Her tongue is dark purple with prominent longitudinal crack lines, a deep central groove, and white coating; her pulses are bounding and slippery, excessive on the right side; her temperature is hot everywhere, especially the top of the head. CBC, chemistry profile, urinalysis are unremarkable, Thyroid panel including autoantibodies-WNL and radiographs of the entire body are unremarkable. Acepromazine, Diazepam, Alprazolam, and Clopiramine had little to no effect during the rage attacks and overly sedated or knocked her out when in a normal state of mind.

Roxanne was diagnosed with Heart Phlegm-Fire *Shen* disturbance and put on high doses of *Zhen Xin San* (Chapter 29), raw food, weekly acupuncture, and behavior modification classes. In less than 2 months they had a happy household.

Example 2

"Luke," a 10-month-old, castrated, male, mixed-breed puppy current on vaccines (RV, DHPPC, BB) presented for purulent nasal and ocular discharge and a productive cough of 1 week duration, getting progressively worse. Luke was febrile, tachycardic, and tachypnic. CBC yielded neutrophilia with a left shift, monocytosis, and lymphopenia; chemistry profile with electrolytes yielded increased ALP, hyponatremia, hypokalemia; urinalysis revealed an elevated microalbuminuria; thoracic radiographs yielded a diffuse interstitial to bronchiolar Pattern. His tongue was dark red and dry; pulses were wiry and fast, with the left pulse weaker than the right; temperature was hot on ears, top of head (CV 20), and at CV 14. Luke was diagnosed with Wind-Heat. This was an Exterior, Excess Heat Pattern moving Interior with Phlegm. He was treated with fluid therapy, a one-time injection of Penn-G, oral aloe liquid, probiotics, a multivitamin with iron, vitamin C, eucalyptus essential oil steam with coupage several times daily, acupuncture, *Yin Qiao San* (Chapter 19), and *Wei Qi Bu* (Chapter 18) to clear Heat, strengthen the Lung, and increase the immune system. Within 2 days Jake was acting like himself; within 5 days he had cleared clinical symptoms; within 2 weeks his blood work was back to normal.

Herbal Medicine is an essential part of total body wellness and can be incorporated into practice with ease and harmony. With a working knowledge of TCVM tenets, a Pattern diagnosis can be made. The diagnosis is based on a cornucopia of information, both in conventional medicine including a history, signalment, and physical exam, as well as a TCVM evaluation including tongue, pulse, temperature, and *Shen*. Knowledge of any other medications or modalities used is also important. When the entire picture has been painted, the finishing touch is the herbal selection. This selection is based on herbal energetics, properties, and administration techniques. Having knowledge of some common mistakes will help prevent them. Knowing some common herbal formulas will allow a practitioner to start an herbal pharmacy with confidence. The last and final step to integrate herbal medicine into practice is to just do it and have fun with it! Your patients will thank you for it!

REFERENCES

1. Xie HS, Preast V. Traditional Chinese Veterinary Medicine—Fundamental Principles. Reddick, FL: Jing Tang, 2005.
2. Li DQ. Prescriptions of Traditional Chinese Medicine. Shanghai: Publishing House of Shanghai University of Traditional Chinese Medicine, 1988.
3. Holmes P. The Traditional Chinese Medicine Materia Medica Clinical Reference and Study Guide. Boulder, CO: Snow Lotus Press, 2002.
4. Zhu M. The Medical Classic of the Yellow Emperor—Translation. Beijing: Foreign Language Press, 2001.
5. Xu XC. The English-Chinese Encyclopedia of Practical Traditional Chinese Medicine—Maintaining Your Health. Beijing: Higher Education Press, 1989.
6. Xu XC. The English-Chinese Encyclopedia of Practical Traditional Chinese Medicine—The Chinese Materia Medica. Beijing: Higher Education Press, 1990.
7. Xie HS. Chinese Veterinary Herbal Handbook. Reddick: Chi Institute of Chinese Medicine, 2004.
8. Shuai XZ. Terminology of Traditional Chinese Medicine. Changsha: Hunan Science & Technology Press, 2005.

36 Clinical Application of Chinese Herbal Medicine for Companion Animals 中药在伴侣动物临床上应用

Constance DiNatale

CARDIOVASCULAR CONDITIONS

The abbreviations used for the herbal remedies in this chapter refer to Chinese herbal suppliers in the United States. See Table 36.1.

Bleeding

Acute trauma with bleeding can be treated with the Chinese patent *Yunnan Bai Yao* (P). Dosing is 1 capsule per 10–20 pounds every few hours in severe cases. The package comes with a single small red pill, which is used in cases of shock. It can be given alone or with the *Yunnan Bai Yao* capsules. This is a useful remedy to have on hand for animals with internal neoplasia that may bleed. A medium-sized dog could take 1–2 capsules twice daily on a short-term basis to prevent bleeding from an abdominal or nasal tumor.

Congestive Heart Failure

Heart herbs may be combined with conventional medication. Herbal formulas such as *Wu Pi Yin* (P, Chapter 23) and *Wu Ling San* (P, Chapter 23) may be helpful for ascites and pulmonary edema when one wants to wean an animal off diuretics.

Heart *Qi* Deficiency Symptoms include shortness of breath, palpitations, panting, fatigue, and weakness. The tongue is pale with a white coating, and the pulse is weak.

Herbal treatment:

Yang Xin Tang (P, Chapter 18)—tonifies Heart *Qi*, invigorates Blood

Heart *Yang* Deficiency Symptoms are the same as for Heart *Qi* Deficiency with cold ears and feet, loose stool, and lethargy. Tongue is pale or lavender, pulse is weak.

Herbal treatment:

Bao Yuan Tang (P, Chapter 18)—tonifies Heart *Qi* and *Yang*

Kidney *Yang* Deficiency The animal has shortness of breath and cough and seeks warmth. There may be watery diarrhea, rear leg edema, ascites, or pulmonary edema. The animal retains excess fluid due to Deficiency of *Yang*. Tongue is lavender and wet; pulses are deep and weak.

Herbal treatment:

Zhen Wu Tang (P, Chapter 22)—warms *Yang*, eliminates Damp, frees urine, invigorates Blood

Heart *Qi*-Blood-*Yin* Deficiency Symptoms are weakness, fatigue, and exercise intolerance. Heart rate is irregular. There is anemia and insomnia. Tongue is pale to red and dry, and pulses are weak or thready.

Herbal treatment:

Zhi Gan Cao Tang (P, Chapter 18)—tonifies and warms *Qi*, tonifies *Yang* and nourishes *Yin* and Blood

DERMATOLOGICAL CONDITIONS

Categories are based on lesion types and locations. For instance, ventral lesions are considered to derive from Dampness. *Xiao Feng San* (P, Chapter 31) may be added to most other formulas to help alleviate itch.

External Wind Symptoms are itching caused by atopic/contact dermatitis or fleas. Pruritis is mild to moderate, primarily upper body, face, and neck. Tongue is red and dry, pulses are fast and wiry.

Table 36.1. Chinese Herbal Suppliers in the USA.

Abbreviation	Herbal Supplier
GF	Golden Flower, Placitas, NM
ITM	Institute for Traditional Medicine, Portland, OR
JT	Jing-Tang Herbal, Reddick, FL
P	Patent, available through many suppliers such as Mayway, Nuherbs, or Jing Tang in the USA

Herbal treatment:

External Wind (JT)—clears External Wind, detoxifies, alleviates itching, cools Blood, activates Blood

Wind-Heat Skin is warm and moderately pruritic. There is erythema, papules, and alopecia. The tongue is red, and pulses are floating and forceful.

Herbal treatment:

1. *Xiao Feng San* (P, Chapter 31)—disperses Wind, clears Heat, cools Blood, relieves itching, eliminates Damp
2. Wind Toxin Formula (JT)—clears Wind and Heat, detoxifies, alleviates itching

Blood Heat Symptoms are severe pruritis with papules, pustules, erythema, plaques, and swelling. Tongue is deep red and dry, pulses are fast.

Herbal treatment:

Wu Wei Xiao Du Yin (P, Chapter 21)—clears Heat, detoxifies, reduces swelling

Damp-Heat Papules, pustules, and vesicles are present with thick discharge and odor. There is restlessness, rubbing, and itching. Lesions may tend toward ventrum. Tongue is red or purple; pulses are fast.

Herbal treatment:

1. Damp Heat Skin (JT)—clears Damp and Heat, detoxifies and cools Blood
2. *Bi Xie Sheng Shi* (P)—clears Damp and Heat, cools Blood, detoxifies

Damp-Heat in Paws Feet are red, swollen, and hot. There may be discharge, odor, and pruritis. Pulse and tongue are as for Damp-Heat.

Herbal treatment:

Four Paws Damp Heat (JT)—clears Damp and Heat, detoxifies, cools Blood

Damp-Heat Lower Burner Signs are as for Damp-Heat, but they are located in the Lower *Jiao* (abdomen, inner thighs, rear limbs).

Herbal treatment:

1. Lower Damp Heat (JT)—clears Damp and Heat, detoxifies
2. *Long Dan Xie Gan Tang* (P, Chapter 21)—clears Heat, drains Damp, cools Blood

Damp-Heat in Genital Area Signs are as for Damp-Heat; lesions are around the genitals.

Herbal treatment:

1. Genital Damp Heat (JT)—clears Damp and Heat, detoxifies, cools Blood
2. *Long Dan Xie Gan Tang* (P, Chapter 21)—clears Heat, drains Damp, cools Blood

Damp-Heat in Ears Symptoms are swelling, erythema, Heat, odor, and discharge from the ears. Tongue and pulse are as above.

Herbal treatment:

1. Ear Damp Heat (JT)—clears Damp and Heat, detoxifies, cools Blood
2. *Long Dan Xie Gan Tang* (P, Chapter 21)—clears Heat, drains Damp, cools Blood

Blood Deficiency Symptoms are dry coat, pads, nose, and skin with dandruff. There is alopecia, pigmentation, and low-grade chronic itch with no odor. Tongue is pale and dry; pulses are deep, thready, and weak.

Herbal treatment:

1. *Bu Xue Xi Feng* (JT)—nourishes Blood, clears Wind, eliminates itch
2. *Si Wu Tang* (P, Chapter 18)—tonifies Blood, moistens Dryness

***Yin* Deficiency** Animal presents as chronic itching, and it is worse at night. Coat and skin are dry with dandruff and alopecia. Animal is thirsty and hot and may have anxiety.

Herbal treatment:

Zhi Bai Di Huang Wan (P, Chapter 18)—tonifies *Yin*, clears Heat

***Yin* and Blood Deficiency** Skin is chronically dry and itchy. There is dandruff and thinning hair. Tongue is dry and pale; pulse is thready and weak.

Herbal treatment:

Dandruff Formula (JT)—nourishes *Yin* and Blood, clears Wind-Heat, relieves itching

Blood Deficiency with Fungus Skin is pruritic, with dandruff and dry coat. Tongue is pale, and pulses are thready and weak.

Herbal treatment:
Ku Shen Si Wu Tang (JT)—kills fungi, nourishes Blood, clears Heat, and stops itching

GASTROINTESTINAL CONDITIONS

Anorexia

Anorexia may have an acute onset, as when one's dietary habits cause indigestion and/or nausea, or may be more chronic, due to weak digestion or disease.

Cold-Damp Onset is acute, with preference for heat. Ears/nose are cold, and there is excess saliva. Tongue is pale/purple with white coating; pulses are deep and slow. There may be a history of eating cold food or water, or of being exposed to an excessively cold environment.

Herbal treatment:
1. *Ping Wei San* (P, Chapter 23)—tonifies Spleen *Qi*, dispels Damp, harmonizes Stomach
2. Happy Earth Formula (JT)—dispels Dampness, strengthens Spleen *Qi*, moves Stomach *Qi* downward

Stomach Heat Symptoms are Heat signs and excessive thirst. There is a foul smell from the mouth. Feces are dry, and urine is dark and scant. Tongue is red and dry with a thick yellow coating. Pulses are fast and surging.

Herbal treatment:
1. *Yu Nü Jian* (P, Chapter 21)—nourishes Stomach *Yin* and clears Heat
2. *Qing Wei San Wan* (P)—drains Fire, cools Blood, tonifies *Yin*

Spleen *Qi* Deficiency The primary symptom is chronic anorexia. The stool may be loose. There is fatigue, weakness, edema, and undigested food in the feces. Tongue is pale, is wet and has a white coating. Pulses are weak and thready.

Herbal treatment:
1. *Jian Pi Wan* (P, Chapter 25)—tonifies Spleen *Qi*, promotes digestion, harmonizes Stomach, dispels food Stasis
2. *Xiang Sha Liu Jun Zi Tang* (P, Chapter 18)—tonifies Spleen *Qi*, descends Stomach *Qi*, promotes appetite

Constipation

Constipation is seen in small animals as either an acute onset, such as with a rapid food change, or chronic, such as with elderly animals or animals with renal or cardiac disease.

Heat Heat has an acute onset, with dry impacted stool with mucus coating. The animal is thirsty and has a foul mouth odor. The tongue is red and dry with a thick yellow coating. Pulses are fast and wiry.

These formulas are very strong and purging, and they should be used only 1–5 days and stopped as soon as a bowel movement occurs. Their coldness damages Spleen *Qi* if used continuously, and caution should be used for deficient animals.

Herbal treatment:
1. *Da Huang Jiang Zhi Wan* (P)—clears Heat, frees the stool, resolves toxins, invigorates Blood, clears and purges the bowels
2. *Da Cheng Qi Tong* (Chapter 32)—clears Heat and purges accumulations through the bowels

Qi Stagnation

The patient is often a Wood animal. The stool is dry and sporadic. There is abdominal bloating and pain. The tongue is purple to red, and pulses are fast and wiry.

Herbal treatment:
Tong Shun Wan (P)—purges accumulations, invigorates Blood, moistens Intestines, frees the stool, clears Heat; used for very stubborn constipation, 1–5 days; use with caution in Deficient animals

***Qi* Deficiency** The constipation is chronic, with small, thin stool. The animal prefers warmth and is generally weak and thin. The tongue is pale; pulses are deep and weak. One may use a combination of products to treat this condition.

Herbal treatment:
Si Jun Zi Tang (P, Chapter 18)—could be used at 1/2 dose, with *Fan Xie Ye* (JT) added short term, also at lowered dosing

Blood/*Yin* Deficiency Constipation is very chronic, with dry stool, such as with megacolon. There is impaction and possibly vomiting. Coat is dry with dorsal strip of flaking. The patient is elderly or weak. The tongue is dry and pale or red; pulses are thready or soft.

Herbal treatment:
1. *Ma Zi Ren Wan* (P, Chapter 32)—moistens Intestines, nourishes Blood, tonifies *Qi*, frees the stool, clears Heat
2. *Dang Gui Cong Rong Tang* (JT, Chapter 32)—moistens large Intestine, resolves impaction

Diarrhea

Heat-Toxin/Damp-Heat Diarrhea is bloody, watery, and/or mucoid with a foul odor. The animal may have a history of dietary indiscretion. It may be large or small Intestine etiology. Ears and nose are hot, with increased thirst and possibly fever. Tongue is deep red with a yellow coating and pulses are rapid. Do not use the following formulas long term. Most will resolve symptoms in days, but treatment may be continued for a few weeks if symptoms are improving.

Herbal treatment:

1. Great Saussurea Coptis (JT)—clears Damp-Heat, moves *Qi*, relieves pain
2. *Xiang Lian Wan* (P)—clears Damp-Heat, moves *Qi* and relieves pain

Liver-Spleen Disharmony Diarrhea is brought on by emotional or environmental stress. This is common in "worriers" when diarrhea results from boarding away from home, changes at home, vaccines, or dietary changes. The tongue is purple or red, and pulses are tight and wiry.

Herbal treatment:

1. *Yue Ju Wan* (Chapter 24)—promotes movement of *Qi*, resolves five Stagnations of *Qi*, Blood, Phlegm, Food, and Heat
2. Bupleurum 12 (ITM)—mediates harmony, disperses *Qi* and moisture

Spleen *Qi* Deficiency Diarrhea is chronic, with light color, undigested food, poor appetite, low body score, and low energy. The tongue is pale and pulses are deep and weak.

Herbal treatment:

1. *Shen Ling Bai Zhu San* (P, Chapter 18)—tonifies Spleen *Qi*, harmonizes Stomach, counters ascent of Stomach *Qi*, dispels Damp, relieves diarrhea
2. Ginseng 18 (ITM)—tonifies *Qi*, drains Damp, regulates *Qi* and warms the center

Kidney *Yang* Deficiency Diarrhea is chronic, especially at nighttime or daybreak. The back is cold. There is low energy and weak limbs. The tongue is pale and pulses are deep and weak.

Herbal treatment:

Si Shen Wan (P, Chapter 28)—warms and tonifies Kidney and Spleen *Yang*

Parvovirus

This represents a combination of Damp-Heat, as well as Deficiency. Diarrhea is bloody with mucus. There is vomiting and anorexia, and treatment is aimed at clearing Damp-Heat, as well as supporting the animal.

Herbal treatment:

Zhi Li Tang (Chapter 21)—clears Damp-Heat, moves *Qi*, relieves pain, nourishes Blood, and tonifies *Qi*. This formula has been used successfully via rectal infusion in cases of severe vomiting.

Hepatitis

Liver disease often responds quickly to TCVM treatment.

Damp-Heat Pattern Liver enzymes are markedly elevated. There may be jaundice. Eyes are watery and red. The tongue is red with a yellow coating; pulses are fast and wiry.

Herbal treatment:

Long Dan Xie Gan Tang (P, Chapter 21)—clears Liver Heat, clears Damp-Heat

Damp-Heat Pattern with Jaundice/Icterus The tongue is yellow with a greasy coating; pulses are fast and wiry.

Herbal treatment:

Artemisia Combination (JT)—eliminates Damp and clears Damp-Heat

Liver *Qi* Stagnation The animal may be aggressive or angry, barks, and overcontrols others. There is stress and failure to adapt. The tongue is purple and pulses are usually wiry.

Herbal treatment:

1. *Xiao Yao San* (P, Chapter 24)—soothes Liver, disperses Liver Stasis, harmonizes Liver and Spleen, moves *Qi*, invigorates Blood and tonifies Spleen
2. *Chai Hu Shu Gan Wan* (P, Chapter 24)—moves Liver Blood, cools Liver Heat, harmonizes Liver and Stomach, counters ascent of Stomach *Qi*, and relieves pain. This formula is more complex than *Xiao Yao San* and addresses more severe gastrointestinal complaints.

Liver *Qi* Stagnation with Heat The animal is irritable, with red eyes, restlessness, and hyperactivity. The tongue is purple or red, and pulses are wiry.

Herbal treatment:

1. Liver Happy (JT)—soothes Liver *Qi*, clears Heat, and resolves Stagnation
2. *Jia Wei Xiao Yao San* (P)—soothes Liver, dispels Liver Stagnation, clears Heat, harmonizes Liver and Spleen, nourishes and invigorates Blood, and tonifies Spleen
3. Bupleurum 12 (ITM)—mediates harmony and disperses *Qi* and moisture

Liver-Kidney *Yin* Deficiency The coat is dull and the animal has increased thirst. The tongue is red and dry and pulses are thready and fast.

Herbal treatment:

Yi Guan Jian (P, Chapter 18)—nourishes Liver *Yin* and clears Heat

Liver Blood Deficiency The coat is dull, pads are dry, and there is possible anemia. There is obvious Deficiency. The tongue is lavender and dry and pulses are thin and deep.

Herbal treatment:

1. *Tang Kuei* 18 (ITM)—nourishes Blood and *Yin*, regulates *Qi* and vitalizes Blood
2. *Si Wu Tang* (P, Chapter 18)—nourishes Blood and invigorates Blood

Inflammatory Bowel Disease

This category encompasses many diseases, from gastroenteritis to enterocolitis. Stronger formulas, such as Great Saussurea Coptis and *Xiang Lian Wan*, contain coptis, which clears Damp-Heat. These formulas tend to be indicated in animals who show positive response to Damp-Heat–clearing drugs such as Metronidazole.

Heat Toxin/Damp-Heat Symptoms are bloody, watery, and/or mucoid feces with a foul odor. Heat signs prevail, with hot ears and nose, increased thirst, and vomiting. The tongue is red with a yellow coating; pulses are deep and rapid.

Herbal treatment:

Great Saussurea Coptis (JT)—clears Damp-Heat, moves *Qi* and relieves pain; use up to 1 month, but may use at 1/2 dose if symptoms improve and then return if the formula is stopped

***Qi*-Blood Stagnation** Diarrhea is chronic with foul odor. The animal is painful, with anorexia and/or vomiting. The tongue is red or purple and the pulses are wiry.

Herbal treatment:

Xiang Lian San (JT)—clears Damp-Heat and strengthens Spleen and Stomach

Liver-Spleen Disharmony Symptoms are chronic diarrhea or vomiting from emotional or environmental stress. Often heat signs are present. The tongue is red and pulses are wiry.

Herbal treatment:

Bupleurum 12 (ITM)—mediates harmony, disperses *Qi* and moisture

Spleen *Qi* Deficiency Diarrhea is chronic with light color, undigested food, poor appetite, low body score, and low energy. The tongue is pale, and pulses are deep and weak.

Herbal treatment:

1. *Shen Ling Bai Zhu San* (P, Chapter 18)—tonifies Spleen *Qi*, harmonizes Stomach, counters ascent of Stomach *Qi*, dispels Damp, relieves diarrhea
2. Ginseng 18 (ITM)—tonifies *Qi*, drains Damp, regulates *Qi* and warms the center

Vomiting

Invasion of the Stomach by External Pathogens Onset of vomiting is sudden, especially with seasonal changes or after travel. There may be aversion to Cold, Wind, or Heat. There is headache (aversion to touching the head), red eyes, possible fever, and abdominal pain. The tongue has a pale coating and pulses are floating and superficial.

Herbal treatment:

1. Happy Earth Formula (JT)—dispels Dampness, strengthens Spleen *Qi*, moves Stomach *Qi* downward
2. *Huo Xiang Zheng Qi Wan* (P, Chapter 23)—dispels pathogenic factors, dispels Damp, harmonizes Middle *Jiao*, relieves diarrhea

These formulas may also be used in chronic cases of Spleen *Qi* Deficiency with Stagnation of food and Damp. There is burping and flatulence with abdominal pain, and it is worse in cold and damp weather.

Food Stagnation Food Stagnation can be from Excess or Deficiency. Excess: Symptoms are sudden onset of vomiting bile or undigested food after eating, loose stool, anorexia, foul odor from mouth, cranial abdominal distress. Heat signs are present. The tongue is red with a greasy, thick coating, and pulses are slippery.

Herbal treatment:

Bao He Wan (P, Chapter 25)—dispels food Stasis, harmonizes Stomach, dispels Damp, promotes appetite

Deficiency Symptoms are vomiting of undigested food, burping, anorexia, loose stool, absence of odor from the mouth. The tongue is pale with a white coating and pulses are deep.

Herbal treatment:

Jian Pi Wan (P, Chapter 25)—dispels food Stasis, harmonizes Stomach, descends *Qi*, tonifies Spleen

Liver *Qi* Stagnation Animal is irritable, with a "hyper" personality, vomits small amounts of food or bile, and has flank and rib pain. There is frequent burping and Heat signs such as red eyes, warm nose and ears. The tongue is purple and pulses are wiry.

Herbal treatment:

1. Liver Happy (JT)—soothes Liver, clears Heat, resolves Stagnation
2. *Chai Hu Shu Gan Wan* (P, Chapter 24)—soothes Liver, invigorates Blood, tonifies Spleen and stops pain

Spleen *Qi-Yang* Deficiency Symptoms are vomiting, loose stool with undigested food, fatigue, anorexia, and edema. Animal seeks warm. There is abdominal discomfort, which is better with massage. The tongue is pale, and pulses are deep and weak.

Herbal treatment:

Eight Gentlemen (JT)—tonifies *Qi*, strengthens Spleen, moves *Qi*, eliminates Damp

Stomach *Yin* Deficiency Vomiting occurs in frequent small amounts. Symptoms can include anorexia, increased thirst, dry stool, abdominal pain, and stress-related ulcers. The tongue is red and pulses are thready and fast.

Herbal treatment:

1. Stomach Happy (JT)—nourishes *Yin*, moves *Qi*, relieves pain
2. *Yu Nü Jian* (P, Chapter 21)—nourishes Stomach *Yin*, clears Heat

HEMATOPOIETIC AND HEMOLYMPHATIC DISORDERS

Anemia/Autoimmune Hemolytic Anemia

These formulas are useful for autoimmune, hemolytic, or chronic diseases that lead to anemia.

Damp-Heat with Blood Deficiency There are Heat signs, low-grade fever, jaundice, tachypnea and tachycardia, depression, and exercise intolerance. This would likely be a hemolytic anemia formula.

Herbal treatment:

Zhu Huang Tang (JT)—clears Heat, clears Damp, tonifies Blood

Blood Deficiency Gums are pale, coat is dry, tendons may be weak or stiff. There is constipation and anxiety or lassitude.

Herbal treatment:

1. *Si Wu Tang* (P, Chapter 18)—nourishes Blood, invigorates Blood
2. *Tang Kuei* 18 (ITM)—nourishes Blood, invigorates Blood
3. Millettia 9 (ITM)—nourishes Blood, vitalizes Blood—Blood Deficiency due to bone marrow suppression
4. *Ji Xue* Formula (GF)—supplements Blood and *Qi*, invigorates Blood, promotes digestion, drains Damp, relieves toxins

***Qi* and Blood Deficiency** This is seen in chronic hemorrhagic anemia or hemolytic anemia. There may be diarrhea or decreased appetite, lethargy, pale gums, and poor coat. The tongue is pale and dry. Pulses are thready and weak.

Herbal treatment:

1. *Gui Pi Tang* (P, Chapter 18)—nourishes Heart Blood, tonifies Spleen *Qi*
2. *Ba Zhen Tang* (P, Chapter 18)—nourishes Liver Blood, tonifies *Qi*

Kidney *Yang* Deficiency There is weakness and lethargy. Extremities and ears are Cold. The tongue is pale and the pulses are deep and weak.

Herbal treatment:

Antler 8 (ITM)—nourishes Marrow, generates Blood, invigorates *Yang*

Ascites and Edema

Ascites is most commonly seen in small animals in cases of Heart or Liver disease or with neoplasia. Edema can been seen after trauma or with poor circulation. The formulas listed may not act as quickly and dramatically as furosamide or spironolactone, but they are safer and can often be helpful in weaning the animal off the drugs or replacing the drugs over time.

Herbal treatment:

1. *Wu Ling San* (P, Chapter 23)—eliminates Damp, frees the movement of water, benefits Kidney and Spleen; useful for abdominal and chest ascites
2. *Wu Pi Yin* (P, Chapter 23)—eliminates Damp, benefits movement of water, tonifies and warms Spleen; made from the peels of the fruits and is therefore more useful for edema of the limbs and joints, though it can also be used for ascites
3. *Zhen Wu Tang* (P, Chapter 22)—warms *Yang*, eliminates Damp, frees movement of urine, invigorates Blood; used when there is Kidney and Spleen *Yang* Deficiency, such as with congestive heart failure or nephritis/nephrosis, leading to edematous limbs, ascites, or swollen joints

ENDOCRINE CONDITIONS

Diabetes

Diabetes in TCVM is seen as a Deficiency Heat disease. It is known as *Xiao-ke*, or emaciation-thirst disease. Incidence of diabetes is increasing in small animal medicine. TCVM may alleviate symptoms and decrease glucosuria. Herbal formulas are safe to use with insulin. TCVM dietary therapy may also dramatically impact the treatment results.

Stomach Heat Middle *Xiao* There is polyphagia, polydipsia, and polyuria. Stool is dry and gums are red. The tongue is red and dry with a yellow coating and pulses are forceful and slippery.

Herbal treatment:
Jade Lady (JT)—nourishes Stomach *Yin*, clears Heat

Kidney *Yin* Deficiency There is polydipsia and polyuria. The animal pants excessively and seeks coolness. The coat, skin, pads, and nose are dry. Tongue is red and dry; pulses are thready and fast.

Herbal treatment:
1. *Xiao Ke Feng* (JT)—nourishes *Yin*, resolves thirst, reinforces Kidney Essence, nourishes Liver Blood
2. Rehmannia 16 (ITM)—moistens dryness, nourishes *Yin*, clears deficient Heat

Kidney *Qi-Yin* Deficiency Signs include polydipsia, polyuria, and dry coat. The animal has muscle atrophy, fatigue, and loose stool. The tongue is red or pale and dry; pulses are thready and fast or deep and weak.

Herbal treatment:
1. *Jiang Tang Cha* (JT)—tonifies *Qi*, nourishes *Yin*, resolves thirst, clears Heat
2. *Yu Quan Wan* (P)—nourishes Kidney, tonifies Spleen, clears Heat, resolves thirst

Cushing's Disease

Herbal medicine can often be used without conventional drugs to treat Cushing's disease. Blood levels for cortisol may remain elevated, but one might expect liver enzymes to decrease and symptoms to regress. Formula categories should be combined, if needed, to treat cases.

***Yin* Deficiency** There is excessive drinking and urination. The coat, skin, and pads are dry. There is bilateral symmetrical alopecia, along with thinning hair. There is excessive panting, especially at night, along with anxiety. Tongue is dry and red, and pulses are thready and rapid.

Herbal treatment:
1. Ophiopogon Formula (JT)—nourishes *Yin*, clears Heat, promotes body fluids
2. Rehmannia 16 (ITM)—moistens dryness, nourishes *Yin*, clears deficient Heat

***Qi* and *Yin* Deficiency** There is polydipsia and polyuria, abdomen is enlarged, and the animal is lethargic. There may be internal organ dysfunction. The coat is dry, and there is excessive panting, especially at night. Tongue is red or pale; pulses are thready and weak.

Herbal treatment:
Rehmannia 11 (JT)—tonifies *Qi*, nourishes *Yin*, restrains urine

Hyperthyroidism

Inappropriate diet may be one of the leading causes of thyroid dysfunction in cats. It can also be seen as a sequelae to chronic illness.

***Qi* Stagnation and Phlegm** There is a thyroid nodule, weight loss, irritability, and depression. Vomit is slimy and the animal resists touch. Tongue is pale red with thin, slimy fur; pulses are wiry or slippery.

Herbal treatment:
1. *Er Chen Tong* (P, Chapter 20) combined with *Xiao Chai Hu Tong* (P)—drains Damp, transforms Phlegm, tonifies Spleen, soothes Liver, clears Liver Heat, moves Liver *Qi*
2. *Hai Zao Yu Hu Tang* (P, Chapter 20)—softens the swelling, moves *Qi*, dissolves Phlegm, breaks up masses

***Yin* Deficiency with Heat** There is a thyroid nodule, tachycardia, weight loss and emaciation. The cat is irritable, hyperactive, and aggressive. There is polyphagia, polydipsia, and polyuria. There are vocalizations, especially at night, vomiting, and constipation. Tongue is red, dry, and small, and pulses are fast.

Herbal treatment:
1. *Zhi Bai Di Huang Wan* (P)—nourishes Kidney *Yin*, clears Heat, subdues deficient Fire floating upward
2. Hyper *Jia Bing* Formula (JT)—tonifies *Yin* and pacifies *Yang*

Hypothyroidism

The most common hypothyroid Patterns encountered in small animals are *Yang/Qi* Deficiency and *Qi/Yin* Deficiency.

***Yang/Qi* Deficiency** Digestion is poor, with chronic loose stools. Extremities are cool, animal seeks warmth, and there is exercise intolerance and fatigue. Tongue is pale and wet with white coating; pulses are deep and weak.

Herbal treatment:
Xiao Ying San (JT)—tonifies Kidney *Qi* or *Yang*, moves Blood, resolves Stagnation

***Qi/Yin*/Blood Deficiency** There is lethargy and exercise intolerance. The skin is dry with truncal bilateral alopecia, alopecia of the chest or ears, and dull coat. The animal may be PU/PD, prone to gastrointestinal problems, and have cool feet and clear urine. Muscles are flaccid and the abdomen is distended. The face has the classic "tragic" look. The tongue is pale and swollen or red and dry; pulses are weak and deep.

Herbal treatment:

Jia Bing Fang (JT)—tonifies *Qi* and nourishes *Yin* and Blood, transforms Phlegm, softens hardness

One may combine various formulas to treat the presenting Pattern. For *Qi*/Blood Deficiency, one might use *Si Wu Tang* with *Si Jun Zi Tang* or could substitute *Liu Wei Di Huang Wan* for *Si Wu Tang* if *Yin* Deficiency was more pronounced than Blood Deficiency. *Xiao Yao San* is a good choice to add when there is Liver *Qi* Stagnation, usually from concurrent drug treatment.

NEOPLASIA

Formulas for cancers are determined by the presenting Pattern of the patient, as well as the general health of the patient. Cancer represents a Stagnation, so an herbal formula to move Stagnation must be chosen. The animal may have an underlying Deficiency, which must be addressed as well. Finally, one may add additional formulas to bring the main formula to a particular area of the body.

Herbal Therapy—General Cancer Formulas:

1. *Wei Qi* Booster (JT)—tonifies *Qi* and Blood, tonifies *Wei Qi*, inhibits cell mutation. Often useful alone for debilitated, deficient animals with cancer, or can be combined with stronger formulas for more aggressive treatment
2. Max's Formula (JT)—softens hardness, clears nodules. Useful in geriatric or deficient animals with weak pulses and pale tongues. Also used for softening lipomas and for lymph node enlargement and lymphoma
3. Stasis Breaker (JT)—breaks Blood Stasis, softens hardness, clears enlargement. This is an aggressive formula for animals with strong constitutions. Pulses are weak or choppy, and the tongue is purple.
4. Chih-ko and Curcuma (ITM)—resolves masses, disperses Blood, regulates *Qi*. It is a moderately strong formula for masses.
5. Prostate Invigorator (JT)—moves Blood, clears Heat, resolves Stagnation, stops pain. Pulse is wiry, tongue is purple. This formula is useful for enlarged, painful prostate or prostate cancer. May be used for anal gland carcinoma or rectal tumors.
6. Bone Stasis Formula (JT)—breaks down Stasis, activates Blood, clears Channel blockage, relieves pain. Combine with Stasis Breaker or Max's Formula for bone cancer.
7. Stasis in the Mansion of Mind (JT)—breaks down Blood Stasis, transforms Phlegm, resolves nodules, relieves pain. Used for brain cancer.
8. Otolith Tablets (ITM)—calms Wind, opens orifices, cleans toxins, removes Phlegm-Damp accumulations. Used for brain tumors, and may be useful poststroke or with GME or head trauma.
9. *Xue Fue Zhu Yu Tang* (P, Chapter 27)—invigorates Blood/*Qi*, resolves Blood Stasis, relieves pain. This formula is useful in cancers with concurrent Blood Deficiency, such as some mast cell tumors. It is not an aggressive formula. It may be combined with Blood tonics.
10. *Shao Fu Zhu Yu Tang* (P, Chapter 27)—invigorates Blood/*Qi*, resolves Blood Stasis, relieves pain. Used for bladder cancer or cancers in the lower abdominal area.
11. Sparghanium 12 (ITM)—vitalizes Blood, regulates *Qi*, resolves masses. This is a nice formula for liver cancer that seems to be tolerated by most animals, despite the strong herbs it contains. Glandulars are also useful in these cancers.

Formulating Cancer Protocols: Take care not to "cookbook" cancer therapy, but to choose combinations thoughtfully. For example, bladder cancer showing signs of severe Damp-Heat in the Lower *Jiao* (straining, bleeding, strong pulses, Heat signs) may benefit from Stasis Breaker combined with *Long Dan Xie Gan Tang*.

For an older, *Yin* deficient animal with bladder cancer one might choose *Liu Wei Di Huang Wan* or *Zhi Bai Di Huang Wan* combined with *Shao Fu Zhu Yu Tang*.

For bone cancer, one may choose Stasis Breaker, *Wei Qi* Booster and 1/2 to a full dose of Bone Stasis for an excess animal, whereas an older, deficient animal may need *Qi* and *Yin* tonics added, along with a milder cancer formula. Often, brain cancers are found in Blood deficient animals and Blood tonics should be added if necessary.

Herbal treatment:

Tang Kuei 18 (ITM) and *Si Wu Tang* (P)—may be used to supplement Blood when treating Blood Deficiency cancers

MUSCULOSKELETAL CONDITIONS

Arthritis

Arthritis is referred to as *Bi* Syndrome in TCVM. *Bi* Syndrome is always seen as a blockage of *Qi* and Blood through the channels. The five main classifications are Cold *Bi*, Wandering *Bi*, Damp *Bi*, Heat *Bi*, and Bony *Bi*. Classification of the different Patterns is based on factors such as acute versus chronic, degree of pain, and temperature preferences.

Painful (Cold) *Bi* Cold invades joints and causes Stagnation. Cold *Bi* tends to be very painful and can affect any joint. Wind and Damp may also be present.

Characteristics of Painful (Cold) *Bi* is onset during, or aggravated by, cold weather, pain more prevalent than stiffness, pain relieved by heat, and aversion to massage.

Herbal treatment aims to move Blood and *Qi*, tonify *Yang*, and eliminate Wind-Damp.

Herbal treatment:

1. *Xiao Huo Luo Dan* (P, Chapter 31)—warms Interior, warms Channels, invigorates Collaterals, moves *Qi* and Blood, relieves pain, dispels Phlegm
2. Dok's Formula (JT)—dissipates Cold, eliminates Wind-Damp, invigorates *Qi* and Blood, tonifies Kidney *Yang*, warms Channels

Wandering (Wind) *Bi* This syndrome is not seen as commonly in animals as in humans. There is invasion of exogenous pathogens, characterized by wandering muscle and joint pain, especially stifles, hocks, carpi, and elbows. There is acute onset, often characterized by fever or chills. One can see this occur concurrently with respiratory or gastrointestinal infections.

Fixed (Damp) *Bi* This syndrome manifests as localized pain that does not move. The body and limbs feel heavy, and stiffness is greater than pain. Movement is difficult. Heat and dryness relieve pain, and Cold and Damp exacerbate pain. The tongue has a greasy, pale coating, and pulses are soft and slow.

Herbal treatment:

1. Coix Formula (JT) drains Damp, dispels Wind-Damp, warms the Channels, relieves pain, strengthens Spleen
2. *Juan Bi Wan* (P)—dispels Wind-Damp, drains Damp, invigorates Blood, warms the Channels and Collaterals, relieves pain
3. *Guan Jie Yan Wan* (P)—drains Damp, dispels Wind-Damp, warms and opens the Channels and Collaterals, relieves pain; especially useful for lower-limb arthritis or sciatica, when accompanied by swelling

Heat *Bi* Heat *Bi* presents as local redness, swelling, and severe pain in one or several joints. There is limitation of movement and possible deformity of joints. The tongue is red, possibly a yellow coating, and the pulses are rapid.

Herbal treatment:

Si Miao Wan (P, Chapter 23)—eliminates Damp, clears Heat, relieves pain

Bony *Bi* Bony *Bi* is divided into two main categories: *Yang* Deficiency, and *Yin* and *Qi* Deficiency

***Yang* Deficiency** is chronic and presents as Cold back and extremities; the animal seeks Warmth, possibly has loose stools, and is better with massage and Heat. The tongue is pale and wet and pulses are deep and weak.

Herbal treatment:

Loranthus Formula (JT)—tonifies Kidney *Yang*, dispels Wind, Cold and Damp, strengthens back and limbs

***Yin* and *Qi* Deficiency** is very chronic. There is dry coat, excessive thirst, and aggravation with warmth. Spine or joints are inflamed, and there is weakness and lethargy. Pulses are thready and weak, and the tongue is dry and red.

Herbal treatment:

Di Gu Pi San (JT)—nourishes *Yin* and *Qi*, clears deficient Heat, dispels Wind-Damp

Disc Disease and Spondylosis

Both of these conditions fall under the category of *Bi* Syndrome. Disc disease is acute and leads to chronic degenerative changes, and spondylosis is chronic and more of a deficient state.

For acute disc disease with paralysis or paresis, use strong Blood-moving herbs. The tongue is purple and pulses are fast.

Herbal treatment:

1. Double P #2 (JT)—moves Blood Stasis, moves *Qi*, relieves pain; for paralysis and paresis due to disc disease
2. Cervical Formula (JT)—same as above, but for cervical area. May be combined with Double P #2 for severe cervical spinal injury due to disc protrusion.

For chronic disc disease and spondylosis, one may use any of the formulas in the arthritis section, as well as the following herbal treatments.

Herbal treatment:

1. *Kang Gu Zeng Sheng Pian* (P)—tonifies *Qi* and *Yang*, benefits Kidney, nourishes Liver, benefits Tendon and Bone, invigorates Blood, relieves pain
2. Liquidamber 18 (ITM)—invigorates Blood, invigorates Meridians and Vessels, dispels Wind-Damp

Weakness/Stroke (*Wei* Syndrome)

Wei syndrome refers to generalized weakness and flaccidity in the absence of pain. This can be an acute or chronic presentation, but there will be a history of Deficiency.

Damp-Heat This presents as obesity, with muscle atrophy and weakness. Patient is panting and warm.

Limbs may be edematous. There is a history of Dampness in the gastrointestinal tract and/or skin. Tongue is greasy and wet; pulses are fast.

Herbal treatment:
Si Miao San (P, Chapter 23)—eliminates Damp, clears Damp-Heat

***Qi-Yang* Deficiency** Animal may be too weak to stand. There is profound weakness, lethargy, and anorexia. Coat is poor, body score is low, and the feet and ears are cool. Tongue is pale and wet; pulses are thready and weak.

Herbal treatment:
Bu Yang Huan Wu Tang (P, Chapter 27)—tonifies *Qi*, nourishes Blood, dredges and opens the Channels and Collaterals

***Qi-Yin* Deficiency** There is weakness of the limbs, emaciation, dry coat, and thirst. Tongue is red and dry or pale and wet; pulses are deep, thready, and weak.

Herbal treatment:
Hindquarter Formula (JT)—tonifies Kidney, strengthens back and hind limbs, moves *Qi*, relieves pain

NEUROLOGICAL CONDITIONS

Epilepsy

Animals with epilepsy often benefit greatly from herbal treatment. If already on pharmaceutical anticonvulsants, animals may still take herbal medications and may then be slowly weaned off pharmaceutical drugs, or to the lowest dose needed to remain seizure free.

Obstruction by Wind-Phlegm Seizures cause loss of consciousness with convulsions, foaming at the mouth, and/or vocalization. There may be loss of bladder and bowel control. Some animals may present with disorientation without seizures, including staring into corners, "fly-catching," following imaginary things around the room, or obsessing with shadows. The tongue is pale or purple with a white, greasy coating, and pulses are wiry and slippery.

Herbal treatment:
1. *Ding Xian Wan* (JT)—expels Phlegm, extinguishes Wind, opens the orifices, stabilizes seizures
2. Gastrodia 9 (ITM)—sedates Internal Wind, resolves Phlegm obstruction

Stagnation of Blood Seizure has sudden onset, with loss of consciousness, convulsion, foaming at the mouth, vocalization, and possible fecal and bladder incontinence. There is a history of head trauma. Disorientation may occur without seizure. The tongue is pale or purple with a white, greasy coating, and the pulses are wiry and slippery.

Herbal treatment:
1. *Ding Xian Wan* (JT)—expels Phlegm, extinguishes Wind, opens the orifices, and stabilizes seizures; may be combined with *Tao Hong Si Wu Tang*.
2. *Tao Hong Si Wu Tang* (P, Chapter 27)—resolves Blood Stasis

Liver Blood Deficiency Seizures are chronic. The coat and footpads are dry and coarse. There may be anemia or low body score and poor stamina. Seizures may present with rigid jaw and neck. The tongue is pale and dry, and pulses are weak and thready.

Herbal treatment:
Bu Xue Xi Feng (JT)—nourishes Blood, clears Internal Wind

Liver/Kidney *Yin* Deficiency Seizures are chronic and coat and nose are dry. The animal may be PU/PD and seek cold. Seizures often occur at night or late afternoon. The tongue is red and pulses are weak, thready, and fast.

Herbal treatment:
Yang Yin Xi Feng (JT)—nourishes Blood and *Yin*, clears Internal Wind

Blood and *Yin* Deficiency Any combination of the former two Patterns.

Herbal treatment:
1. *Tian Ma* Plus II (JT)—nourishes *Yin* and Blood, clears Internal Wind
2. *Tian Ma Gou Teng Wan* (P, Chapter 31)—nourishes *Yin* and Blood, clears Internal Wind

Spleen *Qi* Deficiency with Damp The animal may have a history of vomiting or chronic diarrhea. Dogs may have a "wet mouth" or drool excessively. The tongue is pale with a thin coating, and pulses are wiry and slippery.

Herbal treatment:
Tian Ma Bai Zhu (JT)—clears Internal Wind, strengthens Spleen, eliminates Damp, transforms Phlegm

OPHTHALMOLOGICAL CONDITIONS

Healthy vision relies on healthy liver and kidney function. Liver Blood and *Yin* help moisten the eyes, and Liver Fire can burn up *Yin*, causing redness, sties, or sclerosis of the lens.

Liver Heat with Stagnation The eyelids are swollen and there is ocular discharge. There may be corneal opacity, miosis, and photophobia. The tongue is red or pale, and the pulse is surging or weak.

Herbal treatment:
Jue Ming San (Chapter 21)—clears Liver, eliminates Fire, clears eyes, resolves nebula

Liver Heat The eyelids are swollen and sclera are injected. The conjunctiva are swollen, deep red, and itchy. The eyes are watery. Tongue is red with a yellow coating, and pulses are fast and wiry.

Herbal treatment:
Long Dan Xie Gan Tang (P, Chapter 21)—clears Liver-Heat, drains Damp-Heat

Blood and *Yin* Deficiency The eyes are dry (KCS), red, and itchy. There may be glaucoma, cataract, uveitis, or poor night vision. Tongue is red or pale; pulses are thready and fast.

Herbal treatment:
1. *Ming Mu Di Huang Wan* (P)—nourishes Kidney and Liver *Yin*, nourishes Liver Blood, subdues *Yang*, benefits eyes
2. *Qi Ju Di Huang Wan* (P, Chapter 18)—nourishes Kidney *Yin*, nourishes *Yin* and Blood, benefits the eyes; like *Ming Mu Di Huang Wan*, but less heat clearing; nourishes Kidney and Liver *Yin*, nourishes Blood, benefits the eyes

RESPIRATORY CONDITIONS

Asthma

Asthma refers to difficulty breathing due to narrowing of the respiratory tract from muscle spasm or edema of the bronchial tubes. It may be induced by allergy, infection, autonomic nervous system disorders, psychological processes, and aerosolized irritants.

Lung *Yin* Deficiency The animal has dry coat, emaciation, dry cough, and dry, thick nasal secretions. The animal seeks cold. Pulses are thready and fast. Tongue is red and dry.

Herbal treatment:
1. *Bai He Gu Jin Wan* (P, Chapter 18)—nourishes Lung *Yin*, moistens the Lung, clears Heat, transforms Phlegm
2. Lily Combination (JT)—nourishes *Yin* and moistens Lung, stops cough and asthma

Lung *Qi* Deficiency Asthma is chronic and worse with movement. The voice is weak. There is fatigue, exercise intolerance, and shortness of breath. Tongue is pale and wet; pulses are weak and deep.

Herbal treatment:
Bu Fei San (P, Chapter 18)—tonifies Lung *Qi*, stops cough and asthma

Lung and Kidney *Qi* Deficiency Animal presents with long-term asthma. Breathing is shallow, with loss of breath and is worse with movement. There is exercise intolerance and weakness. Tongue is pale with a thin coating. Pulses are deep and weak.

Herbal treatment:
Hu Xi Cang (P, Chapter 18)—tonifies Lung and Kidney *Qi*, nourishes Lung *Yin*, stops asthma and cough

Cough

There are many Patterns for cough in TCVM, with emphasis placed on the chronicity, loudness, temperature preferences, and thirst.

Wind-Cold Onset is acute, with cold aversion, cold ears and nose, clear nasal discharge, and cough with clear sputum. Tongue is pale and red with thin coating. Pulses are superficial and slow.

Herbal treatment:
1. *Xiao Qing Long Wan* (P, Chapter 19)—dispels pathogenic Wind-Cold, transforms Phlegm, warms Lung, stops cough, descends *Qi*
2. *Zhi Sou San* (Chapter 20) —moistens Lung, transforms Phlegm, stops cough

Wind-Heat Heat signs, fever, and thirst are evident. There is a loud cough with little sputum. Tongue is red with a yellow coating; pulses are superficial and fast.

Herbal treatment:
1. Jade Screen Eight (JT)—tonifies *Qi*, clears Heat, releases exterior
2. *Yin Chiao Chieh Tu Pien* (P)—dispels pathogenic Wind, clears Heat, resolves toxins, benefits throat, relieves thirst, diffuses Lung Heat

Phlegm Heat The cough becomes more chronic. There is a loud, persistent cough. Nasal discharge is yellow and thick. Ears and nose are hot.

Herbal treatment:
Qing Qi Hua Tan Wan (P, Chapter 20)—transforms Phlegm, clears Heat, drains Lung, relieves cough

Phlegm-Damp The cough becomes more chronic. There is little to no nasal discharge. Cough is very loud, wet, and productive. The tongue is wet with a thick, white coating, and the pulse is tight and slow.

Herbal treatment:
Er Chen Tang (P, Chapter 20)—transforms and dispels Phlegm, dries Dampness, harmonizes the Stomach

Lung-Liver Fire This Pattern is often seen in Wood animals, or in some cases of distemper or kennel cough. Cough is painful, with little sputum, or with sticky, difficult-to-expectorate Phlegm. The cough is loud and "barking," not rattling. There is increased thirst, hot ears and nose, and costal pain. Tongue is red to purple, dry, and has a yellow coating. Pulses are wiry and fast.

Herbal treatment:
Ching Fei Yi Huo (P)—clears Lung Heat, eliminates Phlegm, relieves cough; may be combined with antiviral or antibacterial herbs

***Yin* Deficiency** Cough is chronic, weak, and dry, and is worse at night. There is no nasal discharge. Coat and pads are dry and the animal is emaciated. The tongue is red and dry, with no coating. The pulses are thready and weak.

Herbal treatment:
1. *Sha Shen Mai Dong Wan* (P)—nourishes Lung *Yin*, moistens Lung, relieves cough, generates fluid
2. *Bai He Gu Jin Tang* (P)—nourishes Lung *Yin*, moistens Lung, stops cough

Lung *Yin-Qi* Deficiency Cough is long-term chronic, weak, and nonproductive. Coat and pads are dry. There is exercise intolerance and shortness of breath. Tongue may be pale or red, dry or wet. Pulses are thready, deep, and weak.

Herbal treatment:
Bu Fei Wan (P)—the classic version of this formula contains both *Huang Qi* and *Shu Di Huang* in equal amounts, and thus tonifies Lung *Yin* and *Qi* and relieves cough.

Lung *Qi* Deficiency Cough is long-term chronic. There is exercise intolerance, shortness of breath, and fatigue. Tongue is pale and wet; pulses are deep and weak.

Herbal treatment:
Bu Fei San (JT)—the *Jing Tang* formula focuses on tonifying Lung *Qi* and stopping cough and asthma. It does not contain the *Yin* tonics that are in the patent formulas do

Symptomatically, various formulas are available to combine with the previous formulas to alleviate productive coughs.

Herbal treatment:
1. *San She Dan Chuan Bei Yi* (P)—draw up the patent 10 ml vials in a syringe and dispense at 1/4–1 vial up to qid; good for stubborn chronic Phlegm Heat; moistens throat, resolves toxins, transforms Phlegm
2. Fritillaria and Pinellia Syrup (GF)—useful with Hot, productive coughs; thinner and thus easier to use than the traditional patent Loquat and Fritillaria syrup

Upper Respiratory Infection/Nasal Congestion/Discharge

Herbal formulas for upper respiratory issues have the greatest small animal application for cats with oral and bacterial issues and dogs with sinusitis.

Wind Heat There are heat signs such as fever, warm ears, and nose, and injected sclera. Thirst is increased. As symptoms progress, there may be swollen red throat and tonsils, thick yellow nasal discharge, and dry feces. Tongue is red and dry with a yellow coating. Pulses are fast and floating.

Herbal treatment:
1. *Yin Chiao Chieh Tu Pien* (P)—dispels Wind, clears Heat, detoxifies, benefits the throat; useful for early stage feline URTI and for exposure to kennel cough, showing sore throat, watery eyes, and fever
2. *Tuo Ming Tang* (P, JT)—cools Blood, clears Wind Heat, moves Blood; used for allergic rhinitis, sinusitis, and thick nasal discharge
3. *Cang Er Zi Wan* (P)—dispels Wind, eliminates Heat, opens nasal passages

Wind-Cold, Cold Damp There is clear nasal discharge with sneezing and headache. Tongue is pale; pulse is tight.

Herbal treatment:
Xin Yi San (P, Chapter 19)—dispels Wind and Cold, opens nasal passages, dispels turbidity, transforms Phlegm

Phlegm Stagnation Symptoms are thick profuse nasal discharge with odor, sneezing, and frontal headache. Tongue is purple or red; pulses are deep or fast.

Herbal treatment:
Huey's Formula (JT)—clears Wind-Heat and Wind-Cold, opens nasal passages

UROGENITAL CONDITIONS

Female Infertility

Small animals typically display Liver *Qi* Stagnation, Blood Deficiency, and/or *Yin* Deficiency. After commencing herbs, it is wise to go through at least one complete, normal heat cycle before breeding to allow the animal to regain balance and have the best chance for reproductive success.

Liver *Qi* Stagnation There is often a history of gastrointestinal or emotional issues. Heat cycles may be infrequent, the female does not "catch," or she may be nonreceptive or even violent. The tongue is purple or red and the pulses are wiry.

Herbal treatment:

1. Liver Happy (JT)—soothes Liver *Qi,* clears Heat, resolves Stagnation; good for Wood-type dog with anger and heat signs
2. *Xiao Yao San* (P, Chapter 24)—soothes Liver, harmonizes Liver and Spleen, tonifies Spleen and Blood; useful when there is a history of diarrhea, loose stools, or abnormal appetite

Blood Deficiency Coat is dull, and skin is dry and has dandruff. Heat cycles are absent or infrequent. The animal has anxiety or nervousness. There is lethargy and gums are pale. Tongue is lavender and dry; pulses are deep and weak.

Herbal treatment:

1. *Xiao Yao San* (P, Chapter 24)—as above
2. *Si Wu Tang* (P, Chapter 18)—nourishes Blood, invigorates Blood, regulates menses

***Yin* Deficiency** This is a common Pattern in cats, or in conjunction with Liver *Qi* Stagnation in dogs. Coat is dry and dull, skin has dandruff. The animal is polydipsic and is restless in the evening. Heat cycles are short or absent. Tongue is red and dry and pulses are thin and thready.

Herbal treatment:

1. *Liu Wei Di Huang Wan* (P, Chapter 18)—nourishes Kidney and Liver *Yin*, cools deficient Heat, nourishes *Jing*.
2. *Zhi Bai Di Huang Wan* (P, Chapter 18)—nourishes Kidney and Liver *Yin*, cools deficient Heat, nourishes *Jing* (more cooling than *Liu Wei Di Huang Wan*)

Male Infertility

Low libido and low sperm counts are typically due to Kidney *Yang/Jing* Deficiency, and also are due to aging, overuse as a breeding animal, poor genetics, or poor husbandry.

Herbal treatment:

1. *Jin Suo Gu Jing Wan* (P, Chapter 28)—secures *Jing*, benefits Kidney, astringes urine
2. *Yin Yang Huo San* (Chapter 18)—tonifies Kidney *Yang*, nourishes *Yin/Jing*

Prostate Disease

Most prostate issues in small animals occur in older intact male dogs. Prostatitis can have a Damp-Heat Pattern or Spleen *Qi*/Kidney *Qi* Deficiency.

Heat and Damp-Heat There is soreness in the low back. The animal may be polydipsic, and may have trouble urinating or defecating. There may be a history of poor diet or loose stools. Tongue is red and pulses are fast.

Herbal treatment:

1. *Ba Zheng San* (P, Chapter 23)—clears Heat, dispels Damp, benefits movement of urine, relieves pain
2. Prostate Invigorator (JT)—moves Blood, clears Heat, resolves Stagnation, stops pain

Spleen *Qi* Deficiency/Kidney *Qi* Deficiency There is lethargy and exercise intolerance. The urine stream is weak, or animal dribbles urine. There is diarrhea, chronic IBD, or poor appetite. The animal seeks warmth and has cool extremities. The tongue is pale and wet; pulses are deep and weak.

Herbal treatment:

Kai Kit Wan (P)—tonifies *Qi*, tonifies Blood, tonifies Kidney *Yang*, nourishes Kidney *Yin*, invigorates Blood, clears heat, promotes urination

Renal Failure

Renal failure lends itself very well to treatment with Chinese herbs. Herbs in this section specifically treat the Kidney Pattern, and herbs can be chosen from other groups for symptoms such as vomiting, anorexia, or anemia. The following sections summarize the main categories.

Kidney *Qi* Deficiency The animal presents with back weakness and/or rear-end weakness. There is incontinence, dysuria, or stranguria. The tongue is pale and wet, and pulses are deep and weak, especially on the right.

Herbal treatment:

Suo Quan Wan (P, Chapter 28)—warms and consolidates Kidney *Qi*

Kidney *Yang* Deficiency The face is drawn, and the manner is subdued. There is cold aversion, cold extremities, sore lumbar area, and general weakness and debility. Teeth are poor, hearing is diminished, urine is copious, or there is enuresis. There may be limb or ventral abdominal ascites. The tongue is pale and swollen with a pale coating, and pulses are deep and weak, especially on the right side.

Herbal treatment:

1. *Zhen Wu Tang* (P, Chapter 22)—tonifies Heart and Kidney *Yang*, drains Damp
2. *You Gui Wan* (P, Chapter 18)—tonifies Kidney *Yang*, warms *Ming Men* Fire, nourishes Blood, and strengthens tendons and bones

Kidney *Yin* Deficiency There may be dysuria or stranguria. The back is weak and the lumbar area is sore. The animal appears thin with a dull coat. The nose, coat, feces, and skin are dry. There is polydipsia with panting, especially in the late afternoon and at night. The footpads and head are hot, and the skin may be red. Heat signs may be worse in the late afternoon and at night. The tongue is dry and red, and the pulses, especially left, are deep, thready, and weak.

Herbal treatment:

1. *Liu Wei Di Huang Wan* (P, Chapter 18)—benefits Kidney, nourishes Liver *Yin*, cools deficient Heat
2. *Zuo Gui Wan* (P, Chapter 18)—benefits Kidney, nourishes Kidney *Yin*, nourishes *Jing*, strengthens tendons and bones
3. *Zhi Bai Di Huang Wan* (P, Chapter 18)—nourishes Kidney *Yin*, clears Heat; especially useful for excessive false Heat signs, such as severe PU/PD, anxiety, and panting at night

Kidney *Qi* and *Yin* Deficiency The animal has weak or sore low back, exercise intolerance, and lethargy. The coat and pads are dry, and the skin may be red. The tongue is red and dry or pale and wet. Pulses are thready and rapid or deep and weak.

Herbal treatment:

Rehmannia 11 (JT)—tonifies *Qi* and nourishes *Yin*

For an animal that shows signs of Kidney *Yin* and *Yang* Deficiency, one may use *You Gui Wan* in the morning and *Zuo Gui Wan* at night.

Kidney *Jing* Deficiency The animal is born with congenital defects, develops bony abnormalities at a young age, and may have delayed tooth eruption and delayed sexual maturity. There may be cryptorchidism or hermaphroditism. Teeth may decay early and other Kidney *Qi* and *Yin* symptoms may be evident, such as incontinence at a young age. The tongue is pale or red, and pulses are weak.

Herbal treatment:

1. *Yin Yang Huo San* (Chapter 18)—tonifies Kidney *Yang*, nourishes *Yin* and *Jing*; may be warming for some animals
2. *Liu Wei Di Huang Wan* (P)—tonifies Kidney *Yin* and *Jing*, especially, but not necessarily, if Heat signs are evident

Urinary Tract Infection

Herbal remedies are effective for both acute and chronic conditions.

Bladder Damp-Heat There is polyuria, straining to urinate, and licking of the genitals. Urine is dark, bloody, and has a strong odor. The tongue is red with yellow coating. Pulses are slippery and fast.

Herbal treatment:

Ba Zheng San (P, Chapter 23)—clears Heat and Fire, eliminates Damp; may use lower dose long term for chronic cystitis

Bladder Damp-Heat with Kidney or Bladder Stones This has a similar Pattern as above, but stones or crystals are present.

Herbal treatment:

1. Crystal Stone Formula (JT)—clears Heat and Damp, resolves crystals, stops hemorrhage
2. Amber Stone Transforming Formula (GF)—expels stones, dispels Damp-Heat, moves *Qi*, clears Heat, invigorates Blood, stops bleeding and pain

Stone formulas may be dosed lower for deficient animals, and they may be combined with Kidney *Yin* tonics if applicable.

Bladder Damp-Heat with *Yin* Deficiency There is a history of chronic urinary tract infections. There is straining to urinate and increased thirst. Male cats may be prone to mucous plugs. The coat is dry and the animal is thin. Tongue is red and dry and may have a thin coating. Pulses are fast and thready.

Herbal treatment:

Zhu Ling Tang (P, Chapter 23)—clears Damp-Heat, tonifies *Yin*

37 Clinical Application of Chinese Herbal Medicine for Horses
中药在大动物临床上应用

Lisa Trevisanello, Huisheng Xie

MUSCULOSKELETAL CONDITIONS

Lameness

Lameness is a gait abnormality caused by either a structural or a functional disorder of one or more of the limbs, the neck, or the trunk. It is either a manifestation of pain, a mechanical lameness, or a combination of the two. In Traditional Chinese Veterinary Medicine (TCVM), lameness can be caused by *Qi* or Blood Stagnation or a combination of both, which can affect the muscles, tendons, ligaments, or bones. Another cause of lameness is invasion of pathogenic Wind, Cold, and Damp. Pain results from *Qi* and/or Blood Stagnation, and it could be in the Channels or in various tissues (Table 37.1).

***Qi*-Blood Stagnation in the Channels** Traumatic injuries that are lodged in more Exterior areas of the body (muscle and connecting tissues) lead to sprain, strain, swelling, and pain around an area of injury.

Herbal treatment:
Die Da Wan

***Qi*-Blood Stagnation in the Tendons and Ligaments** The Liver dominates and controls the tendons and ligaments. Usually weakness of tendons and ligaments is related to Liver *Yin* and Blood Deficiency.

Herbal treatment:
A combination of *Shen Tong Zhu Yu Tang* and *Hu Qian Wan*

Blood Stagnation in the Bones Blood Stagnation can affect the bones and cause osteophyte, ringbone, intra-articular chip fracture, and calcium overdeposition.

Herbal treatment:
Bone Stasis Formula (JT)[1]

Wind, Cold, and Damp Invasion The pathogenic combination of Wind, Cold, and Damp causes *Qi* and Blood Stagnation and ultimately pain.

Herbal treatment:
1. For severe cases with strong constitution: *Xiao Huo Luo Dan*
2. For weak constitution: *Du Huo Ji Sheng Tang*

Laminitis

Laminitis is a degeneration of the union between the horny and sensitive laminae with areas of ischemia or hemostasis within the laminae. It is a manifestation of a generalized metabolic imbalance.

Table 37.1. TCVM Patterns and herbal treatment of lameness.

TCVM Pattern	Clinical Signs	Herbal Formula
Qi-Blood Stagnation	Pain in the surface and muscles	*Die Da Wan*
Qi-Blood Stagnation with Liver *Yin* or/and Blood Deficiency	Ligament or Tendon injuries	*Shen Tong Zhu Yu Tang* + *Hu Qian Wan*
Blood Stagnation	Osteophyte, intra-articular chip fractures	Bone Stasis (JF)
Wind-Cold-Damp *Bi* Syndrome	Wind-Cold-Damp invasion	For strong constitution: *Xiao Huo Luo Dan* For weak constitution: *Du Huo Ji Sheng Tang*

Damp-Heat Pattern Symptoms are acute onset of founder or laminitis, red or purple tongue, and wiry or fast pulse.

Herbal treatment:
1. A combination of *Yin Chen Hao San* and *Fu Yuan Huo Xue Tang*
2. Hot Hoof II (JT)[1]

***Qi*-Blood Stagnation with *Yin* Deficiency** Chronic laminitis occurs in Cushing's syndrome or equine metabolic syndrome with red tongue and fast pulse.

Herbal treatment:
1. A combination of *Shen Tong Zhu Yu Tang* and *Zuo Gui Wan*
2. Hot Hoof I (JT)[1]

***Qi*-Blood Stagnation with *Yang* Deficiency** Chronic laminitis occurs in Cushing's syndrome or equine metabolic syndrome with pale purple and swollen tongue, and deep and weak pulse.

Herbal treatment:
1. A combination of *Shen Tong Zhu Yu Tang* and *You Gui Wan*
2. Rehmannia 14 (JT)[1]

Exertional Rhabdomyolysis (Tying Up)

Several exertional myopathies can occur in the horse. They are a syndrome of muscle fatigue, pain, or cramping most commonly caused by exercise following a period of inactivity. Most exertional myopathies result in necrosis of striated skeletal muscle and are called "exertional rhabdomyolysis." Exertional rhabdomyolysis is no longer considered a single disease but consists of several different myopathies, with different etiopathology. In the past it was often described as azoturia, tying up, or cording up.

Etiology and Pathology: Exertional rhabdomyolysis is mainly caused by Earth-Water-Wood disharmony. The excessive Wood can overcontrol (*cheng*) the Earth (muscle) leading to *Qi* Stagnation of the muscles. Disorders of Spleen (muscle) can overcontrol the water system (Kidney, Bladder) leading to azoturia. Fearful Water or nervous Wood personality horses seem more prone to tying up. A diet rich in carbohydrates and imbalanced exercise can also lead to *Qi* Stagnation.

***Qi*-Blood Stagnation with Invasion of Wind Damp** The clinical symptoms are muscle pain; muscles firm to palpation; reluctance to move; and short, stiff, stilted gait. Urine can be dark or red-brown. The horse may sweat excessively. The tongue is purple or pale purple. The pulse is wiry.

Herbal treatment:
1. *Shen Tong Zhu Yu Tang* + *Qiang Huo Sheng Shi Tang*
2. Equine Tie-Up (JT)[1]

RESPIRATORY DISEASES

Recurrent Airway Obstruction (Heaves, Chronic Obstructive Pulmonary Disease)

Recurrent airway obstruction (RAO) is an allergic respiratory disease of the horse. Allergen exposure causes bronchoconstriction and production of mucus. It often occurs in susceptible horses that are stabled in an environment with an abundance of dust and molds in the air, beds of straw and hay for feed. The incidence increases with aging. A similar condition (summer pasture–associated obstructive pulmonary disease) can be caused by summer pasture–associated allergies, especially in the southeastern U.S. Table 37.2 summarizes differentiation of patterns and treatment of RAO. In TCVM, the Lung governs *Qi* and respiration; Lung *Qi* Deficiency and an external pathogenic factor invading the body cause weak respiration, dyspnea, and asthma. Patterns of RAO include Lung Heat and *Yin* Deficiency, Lung *Qi* Deficiency, and Lung/Kidney *Qi* Deficiency.

Table 37.2. TCVM Patterns and herbal treatment of recurrent airway obstruction (RAO).

TCVM Pattern	Clinical Signs	Herbal Formula
Lung Heat with *Yin* Deficiency	Dry cough Dry hair coat Dry nasal discharge Cool seeking Flared nostrils Tachypnea Tongue: red and dry Pulse: rapid and thready	*Bai He Gu Jin Tang & Wu Wei Xiao Du Yin*
Lung *Qi* Deficiency	Chronic course of disease Weak cough Tachypnea Fatigue Flared nostrils Tongue: pale, wet Pulse: weak and deep	*Bu Fei San*
Kidney and Lung *Qi* Deficiency	Hypertrophy of the external abdominal oblique muscles (heave line) Flared nostrils Fatigue Wheezing Prolonged expiration Tracheal rattle Crackles Expanded lung fields Tongue: pale, thin coating Pulse: weak and deep	*Hu Xi Cang*

Lung Heat and *Yin* Deficiency If *Zheng Qi* is not strong enough to dispel the pathogen (allergen), Heat invades the Lung. Heat in the Lung further impairs Body Fluids leading to *Yin* Deficiency. The main symptoms are summer pasture–associated allergies, heaves seen only or worse in summer, dry cough, dry hair coat, dry nasal discharge, cool-seeking, flared nostrils, tachypnea, red and dry tongue, and fast pulse.

Herbal treatment:

1. *Bai He Gu Jin Tang* + *Wu Wei Xiao Du Yin*
2. Schisandra 5 (JT)[1]

Lung *Qi* Deficiency Lung *Qi* Deficiency can be caused by chronic cough and dyspnea, grief and sadness, or overwork. Clinical signs include chronic course of disease, weak cough, tachypnea, exercise intolerance, flared nostrils, pale and wet tongue, and weak and deep pulse.

Herbal treatment:
Bu Fei San

Lung and Kidney *Qi* Deficiency A prolonged Lung *Qi* Deficiency might damage the Kidney and lead to the failure of the Kidney to hold down the *Qi*. The main clinical signs include hypertrophy of the external abdominal oblique muscles (heave line), flared nostrils, fatigue, wheezing, prolonged expiration, tracheal rattle, crackles, expanded Lung fields, pale tongue with thin coating, and weak and deep pulse.

Herbal treatment:
Hu Xi Cang

Nasal Congestion and Discharge

In the horse, nasal congestion and discharge may be a sign of viral respiratory infection, secondary bacterial disease, or noninfectious respiratory disease. In TCVM, this syndrome is called *Bi-Yuan*. The nose is the opening orifice of the Lung, and the pathway through which pathogenic *Qi* can enter the Lung. Normal Lung *Qi* maintains an unobstructed respiration, Stagnation of the Lung *Qi* will cause nasal congestion and discharge (Table 37.3).

Table 37.3. TCVM Patterns and herbal treatment of nasal discharge and congestion.

TCVM Pattern	Clinical Signs	Herbal Formula
Wind-Cold	Nasal congestion with clear discharge Sneezing Tongue: pale Pulse: slow	*Xin Yi San*
Allergy Wind-Heat	Allergic rhinitis Sinusitis Sneezing Nasal congestion with thick discharge Tongue: red Pulse: fast	*Tuo Min Fang*
Phlegm Stagnation	Sinusitis with accumulation of pus Yellow, thick nasal discharge with pus Tongue: red or purple Pulse: deep	Huey's Formula
Damp-Heat	Yellow, thick nasal discharge with odor and pus Ulcer on gums or tongue Obesity Anorexia or polyphagia Loose stool Tongue: red or purple with greasy coating Pulse: rapid	*Huang Lian Jie Du Tang*

Wind-Cold Wind is often the primary pathogen to enter the body. It usually carries other pathogens into the body. Wind tends to affect the upper and superficial parts of the body. Exogenous Wind invades the body from the external environment. Wind associated with Cold can invade the body entering the nose and skin. It causes Stagnation of the Lung *Qi*. Sneezing and nasal discharge are the *Wei Qi* and Lung *Qi* responses to try to dispel the pathogen. The clinical signs include nasal congestion with clear discharge, sneezing, pale tongue, and slow superficial pulse.

Herbal treatment:
Xin Yi San

Wind Heat Wind can combine with Heat and invade the body as Wind-Heat pathogen. The main clinical signs are allergic rhinitis, sinusitis, sneezing, nasal congestion with thick discharge, red tongue, and fast pulse.

Herbal treatment:

1. *Ju Hua Cha Tiao San*
2. *Tuo Min Fang* (JT)[1]

Phlegm Stagnation Phlegm is a pathological form of Body Fluid. It can be caused by exogenous Heat or Cold affecting the Lung, Spleen, or Kidney. The Lung is the major system affected by Phlegm. The main clinical signs are sinusitis with accumulation of pus, yellow, thick nasal discharge with pus, red or purple tongue, and deep pulse.

Herbal treatment:

1. *Pi Ji Xiao Du Yin*
2. Huey's Formula (JT)[1]

Damp-Heat Damp tends to obstruct the *Qi* flow and is difficult to remove from the body. When Damp combines with Heat and enters the Lung, it can cause thick nasal discharge. The clinical signs include yellow, thick nasal discharge with odor and pus; ulcer on gums or tongue; obesity; anorexia or polyphagia; diarrhea; red or purple tongue with greasy coating; and fast pulse.

Herbal treatment:
1. *Huang Lian Jie Du Tang*
2. Nasal Damp Heat (JT)[1]

Exercise-Induced Pulmonary Hemorrhage

Exercise-induced pulmonary hemorrhage (EIPH) is a consequence of strenuous exercise and occurs in equine athletes. Approximately 5% of horses with EIPH exhibit epistaxis. In most cases, hemorrhage is detected through endoscopic observation of the tracheobronchial airways or cytologic examination of bronchoalveolar lavage. In TCVM, strenuous exercise and a stressful environment (traveling, pollution, stall confinement, training and racing, shows, and medications) generate Heat and cause Liver *Qi* Stagnation that, over time, will produce more Heat. This is compounded by racehorses being Fire or Wood animals that generate excess Heat. The excessive Heat can induce EIPH. The clinical signs include blood within the airways, epistaxis, poor performance, red tongue, and fast pulse.

Herbal treatment:
1. *Yunnan Bai Yao*
2. Single Immortal (JT)[1]
3. For prevention: *Qing Fei San*

GASTROINTESTINAL DISORDERS

Gastric Ulcers

Gastric ulceration is a widespread condition in horses and foals. It affects up to 90% of racehorses. In foals, the overall prevalence of mild gastric ulcers is around 50%.[2–5] In TCVM, stress caused by competition, environment, imbalanced diet, or a systemic disease can cause Liver *Qi* Stagnation. A stagnant Liver *Qi* will eventually transform into Heat or Fire. Chronic inflammation impairs Body Fluids, and when associated with Heat, leads to Stomach *Yin* Deficiency and gastric ulcers.

Stomach *Yin* Deficiency This is a main Patterns of gastric ulcers in horses. Most signs of ulcers are nonspecific colic, poor appetite, weight loss, poor performance, poor body condition, attitude changes, dry nose and mouth, cool-seeking behavior, red tongue, and thready, fast pulse. In foals, clinical signs include diarrhea, bruxism, poor growth, frequently interrupted nursing, dorsal recumbency, and salivation.

Herbal treatment:
1. *Mai Wei Di Huang Wan*
2. Stomach Happy (JT)[1]

If the patient is presented with Liver *Qi* Stagnation (strong Wood constitution, easily irritable, purple tongue, and wiry pulse), add *Chai Hu Shu Gan Wan*. If Spleen *Qi* Deficiency (watery diarrhea, pale tongue, and weak pulse) is presented, add *Xiao Yao Wan*.

Diarrhea

Diarrhea is an increase in the water content of the feces or frequency of defecation. In less than 50% of cases a definitive cause can be determined in conventional medicine.[4,5] Although diarrhea in adult horses can be acute or chronic, it is considered chronic if it persists for over a month. Acute diarrhea can be caused by infectious agents including *Salmonella enteritica*, *Neorickettsia* (previously known as *Ehrlichia*) *risticii*, *Clostridium difficile*, and *Clostridium perfringens*. Other causes are ingestion of toxic agents or sand. The use of antimicrobials and NSAIDs can alter the intestinal flora and the fermentation process in the colon and cause diarrhea. Chronic diarrhea can be a nonspecific response to inflammatory or neoplastic conditions involving the intestine or diseases of another organ system, such as congestive heart failure and chronic Liver diseases (Table 37.4).

In TCVM, the major organs involved in diarrhea are the Spleen and Stomach. The Spleen transports and transforms food and drink, nourishing the entire body. Normally, the Spleen *Qi* always ascends. The Stomach receives and decomposes food. Stomach *Qi* always descends to the small intestine. Consequently, the Stomach and Spleen act together in the absorption and digestion processes. Many pathogens can damage the Spleen and the *Qi* flow between the Stomach and Spleen, leading to gastrointestinal disorders such as diarrhea.

Damp-Cold Pattern Cold weather, a sudden change in diet, drinking cold water, or other stressful environmental changes can cause Stomach Cold or a Cold-Damp Patterns. The clinical signs include colic, cold ear/nose, pale or purple and wet tongue, and deep and slow pulse.

Herbal treatment:
Wei Ling San

Heat Toxin or Damp-Heat Pathogens Heat Toxin diarrhea generally has an acute course and can be caused by invasion of the Stomach by a Damp-Heat pathogen, such as *Salmonella enteritica*, *Neorickettsia risticii*, *Clostridium difficile*, and *Clostridium perfringens*. But it can also occur as a nonspecific enterocolitis. The clini-

Table 37.4. TCVM Patterns and herbal treatment of diarrhea.

TCVM Pattern	Clinical Signs	Herbal Formula
Cold-Damp	Diarrhea after stressful environmental changes Sudden changes in diet Drinking too much cold water Colic Cold ear/nose Tongue: pale or purple and wet Pulse: deep and slow	*Wei Ling San*
Heat-Toxin (Damp-Heat)	Bloody/watery diarrhea Colitis, enterocolitis, Potomac fever Salmonellosis and nonspecific gastroenteritis Thirst Hot ear/nose Tongue: deep red with yellow coating Pulse: deep and rapid	*Yu Jin San*
Liver *Qi* Stagnation	Diarrhea due to stressful work or environment or gastric ulcer Racehorses are predisposed Tongue: purple or red Pulse: taut-string or wiry	*Xiao Yao San*
Food Stagnation	Soft or watery diarrhea with undigested grain Anorexia Abdominal fullness and pain Tongue: red with a thick coating Pulse: deep	*Bao He Wan*
Spleen *Qi* Deficiency	Chronic watery diarrhea Anorexia Loss of body weight Fatigue Poor performance Tongue: pale or yellow Pulse: deep and weak	*Shen Ling Bai Zhu San*
Kidney *Yang* Deficiency	Prolonged diarrhea Diarrhea at night or early morning Cold and painful back Rear weakness and stiffness Tongue: pale Pulse: deep and weak	*Si Shen Wan*
Diarrhea in Foal	Soft to watery diarrhea due to bacteria, viruses, parasites, or other pathogenic factors Tongue: Pale or purple Pulse: Thready and fast	*Wu Mei San*

cal signs are bloody/watery diarrhea, increased thirst, hot ear and nose, deep-red tongue with yellow coating, and deep and fast pulse.

Herbal treatment:
Yu Jin San

Liver Qi Stagnation Stress caused by competition, environment, imbalanced diet, or a systemic disease can cause Liver *Qi* Stagnation . A stagnant Liver *Qi* will eventually transform into Heat and may invade the Spleen leading to gastric ulcers or diarrhea. The main clinical signs are diarrhea due to stressful work or environment or gastric ulcers (racehorses being predisposed), purple or red tongue, and wiry pulse.

Herbal treatment:
Xiao Yao San

Food Stagnation Stomach *Qi* normally descends to the small intestine. Overfeeding can obstruct the normal flow of *Qi* and cause Food Stagnation . The clinical signs are soft or watery diarrhea with undigested grain, anorexia, abdominal fullness and pain, red tongue with a thick coating, and deep pulse.

Herbal treatment:
Bao He Wan

Spleen *Qi* Deficiency When Spleen *Qi* is deficient, the Spleen cannot transport and transform the food and fails to ascend, causing chronic diarrhea. The main clinical signs are chronic watery diarrhea, anorexia, loss of body weight, fatigue, poor performance, pale or yellow tongue, and deep and weak pulse.

Herbal treatment:
Shen Ling Bai Zhu San

Kidney *Yang* Deficiency Normally, Kidney *Yang* should warm the Spleen. If the Kidney is deficient, it fails to support the Spleen *Yang*, and the Spleen cannot digest and absorb water and food. This will lead to prolonged diarrhea. The clinical signs are prolonged diarrhea, diarrhea at night or early morning (daybreak diarrhea), cold and painful back, rear weakness and stiffness, pale tongue, and deep and weak pulse.

Herbal treatment:
Si Shen Wan

Diarrhea in Foals Diarrhea in foals can be caused by an invasion of the Stomach by Heat-Toxin from pathogens such as *Salmonella* spp, *Escherichia coli, Klebsiella* spp, and *Clostridium* spp, rotavirus, and parasites. The clinical signs are soft to watery diarrhea due to bacteria, viruses, parasites, or other pathogenic factors, pale or purple tongue, and thready and fast pulse.

Herbal treatment:
Wu Mei San

Abdominal Pain (Colic)

The term "colic" means abdominal pain. It is a broad term indicating clinical signs of abdominal pain in the horse and it refers to conditions of different etiologies and severity. In TCVM, abdominal pain results from the Stagnation of *Qi* in the abdomen, which can be caused by disorders of the *Zang-Fu* organs. The five main patterns seen are Cold, Damp-Heat, *Qi* Stagnation, Blood Stagnation, and Food Stagnation (Table 37.5).

Table 37.5. TCVM Patterns and herbal treatment of abdominal pain.

TCVM Pattern	Clinical Signs	Herbal Formula
Cold Pattern	Acute onset of abdominal pain Intermittent abdominal pain Pawing with a front foot Looking at the flank region Raising a rear leg or kicking at the abdomen Lying down Rolling from side to side Soft or watery feces Borborygmus Cold ears Tongue: purple or pale Pulse: slow and deep	*Ju Pi San*
Damp-Heat Pattern	Acute onset of abdominal pain Intermittent abdominal pain Fever Increased thirst Diarrhea with mucous and foul smell Dark urine Tongue: deep red with yellow, greasy coating Pulse: Surging and rapid	*Yu Jin San*
Qi Stagnation	Subacute onset of colic Bloat, gaseous bowel movement Abdominal fullness Anorexia Tongue: purple or red Pulse: fast or wiry	*Xiao Zhang San*
Blood Stagnation	Colic worse during/after work Tongue: purple Pulse: fast or weak	*Shao Fu Zhu Yu Tang*
Food Stagnation	Acute onset of abdominal pain Tongue: deep red with yellow, thick coating Pulse: deep	*Ma Jia Wan*

Cold Pattern Cold weather or ingestion of cold food or cold water can cause *Qi* and Blood Stagnation in the gastrointestinal tract. This Patterns can be associated with enterospasm. The clinical signs are acute onset of abdominal pain or intermittent abdominal pain, pawing with a front foot, looking at the flank region, raising a rear leg or kicking at the abdomen, lying down, rolling from side to side, soft or watery feces, cold ears, purple or pale tongue, and slow and deep pulse.

Herbal treatment:
Ju Pi San

Damp-Heat Pattern Pathogenic Damp-Heat leads to *Qi* Stagnation and pain. It can be caused by hot and humid weather, some medications, toxins, and a diet high in carbohydrates. This Patterns can be associated with enteritis. The main clinical signs are acute onset of abdominal pain, intermittent abdominal pain, pawing with a front foot, looking at the flank region, raising a rear leg or kicking at the abdomen, lying down, rolling from side to side, fever, increased thirst, diarrhea with foul smell, dark urination, deep-red tongue with yellow and greasy coating, and surging and rapid pulse.

Herbal treatment:
Yu Jin San

***Qi* Stagnation Pattern** The clinical signs are subacute onset of colic, pawing with a front foot, looking at the flank region, raising a rear leg or kicking at the abdomen, lying down, rolling from side to side, bloat, gaseous bowel movement, abdominal fullness, anorexia, purple or red tongue, and fast or wiry pulse.

Herbal treatment:
Xiao Zhang San

Blood Stagnation Clinical signs are colic that is worse during or after work, pawing with a front foot, looking at the flank region, raising a rear leg or kicking at the abdomen, lying down, rolling from side to side, purple tongue, and fast or weak pulse.

Herbal treatment:
Shao Fu Zhu Yu Tang

Food Stagnation Clinical signs are acute onset of abdominal pain, pawing with a front foot, looking at the flank region, raising a rear leg or kicking at the abdomen, lying down, rolling from side to side, and deep-red tongue with yellow and thick coating, deep pulse.

Herbal treatment:
Ma Jia Wan

ENDOCRINE DISEASES

Equine Metabolic Syndrome and Equine Cushing's Syndrome

Equine Metabolic Syndrome (EMS) is a cluster of problems that include obesity, insulin resistance, and laminitis. Tests for pituitary dysfunction generally yield negative results in these EMS horses. Equine Cushing's Syndrome refers to adenomas or adenomatous hypertrophy of the pituitary gland (pars intermedia). Horses suffering from both EMS and Cushing's Syndrome can be divided into four TCVM patterns: *Qi* Deficiency and Damp, *Yin* Deficiency, *Qi-Yin* Deficiency, and *Yang* Deficiency (Table 37.6).

***Qi* Deficiency and Damp** The clinical signs are poor performance, poor or slow shedding, obesity, pale and wet tongue, and deep pulse.

Herbal treatment:
Liu Jun Zi Tang

***Yin* Deficiency** The clinical signs include polyuria (PU), polydipsia (PD), polyphagia, dry hair coat and skin, with thinning hair or alopecia, dry hooves, excessive panting mostly at night, dry and red tongue, and thready and fast pulse.

Table 37.6. TCVM Patterns and herbal treatment for Equine Metabolic Syndrome and Cushing's Syndrome.

TCVM Pattern	Clinical Signs	Herbal Formula
Qi Deficiency and Damp	Poor performance Poor or slow shedding Obesity Tongue: pale and wet Pulse: deep	*Liu Jun Zi Tang*
Yin Deficiency	Polyphagia Dry haircoat, skin, and hooves Hair thinning PU/PD Excessive panting, mostly at night Tongue: dry and red Pulse: thready and rapid	*Zuo Gui Wan*
Qi and *Yin* Deficiency	PU/PD Pendulous abdomen or ascites Pulmonary edema Congestive heart failure Enlarged liver Excessive panting, mostly at night Tongue: pale or red Pulse: thready and weak	*Xiao Ke Fang*
Yang Deficiency	PU/PD Pendulous abdomen or ascites Pulmonary edema Congestive heart failure Enlarged liver Warm-seeking Hirsutism Chronic/recurrent laminitis Tongue: swollen and pale Pulse: deep and weak	*You Gui Wan*

Herbal treatment:
1. *Zuo Gui Wan*
2. *Mai Men Dong* (JT)[1]

***Qi-Yin* Deficiency** The clinical signs are PU, PD, muscle wasting, pendulous abdomen or ascites, pulmonary edema, congestive heart failure, enlarged Liver, excessive panting mostly at night, pale or red tongue, thready and weak pulse.

Herbal treatment:
1. *Xiao Ke Fang*
2. Rehmannia 11 (JT)[1]

***Yang* Deficiency** The clinical signs are PU, PD, muscle wasting, pendulous abdomen or ascites, pulmonary edema, congestive heart failure, enlarged Liver, warm-seeking, hirsutism, chronic/recurrent laminitis, swollen and pale tongue, and deep and weak pulse.

Herbal treatment:
1. *You Gui Wan*
2. Rehmannia 14 (JT)[1]

REPRODUCTIVE PROBLEMS

Female Infertility

Infertility is the failure to produce a normal number or any offspring. In females, anestrus, irregular estrus, or silent estrus are caused by dysfunction of the ovaries or the hypothalamus-pituitary axis. In TCVM, the reproductive system is regulated by the Kidney, Liver, and *Ren* and *Chong* Channels. Mare infertility can be divided into four patterns: Kidney *Qi-Yang* Deficiency, Kidney *Jing* Deficiency, Kidney-Liver *Yin* Deficiency, and Liver *Qi*-Blood Stagnation (Table 37.7).

Kidney *Qi-Yang* Deficiency The clinical signs are anestrus, prolonged diestrus, anovulatory follicles, silent estrus, or irregular estrous cycle, poor body condition, emaciation, depression, lack of strength, poor performance, cold back and extremities, pale tongue with thin coating, and deep and weak pulse.

Herbal treatment:
Di Huang Yin Zi

Kidney *Jing* Deficiency Clinical signs are anestrus, irregular estrous cycle, failure to conceive, weakness in the back, fatigue, premature aging, poor skeletal development, deep-red or pale swollen tongue, and deep, weak, and thready pulse.

Herbal treatment:
Yin Yang Huo San

Kidney-Liver *Yin* Deficiency Clinical signs are anestrus, irregular estrous cycle, failure to conceive, vaginal thick and yellow discharge, weakness in the back, fatigue, dry hair coat, skin or hooves, purple red tongue, and deep, weak, thready pulse.

Herbal treatment:
Yi Guan Jian

Liver *Qi* Blood Stagnation Clinical signs are cystic ovaries, anestrus, short luteal phase or irregular estrous cycle, vaginal thick discharge, intolerance to pressure on the abdomen, purple tongue with a thin coating, and wiry pulse.

Herbal treatment:
1. *Tao Hong Si Wu Tang*
2. Lotus Formula (JT)[1]

Table 37.7. TCVM Patterns and herbal treatment of infertility.

TCVM Pattern	Clinical Signs	Herbal Formula
Kidney *Qi–Yang* Deficiency	Anestrus, prolonged diestrus Anovulatory follicles, silent estrus Irregular estrous cycles Poor body condition, emaciation, depression Lack of strength, poor performance Cold back and extremities Tongue: pale with thin coating Pulse: deep and weak	*Di Huang Yin Zi*
Kidney *Jing* Deficiency	Anestrus Irregular estrous cycles Failure to conceive Weakness in the back, fatigue Premature aging Poor skeletal development Tongue: deep red, or pale and swollen Pulse: deep, weak, and thready	*Yin Yang Huo San*
Kidney-Liver *Yin* Deficiency	Anestrus, irregular estrous cycle Failure to conceive Vaginal thick and yellow discharge Weakness in the back, fatigue Dry haircoat, skin, or hooves Tongue: purple red Pulse: deep, weak, and thready	*Yi Guan Jian*
Liver *Qi*-Blood Stagnation	Cystic ovaries Anestrus, short luteal phase, or irregular estrous cycle Vaginal thick discharge Intolerance to pressure on the abdomen Tongue: purple with a thin coating Pulse: wiry	*Tao Hong Si Wu Tang*

Male Infertility

In general, infertility problems in males are caused by disorders of spermatozoa (poor quality, low count), lack of libido, and inability to mate. TCVM patterns of male infertility are Kidney *Jing-Yang* Deficiency and Liver *Qi* Stagnation.

Kidney *Jing-Yang* Deficiency Male reproductive function depends on both Kidney *Yang* and Kidney *Jing*. Poor quality and quantity of spermatozoa in stallions is related to Kidney *Yang* and *Jing* Deficiency. The clinical signs are impotence, poor sperm quality, low sperm counts, cold back and extremities, pale and swollen tongue, and weak and deep pulse.

Herbal treatment:
You Gui Wan

Liver *Qi* Stagnation A stressful environment, competition, travel, stall confinement, and use of drugs often result in Liver *Qi* Stagnation. Chronic Liver *Qi* Stagnation can disturb the *Shen* (mind) and lead to sexual behavior dysfunctions, such as lack of libido. The clinical signs are Wood type personality, lack of libido, sexual behavior dysfunction, purple tongue, and wiry pulse.

Herbal treatment:
1. *Chai Hu Shu Gan San* + *Suan Zao Ren Tang*
2. Shen Calmer (JT)[1]

Endometritis

In TCVM, endometritis belongs to a syndrome called *Dai Xia Bing*, which means genital discharge. Infertility in mares is often related to endometritis. Although it can be caused by numerous bacterial pathogens, the most common etiologic agent of endometritis is *Streptococcus zooepidemicus*. *Dai Xia Bing* can be divided into *Qi* Deficiency and Damp-Heat patterns (Table 37.8).

Damp-Heat Pattern When Damp-Heat from the environment invades the body, it moves into the lower *Jiao* and accumulates in the uterus, causing an acute onset of endometritis. The clinical signs are acute onset of endometritis; loss of appetite; dark urine; heavy amount of yellow, thick, and sticky discharge with foul odor; diarrhea with mucous and foul odor; dark urination; red tongue with yellow/greasy coating; and slippery-wiry or soft-fast pulse.

Herbal treatment:
1. *Long Dan Xie Gan Tang*
2. Phellodendron and Plantago (*Bai Che San*) (JT)[1]

***Qi* Deficiency** A stressful environment, overwork, or chronic inflammation leads to Spleen *Qi* Deficiency. The Spleen fails to transport Damp, which accumulates in the uterus causing chronic endometritis. The clinical signs are chronic endometritis, fatigue, poor appetite, medium amount of thin white or yellow discharge without foul odor, pale and wet tongue, and weak pulse.

Herbal treatment:
Wan Dai Fang

Table 37.8. TCVM Patterns and herbal treatment of endometritis.

TCVM Pattern	Clinical Signs	Herbal Formula
Damp-Heat Pattern	Acute onset of endometritis Loss of appetite Dark urine Heavy amount of yellow, thick and sticky discharge with foul odor Diarrhea with mucous, foul smell, dark urine Tongue: Red with yellow/ greasy coating Pulse: Slippery-wiry or soft-rapid	Phellodendron and Plantago (*Bai Che San*) (JT)
Qi Deficiency Pattern	Chronic course of endometritis Fatigue Poor appetite Medium amount of thin white or yellow discharge without foul odor Tongue: pale, wet Pulse: weak	*Wan Dai Fang*

NEUROLOGIC DISORDERS

Laryngeal Hemiplegia

Laryngeal hemiplegia is characterized by paralysis of the left arytenoid cartilage and vocal fold, most commonly where the arytenoid cartilage does not move away from the midline during inspiration. The clinical signs are exercise intolerance and a respiratory noise, particularly during inspiration and exercise (also called "roaring"). Laryngeal paralysis is the result of the progressive degeneration or damage of the distal portion of the recurrent laryngeal nerve, which causes neurogenic atrophy of the laryngeal musculature, particularly the cricoarytenoideus dorsalis muscle. Asynchronous, asymmetrical, or incomplete arytenoid cartilage abduction noted during the different stages of progressive degeneration of the recurrent laryngeal nerve prior to paralysis is referred to as laryngeal hemiparesis.

TCVM Pattern: *Qi* Deficiency with Kidney *Jing* Deficiency

Herbal treatment:
Si Jun Zi Tang + *Yin Yang Huo San*

Equine Protozoal Myeloencephalitis (EPM)

Equine protozoal myeloencephalitis (EPM) is a neurologic disease caused by a protozoan, *Sarcocystis neurona*. Horses are a dead-end host when they become infected by ingestion of sporocysts. *Sarcocystis neurona* enters the body when *Zheng Qi* is not strong enough and invades the CNS where they cause *Qi* and Blood Stagnation. The main clinical signs are weakness, ataxia, muscle atrophy, pale-purple tongue, and deep and weak pulse.

TCVM Pattern: *Qi* Deficiency with parasite invasion

Herbal treatment:
Qing Hao San

Cervical Stenotic Myelopathy (Wobbler Syndrome)

Cervical stenotic myelopathy is one of a group of diseases grouped under the Wobbler Syndrome. It results from spinal cord compression at the cervical level, and it is characterized by an abnormal gait with the pelvic limbs usually affected more severely. Cervical stenotic myelopathy affects mostly largebreed, rapidly growing horses, particularly thoroughbreds. Males are more commonly affected than females. It appears to be inherited, and overfeeding is a contributory factor. In TCVM, cervical stenotic myelopathy is treated like cervical *Bi* syndrome. *Bi* syndrome refers to pain and stiffness. The main clinical signs are cervical pain or stiffness, ataxia (hind or/and thoracic limbs), purple tongue, and wiry pulse.

TCVM Pattern: *Qi*-Blood Stagnation

Herbal treatment:
1. *Da Huo Luo Dan*
2. Cervical Formula + Double P#2 (JT)[1]

MISCELLANEOUS DISEASES

Ophthalmic Diseases

Equine recurrent uveitis is the most common cause of blindness in horses. This syndrome is characterized by episodes of inflammation of the uveal tract followed by periods of quiescence. Usually, the inflammatory events lead to secondary changes, such as conjunctivitis, keratitis, keratoconjunctivitis sicca, and corneal ulcers. In TCVM, the Liver is usually involved in the development of ophthalmic diseases. Heat can invade the body, accumulate in the Liver and be transmitted upward to the eye. The Liver can also be affected by stress or emotional factors leading to Liver *Yang* rising upward to the eyes. In TCVM, ophthalmic diseases can be the consequence of two patterns: Liver Heat with Stagnation, Liver-Kidney *Yin* Deficiency (Table 37.9).

Liver Heat with Stagnation Clinical signs are conjunctivitis or keratitis, red eyes, swollen eyelids, ocular discharge varying from clear and watery to mucoid, photophobia, opacity of the cornea, red or purple tongue, and fast or weak pulse.

Herbal treatment:
Jue Ming San

Table 37.9. TCVM Patterns and herbal treatment of ophthalmic diseases.

TCVM Pattern	Clinical Signs	Herbal Formula
Liver Heat with Stagnation Pattern	Conjunctivitis or keratitis Red eyes Swollen eyelids Ocular discharge varying from clear and watery to mucoid Photophobia Miosis Opacity of the cornea Tongue: red or purple Pulse: Surging fast or weak and deep	*Jue Ming San*
Liver-Kidney *Yin* Deficiency Pattern	Atrophied pupil Thick mucoid ocular discharge Corneal opacity Atrophied, yellow or gray sclera Tongue: deep red Pulse: deep, weak	*Qi Ju Di Huang Wan*

Liver-Kidney *Yin* Deficiency Clinical signs are atrophied pupil; thick mucoid ocular discharge; corneal opacity; atrophied, yellow or grey sclera; deep-red tongue; and deep and weak pulse.

Herbal treatment:
Qi Ju Di Huang Wan

Anhidrosis

Anhidrosis, or the inability to sweat, is a common problem in horses. The condition develops most frequently in horses stabled and trained where temperatures and humidity stay high for lengthy periods of time. It is also described as "dry coat" or "nonsweating" disease. In TCVM, sweating is regulated by the Heart, Lung, and Triple Burner (Triple Heater). Since sweat comes from the Body Fluids, a component of Blood, the Heart controls perspiration because it dominates the Blood. Regulating the opening and closing mechanism of skin pores (sweat glands) is part of the ascending function of the Lung. The TB is the general pathway of Body Fluids. Normal *Qi* flow of the Heart, Lung, and TB is interrupted by the invasion of the pathogen, Summer Heat, leading to anhidrosis. If the pathogen continues invading the body, it can damage Body Fluids and the Heart *Yin* and Blood, leading to Heart *Yin* and Blood Deficiency. Fire/Heat can damage the Lung and create Lung *Qi* Deficiency; this can cause failure of the skin pores to open, resulting in anhidrosis. The main clinical signs are dry coat; nonsweating; fatigue; reduced performance; panting; poor stamina and exercise tolerance; dry, pale, or red tongue; and fast pulse. Horses may develop Heat overload and collapse during strenuous exercise.

TCVM Diagnosis: Summer Heat or Damp-Heat

Herbal treatment:
1. *Xiang Ru San*
2. *New Xiang Ru San*

Urticaria (Hives)

Urticaria is characterized by the acute onset of localized edema or swelling in multiple sites on the skin surface. Urticaria is generally allergic in origin and can be caused by bites of insects, administration of medications, or contact with chemicals. Occasionally, hives are secondary to GI conditions. Urticaria can be caused by either an external invasion of Wind and Heat (exogenous hives) or by accumulation of Heat in the Lung and Heart (endogenous hives). The main clinical signs are pruritus with elevated, round, flat-topped 1–20 cm diameter skin lesions, red tongue, and surging and rapid pulse.

Herbal treatment:
1. *Xiao Huang San*
2. Lung Wind *Huang* (JT)[1]

REFERENCES

1. Huisheng Xie. Chinese Veterinary Herbal Handbook, 2nd Edition (Vanessa Preast (ed). Reddick, FL: Chi Institute of Chinese Medicine, 2008.
2. Bell RJ, et al. The prevalence of gastric ulceration in racehorses in New Zealand. New Zealand Veterinary Journal 2007;55(1):13–18.
3. McClure SR, et al. Gastric ulcer development in horses in a simulated show or training environment. JAVMA 2005;227(5):775–778.
4. Kahn, CM (ed). The Merck Veterinary Manual, 9th Edition. Whitehouse Station, NJ: Merck & Co., Inc., 2008.
5. Smith, BP. Large Animal Internal Medicine. St. Louis, MO: Mosby, 1996.

Note: The herbal products can be obtained at Dr. Xie's Jing-tang Herbal (JT) (Reddick, FL); Golden Flower Chinese Herbs (Placitas, NM); Honso (Phoenix, AZ); Institute of Traditional Medicine (ITM) (Portland, OR) Mayway Herbal (Oakland, CA); and Treasure of the East (Ithaca, NY).

Appendix A Chronicle of Chinese History and Traditional Chinese Veterinary Medicine (TCVM)

TCVM Around the World

6,000–5,000 BCE	New Stone Age	The stone needles (*Bian Shi*), which were unearthed in 1963 in Toudaowa of Duolun in Inner Mongolia, are the first known acupuncture tools.
2070–1046 BCE	*Xia-Shang* Dynasty	*Xia* is China's legendary first Dynasty. Emperor Yu is credited with flood control and irrigation systems.
		Jia Gu Wen, the first Chinese written language, evolved during this period. Ancient Chinese characters were written on animal bones and turtle shells.
		According to pictographic characters inscribed on bones, surgical methods for castration in animals had been developed by this time.
		Chinese medicines such as bunge, cherry seed and peach pit were used during this period. These medicines were excavated from the *Gaocheng* ruins of the *Hebei* Province.
		Bronze knives and needles were available for castration and acupuncture.
		The pigsty, cowshed, stable, and sheepfold came into use.
1046–221 BCE	*Zhou* Dynasty	Five Elements, *Zang-fu*, and Eight Principles theories evolved during this time.
		Confucius, *Lao Zi*, and *Yi Jing* promoted philosophical movements that became part of the Hundred Schools of Thought.
		According to *Zhou Li Tian Guan*, a *Zhou* Dynasty history book, full-time veterinarians could be found treating animal disease during this time.
		Zhou Li (*The Rites of Zhou Dynasty*), *Shi Jing* (*The Book of Songs*) and *Shan Hai Jing* (*The Book of Mountains and Rivers*) described more than 100 Chinese medicines.
		Li Ji (*The Book of Rites*) describes some serious domestic animal diseases and records information about collecting medical herbs in summer.
		Huang Di Nei Jing (*Yellow Emperor's Classic of Internal Medicine*) was written during this period. This text documented the basic theories of Traditional Chinese Medicine and Traditional Chinese Veterinary Medicine by presenting a collection of experiences of ancient Chinese people as they struggled against disease.
		Several well-known veterinarians lived during this time: Zao Fu, Bo Le, Wang Liang.
		Veterinarians specializing in equine diseases emerged.
		The books during this period recorded a variety of domestic animal diseases, including boils, weakness, wounds, and sudden death in cattle and horses.
221–207 BCE	*Qin* Dynasty	The First Emperor unified the language, money, and measurements.
		Construction began on the Great Wall, and it was later rebuilt and expanded several more times.
		Jiu Yuan Lu (*Animal & Veterinary Medical Laws*), the first book about veterinary medical laws, was written during this period.
206 BCE–220 CE	*Han* Dynasty	Paper was invented in China during this period, which is about 1400 years earlier than it was used in Western civilization.
		Sima Qian (145–187 BCE) wrote *Shi Ji* (*Historical Records*).
		The animal husbandry laws became known as *Jiu Lu*.
		Shen Nong Ben Cao Jing (*Shen Nong's Book of Medical Herbs*), the first *Materia Medica* (containing 365 herbs), was written during this period.
		Zhang Zhong-Jing (150–219 CE) wrote *Shang Han Za Bing Lun* (*Treatise on Cold-Induced Disorders*).

TCVM Around the World

		Veterinary prescriptions for oral medications were written upon bamboo slips.
		Leather horseshoes and hoof trimming were used to prevent hoof diseases.
		Veterinarians specializing in cattle diseases emerged.
		A set of nine different types of metal needles discovered by modern scientists is attributed to this period.
		Buddhism was introduced but didn't become popular in China until the *Tang* Dynasty (618–907 CE).
		Some books record using a combination of acupuncture and herbal medicine to treat animal diseases.
		Understanding of epidemic diseases expanded during this time, and some Chinese characters were created to represent these diseases.
220–280 CE	Three Kingdoms	Hua Tuo lived during this time. Hua-tuo-jia-ji points are named after this famous physician who discovered their usefulness. He also developed *Ma Fei San* (herbal anesthetic formula) for general anesthesia to assist with abdominal surgery.
265–581 CE	*Jin* to *Southern-Northern* Dynasties	Ge Hong wrote *Zhou Hou Bei Ji Fang* (*Pocket Book for Emergency Therapies*) around 281–341 CE. This book described animal disease treatments and rectal palpation methods.
		Bo Le Liao Ma Jing (*Bole's Classics on Treatment of Equine Diseases*) was published around 502–557 CE
		Jia Si-Xie wrote *Qi Min Yao Shu* (*Basic Techniques for Farmers*) around 533–544 CE. This text explained more advanced animal husbandry and veterinary medical techniques.
		In 562, the Chinese government sent the book *Ming Tang Tu* (*Canon of Equine Acupuncture*) along with 160 other medical books to Mikado in Japan.
581–618 CE	*Sui* Dynasty	The *Sui* court government established the *Tai Pu Si* (Institute of Veterinary Medicine). This government branch was in charge of animal husbandry and veterinary medicine and employed 120 veterinarians. Veterinary medicine began to branch out as more specific books on diagnosis, treatment, medicinal herbs, acupuncture, and moxibustion were published.
		Books published during this period include: *Liao Ma Fang* (*Prescriptions for Horse*), *Bo Le Zhi Ma Za Bing Jing* (*Treatise on Treatment for Sick Horses* by *Bo Le*), *Yu Ji Liao Ma Jing (Classics on Treatment of Equine Diseases* by *Yu Ji*), *Liao Ma Jing (Classics on Treatment of Equine Diseases)*, *Zhi Ma Jing Tu (Classics on Treatment of Equine Diseases with Pictures)*, *Ma Jing Kong Xue Tu (Atlas of Equine Meridians and Acupuncture Points)*, *Zhi Ma Niu Tuo Luo Deng Jing (The Classics on Treatment of Diseases in Horses, Cattle, Camel and Mule)*.
618–907 CE	*Tang* Dynasty	A comprehensive Veterinary Medical Education System was established. From 705 to 707 CE, there were 600 veterinarians, 4 veterinary teachers, and 100 veterinary students in *Tai Pu Si* (a government-funded educational institute).
		The *Tang* court government organized authors to write *Xin Xiu Ben Cao* (*Newly Revised Materia Medica*), which was published in 659 CE. This book described 850 Chinese herbal medicines and became China's first pharmacopeia for human and veterinary medicine.
		Li Shi, a former government official, wrote *Si Mu An Ji Ji* (*A Collection of Equine Medicine*) around 783–845 CE. The text systematically described the basic theories, diagnostics, and treatment techniques of TCVM. It also included the whole text of *Bo Le Zhen Jing* (*Bo Le's Canon of Veterinary Acupuncture*).
		The Japanese government sent Ping Zhong Guo to China to learn TCVM in 804 CE.
960–1279 CE	*Song* Dynasty	*Bing Ma Jian* (Equine Hospital) was established by the *Song* court government in 1007. It was the first government-funded animal hospital to treat sick horses near the capital.
		Movable type printing was first invented in China in 1045, which is 400 years earlier than Gutenberg's movable type invention in the West.
		In 1103 CE, the Song court government established *Pi Bao Suo* (Institute of Pathological Necropsy) to perform animal postmortem examinations.
		Yao Mi Ku (Government-funded Herbal Inventory and Dispensary) was the first veterinary dispensary.
		During this time, a famous veterinarian named Chang Shun lived in *Yang Cheng* of the *Shanxi* Province. He won the *Song* Court's highest award (*Guang Chan Hou*) in 1120 CE for successfully treating skin problems in war horses using a topical herbal medication.
		Around 1086–1110, Wan Yu wrote *Fan Mu Cuan Yan Fang* (*Collection of Effective Prescriptions for Equine Diseases*), which details herbal formulas and acupuncture techniques for common Spleen, Liver, Heart, Lung, and Kidney diseases.
1279–1368 CE	*Yuan* Dynasty	*Quan Ji Tong Xuan Lun* (*Treatment of Sick Horses*) was written by Bian Bao or Bian Guangou. This book describes visceral organ pathology and common animal disease treatments.

TCVM Around the World

1368–1644 CE	*Ming* Dynasty	In 1438 CE, the *Ming* Court government established a mandatory quota for veterinary training among horse caretakers. Every head caretaker of 25 horses (later 50 horses) should select two or three clever young men to study veterinary medicine and become veterinarians to treat horse diseases. In 1578 CE, Li Shi-Zhen (1518–1593) wrote *Ben Cao Gang Mu* (*Compendium of Materia Medica*) based on 30 years of personal experience and his review of more than 800 books, including veterinary medical texts. This text described 1,892 Chinese herbs and 11,096 Chinese herbal formulas. *Ma Shu* (*The Book of Horses*), written by Yang Shi-Qiao in 1594 CE, contains substantial quantities of information about treating equine diseases. Yu Ben-Yuan and Yu Ben-Heng published *Yuan Heng Liao Ma Ji* (*Yuan-Heng's Therapeutic Treatise of Horses*) in 1608. This representative work of traditional Chinese veterinary medicine spread widely throughout China. In 1633 CE, two Korean authors, Zhao Jun and Jin Shi-Heng, wrote the book *Xin Bian Ji Cheng Ma Yi Fang Niu Yi Fang* (*New Collection of Prescriptions for Horses and Cattle*) in the Chinese language. Many books published during this time described castration in horses, cattle, sheep, pigs, dogs, and chickens.
1644–1911 CE	*Qing* Dynasty	Li Yu-Shu revised the book *Yuan Heng Liao Ma Ji* in 1736 CE. This new version had a preface by Xu Keng and it has become the most popular text in use today. *Chuan Ya Shou Yi Fang* (*Compiled Veterinary Formulas*), written by Zhao Xue-Min in 1758 CE, contains the most popular herbal formulas for treating horses, cattle, goats, sheep, dogs, cats, deer, elephants, camels, chickens, birds, goldfish, and turtles. In 1785 CE, Guo Huai-Xi annotated the earlier work *Yuan Heng Liao Ma Ji* and published it as *Ma Niu Tuo Jing Da Quan* (*The Complete Collection of Diseases of Horses, Cattle and Camels*). Fu Shu-Feng wrote the two-volume book *Yang Geng Ji* (*A Collection on Management of Cattle*) in 1800. The first volume discusses acupuncture using 40 acupoints and 20 special techniques. The second volume discusses Chinese herbal medicine. *Niu Yi Jin Jian* (*Golden Mirror of Bovine Medicine*), published in 1815, contains 148 segments. It discusses Zang-fu physiology and pathology as well as treating common cattle diseases. *Hou Shou Ci Zhou* (*Human Care of Animals*) written by Li Nan-Hui in 1873, contains over 700 herbal formulas. It explains, in detail, the disease Patterns in various species including yellow cattle, buffalo, pigs, horses, sheep, dogs, and cats. *Zhu Jin Da Quan* (*Complete Collection of Swine Diseases*) was a unique book about swine medicine that described therapeutics for 48 kinds of pig diseases. *Ju Bing Ji* (*A Collection of Diseases in Foals*), published in 1909 (unknown author), discusses 70 diseases in foals and 16 diseases in mares. Other TCVM books published during *Qing* Dynasty include *Bao Du Ji* (*Treatise on Calf Diseases*), *Niu Jing Pei Yao Yi Fang* (*Essential Prescriptions for Cattle Diseases*), and *Niu Ji Da Quan* (*Complete Collection of Bovine Diseases*), also called *Da Wu Jing*. *Bei Yang* Equine Medical School was established in Baoding, *Hebei* province in 1904. Western Veterinary Medicine was formally introduced in China at that time.
1911–1949 CE	Republic of China	*Zhi Luo Ma Liang Fang* (*Herbal Formulas for the Treatment of Mules and Horses*), written by *Qi* Jia-Ben in 1933, contains 130 herbal formulas. Formal college training in Traditional Chinese Veterinary Medicine was offered at the North China University in 1947.
1949 CE–present day	People's Republic of China	Hebei TCVM School was established in 1956. This was the first TCVM 3-year program. China National Society of TCVM was founded in 1956. The China Ministry of Agriculture *Lanzhou* Institute of TCVM Institute was founded in 1958. *Si Chuan* College of Animal Science and Veterinary Medicine was founded in 1979. This was the first DVM program with a TCVM specialty. Similar programs were also started in other Veterinary Medical Schools, including Beijing Agricultural University, Nanjing Agricultural University, People's Liberation Army (PLA) Veterinary University, Northeast Agricultural University, Central China Agricultural University. Two professional journals about Traditional Chinese Veterinary Medicine have been published regularly and distributed nationally. The *Chinese Journal of Traditional Veterinary Science* was founded in Jiangxi in 1957, and the *Journal of Traditional Chinese Veterinary Medicine* was founded in Lanzhou in 1982. About 100 books on TCVM have been published since 1949. Various studies on TCVM have been funded by the central and provincial government in China. Over 1,500 peer-reviewed research papers have been published on the topic.

TCVM Around the World	
USA	The International Veterinary Acupuncture Society (IVAS) was formed in the USA in 1974 CE.
	The Chi Institute of Traditional Chinese Veterinary Medicine (Chi Institute) was established in Reddick, Florida, USA, in 1998 CE. It becomes the leading school for providing TCVM Continuing Education programs in acupuncture, herbal medicine, Tui-na, and food therapy.
	The National Center for Complementary and Alternative Medicine was founded by the NIH in 1998 to study the effects of acupuncture and other modalities. It received $125,471,000 in 2009.
	University of Florida (UF) has offered an acupuncture service to clients since 1999 and has also offered training for veterinary students and interns: 1) a 2-credit elective Complementary and Alternative Medicine (VEM 5208) since 1999, 2) a 2-week Acupuncture Clinical Rotation elective (VEM 5876) for junior and senior veterinary professional students since 2001, and 3) Acupuncture Internship Programs since 2004.
	Other Veterinary Medical Schools offering acupuncture or other Complementary and Alternative Veterinary Medicine (CAVM) services for clients include Colorado State University (CSU), University of Minnesota (UM), and UC Davis. Schools other than UF offering elective courses in acupuncture or CAVM include CSU, UM, UC Davis, Washington State University, Virginia Tech, and North Carolina State.
Japan and Korea	Around 482–507 CE, the Japanese Emperor sent some Japanese citizens to China to learn TCVM.
	The Chinese government sent the book *Ming Tang Tu* (*Canon of Equine Acupuncture*) with 160 other medical books to Mikado of Japan in 562 CE.
	Numerous Japanese went to China to learn TCVM during *Sui* Dynasty (581 to 618 CE).
	Korean monks went to Japan to learn equine TCVM in 595 CE.
	The Japanese government sent Ping Zhong Guo to China to learn TCVM in 804 CE.
	In 1633 CE, two Korean authors Zhao Jun and Jin Shiheng wrote the book *Xin Bian Ji Cheng Ma Yi Fang Niu Yi Fang* (*New Collection of Prescriptions for Horses and Cattle*) in the Chinese language.
Europe	Acupuncture was introduced into France by the Jesuits serving in Chinese courts during the 16th and 17th centuries. The Jesuit PP Harvieu published a book on acupuncture in 1671.
	In 1683, Wilhelm Ten Rhyne, a Dutch physician, introduced acupuncture to London.
	Acupuncture was taught in French veterinary medical programs in Lyon & Alfort in 1761.

Appendix B Map of China and the Top Provinces/Regions Where Herbs Are Produced

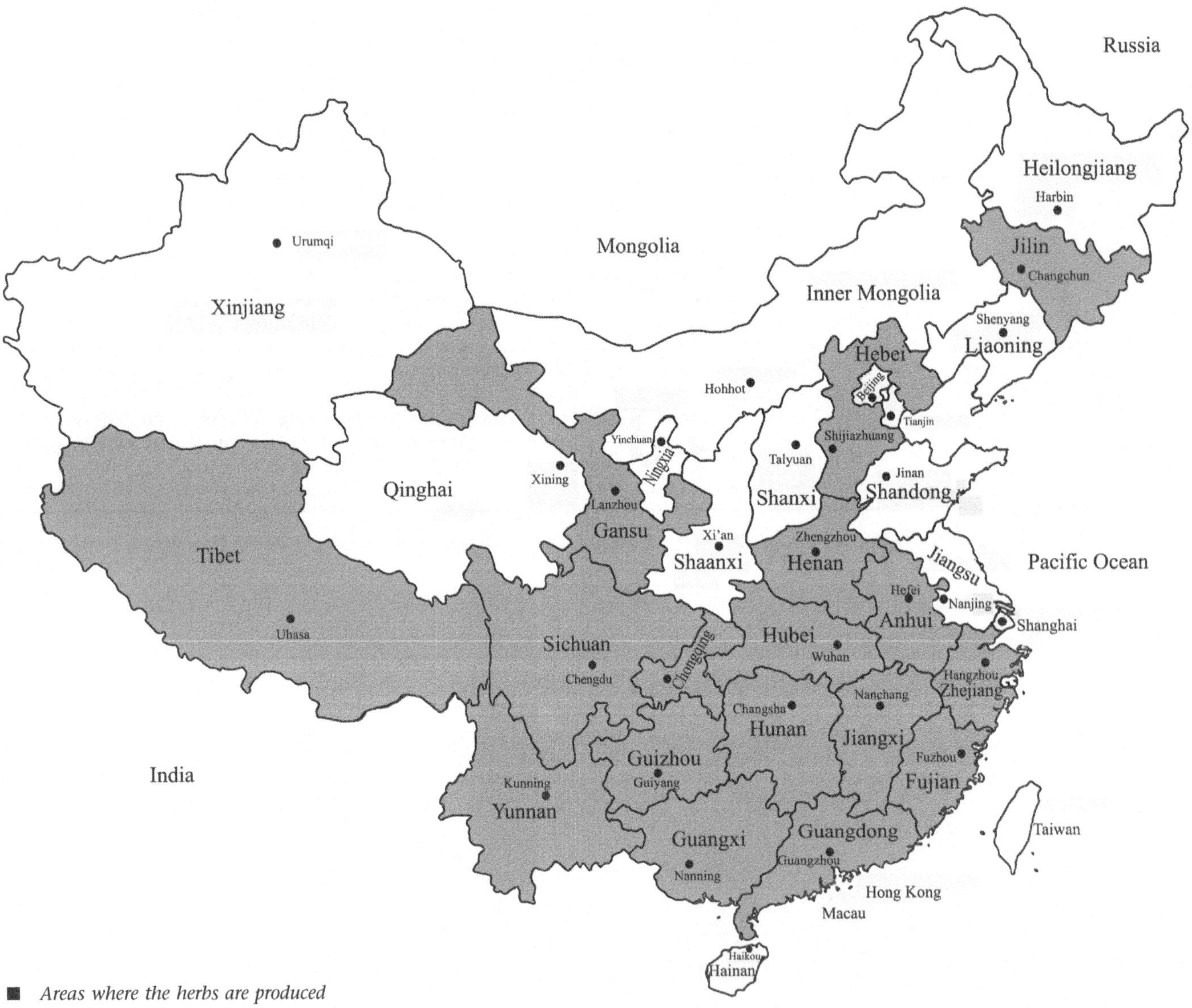

■ *Areas where the herbs are produced*

Total territorial Size: 9,602,716 km^2

- 4 municipality regions: Beijing, Shanghai, Tianjin, and Chongqing
- 23 provinces
- 5 autonomous Regions: Xinjiang, Tibet, Ningxia, Inner Mongolia and Guangxi
- 2 special administrative regions: Hong Kong and Macau

Population: 1.3 billion

Appendix C Guide to Pronunciation of TCVM Terms

This reference explains the pronunciation and translation of the most commonly used Chinese words. The first item in italics is the Chinese word written in English (*Pin-Yin*). The parentheses contain a word or two representing how the Chinese word sounds followed by the Chinese word as a symbol. The word after the equal sign is the meaning of that Chinese word.

Ba (bah 八) = 8
Bai (buy 白) = white
Bi (bee 鼻) = nose
Biao (bi-ow 表) = Exterior
Bian Zheng (bian tzeng 辨证) = Pattern Differentiation
Biao Ben (Piao ben 标本) = Manifestation and Root
Bu Fa (boo fa 补法) = tonification
Chang Xia (chang sheah 长夏) = later summer
Chen mai (chen my 沉脉) = deep pulse
Chi mai (chuh my 迟脉) = slow pulse
Chun (choon 春) = spring
Da chang (da chang 大肠) = Large Intestine
Da Qi (da chee 大气) = inhaled air
Dan (dan 胆) = Gallbladder
Dan (dan 丹) = pill
Dong (dong 冬) = winter
Er (arr 耳) = ears
Er (arr 二) = 2
Fei (fay 肺) = Lung
Feng (fung 风) = Wind
Fu (foo 腹) = abdomen
Fu mai (foo my 浮脉) = floating pulse
Gan (gan 肝) = Liver
Gen (gen, 根) = root
Gou (go 狗) = dog
Gu Qi (goo chee 谷气) = food *Qi*
Han (han 寒) = Cold
Hei (hay 黑) = black
Hong (hong 红) = red
Hua (hooah 花) = flower
Hua mai (Hoo-ah my 滑脉) = slippery pulse
Huang (hwang 黄) = yellow
Huo (hoo-ah 火) = Fire
Jiao Nang (jeow nang 胶囊) = capsule
Jin (jin 金) = Metal
Jing (jing 精) = Essence
Jing (jing 颈) = cervical
Jing Luo (jing loo-oh 经络) = Meridian system
Jing Luo Qi (jing loo-oh chee 经络气) = Channel/ Meridian *Qi*
Jing Mai (jing my 经脉) = Channel, Main Meridian
Jin ye (jin-yea 津液) = body fluid
Jiu (Joe 九) = 9
Jue Yin (jew-eh yin 厥阴) = disappearing *Yin*
Kou (kou 口) = mouth
Li (Lee 里) = Interior
Liu (lee-oo 六) = 6
Lu (lew) = green
Luo Mai (loo-oh my 络脉) = Branch Meridian
Ma (mah 马) = horse
Mai (my 脉) = vessel, channel
Mao (maow 猫) = cat
Mao (mao 毛) = hair
Mu (moo 木) = Wood
Niao (neow 鸟) = birds
Niu (new 牛) = cows
Pang-guang (pang gwang 膀胱) = urinary bladder
Pi (pee 皮) = skin
Pi (pee 脾) = Spleen
Qi (chee 七) = 7
Qi (chee 气) = *Qi*
Qing Qi (ching chee 清气) = cosmic *Qi*
Qiu (chew 秋) = fall
Re (thuh 热) = Heat

Ri (the 日) = sun
San (sahn, 散) = powder
San (san 三) = 3
San Jiao (sahn jeow 三焦) = Triple Heater
Se mai (suh my 涩脉) = choppy pulse
Shan (shan 山) = mountain
Shao Yang (shaow yang 少阳) = little *Yang*, small *Yang*
Shao Yin (Shaow yin 少阴) = little *Yin*, small *Yin*
She (shuh 舌) = tongue
Shen (shen 神) = mind/spirit
Shen (shen 肾) = Kidney
Shi (shuh 湿) = Damp
Shi (shuh 实) = Excess
Shi (shur 十) = 10
Shou (show 手) = hand
Shou yi (show ee 兽医) = veterinarian
Shu (shew 暑) = Summer Heat
Shu mai (shoo my 束脉) = rapid pulse
Shu Xue (shoo shu-eh 俞穴) = acupuncture point
Shui (Schwee 水) = Water
Si (suh 四) = 4
Tai Yang (tie yang 太阳) = great *Yang*
Tai Yin (Tie yin 太阴) = great *Yin*, supreme *Yin*
Tang (tahng, 汤) = Decoction
Tou (Tow 头) = head
Tu (too 土) = Earth
Wan (wahn, 丸) = teapill
Wei (wey 尾) = tail
Wei (wey 胃) = Stomach
Wei Qi (wei chee 卫气) = Defensive *Qi*
Wu (woo 五) = 5
Xi mai (shee my 细脉) = thin pulse
Xia (sheah 夏) = summer
Xiao chang (sheow chang 小肠) = Small Intestine
Xie Fa (shay fa 泻法) = sedation
Xie Qi (shay chee 邪气) = Pathogenic *Qi*
Xin (sheen 心) = Heart
Xin Bao (sheen bao 心包) = Pericardium
Xiong (shee-ong 胸) = thoracic
Xu (Shew 虚) = Deficiency
Xuan mai (shwan my 玄脉) = wiry pulse
Xue (shu-eh 血) = Blood
Yan (yan 眼) = eyes
Yang Ming (yang ming 阳明) = brightest *Yang*
Yao (yao 腰) = lumbar
Yi (eee 一) = 1
Ying Qi (ying chee 营气) = nutrient *Qi*
Yuan Qi (yuan chee 元气) = Source *Qi*
Yue (yoo-eh 月) = moon
Zang Fu Qi (tzang fu chee 脏腑气) = Organ *Qi*
Zao (tzaow 燥) = Dryness
Zheng Qi (tzeng chee 正气) = Healthful *Qi*
Zhong Qi (chong chee 中气) = Central *Qi*
Zhong Shou Yi (chong show ee 中兽医) = TCVM
Zhu (tsoo 猪) = pigs
Zi (tzuh 子) = Seed
Zi She (tzuh shuh 紫舌) = purple tongue
Zong Qi (tzong chee 宗气) = Ancestral *Qi* (*Da Qi* + *Gu Qi*)
Zu (tzoo 足) = foot

Appendix D Glossary

Bi Zheng (闭证 Closed Syndrome): *Bi* refers to closed or unconscious. *Zheng* is syndrome or Pattern of a disease. *Bi Zheng* refers to loss of consciousness when the *Qiao* organs are closed due to pathogenic Excessive Heat or excessive Cold Phlegm. The orifices are called *Qiao*. *Qiao* organs include the nose, ears, brain, eyes, and skin. When *Qiao* organs are open, the body has normal senses and perception. When *Qiao* organs are closed, *Bi Zheng* results and the animal loses consciousness. However, unlike *Tuo Zheng*, the patient maintains control of limbs, defecation, and urination.

Bian Zheng (辨证 Pattern Differentiation): *Bian* is differentiation and identification. *Zheng* is a type or Pattern of illness. *Bian Zheng* indicates that the TCVM diagnostic system relies upon Pattern differentiation. The most common *Zheng*s are Excess Heat, Interior Cold, *Qi*-Blood Stagnation, *Yin* Deficiency, Blood Deficiency, *Qi* Deficiency, and *Yang* Deficiency.

Biao Ben (标本 Manifestation and Root): The Manifestation (*Biao*) and the Root (*Ben*) represent two aspects of one entity. In general, the Root is the primary aspect of a disease, and the Manifestation is the symptom(s) caused by the Root. For example, Kidney *Qi* Deficiency is the root, and weakness in the hind end and urinary incontinence are the manifestations. Spleen (GI) Damp Heat is the Root, and Bloody/mucous/smelly diarrhea is the Manifestation. During the clinical course of a disease, the original or the primary condition is the Root, and the complication or secondary condition is the Manifestation. Regarding the location of a lesion, the internal organ is the Root, and the external surface is the Manifestation.

Biao Zheng (表证 Exterior Pattern): *Biao* here refers to the skin, hair, muscles, and space between them, as well as the superficial portion of the Meridians and Collaterals. *Biao Zheng* is the Exterior Pattern in which the clinical signs are located in superficial skin, hair, muscles, or Meridian pathways. External attack by exogenous pathogens (Wind-Cold or Wind-Heat) is often the cause. The common clinical signs supporting an Exterior Pattern diagnosis include the following: 1) the patient is in the early stage of disease, 2) the signs are acute in onset and the illness is of short duration, 3) the tongue usually has a thin coating, and 4) the pulse is usually floating (or superficial). This Pattern is paired with the Interior Pattern (*Li Zheng*).

Fu (腑 *Fu* Organs): *Fu* are the *Yang* internal organs, including Stomach, Large Intestine, Small Intestine, Bladder, Gallbladder, and *San Jiao* (Triple Heater). The main actions of *Fu* organs are to receive and digest food and to transport and excrete wastes. The *Fu* organs are hollow.

Gu Qi (谷气 Food *Qi*, or Food Essence): Food enters the Stomach where it is broken down. The food is then transformed into *Gu Qi* (Food Essence) by the Spleen. The *Gu Qi* rises into the chest to the Lung where it combines with *Qing Qi* in the Lung to form *Zong Qi*. Thus, *Gu Qi* is a substance produced by the Spleen's activity. This function of the Spleen occurs in an ascending direction. The Spleen should always send *Gu Qi* up to the Lung. In this way, the Spleen is a major source of *Qi* after birth, and it also controls the ascending movement of *Qi*. If the Spleen *Qi* descends, the food may not be transformed properly and thus results in diarrhea.

Li Zheng (里证 Interior Pattern): *Li* means Interior, which refers to the *Zang-Fu* organs. *Li Zheng* is Interior Pattern, in which one or more of the internal organs are affected. It is often caused by chronic exposure to exogenous pathogens, internal emotional stress, improper training, or an inappropriate feeding program. An Interior Pattern diagnosis is typically made when the patient is at a later disease stage after a longer course of illness. There is usually a thick coating or no coating of the tongue, and the pulse is deep. Common Interior Patterns include Interior Excess Heat, Interior Excess Cold, *Yang* Deficiency, *Yin* Deficiency, *Qi* Deficiency, and Blood Deficiency.

***Qi* Stage/Phase** (气分病证): *Qi* Stage or *Qi* Phase is one of the *Wei Qi Ying Xue* Patterns, or the Four Stages. In this Pattern, the exogenous Warm Pathogenic factors (Heat) are lodged in the Lung, Stomach, and Large Intestine. The main clinical signs of this Pattern are high fever, tachypnea or dyspnea, cough, excessive thirst, excessive sweating in horses or panting in dogs, gingivitis, stomatitis or halitosis, constipation, red tongue, and an excessive pulse. The typical classical herbal formula for this Pattern is *Bai Hu Tang* (White Tiger Decoction).

Qing Qi (清气 Cosmic *Qi*): *Qing Qi* is sometimes called universal clean air (*Kong Qi*). It is the abundant, mostly invisible energy of the Universe made up of air, light, electromagnetic forces, and various energetic particles in space and the atmosphere. It is inhaled by the Lung. Combined with *Gu Qi* (Food *Qi*), it forms *Zong Qi* in the chest.

San Jiao (三焦 Triple Burner): *San* is three. *Jiao* refers to burner, heater, or warmer. Thus, *San Jiao* (SJ) is translated as Triple Burner (TB), Triple Heater (TH), or Triple Warmer (TW). *San Jiao*'s exact nature and form have been disputed for centuries. Generally, there are four meanings of *San Jiao*: 1) It is a Channel pathway on the body surface (commonly called the Triple Heater Meridian, TH), and its Channel connects with the Pericardium. 2) It is considered one of the six *Fu* organs, and it shares an external-internal relationship with the Pericardium. 3) It is the general pathway for distribution of *Yuan Qi* (Source *Qi*) and Body Fluid. 4) The most common meaning of *San Jiao* refers to three parts of the body: the *Shang Jiao* (Upper Burner), the *Zhong Jiao* (Middle Burner), and the *Xia Jiao* (Lower Burner).

Shang Jiao (上焦 Upper Burner): *Shang Jiao* refers to the region from the head to the chest and mainly includes the Lung and Heart. It primarily governs respiration and the blood vessels, and it distributes the nutrients from food and water to the body. Its two main internal organs are the Heart and Lung.

Tan (痰 Phlegm): *Tan* (Phlegm) is a turbid, thick, and damp material. It is a pathological product of *Zang-Fu* organ dysfunction. *Tan* (Phlegm) often results when the body fluids fail to circulate adequately and properly and then congeal due to Heat, Cold, Damp, or Spleen *Qi* Deficiency.

Tuo Zheng (脱证 Abandoned Syndrome): *Tuo* refers to abandoned. *Tuo Zheng* refers to Abandoned, Collapsing, or Flaccid Syndrome. *Tuo Zheng* is often caused by excessive blood loss, shock, excessive loss of Body Fluids, or coma. The main clinical signs of *Tuo Zheng* are loss of consciousness, excessive sweating, cold extremities, fecal and urinary incontinence, flaccidity, open mouth and eyes, and a frail or faint pulse. *Tuo Zheng* is severe Deficiency of *Qi*, *Yuan Qi*, or *Yang Qi*. This is different from *Bi Zheng*, which is caused by Excess Heat or Excess Cold Phlegm.

Wei Qi (卫气 Defensive *Qi*): *Wei Qi*, referring in concept to the immune system, is an important part of *Zheng Qi*. *Wei Qi* is a defense system of white blood cells, antibodies, and other substances used to fight infections and reject foreign proteins. *Wei Qi* is derived from *Gu Qi* (Food *Qi*). It circulates in superficial, extravascular parts of the body; protects the integument and musculature against the external attack of pathogens: controls the opening and closing of pores; and regulates body temperature. It is also known as Defensive *Yang* or *Wei Yang* because it is part of the body's *Yang Qi*. *Wei Qi* is also able to recognize "self" cells from "nonself" cells by markers found on the surface of every cell in the body. Consequently, the "normal" *Wei Qi* attacks only foreign invaders (viruses, bacteria and fungi). However, *Wei Qi* can be abnormal, either by not doing its job (Deficiency) or by doing it too much (Excess). For example, Deficient *Wei Qi* occurs in FIV, SIV, and HIV and all conditions that cause an acquired immunodeficiency syndrome (AIDS) specific to that species. In such cases, the deficient *Wei Qi* fails to protect the body, leaving it vulnerable and open to attack by an opportunistic infection. On the other hand, Excessive *Wei Qi* can overreact to the foreign pathogens (pollens) and lead to allergy. *Wei Qi* is also associated with the body's ability to identify abnormal tissue. When *Wei Qi* is deficient, the T-cells fail to check the tissues for mutations and abnormal cells (*Yin* substances). Thus, the body fails to move the *Yin* substances, and these substances accumulate, eventually forming tumors or cancer.

***Wei Qi Ying Xue* Pattern** (卫气营血病证, Four Stage/Phase Pattern): *Wei* (Defense), *Qi*, *Ying* (Nutrient), *Xue* (Blood) Pattern, or the Four Stages, was created by Ye Tianshi in 1746. This system is used when the initial symptoms of disease include acute febrile conditions (Excess Heat). *Wei Qi Ying Xue* can identify the Patterns of acute febrile diseases that are commonly seen in veterinary practice. Acute febrile diseases usually occur when the *Zheng* Qi (Anti-Pathogenic *Qi*) is not strong enough to prevent the *Xie Qi* (Pathogenic *Qi*) from invading the body. These diseases are characterized by their abrupt onset and their tendency to injure *Yin*,

Body Fluid, and Blood. In addition to generalizing the clinical appearance of febrile diseases, the *Wei* (Defense), *Qi*, *Ying* (Nutrient), and *Xue* (Blood) represent four different stages of a disease's pathological development. They measure the depth and severity of a disease. The most superficial is the *Wei* (Defense) Stage. The next level is the *Qi* Stage, and deeper still is the *Ying* (Nutrient) Stage. The deepest level is the *Xue* (Blood) Stage. *Wei* (Defense) and *Qi* Patterns are mild and superficial, but *Ying* (Nutrient) and *Xue* (Blood) Patterns are deep and severe.

***Wei* Stage/Phase** (卫分病证): *Wei* Stage or *Wei* Phase is one of the *Wei Qi Ying Xue* Patterns, or the Four Stages. In this Pattern, the exogenous Wind-Heat is lodged in the superficial body surface, muscle, and joints. The main clinical signs of this Pattern are severe fever, sore throat, thick nasal discharge, cough, red tongue, and fast pulse. The typical classical herbal formula for this Pattern is *Yin Qiao San*.

Xia Jiao (下焦 Lower Burner): *Xiao Jiao* (Lower Burner) refers to the region from the umbilicus to the rear feet, and mainly includes the Kidney.

Xie Qi (邪气, Pathogenic *Qi*): *Xie Qi* refers to the six pathogenic factors and includes the Six Excessive or Noxious *Qi* (Wind, Cold, Heat, Summer Heat, Dryness, and Damp). These factors invade the body through the skin, mouth, or nose. Diseases due to the Six Excessive *Qi* are closely related to the nature of an individual's environment and the weather, especially seasonal changes. For example, a Heat Pattern mostly occurs in the summer, a Cold Pattern in the winter, and a Damp Pattern in late summer. However, things are not always that simple. The Six Excessive *Qi* may also cause disease in much more complex ways. Under certain circumstances, one type of Excessive *Qi* can even transform into another. It is possible for a Cold Pattern to occur in the summer. Also, an Extreme Heat Pattern can change into Wind, or an Extreme Wind Pattern may transform into Dryness. Each of the Six Excessive *Qi* may affect the body singly or in combination. For instance, Summer Heat alone causes sunstroke, but the common cold is due to a combination of Wind and Cold. The Six Excessive *Qi* usually invade the body from the exterior via the skin, mouth, or nose.

***Xue* Stage/Phase** (血分病证, Blood Stage Pattern): This is the deepest and most severe of the *Wei Qi Ying Xue* Patterns. It is associated with Liver and Kidney pathology. The main clinical signs are fever, coma, petechiae and ecchymosis, rash, bloody urine or feces, seizure, a deep-red tongue, and a thin or rapid pulse. The typical classical herbal formula for the treatment of *Xue* Stage is *Xi Jiao Di Huang Tang*.

Ying Qi (营气 Nutrient *Qi*). *Ying Qi* is derived from *Gu Qi* (Food *Qi*). It circulates in the blood vessels, produces Blood, and nourishes the whole body. Hemoglobin and other serum proteins are a part of *Ying Qi*. It is also called *Ying Xue* (Nutrient Blood or *Ying* Blood) due to its association with Blood and its flow within blood vessels.

***Ying* Stage/Phase** (营分病证, Nutrient Stage Pattern): This is one of the *Wei Qi Ying Xue* Patterns. It is involved with the central nervous system, *Shen*, Heart, and Pericardium. The main clinical signs are seizure, restlessness, delirium or dementia, prolonged high fever (especially at night), tachypnea, asthma, petechiae or macules in the skin or mucosa, a deep red tongue, and a thready and rapid pulse. The typical classical herbal formula for the treatment of this Pattern is *Qing Ying Tang*.

Ying Wei (营卫, Nutrient and Defense): *Ying* refers to *Ying Qi*, and *Wei* refers to *Wei Qi*. *Ying Qi* produces Blood and nourishes the whole body, and *Wei Qi* protects the body against the external attack of pathogens. *Ying* and *Wei* have a close relationship. *Wei* circulates in superficial, extravascular parts of the body and protects the deeper *Ying*. *Ying* circulates in the blood vessels and cools and restrains *Wei*. The *Wei Qi*, as the "soldier" of the immune system, requires the weapons and guidance provided by the *Ying Qi* in order to function effectively. Without the *Ying*'s weapons, *Wei* will fail in its efforts to defend the body. *Ying* and *Wei* are also like brother and sister. Being the young brother, *Wei* protects the elder sister (*Ying*). Without *Wei*'s protection, *Ying* is easily attacked by exogenous pathogens. Being the elder sister, *Ying* restrains and cools the excessive actions of brother *Wei*. Without Ying's restraint, *Wei* will overreact to exogenous pathogens (leading to allergies) or to the body's own tissues (leading to autoimmune diseases). Therefore, the key treatment principle for these conditions is to balance *Ying* and *Wei*.

Ying Xue (营血 Nutrient and Blood): *Ying Qi* circulates in the blood vessels, produces Blood and nourishes the whole body. Hemoglobin and other serum proteins are a part of *Ying Qi*. Because *Ying* has a close association with *Xue* (Blood) and it flows within blood vessels, *Ying* (Nutrient) and *Xue* (Blood) are together called *Ying Xue* (Nutrient Blood or *Ying* Blood).

Zang (脏): *Zang*, or *Zang* organs, include the Liver, Heart, Spleen, Lung, and Kidney. The Pericardium is generally considered the sixth *Zang* organ. The *Zang* organs are solid. The *Zang* organs mainly function to manufacture and store essential substances, including *Qi*, Blood, and Body Fluid.

Zang-Fu (脏俯): *Zang-Fu* is the general term for the body's internal organs. This includes the five *Zang* organs (sometimes described as the six *Zang* organs), the six *Fu* organs, and the extraordinary *Fu* organs. The Liver, Heart, Spleen, Lung, and Kidney are the five *Zang* organs. The Pericardium is generally considered the sixth Zang organ. The six *Fu* organs include the Gallbladder, Stomach, Small Intestine, Large Intestine, Urinary Bladder, and *San Jiao* (Triple Heater). The brain, marrow, bones, vessels, Gallbladder and uterus are known as the extraordinary *Fu* organs. A *Yin* and *Yang*, as well as an Exterior and Interior, relationship exists between the *Zang* organs and the *Fu* organs. The *Zang* organs are the Interior or *Yin* organs, and the *Fu* organs are the Exterior or *Yang* organs. *Zang* and *Fu* organs may be thought of in pairs. The *Zang* organs are the "wives," and the *Fu* organs are their "husbands." *Zang* and *Fu* organs work together and support each other, but they are functionally and anatomically different from each other. Despite the differences in form and function between the *Zang* and *Fu* organs, they are still connected to each other and to the entire body. The Meridians and Collaterals form the structural and functional connections within the body. The Meridians join individual *Zang* and *Fu* organs into husband-wife pairs. The *Zang-Fu* organs are also joined to the five sense organs. In the end, every part of the body is combined into a whole.

Zheng (证 Pattern): The *Zheng* is a subtle, but major difference between TCVM and conventional Western medical disease diagnosis. Western medicine tends to view the body as a mechanical system for which the doctor needs to run diagnostic tests to find, then fix, the damaged part. However, TCVM has a more energetic and holistic view of the body. TCVM takes all symptoms into consideration in order to identify a special *Zheng*, or Pattern of disease, and then it uses this Pattern to select treatments that can help bring the body back into balance. For example, consider two horses with bloody diarrhea. The first horse is a 2-year-old thoroughbred filly that presents with profuse hemorrhagic diarrhea. The bloody diarrhea began about 3 days ago. The fecal cultures were positive for *Salmonella* species. The horse also had a red tongue and rapid pulse. Conventional Western practitioners may diagnose the disease as *Salmonella* colitis, but TCVM practitioners recognize an Excess Heat Pattern because of the red tongue, rapid pulse, young age, and acute onset. The other horse, an 18-year-old thoroughbred mare, presents with a 21-day history of bloody diarrhea. The fecal test was also positive for *Salmonella* species, and the mare had a pale tongue and weak pulse. Just as in the first case, conventional Western practitioners diagnosed *Salmonella* colitis. The TCVM practitioners, however, diagnose Spleen *Qi* Deficiency based upon her pale tongue, weak pulse, old age and chronic diarrhea. Even though these two cases have the same Western diagnosis and treatment protocols, different TCVM treatments are given to the two horses because they each have a totally different TCVM diagnosis (Pattern). Horse 1 (Excess Heat Pattern) should be treated with herbal formula *Yu Jin San* and acupoints GV-14, LI-4, LI-11 and ST-44 to clear Heat from the GI tract. Horse 2 (Spleen *Qi* Deficiency Pattern) should be treated with herbal medicine *Shen Ling Bai Zhu San* and acupoints BL-20, BL-21, ST-36, and SP-6 to tonify the *Qi* of the Spleen.

Zheng Qi (正气 Antipathogenic *Qi*): *Zheng Qi* (Antipathogenic *Qi*), including *Wei Qi* (Defensive *Qi*), refers to the body's functional activity and ability to resist diseases. It includes defensive ability, adaptability, and ability to maintain homeostasis. It is the whole body's power to kill and/or resist any *Xie Qi* (Pathogenic *Qi*). *Xie Qi* refers to all the various causative factors of disease. *Qi* Flow (*Qi Ji*), which includes *Zheng Qi*, normally circulates through the whole body with Ascending, Descending, Inward, and Outward Movements. There are three aspects of the *Zheng Qi*, which relate to the body's defensive ability, adaptability, and ability to maintain homeostasis: (1) *Zheng Qi* is involved in the body's ability to resist pathogens. This function also includes Wei *Qi*. (2) *Zheng Qi* assists the body in maintaining the *Yin* and *Yang* balance. This includes Ying *Qi*, *Wei Qi*, Blood, Body Fluid, *Yin*, and *Yang*. (3) *Zheng Qi* is important in the body's will to live. This includes *Shen*, *Yuan Qi*, and *Jing*.

Zhong Jiao (中焦 Middle Burner): *Zhong Jiao* refers to the region from the chest to the umbilicus, and mainly refers to the Spleen and Stomach.

Zong Qi (宗气, Pectoral *Qi*, Gathering *Qi*, Ancestral *Qi*, Chest *Qi*): *Zong Qi* is formed by combining *Gu Qi* (Food *Qi*) and *Qing Qi* (Cosmic *Qi*) and is gathered and stored in the chest. It promotes the Lung's respiratory function (control of respiration) and promotes the Heart's circulatory function (governing Blood and vessels). *Zong Qi* is related to the voice, to respiration, and to the circulation of *Qi* and Blood.

Appendix E
Forms of Herbal Medicine Available in the U.S. Market

Form	Herbal Suppliers
Raw herbs	Dr. Xie's Jing-tang Herbal Mayway nuherbs Co. Spring Wind
Extract granules	Blue Light Dr. Xie's Jing-tang Herbal Qualiherb South Mountain Sun Ten
Alcohol extracts	Kan Herb Co. Zand Chinese Classics
American-made Chinese herbal products	Dr. Xie's Jing-tang Herbal Golden Flower Health Concerns K'an Herb Co. Seven Forest
Chinese-made patent medicines	Dr. Xie's Jing-tang Herbal Mayway nuherbs Co.
Chinese-American patent medicine	Dr. Xie's Jing-tang Herbal Kan Herb Co. Mayway (Plum Flower Brand) nuherbs Co. (Nü Herb Patent Medicines)

Appendix F
Herbal Suppliers

Herbal Suppliers	Contact Information
Bio Essence Corporation	Min Tong 1030 Ohio Avenue Richmond, CA 94804 Tel: 510-215-5588 Fax: 1-800-875-0798 info@bioessence.com www.bioessence.com
Blue Light	Treasure of the East 631 West Buffalo Street Ithaca, NY 14850 Tel: 888-BLUE-LIT 888-258-3548 Fax: 888-666-9888 info@treasureofeast.com www.treasureofeast.com
Crane Herb Company	745 Falmouth Road Mashpee, MA 02649 Tel: 508-539-1700 Fax: 508-539-2369 info@craneherb.com www.craneherb.com
Dr. Xie's Jing-tang Herbal	9700 West Hwy 318 Reddick, FL 32686 Tel: 800-891-1986 Fax: 866-700-8772 admin@tcvm.com www.tcvmherbal.com Free consultation Veterinary products only
Golden Flower Chinese Herbs	2724 Vassar Place NE Albuquerque, NM 87107 Tel: 800-729-8509 Fax: 866-298-7541 www.gfcherbs.com
Health Concerns	8001 Capwell Drive Oakland, CA 94621 Tel: 800-233-9355 www.healthconcerns.com

Herbal Suppliers	Contact Information
K'an Herb Company	6001 Butler Lane Scotts Valley, CA 95066 Tel: 831-438-9450 Fax: 831-438-9457 info@kanherb.com www.kanherb.com
Mayway USA	1338 Mandela Parkway Oakland, California 94607 Tel: 800-262-9929 Fax: 800-909-2828 www.mayway.com
nuherbs Co.	3820 Penniman Avenue Oakland, Ca, 94619 Tel: 800-233-4307 Fax: 800-550-1928 www.nuherbs.com
Qualiherb	116 Pleasant Street Suite 328 Easthampton, MA 01027 Tel: 888-884-8355 Fax: 413-529-1099 www.qualiherb.com
Institute of Traditional Medicine (ITM)	Seven Forests 2017 SE Hawthorne Boulevard Portland, OR 97214 Tel: 800-544-7504 www.itmonline.org
Spring Wind	2325 Fourth Street Suite 6 Berkeley, CA 94710 Tel. 800-588-48883 customerservice@springwind.com http://www.springwind.com
Sun Ten Laboratories	9250 Jeronimo Road Irvine, California 92618 Tel: 800-715-7846 Fax: 949-587-8914 www.sunten.com
Zand Chinese Formulas	1441 West Smith Road Ferndale, WA 98248 Tel: 800-241-0859 Fax: 360-384-1140 www.zand.com

Index